Robot-Assisted Radical Prostatectomy

Shancheng Ren • Senthil Nathan
Nicola Pavan • Di Gu
Ashwin Sridhar • Riccardo Autorino
Editors

Robot-Assisted Radical Prostatectomy

Advanced Surgical Techniques

Springer

Editors
Shancheng Ren
Changzheng Hospital
Shanghai, China

Nicola Pavan
Urology Clinic, Medical, Surgical and Health Sciences Department
University of Trieste
Trieste, Italy

Urology Clinic, Department of Surgical Oncological and Stomatological Sciences
University of Palermo
Palermo, Italy

Ashwin Sridhar
Urology
University College London Hospital NHS Trust
Hatfield, UK

Senthil Nathan
Institute of Urology
University College London
London, UK

Di Gu
The First affiliated Hospital of Guangzhou Medical University
Guangzhou, China

Riccardo Autorino
Department of Urology
Rush University Medical Center
Chicago, IL, USA

ISBN 978-3-031-05854-7 ISBN 978-3-031-05855-4 (eBook)
https://doi.org/10.1007/978-3-031-05855-4

This Springer imprint is published by the registered company Springer Nature Switzerland AG
The registered company address is: Gewerbestrasse 11, 6330 Cham, Switzerland

Preface

Most of us have heard the statement "*We shot at the heart and hit the prostate*". Robotic surgery has certainly represented the most striking technological innovation in the surgical field over the past 20 years, and urology as specialty has led the field in the implementation of this technology on large scale worldwide. Robotic-assisted laparoscopic radical prostatectomy (RALP) has become de facto the new standard for the surgical treatment of prostate cancer, the most common cancer in the male population. In the USA, over 80% of radical prostatectomy procedures are nowadays done robotically, and similar figures have been reached worldwide. Thus, not surprisingly, the field of robotic surgery has been largely fueled by this single surgical procedure. Many years have gone by since the first pioneering reports of radical prostatectomy procedures by Dr. Abbou and Dr. Vallancien in Paris and Dr. Binder in Frankfurt, soon followed by the establishment of the first structured robotic prostate surgery program by Dr. Menon in Detroit. Over 5000 daVinci systems are now installed worldwide, and currently available robotic platforms are undeniably much better than the one used by those pioneers, and this has made the procedure safer, easier to learn and more reproducible. Moreover, new robotic systems are coming to the market, and upcoming competition will drive further innovation. As robotic surgical technology evolved, many advances were made in terms of knowledge of the surgical anatomy, building on the foundations of early studies reported by Dr. Walsh in the 1980s, and further advances brought by laparoscopic surgery in the early 2000s. A better understanding of prostate cancer biology allowed to improve patient selection. Modern diagnostic pathways with the introduction of MRI-based biopsy techniques allowed to better risk-stratify patients and aid surgical planning. All this translated into never-ending refinements of surgical techniques and, ultimately, into improved outcomes.

The idea behind this book was to provide a comprehensive high yield and user-friendly educational tool for urologists and trainees alike. With this aim in mind, we asked opinion leaders across the globe to contribute with state-of-the-art chapters on a variety of topics related to the ever-evolving field of robotic prostate cancer surgery. We would like to thank these esteemed colleagues and their teams for their outstanding work, which is testament to their commitment to foster future generations of robotic urologic surgeons and, ultimately, to their dedication to provide better care to prostate cancer patients. This effort is even more valuable if one considers this book was conceived and prepared in the middle of a pandemic that has unfortunately changed our lives. We are confident to have accomplished what we initially planned; enjoy the reading!

Sincerely,

Chicago, IL, USA	Riccardo Autorino
Guangzhou, China	Di Gu
London, UK	Senthil Nathan
Trieste, Trieste, Italy	Nicola Pavan
Shanghai, China	Shancheng Ren
Hatfield, UK	Ashwin Sridhar

Contents

Part I

Introduction to RALP

A Historical Perspective of RALP

1

Giacomo Rebez and Maria Carmen Mir

Introduction

In the current chapter we endeavored to provide the reader with a historical perspective on the milestones for RARP further envisioning future technological improvements.

Brief History of Radical Prostatectomy

Radical prostatectomy was initially described over a 100 years ago: the first perineal prostatectomy was accomplished by Proust in France in 1901. In the USA, in 1904, 4 years later, Young [1] begun to perform the surgery on patients affected by prostate cancer. Mortality and morbidity, often related to a lack of medical technology, were relevant during the early years with 30% mortality rates [2]. From the late 1940s improvements in technique and technologies were made; Millin's retropubic prostatectomy was used for prostate cancer by Memmelaar and others. In the last four decades we have achieved the highest standard of surgical interventions through improved disease staging, better patient's selection, and improvement in medical technology [3]. In the late 1980s the open "anatomic" RP was described by Walsh [4]. The early control of Santorini's plexus, and the possibility to spare the neurovascular bundles, facilitating functional recovery turned this surgery the gold standard in the 80s, leading to the abandonment of perineal prostatectomy. Later on, the new standard was challenged by laparoscopic RP (LRP), which was developed as a "minimally-invasive" alternative in the early 1990s. Schuessler et al. [5] reported the first LRP, however, later the surgery was abandoned due to its technical challenges and surgical time. The challenge of laparoscopy moved across the Atlantic Ocean to France, where Guillonneau and Vallancien and others described the standardized Montsouris technique [6]. LRP proved to provide similar oncological and functional results as open RP, although this was initially hotly disputed. However, LRP implies a rather long learning curve. For this reason, its adoption was not universal, and many urologists stuck to the still "gold standard" of open RP [7] until the early 2000s when robotic surgery was introduced in urology.

G. Rebez
Department of Urology, University of Trieste, Trieste, Italy

M. C. Mir (✉)
Fundacion Instituto Valenciano Oncologia, Valencia, Spain

Robotic Surgery Historical Perspective

The first industrial robot was developed in 1937, while [8] the history of robotics in surgery begins with the Puma 560, a robot used in 1985 by Kwoh et al. [9] to perform brain biopsies. This system eventually led to the development of PROBOT, a robot designed specifically for transurethral resection of the prostate [10]. Concomitantly, Integrated Surgical Supplies Ltd of Sacramento, CA, developed [11] a surgical robot able to precisely core out the femoral shaft with 96% precision, whereas a standard surgery provided only 75% accuracy. It was named RoboDoc and it was [11] the first surgical robot approved by the FDA. A group of researchers at the National Air and Space Administration (NASA), working on virtual reality, became interested in using this new information on robotic surgery to develop telepresence surgery. In the late 1980s, the concept of telesurgery became one of the main driving forces behind the development of surgical robots. In the early 1990s, several of the scientists from the NASA-Ames team joined the Stanford Research Institute (SRI). Working with SRI's other roboticists and virtual reality experts, these scientists developed a dexterous tele manipulator for hand surgery. The US Army became interested in the possibility of decreasing wartime mortality by "bringing the surgeon" to the wounded soldier—through telepresence [11–13]. With funding from the US Army, a system was devised whereby a wounded soldier could be loaded into a vehicle with robotic surgical equipment and be operated on remotely by a surgeon at a nearby Mobile Advanced Surgical Hospital (MASH). This system,

S. Ren et al. (eds.), *Robot-Assisted Radical Prostatectomy*, https://doi.org/10.1007/978-3-031-05855-4_1

it was hoped, would decrease wartime mortality by preventing wounded soldiers from exsanguinating before they reached the hospital. During the research several of the surgeons and engineers working on surgical robotic systems for the Army eventually formed commercial ventures that lead to the introduction of robotics to the civilian surgical community [12]. Especially, Computer Motion, Inc. of Santa Barbara, employed seed money provided by the Army to develop the Automated Endoscopic System for Optimal Positioning (AESOP), a robotic arm controlled by the surgeon voice commands to manipulate an endoscopic camera. Shortly after AESOP was marketed, Integrated Surgical Systems (now Intuitive Surgical) of Mountain View, CA, licensed the SRI Green Telepresence Surgery system. That system after an extensive redesign will be reintroduced later as the Da Vinci surgical system. In 1996 Buess and Schurr pioneered the first tele-surgical laparoscopic porcine cholecystectomy using the ARTEMIS-System [14]. Despite various promising experimental trials in abdominal and cardiac surgery, the device never made it beyond the experimental state [15]. The first clinically used robot was ZEUS (Computer Motion, USA) with the surgeon seated at an open console on a high-backed chair with arm-rests controlling instruments of two robotic arms by use of chop-stick-like handles [16]. The right and left robotic arms replicate the arms of the surgeon, and the third arm was a voice-controlled robotic endoscope for visualization AESOP [17]. The system used both straight shafted endoscopic instruments similar to conventional endoscopic instruments and jointed instruments with articulating end-effectors and 4 degrees of freedom (jaw, pitch, insertion, rotation). The ZEUS system was developed for cardiovascolar surgery [16] and was rarely used in Urology [18]. The da Vinci Surgical system (Intuitive Surgical, Sunnyvale, United States) was also initially designed for robot-assisted coronary artery surgery [19]. The da Vinci and Zeus systems were very similar in their capabilities but different in their approaches to robotic surgery. Both systems were composed of master–slave surgical robot with multiple arms operated remotely from a console with video assisted visualization and computer enhancement [13]. The tele-presence effect was abandoned due to the long-distance transmission delay and FDA approved Da Vinci platform in 2000. From 2004 to 2016, there was no active opponent for Intuitive Surgical based on the fact, that Intuitive acquired Computer Motion, assigning all patents concerning the principle of ZEUS. Intuitive built a practically insurmountable competitive moat blocking the entrance of other companies into the market by developing a superior product, protecting its intellectual portfolio, and gaining surgeons' trust [20]. In 2019 some of the key-patents of Da Vinci 2000 and ZEUS expired enabling other companies to enter the market. Currently, other than the da Vinci systems, five robotic surgical systems are commercially available: Senhance has regulatory approval for human use in the USA, Europe, and Japan; Versius and Avatera hold a CE Mark certification for use in Europe, whereas Revo-I and Hinotori are available in the Korean and Japanese markets, respectively.

Major Technical Improvements for RARP Overtime

In 2000, the first robotic prostatectomy was performed at the Department of Urology of Frankfurt University in Germany [21] by Binder and Kramer while Abbou in France published a case report on his first RALP in the same year [22]. Then in the US, in 2002, Menon et al. [23] published the first prospective trial comparing the results of RALP with those of open retropubic RP achieving a breakthrough in urologic surgery subsequently obtaining the FDA approval for the use of the system for prostatic surgery. The first robotic technique was described in 2003, by Menon et al. [24]: the Vattikuti Institute Prostatectomy (VIP). The main principles of the VIP included development of the extraperitoneal space, lymph node dissection if indicated, incision of the endopelvic fascia, dorsal vein complex control, bladder neck transection, posterior dissection, control of the lateral pedicles, release of the neurovascular bundles, retrograde apical dissection, division of the dorsal venous complex and urethra, vesical-urethral anastomosis, specimen retrieval, and completion. This technique incorporated an incremental nerve preservation, the "Veil of Aphrodite" with the development and preservation of the lateral prostatic fascia (i.e., veil of Aphrodite). It involves the releasing of cavernous nerve tissue extending along the posterolateral aspects of the prostate bilaterally, up to the fibrous stroma of the dorsal vein complex anteriorly overlying the apex of the prostate.

Excellent oncological and functional outcomes were reported by many authors [23, 25–27] leading to an expansion in the application of RARPs worldwide. Since the initial introduction of RALP, various groups have reported modifications to the original VIP technique (see Fig. 1.1). The Van Velthoven anastomosis, consisting of a double-running suture, was reported for both laparoscopic and robotic prostatectomy in 2003 [28] and is now a standard technique used in RALP. The preservation of the high lateral prostatic fascia, reported by Kaul et al. [29]; led to improved potency rates, probably related to intra-operative tension reduction on the neurovascular bundles. The avoidance of thermal injury of the neurovascular bundle has been highlighted by many authors [30], with short-term results showing a difference in potency rates between cautery and non-cautery techniques.

The Rocco stitch was first described in radical retropubic prostatectomy by Rocco in 2007 [31] and has been reported by Tewari et al. [32] for its use in RALP. This is a posterior

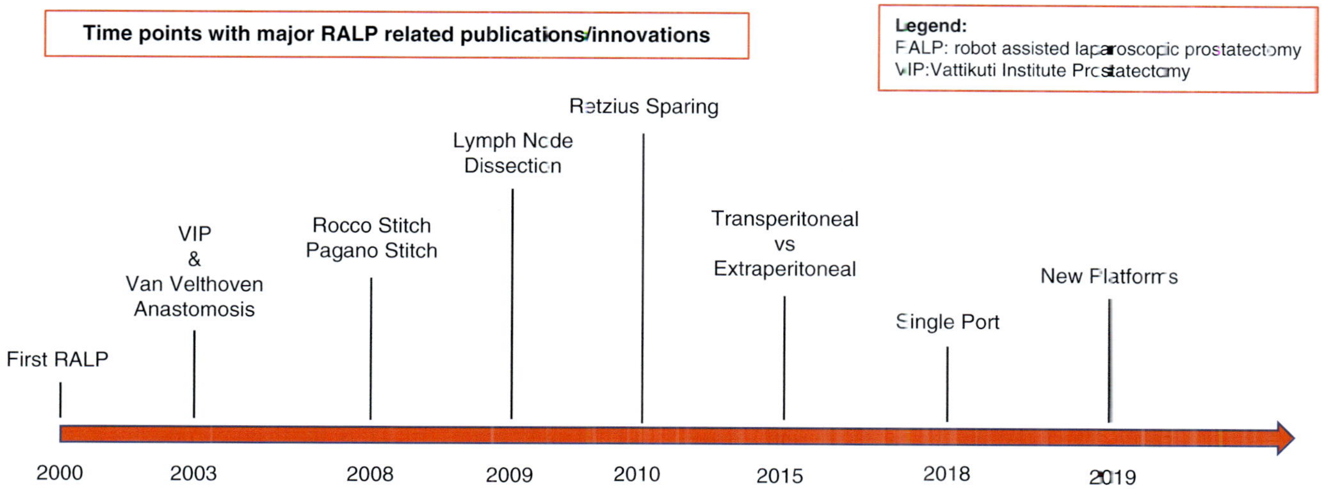

Fig. 1.1 Time points with major RALP related publications/innovations. *RALP* robot assisted laparoscopic prostatectomy. *VIP* Vattikuti Institute Prostatectomy

reconstruction to support the urethral sphincter, and it has been used in combination with the Pagano stitch, which adds further reinforcement to the posterior bladder neck. Tewari et al. [32] reported an earlier return to total urinary continence with 83% continence rate at 6 weeks.

The Retzius sparing (or Bocciardi approach) robot assisted radical prostatectomy RS-RARP was described in 2010. The anatomic rationale of this technique stems from the preservation of the anterior structures involved in continence and potency preservation, such as pubo-vesical ligaments, puboprostatic fascia, NVBs, accessory pudendal artery, and dorsal vein complex. This approach encompasses incising the parietal peritoneum at the anterior surface of the vesicorectal pouch, at the level of the seminal vesicles. After having dissected the vasa deferentia and the seminal vesicles and retracted them by means of two sutures placed transabdominally, dissection of the prostate is carried out in an antegrade fashion [33]. The Denonvilliers fascia is separated by the posterolateral surface of the prostate, and the prostatic apex is reached. The RCT by Dalela et al. [34] showed an earlier return to continence with the Retzius-sparing RARP (RS-RARP) technique than with the anterior approach (71%—48% 1 week after catheter removal).

The distinction between an ascending, retrograde dissection and a descending, antegrade dissection is still debated [35]. Extraperitoneal approach (EP) and transperitoneal approach (TP) were developed in the early years, but the use of the transperitoneal approach vastly outnumbers the extraperitoneal. There are advantages in extraperitoneal approach since it does not violate the peritoneal cavity, which might be useful especially in obese patients, those who have had abdominal procedures in the past and those with bowel diversion. One distinct disadvantage of the EP approach is the limited space available for robotic movements which might be a limitation for performing extended pelvic lymph node dissection. The rational of use behind TP approach is its fast performance and shorter learning-curve. However, in experienced hands, one is able to do a very comparable job. Though the TP approach would continue to be the premium approach for robotic and laparoscopic radical prostatectomy, the EP approach has its indications and might be a useful skill. Only two RCTs have evaluated the extraperitoneal versus transperitoneal approach [36, 37]. Both trials, even if limited by their small sample size, demonstrated similar outcomes of the two approaches, with one showing reduced time to solid diet when the extraperitoneal approach was chosen [30]. Among the newest robotic approaches there is the partial resection of the prostate, thanks to the advances in the mpMRI field [38, 39]. Regarding the partial prostatectomy techniques, functional outcomes are expected to be optimal in a few selected patients. Potentially, in addition to RCTs, a novel definition of PSA response after the procedure would likely be required in an effort to assess the oncological success of the procedure.

The use of extended pelvic lymph node dissection (PLND) has been demonstrated in RALP and was shown to be feasible with respect to both surgical technique and number of lymph nodes removed [40]. The indications and clinical benefit of this in open, laparoscopic, or robotic-assisted approaches remain unclear, although an increased number of positive nodes are found when extended PLND is performed [41]. Refinements in the mostly transabdominal technique, improvements in nerve-preservation, technical developments (fourth arm), and the development of the extraperitoneal approach, brought more complexity but also improved results and reduced complications with RALP.

Single Port Robotic Radical Prostatectomy

Single port (SP) robotic assisted laparoscopic surgery was approved by the FDA for urologic surgery in 2018. The system enables a camera and three separate instruments, with fully wristed motions, to be placed through a single 25 mm port. It was designed to perform complex surgery in narrow deep spaces [42] providing benefit in select clinical situations over the conventional four-arm da Vinci robotic systems. The experience of the authors with the SP system includes mainly radical prostatectomies through the trans perineal and Retzius-sparing approaches. Both procedures could be safely performed without conversion and acceptable operative time. The latest review on single port surgery showed similar intraoperative and perioperative outcomes to those obtained with the standard multiport da Vinci system [43].

The handling of the robotic instruments through the console is similar to the previous da Vinci systems. The downside is the working space of the assistant's instruments which is limited owing to collisions with the bulky multichannel port and extracorporeal robotic arm. According to Lenfant, patients with high-risk localized prostate cancer and limited treatment options due to a complex abdominal surgical history (i.e., frozen pelvis) may be suitable candidates for single-port radical perineal prostatectomy [44]. The costs for SP and MP prostatectomy are comparable. The higher SP cost for consumable surgical materials is offset by the lower cost associated with hospitalization, which was largely due to a shorter hospital stay after SP surgery. Moreover, a comparative study between pure single-site single-port extraperitoneal prostatectomy and multi-port showed a shorter length of stay as well as a decreased need for postoperative pain medication and narcotic administration for single port, with comparable postoperative complication and readmission rate [45].

Consequently, the SP system appears to be an option, with an easy learning curve for expert robotic surgeons, allowing minimally invasive treatment in few selected patients.

Currently Available Platforms for Radical Prostatectomy

Da Vinci XI/DaVinci X

Da Vinci surgical platform will be described in detail on a full chapter. Briefly, in 2014, Intuitive Surgical launched the Da Vinci XI-system with an 8 mm-3D-HD-camera that can be moved at all four ports, especially helpful during a kidney surgery. The robotic arms are finer than Si model, to minimize instrument clashing, and the OR-table can be moved while the robotic arms are connected [46]. Additionally, the system can provide a feature in combination with a specific OR-table (Trumpf-Medical, Germany), which enables to move the table without the need to undock the arms. Recently, the company introduced the X-system, a new version of the robot designed to be a little easier on the budget, while still providing most of the abilities of the flagship model. The da Vinci X takes the thinner, more capable arms and instruments of the Xi and moves them onto a cart like the Si model. That means the system sacrifices some of the versatility of the higher-end model, like the ability to perform procedures in several parts of the body at once, but that's the trade-off for the lower price [46]. Thus, the main purpose for introduction of this device is to reduce the costs for those hospitals, where General Surgery does not play an important role with respect to robotics, because it seems to be very useful for urologic and gynecologic applications.

Versius

The Versius surgical system (Cambridge Medical Robotics Ltd., Cambridge, UK) received the European CE Mark in March 2019. It was created following the idea of independent robotic arms with separate functional units [47]. With an open console and advanced robotic joints, it provides a more human-like range of arm movements. A haptic feedback system, which is a relevant innovation, is featured in this platform. Moreover, the surgeon can choose to operate in a sitting or a standing position while controlling the system through joystick handles. The company adopted a different marketing strategy in the form of a managed-service contract system [48] without an upfront capital payment. A recent study on the feasibility of the Versius platform for renal and prostate procedures in a preclinical setting reported that the system is ready to be tested in live human studies [49].

Revo-i

The Revo-i (Meere Company Inc., Yongin, Korea) surgical platform is a master–slave system, which received approval for human use from the Korean Ministry of Food and Drug Safety in August 2017. The system, which is quite similar to da Vinci Si system, consists of a control console, a four-arm robotic cart, a vision cart with high-definition quality, and multi-use endoscopic instruments [50, 51]. The 3D endoscope is 10 mm in diameter. The instruments are fully wristed, providing 7 degrees of freedom, with a 7.4 mm diameter, and are reusable for up to 20 times [52]. The safety and feasibility of fallopian tube reconstruction, cholecystectomy, and partial nephrectomy were assessed in animal preclinical studies [53–55]. In 2018 the first human trial using Revo-i in Retzius-sparing robot-assisted radical prostatectomy (RS-RARP) reported promising results [52]. Further studies are needed to gain more solid results, but the platform seems to be valid, and would probably be a strong competitor for Da Vinci system.

Senhance (Telelap ALF-X)

In October 2017 FDA-approved ALF-X (Senhance; TransEnterix®, Morrisville, USA) is a new multiport robotic system. It was first developed by an Italian company (Sofar, Milan, Italy) and received the CE Mark certification in 2016 for all abdominal and noncardiac thoracic procedures. In October 2017, Senhance received the FDA clearance; however, they did not include urologic procedures [56]. The surgeon is ergonomically seated in an open console, called the "cockpit," and a monitor provides 3D high-definition visualization thanks to polarized glasses. The camera manipulation is controlled by the surgeon's eye movements through an infrared eye-tracking system [57]. The advantages are totally independent surgical arms, haptic feedback, and eye tracking systems [58, 59] while the downsides are the need of polarized glasses and a spacious operative room for the independent surgical arms. The use of Senhance for extraperitoneal radical prostatectomy [60] and different urological procedures was described in eastern Europe [61]. Further solid clinical trials are needed to better assess the performance of this platform on urologic surgeries.

Even though the da Vinci system brought to the market many different robots with significant developments for each generation, there has been no significant improvement in the console. The closed console design envelops the face of the surgeon and decreases the awareness of the surrounding operative theatre. The communication is mainly verbal through the microphone of the console and the speakers of the system, and an experienced surgical team with excellent communication skills is needed. Two platforms, Senhance and Versius, offer an open-console design, allowing verbal and nonverbal communication between the surgeon and the surgical team [58, 62] but also Avatera system features an microscope like eyepiece that provides an easier communication [63]. Haptic feedback is one of the biggest flaws of the da Vinci platform, which hopefully will be assessed in the future. Robotic surgeons have compensated for this limitation by developing a "pseudo-haptic" ability, which relies on optical cues to assess the tension on tissues [64]. The haptic feedback is featured in Senhance and Versius thanks to a mechanism that translate the force and its direction applied from the tips of the instruments on tissues in counter-movements in console handles [60]. The haptic feedback could provide additional advantages like improved tissue manipulation and might reduce the learning curve of robotics [65]. All new companies attempted to reduce the instruments' diameter of their platforms to promote less tissue trauma and invasiveness and move toward better cosmesis. Revo-I utilizes 7.4-mm instruments, but the port size remains at 8 mm [20]. Versius and Avatera use instruments of 5 mm in diameter [49, 63]. Senhance, except for the 5-mm instruments, offers the option of micro laparoscopy with 3-mm instruments, although the lack of articulation is a significant drawback [66]. The question is, even if most of these new robotic systems receive FDA/CE mark approval, how many of them will commercially succeed. Unavoidably, each emerging system has to compete with the existing gold standard while generating data to evaluate potential safety and efficiency. New companies have carefully studied the features lacking in the established system, in the attempt to implement new technologies to try to improve the capabilities of the existing platform.

Future Perspectives on Robot-Assisted Radical Prostatectomy

As a result of several factors such as improvements of early continence and potency rates, short learning curve, improved surgeon/console ergonomics, market-driven forces and the patients "choice", the robotic system is likely to gain even more popularity in the foreseeable future. The hegemony of the da Vinci surgical systems is subject to change as a handful of platforms for robot-assisted laparoscopic surgical procedures are available in the market worldwide. The innovation of robotic surgery is still growing; new robotic systems are in the process of development and will approach the market, hopefully bringing new features and reducing costs. For example, the adoption of a glasses-free 3D display technology will be an innovative step. Among the new technologies a DROP-IN gamma probe was recently introduced to implement radio guided surgery [67]. Through enhanced maneuverability and surgical autonomy, the DROP-IN promotes the implementation of radio guided lymphadenectomy compared to traditional laparoscopic guide. This new feature is probably going to be implemented in the future.

As surgeons we are looking forward to welcoming new platforms and technologies that will improve patient care in a cost-effective manner. As more surgeons perform RALP and more platforms will be available, it is likely that further modifications of surgical technique will be made to improve both oncological and functional outcomes. Further developments may reduce the number of ports and implement the integrated use of three-dimensional reconstructions of prostate MRI during surgery. Recent advances in 3D reconstruction from digitalized images have made possible to provide intraoperative surgical navigation. The 3D elastic augmented reality of Porpiglia et al. [68] approximate the deformation of the target organ creating a virtual overlapping of MRI imaging during RALP. The accuracy offered by this technology is now allowing for "real-time" intraoperative tailoring of the robotic procedure to the specific anatomy of the patient and the specific location of the cancer.

Conclusions

RALP has already proven an excellent performance and has brought surgery into the digital age. Robotic technology has revolutionized surgery by facilitating and expanding laparoscopic procedures, advancing surgical technology, changing the mentoring and the surgical techniques. Technology has been expanding the treatment modalities beyond the limits of human abilities. Telesurgery is still under validation even if not yet widely available in clinical practice due to long distance errors. Robotic is here to stay and will likely be improved in the foreseeable future. Open markets will turn these technologies making them available worldwide.

References

1. Sohn M, Hubmann R, Moll F, Hatzinger M. Von den Anfängen bis DaVinci. Aktuelle Urol. 2012;43:228–30.
2. Sharma NL, Shah NC, Neal DE. Robotic-assisted laparoscopic prostatectomy. Br J Cancer. 2009;101:1491–6.
3. John H, Wiklund P. Robotic urology. 3rd ed. Cham: Springer Nature Switzerland AG; 2018. https://doi.org/10.1007/978-3-319-65864-3.
4. Walsh PC. Radical prostatectomy in locally confined prostatic carcinoma. Prog Clin Biol Res. 1990;359:199–207.
5. Schuessler WW, Schulam PG, Clayman RV, Kavoussi LR. Laparoscopic radical prostatectomy: initial short-term experience. Urology. 1997;50:854–7.
6. Hemal AK, Menon M. Robotics in urology. Curr Opin Urol. 2004;14:89–93.
7. Hakenberg OW. A brief overview of the development of robot-assisted radical prostatectomy. Arab J Urol. 2018;16:293–6.
8. Jain S, Gautam G. Robotics in urologic oncology. J Minim Access Surg. 2015;11:40–4.
9. Kwoh YS, Hou J, Jonckheere EA, Hayati S. A robot with improved absolute positioning accuracy for CT guided stereotactic brain surgery. IEEE Trans Biomed Eng. 1988;35:153–60.
10. Lanfranco AR, Castellanos AE, Desai JP, Meyers WC. Robotic surgery: a current perspective. Ann Surg. 2004;239:14–21.
11. Satava RM. Surgical robotics: the early chronicles. Surg Laparosc Endosc Percutan Tech. 2002;12:6–16.
12. Satava RM. Virtual reality and telepresence for military medicine. Comput Biol Med. 1995;25:229–36.
13. George EI, Brand TC, LaPorta A, Marescaux J, Satava RM. Origins of robotic surgery: from skepticism to standard of care. JSLS. 2018;22(4):e2018.00039. https://doi.org/10.4293/JSLS.2018.00039.
14. Schurr MO, Arezzo A, Buess GF. Robotics and systems technology for advanced endoscopic procedures: experiences in general surgery. Eur J Cardiothorac Surg. 1999;6(Suppl 2):S97–S105. https://doi.org/10.1016/S1010-7940(99)00281-X.
15. Rininsland H. ARTEMIS. A telemanipulator for cardiac surgery. Eur J Cardiothorac Surg. 1999;16(Suppl 2):S106–11. https://doi.org/10.1016/S1010-7940(99)00282-1.
16. Reichenspurner H, Damiano RJ, Mack M, Boehm DH, Gulbins H, Detter C, Meiser B, Ellgass R, Reichart B. Use of the voice-controlled and computer-assisted surgical system zeus for endoscopic coronary artery bypass grafting. J Thorac Cardiovasc Surg. 1999;118:11–6.
17. Kavoussi LR, Moore RG, Adams JB, Partin AW. Comparison of robotic versus human laparoscopic camera control. J Urol. 1995;154:2134–6.
18. Luke PPW, Girvan AR, Al Omar M, Beasley KA, Carson M. Laparoscopic robotic pyeloplasty using the Zeus Telesurgical System. Can J Urol. 2004;11:2396–400.
19. Mohr FW, Falk V, Diegeler A, Autschbach R. Computer-enhanced coronary artery bypass surgery. J Thorac Cardiovasc Surg. 1999;117:1212–4.
20. Rassweiler JJ, Autorino R, Klein J, et al. Future of robotic surgery in urology. BJU Int. 2017;120:822–41.
21. Binder J, Kramer W. Robotically-assisted laparoscopic radical prostatectomy. BJU Int. 2001;87:408–10.
22. Abbou CC, Hoznek A, Salomon L, Lobontiu A, Saint F, Cicco A, Antiphon P, Chopin D. Remote laparoscopic radical prostatectomy carried out with a robot. Report of a case. Prog Urol. 2000;10:520–3.
23. Menon M, Tewari A, Baize B, Guillonneau B, Vallancien G. Prospective comparison of radical retropubic prostatectomy and robot-assisted anatomic prostatectomy: The Vattikuti Urology Institute experience. Urology. 2002;60:864–8.
24. Menon M, Tewari A, Peabody J, Baize B, Hemal A, Sarle R, Shrivastava A. Vattikuti Institute prostatectomy: technique. J Urol. 2003;169:2289–92.
25. Tewari A, Peabody J, Sarle R, Balakrishnan G, Hemal A, Shrivastava A, Menon M. Technique of da Vinci robot-assisted anatomic radical prostatectomy. Urology. 2002;60:569–72.
26. Shrivastava A, Baliga M, Menon M. The Vattikuti Institute prostatectomy. BJU Int. 2007;99:1173–89.
27. Menon M, Tewari A, Peabody JO, Shrivastava A, Kaul S, Bhandari A, Hemal AK. Vattikuti Institute prostatectomy, a technique of robotic radical prostatectomy for management of localized carcinoma of the prostate: experience of over 1100 cases. Urol Clin North Am. 2004;31:701–17.
28. Van Velthoven RF, Ahlering TE, Peltier A, Skarecky DW, Clayman RV. Technique for laparoscopic running urethrovesical anastomosis: the single knot method. Urology. 2003;61:699–702.
29. Kaul S, Bhandari A, Hemal A, Savera A, Shrivastava A, Menon M. Robotic radical prostatectomy with preservation of the prostatic fascia: a feasibility study. Urology. 2005;66:1261–5.
30. Ahlering TE, Skarecky D, Borin J. Impact of cautery versus cautery-free preservation of neurovascular bundles on early return of potency. J Endourol. 2006;20:586–9.
31. Rocco B, Gregori A, Stener S, Santoro L, Bozzola A, Galli S, Knez R, Scieri F, Scaburri A, Gaboardi F. Posterior reconstruction of the rhabdosphincter allows a rapid recovery of continence after transperitoneal videolaparoscopic radical prostatectomy. Eur Urol. 2007;51(4):996–1003. https://doi.org/10.1016/j.eururo.2006.10.014.
32. Tewari A, Jhaveri J, Rao S, et al. Total reconstruction of the vesico-urethral junction. BJU Int. 2008;101:871–7.
33. Martini A, Falagario UG, Villers A, et al. Contemporary techniques of prostate dissection for robot-assisted prostatectomy. Eur Urol. 2020;78:583–91.
34. Dalela D, Jeong W, Prasad MA, et al. A pragmatic randomized controlled trial examining the impact of the Retzius-sparing approach

on early urinary continence recovery after robot-assisted radical prostatectomy. Eur Urol. 2017;72:677–85.
35. Rassweiler J, Wagner AA, Moazin M, Gözen AS, Teber D, Frede T, Su LM. Anatomic nerve-sparing laparoscopic radical prostatectomy: comparison of retrograde and antegrade techniques. Urology. 2006;68:587–91.
36. Stewart LA, Clarke M, Rovers M, Riley RD, Simmonds M, Stewart G, Tierney JF. Preferred reporting items for a systematic review and meta-analysis of individual participant data: the PRISMA-IPD statement. JAMA. 2015;313(16):1657–65. https://doi.org/10.1001/jama.2015.3656.
37. Akand M, Erdogru T, Avci E, Ates M. Transperitoneal versus extraperitoneal robot-assisted laparoscopic radical prostatectomy: a prospective single surgeon randomized comparative study. Int J Urol. 2015;22:916–21.
38. Abdollah F, Jeong W, Dalela D, Palma-Zamora I, Sood A, Menon M. Menon-precision prostatectomy (MPP): an idea, development, exploration, assessment, long-term follow-up (IDEAL) stage 1 study. Eur Urol Suppl. 2019;18:e622.
39. Villers A, Puech P, Flamand V, et al. Partial prostatectomy for anterior cancer: short-term oncologic and functional outcomes. Eur Urol. 2017;72:333–42.
40. Feicke A, Baumgartner M, Talimi S, Schmid DM, Seifert HH, Müntener M, Fatzer M, Sulser T, Strebel RT. Robotic-assisted laparoscopic extended pelvic lymph node dissection for prostate cancer: surgical technique and experience with the first 99 cases. Eur Urol. 2009;55:876–84.
41. Bhatta Dhar N, Burkhard FC, Studer UE. Role of lymphadenectomy in clinically organ-confined prostate cancer. World J Urol. 2007;25:39–44.
42. Billah MS, Stifelman M, Munver R, Tsui J, Lovallo G, Ahmed M. Single port robotic assisted reconstructive urologic surgery-with the da Vinci SP surgical system. Transl Androl Urol. 2020;9:870–8.
43. Checcucci E, De Cillis S, Pecoraro A, et al. Single-port robot-assisted radical prostatectomy: a systematic review and pooled analysis of the preliminary experiences. BJU Int. 2020;126:55–64.
44. Lenfant L, Garisto J, Sawczyn G, Wilson CA, Aminsharifi A, Kim S, Schwen Z, Bertolo R, Kaouk J. Robot-assisted radical prostatectomy using single-port perineal approach: technique and single-surgeon matched-paired comparative outcomes. Eur Urol. 2021;79:384–92.
45. Lenfant L, Sawczyn G, Aminsharifi A, Kim S, Wilson CA, Beksac AT, Schwen Z, Kaouk J. Pure single-site robot-assisted radical prostatectomy using single-port versus multiport robotic radical prostatectomy: a single-institution comparative study. Eur Urol Focus. 2021;7(5):964–72. https://doi.org/10.1016/j.euf.2020.10.006.
46. Intuitive | Robotic Assisted Systems | da Vinci Robot. https://www.intuitive.com/en-us/products-and-services/da-vinci/systems. Accessed 19 Apr 2021.
47. Almujalhem A, Rha KH. Surgical robotic systems: what we have now? A urological perspective. BJUI Compass. 2020;1:152–9.
48. Peters BS, Armijo PR, Krause C, Choudhury SA, Oleynikov D. Review of emerging surgical robotic technology. Surg Endosc. 2018;32:1636–55.
49. Thomas BC, Slack M, Hussain M, Barber N, Pradhan A, Dinneen E, Stewart GD. Preclinical evaluation of the versius surgical system, a new robot-assisted surgical device for use in minimal access renal and prostate surgery. Eur Urol Focus. 2021;7:444–52.
50. Gosrisirikul C, Don Chang K, Raheem AA, Rha KH. New era of robotic surgical systems. Asian J Endosc Surg. 2018;11:291–9.
51. revo. http://revosurgical.com/#/main.html. Accessed 19 Apr 2021.
52. Chang KD, Abdel Raheem A, Choi YD, Chung BH, Rha KH. Retzius-sparing robot-assisted radical prostatectomy using the Revo-i robotic surgical system: surgical technique and results of the first human trial. BJU Int. 2018;122:441–8.
53. Kim DK, Park DW, Rha KH. Robot-assisted partial nephrectomy with the REVO-I robot platform in porcine models. Eur Urol. 2016;69:541–2.
54. Abdel Raheem A, Troya IS, Kim DK, Kim SH, Won PD, Joon PS, Hyun GS, Rha KH. Robot-assisted Fallopian tube transection and anastomosis using the new REVO-I robotic surgical system: feasibility in a chronic porcine model. BJU Int. 2016;118:604–9.
55. Lim JH, Lee WJ, Park DW, Yea HJ, Kim SH, Kang CM. Robotic cholecystectomy using Revo-i Model MSR-5000, the newly developed Korean robotic surgical system: a preclinical study. Surg Endosc. 2017;31:3391–7.
56. Rao PP. Robotic surgery: new robots and finally some real competition! World J Urol. 2018;36:537–41.
57. Bozzini G, Gidaro S, Taverna G. Robot-assisted laparoscopic partial nephrectomy with the ALF-X robot on pig models. Eur Urol. 2016;69:376–7.
58. Gidaro S, Buscarini M, Ruiz E, Stark M, Labruzzo A. Telelap Alf-X: a novel telesurgical system for the 21st century. Surg Technol Int. 2012;22:20–5.
59. Senhance Surgical System | Digital Laparoscopy | A New Era in MIS. https://www.senhance.com/. Accessed 19 Apr 2021.
60. Kaštelan Ž, Knežević N, Hudolin T, Kuliš T, Penezić L, Goluža E, Gidaro S, Ćorušić A. Extraperitoneal radical prostatectomy with the Senhance Surgical System robotic platform. Croat Med J. 2019;60:556–7.
61. Samalavicius NE, Janusonis V, Siaulys R, Jasėnas M, Deduchovas O, Venckus R, Ezerskiene V, Paskeviciute R, Klimaviciute G. Robotic surgery using Senhance® robotic platform: single center experience with first 100 cases. J Robot Surg. 2020;14:371–6.
62. Next-generation robot revealed to the world for the first time Robotics Research. https://www.roboticsresear.ch/articles/15309/next-generation-robot-revealed-to-the-world-for-the-first-time. Accessed 20 Apr 2021.
63. avatera system—avateramedical. https://www.avatera.eu/en/avatera-system. Accessed 20 Apr 2021.
64. Hagen ME, Meehan JJ, Inan I, Morel P. Visual clues act as a substitute for haptic feedback in robotic surgery. Surg Endosc Other Interv Tech. 2008;22 1505–8.
65. Saracino A, Deguet A, Staderini F, Boushaki MN, Cianchi F, Menciassi A, Sinibaldi E. Haptic feedback in the da Vinci Research Kit (dVRK): a user study based on grasping, palpation, and incision tasks. Int J Med Robot. 2019;15(4):e1999. https://doi.org/10.1002/rcs.1999.
66. Montlouis-Calixte J, Ripamonti B, Barabino G, Corsini T, Chauleur C. Senhance 3-mm robot-assisted surgery: experience on first 14 patients in France. J Robot Surg. 2019;13:643–7.
67. Dell'Oglio P, Meershoek P, Maurer T, Wit EMK, van Leeuwen PJ, van der Poel HG, van Leeuwen FWB, van Oosterom MN. A DROP-IN gamma probe for robot-assisted radioguided surgery of lymph nodes during radical prostatectomy. Eur Urol. 2021;79:124–32.
68. Porpiglia F, Checcucci E, Amparore D, et al. Three-dimensional elastic augmented-reality robot-assisted radical prostatectomy using hyperaccuracy three-dimensional reconstruction technology: a step further in the identification of capsular involvement. Eur Urol. 2019;76:505–14.

Surgical Anatomy of the Prostate

2

Anthony J. Costello and Daniel M. Costello

Before 1980 retropubic radical prostatectomy was a very hazardous operation for the patient. After the description of the retropubic approach by Millen in 1948 this was the way radical prostatectomy was performed by the open method [1]. Previously the perineal prostatectomy had been popularised by Hugh Hampton Young but was abandoned in favour of the Millens approach which was a more familiar operative technique for the urologist than the perineal operation [2]. It was certainly daunting for the surgeon but it was the patient who suffered the almost inevitable consequence of loss of erectile function, with at least 50% chance of being incontinent of urine. The surgery could be performed, but the quality of life outcomes and cancer outcomes were very poor. The surgical textbook Bailey and Love which the author used in the 1970s as a medical student, stated that surgery for prostate cancer has been tried without much success and the disease is eventually fatal within 3 years [3].

The anatomical insights published by Patrick Walsh and Peter Donker in the 1982 which allowed identification and preservation of the neurovascular bundles during open radical prostatectomy [4]. The operation was performed with consistent bleeding from the dorsal vein complex which was not secured at the beginning of the operation. Walsh reported in 1980 that the dorsal vein could be suture-ligated preventing the significant bleeding, which occurred from simply cutting the dorsal vein and using a balloon catheter tamponade. Walsh reported the ability to tie the dorsal vein and secure it the surgeon simply cut the dorsal vein causing severe haemorrhage [5]. A number of other techniques were used in an attempt to control the dorsal venous bleeding including excision of the anterior pubic bone to improve access to the prostatic apex. A large catheter was placed to post operatively intraoperatively balloon inflated to 30 mL and heavy traction was applied to the dorsal vein complex. This traction also caused ischaemia of the skeletal muscle of the urinary sphincter and this clearly will contribute to poor sphincter function following radical prostatectomy. This report by Walsh rendered radical retropubic prostatectomy a much safer operation and almost certainly help improve continence post prostatectomy by controlling the bleeding and avoiding ischaemia of the striated muscle of the external sphincter from prolonged catheter balloon tamponade. The anastomosis between the urethra and bladder once the prostate was removed was able to be fashioned without being obscured by a constant venous bleeding. The surgeon was able to see where sutures were to be placed in the urethra and bladder neck and potentially avoid pudendal nerve damage in this apical area. The pudendal nerve emerges from levator ani at the apex of the prostate and line sutures placed in an area could have caused damage to the pudendal nerve and thus compromise post-operative urinary continence. Careful dissection with visualisation of the neurovascular bundles was combined with careful the dissection of the external rhabdosphincter with much improved quality of life outcomes of potency and continence.

This chapter on surgical anatomy of the prostate for the robotic radical prostatectomist will concentrate principally on three key anatomical issues, potency, continence and cancer control and how anatomy guides us to achieve the best possible outcomes in these three domains.

The advent of PSA testing in the 1980s Catalona gave a 7–9 year lead time for diagnosis of early prostate cancer [6]. Prostate cancer could be diagnosed before it became palpable and was generally located inside the prostate. Prior to

A. J. Costello (✉)
Department of Urology, Royal Melbourne Hospital, Melbourne, VIC, Australia

The Australian Medical Robotics Academy, Melbourne, VIC, Australia

Department of Surgery, The University of Melbourne, Melbourne, VIC, Australia

The Australian Prostate Centre, Melbourne, VIC, Australia
e-mail: tony@tonycostello.com.au

D. M. Costello
Department of Urology, Royal Melbourne Hospital, Melbourne, VIC, Australia

Department of Surgery, The University of Melbourne, Melbourne, VIC, Australia

S. Ren et al. (eds.), *Robot-Assisted Radical Prostatectomy*, https://doi.org/10.1007/978-3-031-05855-4_2

1990 when PSA testing became accepted and urologists realised that PSA below 10 meant almost certainly organ confined disease. Before 1980 prostate cancer was diagnosed after digital rectal palpation and discovery of a lump or mass in the prostate. This induration was then biopsied using a finger-guided needle in the rectum. Prostate cancer when palpable is usually advanced. Most men who underwent surgery to remove the prostate had their operation on an already advanced prostate cancer. Cure of the prostate cancer was unlikely because of late diagnosis when cancer was probably metastatic at diagnosis.

Muller's Description of the Neurovascular Bundles and Their Significance 1836

Surgeons in the twentieth century were unaware of the anatomical dissections of Dr. Johannes Muller [7]. Muller dissected the cavernous nerves and in 1836 and described them in a published work. This was later published in Gray's anatomy in 1858 the first edition of that textbook. Dr. Robert Myers who has made a life's work observing and reporting anatomical insights of the periprostatic and prostatic anatomy described these findings and commented on the work of Walsh and others in the most recent addition of Gray's anatomy Chapter 75 2015. Muller's discovery of the major and minor cavernous nerves was reported in the first edition of Gray's Anatomy in 1858. It was interesting that Henry Gray illustrated the course of the autonomic nerves from pelvic plexus to prostatic plexus with continuation of the nerves supplying the erectile structures of the penis without attribution to Muller. Perhaps the reason Muller's fine work remained unrecognised was that it was published in German and not translated into English or any other language. Surgeons in English-speaking countries or those who were not fluent in the German language were unaware of Muller's work. It was not until Walsh and Donker in an elegant series of the sections dissections described neurovascular bundle anatomy 1982 [4]. This paper was truly ground-breaking as the operation clearly could be performed in 1836. The operation of radical prostatectomy was only popularised in the twentieth century. Walsh's insights on neuromuscular bundle anatomy were then understood by surgeons performing the retropubic prostatectomy (Fig. 2.1).

The Walsh Donker Contribution to Understanding of the Neurovascular Bundle Anatomy

The anatomical insights published by Patrick Walsh and Peter Donker in 1982 allowed surgeons to understand that neurovascular bundle could be visualised and preserved at

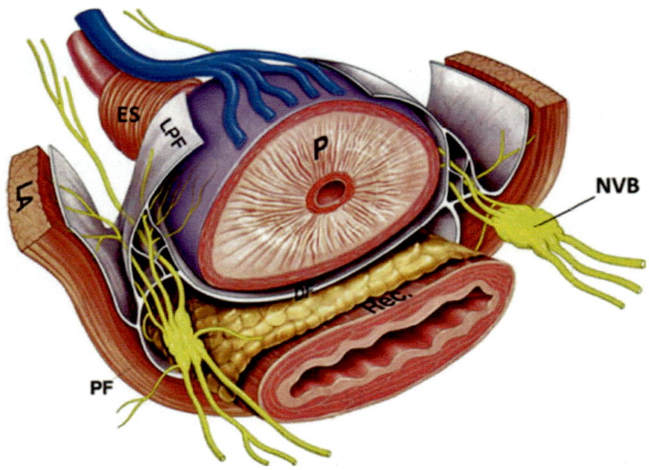

Fig. 2.1 Prostate and neurovascular bundle encased in fascial layers. *P* prostate, *NVB* neurovascular bundle, *LA* levator ani, *PF* prostatic fascia, *ES* external sphincter, *DF* Denonvilliers fascia, *Rec* rectum, *LPF* lateral prostatic fascia

retropubic prostatectomy. Before these anatomical dissections were performed, surgeons were unaware of the existence of the bilateral neurovascular bundles and simply cut or excised the nerves during the section. The accepted belief at that time was that the nerves ran through the prostate. Thus removing the prostate caused certain impotence. Division or excision of the neurovascular bundles made almost certain the patient would be impotent following the operation. Patients do suffer erectile dysfunction early after robotic radical prostatectomy and probably 50% recover potency over time [8]. The likely cause of the early erectile dysfunction following prostatectomy is neurapraxia with traction on the neurovascular bundles causing at least temporary loss of potency. Other mechanisms of nerve injury are except excessive use of diathermy surgical division surgical excision and vascular injury. The nerves in the neurovascular bundle are 0.02–0.4 mm in diameter. The human hair is 0.2 mm in diameter. Even a small amount of traction could cause neurapraxia in such delicate and thin nerve fibres. Walsh demonstrated that the neurovascular bundle ran in the groove between the rectum and the prostate and if it was preserved there was a real possibility of erectile recovery after surgery.

In the 1988 Dr. McNeal and Dr. Stamey from Stanford University described zonal anatomy of the prostate [9]. They described two anatomically and pathologically important zones from a surgical point of view. Their description of the transition zone and the peripheral zone in the prostate informed us that prostate cancer develops generally in the peripheral zone away from the urethra and the transition zone is the site of benign prostatic hypertrophy. Stamey also popularised transrectal ultrasound imaging of the prostate which was then combined with a targeted transrectal ultrasound-guided needle biopsy to improve accuracy of diagnosis [10]. The 1980s heralded a huge improvement in diagnosis, transrectal ultrasound guided biopsy (Stamey) surgical technique (Walsh) and PSA levels (Catalona) for oncologic and quality of life outcomes for radical retropubic prostatectomy [6, 9, 11].

The Royal Melbourne Hospital Anatomic Studies of the NVB and Urinary Sphincter 2004–2018

The work of Walsh and Donker published 1982, completely altered the way urologists approached the technique of radical retropubic prostatectomy. It was now possible to dissect and preserve the neurovascular bundles. There were reports in 1991 of animal experimentation with rats with nerve grafting was performed after the single erectile nerve in the rat model had been excised to examine whether the rat regained potency [12]. In 2001 Kim published paper on bilateral nerve grafting during radical retropubic prostatectomy with extended follow-up [13]. In this article they described removing the sural nerve from the foot of the patient and fixing the nerve in the prostatic bed between the membranous urethra and vascular pedicle of the prostate. This report suggested potency restoration using this technique. The Senior Author was confused by the finding that one could take a somatic nerve the sural nerve, imbed it in the area of parasympathetic and sympathetic autonomic nerves and bring about nerve regrowth with restoration of potency. This article was viewed with the degree of scepticism in our department. This stimulated our team to conduct detailed anatomical dissections to define the anatomy of the neurovascular bundle and at the same time examine the potential of sural nerve grafting onto autonomic nerves. Our sections were concentrated on defining the compartmental structure of the neurovascular bundle, the number of nerves which constituted the neurovascular bundle and the levels at which they ran [14].

We commenced anatomical dissection in anatomy Department at the University Melbourne medical school in 2003. Twelve fixed male human adult cadaver's were dissected [14, 15]. The neurovascular bundle was bilaterally detected on each cadaver and its anatomical relationship to surrounding pelvic structures was documented photographically. Four cadaver specimens were hemisected and eight cadaver specimens were prepared en-bloc by pelvic resection. The branches of the pelvic plexus autonomic nerves were fastidiously dissected under six times magnification. The constituents of the neurovascular bundle were traced from the tips of the seminal vesicles to their target organs which included seminal vesicles prostate rectum and cavernous tissue (Fig. 2.2). We recorded and documented the relationship of the neurovascular bundles to the surrounding pelvic structures. Particular care was taken in describing the relationship of the neurovascular bundle to the rectum posterolateral prostate seminal vesicles and urethral apex. The sectioning enabled a description of all the branches of the autonomic nerve supply prostate.

The neurovascular bundle is comprised of sympathetic and parasympathetic components. These autonomic contributions originate from the hypogastric nerve at T12-L1, which is sympathetic, which joins the parasympathetic contribution S2–S4 at the level of the base of the prostate below the 9 o'clock area. The majority of the autonomic nerves are in fascial compartments below the 9 o'clock level. The number of nerves identified very between 6 and 16. Cavernosal nerves were traced to the proximal corpora cavernosa. There were 24 dissections in 12 pairs. The pelvic plexus was 0.5–2 cm inferior to the level of the tip of the seminal vesical. These nerves were noted to be in three or four individual

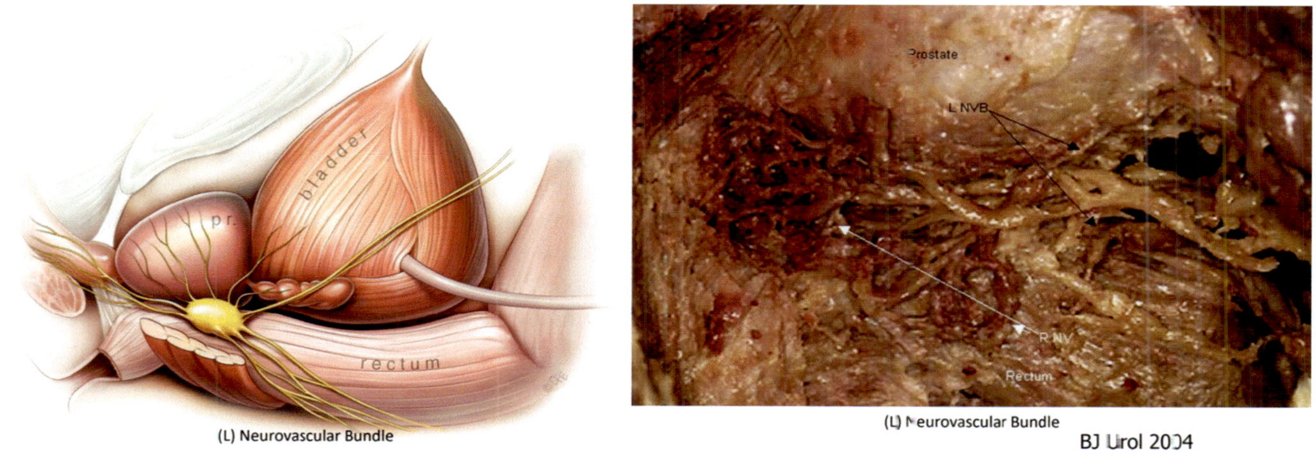

Fig. 2.2 Schematic and acutal dissection of neurovascular bundle. Note ganglion where sympathetic and parasympathetic nerves join is at the base of the prostate

fascial compartments. There was a 3 cm separation between anterior and posterior nerves. Most of the neurovascular bundle travelled posterior to the seminal vesical. Nerves converge into several ganglia between base and mid prostate level to form a dense neurovascular bundle and this is where the parasympathetic nerve supply enters the neurovascular bundle. The nerves in diverge again at the prostatic apex and course in an upwards direction from the 9 o'clock level. Our dissection confirmed that the course true of the cavernosal nerves was in the posterolateral groove between prostate and rectum with the autonomic nerves generally in a separate fascial compartment.

Nerves travel intimately with vasculature both venous and arterial. We observed that there were nerves running in the neurovascular bundle which innovated rectum, prostate and levator ani muscle as well others continuing distally into the corpora cavernosa. The nerves which entered the posterior aspect of the prostate were intimately associated with a arteries and veins of the prostate. The significance of this work was the discovery and the description of the course, number of nerves and the distinct fascial compartments within the neurovascular bundle. The constituents of the neurovascular bundle were in three to four fascial compartments. The compartment containing the cavernous nerves ran below nerves to the prostate (Fig. 2.3).

Superolaterally there is a component of nerves which travel to levator ani. This anatomical insights was important in surgical dissection because we found that there is a 3–5 mm gap between the cavernous nerve compartment and the capsule of the prostate. In principle this could allow dissection 3–5 mm away from the prostate capsule whilst still facilitating preservation of the cavernous nerves in neurovascular bundles. The concept of having to excise the whole neurovascular bundle because of a palpable abnormality in the prostate on digital rectal exam is probably incorrect. Epstein and Walsh described in multiple histological examinations of removed prostate that the average capsular penetration is 3 mm of cancer through the prostatic capsule [16]. Hence the concept of incremental nerve sparing can been feasible as it appears anatomically valid. Before our report in previous publications the terms neurovascular bundle and cavernosal nerves were often used synonymously. We have also have shown using specific collagen stains for the fascial layers around the prostate, the compartmental architecture of the neurovascular bundle. There is a separate discrete compartment for the cavernous nerves. As previously discussed, the concept of laying a somatic sural nerve in this region and expect parasympathetic and sympathetic growth along this nerve conduit to restore potency seems scientifically difficult to reconcile [13].

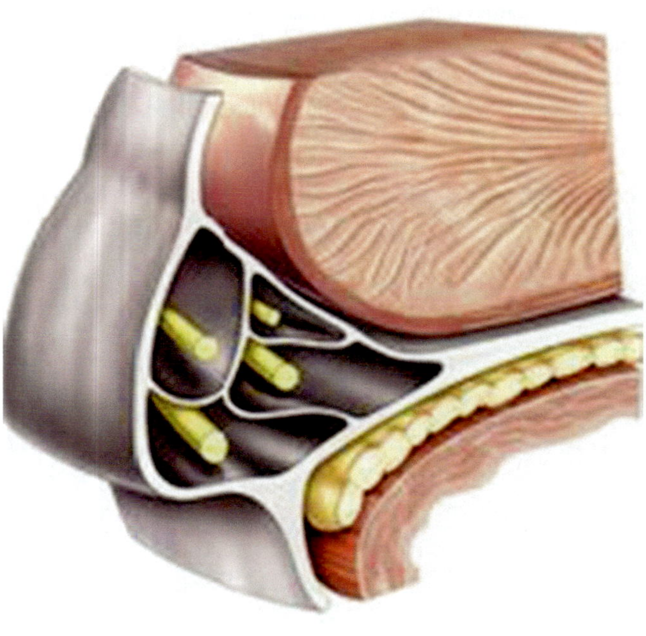

Fig. 2.3 Schematic of the neural compartments cavernous nerves posterior medial below the prostatic nerve compartment

In further anatomical studies in our department published by Clareborough we examined the precise localisation of the sympathetic and parasympathetic nerves in the neurovascular bundle in their particular compartment [15]. By using specific antibodies to parasympathetic nerve, Nitric Oxide, we could identify the parasympathetics, and using tyrosine hydroxylase could identify the sympathetic nerves. Somatic nerves were stained separately. Findings showed that at the prostate base the parasympathetic nerves counted for 43% of all the nerve fibres present this increased to 45% of the prostatic apex. There are only very few nerves in the NVB between 4% and 6% of the total number of nerves between the base mid prostate regions which are above the level of 9 o'clock (Fig. 2.4). Key findings relate to the fact that most of the autonomic nerves run below the 9 o'clock level until the apex of the prostate when they swing anteromedially adjacent to the urethra. The importance of this discovery for the surgeon performing robotic prostatectomy is that the apex of the prostate is where it is likely most damage can be done to the neurovascular bundle by less than meticulous technique in dissection. The autonomic nerves, parasympathetic and sympathetic swing anteriorly and medially sub pubically to enter the cavernous tissue of the penis (Fig. 2.4). It is most important for the robotic prostatectomist to understand this anteromedial direction of the cavernous nerves at the apex. Great care in the dissection must occur at the apical area, given that the parasympathetic and sympathetic autonomic nerves are in close proximity anteriorly at the apex. The pudendal nerve branches emerge from the levator ani at this position about 5 mm away. The pudendal nerve also can be damaged here by inadvertent wider dissection. Thus both potency via the

Illustration 5 – Apical dissection

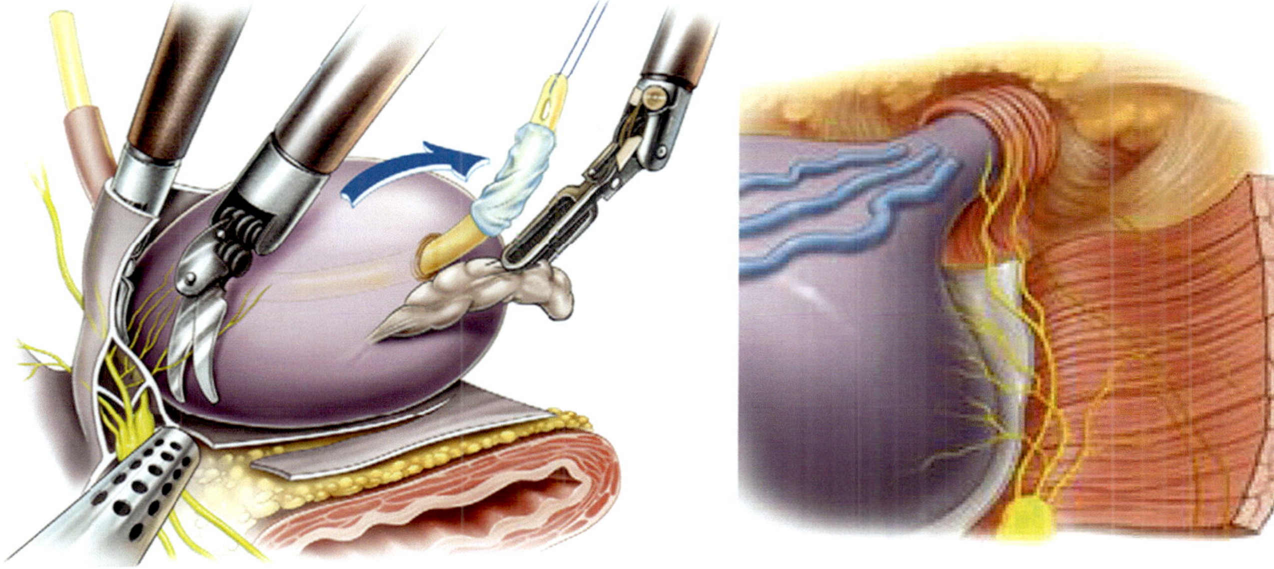

Fig. 2.4 Apical dissection. Text care at the apex where the autonomic nerves swing anteromedially. Note the proximity of cavernous nerves at the prostatic apex as they swing anteromedially on the urethra. The pudendal nerve pierces the levator in close proximity (shown in figure on the right)

autonomic nerves and continence via pudendal nerve branches can be impaired if dissection in this area is excessive. The concept of a high fascial release or release of what was called the Veil of Aphrodite, the fascial layers which drape over the anterior prostate was popularised by Menon 2004 in his early description of technique of robotic radical prostatectomy [17]. Although we have shown that there are very few parasympathetic and sympathetic nerves are above the 9 o'clock level at this point of dissection (base of prostate to mid prostate) it may be that high fascial release in this area allows for less traction on the neurovascular bundle and avoids neuropraxia to these nerves [15].

The Anatomy of the Urinary Sphincter and Implications for Radical Prostatectomy and Continence Preservation

There are several key aspects to understanding the anatomy of the external striated muscle of the urinary sphincter in the male. Firstly the nerve supply to the sphincter is via the pudendal nerve which runs in the space between levator ani and obturator internus. The external sphincter is the principal muscle involved in maintenance of urinary continence. The so-called passive sphincter is the smooth muscle of the bladder neck and urethra. The urethral smooth muscles function is by coaption of the smooth muscle and mucosa which will maintain passive continence. Any exertion by the individual will cause the fast and slow twitch fibres of the external striated sphincter to contract and thus prevent stress urinary incontinence. The control of the urinary sphincter neurologically is by the pudendal nerve, which is a somatic nerve S2/3. There is no contribution to continence of the external sphincter by the autonomic nervous system. Careful nerve sparing surgery is probably not related to maintenance of post prostatectomy urinary continence It is preservation of the pudendal nerve a somatic nerve which maintains continence post prostatectomy. A meta analysis of the relationship between nerve sparing had radical prostatectomy and continence preservation was published by Reeves et al. in 2015 demonstrating no relationship between continence and nerve sparing [18].

Mechanism of Striated Sphincter Contraction

Contraction of the skeletal muscle of the horseshoe shaped sphincter around the membranous urethra brings the anterior wall of the urethra to the posterior wall at the level of the membranous diaphragm. Denonvilliers fascia and rectourethralis form a rigid posterior plate against which compression of the pliable urethral wall produces a transversely softened and occluded urethral lumen. In fact there are forces which are transmitted by several pairs of the skeletal muscle. These include the contribution from levator ani which seems to be a separate horseshoe shaped muscle discrete from levator ani, as well as contraction of puborectalis and the bulbocavernosus muscles. At surgery when dissecting in the area of the apex of the prostate it does appear that there is a separate muscle beyond the distal limit of a levator ani which makes up the striated horseshoe-shaped skeletal muscle sphincter innervated by the pudendal nerve. This striated muscle is often described as part of the levator ani. The anatomy of urinary continence was elegantly described and illustrated by Stafford and his group in the Journal Urology in 2013 [19]. For a comprehensive review of urethral sphincter function, Koraitim published a scholarly article the Journal of urology 2008 [20]. This manuscript is as a very helpful reference article for insights into the understanding of anatomy and function of the male external genitourinary sphincter.

Anatomical Insights Regarding the Modifications in Robotic Surgery Without Evidence of Benefit

As previously discussed autonomic nerve sparing is not anatomically associated with continence outcomes. Post prostatectomy, men can be totally potent but incontinent and vice versa, a man patient can be potent and be incontinent. There are separate neural inputs, the neurovascular bundle being autonomic both parasympathetic and sympathetic and the striated external sphincter being supplied by the somatic pudendal nerve S2 and S3.

Preservation of Urethral Smooth Muscle

As described in Nature Reviews Urology 2020 preservation of the smooth muscle of the urethra has been postulated to be linked to restoration of post-operative continence following radical prostatectomy [21]. As stated above, the smooth muscle of the urethral sphincter supplies only passive continence and urinary continence is mediated by the pudendal nerve innovation of striated muscle. Unless urethral preservation length correlates with improved preservation of skeletal muscle fibres, which draped over the anterior prostate, there is no anatomical basis to contend that preservation of urethral smooth muscle improves post-operative continence following radical prostatectomy.

Suburethral Plication Stitch (The Rocco Stitch)

Several studies have suggested that a plication stitch placed suburethrally at the apex of the prostate beyond the fusion of the Denonvilliers fascia and the posterior median raphe of the urethra will improve post-operative urinary continence. If this is done the needle must be placed carefully because there is certain degree of risk of nerve entrapment of the neurovascular bundle and potentially the pudendal nerve. In subsequent studies comparing plication stitch versus no plication stitch there has been no long-term difference in continence outcomes [8]. The deployment of the stitch however does have utility as it draws the bladder neck distally to approximate the urethra and makes for a neater vesicourethral anastomosis.

Seminal Vesical Sparing Prostatectomy

There were reports that seminal vesical sparing led to improved post-operative continence and potency after radical prostatectomy. This surgical maxim has been anecdotal not in published literature. No specific report in the literature supports this claim, which has been handed down for decades. A randomised controlled trial in 2017 reported no difference in the functional outcomes in sexual and urinary scores surgical margin status or PSA recurrence between the two groups [22]. The authors concluded that seminal vesical sparing prostatectomy was of little use. This conclusion is supported by the studies performed by our group at the Royal Melbourne Hospital in 2004, which demonstrated that the hypogastric nerve and the parasympathetic nerve are not in close proximity to the tips of the seminal vesicles. The S2–S4 contribution of the parasympathetic nerves joined the ganglia at or below the base of the prostate, away from the seminal vesicles. The dissection of the seminal vesicles is unlikely to compromise autonomic function.

Summary and Conclusion

The fundamental anatomical insights necessary for the robotic prostatectomist relate to the knowledge of several key structures in pelvic anatomy. These are, anatomy and fascial compartments of the neurovascular bundle, the striated muscle sphincter and the course of the pudendal nerve. In this chapter, we highlight the importance of dissection at the prostatic apex where it is most likely that inadvertent damage to autonomic nerves for erectile function, and injury to the nerves for control of continence of the striated external sphincter can occur.

References

1. Millin T. Retropubic prostatectomy. J Urol. 1948;59(3):267–80.
2. Young HH. VIII. Conservative perineal prostatectomy: the results of two years' experience and report of seventy-five cases. Ann Surg. 1905;41(4):549–57.
3. Harding Rains AJC. Bailey & Love's short practice of surgery. 14th ed. London: HK Lewis; 1998.

4. Walsh PC, Donker PJ. Impotence following radical prostatectomy: insight into etiology and prevention. J Urol. 1982;128(3):492–7.
5. Reiner WG, Walsh PC. An anatomical approach to the surgical management of the dorsal vein and Santorini's plexus during radical retropubic surgery. J Urol. 1979;121(2):198–200.
6. Hudson MA, Bahnson RR, Catalona WJ. Clinical use of prostate specific antigen in patients with prostate cancer. J Urol. 1989;142(4):1011–7.
7. Müller J. Über die organischen Nerven der erectilen männlichen Geschlechtsorgane des Menschen und der Säugethiere. Berlin: F Dümmler; 1836.
8. Ficarra V, Novara G, Ahlering TE, Costello A, Eastham JA, Graefen M, et al. Systematic review and meta-analysis of studies reporting potency rates after robot-assisted radical prostatectomy. Eur Urol. 2012;62(3):418–30.
9. McNeal JE, Redwine EA, Freiha FS, Stamey TA. Zonal distribution of prostatic adenocarcinoma. Correlation with histologic pattern and direction of spread. Am J Surg Pathol. 1988;12(12):897–906.
10. Ragde H, Aldape HC, Bagley CM Jr. Ultrasound-guided prostate biopsy. Biopty gun superior to aspiration. Urology. 1988;32(6):503–6.
11. Walsh PC. Radical prostatectomy for the treatment of localized prostatic carcinoma. Urol Clin North Am. 1980;7(3):583–91.
12. Burgers JK, Nelson RJ, Quinlan DM, Walsh PC. Nerve growth factor, nerve grafts and amniotic membrane grafts restore erectile function in rats. J Urol. 1991;146(2):463–8.
13. Kim ED, Nath R, Slawin KM, Kadmon D, Miles BJ, Scardino PT. Bilateral nerve grafting during radical retropubic prostatectomy: extended follow-up. Urology. 2001;58(6):983–7.
14. Costello AJ, Brooks M, Cole OJ. Anatomical studies of the neurovascular bundle and cavernosal nerves. BJU Int. 2004;94(7):1071–6.
15. Clarebrough EE, Challacombe BJ, Briggs C, Namdarian B, Weston R, Murphy DG, et al. Cadaveric analysis of periprostatic nerve distribution: an anatomical basis for high anterior release during radical prostatectomy? J Urol. 2011;185(4):1519–25.
16. Epstein JI, Walsh PC, Carmichael M, Brendler CB. Pathologic and clinical findings to predict tumor extent of nonpalpable (stage T1c) prostate cancer. JAMA. 1994;271(5):368–74.
17. Menon M, Tewari A, Peabody JO, Shrivastava A, Kaul S, Bhandari A, et al. Vattikuti Institute prostatectomy, a technique of robotic radical prostatectomy for management of localized carcinoma of the prostate: experience of over 1100 cases. Urol Clin North Am. 2004;31(4):701–17.
18. Reeves F, Preece P, Kapoor J, Everaerts W, Murphy DG, Corcoran NM, et al. Preservation of the neurovascular bundles is associated with improved time to continence after radical prostatectomy but not long-term continence rates: results of a systematic review and meta-analysis. Eur Urol. 2015;68(4):692–704.
19. Stafford RE, Ashton-Miller JA, Constantinou CE, Hodges PW. A new method to quantify male pelvic floor displacement from 2D transperineal ultrasound images. Urology. 2013;81(3):685–9.
20. Koraitim MM. The male urethral sphincter complex revisited: an anatomical concept and its physiological correlate. J Urol. 2008;179(5):1683–9.
21. Costello AJ. Considering the role of radical prostatectomy in 21st century prostate cancer care. Nat Rev Urol. 2020;17(3):177–88.
22. Gilbert SM, Dunn RL, Miller DC, Montgomery JS, Skolarus TA, Weizer AZ, et al. Functional outcomes following nerve sparing prostatectomy augmented with seminal vesicle sparing compared to standard nerve sparing prostatectomy: results from a randomized controlled trial. J Urol. 2017;198(3):600–7.

3 Robotic Training for RALP

Nicholas Raison and Prokar Dasgupta

Introduction

The structure and delivery of surgical training has undergone significant changes in recent years and continues to evolve. Changes have been driven by both external (economic, social and regulatory changes) and internal factors such as developments in the standards and constitution of medical education. Training programmes have been adapted to these new demands, partly as a result of the growing body of evidence supporting the use of simulation training. There has also been greater acceptance by the medical community of modern educational practices and recognition of the importance of focussed training over simpler time based models which rely predominantly on experience [1]. This has resulted in the expansion of competency based medical training which has been adopted by medical boards around the world. Across the majority of surgical specialities, rationalisation of the existing teaching frameworks with the newer models of competency and simulation-based training have resulted in gradual but major adaptions to existing programmes.

The relatively recent introduction of robotic surgery offers a unique opportunity to build effective training systems and embed evidence-based practices for training and assessment. Clinicians are recognising the important of establishing standards for practice to maintain patient safety. Increasingly training programmes are directed towards ensuring that surgeons can demonstrate minimum competency standards [2, 3]. The impact of learning curves on patient safety are also increasingly viewed as unacceptable, further driving the need for standardised and safe training programmes. This community of surgeons in leading the inclusion of simulation into education curricula and have embraced the need for a national and international standard for training [4].

The Halstedian system of a structured residency programme has been used for over a century. Whilst being criticised for the long, onerous hours especially in surgery, it remains an effective model for clinical training. Out of the Halstedian model of surgical apprenticeship, a three-stage process was broadly adopted for surgical skill acquisition. Initially trainees would just observe a number of surgical procedures. In the second stage they would perform the techniques under close supervision. Finally, in the third stage they would undertake a more independent role as the main surgeon. Whilst not an accurate description, this process is widely known by the phrase "see 1, do 1, teach 1".

Towards the end of the twentieth century various factors meant that this training model was increasingly questioned. Overly long working hours, even in medicine, were deemed unacceptable both for the health of the workers as well as concerns over errors and safety. Changes were made in the permitted working hours most significantly in Europe with the introduction of the European Working Time Directive. This limited workers to 48 h per week with further controls on rest periods. Similarly, working hours were reduced in the USA with guidelines limiting resident to 80 h per week. Another major factor on surgical training were the increasing concerns over medical errors and complications. Expectations for zero-complication surgery have led to the expansion of safeguards, standardisation of practices and ever-greater scrutiny of surgical outcomes. Publication of the report "To Err is Human" which highlighted that 10% of hospital patients suffered a complication led to increasing evaluation of clinical training [5]. This issue has been highlighted in the UK by the publication of surgical outcomes for a number of specialities. As a result, the effect of learning curves on sur-

N. Raison (✉)
Simulation Unit, MRC Centre for Transplantation, NIHR Biomedical Research Centre, Guy's Hospital, King's College London, London, UK
e-mail: nicholas.raison@kcl.ac.uk

P. Dasgupta
Simulation Unit, MRC Centre for Transplantation, NIHR Biomedical Research Centre, Guy's Hospital, King's College London, London, UK

Department of Urology, Guy's and St Thomas' NHS Trust, London, UK

S. Ren et al. (eds.), *Robot-Assisted Radical Prostatectomy*, https://doi.org/10.1007/978-3-031-05855-4_3

gical outcomes, specifically with regards to trainees, has been carefully scrutinised.

The importance of having a dedicated environment for surgical training, where possible, outside the operating room to promote safe clinical practice and efficient learning, is increasingly being realised. Likewise, the importance of focussed training. Achieving aptitude in everyday tasks to an acceptable level such as learning to drive or play recreational golf is relatively easy to achieve with limited training and practise. It has been estimated to take less than 50 h for most skills. At this stage, an automated state is reached in which the task can be executed relatively smoothly with infrequent errors. In contrast development of expertise rather than just aptitude in a particular skill or field is not solely a product of the length of experience or training. Success is reliant on continued engagement in focussed deliberate practice [6].

Simulation training is the key to addressing these problems. There is already a considerable breadth of literature evaluating the potential of simulation training in surgical education. In the initial stages of the learning curve, simulation enables surgeons to gain the relevant experience before encountering their first "live patient". Further along the curve, simulators provide the opportunity for deliberate practice, focussing practice on areas of weakness. Like an international violinist who will spend countless hours practicing difficult pieces, the surgeon is able to hone his skill outside the operating room. A number of high-quality systematic reviews have analysed effectiveness of simulation-based training. There is consistent evidence to support the use of simulation over no training although most data related to direct effects such as improvement in technical proficiency on the simulator [7, 8]. Significantly fewer studies evaluated downstream effects of surgical simulation but pooled analyses have shown that simulation training can result in significant improvements in operating room performance. Data on effects on patient outcomes is extremely limited.

Robot assisted laparoscopic surgery (hitherto referred to as robotic surgery) entered general surgical practice following the US Food and Drug Administration (FDA) approval of robotically assisted surgical devices for human surgery in 2000. At the time of writing, the Da Vinci surgical robot (Intuitive Surgical, Sunnyvale, CA, USA) remains the most commonly used surgical robot world-wide although other robots such the Versius system produced by CMR (CMR Surgical, Cambridge, UK) are rapidly gaining popularity. The Da Vinci surgical robot offers the surgeon a number of unique benefits such 3D vision, 7 degrees of freedom of laparoscopic instruments, tremor damping, motion amplification and camera stability (Fig. 3.1). It is argued such advantages makes the Da Vinci surgical robot superior to open and laparoscopic approaches particularly in delicate surgery such as radical prostatectomy.

Simulation Training Tools for Robot Assisted Radical Prostatectomy

A wide variety of simulation tools are now available for robotic surgical training. These can be broadly divided into dry lab (synthetic models and virtual reality (VR) simula-

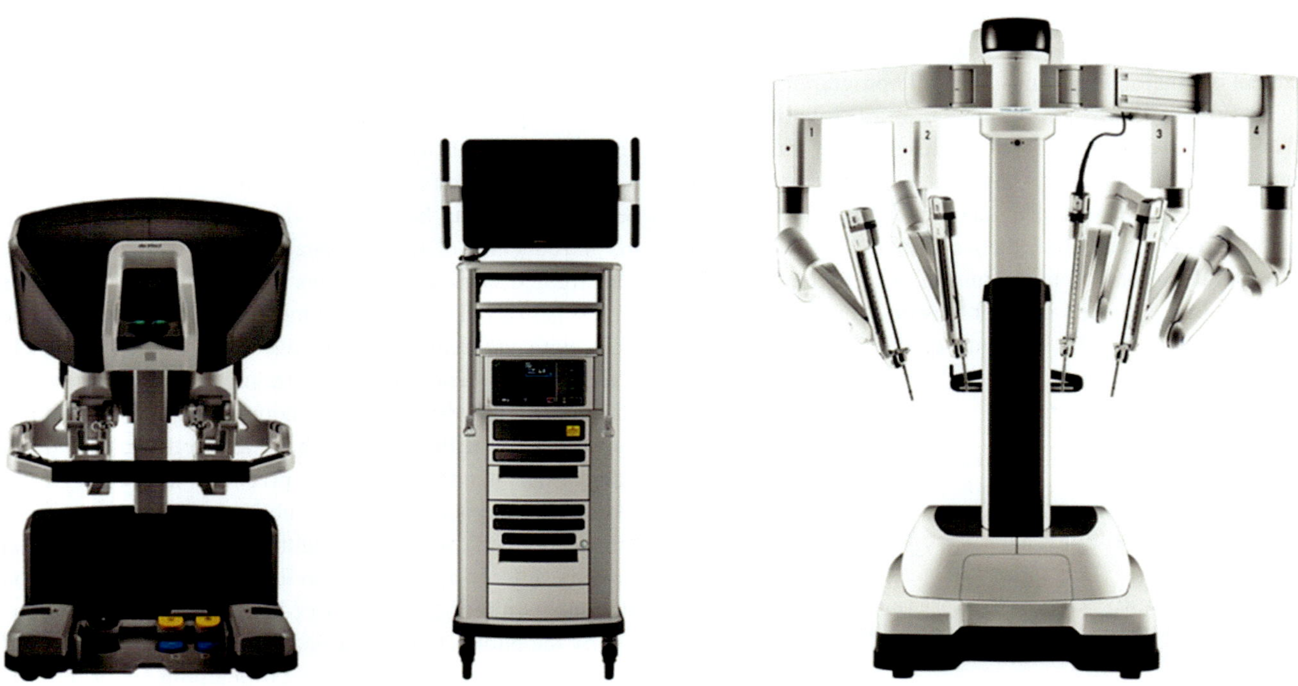

Fig. 3.1 The Da Vinci surgical robot

tors) and wet lab tools such as live animal, human cadaveric and animal cadaveric models. Historically dry lab models have predominantly been used for basic skill training although they are also being applied to more advanced procedural skill training. For example, both synthetic and VR models have been developed for practicing the urethrovesical anastomosis. Wet lab simulation in the form of cadaveric or live animal models, as well as being one of the oldest "simulation" tools, represent the highest fidelity simulation available for training and is most commonly used for more advanced skills training.

Establishing routine non-technical skill (NTS) training for surgery has been relatively slow in comparison to other high-risk industries such as the aviation. Nevertheless, there is now widespread recognition of the importance of NTS alongside technical skills training. Major procedures like robotic surgery demand a variety of professionals working together with overlapping but differing skill sets, complex anaesthetic and surgical inventions and involve complex technology. Training of NTS may incorporate a number of different techniques such as lectures or demonstrations but simulated exercises are most commonly used. Whilst simulated tasks are important like in technical simulation, feedback and discussion of the performance forms a central component of the training process. Rating systems are important to support structured feedback as well as assessment of trainees.

Virtual Reality Simulation

VR was first applied to surgical training with the development of a general abdominal simulator by Dr. Satava in 1991. VR simulation remains one of the most technologically advanced methods for surgical training. It has been enthusiastically embraced by units around the world but for a long period of time the medical community resisted its integration. Numerous high-quality studies demonstrating its effectiveness have helped to overcome this scepticism. A landmark study showed that VR training results in significantly better operating room performances for laparoscopic cholecystectomy [9]. VR simulation training has successfully been applied to a wide variety of surgical specialities. In all cases VR simulation was found to be at least as effective as other training modalities or traditional surgical training.

A relatively large number of VR simulators have been developed for robotic training but importantly have undergone varying levels of validation [10]. The principal VR simulators available for robotic surgery are the Robotic Surgical Simulator (ROSS) (Simulated Surgical Systems, USA), the dV-Trainer (Mimic Technologies, USA), SimSurgery Educational Platform (SEP) Robot (SimSurgery, Norway), da Vinci Skills Simulator (dVSS) (Intuitive Surgical, USA), ProMIS (CAE Healthcare, Canada) and RobotiX Mentor (3D Systems Healthcare, Littleton, USA formerly Simbionix, Israel). Both simulator hardware and software vary considerably between the different models. The dVSS is the only simulator to work directly with the da Vinci robot. The dVSS backpack is attached directly onto the console, enabling the user to practice operating on the da Vinci robot in a virtual environment. All the others are standalone simulators. Whilst mimicking the Da Vinci robot, the standalone dV-Trainer hand controls differ from those of the da Vinci system, with the master controllers connected via two tension cables as opposed to the jointed arms of the da Vinci robot. Likewise, the RobotiX Mentor, released in 2014, uses free-floating hand controls but otherwise closely replicates the Da Vinci systems (Fig. 3.2). The SEP robot uses two motion-tracked hand controls that mimic rather than replicate robotic control arms. Like the da Vinci robot, a clutch is incorporated, but the video feed is displayed by a 2D screen as opposed to the 3D video provided by the above simulators. Importantly a number of studies have reported evidence to support the consequences of VR robotic training. Notably Culligan et al. demonstrated that completing a training programme using the dVSS simulator led to successful completion of a supravesical hysterectomy equivalent to experienced robotic surgeons measured by blood loss, operative time and technical skills evaluation [11].

A number of VR simulators have been developed for radical prostatectomy training specifically. These range from more basic generic training modules to full procedure specific simulations. Tubes 3 module from Mimic (Mimic Technologies, Seattle, WA, USA) offer procedure specific training for UVA. Tube 3 simulates the running anastomosis technique that uses double-armed needles between the bladder neck and urethra. Procedure specific VR training modules have been developed for a number of simulators. Of the six VR simulators available for robotic surgery, procedural training is available for three (RoSS, the dV-Trainer, the RobotiX Mentor). Prostatectomy, cystectomy, and lymph node dissection training is available for the RoSS simulator. Mimic have developed an alternative system called Maestro which provides procedure-specific training through manipulation of a 3D anatomical video. It should be noted that the programme does not allow full procedural training. The most advanced system is available on the RobotiX Mentor. This programme offers training for radical prostatectomy. A number of initial validation studies have been undertaken with one showing that structured procedural VR simulation is effective for robotic training with technical skills successfully transferred to a clinical task in cadavers [12]. The RobotiX Mentor software is also available as part of the SimNow simulation program from da Vinci (Intuitive Surgical Inc.).

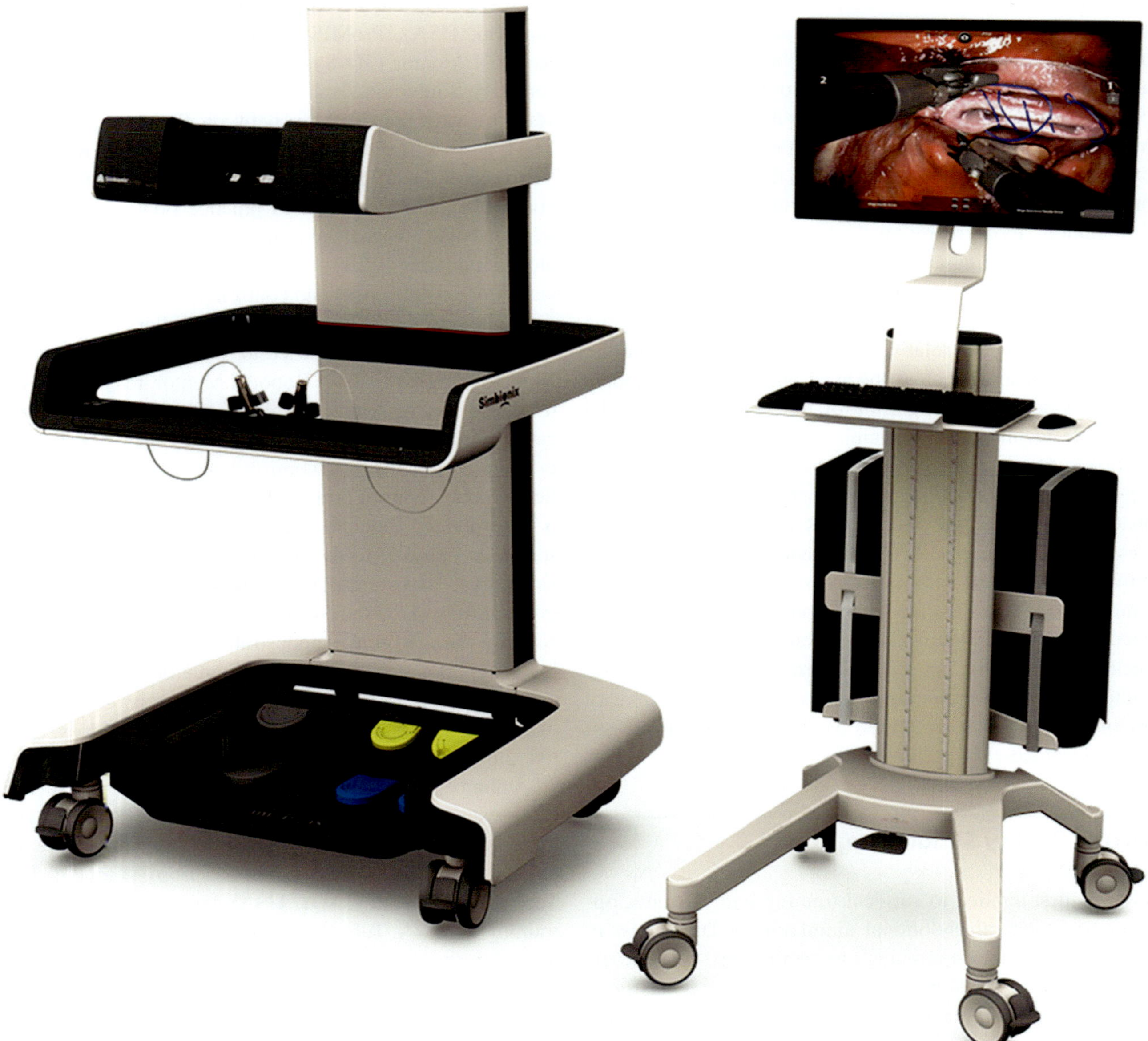

Fig. 3.2 RobotiX Mentor (3D Systems Healthcare, Littleton, USA formerly Simbionix, Israel)

Dry Lab Simulation Training

Dry lab models are widely used in surgical simulation particularly for open and laparoscopic training. In laparoscopic surgery box trainers (dry-lab simulation models) have been shown to be largely equivalent to VR simulation. They allow training using actual instruments and provide realistic haptic feedback. However they lack the objective performance assessment provided by VR simulation. The major advantages of dry lab models are that they offer relatively low cost, effective training especially for basic skills that is easily accessible.

For robotic surgery, a number of dry-lab models have been developed for use with the da Vinci Surgical System but only two basic skills models have been formally validated. Anecdotally most dry lab training is undertaken using basic skills models such as suture pads. A set of three dry-lab models were reverse engineered from the Mimic Msim VR software. Similarly Goh et al. developed four training exercises (suturing, dissection, peg transfer, and needle driving) for robot-assisted radical prostatectomy (RARP) [13]. Validation in both cases extended only to expert novice comparisons. Several procedure specific models have also been described in the literature albeit not for radical prostatectomy. The

SIMPLE partial nephrectomy model was developed using 3D printing comparisons between performances on the model and in live surgery were shown to be equivalent demonstrating relationships with other variables.

Wet Lab Simulation Training

Both live animals and cadaveric human tissues provide unique opportunities for training. Anatomical fidelity and the ability to train complex procedure specific skills together with complication management mean that they continue to form an important component of surgical training. Aside from ethical concerns, further disadvantages are the extensive facilities and costs necessary to provide such training. Ex-vivo and live animal models have undergone limited assessment in the literature to date.

For robotic surgery, whilst live animal training is regularly provided by numerous centres across Europe and the US, there has been limited validation of training using either live animals or cadavers. Limited assessment of the use of live porcine models for robotic surgery has been undertaken and shows beneficial outcomes although the level of evidence remains low [14]. Live porcine models forms part of the European Association of Urology (EAU) robotic training curriculum. Although specific data pertaining to their use as wet lab models are not available, the curriculum was shown to be effective overall good educational impact and acceptability [15]. This programme offers training for radical prostatectomy (Fig. 3.3).

Similarly, cadavers have been using in surgical training around the world for many centuries, in many areas it remained proscribed forcing the ardent surgeon and anatomist to obtain specimens by various nefarious, if not illegal methods. Indeed, in the UK, it was not until 2006 that the Human Tissue Act 2004 came into force allowing surgical procedures to be performed on human cadavers. Prior to this, anatomical dissection was permitted but any rehearsal of surgical techniques was strongly prohibited. This relaxation of the statute enabled the development of cadaveric training programmes in the UK for both surgeons and the many other healthcare professionals who continue to benefit from cadaveric simulation training. Following enactment, there was a rapid growth in cadaveric simulation training programmes within the UK.

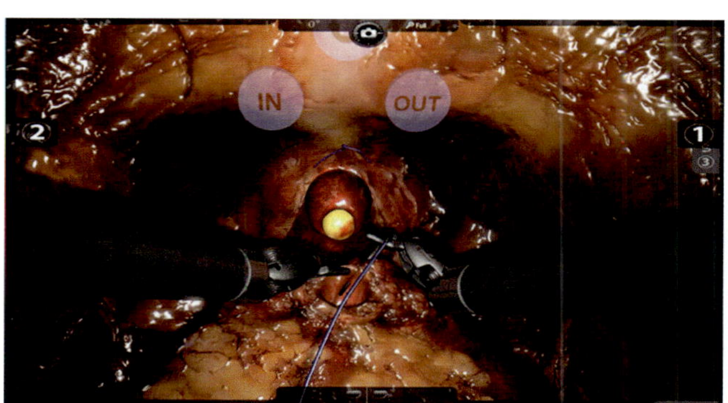

Fig. 3.3 Radical prostatectomy training module, RobotiX Mentor (3D Systems)

Although most anatomical dissection is performed on embalmed cadavers, the reduction in the tissue quality caused by the embalming process and the resultant rigidity largely precludes the use of embalmed cadavers for surgical training. Fresh frozen cadavers are used most commonly for surgical training. Specimens are immediately frozen to preserve tissue quality and then defrosted prior to the teaching event. This technique provides relatively realistic tissues but does come with a number of disadvantages. Principally specimens must be used within a 24–48 h following thawing otherwise tissue start to decompose. Nevertheless, it is frequently noted by participants that cadavers develop an unpleasant odour over the course of a training session which can be very off-putting. The very limited shelf life of cadavers also greatly limits their utility and necessitates cold storage facilities which all result in increased costs. An alternative approach is Thiel embalming. This technique uses very low concentrations of formaldehyde alongside glycol and other salts. This form of "soft" embalming preserves tissue texture and colour whilst avoiding the need for refrigeration or other special storage. Studies have demonstrated overall good fidelity of Thiel embalmed tissues compared to live or cadaveric tissue. Preservation of tissues with the Thiel technique also means that specimens can be reused. The drawbacks of this technique are firstly that costs of preparing the specimens are higher than either standard embalming or fresh frozen and some tissues such as brain, eyes are not amenable to the technique.

The unique benefit of human cadaveric training, irrespective of the preservation technique is that it accurately imitates real life operating and offers an excellent platform for training specific procedural skills. It is often considered the gold standard for simulation training as it most closely models live patients. The value cadaveric training has been shown for a number of modalities such as laparoscopy, endourology and open surgery. Studies have investigated the role of cadaveric training for procedural skills training however data are predominantly only qualitative [16]. The importance of the tissue quality and tissue planes have been highlighted as important factors missing in even high-fidelity VR simulation. Similar findings have been found to a more limited extent in robotic surgery [17].

Assessment and Training

Technical skills assessment is an important component of simulation. Effective training requires more than just repetitive practice. A central concept for effective training is deliberate practice. Introduced by Ericsson deliberate practice is characterised by a highly structured, goal orientated approach to training. It is based on a number of key principles; motivated learners; repetitive performance of a particular task; well define objectives addressing relevant skills or topics; effective assessment with reliable data, informative feedback and performance evaluation [1]. Ericsson demonstrated that specialised training and feedback provide the optimum conditions for nurturing performance improvement. Studies have demonstrated the effectiveness of deliberate practice and shown it be substantially superior to traditional methods of clinical training in a range of disciplines. A critical component of mastery learning and deliberate practice is accurate performance evaluation. Assessment before and after training is important to ensure that the necessary standards have been achieved and that training has been successful. Evaluation is also important for training in itself: feedback to learners helps to direct their learning, aids motivation and provides a standard against which progression can be checked.

A variety of assessment tools are available to the robotic surgeon. Validated global rating scales (GRS) are frequently used. For robotic surgery the Global Evaluative Assessment of Robotic Skills (GEARS) tool by Goh et al. is most widely used and validated [18]. Uniquely GEARS score have been shown to predict continence after robotic prostatectomy [19]. The major disadvantage of GRS is the need for expert reviewers to assess and mark performance, greatly limiting their application to routine training. A variety of approaches to avoiding the need for the labour intensive have been trialled. An innovative approach that does offer great potential is the use of lay members of the public to assess proficiency. Crowd-Sourced Assessment of Technical Skills (C-SATS) which uses an online to recruit large numbers of untrained "crowd workers" has been used in various fields such as laparoscopy and robotics. Whilst crowd-source GEARS scores have been shown to correlate with experts, limitations will likely prevent its use in summative assessment [20].

Checklists, whilst offering a more structured approach to assessment are used less frequently as they are more specific and, arguably, difficult to use. Lovegrove et al. used an innovative approach to developing a comprehensive checklist for robotic prostatectomy training [21]. Using Healthcare Failure Mode and Effect Analysis (HFMEA) to identify the key, hazardous steps in robotic radical prostatectomy, the authors developed a detailed checklist for the procedure. Assessment of trainees using this checklist allowed learning curves for each of the key steps to be plotted.

Non-Technical Skills Training

Recognition of the vital importance of NTS has resulted in the development of various NTS behavioural rating systems for surgery. Separate systems have been developed for assessment of the entire surgical team as well as individual team members such as surgeons, anaesthetists and scrub practitioners. To be effective such rating systems must accurately capture relevant behaviours and notably there is significant overlap in the NTS that the various tools identify and measure. These similarities help to demonstrate the generalisability of NTS across both surgical specialities and surgical teams. Established systems such as Non-Technical Skills for Surgeons (NOTSS) taxonomy have also been applied to a variety of surgical specialties and environments outside the operating such as critical care. Alongside a validated behavioural rating system, trained faculty with experience of NTS assessment are also important. The participants themselves must also be motivated and understanding of the learning process.

Robotic surgery demands significant adaptations to the standard operating room (OR) environment including team interaction. As a result, proficiency in robotic surgery requires specialist training in both technical and non-technical skills. Despite this, only recently have robotic surgical curricula begun to incorporate NTS. Furthermore, whilst generic systems such as NOTSS can be used in robotic surgery, the unique environment presents its own NTS challenges. In response specific rating systems for robotic surgery such as the ICARS and RAS-NOTECHS have been developed [22, 23]. Further work is required on developing dedicated training programmes for developing NTS in robotic surgery.

The Future for Simulation Training

Surgical training has already been greatly transformed by the introduction of simulation training but there is scope for further improvement. The shift towards competency-based training is likely to increase. Focussing on technical skills performance rather than time-based programmes aims to improve training outcomes. Simulation will play a central role both as training tools and in the assessment of trainees to ensure technical and non-technical competencies have been achieved. A number of robotic skills curricula such as the European Association of Urology Robotic Training

Curriculum which provide a full structured programme for radical prostatectomy have already been developed. This includes theoretical sessions, skills training (dry and wet simulation), observation, and console mentoring to guide trainees from novice to competent surgeon. Such structure training is likely to be increasingly used to demonstrate proficiency and the ability to operate independently.

Incorporation of simulation tools in the ongoing assessment and accreditation of robotic surgeons is also likely to grow in the future. There has been some application of licensing practices in American Hospital but the adoption of national and even international standards is likely to emerge in the future.

VR simulation tools are likely to continue to play an increasing role as the fidelity of procedural VR continues to improve. Whilst generic simulators will always be important for basic skills training, the possibility of full procedural training will mean that a wider variety of operations and advanced procedural skills will be able to be trained and assessed using VR simulators. The major exception to this is non-technical skills training in which the importance of physical training for the whole team is unlikely to be replaced.

Automated performance metrics is another exciting area of development. Currently aside from automatic metrics produced by VR simulators, assessing performance remains labour intensive requiring experienced, expert surgeons to assess performance using validated scoring schema. Initial work has shown than algorithms can be trained to distinguish good and bad performances using various data including video feeds, instrument tracking (accelerometers, force-torque monitors) and system metrics (endowrist movements, camera usage). These have been shown to be able to distinguish between different levels of expertise with correlation to clinical outcomes. Other technologies have been used to develop to utilise automatic anatomical and instrument identification during radical prostatectomy surgery and other procedures. Machine learning algorithms have been trained to use this data to predict a surgeons expertise [24]. As this technology matures it will allow both greater objective assessment of training and offer surgeons ongoing live feedback to help improve outcomes.

Conclusion

Training programmes in surgery have undergone major transformation in recent years with the application of modern education practices and wider implementation of training tools such as simulators. Robotic surgery in particular has seen wide spread adoption of simulation-based training and there are now a variety of simulation tools and programmes available. Whilst other areas of surgery take up similar approaches, new technologies such as machine learning are already been applied to robotic radical prostatectomy training to drive further improvements.

References

1. Ericsson KA, Krampe RT, Tesch-Romer C. The role of deliberate practice in the acquisition of expert performance. Psychol Rev. 1993;100(3):363–406.
2. Leung WC. Competency based medical training: review. BMJ. 2002;325(7366):693–6.
3. Shaughnessy AF, Torro JR, Frame KA, Bakshi M. Evidence-based medicine and life-long learning competency requirements in new residency teaching standards. Evid Based Med. 2016;21(2):46–9.
4. Ahmed K, Khan R, Mottrie A, Lovegrove C, Abaza R, Ahlawat R, et al. Development of a standardised training curriculum for robotic surgery: a consensus statement from an international multidisciplinary group of experts. BJU Int. 2015;116(1):93–101.
5. Vincent C, Neale G, Woloshynowych M. Adverse events in British hospitals: preliminary retrospective record review. BMJ. 2001;322(7285):517–9.
6. Ericsson KA. Deliberate practice and the acquisition and maintenance of expert performance in medicine and related domains. Acad Med. 2004;79(10 Suppl):S70–81.
7. Sturm LP, Windsor JA, Cosman PH, Cregan P, Hewett PJ, Maddern GJ. A systematic review of skills transfer after surgical simulation training. Ann Surg. 2008;248(2):166–79.
8. Cook DA, Hatala R, Brydges R, Zendejas B, Szostek JH, Wang AT, et al. Technology-enhanced simulation for health professions education: a systematic review and meta-analysis. JAMA. 2011;306(9):978–88.
9. Grantcharov TP, Kristiansen VB, Bendix J, Bardram L, Rosenberg J, Funch-Jensen P. Randomized clinical trial of virtual reality simulation for laparoscopic skills training. Br J Surg. 2004;91(2):146–50.
10. Abboudi H, Khan MS, Aboumarzouk O, Guru KA, Challacombe B, Dasgupta P, et al. Current status of validation for robotic surgery simulators—a systematic review. BJU Int. 2013;111(2):194–205.
11. Culligan P, Gurshumov E, Lewis C, Priestley J, Komar J, Salamon C. Predictive validity of a training protocol using a robotic surgery simulator. Female Pelvic Med Reconstr Surg. 2014;20(1):48–51.
12. Raison N, Harrison P, Abe T, Aydin A, Ahmed K, Dasgupta P. Procedural virtual reality simulation training for robotic surgery: a randomised controlled trial. Surg Endosc. 2021;35(12):6897–902.
13. Goh A, Joseph R, O'Malley M, Miles B, Dunkin B. 1336 development and validation of inanimate tasks for robotic surgical skills assessment and training. J Urol. 2010;183(4S):e516.
14. Raison N, Poulsen J, Abe T, Aydin A, Ahmed K, Dasgupta P. An evaluation of live porcine simulation training for robotic surgery. J Robot Surg. 2021;15(3):429–34.
15. Volpe A, Ahmed K, Dasgupta P, Ficarra V, Novara G, van der Poel H, et al. Pilot validation study of the European Association of Urology robotic training curriculum. Eur Urol. 2015;68(2):292–9.
16. Gilbody J, Prasthofer AW, Ho K, Costa ML. The use and effectiveness of cadaveric workshops in higher surgical training: a systematic review. Ann R Coll Surg Engl. 2011;93(5):347–52.
17. Blaschko SD, Brooks HM, Dhuy SM, Charest-Shell C, Clayman RV, McDougall EM. Coordinated multiple cadaver use for minimally invasive surgical training. JSLS. 2007;11(4):403–7.
18. Goh AC, Goldfarb DW, Sander JC, Miles BJ, Dunkin BJ. Global evaluative assessment of robotic skills: validation of a clinical assessment tool to measure robotic surgical skills. J Urol. 2012;187(1):247–52.

19. Goldenberg MG, Goldenberg L, Grantcharov TP. Surgeon performance predicts early continence after robot-assisted radical prostatectomy. J Endourol. 2017;31(9):858–63.
20. Ghani KR, Miller DC, Linsell S, Brachulis A, Lane B, Sarle R, et al. Measuring to improve: peer and crowd-sourced assessments of technical skill with robot-assisted radical prostatectomy. Eur Urol. 2016;69(4):547–50.
21. Lovegrove C, Novara G, Mottrie A, Guru KA, Brown M, Challacombe B, et al. Structured and modular training pathway for robot-assisted radical prostatectomy (RARP): validation of the RARP assessment score and learning curve assessment. Eur Urol. 2016;69(3):526–35.
22. Raison N, Wood T, Brunckhorst O, Abe T, Ross T, Challacombe B, et al. Development and validation of a tool for non-technical skills evaluation in robotic surgery—the ICARS system. Surg Endosc. 2017;31(12):5403–10.
23. Schreyer J, Koch A, Herlemann A, Becker A, Schlenker B, Catchpole K, et al. RAS-NOTECHS: validity and reliability of a tool for measuring non-technical skills in robotic-assisted surgery settings. Surg Endosc. 2022;36(3):1916–26.
24. Chen J, Remulla D, Nguyen JH, Aastha D, Liu Y, Dasgupta P, et al. Current status of artificial intelligence applications in urology and their potential to influence clinical practice. BJU Int. 2019. https://doi.org/10.1111/bju.14852.

Part II

Imaging in RALP

Magnetic Resonance Imaging in Prostate Cancer

4

Martina Pecoraro, Emanuele Messina, Giorgia Carnicelli, Claudio Valotto, Vincenzo Ficarra, Gianluca Giannarini, and Valeria Panebianco

Introduction

Historical Notes

The diagnostic potential of magnetic resonance imaging (MRI) was largely unrecognized when the first scans were performed back in the 1980s [1]. MRI was mainly used in the research setting to explore prostate gland anatomy and cancer spectroscopic characteristics. Still, the additional information derived from MR images did not outweigh the costs associated with scanning, hence why applying it to the clinical practice was considered rather unrealistic. The usefulness of MRI in prostate cancer (PCa) diagnosis became evident only 30 years later, when researchers started integrating imaging data from different MRI modalities in a single reading, the so-called "multiparametric acquisition" [2], mostly thanks to technology advances. In 2011, the first consensus meeting was published on the use of multiparametric MRI (mpMRI) in the clinical practice [3]. Another breakthrough came 1 year later, with the release of the first standardized algorithm for the reporting of prostate lesions at mpMRI, the "*Prostate Imaging Reporting and Data System*" (PI-RADS). PI-RADS provided a universal language that urologists and radiologists can now use worldwide for assessing PCa risk and for guiding therapy [2]. In the past decade, two other versions of PI-RADS have been released, and the acquisition technique has impressively advanced, so that mpMRI currently represents the state-of-the-art imaging in the workup of men at risk for PCa [4, 5]. The outstanding evolution of mpMRI and PI-RADS reporting is gradually shifting the workup of PCa from an approach based on conventional clinical parameters to an imaging-centered strategy.

MRI in Prostate Cancer

Current international guidelines recommend that all men at risk for PCa undergo mpMRI compliant with PI-RADS scoring [4], given its very high negative predictive value in excluding clinically significant PCa (csPCa) [6, 7]. The category at risk comprises men with PSA levels >3 ng/mL and those with a positive digital rectal examination (DRE). Additional factors identifying subjects at risk are the familiarity for PCa, inherited predisposing mutations (BRCA1 and BRCA2 being the most frequent) and African-Caribbean ethnicity. mpMRI allows to stratify the risk of csPCa in these patients, ultimately directing them to either biopsy, preferably MRI directed biopsy (MRDB), or follow-up [5]. As part of the evaluation, the radiologist should collect clinical data at the time of MRI acquisition, the most important being the latest PSA measurements, reports of previous biopsies, imaging exams performed and findings during the clinical examination. This information should not interfere with PI-RADS category assignment; however, it may help decide the appropriate diagnostic and therapeutic strategy. For this purpose, it is fundamental that a good communication exists between the referring urologist and the radiologist, and that a multidisciplinary management is pursued [4 8].

Gianluca Giannarini and Valeria Panebianco are joint senior authorship.

M. Pecoraro · E. Messina · G. Carnicelli · V. Panebianco
Department of Radiological Sciences, Oncology and Pathology, Sapienza University of Rome, Rome, Italy
e-mail: emanuele.messina@uniroma1.it; valeria.panebianco@uniroma1.it

C. Valotto · G. Giannarini (✉)
Urology Unit, "Santa Maria della Misericordia" University Hospital, Udine, Italy
e-mail: claudio.valotto@asufc.sanita.fvg.it

V. Ficarra
Urologic Section, Department of Human and Pediatric Pathology "Gaetano Barresi", University of Messina, Messina, Italy
e-mail: vincenzo.ficarra@unime.it

S. Ren et al. (eds.), *Robot-Assisted Radical Prostatectomy*, https://doi.org/10.1007/978-3-031-05855-4_4

Prostate MRI

Prostate Anatomy and MRI Semiology

The prostate gland is a chestnut-shaped pelvic organ located between the bladder neck and the urogenital diaphragm. It lies in close relation with the rectum, the bladder, the urethra, which crosses it for its entire length, and the seminal vesicles. In the young adult, it measures approximately 20–30 mL, with an average size of 3 × 4 × 2 cm. According to the conventional model, the prostate can be divided into three segments on the coronal plane: the base cranially, the mid-gland segment and the apex caudally. On the axial plane, four different anatomic zones can be identified:

(a) peripheral zone (PZ)—outer posterior, lateral, and apex regions of the prostate, showing a relatively hyperintense signal intensity (SI) on T2-weighted imaging (T2WI); 70% cancers arise in this region, due to the high percentage of glandular tissue;
(b) central zone (CZ), bilaterally symmetric low-SI tissue on T2WI and apparent diffusion coefficient (ADC) images encircling the ejaculatory ducts;
(c) transition zone (TZ), composed by a varying number of hyperplastic nodules and intervening tissue showing heterogeneous SI on T2WI; 20–30% cancers arise in this region;
(d) anterior fibromuscular stroma (AFMS), bilaterally symmetric shape ("crescentic") and with symmetric low SI (like that of obturator or pelvic floor muscles) on T2WI, ADC, and high b-value diffusion-weighted imaging (DWI).

The prostate is almost entirely bounded by the prostatic capsule, which appears as a thin hypointense ring in the morphologic sequences. Owing to the dimensions of the field of view (FOV), mpMRI acquisition allows to assess also the pelvic nearby structures, including regional lymph nodes and iliac vessels.

A sector map of the prostate is used as reference model for reporting the imaging findings, consisting of 41 sectors including the seminal vesicles. This standardized segmentation scheme was purposely designed in the PI-RADS v2.1 guidelines [8].

MRI Acquisition Protocol

According to PI-RADS v2.1 standards of practice, a high field MRI scan is required (3 T/1.5 T), however a 3 T scan is preferred to achieve better signal-to-noise ratio (SNR) and high spatial resolution. The use of multi-channel surface phased-array body coils and strong gradients is recommended to increase image quality. The use of surface phased-array coils is preferred to endo-rectal coils. No consensus exists on patient preparation. Notably, the presence of stool or air in the rectum might cause artefactual distortion of functional images, reducing the quality of the exam, thus the use of micro-enema might be considered. To reduce motion artefacts, antispasmodic agents could be administered during the examination, if no contraindications exist.

Acquisition protocol consists of morphologic T2WI, functional DWI and dynamic contrast enhanced (DCE) imaging [8]. Acquisition of at least one pulse sequence with a large FOV is recommended to evaluate pelvic nodes up the aortic bifurcation, for detecting the presence of hemorrhage within the prostate and seminal vesicles, and for the assessment of bone lesions.

T2-Weighted Imaging

T2WI consists of multiplanar Fast Recovery Fast Spin Echo (FRFSE) sequences that allow to depict the morphology and topography of the prostate gland thanks to the excellent spatial resolution that they provide. On T2WI, the PZ generally appears more hyperintense with respect to the TZ, and the boundary between the two is well demarcated. This sequence allows for accurate delineation of all lesions, which tend to appear hypointense with respect to the surrounding tissue. Characteristics of malignant prostate lesions are an irregular contour, pseudo-nodular or plaque like morphology, marked hypointensity, and distortion of the surrounding parenchyma. Evidence of interruption or displacement of the prostate capsule (capsular bulging) are signs indicative of csPCa, and have value in the pretreatment planning [8, 9].

Diffusion-Weighted Imaging and Apparent Diffusion Coefficient Map

DWI is an Echo Planar Imaging (EPI) and relies on the study of micro-architectural alterations. By depicting the random or *Brownian* motion of water molecules within an examined region, DWI allows to distinguish pathologic from disease-free tissue. Images are acquired using multiple "b-values"; these generally range from 0–800–1000 to 2000 s/mm^2. High b-values (defined as b value >1400 s/mm^2) allow to accurately detect foci of pathologic tissue, and to better characterize the lesions identifiable at morphologic imaging. Malignant prostate lesions tend to display high restriction patterns on DWI, thus appearing hyperintense with regard to the surrounding dark background [8, 10]. DWI also allows for the elaboration of ADC maps. These can be seen as negative images of DWI images: lesions with high degree of restriction appear hypointense, in contrast to the bright background. The ADC map provides additional information to DWI, it allows for quantitation of the degree of restriction within a region of interest (ADC ratio and ADC numeric values), and, more importantly, can be used to further confirm or to exclude the malignant nature of a lesion [10]. While malignant lesions appear markedly hyperintense on DWI, and hypointense in the ADC map, this correspondence is not found for inflammatory or cystic lesions [8]. As a drawback of this imaging modality, spatial resolution is poor, and yields only dark-field images with no clearly recognizable anatomic landmarks. In addition, DWI is highly susceptible to signal artifacts, mostly due to air in the rectum, and presence of local (femoral) prosthetic joints [11].

Dynamic Contrast Enhanced Imaging

DCE imaging is a T1WI Gradient-Echo sequences acquired after administration of a body weight-adjusted intravenous bolus of contrast medium (0.1 mmol/kg) using a temporal resolution of ≤15 s. DCE imaging depicts the kinetics of contrast flow, and thus the vascularization of a given tissue [12]. Malignant prostate lesions tend to display early and focal increased enhancement, appearing hyperintense on DCE imaging [8]. Of note, inflammatory lesions also display enhanced uptake, which may be misleading especially for unexperienced readers. In PI-RADS v2.1 recommendations, DCE imaging has a marginal role in PCa detection, since it only helps assess equivocal foci in the PZ of the gland. Nonetheless, different investigations reported that DCE may assist in the detection of csPCa (e.g. less experienced readers, degraded DWI) as "safety net" to increase the sensitivity of the technique [13, 14].

Prostate MRI Scoring and Reporting

Principles of Prostate MRI Reporting

According to the standards set in PI-RADS v2.1 guideline, a structured prostate MRI report should include prostate gland volume, serum PSA level and PSA density (serum PSA level divided by prostate volume, expressed in ng/mL^2). Prostate gland volume is usually calculated using the ellipsoid formula. Single-lesion evaluation involves measuring the maximum diameters, locating the lesion within the sector map, and describing its morphology (either band-like, plaque-like, triangular, or pseudo-nodular). Every lesion is assigned a PI-RADS score, depending on its morphologic and functional imaging characteristics. Up to four lesions can be reported in a single evaluation, identifying the most significant one as the index lesion [8]. Along with these data, it is suggested to report the indications to perform the exam, which can range from early PCa detection (elevated serum PSA levels, DRE abnormalities or strong familiarity), to active surveillance of low-risk disease, to post-therapy evaluation. The structured report should also include the assessment of prostate capsule integrity and morphology, of nearby lymph nodes and structures (seminal vesicles, bladder, rectum, bones). Any concomitant genitourinary/pelvic pathology found at imaging should be accurately described.

PI-RADS Category Assignment

PI-RADS v2.1 is currently the gold standard scoring for prostate MRI image assessment and reporting, recommended by the EAU guidelines [4]. PI-RADS is a standardized five-tier scoring system expressing the likelihood of radiological lesions being csPCa. According to the system:

- PI-RADS 1 category expresses very low risk of csPCa (csPCa is highly unlikely)
- PI-RADS 2 category expresses low risk of csPCa (csPCa is unlikely)
- PI-RADS 3 category expresses intermediate risk of csPCa (the presence of csPCa is equivocal)
- PI-RADS 4 category expresses high risk of csPCa (csPCa is likely)
- PI-RADS 5 category expresses very high risk of csPCa (csPCa is highly likely)

The score is obtained by combining the single scores from the three different imaging sequences. A standardized reporting scheme is applied to T2WI, to DWI/ADC and to DCE imaging separately. Each sequence is evaluated and scored from 1 to 5 (Figs. 4.1 and 4.2). A specific algorithm is then applied to draw an overall PI-RADS score from all single sequence scores. Scoring varies depending on the location of the lesion: in the PZ the dominant sequence is the DWI; in the TZ instead, the dominant sequence is T2WI [8].

Scoring and Reporting of Peripheral Zone Findings

In the PZ the assessment of prostate lesions relies mainly on DWI and ADC map. The underlying rationale is that PZ can be involved in several different pathologies other than PCa (e.g., fibrosis, inflammatory processes, and chronic prostatitis). These may all display a similar appearance on T2WI, hence the assessment of csPCa cannot be made on the ground of the sole morphology but must rely on DWI evaluation. DCE imaging play a more marginal role in PI-RADS category assignment. The scoring of a lesion is marked as only either positive or negative for contrast enhancement and serves as complementary in the evaluation of undetermined lesion or when the acquisition of DWI sequences is inade-

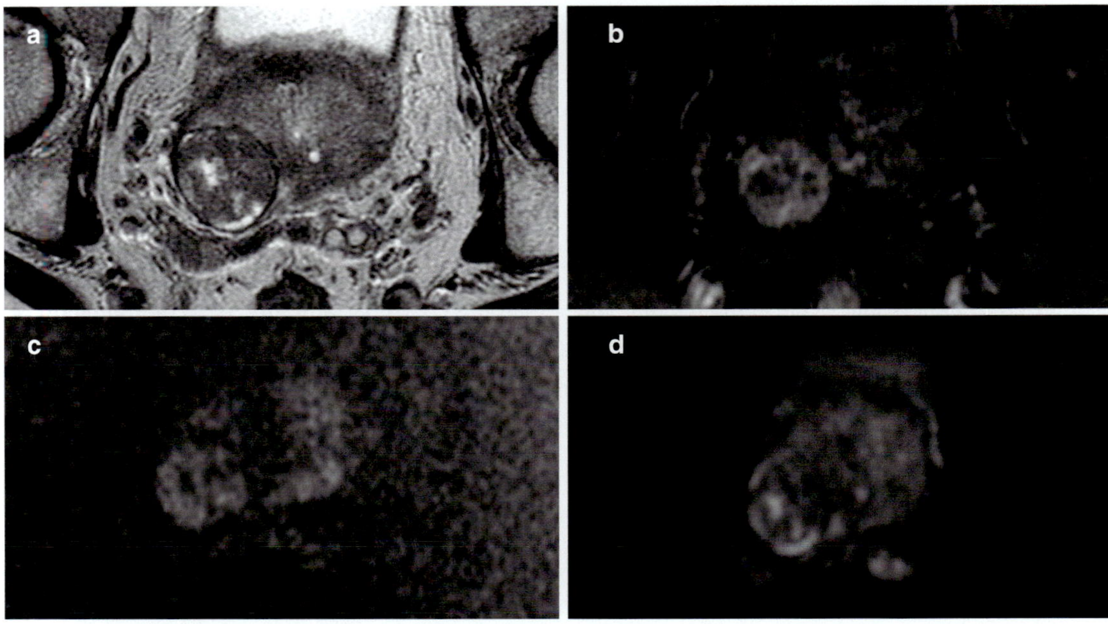

Fig. 4.1 Multiparametric MRI of a 57-year-old-man with elevated serum PSA level (5.4 ng/ml). (**a**) T2WI shows a heterogeneous ectopic nodule extending toward the right peripheral zone at the mid-base of the gland. (**b**) DCE imaging shows early contrast enhancement of the nodule. (**c**, **d**) DWI and ADC map show mild hyperintensity of the nodule in both sequences. The final assigned PI-RADS category was 2. *PSA* prostate specific antigen, *T2WI* T2 weighted imaging, *DCE* dynamic contrast enhancement, *DWI* diffusion-weighted imaging, *ADC* apparent diffusion coefficient, *PI-RADS* prostate imaging reporting and data system

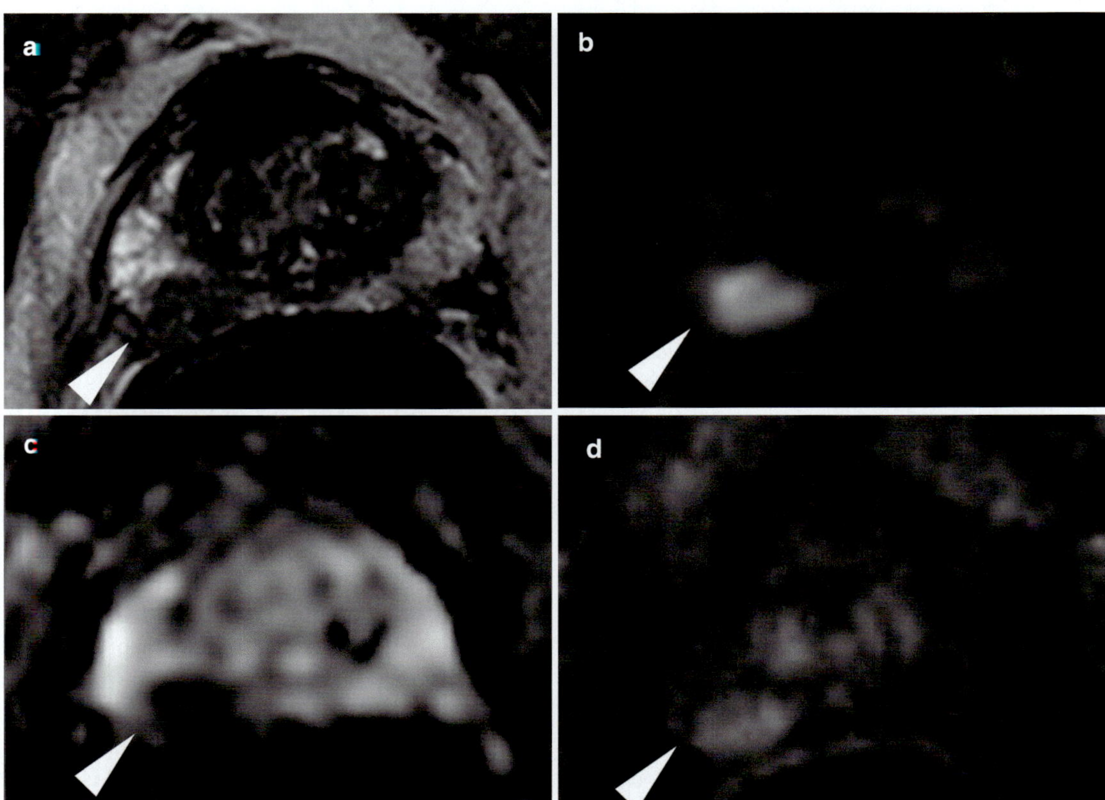

Fig. 4.2 Multiparametric MRI of a 72-year-old-man with elevated serum PSA level (5.9 ng/ml) and family history. (**a**) T2WI shows a hypointense nodule at the right mid posterolateral peripheral zone (size <1.5 cm, between 7- and 9-o-clock position). (**d**) DCE MRI shows mild early contrast enhancement of the nodule. (**b**, **c**) DWI and ADC map show marked hyperintensity and marked hypointensity respectively. The final assigned PI-RADS category was 4. *PSA* prostate specific antigen, *T2WI* T2 weighted imaging, *DCE* dynamic contrast enhancement, *DWI* diffusion-weighted imaging, *ADC* apparent diffusion coefficient, *PI-RADS* prostate imaging reporting and data system

quate. Specifically, when early contrast enhancement is present, the lesion classified as PI-RADS 3 will be upgraded to PI-RADS 4 category [8]. Characteristics of MRI findings for each PI-RADS category assignment of the PZ are displayed in Table 4.1.

Scoring and Reporting of Transition Zone Findings

TZ is characterized by the presence of multiple hyperplastic nodules and intervening stroma, appearing as well-defined nodules of variable signal intensities at MRI. Malignant nodules may develop in the context of this nodular heterogeneous background, making the diagnosis of csPCa in the TZ rather difficult, especially to unexperienced eyes. Benign hyperplastic nodules can be accurately differentiated from csPCa in virtue of some of their morphologic characteristics. For this reason, T2WI is the dominant sequence for the PI-RADS assessment of TZ lesions. In TZ, lesions corresponding to csPCa are characterized by marked hypointensity compared to the surrounding benign hyperplastic nodules; the margins are typically ill-defined and infiltrative, and a proper nodular capsule cannot be recognized. Malignant lesions may display lenticular or plaque-like morphology, and often grow in the intervening tissue between adjacent benign hyperplastic nodules. DWI assessment in the TZ is less reliable than in the PZ. Hyperplastic nodules often display restriction at DWI, which however is less marked than that of csPCa lesions. DWI is used as complementary evaluation of TZ lesions, and is particularly useful in case of diagnostic uncertainty, and in the setting of equivocal PI-RADS 3 lesions. DCE imaging, instead, has limited utility in TZ PI-RADS scoring, due to the fact that hyperplastic nodules are functionally active and often display enhanced contrast uptake. Characteristics of MRI findings for each PI-RADS category assignment of the TZ are displayed in Table 4.1.

Table 4.1 Summary table describing PI-RADS v2.1 scoring assessment categories for peripheral and transition zone findings at T2-weighted and diffusion-weighted imaging

Score	Peripheral zone—T2WI	Transition zone—T2WI
1	Uniform hyperintense signal intensity (normal)	Normal appearing TZ (rare) or a round, completely encapsulated nodule ("typical nodule")
2	Linear or wedge-shaped hypointensity or diffuse mild hypointensity, usually indistinct margin	Mostly encapsulated nodule OR a homogeneous circumscribed nodule without encapsulation. ("atypical nodule") OR a homogeneous mildly hypointense area between nodules
3	Heterogeneous signal intensity or non-circumscribed, rounded, moderate hypointensity Includes others that do not qualify as 2, 4 or 5	Heterogeneous signal intensity with obscured margins Includes others that do not qualify as 2, 4 or 5
4	Circumscribed, homogeneous moderate hypointense focus/mass confined to prostate and <1.5 cm in greatest dimension	Lenticular or non-circumscribed, homogeneous, moderately hypointense, and <1.5 cm in greatest dimension
5	Same as 4, but ≥1.5 cm in greatest dimension or definite extraprostatic extension/invasive behavior	Same as 4 but ≥1.5 cm in greatest dimension or definite extraprostatic extension/invasive behavior

	Peripheral zone/Transition zone—DWI
1	No abnormality (i.e., normal) on ADC and high b-value DWI
2	Linear/wedge shaped hypointense on ADC and/or linear/wedge shaped hyperintense on high b-value DWI
3	Focal (discrete and different from the background) hypointense on ADC and/or focal markedly hyperintense on high b-value DWI; may be markedly hypointense on ADC or markedly hyperintense on high b-value DWI, but not both
4	Focal markedly hypointense on ADC and markedly hyperintense on high b-value DWI; <1.5 cm in greatest dimension
5	Same as 4 but ≥1.5 cm in greatest dimension or definite extraprostatic extension/invasive behavior

Scoring and Reporting of Central Zone and Anterior Fibromuscular Stroma Findings

Occasionally, encountered lesions appear to originate in the CZ or involve the AFMS, and warrant special consideration. Most PCa foci found in the CZ usually arise in either the adjacent PZ or TZ and extend into the CZ. Focal early enhancement and/or asymmetry between the right and left CZ onT2W, DWI/ADC is a finding that may indicate the presence of PCa, according to PI-RADS v2.1 [8].

PCa only rarely primarily originates in the AFMS, therefore when reporting a suspicious lesion in the AFMS, criteria for either the PZ or the TZ should be applied. Abnormalities with increased SI relative to the pelvic muscles on T2WI, high signal intensity on high b-value DWI, low signal on ADC and early enhancement can raise the suspicion of AFMS neoplastic involvement [15].

Reporting Pitfalls in Prostate MRI

Several benign prostate diseases and anatomic variants may display imaging features that closely resemble PCa, leading to false positives and incorrect PI-RADS category assignment [11, 16].

Pitfalls Related to Prostate Benign Diseases

Benign diseases and conditions of the prostate include benign prostatic hyperplasia (BPH), chronic and acute prostatitis, abscesses, cystic lesions, calcifications, hemorrhage and atrophic gland changes.

BPH generally presents as well-encapsulated nodules of variable intensity, with stromal nodules showing moderate/marked hyperintensity. Because of their functional characteristics, BPH lesions may display early contrast enhancement on DCE and moderate restriction on DWI/ADC. Ectopic BPH nodules (BPH nodule extending through the peripheral zone of the gland) may constitute diagnostic difficulties especially to unexperienced readers, however lesion morphology along with the presence of a well-delineated capsule constitute important clues to recognize this pitfall [11].

The multi-faceted nature of chronic prostatitis produces a variety of atrophic and inflammatory changes which may be mistaken for cancer [17]. Lesions appear hypointense on T2WI sequences, sometimes with irregular margins or producing parenchymal distortion. The morphologies generally associated are band-like and triangular, but virtually all presentations are reported. Often lesions are multiple, restriction at DWI can be mild-to-moderate, and contrast enhancement is sometimes found, although rather delayed and diffuse [11, 18]. In some cases, the stigmata of long-standing chronic prostatitis can appear as a diffuse gland change, better defined with the term "dirty gland". This pattern can make the assessment of the prostate gland more difficult, hampering the detection of significant lesions.

Acute prostatitis also can produce focal and diffuse gland changes with unpredictable presentation. These range from diffuse signal alterations to variable areas of hypointensity on T2WI, with or without focal abscesses. Early contrast enhancement is often present, and can involve the gland diffusely, producing a so-called *Halloween sign* (due to its similarity with a "Jack-o-Lantern") [19]. Because of the diagnostic challenge represented by prostatitis-related changes, the evaluation of serum PSA levels and the follow-up of lesions over time after antimicrobial therapy constitute extremely helpful tools for the clinical radiologist.

Hemorrhage may be encountered in the post-biopsy settings, in acute prostatitis, or as incidental finding. It appears as a marked hyperintensity on T1-weighted imaging (T1WI), produced by the paramagnetic effect of methemoglobin, and a corresponding hypointensity on T2WI. Post-biopsy changes may persist for longer than 4 months from the procedure [11, 19].

Periurethral calcifications are a frequent finding especially in older subjects. Due to their physical properties, calcifications appear as markedly hypointense, minute lesions within the prostate gland. These changes may appear as hypointensity in the ADC map, however no restriction on DWI or hypointensity on T1WI matches this finding.

Pitfalls Related to Anatomic Variants

Among the pitfalls associated to prostate anatomy, one of the most frequently encountered is produced by the hyperplastic gland stroma compressing the adjacent peripheral zone. When central zone hyperplastic nodules impinge on the PZ, peripheral symmetric hypointensity appear in the posterolateral PZ, resembling multiple neoplastic foci. This pitfall goes under the name of *moustache sign* and can be differentiated from PCa for its symmetric and regular appearance, and from the typical mid-gland/base localization. When instead a single large adenoma compresses the PZ, this produces a similar single hypointense lesion, also known as *moustache-like sign.* Other similar pitfalls can result from the presence of hyperplastic nodules, or a hyperplastic central zone impinging on the PZ, near the veru montanum. This imaging finding is also known as *teardrop* sign, and it appears as a moderately hypointense lesion involving paramedian and median PZ. Other important imaging findings which may be challenging to distinguish from PCa are produced by a hypertrophic periprostatic neurovascular plexus: this may appear as a markedly hypointense lesion, sometimes displaying mass-like morphology, involving the PZ in the pericapsular area [11, 18]. This pitfall is frequently found in men with active inflammation and is produced by engorgement of the venous plexus surrounding the PZ. Other misleading anatomic variants may be represented by a thickened capsule separating the PZ from the TZ, sometimes referred as surgical pseudocapsule [19].

Issue to Address and New Strategies

mpMRI has undergone an outstanding evolution in the last decade, gaining a central role in PCa diagnosis. The increasing utilization of this technique on one side has brought new challenges to overcome, the first being the increasing demand for prostate MRI scans. The major challenge in the horizon of prostate mpMRI resides in the standardization of image quality across the world [20]. Until a few years ago prostate MRI was considered a *niche* diagnostic technique, performed only in high-volume centers and by top-level experts in the field. In few years, the landscape of PCa diagnosis has dramatically changed. mpMRI and PI-RADS are now considered the gold-standard for the workup of PCa and there are growing concerns about the lack of availability of qualified radiologists that would allow to face the upcoming large demand of prostate MRI.

Therefore, new strategies are being proposed, notably, the use of MRI without contrast medium (commonly referred to as "biparametric MRI") is investigated to push toward a more personalized, less invasive, and highly cost-effective diagnostic workup. In regard to the diagnostic yield of unenhanced biparametric MRI, meta-analysis studies show that this technique has comparable accuracy to mpMRI, with non-statistically significant differences [13, 20–22]. The PI-RADS committee recently recommended the use of risk grouping for the risk assessment of biopsy naïve men for whom contrast medium injection is advisable and for guiding biopsy and/or focal treatment. However, the detection of a higher number of clinically insignificant cancers implies the need of the definition of patient subgrouping where the benefits and harms of contrast enhancement are aligned to their clinical priorities [23].

MRI image quality and reader expertise are of paramount importance to ensure high performance to the MRI-based diagnostic pathway. Recently, the Prostate Imaging—Quality (PI-QUAL) from the PRECISION trial, was created to offer clinicians a scoring system for evaluating and reporting the quality of their prostate MRI scans [24]. Also, consensus statements from the ESUR/ESUI working group were released on MRI images quality. Recommendations included to check and report on image quality, to visually assess images adequacy for determining diagnostic acceptability, to control image quality at 6 months intervals or in 5% of studies, and to standardize ADC measurements on phantom [25].

Among the most promising upcoming applications for non-contrast prostate MRI, the opportunistic PCa screening covers a main position [26, 27]. Indeed, the need for a more sensitive test to early diagnose csPCa follows the lack of recommendations for serum PSA thresholds in international guidelines.

The Novel MRI-Based Pathway for Prostate Cancer Detection

In the past, prostate biopsies used to be performed by systematic sampling of the entire gland, bilaterally from apex to base, with a minimum of 8–10 cores. This whole-gland approach carried important inaccuracies. Currently, it is widely accepted that increasing the number of cores does not increase the rate of cancer detection, nor the negative predictive value of the test [28]. Targeting specific lesions can be performed by MR-directed biopsy (MRDB) with different techniques: the visual cognitive biopsy, the software-assisted MRI-TRUS fusion biopsy and the MRI-guided in-bore biopsy. MRDB in the setting of the MRI pathway has demonstrated a high diagnostic performance. A Cochrane meta-analysis of 18 studies on MR-guided targeted biopsy reports a pooled sensitivity of over 70% and a pooled specificity of 96% in detecting csPCa [29]. The most valuable strength of targeted biopsy resides in its negative predictive value (NPV): MRDB can exclude the presence of csPCa with >90% accuracy [7].

Owing to its high diagnostic yield, the mpMRI and its "pathways" have been recognized as "state-of-the-art" management tools and the most cost-effective exams for PCa workup. Men referred for early PCa detection patients follow a precise protocol in which PI-RADS-compliant mpMRI serves as triage test for stratifying their risk and establishing the most appropriate treatment. The MRI pathway involves the identification of prostate lesions carrying the highest probability of being csPCa and allocating these to subsequent targeted biopsy. Compared to the traditional systematic approach, this protocol has significantly improved the rate of csPCa detection (12% higher rate), at the same time reducing the rate of insignificant cancer diagnosis by over 40% [29]. Its accuracy has been evaluated in four major prospective multicenter trials (the PRECISION trial [30], the MRI-FIRST trial [31], the 4M study and the PROMIS trial [32, 33]), and further validated in subsequent metanalyses [7, 29, 34]. The MRI pathway not only constitutes a strategy for early csPCa detection, but it provides accurate risk estimation. It can be used, in fact, for guiding subsequent follow-up (in intermediate risk-patients), or for avoiding further useless diagnostic procedures (low-risk patients) [5].

The MRI-pathway has been largely validated in the re-biopsy settings, however the evidence so far gathered is still not sufficient for endorsing its use alone in biopsy naïve patients [4, 29]. According to current EAU guidelines, mpMRI can be used in two possible pathways for the early detection of PCa [4]:

(a) the MRI pathway in which a targeted biopsy only is performed, if significant lesions are detected on mpMRI. This pathway is recommended in patients with prior negative biopsies and persistent PCa suspicion;
(b) the combined pathway, where pre-biopsy MRI is performed, and if relevant foci are detected both systematic and MRI-targeted biopsies are performed. This approach is currently recommended in biopsy-naïve patients.

Overall the MRI pathway has brought revolutionary advances in PCa diagnosis, but there is still space for improvement: despite its high NPV, this technique is estimated to miss roughly 10% clinically significant cancers, and the positive predictive value is still prone to wide variability [29].

Other Applications of MRI in Prostate Cancer

MRI for Local Staging and Therapy Planning

Multiparametric MRI is fairly accurate in assessing locally invasive disease and constitutes a key diagnostic exam for estimating patient prognosis and for therapeutic planning. T1WI sequences and morphologic imaging allow for the accurate assessment of pelvic lymph nodes, and can distinguish between organ confined from locally advanced disease [4, 9].

In comparison to TNM staging, nomograms and other traditionally used prognostic tools, mpMRI has demonstrated an overall higher performance [35]. T2WI sequences in particular carry a high specificity (>95%) for detecting extraprostatic extension (EPE), seminal vesicle invasion (SVI) and overall T3-stage disease (periprostatic invasion, including periprostatic fat, the neurovascular bundle and prostatic capsule). The weak point of mpMRI however resides in the sensitivity for locally extensive disease (approximately 50%). Assessing EPE, in particular, can be difficult when the disease is minimally invasive, and is largely dependent on image quality (3 T machines are preferred to 1.5 T), patient anatomy and reader experience [35, 36]. Accurate local staging and assessment of microscopic EPE therefore still relies on definitive histology after radical prostatectomy. Although guidelines consider mpMRI as second-line investigation for the local staging, the use of this technique is recommended as pivotal step in therapy planning [4]. Prostate MRI finds important applications in the pre-surgical phase. It is fundamental in determining which patients are candidates to surgery, and it aids in planning surgical strategies for neurovascular bundle preservation [9, 37]. The introduction of robotic-assisted surgery has allowed to dramatically improve the functional outcomes of PCa patients, reducing the risk of side effects such as erectile dysfunction and urinary incontinence. With regard to robotic-assisted radical prostatectomy, mpMRI has shown to have a significant impact on treatment decision, leading to change the surgical strategy in up to 50% of cases, and reducing functional morbidity [38, 39]. mpMRI-based assessment of T3 disease and EPE has recently been validated in a study as independent predictor of negative margin resection, and of nerve sparing utilization [40]. Information obtained from preoperative mpMRI also has important prognostic value, and correlates accurately with the occurrence of disease relapse. Among the novel applications, mpMRI has been used also in the setting of neoadjuvant therapy of locally invasive PCa with aggressive phenotype. Recent studies demonstrate its efficacy in estimating residual cancer burden (RCB) and response to treatment, subsequent guiding the surgical therapeutic strategy [41, 42]. In conclusion mpMRI allows to tailor therapies more accurately, and may be introduced as fundamental tool in guiding novel techniques such as partial gland ablation and focal therapy, and modulating radiation doses in radiotherapy [38].

MRI for Disease Monitoring

MRI has important applications also in the setting of active surveillance (AS) and assessment of patients with biochemical recurrence after whole-gland therapies.

Serial mpMRI is a key part of the follow-up protocol, together with clinical evaluation including PSA kinetics, and repeat prostate biopsy [4]. Multiple studies demonstrate that MRI-visible lesions are more likely to be upgraded, and that a correlation exists between radiological evolution and pathological progression [43]. Any suspicious finding at follow-up mpMRI should prompt a repeat biopsy, and any rise in PSA level or new clinical finding should be followed by mpMRI evaluation [4, 44]. Current guidelines recommend that MR-directed targeted biopsy combined with systematic sampling be used to confirm disease progression and initiate active treatment [4, 45]. On the other hand, serial mpMRI is being evaluated for its potential as tool to better stratify the risk of patients in AS, and could be used to select those lower-risk cases in whom a repeat biopsy can be safely avoided [46, 47]. For the purpose of optimal risk assessment and better tailoring of the therapeutic strategy, the *Prostate Cancer Radiological Estimation of Change in Sequential Evaluation (PRECISE)* recommendations have been released in 2017 [48]. According to these recommendations, lesions evaluated on serial mpMRI are assigned a score from 1 to 5, which summarizes the radiological evolution during the follow-up time (Figs. 4.3 and 4.4). As additional tool, the quantitative estimation of the ADC ratio of radiological lesions on follow-up mpMRI has been shown to significantly correlate with disease progression. Progression to csPCa was associated with a significant reduction in the values of normalized ADC and ADC [49].

In patients experiencing biochemical recurrence, detection of local recurrence of PCa is crucial for proper patient management. Indeed, it is essential to provide a stepwise, multimodal approach that allows local and systemic restaging of PCa, strictly depending on clinical priority. In this setting, the role mpMRI becomes increasingly important for the detection of PCa local recurrence. mpMRI is a suitable modality to identify the presence of benign or malignant pathology at the level of prostatic bed after radical prostatectomy, namely to distinguish expected post-therapy changes (e.g. distorted anatomy, fibrosis, artifacts from clips) from local recurrence, and to evaluate local tumor recurrence after radiation therapy [50–59]. A panel of international experts have recently released a standardized method to promote standardization and reduce variations in the acquisition, interpretation, and reporting of MRI for PCa recurrence and to guide therapy, called the *Prostate MR Imaging for local*

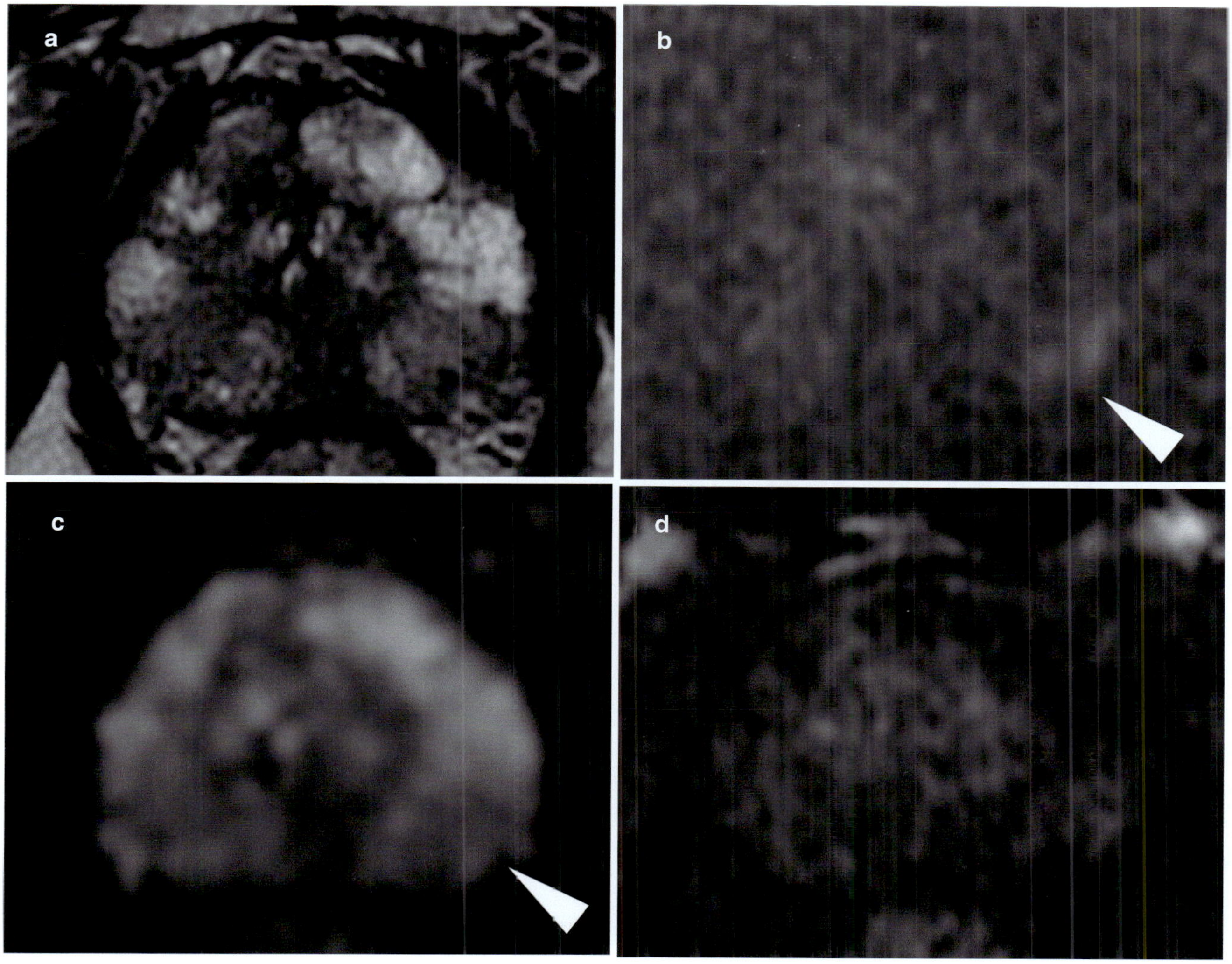

Fig. 4.3 Multiparametric MRI of a 71-year-old man with Grade Group 1 prostate cancer enrolled in an active surveillance program. (**a**) T2WI shows bilateral band-like non-focal alterations (4-o-clock position); (**d**) DCE-MRI does not show significant post-contrast enhancement. (**b**) DWI shows mild hyperintensity at the left postero-lateral peripheral zone (4-o-clock position) with no corresponding and hypointensity on ADC map (**c**). The final assigned PI-RADS category was 3, and the patient initiated scheduled clinical visits and serial PSA testing. *PSA* prostate specific antigen, *T2WI* T2 weighted imaging, *DCE* dynamic contrast enhancement, *DWI* diffusion-weighted imaging, *ADC* apparent diffusion coefficient, *PI-RADS* prostate imaging reporting and data system

Recurrence Reporting (PI-RR) [60]. PI-RR uses a 5-point scoring system that indicates the level of suspicion for presence of PCa recurrence on mpMRI (Figs. 4.5 and 4.6). Pending clinical validation, PI-RR might be used as a clinical guide to improve the care of men with recurrent PCa by providing a better diagnosis and more patient-tailored treatment.

Conclusions

Prostate MRI has a leading role in the diagnostic pathway of PCa, providing a highly accurate detection of csPCa, directing targeted prostate biopsies and guiding therapy. Prostate MRI requires high image quality and reader expertise to reach its diagnostic potential, and the introduction of novel, individualized, risk-stratification strategies are warranted to meet the increasing demand for MRI-based pathways for both diagnosis and management of PCa. Artificial intelligence-based tools might be explored to ameliorate some critical issues of prostate MRI such as inter-reader agreement, accuracy of less experienced readers, and image reporting time. This becomes paramount when biparametric MRI is proposed as a screening tool. MRI has also shown utility as a tool for local staging and treatment planning as well as for monitoring patients under active surveillance and after radical treatment with curative intent at the time of biochemical recurrence.

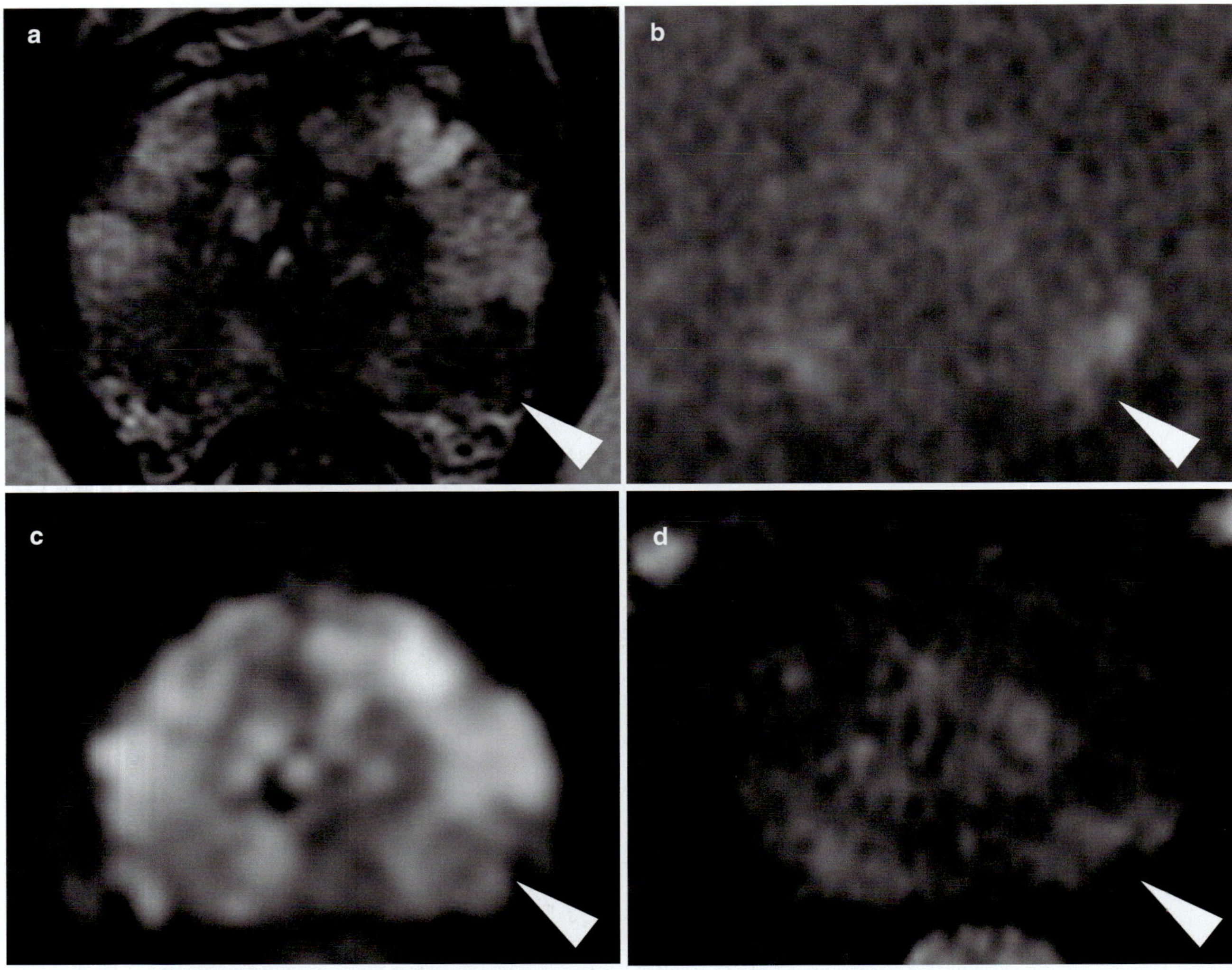

Fig. 4.4 Surveillance multiparametric MRI of the same patient as in Fig. 4.3 after 1 year from initial MRI. The previous PI-RADS 3 lesion on the left showed more marked alterations on (**a**) T2, and on (**b**, **c**) DWI/ADC map with corresponding focal enhancement on DCE (**d**), classified as PI-RADS 4. On the right lobe, a new lesion scored as PI-RADS 4 was detected. The final assigned PRECISE score was 5 due to increase in size and higher conspicuity of the lesion on the left and the new lesion on the right. *PSA* prostate specific antigen, *T2WI* T2 weighted imaging, *DCE* dynamic contrast enhancement, *DWI* diffusion-weighted imaging, *ADC* apparent diffusion coefficient, *PI-RADS* prostate imaging reporting and data system

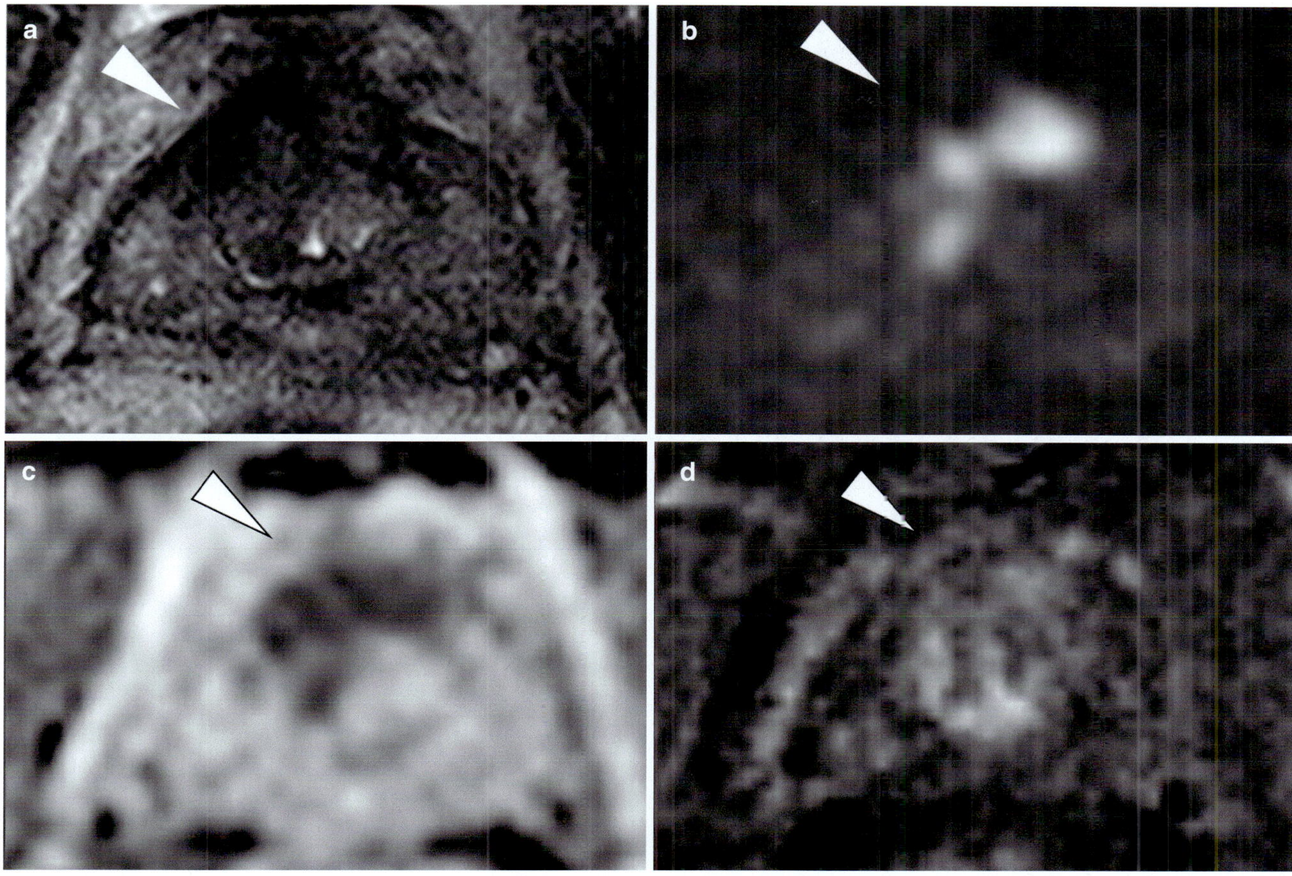

Fig. 4.5 Multiparametric MRI of a 63-year-old man treated with radiation therapy for Grade Group 3 prostate cancer in 2014, and presenting with a rising serum PSA value (1.06 ng/ml) in 2022. (**a**) T2WI shows a focal hypointensity area at the mid anterior right transitional zone. (**b**, **c**) DWI and ADC map show hyperintensity at high b values and hypointensity of the same focal area, respectively. (**d**) DCE-MRI shows partial early enhancing focal area. The final assigned PI-RR score was 5 (primary tumor location unknown but matching of DWI/ADC and DCE). *PSA* prostate specific antigen, *T2W* T2 weighted imaging, *DCE* dynamic contrast enhancement, *DWI* diffusion-weighted imaging, *ADC* apparent diffusion coefficient, *PI-RADS* prostate imaging reporting and data system, *PI-RR* prostate imaging for local recurrence reporting

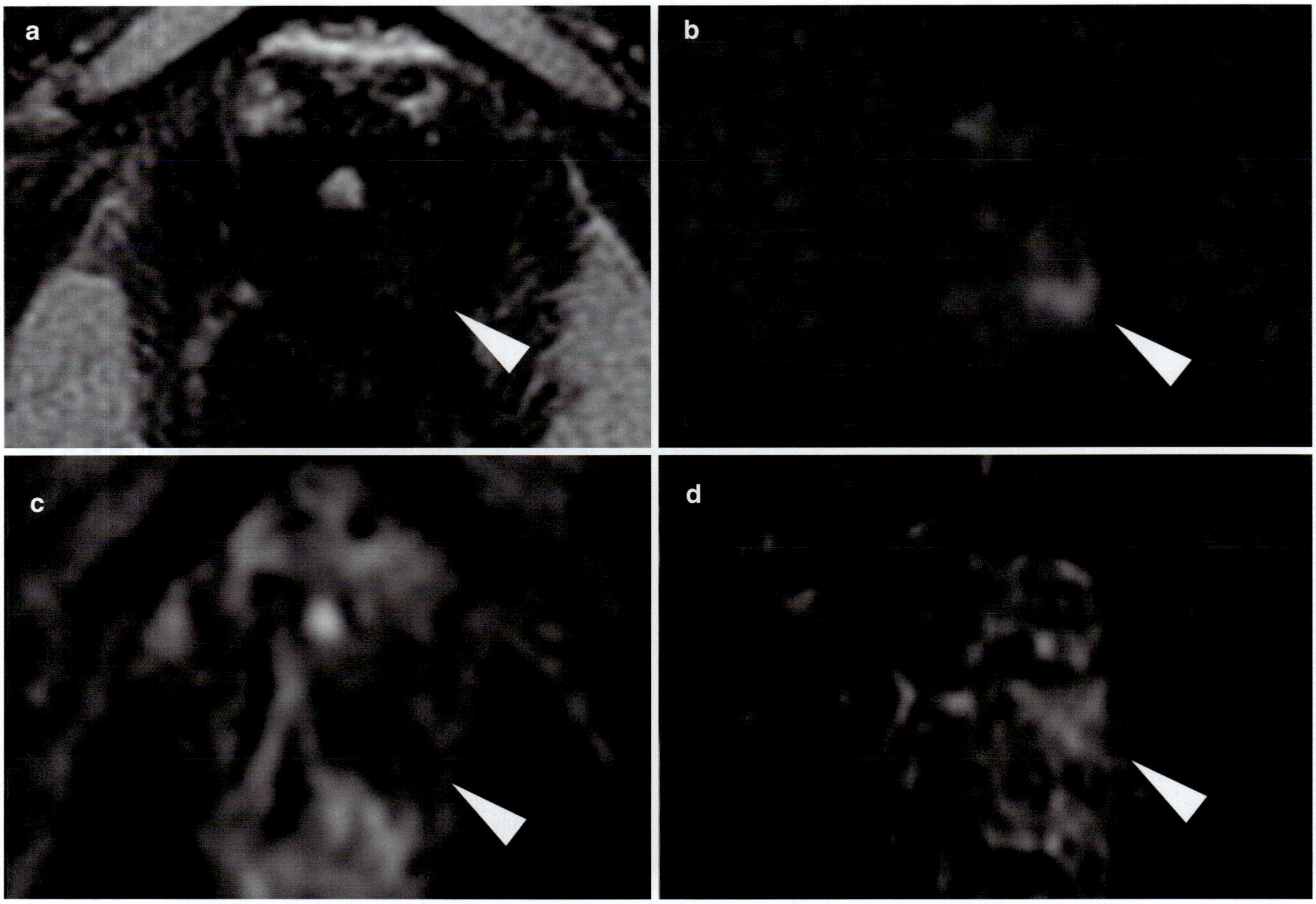

Fig. 4.6 Multiparametric of a 74-year-old man treated with radical prostatectomy for Grade Group 2 pT2c pN0 prostate cancer in 2010, and presenting with a rising serum PSA value (0.48 ng/ml) in 2022. (**a**) T2WI shows an asymmetric focal hyperintensity in the perianastomotic area at the same side of primary tumor (white arrow, 4-o-clock position). (**b**, **c**) DWI and ADC map show marked hyperintensity and marked hypointensity, respectively. (**d**) DCE-MRI confirms an early enhancing focal area after contrast injection (white arrow). The final assigned PI-RR score was 5. *PSA* prostate specific antigen, *T2WI* T2 weighted imaging, *DCE* dynamic contrast enhancement, *DWI* diffusion-weighted imaging, *ADC* apparent diffusion coefficient, *PI-RADS* prostate imaging reporting and data system, *PI-RR* prostate imaging for local recurrence reporting

References

1. Steyn JH, Smith FW. Nuclear magnetic resonance imaging of the prostate. Br J Urol. 1982;54(6):726–8.
2. Giganti F, Rosenkrantz AB, Villeirs G, Panebianco V, Stabile A, Emberton M, et al. The evolution of MRI of the prostate: the past, the present, and the future. Am J Roentgenol. 2019;213(2):384–96.
3. Dickinson L, Ahmed HU, Allen C, Barentsz JO, Carey B, Futterer JJ, et al. Magnetic resonance imaging for the detection, localisation, and characterisation of prostate cancer: recommendations from a European consensus meeting. Eur Urol. 2011;59(4):477–94.
4. Mottet N, Bellmunt J, Briers E, Bolla M, Bourke, Cornford P, et al. EAU-ESTRO-ESUR-SIOG guidelines on prostate cancer. Edn. presented at the EAU annual congress Amsterdam 2020. Arnhem: EAU Guidelines Office; 2020.
5. Van Poppel H, Hogenhout R, Albers P, van den Bergh RCN, Barentsz JO, Roobol MJ. Early detection of prostate cancer in 2020 and beyond: facts and recommendations for the European Union and the European Commission. Eur Urol. 2021;79(3):327–9.
6. Panebianco V, Barchetti G, Simone G, Del Monte M, Ciardi A, Grompone MD, et al. Negative multiparametric magnetic resonance imaging for prostate cancer: what's next? Eur Urol. 2018;74(1):48–54.
7. Sathianathen NJ, Omer A, Harriss E, Davies L, Kasivisvanathan V, Punwani S, et al. Negative predictive value of multiparametric magnetic resonance imaging in the detection of clinically significant prostate cancer in the prostate imaging reporting and data system era: a systematic review and meta-analysis. Eur Urol. 2020;78(3):402–14.
8. Padhani AR, Weinreb J, Rosenkrantz AB, Villeirs G, Turkbey B, Barentsz J. Prostate Imaging-Reporting and Data System Steering Committee: PI-RADS v2 status update and future directions. Eur Urol. 2019;75(3):385–96.
9. Margolis DJA. Multiparametric MRI for localized prostate cancer: lesion detection and staging. Biomed Res Int. 2014;2014:1–11.
10. Meyer H-J, Wienke A, Surov A. Discrimination between clinical significant and insignificant prostate cancer with apparent diffusion coefficient—a systematic review and meta analysis. BMC Cancer. 2020;20(1):482.
11. Panebianco V, Giganti F, Kitzing YX, Cornud F, Campa R, De Rubeis G, et al. An update of pitfalls in prostate mpMRI: a practical approach through the lens of PI-RADS v. 2 guidelines. Insights Imaging. 2018;9(1):87–101.

12. Wei C, Jin B, Szewczyk-Bieda M, Gandy S, Lang S, Zhang Y, et al. Quantitative parameters in dynamic contrast-enhanced magnetic resonance imaging for the detection and characterization of prostate cancer. Oncotarget. 2018;9(22):15997–6007.
13. Schoots IG, Barentsz JO, Bittencourt LK, Haider MA, Macura KJ, Margolis DJA, et al. PI-RADS Committee position on MRI without contrast medium in biopsy-naive men with suspected prostate cancer: narrative review. Am J Roentgenol. 2021;216(1):3–19.
14. Zawaideh JP, Sala E, Shaida N, Koo B, Warren AY, Carmisciano L, et al. Diagnostic accuracy of biparametric versus multiparametric prostate MRI: assessment of contrast benefit in clinical practice. Eur Radiol. 2020;30(7):4039–49.
15. Turkbey B, Rosenkrantz AB, Haider MA, Padhani AR, Villeirs G, Macura KJ, et al. Prostate imaging reporting and data system version 2.1: 2019 update of prostate imaging reporting and data system version 2. Eur Urol. 2019;76(3):340–51.
16. Panebianco V, Barchetti F, Barentsz J, Ciardi A, Cornud F, Futterer J, et al. Pitfalls in interpreting mp-MRI of the prostate: a pictorial review with pathologic correlation. Insights Imaging. 2015;6(6):611–30.
17. Wang X, Liu W, Lei Y, Wu G, Lin F. Assessment of prostate imaging reporting and data system version 2.1 false-positive category 4 and 5 lesions in clinically significant prostate cancer. Abdom Radiol (NY). 2021;46(7):3410–7. https://doi.org/10.1007/s00261-021-03023-w.
18. Thomas S, Oto A. Multiparametric MR imaging of the prostate. Radiol Clin North Am. 2018;56(2):277–87.
19. Labra WA, Zúñiga GÁ. Pitfalls en RM de Próstata Multiparamétrica. Rev Chil Radiol. 2019;25(4):128–40.
20. Woo S, Suh CH, Kim SY, Cho JY, Kim SH. Diagnostic performance of prostate imaging reporting and data system version 2 for detection of prostate cancer: a systematic review and diagnostic meta-analysis. Eur Urol. 2017;72(2):177–88.
21. Kang Z, Min X, Weinreb J, Li Q, Feng Z, Wang L. Abbreviated biparametric versus standard multiparametric MRI for diagnosis of prostate cancer: a systematic review and meta-analysis. Am J Roentgenol. 2019;212(2):357–65.
22. Alabousi M, Salameh J-P, Gusenbauer K, Samoilov L, Jafri A, Yu H, et al. Biparametric vs multiparametric prostate magnetic resonance imaging for the detection of prostate cancer in treatment-naïve patients: a diagnostic test accuracy systematic review and meta-analysis. BJU Int. 2019;124(2):209–20.
23. Schoots IG, Barentsz JO, Bittencourt LK, Haider MA, Macura KJ, Margolis DJA, et al. PI-RADS Committee position on MRI without contrast medium in biopsy naive men with suspected prostate cancer: a narrative review. Am J Roentgenol. 2021;216(1):3–19.
24. Giganti F, Allen C, Emberton M, Moore CM, Kasivisvanathan V. Prostate imaging quality (PI-QUAL): a new quality control scoring system for multiparametric magnetic resonance imaging of the prostate from the PRECISION trial. Eur Urol Oncol. 2020;3(5):615–9.
25. de Rooij M, Israël B, Tummers M, Ahmed HU, Barrett T, Giganti F, et al. ESUR/ESUI consensus statements on multi-parametric MRI for the detection of clinically significant prostate cancer: quality requirements for image acquisition, interpretation and radiologists' training. Eur Radiol. 2020;30(10):5404–16. https://doi.org/10.1007/s00330-020-06929-z.
26. Panebianco V, Pecoraro M, Fiscon G, Paci P, Farina L, Catalano C. Prostate cancer screening research can benefit from network medicine: an emerging awareness. npj Syst Biol Appl. 2020;6(1):13.
27. Eldred-Evans D, Burak P, Connor MJ, Day E, Evans M, Fiorentino F, et al. Population-based prostate cancer screening with magnetic resonance imaging or ultrasonography: the IP1-PROSTAGRAM study. JAMA Oncol. 2021;7(3):395–402. https://jamanetwork.com/journals/jamaoncology/fullarticle/2776224.
28. Da Silva V, Cagiannos I, Lavallée LT, Mallick R, Witiuk K, Cnossen S, et al. An assessment of Prostate Cancer Research International: Active Surveillance (PRIAS) criteria for active surveillance of clinically low-risk prostate cancer patients. CUAJ. 2017;11(8):238–43.
29. Drost F-JH, Osses DF, Nieboer D, Steyerberg EW, Bangma CH, Roobol MJ, et al. Prostate MRI, with or without MRI-targeted biopsy, and systematic biopsy for detecting prostate cancer. Cochrane Database Syst Rev. 2019;4(4):CD012663. https //doi.org/10.1002/14651858.CD012663.pub2.
30. Kasivisvanathan V, Rannikko AS, Borghi M, Panebianco V, Mynderse LA, Vaarala MH, et al. MRI-targeted or standard biopsy for prostate-cancer diagnosis. N Engl J Med. 2018;378(19):1767–77.
31. Rouvière O, Puech P, Renard-Penna R, Claudon M, Roy C, Mège-Lechevallier F, et al. Use of prostate systematic and targeted biopsy on the basis of multiparametric MRI in biopsy-naive patients (MRI-FIRST): a prospective, multicentre, paired diagnostic study. Lancet Oncol. 2019;20(1):100–9.
32. van der Leest M, Cornel E, Israël B, Hendriks R, Padhani AR, Hoogenboom M, et al. Head-to-head comparison of transrectal ultrasound-guided prostate biopsy versus multiparametric prostate resonance imaging with subsequent magnetic resonance-guided biopsy in biopsy-naïve men with elevated prostate-specific antigen: a large prospective multicenter clinical study. Eur Urol. 2019;75(4):570–8.
33. Ahmed HU, El-Shater Bosaily A, Brown LC, Gabe R, Kaplan R, Parmar MK, et al. Diagnostic accuracy of multi-parametric MRI and TRUS biopsy in prostate cancer (PROMIS): a paired validating confirmatory study. Lancet. 2017;389(10071):815–22.
34. Kasivisvanathan V, Stabile A, Neves JB, Giganti F, Valerio M, Shanmugabavan Y, et al. Magnetic resonance imaging-targeted biopsy versus systematic biopsy in the detection of prostate cancer: a systematic review and meta-analysis. Eur Urol. 2019;76(3):284–303.
35. Caglic I, Kovac V, Barrett T. Multiparametric MRI—local staging of prostate cancer and beyond. Radiol Oncol. 2019;53(2):159–70.
36. de Rooij M, Hamoen EHJ, Witjes JA, Barentsz JO, Rovers MM. Accuracy of magnetic resonance imaging for local staging of prostate cancer: a diagnostic meta-analysis. Eur Urol. 2016;70(2):233–45
37. Marenco J, Orczyk C, Collins T, Moore C, Emberton M. Role of MRI in planning radical prostatectomy: what is the added value? World J Urol. 2019;37(7):1289–92.
38. Duvnjak P, Schulman AA, Holtz JN, Huang J, Polascik TJ, Gupta RT. Multiparametric prostate MR imaging: impact on clinical staging and decision making. Radiol Clin North Am. 2018;56(2):239–50.
39. Schiavina R, Bianchi L, Borghesi M, Dababneh H, Chessa F, Pultrone CV, et al. MRI displays the prostatic cancer anatomy and improves the bundles management before robot-assisted radical prostatectomy. J Endourol. 2018;32(4):315–21.
40. Radtke JP, Hadaschik BA, Wolf MB, Freitag MT, Schwab C, Alt C, et al. The impact of magnetic resonance imaging on prediction of extraprostatic extension and prostatectomy outcome in patients with low-, intermediate- and high-risk prostate cancer: try to find a standard. J Endourol. 2015;29(12):1396–405.
41. Karzai F, Walker SM, Wilkinson S, Madan RA, Shih JH, Merino MJ, et al. Sequential prostate magnetic resonance imaging in newly diagnosed high-risk prostate cancer treated with neoadjuvant enzalutamide is predictive of therapeutic response. Clin Cancer Res. 2021;27(2):429–37.
42. Fennessy FM, Fedorov A, Vangel MG, Mulkern RV, Tretiakova M, Lis RT, et al. Multiparametric MRI as a biomarker of response to neoadjuvant therapy for localized prostate cancer—a pilot study. Acad Radiol. 2020;27(10):1432–9.

43. Schoots IG, Petrides N, Giganti F, Bokhorst LP, Rannikko A, Klotz L, et al. Magnetic resonance imaging in active surveillance of prostate cancer: a systematic review. Eur Urol. 2015;67(4):627–36.
44. Lam TBL, MacLennan S, Willemse P-PM, Mason MD, Plass K, Shepherd R, et al. EAU-EANM-ESTRO-ESUR-SIOG prostate cancer guideline panel consensus statements for deferred treatment with curative intent for localised prostate cancer from an international collaborative study (DETECTIVE study). Eur Urol. 2019;76(6):790–813.
45. Schoots IG, Nieboer D, Giganti F, Moore CM, Bangma CH, Roobol MJ. Is magnetic resonance imaging-targeted biopsy a useful addition to systematic confirmatory biopsy in men on active surveillance for low-risk prostate cancer? A systematic review and meta-analysis. BJU Int. 2018;122(6):946–58.
46. Schoots IG, Moore CM, Rouvière O. Role of MRI in low-risk prostate cancer: finding the wolf in sheep's clothing or the sheep in wolf's clothing? Curr Opin Urol. 2017;27(3):238–45.
47. Klotz L, Loblaw A, Sugar L, Moussa M, Berman DM, Van der Kwast T, et al. Active surveillance magnetic resonance imaging study (ASIST): results of a randomized multicenter prospective trial. Eur Urol. 2019;75(2):300–9.
48. Moore CM, Giganti F, Albertsen P, Allen C, Bangma C, Briganti A, et al. Reporting magnetic resonance imaging in men on active surveillance for prostate cancer: the PRECISE recommendations—a report of a European School of Oncology Task Force. Eur Urol. 2017;71(4):648–55.
49. Giganti F, Pecoraro M, Fierro D, Campa R, Del Giudice F, Punwani S, et al. DWI and PRECISE criteria in men on active surveillance for prostate cancer: a multicentre preliminary experience of different ADC calculations. Magn Reson Imaging. 2020;67:50–8.
50. Morgan VA, Riches SF, Giles S, Dearnaley D, deSouza NM. Diffusion-weighted MRI for locally recurrent prostate cancer after external beam radiotherapy. Am J Roentgenol. 2012;198(3):596–602.
51. Barchetti F, Panebianco V. Multiparametric MRI for recurrent prostate cancer post radical prostatectomy and postradiation therapy. Biomed Res Int. 2014;2014:1–23.
52. Casciani E, Polettini E, Carmenini E, Floriani I, Masselli G, Bertini L, et al. Endorectal and dynamic contrast-enhanced MRI for detection of local recurrence after radical prostatectomy. Am J Roentgenol. 2008;190(5):1187–92.
53. Roy C, Foudi F, Charton J, Jung M, Lang H, Saussine C, et al. Comparative sensitivities of functional MRI sequences in detection of local recurrence of prostate carcinoma after radical prostatectomy or external-beam radiotherapy. Am J Roentgenol. 2013;200(4):W361–8.
54. Dinis Fernandes C, Dinh CV, Walraven I, Heijmink SW, Smolic M, van Griethuysen JJM, et al. Biochemical recurrence prediction after radiotherapy for prostate cancer with T2w magnetic resonance imaging radiomic features. Phys Imaging Radiat Oncol. 2018;7:9–15.
55. Abd-Alazeez M, Ramachandran N, Dikaios N, Ahmed HU, Emberton M, Kirkham A, et al. Multiparametric MRI for detection of radiorecurrent prostate cancer: added value of apparent diffusion coefficient maps and dynamic contrast-enhanced images. Prostate Cancer Prostatic Dis. 2015;18(2):128–36.
56. Notley M, Yu J, Fulcher AS, Turner MA, Cockrell CH, Nguyen D. Diagnosis of recurrent prostate cancer and its mimics at multiparametric prostate MRI. Br J Radiol. 2015;88(1054):20150362.
57. Panebianco V, Barchetti F, Sciarra A, Musio D, Forte V, Gentile V, et al. Prostate cancer recurrence after radical prostatectomy: the role of 3-T diffusion imaging in multi-parametric magnetic resonance imaging. Eur Radiol. 2013;23(6):1745–52.
58. Maurer T, Eiber M, Fanti S, Budäus L, Panebianco V. Imaging for prostate cancer recurrence. Eur Urol Focus. 2016;2(2):139–50.
59. De Visschere PJL, Standaert C, Fütterer JJ, Villeirs GM, Panebianco V, Walz J, et al. A systematic review on the role of imaging in early recurrent prostate cancer. Eur Urol Oncol. 2019;2(1):47–76.
60. Panebianco V, Villeirs G, Weinreb JC, Turkbey BI, Margolis DJ, Richenberg J, et al. Prostate magnetic resonance imaging for local recurrence reporting (PI-RR): international consensus-based guidelines on multiparametric magnetic resonance imaging for prostate cancer recurrence after radiation therapy and radical prostatectomy. Eur Urol Oncol. 2021;4(6):868–76.

PET/CT for Detection of Biochemical Recurrence Post Radical Prostatectomy

5

Victoria Jahrreiss, Bernhard Grubmüller, Sazan Rasul, and Shahrokh F. Shariat

Introduction

Prostate cancer (PCa) is the most common cancer in men in developed countries, and the second most cause of cancer death. Radical prostatectomy is often the primary treatment choice for the large majority of patients today, diagnosed with clinically non metastatic disease [1]. RP leads to durable local disease control with ever improving functional outcomes [2–5].

After primary treatment of clinically non-metastatic prostate cancer with curative intent, a substantial number of patients are diagnosed with cancer recurrence, mostly detected by rising prostate specific antigen (PSA) serum levels without clinical evidence of metastases. 27–57% of patients who undergo radical prostatectomy for clinically non-metastatic prostate cancer eventually experience BCR. Patients with BCR are at higher risk of developing local or distant recurrent disease [6–8]. Biochemical failure can precede metastatic disease by years [9]. Salvage treatments in these patients can provide disease control and thereby prolong survival [10–15]. Patients with distant recurrences are often treated with androgen deprivation therapy (ADT), while patients with local recurrence are offered radiation therapy alone or with ADT [10, 16]

Identifying patients who will profit from salvage treatments, while avoiding overtreatment for others poses a challenge in clinical management. As disease control is highly depended on the site and extent of recurrence, accurate and sensitive imaging is of utmost importance in these cases.

Conventional imaging techniques have shown limited accuracy for the assessment and detection of disease recurrence in prostate cancer patients after primary treatment. Functional molecular imaging modalities, on the other hand, offer additional information by depicting molecular and cellular processes of cancer recurrences [17].

Abdominopelvic Contrast-Enhanced Computerized Tomography (CT) Scan/Bone Scan

A PSA threshold of >0.4 ng/mL has been found to most accurately predict systemic progression after RP [18, 19]. Furthermore, radiation therapies show the highest efficacy at PSA values <0.5 ng/mL [15, 20]. However, most imaging modalities have limited sensitivity in detecting disease, as well as distinguishing between local and distant recurrence at these thresholds. Studies found that abdominopelvic contrast-enhanced CT scans were positive in only 11–14% of patients with BCR [21–23]. Likewise, less than 5% of patients with BCR after RP had positive bone scans, when PSA values where below 7 ng/mL [23, 24].

V. Jahrreiss · B. Grubmüller
Department of Urology, Comprehensive Cancer Center, Medical University of Vienna, Vienna, Austria
e-mail: victoria.jahrreiss@meduniwien.ac.at; bernhard.grubmueller@meduniwien.ac.at

S. Rasul
Division of Nuclear Medicine, Department of Biomedical Imaging and Image-Guided Therapy, Medical University of Vienna, Vienna, Austria
e-mail: sazan.rasul@meduniwien.ac.at

S. F. Shariat (✉)
Department of Urology, Comprehensive Cancer Center, Medical University of Vienna, Vienna, Austria

Institute for Urology and Reproductive Health, Sechenov University, Moscow, Russia

Department of Urology, Weill Cornell Medical College, New York, NY, USA

Department of Urology, University of Texas Southwestern, Dallas, TX, USA

Department of Urology, Second Faculty of Medicine, Charles University, Prague, Czech Republic

Karl Landsteiner Institute of Urology and Andrology, Vienna, Austria

Division of Urology, Department of Special Surgery, Jordan University Hospital, The University of Jordan, Amman, Jordan

S. Ren et al. (eds.), *Robot-Assisted Radical Prostatectomy*, https://doi.org/10.1007/978-3-031-05855-4_5

PET CT

The development of molecular imaging modalities, using different tracers in positron emission tomography (PET), has led to improvements in the detection of recurrences in patients with BCR after RP [25]. PET imaging provides additional information by visualizing metabolic tumor activities [17]. Depending on the disease entity, different tracers are used. Most applied tracers in prostate cancer patients are: fluciclovine, choline, and prostate-specific membrane antigen.

Choline PET/CT

Choline facilitates the synthesis of the phospholipids in the cell membrane and modulates transmembrane signaling. In tumor cells choline-kinase activity is upregulated, due to their enhanced proliferation [17]. Moreover, C-Choline shows minimal background activity on imaging in the pelvic area, making it a suitable isotope in PET/CT diagnostics for recurrent PCa [26]. Choline PET/CT has a higher sensitivity and specificity for detecting bone metastases compared to the bone scan. However, its sensitivity is highly depended on PSA levels and its detection of lymph node metastases is limited due to the low sensitivity of the imaging modality [27–30]. At PSA levels below 1 ng/mL detection rates are between 5% and 24%, whereas detection rates rise to 67–100% at PSA levels above 5 ng/mL in patients with BCR [31–33]. Even though imaging with choline PET/CT provides better detection of PCa recurrence compared to contrast-enhanced CT and bone scan, there is still a need for more accurate imaging, especially at lower PSA levels [34, 35].

Fluoride PET and Fluciclovine PET/CT

Fluciclovine is adopted into prostate cancer cells by different the amino acid transporters and therefore functions as a suitable tracer for the detection of recurrences in prostate cancer patients with BCR [36]. Compared to choline PET/C, ^{18}F-Fluciclovine PET/CT has shown higher sensitivity in the detection and localization of recurrences in patients with BCR. Similarly, to choline PET/CT, sensitivity of fluciclovine PET/CT is dependent on the patient's PSA levels [37].

18F-NaF PET/CT is a bone seeking agent, that mainly reflects osteoblastic activity. It has shown higher sensitivity in the detection of bone metastases than bone scan in detecting bone metastases [38], however its specificity is low. Additionally, 18F-NaF PET/CT fails to detect soft tissue metastases [39].

PSMA-PET/CT

Prostate-specific membrane antigen (PSMA) is transmembrane glycoprotein which is overexpressed in prostate cancer cells. Consequently, PSMA acts as a promising tracer in prostate cancer specific imaging [40]. A number of radiolabeled tracers for PSMA PET imaging have been reviewed. While most studies assess imaging with 68Ga-PSMA-11, there is no conclusive data on the differences of tracers at the moment [41]. Compared to choline PET/CT, PSMA PET/CT has shown significantly higher specificity and sensitivity, especially at PSA levels below 1 ng/mL [25, 42, 43]. However, detection rates of the PSMA PET/CT are dependent on PSA levels too and improve with increasing PSA. In a prospective study detection rates were 38% for PSA level below 0.5 ng/mL ($n = 136$), 57% for PSA levels between 0.5 and 1.0 ng/mL ($n = 79$), 84% for PSA levels between 1.0 and 2.0 ng/mL ($n = 89$), 86% for PSA levels between 2.0 and 5.0 ng/mL ($n = 158$), and 97% for PSA 5.0 ng/mL and higher ($n = 173$, $P < 0.001$) [44].

Conclusion

With the high rate of BCR after RP and the effective treatment options for these patients, there is an urgent need for accurate imaging modalities that allow personalized shared decision making in the salvage setting. PET imaging has ushered with the new tracers the age of targeted therapy in the BCR setting. PSMA PET currently is the imaging technique with the highest sensitivity for detection of recurrences in PC patients with BCR after RP, especially at low PSA levels. Therefore, guidelines recommend performing a PSMA PET/CT in these patients, if the results will influence further treatment decisions [16]. Alternatively, fluciclovine PET/CT or choline PET/CT can be performed at PSA levels of 1 ng/mL or higher, if PSMA PET/CT is not available (Table 5.1).

Table 5.1 Diagnostic performance of different imaging modalities in patients with biochemical recurrence after radical prostatectomy

Authors	Imaging modality	N population size	PSA level median	Sensitivity (%)	Specificity (%)	Positive predictive value (%)	Negative predictive value (%)
Tilki et al. [34]	18F-FEC PET/CT	156	6.0 ng/mL (IQR 1.7–9.4 ng/mL)	39.7	95.8	75.7	83.0
Poulsen et al. [45]	FCH PET/CT	25	>10 ng/mL	100	95	75	100
Graute et al. [35]	[^{18}F]fluorocholine PET/CT	82	4.4 ng/mL (range 0.03–36.0 ng/mL)	82	74	n.a.	n.a.
Nanni et al. [37]	(11)C-choline PET/CT	89	3.35 ng/mL (range 0.20–20.72)	32	40	90	3
Beheshti et al. [39]	18F fluorocholine PET/CT	38	Mean 55 ± 64 ng/mL	74	99	n.a.	n.a.
Fendler et al. [44]	68Ga-PSMA-11 PET/CT		2.1 (range 0.1–1154.0)	92	n.a.	84	n.a.
Abufaraj et al. [46]	[68Ga]Ga-PSMA-11 PET/CT(MRI)	65	1.4 ng/mL (IQR 0.8–2.9 ng/mL)	72–100	96–100	95–100	93-100

References

1. Lughezzani G, Briganti A, Karakiewicz PI, Kattan MW, Montorsi F, Shariat SF, et al. Predictive and prognostic models in radical prostatectomy candidates: a critical analysis of the literature. Eur Urol. 2010;58(5):687–700.
2. Novara G, Ficarra V, Rosen RC, Artibani W, Costello A, Eastham JA, et al. Systematic review and meta-analysis of perioperative outcomes and complications after robot-assisted radical prostatectomy. Eur Urol. 2012;62(3):431–52.
3. Novara G, Ficarra V, Mocellin S, Ahlering TE, Carroll PR, Graefen M, et al. Systematic review and meta-analysis of studies reporting oncologic outcome after robot-assisted radical prostatectomy. Eur Urol. 2012;62(3):382–404.
4. Trinh QD, Bjartell A, Freedland SJ, Hollenbeck BK, Hu JC, Shariat SF, et al. A systematic review of the volume-outcome relationship for radical prostatectomy. Eur Urol. 2013;64(5):785–98.
5. Sari Motlagh R, Abufaraj M, Yang L, Mori K, Pradere B, Laukhtina E, et al. Penile rehabilitation strategy after nerve sparing radical prostatectomy: a systematic review and network meta-analysis of randomized trials. J Urol. 2021;205(4):1018–30.
6. Rosenbaum E, Partin A, Eisenberger MA. Biochemical relapse after primary treatment for prostate cancer: studies on natural history and therapeutic considerations. J Natl Compr Canc Netw. 2004;2(3):249–56.
7. Simmons MN, Stephenson AJ, Klein EA. Natural history of biochemical recurrence after radical prostatectomy: risk assessment for secondary therapy. Eur Urol. 2007;51(5):1175–84.
8. Van den Broeck T, van den Bergh RCN, Arfi N, Gross T, Moris L, Briers E, et al. Prognostic value of biochemical recurrence following treatment with curative intent for prostate cancer: a systematic review. Eur Urol. 2019;75(6):967–87.
9. Pound CR, Partin AW, Eisenberger MA, Chan DW, Pearson JD, Walsh PC. Natural history of progression after PSA elevation following radical prostatectomy. JAMA. 1999;281(17):1591–7.
10. Miura N, Pradere B, Mori K, Mostafaei H, Quhal F, Misrai V, et al. Metastasis-directed therapy and prostate-targeted therapy in oligometastatic prostate cancer: a systematic review. Minerva Urol Nefrol. 2020;72(5):531–42.
11. Bravi CA, Fossati N, Gandaglia G, Suardi N, Mazzone E, Robesti D, et al. Long-term outcomes of salvage lymph node dissection for nodal recurrence of prostate cancer after radical prostatectomy: not as good as previously thought. Eur Urol. 2020;78(5):661–9.
12. Stephenson AJ, Shariat SF, Zelefsky MJ, Kattan MW, Butler EB, Teh BS, et al. Salvage radiotherapy for recurrent prostate cancer after radical prostatectomy. JAMA. 2004;291(11):1325–32.
13. Fossati N, Robesti D, Karnes RJ, Soligo M, Boorjian SA, Bossi A, et al. Assessing the role and optimal duration of hormonal treatment in association with salvage radiation therapy after radical prostatectomy: results from a multi-institutional study. Eur Urol. 2019;76(4):443–9.
14. Fossati N, Karnes RJ, Colicchia M, Boorjian SA, Bossi A, Seisen T, et al. Impact of early salvage radiation therapy in patients with persistently elevated or rising prostate-specific antigen after radical prostatectomy. Eur Urol. 2018;73(3):436–44.
15. Briganti A, Karnes RJ, Joniau S, Boorjian SA, Cozzarini C, Gandaglia G, et al. Prediction of outcome following early salvage radiotherapy among patients with biochemical recurrence after radical prostatectomy. Eur Urol. 2014;66(3):479–86.
16. Cornford P, van den Bergh RCN, Briers E, Van den Broeck T, Cumberbatch MG, De Santis M, et al. EAU-EANM-ESTRO-ESUR-SIOG guidelines on prostate cancer. Part II—2020 update: treatment of relapsing and metastatic prostate cancer. Eur Urol. 2021;79(2):263–82.
17. Sutinen E, Nurmi M, Roivainen A, Varpula M, Tolvanen T, Lehikoinen P, et al. Kinetics of [(11)C]choline uptake in prostate cancer: a PET study. Eur J Nucl Med Mol Imaging. 2004;31(3):317–24.
18. Stephenson AJ, Kattan MW, Eastham JA, Dotan ZA, Bianco FJ Jr, Lilja H, et al. Defining biochemical recurrence of prostate cancer after radical prostatectomy: a proposal for a standardized definition. J Clin Oncol. 2006;24(24):3973–8.
19. Toussi A, Stewart-Merrill SB, Boorjian SA, Psutka SP, Thompson RH, Frank I, et al. Standardizing the definition of biochemical recurrence after radical prostatectomy-what prostate specific antigen cut point best predicts a durable increase and subsequent systemic progression? J Urol. 2016;195(6):1754–9.

20. Wiegel T, Lohm G, Bottke D, Höcht S, Miller K, Siegmann A, et al. Achieving an undetectable PSA after radiotherapy for biochemical progression after radical prostatectomy is an independent predictor of biochemical outcome—results of a retrospective study. Int J Radiat Oncol Biol Phys. 2009;73(4):1009–16.
21. Beresford MJ, Gillatt D, Benson RJ, Ajithkumar T. A systematic review of the role of imaging before salvage radiotherapy for post-prostatectomy biochemical recurrence. Clin Oncol (R Coll Radiol). 2010;22(1):46–55.
22. Johnstone PA, Tarman GJ, Riffenburgh R, Rohde DC, Puckett ML, Kane CJ. Yield of imaging and scintigraphy assessing biochemical failure in prostate cancer patients. Urol Oncol. 1997;3(4):108–12.
23. Kane CJ, Amling CL, Johnstone PA, Pak N, Lance RS, Thrasher JB, et al. Limited value of bone scintigraphy and computed tomography in assessing biochemical failure after radical prostatectomy. Urology. 2003;61(3):607–11.
24. Gomez P, Manoharan M, Kim SS, Soloway MS. Radionuclide bone scintigraphy in patients with biochemical recurrence after radical prostatectomy: when is it indicated? BJU Int. 2004;94(3):299–302.
25. Grubmüller B, Baltzer P, D'Andrea D, Korn S, Haug AR, Hacker M, et al. (68)Ga-PSMA 11 ligand PET imaging in patients with biochemical recurrence after radical prostatectomy - diagnostic performance and impact on therapeutic decision-making. Eur J Nucl Med Mol Imaging. 2018;45(2):235–42.
26. de Jong IJ, Pruim J, Elsinga PH, Vaalburg W, Mensink HJ. Visualization of prostate cancer with 11C-choline positron emission tomography. Eur Urol. 2002;42(1):18–23.
27. Fuccio C, Castellucci P, Schiavina R, Guidalotti PL, Gavaruzzi G, Montini GC, et al. Role of 11C-choline PET/CT in the re-staging of prostate cancer patients with biochemical relapse and negative results at bone scintigraphy. Eur J Radiol. 2012;81(8):e893–e6.
28. Shen G, Deng H, Hu S, Jia Z. Comparison of choline-PET/CT, MRI, SPECT, and bone scintigraphy in the diagnosis of bone metastases in patients with prostate cancer: a meta-analysis. Skeletal Radiol. 2014;43(11):1503–13.
29. Brogsitter C, Zöphel K, Kotzerke J. 18F-choline, 11C-choline and 11C-acetate PET/CT: comparative analysis for imaging prostate cancer patients. Eur J Nucl Med Mol Imaging. 2013;40(Suppl 1):S18–27.
30. Treglia G, Ceriani L, Sadeghi R, Giovacchini G, Giovanella L. Relationship between prostate-specific antigen kinetics and detection rate of radiolabelled choline PET/CT in restaging prostate cancer patients: a meta-analysis. Clin Chem Lab Med. 2014;52(5):725–33.
31. Soyka JD, Muster MA, Schmid DT, Seifert B, Schick U, Miralbell R, et al. Clinical impact of 18F-choline PET/CT in patients with recurrent prostate cancer. Eur J Nucl Med Mol Imaging. 2012;39(6):936–43.
32. Ceci F, Herrmann K, Castellucci P, Graziani T, Bluemel C, Schiavina R, et al. Impact of 11C-choline PET/CT on clinical decision making in recurrent prostate cancer: results from a retrospective two-centre trial. Eur J Nucl Med Mol Imaging. 2014;41(12):2222–31.
33. Mitchell CR, Lowe VJ, Rangel LJ, Hung JC, Kwon ED, Karnes RJ. Operational characteristics of (11)c-choline positron emission tomography/computerized tomography for prostate cancer with biochemical recurrence after initial treatment. J Urol. 2013;189(4):1308–13.
34. Tilki D, Reich O, Graser A, Hacker M, Silchinger J, Becker AJ, et al. 18F-fluoroethylcholine PET/CT identifies lymph node metastasis in patients with prostate-specific antigen failure after radical prostatectomy but underestimates its extent. Eur Urol. 2013;63(5):792–6.
35. Graute V, Jansen N, Übleis C, Seitz M, Hartenbach M, Scherr MK, et al. Relationship between PSA kinetics and [18F] fluorocholine PET/CT detection rates of recurrence in patients with prostate cancer after total prostatectomy. Eur J Nucl Med Mol Imaging. 2012;39(2):271–82.
36. Chu CE, Alshalalfa M, Sjöström M, Zhao SG, Liu Y, Chou J, et al. Prostate-specific membrane antigen and fluciclovine transporter genes are associated with variable clinical features and molecular subtypes of primary prostate cancer. Eur Urol. 2021;79(6):717–21.
37. Nanni C, Zanoni L, Pultrone C, Schiavina R, Brunocilla E, Lodi F, et al. (18)F-FACBC (anti1-amino-3-(18)F-fluorocyclobutane-1-carboxylic acid) versus (11)C-choline PET/CT in prostate cancer relapse: results of a prospective trial. Eur J Nucl Med Mol Imaging. 2016;43(9):1601–10.
38. Beer AJ, Eiber M, Souvatzoglou M, Schwaiger M, Krause BJ. Radionuclide and hybrid imaging of recurrent prostate cancer. Lancet Oncol. 2011;12(2):181–91.
39. Beheshti M, Vali R, Waldenberger P, Fitz F, Nader M, Loidl W, et al. Detection of bone metastases in patients with prostate cancer by 18F fluorocholine and 18F fluoride PET-CT: a comparative study. Eur J Nucl Med Mol Imaging. 2008;35(10):1766–74.
40. Afshar-Oromieh A, Haberkorn U, Schlemmer HP, Fenchel M, Eder M, Eisenhut M, et al. Comparison of PET/CT and PET/MRI hybrid systems using a 68Ga-labelled PSMA ligand for the diagnosis of recurrent prostate cancer: initial experience. Eur J Nucl Med Mol Imaging. 2014;41(5):887–97.
41. Giesel FL, Will L, Lawal I, Lengana T, Kratochwil C, Vorster M, et al. Intraindividual comparison of (18)F-PSMA-1007 and (18) F-DCFPyL PET/CT in the prospective evaluation of patients with newly diagnosed prostate carcinoma: a pilot study. J Nucl Med. 2018;59(7):1076–80.
42. Afshar-Oromieh A, Zechmann CM, Malcher A, Eder M, Eisenhut M, Linhart HG, et al. Comparison of PET imaging with a (68) Ga-labelled PSMA ligand and (18)F-choline-based PET/CT for the diagnosis of recurrent prostate cancer. Eur J Nucl Med Mol Imaging. 2014;41(1):11–20.
43. Morigi JJ, Stricker PD, van Leeuwen PJ, Tang R, Ho B, Nguyen Q, et al. Prospective comparison of 18F-fluoromethylcholine versus 68Ga-PSMA PET/CT in prostate cancer patients who have rising PSA after curative treatment and are being considered for targeted therapy. J Nucl Med. 2015;56(8):1185–90.
44. Fendler WP, Calais J, Eiber M, Flavell RR, Mishoe A, Feng FY, et al. Assessment of 68Ga-PSMA-11 PET accuracy in localizing recurrent prostate cancer: a prospective single-arm clinical trial. JAMA Oncol. 2019;5(6):856–63.
45. Poulsen MH, Bouchelouche K, Gerke O, Petersen H, Svolgaard B, Marcussen N, et al. [18F]-fluorocholine positron-emission/computed tomography for lymph node staging of patients with prostate cancer: preliminary results of a prospective study. BJU Int. 2010;106(5):639–43. discussion 44.
46. Abufaraj M, Grubmüller B, Zeitlinger M, Kramer G, Seitz C, Haitel A, et al. Prospective evaluation of the performance of [(68)Ga]Ga-PSMA-11 PET/CT(MRI) for lymph node staging in patients undergoing superextended salvage lymph node dissection after radical prostatectomy. Eur J Nucl Med Mol Imaging. 2019;46(10):2169–77.

6 Augmented Reality in RALP

Francesco Porpiglia, Stefano Granato, Michele Sica, Paolo Verri, Daniele Amparore, Enrico Checcucci, and Cristian Fiori

Introduction

By Augmented Reality (AR) we mean a system able of acquiring a real scene enriching it with additional virtual information, both graphic and textual. In augmented reality, the user is therefore provided with information generated by software capable of improving the perception of reality, unlike what happens in virtual realities where all environmental information is not real. It must be processed in an optimal manner so that the user has the perception of a single scene in which real and virtual tools coexist.

AR can be used in several fields of application: from music to sport, from architecture to entertainment up to medicine. AR adds a new dimension to entertainment allowing the people from the audience to become active participants of the show instead of passive viewers, bringing interactivity and engagement in the show merging the real world with the virtual one. It is estimated that by 2026, AR apps and hardware will be an $80–162 billion market.

Focusing on application of AR in medicine, many fields can be interested: from anatomical and physiological education to histopathology. For this last field, through some dedicated software it is in fact possible to recognize some malignant characteristics of the tissues that are analyzed; Augmented Reality Microscope can be integrated with a traditional pathology workflow, which involves focusing on different parts of the slides under the microscope, moving the field of view around, zooming in and out, and iteratively making and improving diagnostic decisions.

Even if many examples can be made about the application of AR in medicine scenarios, surgery remains its greatest field of application.

As already said AR overlays digitally created content into the user's real-world environment with the aim of enhancing real-word features. A visor and a smartphone or tablet provide spatial registration that can allow geometric persistence concerning placement and orientation within the real world. In this context, a real scene can be defined as the result of an optical projection of the real world onto an imaging sensor, as happens during surgical procedures with endoscopic view.

The main principle of a basic AR system is to superimpose a computer-generated image on a real-world imagery captured by a camera and displaying the combination of these on a computer, tablet PC, or a video projector. Another possibility is to use a special head-mounted display (HMD, sometimes referred to as "smart glasses"), which use special projectors, head tracking, and depth cameras to display digital images on the glass, effectively creating the illusion of augmented reality. Holograms can be visible to different users at the same time and from different angles with proper spatial registration. In 2015 Microsoft presented the HoloLens which allows one to see and interact with holographic 3D virtual objects via voice, gaze, and gestures, in a real environment.

At present, the applications of AR are limited by the essential requisite of preoperative 3D reconstructions of medical images.

3D Reconstruction in Precision Surgery

The concept of "precision surgery" is nowadays intrinsic in the management of the genitourinary cancers. A detailed case-specific understanding of the surgical anatomy represents the key point for a tailored treatment planning. In this setting, the 3D reconstruction of the standard two-dimension cross-sectional imaging has known increasing diffusion as it allows a better representation and understanding of the surgical anatomy. Such technology is perceived as a useful tool in the surgical planning, the surgeon's training and the patient's counselling, because avoids the "building in mind" process

F. Porpiglia (✉) · S. Granato · M. Sica · P. Verri · D. Amparore
E. Checcucci · C. Fiori
Division of Urology, Department of Oncology, School of Medicine, San Luigi Gonzaga Hospital, University of Turin, Turin, Italy
e-mail: francesco.porpiglia@unito.it; daniele.amparore@unito.it; cristian.fiori@unito.it

S. Ren et al. (eds.), *Robot-Assisted Radical Prostatectomy*, https://doi.org/10.1007/978-3-031-05855-4_6

of the two-dimension cross-sectional imaging. It allows a better comprehension of anatomy, vascularization and position of the organs, key steps in the surgical management of many urological malignancies, such as prostate cancer [1].

The creation of virtual prostate models is mainly based on the use of 2D multi-parametric magnetic resonance images (mp-MRI—1 mm thickness) which are evaluated by a bioengineer using a DICOM viewer. In the past, the automatic rendering of 2D images allowed to obtain low quality 3D reconstructions not so useful for an accurate preoperative planning or intraoperative navigation. Nowadays, thanks to technological innovations, the development of dedicated software and the collaboration between bioengineers, radiologists, and urologists, it has been possible to obtain high-definition 3D models [2].

The first segmentation process is performed semi-automatically by dedicated software. At the end of the process the three-dimensional reconstruction obtained is usually refined by a biomedical engineer under the supervision of the urologist. The aim is to obtain an hyperaccurate 3D model (HA3D™—Fig. 6.1), a detailed reproduction of the prostate and the surrounding structures: the virtual model is always focused on the tumor location relatively to the prostate capsule, in order to enhance the location of tumor extracapsular extension, and on the shape and location of neurovascular bundles, in order to have a clear idea of the tissues to spare during the surgery. Final steps of the process are the creation of a transcription code for the visualization of the HA3D reconstruction in an interactive 3D-PDF format to improve the understanding of the relationships between the tumor and the surrounding structures and the conversion of each part in stereo-lithography (STL) format [3, 4].

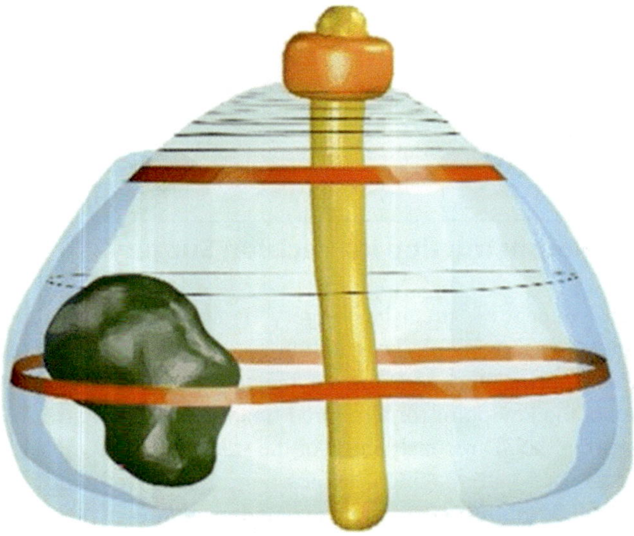

Fig. 6.1 Prostate Hyper-accuracy 3D (HA3D™) reconstruction used intraoperatively for cognitive procedures

Virtual 3D models allow the surgeon to simplify the planning and management of the treatment, reducing the risk of intra- and post-operative complications. Furthermore, they allow to influence the preoperative decision-making process during cognitive surgical procedures, thanks to the virtual reconstruction on a 2D screen, available for consultation both before and during surgery [5, 6].

Augmented Reality RALP

Virtual 3D models can be used in augmented reality surgical procedures thanks to a specific system able to overlay virtual data over the real anatomical view of the organ of interest as taken by the endoscopic camera during surgery. The software can display the 3D model of the patient's organ and control its translation, rotation and scale transformation values. All transformations were applied starting from a specific landmark to accurately reproduce movements and rotations of the real organ during the robotic procedure: for the prostate the apex of the organ. The tracking of prostate can be done by a professional operating the software application and using dedicated input devices to overlay the 3D model to the patient's organ in real time. A six-degrees-of-freedom device is considered the most appropriate for this tracking task, with the possibility to pan, zoom and rotate the 3D model with one hand only. To maximize the surgeon's awareness about the intraoperative environment, the software application allows isolation of specific parts of the 3D model, modifying their transparency value to give a flexible control of the displayed surfaces [7].

In 2018, Porpiglia et al. published their initial experiment with AR during robot-assisted RP, using a software-based integration of rendered prostate virtual models inside the da Vinci surgeon console. Sixteen patients with cT2 prostate cancer underwent an intrafascial nerve-sparing technique, whereas 14 with cT3 tumours underwent standard nervesparing technique together with selective biopsies at the suspected extra-capsular extension. The positive surgical margin rate was 30%, but no positive surgical margins were found in pT2 tumours. Selective biopsies guided by AR confirmed suspected extra-prostatic disease in 11 of 14 biopsies (78%). Finally, the authors scanned the prostate specimens, recording a mismatch between the 3D reconstruction and the scanned prostate from 1 to 5 mm. The same group recently published an update of these experiments. Eleven patients had cT2 vs. 19 cT3 at preoperative MRI. In all the cases, the final pathology examination confirmed the location of the index lesion as indicated by 3D reconstruction. Noteworthy is that 15 out of 19 patients with suspected extra-capsular extension at preoperative MRI had confirmed pT3a stage (79%). In such cases, 11 out of 15 patients (73.3%) were found to have cancer cells at the neurovascular bundle adjacent to the extra-capsular extension. They concluded that this technology, when tested by expert prostate cancer surgeons, has a high rate of success, especially in key steps of the intervention [7, 8].

Elastic Augmented Reality RALP

In order to obtain a correct overlay of the images, we must consider that tissues and organs, during surgical maneuvers, are subjected to forces that could modify their appearance and shape. Due to their own elasticity, they are continuously subjected to traction and rotation forces that make a rigid 3D model inadequate for optimal anatomical overlap.

To overcome this problem, recent technological innovations have led to the development of the concept of elastic augmented reality: using parametric transformation formulas, it is possible to twist, bend, stretch, and tape the model to create more functional and dynamic overlapping, which may be used during the intervention, especially in the nerve-sparing phase, in which the prostate shape is deformed by the traction exerted by the robotic arms (Fig. 6.2) [9].

In this scenario, Porpiglia ed. al., in 2019, introduced the 3D elastic AR RARP thanks to the application of nonlinear parametric deformations, namely "bend" and "stretch", to approximate the deformation of the target organ. The two deformers chosen turned out to be accurate in estimating prostate deformations during surgery. In fact, despite the traction exercised on the prostate by the robotic arms, thanks to the elastic 3D overlapping model, the lesion and CI location were correctly identified during the dynamic nerve-sparing phase (100% of correct lesion identification). Forty patients prospectively enrolled underwent robotic prostatectomy: 20 of them underwent 3D elastic augmented reality guidance, while the other 20 underwent 2D MRI guidance, placing a metallic clip at the level of suspicious extracapsular tumor extension. The pathological analysis evaluated the

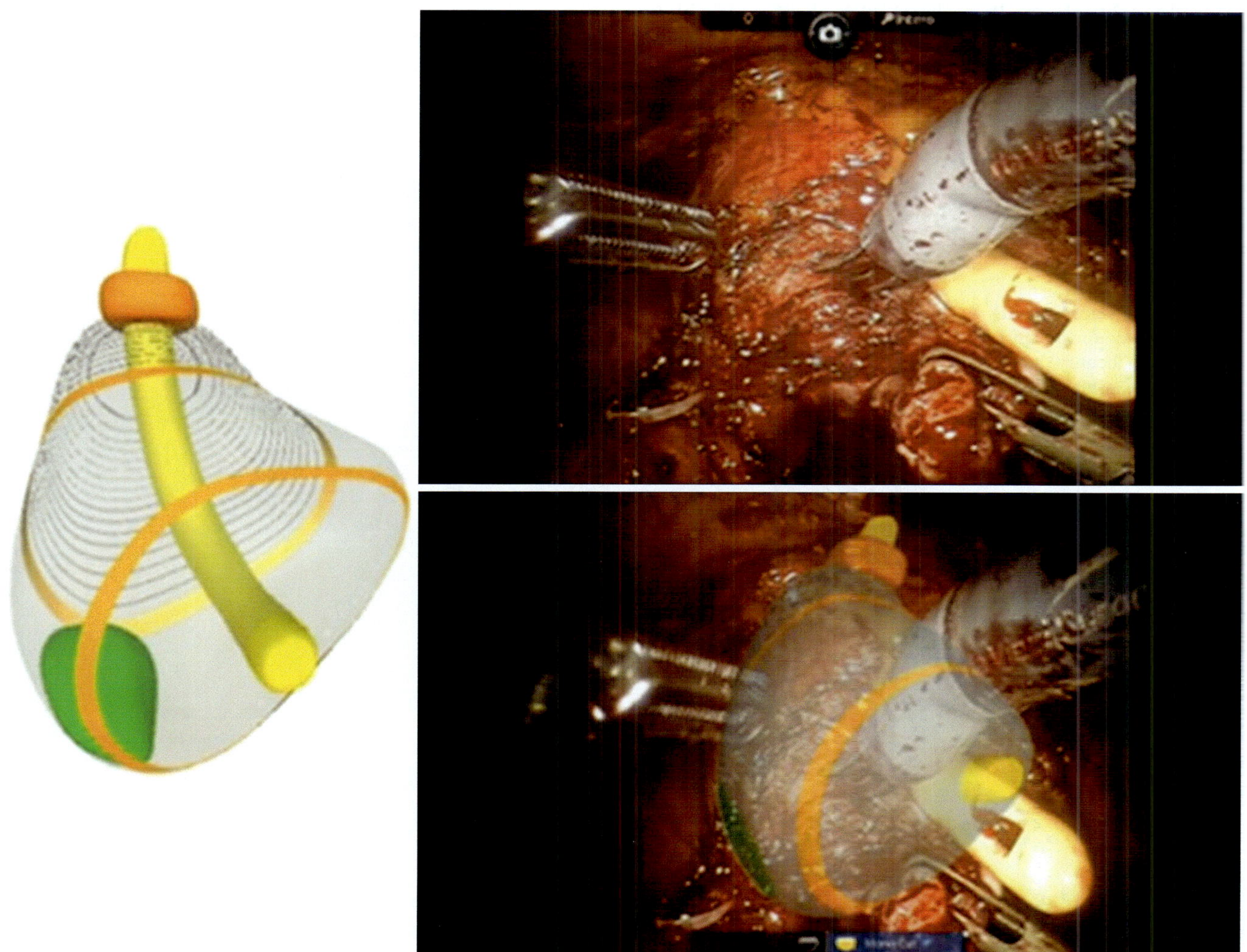

Fig. 6.2 3D Elastic Augmented Reality RALP: the 3D model allows to visualize the tumour location in a dynamic phase of the intervention

presence of tumor at the level of the clip, confirming a statistically significant difference ($p = 0.002$) in favor of elastic augmented reality technology [9, 10].

Automatic Augmented Reality RALP

Even if great steps forward have been made in the last few years, with the introduction of real-time AR procedures and then with the introduction of elastic models able to dynamically chase the real organs, we are still just at the beginning of the development of this technology.

In the near future, the possibility to automatically track organ movements during the procedure will permit automatic overlap of the virtual model to real anatomy. To achieve this goal, different approaches have been proposed, following two main strategies. The first is the application of endoscopic markers that can be detected by the AR software and then, thanks to this information, the models can be overlapped. The second approach, technically more challenging and time consuming, is a markerless strategy based on machine learning algorithms [11].

The first strategy consists of identifying some intraoperative landmarks that can be used to link a virtual landmark (created together with the 3D prostate virtual model). Once the landmarks are identified, a software to automatically link the two landmarks (the real one and the virtual one) has to be developed. For this purpose, the landmark can be an anatomical structure or an extracorporeal landmark introduced into the abdominal cavity in order to be clearly identified by the software. With this purpose, the work recently published by Porpiglia et al. was focused on the final part of the robot-assisted radical prostatectomy, when the prostate has been removed from its place, and a catheter is introduced in the operative environment. Such an evident artificial reference object allows for a specific tracking method less costly from a computational point of view, with respect to the feature detection strategy of identification of the anatomical structure of the prostate, as proven by preliminary tests [12].

Once the automatic augmented reality overlay is performed, is possible to see the position of the tumor lesion projected at the level of the prostatic lodge, and then send back to Da Vinci remote console monitor in real time (Fig. 6.3). After that, is possible to zoom-in or -out the endoscopic camera view and the model automatically modulates its scale and remains anchored properly. Then the transparency of the model can be changed, and the

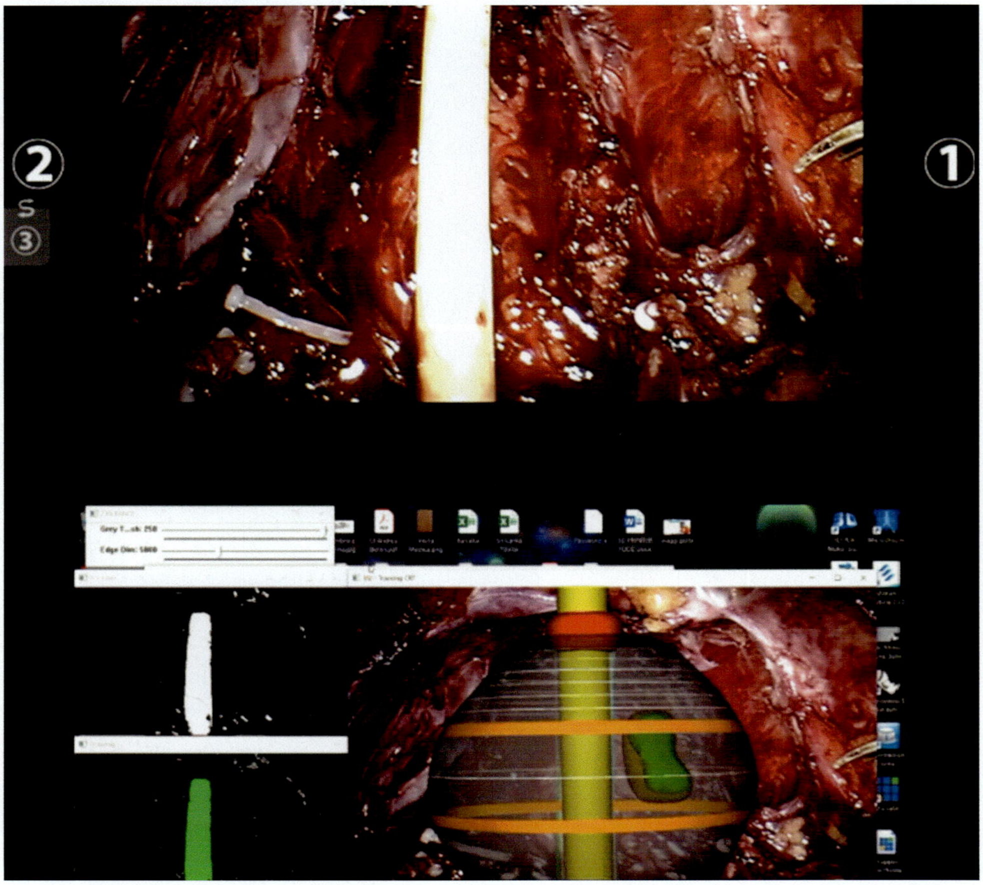

Fig. 6.3 3D Automatic Augmented Reality RALP: in final steps of prostatectomy, when the prostate has been removed from its place, a catheter is introduced and 3D virtual model automatically overlapped to identify the tumour extracapsular extension (ECE) at the level of preserved neurovascular bundles (NVBs)

prostate and intraparenchymal portion of the tumor hidden, leaving projected on the in-vivo anatomy only the catheter and the extracapsular portion of the tumors. At this point a selective biopsy is performable at the level of the preserved neurovascular bundle where the automatic augmented reality images indicated the suspicious contact [12, 13].

In two recent studies Porpiglia evaluate the accuracy of the new automatic augmented reality system in order to identify the tumour extracapsular extension (ECE) at the level of preserved neurovascular bundles (NVBs) during robot assisted radical prostatectomy (RARP). Ten patients candidated to RARP were enrolled with suspicious ECE at preoperative high-resolution multi-parametric magnetic resonance imaging (mpMRI, 1-mm slices) according to dedicated protocol. The obtained 3D reconstruction was overlapped to endoscopic in-vivo anatomy and sent back to DaVinci robotic console. A metallic clip was placed at the level of suspected ECE as indicated by the virtual images. In eight cases the final pathology (pT3) confirmed the presence of ECE. At macroscopic assessment the presence of ECE at the level of metallic clip was recorded in 100% of the cases; then the microscopic evaluation confirmed the cancer presence in all the cases and revealed a mean length of ECE of 4 mm, demonstrating that the 3D virtual images, automatically anchored to the catheter, are able to correctly identify the location of ECE at the level of NVBs [13].

Conclusions

3D virtual technology has entered daily practice in some specialist clinics, especially for the management of urological malignancies, including prostate cancer. It is perceived as a useful tool for surgical planning, physician education/training, and patient counselling. Moreover, the integration of robotic platforms with 3D models and the possibility of performing augmented reality surgeries increase the surgeon's confidence in treating the disease, with a potential benefit in terms of precision and tailoring of the procedures. Further researches are needed to reach the next stage of evolution of such technology, and to maximize its potential applications.

References

1. Autorino R, Porpiglia F, Dasgupta P, et al. Precision surgery and genitourinary cancers. Eur J Surg Oncol. 2017;43(5):893–908. https://doi.org/10.1016/j.ejso.2017.02.005.
2. Veneziano D, Amparore D, Cacciamani G, et al. Climbing over the barriers of current imaging technology in urology. Eur Urol 2020;77(2):142–3. https://doi.org/10.1016/j.eururo.2019.09.016.
3. Checcucci E, Amparore D, De Luca S, Autorino R, Fiori C, Porpiglia F. Precision prostate cancer surgery: an overview of new technologies and techniques. Minerva Urol Nefrol. 2019;71(5):487–501. https://doi.org/10.23736/S0393-2249.19.03365-4.
4. Porpiglia F, Amparore D, Checcucci E, et al. Current use of three-dimensional model technology in urology: a road map for personalised surgical planning. Eur Urol Focus. 2018;4(5):652–6. https://doi.org/10.1016/j.euf.2018.09.012.
5. Checcucci E, Amparore D, Pecoraro A, et al. 3D mixed reality holograms for preoperative surgical planning of nephron-sparing surgery: evaluation of surgeons' perception. Minerva Urol Nephrol. 2019;73:367–75. https://doi.org/10.23736/S0393-2249.19.03610-5.
6. Parikh N, Sharma P. Three-dimensional printing in urology: history, current applications, and future directions. Urology. 2018;121:3–10. https://doi.org/10.1016/j.urology.2018.08.004.
7. Porpiglia F, Fiori C, Checcucci E, Amparore D, Bertolo R. Augmented reality robot-assisted radical prostatectomy: preliminary experience. Urology. 2018;115:184. https://doi.org/10.1016/j.urology.2018.01.028.
8. Checcucci E, Amparore D, Fiori C, et al. 3D imaging applications for robotic urologic surgery: an ESUT YAUWP review. World J Urol. 2020;38(4):869–81. https://doi.org/10.1007/s00345-019-02922-4.
9. Porpiglia F, Checcucci E, Amparore D, et al. Three-dimensional elastic augmented-reality robot-assisted radical prostatectomy using hyperaccuracy three-dimensional reconstruction technology: a step further in the identification of capsular involvement. Eur Urol. 2019;76(4):505–14. https://doi.org/10.1016/j.eururo.2019.03.037.
10. Porpiglia F, Bertolo R, Checcucci E, et al. Development and validation of 3D printed virtual models for robot-assisted radical prostatectomy and partial nephrectomy: urologists' and patients' perception. World J Urol. 2018;36(2):201–7. https://doi.org/10.1007/s00345-017-2126-1.
11. Porpiglia F, Checcucci E, Amparore D, et al. Augmented-reality robot-assisted radical prostatectomy using hyper-accuracy three-dimensional reconstruction (HA3DTM) technology: a radiological and pathological study. BJU Int. 2019;123(5):834–45. https://doi.org/10.1111/bju.14549.
12. Porpiglia F, Bertolo R, Amparore D, et al. Augmented reality during robot-assisted radical prostatectomy: expert robotic surgeons' on-the-spot insights after live surgery. Minerva Urol Nephrol. 2018;70(2):226–9. https://doi.org/10.23736/S0393-2249.18.03143-0.
13. Andras I, Mazzone E, van Leeuwen FWB, et al. Artificial intelligence and robotics: a combination that is changing the operating room. World J Urol. 2020;38(10):2359–66. https://doi.org/10.1007/s00345-019-03037-6.

Part III

Transperitoneal RALP Anterior Approach

The Bladder Neck Management

7

Walter Artibani, Giovanni Enrico Cacciamani, Alessandro Crestani, and Angelo Porreca

Introduction

Bladder neck management represents one of the crucial steps during the robotic-assisted radical prostatectomy (RARP). The correct Identification of its anatomical landmarks guides the surgeon during the surgical procedure to achieve a proper dissection and, therefore, contribute to perform a watertight anastomosis with the urethral stump [1].

A correct bladder neck management might have a role in the continence recovery after RARP. Anterior, lateral, and bladder neck preserving techniques have been extensively described in terms of surgical and functional pros and cons. However, the debate about which approach should be used is still open. The presence of prostate median lobe or previous transurethral resection or laser enucleation (TURP, HoLEP, ThuLEP) could make challenging the bladder neck management. A detailed description of the desirable approaches to use could guide neophyte surgeons approaching this surgical procedure.

This book chapter will discuss the most commonly used approaches for bladder neck dissection step by step.

Anatomical Considerations and Landmarks

Anatomical landmarks of the bladder neck have been described for guiding the surgeons in performing the so-called anatomical radical prostatectomy [2, 3]. The tissue that covers the prostate in part constitutes an extension of the anterior wall of the bladder beyond the bladder neck (the detrusor apron) [4, 5]. This structure covers the prostate's anterior surface, bladder neck, and the limits between the base of the prostate and bladder neck. Laterally to the anterior apron and bladder neck, a triangular "fatty" space is bounded by detrusor of bladder neck medially, prostate base caudally, and prostate pedicle/neurovascular bundle laterally. The dissection of this space exposes the anterior surface of seminal vesicles that represents the deep boundary of dissection and are covered by a fibromuscular fascia.

This anatomical structure is frequently defined as the anterior aspect of Denonvilliers' fascia. Indeed, some authors described this fascia as a muscular structure with the longitudinal disposition of the fibers tented between the outer layer of the bladder muscle and the prostate base. However, this structure is not the anterior layer of Denonvilliers' fascia. Instead, it corresponds to the posterior longitudinal fascia of the detrusor muscle externally stuffed by the bladder adventitia [6]. This concept was further developed by Tewari et al. that focused their attention on a "retrotrigonal layer" consisting of some vertically oriented fibers located posterior to the bladder neck, extending from the trigone (superiorly) to the base of the prostate (inferiorly). Finally, Walz et al. [2] proposed a different and intuitive terminology to describe this structure: the vesicoprostatic muscle, and this, in our opinion, should be the preferred term.

Laterally, the retrotrigonal layer is extended to the proximal neurovascular pedicles and the effacing detrusor fibers on the prostatic capsule. The thickness of this layer is variable, with the superior aspect adjacent to the bladder being the thickest and the inferior element at the prostatic base being the thinnest. Histologically it is principally composed of smooth muscular fibers interposed by small areas of connective tissue with rare fascicles of nerves [7].

W. Artibani · A. Crestani
Department of Robotic Urological Surgery, Abano Terme Hospital, Abano Terme, Italy
e-mail: walter.artibani@univr.it

G. E. Cacciamani (✉)
Department of Urology, Urology Institute, University of Southern California, Los Angeles, CA, USA
e-mail: giovanni.cacciamani@med.usc.edu

A. Porreca
Department of Urology, Istituto Oncologico Veneto, Treviso, Italy

S. Ren et al. (eds.), *Robot-Assisted Radical Prostatectomy*, https://doi.org/10.1007/978-3-031-05855-4_7

Anterior Approach to the Bladder Neck

Prostate Defatting

The periprostatic fat is easily detachable from the anterior and lateral surface of the prostate, continuing cranially. It is adherent to the bladder wall when it becomes pericystium and is anchored by perivesical veins, which must be coagulated and divided. The boundary between detachable fat and adherent fat already gives an indirect idea of the boundary between the anterior bladder wall and prostate.

Tips for Bladder Neck Identification

First, grasping the bladder wall puts in tension and subtends the detrusor apron, which continues in front of the prostate towards the membranous urethra.

Second, moving the inflated Foley balloon alternately towards the prostate and towards/inside the bladder gives an idea of the bladder base and the insertion of the bladder wall on the anterolateral surface of the prostate; of note, in case of prostatic hypertrophy that lifts the bladder floor or middle lobe, the balloon is deflected asymmetrically and can be misleading.

Third, pinching allows an "optical palpation" of the bladder and prostate (Fig. 7.1a).

Anterior Incision of the Bladder Neck

Perform a median incision of the detrusor apron, horizontal or inverted "V" (Fig. 7.1b, c), making visible the longitudinal muscle fibers of the detrusor. The choice of the precise site of section (higher or lower) is dependent according to the oncological status of the prostatic base: very close to the prostate in case of oncological negativity, further towards the bladder in case of possible doubt of involvement of the bladder neck. As the section is deepened with the tip of the monopolar scissor, the cranial grip with the fourth arm is improved to increase the tension; a further tensioning effect is obtained with the Maryland or the Prograsp® in a flat position.

There are veins with a longitudinal course in the central area of the section (from the dorsal vascular complex to the bladder wall) that can be easily coagulated. The more the section goes sideways, the larger veins can be encountered, and therefore it could require control of bleeding. These lateral veins are avoidable with the inverted "V" incision. The remaining part of the plane is avascular until it reaches the vesicourethral mucosa. Minor bleeding then occurs, which indicates that the mucosa has been approximated (Fig. 7.1d). The mucosa is now is dissected, and the bladder catheter is visible. The incision of the anterior half-circumference of the bladder neck is now completed.

Examination of the Bladder Neck

The catheter balloon is deflated, and the catheter is withdrawn and attracted to the operative field, clamped with the fourth arm, and pushed upwards in the direction of the abdominal wall. Outside, a counter-traction is applied to the external portion of the catheter (Fig. 7.1e). This double traction, internal and external, raises the prostate and highlights the open bladder neck and its posterior lip (Fig. 7.2a, b). In addition, the table aid clamps the anterior bladder wall and subtends it cranially. These combined traction maneuvers on the prostate and bladder help to expose the bladder neck.

The bladder neck and trigone are now visually explored as follow:

- Opening the Maryland or Prograsp® inserted into the bladder facilitates the exploration.
- The ureteral orifices and the interureteric line are identified.
- The thickness of the bladder wall is assessed.
- The conformation of the trigone is evaluated: regular flat; raised from the middle lobe; with an anterior notch towards the prostate (this last information is important because a common mistake of the beginner is to violate the trigone in section maneuvers between trigone and prostate).
- The border-line between the prostate and bladder is outlined in cases where a TURP or a HoLEP/ThuLEP has been previously performed.

Posterior Incision of the Bladder Neck

The posterior portion of the bladder neck is now incised (Fig. 7.2c, d), and the vesicoprostatic plane is developed by dissecting the vesicoprostatic muscle getting access to the vas deferens and the seminal vesicles:

- The incision of the posterior lip can start from the center towards the outside or from the outside towards the mid-line.
- The bladder wall must be sectioned full thickness.
- The incision is deepened on the sides of the neck until the yellowish fatty tissue of the vesicular fossa is visible.

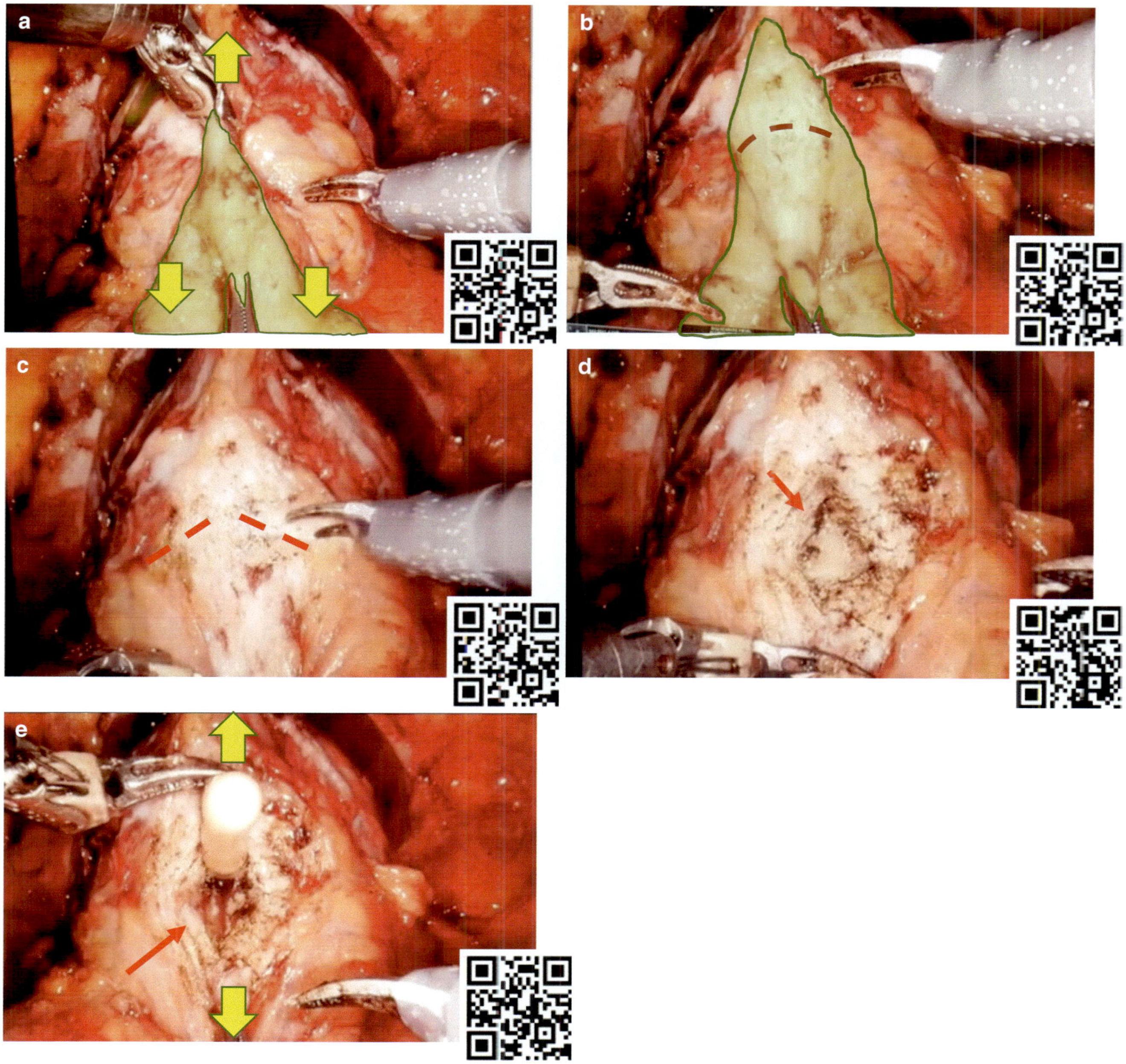

Fig. 7.1 Anterior approach for management of the bladder neck. A linked video-clip is available scanning the QRcode on the right. For Apple users: Open the Camera app from your device's. Hold your device so that the QR code appears in the Camera app's viewfinder. Your device recognizes the QR code and shows a notification. Tap the notification to open the link associated with the QR code. For Android users: download a QRcode scanner app and follow the above instructions

- Release the catheter that was kept in tension, withdrawing it into the urethra and clamp the posterior base of the prostate, attracting it cranially, thus putting tension on the vesicourethral muscle fibers.
- During the vesicourethral muscle section, the incision direction is oblique towards the prostate, not towards the bladder (this avoids violation of the trigone) (Fig. 7.2d).
- Once the vesicoprostatic muscle is dissected, the access to the vas deferens and the seminal vesicles is gained.

Of note, the bladder wall extends over the prostate both anteriorly and posteriorly. The anterior parietal extension corresponds to the detrusor apron, and it is necessary to incise it to reach the anterior portion of the bladder neck. The posterior parietal extension corresponds to the vesicoprostatic muscle, referred to in the past as the anterior leaflet of Denonvillier's fascia [2, 3] and must be dissected to have access to the vas deferens and seminal vesicles.

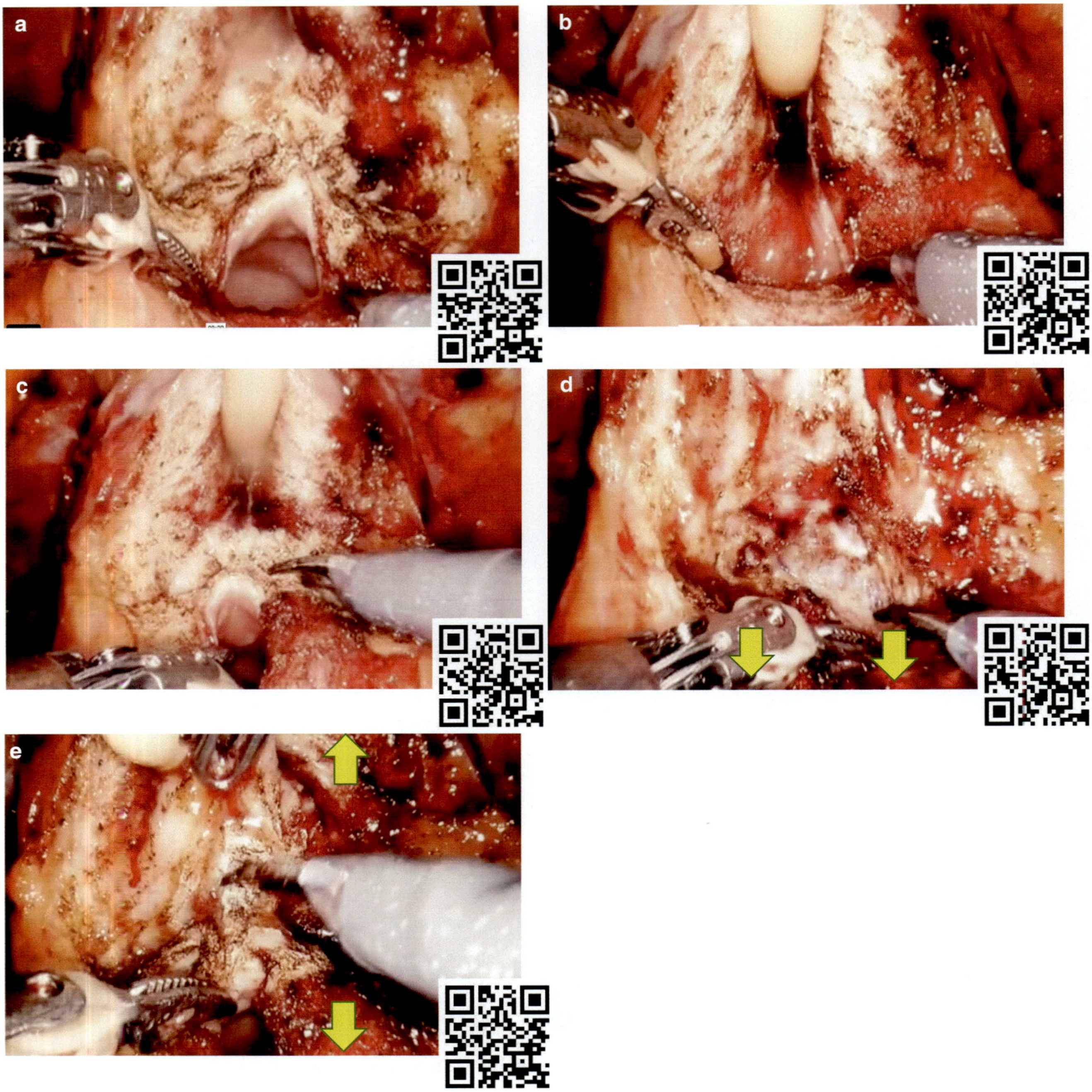

Fig. 7.2 Anterior approach for management of the bladder neck. A linked video-clip is available scanning the QRcode on the right. For Apple users: Open the Camera app from your device's. Hold your device so that the QR code appears in the Camera app's viewfinder. Your device recognizes the QR code and shows a notification. Tap the notification to open the link associated with the QR code. For Android users: download a QRcode scanner app and follow the above instructions

In the case of a Retzius sparing surgical approach according to the Bocciardi technique [8–11] the technique is performed backward: first of all, it is necessary to dissect the vesicoprostatic muscle to have access to the posterior portion of the neck, while the detrusor apron will then be fully preserved anteriorly.

Preservation of Bladder Neck

In selected and oncologically adequate cases, it is possible to preserve the bladder neck and theoretically the so-called "genital sphincter." The technique is similar to that described so far, except that the search for contact with the prostate is maximum. By delicately following the profile of the prostatic base, the bladder neck and part of the proximal prostatic urethra are circumnavigated and circumferentially delimited before dissecting it. It is still controversial whether neck preservation leads to improvement in terms of early recovery to continence. It certainly gives an advantage in having two congruent orifices for a head-to-head anastomosis with the urethral stump.

Lateral Approach to the Bladder Neck

The catheter balloon previously filled to 10 mL is deflated or wholly inserted into the bladder to better identify the limits between the bladder neck and the prostate base. The anterior apron is transversely incised with monopolar scissor until the longitudinal fibers of the bladder neck and urethra are visualized with attention to don't injure the base of the prostate.

Exposition of the "Lateral Triangle"

Identified this boundary, a gentle laterally traction of the bladder neck from left to right with the fourth arm (if placed on the right side) is performed to expose the left triangle between the base of the prostate, bladder neck, and prostate pedicles/neurovascular bundles (Fig. 7.3). This traction is maintained during dissection.

Dissection to the Seminal Vesicle

Next, blunt, athermal dissection of fatty tissue is performed using Maryland bipolar forceps and monopolar scissor until the anterior surface of the left seminal vesicle. During this step, the assistant, with a suction device, maintains the dissection plane at the apex of the triangle created (Fig. 7.4).

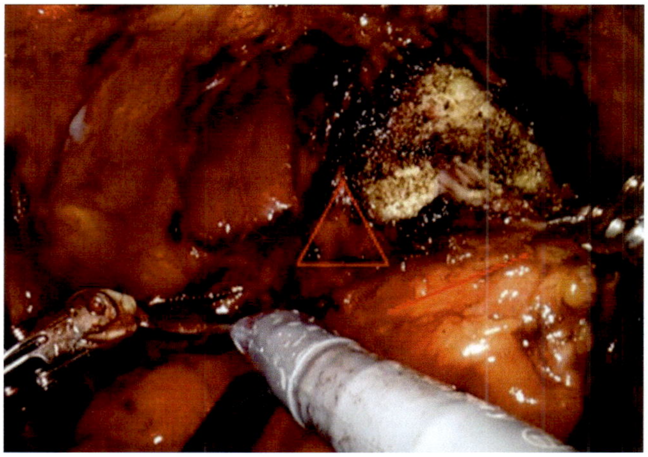

Fig. 7.3 Lateral traction of bladder neck with the fourth arm, exposure of "fatty triangle"

Opening of the Bladder Neck

Once it reaches the plane of the seminal vesicles, the anterior wall of the bladder neck could be opened, and the foley catheter anteriorly tractioned better to expose the posterior wall of the bladder neck and to incise it (Fig. 7.5).

Separation of the Bladder Neck from the Prostate

Subsequent, with attention to maintaining the retrotrigonal layer on the bladder neck side, lateral traction with the right arm allows separating the bladder neck from the prostate base (Fig. 7.6). During this step, the use of a 30° camera will enable us to visualize better the plane of dissection between the ret-

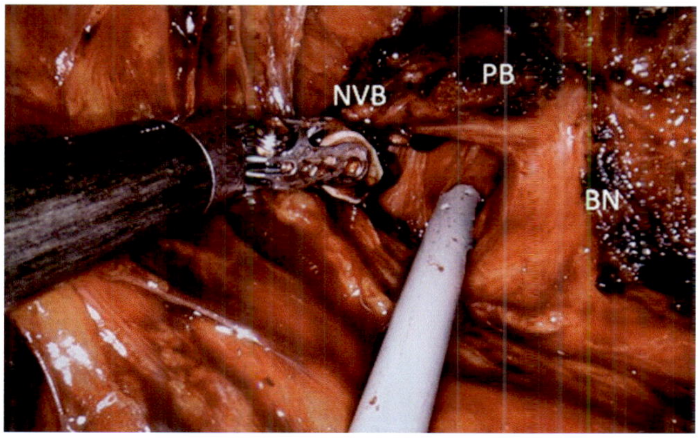

Fig. 7.4 Left triangle between bladder neck (BN), prostate pedicle/neurovascular bundle (NVB), and the base of the prostate (PB)

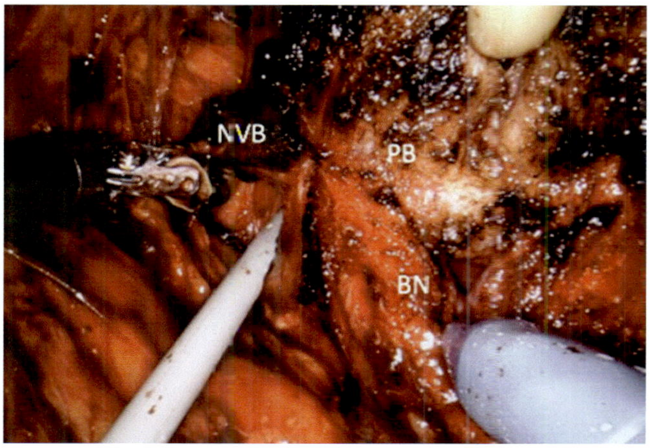

Fig. 7.5 Section of the anterior wall of the bladder neck (BN)

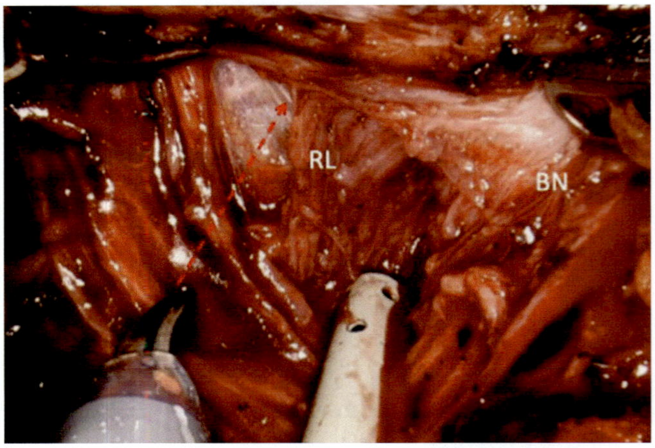

Fig. 7.6 Dissection of the bladder neck maintaining retro trigonal layer (RL) of the right side over the trigone

rotrigonal layer, seminal vesicles, and the base of the prostate, decreasing the risk of trigonal damages. Once completed, the detachment of the bladder neck from the base of the prostate the traction with the fourth arm on bladder neck can release and seminal vesicles can be dissected and isolated.

References

1. Artibani W, Cacciamani G. The apical dissection. In: John H, Wiklund P, editors. Robotic urology. Cham: Springer International; 2018. p. 355–61.
2. Walz J, et al. A critical analysis of the current knowledge of surgical anatomy related to optimization of cancer control and preservation of continence and erection in candidates for radical prostatectomy. Eur Urol. 2010;57(2):179–92.
3. Walz J, et al. A critical analysis of the current knowledge of surgical anatomy of the prostate related to optimisation of cancer control and preservation of continence and erection in candidates for radical prostatectomy: an update. Eur Urol. 2016;70(2):301–11.
4. Myers RP. Practical surgical anatomy for radical prostatectomy. Urol Clin North Am. 2001;28(3):473–90.
5. Myers RP. Detrusor apron, associated vascular plexus, and avascular plane: relevance to radical retropubic prostatectomy—anatomic and surgical commentary. Urology. 2002;59(4):472–9.
6. Secin FP, et al. The anterior layer of Denonvilliers' fascia: a common misconception in the laparoscopic prostatectomy literature. J Urol. 2007;177(2):521–5.
7. Tewari A, et al. Identification of the retrotrigonal layer as a key anatomical landmark during robotically assisted radical prostatectomy. BJU Int. 2006;98(4):829–32.
8. Checcucci E, et al. Retzius-sparing robot-assisted radical prostatectomy vs the standard approach: a systematic review and analysis of comparative outcomes. BJU Int. 2020;125(1):8–16.
9. Galfano A, et al. Retzius-sparing robot-assisted radical prostatectomy: early learning curve experience in three continents. BJU Int. 2021;127(4):412–7.
10. Galfano A, et al. Beyond the learning curve of the Retzius-sparing approach for robot-assisted laparoscopic radical prostatectomy: oncologic and functional results of the first 200 patients with ≥1 year of follow-up. Eur Urol. 2013;64(6):974–80.
11. Secco S, et al. Technical features and the demonstrated advantages of the Retzius sparing robotic prostatectomy. Arch Esp Urol. 2019;72(3):247–56.

Extrafascial (No-Nerve Sparing)

8

Dan Xia, Shuo Wang, Taile Jing, and Di Gu

Introduction

Advances in task-specific surgical instrumentation, optics, digital video equipment, and computer and robotic technology opened a new frontier for minimally invasive laparoscopic prostatectomy. Since the da Vinci system introduction in the United States in 2000, robotic-assisted laparoscopic radical prostatectomy (RALRP) has rapidly grown in popularity with surgeons and patients alike. With rapid dissemination of robotic platforms into large tertiary referral centers and community hospitals, RALRP has become the dominant surgical approach for radical prostatectomy in the United States [1, 2]. Thanks to the vision magnification and the millimetric instruments, more detailed understanding of precise periprostatic anatomy has been achieved [3, 4]. Anatomical studies ultimately translated into better tumor control and higher level of function preservation during prostatectomy. This chapter highlights the extra-fascial techniques for robot-assisted radical prostatectomy, describing the anatomical findings, surgical techniques and summarizing the current evidence supporting its implementation.

Fascia of the Prostate

Endopelvic Fascia

The endopelvic fascia includes the parietal endopelvic fascia and the visceral endopelvic fascia [4]. The visceral component of the endopelvic fascia covers the pelvic organs including prostate, bladder, and rectum, and it is fused with the anterior fibromuscular stroma of the prostate at the upper ventral aspect of the gland [4–6] (Fig. 8.1a). Along the pelvic sidewall at the lateral aspect of the prostate and bladder, the parietal and the visceral components of the endopelvic fascia are fused [4–6]. As a fascial condensation, this fusion is often recognizable as a whitish line and named the fascial tendinous arch of the pelvis (FTAP) [4] (Fig. 8.1a). It stretches from the pubovesical/puboprostatic ligaments (PV/PPLs) to the ischial spine. The parietal endopelvic fascia includes fascia of the levator ani muscle (Fig. 8.1a). The incision of this fascia immediately lateral to the fascial tendinous arch incises the levator ani fascia (LAF) and leaves the muscle fibers of the levator ani bare and the LAF adherent to the prostate [4, 7–9].

Anterior Periprostatic Fascia

This periprostatic fascia (PPF) is not a discrete single-layered structure stretching over the lateral surface of the prostate [4, 8]. Often it is ordered in several layers over the prostate and consists of both collagenous and adipose tissue elements [5]. The anterior periprostatic fascia as visceral endopelvic fascia is associated with the anterior surface of the prostate from approximately the 10-o'clock to 11-o'clock positions to the 1-o'clock to 2-o'clock positions, where it covers the detrusor apron, dorsal vascular complex, and is fused in the midline with the anterior fibromuscular stroma of the prostate [3, 4] (Fig. 8.1).

Lateral Periprostatic Fascia

Lateral periprostatic fascia, on the posterolateral prostate, extend from the anterior surface of the prostate posteriorly or dorsally to embrace or meet the neurovascular bundle (NVB) with the outer LAF passing lateral to the NVB to eventually become the pararectal fascia, which separates the rectum from the levator ani [4, 6, 8, 10] (Fig. 8.1a).

D. Xia (✉) · S. Wang · T. Jing
The First Affiliated Hospital, School of Medicine, Zhejiang University, Hangzhou, China
e-mail: shuowang11@zju.edu.cn

D. Gu
The First Affiliated Hospital of Guangzhou Medical University, Guangzhou, China

S. Ren et al. (eds.), *Robot-Assisted Radical Prostatectomy*, https://doi.org/10.1007/978-3-031-05855-4_8

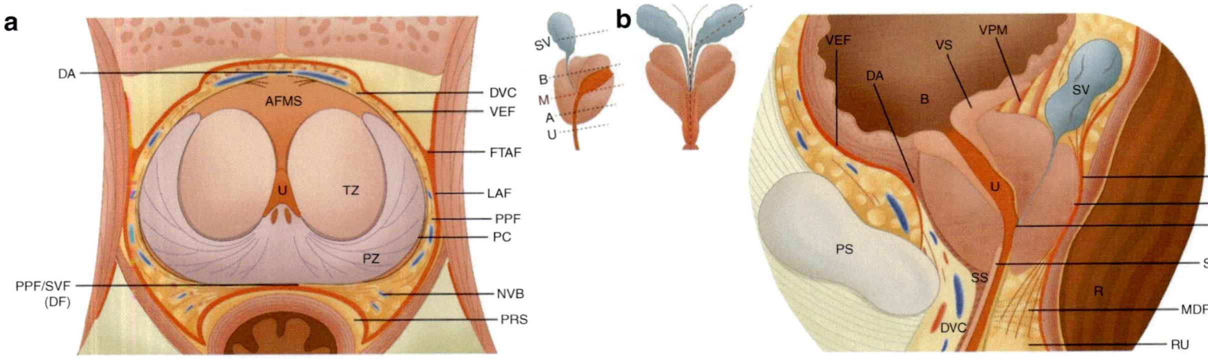

Fig. 8.1 (**a**) Axial section of prostatic and periprostatic fascia at mid-prostate. (**b**) Midline sagittal section of prostate, bladder, urethra, and striated sphincter. *A* apex, *AFMS* anterior fibromuscular stroma, *B* bladder, *DA* detrusor apron, *DF* Denonvilliers fascia, *DVC* dorsal vascular complex, *FTAP* fascial tendinous arch of pelvis, *LAF* levator ani fascia, *M* midprostate, *NVB* neurovascular bundle, *PC* pseudocapsule, *PPF* periprostatic fascia, *PPF/SVF* posterior prostatic fascia/seminal vesical fascia, *PRS* perirectal space, *PZ* peripheral zone, *R* rectum, *SV* seminal vesicle, *TZ* transition zone, *U* urethra, *VEF* visceral endopelvic fascia. *CS* colliculus seminalis (verumontanum), *MDR* medial dorsal raphe, *PC* pseudocapsule of prostate, *PS* pubic symphysis, *RU* rectourethralis muscle, *SMS* smooth muscle sphincter, *SS* striated sphincter, *VEF* visceral endopelvic fascia, *VS* vesical sphincter, *VVPM* vesicoprostatic muscle. (This figure is modified from Walz, J's papers [3, 4])

Posterior Prostatic Fascia and Seminal Vesicles Fascia (Denonvilliers' Fascia)

The posterior surface of the prostate and the seminal vesicles are tightly covered by a continuous layer of posterior prostatic fascia (pPF) and seminal vesicles fascia (SVF), also known as Denonvilliers' fascia [4, 9, 11]. The cephalad origin of the pPF/SVF is found anterior to the caudal end point of the peritoneal cul-de-sac (rectovesical pouch) [4]. The pPF/SVF then extends distally to the apex of the prostate to end at the prostatourethral junction in a terminal plate in continuity with the central perineal tendon, which consists of collagenous, elastic, and numerous muscle fibers and varies from a fragile translucent layer to a dense single-layered membrane [4, 12, 13]. Muraoka et al. investigated that although its configuration appeared to be a firm membranous structure, it was actually recognized as a fascicle of multiple leaves with interlacing branches, with multiple leaves mainly ventrally, and a disorderly, loose connective tissue mainly dorsally [3, 14]. They found a fusion between the pPF/SVF and the pseudocapsule near the base of the prostate at the insertion of the seminal vesicles [14]. The pPF/SVF extended and dispersed laterally into the neurovascular bundle (NVB), and periprostatic nerves ran between multiple leaves and appeared embedded in the fascial complex between pPF/SVF leaves and the pseudo-capsule [3] (Fig. 8.1).

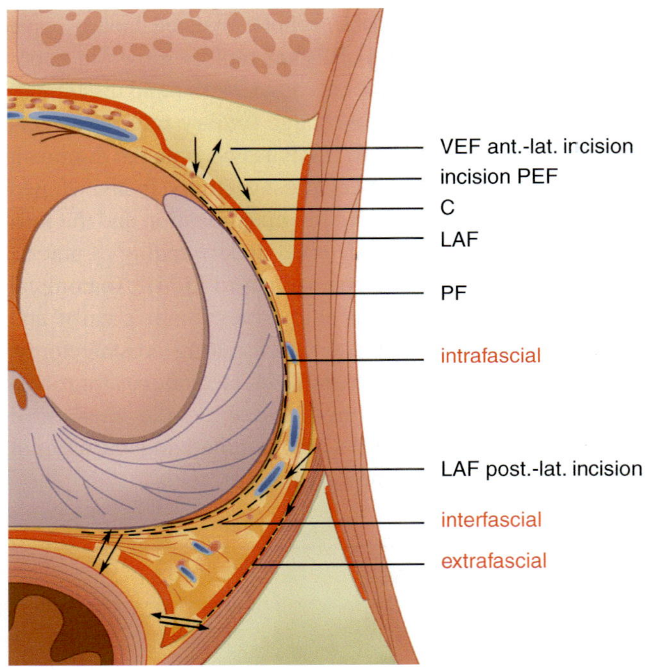

Fig. 8.2 Axial section of prostate and periprostatic fascias at midprostate with three different dissection planes (intrafascial, interfascial and extrafascial) demonstrated. This schematic figure (prostate rotated counterclockwise) shows the classical posterolateral release of interfascial dissection. *C* capsule of prostate, *FTAP* fascial tendinous arch of pelvis, *LAF* levator ani fascia, *NVB* neurovascular bundle, *PEF* parietal endopelvic fascia, *PF* prostatic fascia, *VEF* visceral endopelvic fascia. (This figure is modified from Walz, J's papers [3, 4])

Prostate Capsule

The prostate itself is surrounded by a capsule-like structure, which represents its outer limits [4]. This structure is not a clear capsule in an anatomical sense, but a layer of fibrous muscle bundles, mainly smooth muscle, which is an integral part of the prostate matrix [4, 15, 16]. At its apex, the prostate stroma blends with the muscle fibers of the urinary sphincter and at the base with the smooth muscle fibers of the bladder detrusor, so the prostate capsule cannot be identified at either the apex or the base of the prostate [4, 15, 17] (Fig. 8.2).

Neurovascular Bundle

The neurovascular bundle (NVB), situated between the fascial layers covering the prostate, is composed of numerous nerve fibers superimposed on a scaffold of veins, arteries, and variable amounts of adipose tissue surrounding almost the entire lateral and posterior surfaces of the prostate [3, 4] (Fig. 8.2). Takenaka et al. demonstrated a spray-like distribution of the nerves on the lateral and anterolateral surface of the prostate which was firstly described by Muller and draw a conclusion that the NVB is not a distinct structure but consists of multiple finely dispersed fibers [18]. Several studies demonstrated that only two thirds of all nerves on the lateral aspect are present in the posterolateral location, and the remaining third lie on the anterolateral surface [4, 10, 19, 20]. Many reports showed that preserving the NVB to the prostate could contribute to preservation of postoperative sexual function and early return of postoperative continence [4, 21, 22].

Surgical Technique

Patient Position and Trocar Placement

After induction of general anesthesia, the patient is placed in the steep Trendelenburg position with the arms and hands carefully tucked and padded to avoid injury to the median and ulnar nerves. The patient's legs are spread apart to allow for access to the rectum and perineum during vesicourethral anastomosis.

The Da Vinci Xi robotic surgical system (Intuitive Surgical Inc., Sunnyvale, CA, USA) is the predominant system in use today. For a transperitoneal approach, pneumoperitoneum is established using either a Veress needle inserted at the base of the umbilicus or an open Hasson technique. Trocar configuration is shown in Fig. 8.3. Arm 3 metal 8 mm trocar is initially placed above the umbilicus for insertion of the stereo-endoscope. Three other 8 mm metal robotic trocars are placed under direct laparoscopic view while the assistant provides retraction, suction, and irrigation and pass clips and sutures via the 12 mm trocars placed along the patient's right side.

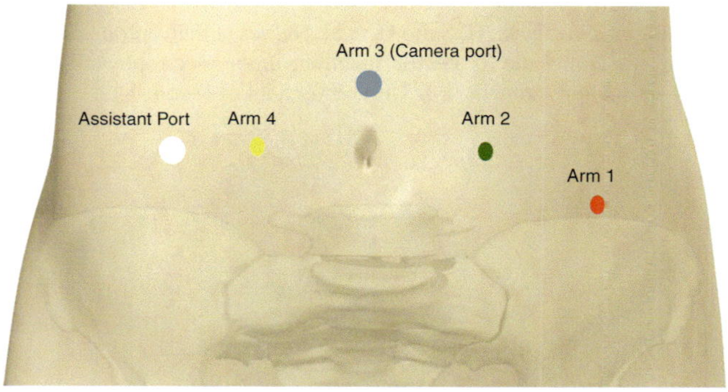

Fig. 8.3 Demonstration of Port Placement: Arm 3 8 mm metal trocar is initially placed above the umbilicus for insertion of the stereo-endoscope. Three other metal robotic 8 mm trocars are placed under direct laparoscopic view while the assistant provides retraction, suction, and irrigation and pass clips and sutures via the 12 mm trocars placed along the patient's right side

Extra-Fascial Dissection

Extra-fascial dissection is a dissection carried lateral to the LAF and posterior to the pPF/SVF [3, 4] (Fig. 8.2a, purple line). Firstly, endopelvic fascia needs to be dissected from the outside of FTAP (Fig. 8.4) and closing to the LAF to confirm the anterior rectal fat on the posterolateral side of the prostate (Fig. 8.2b). As for posterior prostatic fascia, it should be separated closing to the anterior Denonvilliers fascia in the perirectal space from the rear center section to both sides until to meet the anterior rectal fat on the posterolateral side of the prostate (Figs. 8.2a and 8.5). In this case, the NVB along the posterolateral side of the prostate was completely removed, and LAF, PF and pPF/SVF remained on the prostate [4]. Compared with intra-fascial and inter-fascial dissections, this approach leads to the larg-

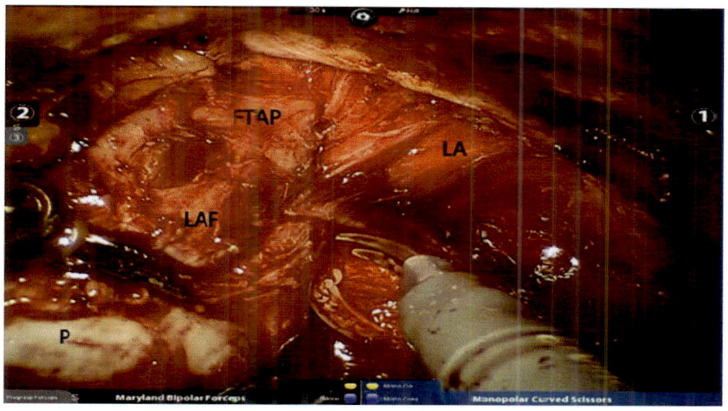

Fig. 8.4 *FTAP* fascial tendinous arch of pelvis, *LAF* levator ani fascia, *LA* levator ani, *P* prostate

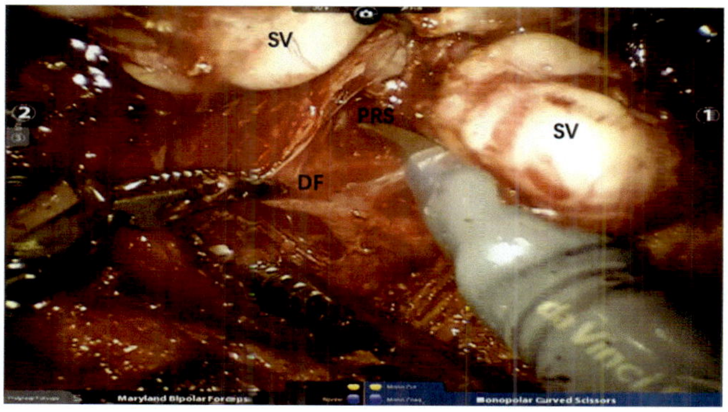

Fig. 8.5 Dissection of posterior prostatic fascia: *DF* Denonvilliers fascia, *PRS* perirectal space, *SV* seminal vesicle

est number of resection of periprostatic tissue (Fig. 8.2). Therefore, it is the safest complete tumor resection with negative margin, but it may be accompanied by complete erectile dysfunction [4].

Conclusion

Wide adaption of RALRP within the urological community has resulted in numerous novel approaches and cut-off edge techniques with the aims of preserving urine continence and sexual function while maintaining oncological success. Performing extra-fascia dissection during RALRP is the standard technique for urologists. This technique is useful on patients with locally advanced disease in oncological control. In this chapter, we summarized the current evidence concerning the prostatic fascia anatomy and briefly described the surgical extra-fascia techniques. Continued development of anatomical concepts and surgical approaches are still on the horizon. Indeed, we want to emphasize that the appropriate technique is tailored to patient's individual anatomy and takes into consider of tumor stage and function preservation.

References

1. Binder J, Kramer W. Robotically-assisted laparoscopic radical prostatectomy. BJU Int. 2001;87(4):408–10.
2. Trinh QD, Sammon J, Sun M, et al. Perioperative outcomes of robot-assisted radical prostatectomy compared with open radical prostatectomy: results from the nationwide inpatient sample. Eur Urol. 2012;61(4):679–85.
3. Walz J, Epstein JI, Ganzer R, et al. A critical analysis of the current knowledge of surgical anatomy of the prostate related to optimisation of cancer control and preservation of continence and erection in candidates for radical prostatectomy: an update. Eur Urol. 2016;70(2):301–11.
4. Walz J, Burnett AL, Costello AJ, et al. A critical analysis of the current knowledge of surgical anatomy related to optimization of cancer control and preservation of continence and erection in candidates for radical prostatectomy. Eur Urol. 2010;57(2):179–92.
5. Kiyoshima K, Yokomizo A, Yoshida T, et al. Anatomical features of periprostatic tissue and its surroundings: a histological analysis of 79 radical retropubic prostatectomy specimens. Jpn J Clin Oncol. 2004;34(8):463–8.
6. Takenaka A, Hara R, Soga H, Murakami G, Fujisawa M. A novel technique for approaching the endopelvic fascia in retropubic radical prostatectomy, based on an anatomical study of fixed and fresh cadavers. BJU Int. 2005;95(6):766–71.
7. Burnett AL, Mostwin JL. In situ anatomical study of the male urethral sphincteric complex: relevance to continence preservation following major pelvic surgery. J Urol. 1998;160(4):1301–6.
8. Costello AJ, Brooks M, Cole OJ. Anatomical studies of the neurovascular bundle and cavernosal nerves. BJU Int. 2004;94(7):1071–6.
9. Myers RP. Practical surgical anatomy for radical prostatectomy. Urol Clin North Am. 2001;28(3):473–90.
10. Kourambas J, Angus DG, Hosking P, Chou ST. A histological study of Denonvilliers' fascia and its relationship to the neurovascular bundle. Br J Urol. 1998;82(3):408–10.
11. Dasgupta P. Anatomic considerations during radical prostatectomy. Eur Urol. 2010;57(2):193–5.
12. Lindsey I, Guy RJ, Warren BF, Mortensen NJ. Anatomy of Denonvilliers' fascia and pelvic nerves, impotence, and implications for the colorectal surgeon. Br J Surg. 2000;87(10):1288–99.
13. Villers A, McNeal JE, Freiha FS, Boccon-Gibod L, Stamey TA. Invasion of Denonvilliers' fascia in radical prostatectomy specimens. J Urol. 1993;149(4):793–8.
14. Muraoka K, Hinata N, Morizane S, et al. Site-dependent and inter-individual variations in Denonvilliers' fascia: a histological study using donated elderly male cadavers. BMC Urol. 2015;15:42.
15. Ayala AG, Ro JY, Babaian R, Troncoso P, Grignon DJ. The prostatic capsule: does it exist? Its importance in the staging and treatment of prostatic carcinoma. Am J Surg Pathol. 1989;13(1):21–7.
16. McNeal JE. The prostate and prostatic urethra: a morphologic synthesis. J Urol. 1972;107(6):1008–16.
17. Epstein JI. Pathologic assessment of the surgical specimen. Urol Clin North Am. 2001;28(3):567–94.
18. Takenaka A, Murakami G, Soga H, Han SH, Arai Y, Fujisawa M. Anatomical analysis of the neurovascular bundle supplying penile cavernous tissue to ensure a reliable nerve graft after radical prostatectomy. J Urol. 2004;172(3):1032–5.
19. Eichelberg C, Erbersdobler A, Michl U, et al. Nerve distribution along the prostatic capsule. Eur Urol. 2007;51(1):105–10; discussion 10–1.
20. Lunacek A, Schwentner C, Fritsch H, Bartsch G, Strasser H. Anatomical radical retropubic prostatectomy: 'curtain dissection' of the neurovascular bundle. BJU Int. 2005;95(9):1226–31.
21. Srivastava A, Chopra S, Pham A, et al. Effect of a risk-stratified grade of nerve-sparing technique on early return of continence after robot-assisted laparoscopic radical prostatectomy. Eur Urol. 2013;63(3):438–44.
22. Kaiho Y, Nakagawa H, Saito H, et al. Nerves at the ventral prostatic capsule contribute to erectile function: initial electrophysiological assessment in humans. Eur Urol. 2009;55(1):148–54.

9 Posterior Approach to Seminal Vesicles

William R. Visser and Lance J. Hampton

Introduction

Variations in anatomy and patient body habitus affect surgical technique in all urologic procedures. This is magnified during radical prostatectomy due to limited working space within the pelvis and differences in the anatomy of the prostatic lobes between patients. The posterior approach for seminal vesicle (SV) dissection was first described for pure laparoscopy and was termed the Montsouris technique [1]. With development and implementation of the surgical robot, surgeons were able to implement this during transperitoneal robotic assisted radical prostatectomy. While dissection technique is surgeon dependent and largely a matter of preference, the posterior approach allows for improved visualization and identification of the SVs initially and improves efficiency of the SV dissection [2].

Surgical Technique

Robotic System and Port Placement

The Da Vinci Xi robotic surgical system (Intuitive Surgical Inc., Sunnyvale, CA, USA) is the predominant system in use today. Robotic port placement and patient positioning are the same regardless to the approach to the seminal vesicle dissection. We use all four robotic arms for all of our prostatectomies and two assistant ports (12 mm Airseal port in the right lower quadrant and a 5 mm port in the right upper quadrant). Patients remain in supine position with 20° of Trendelenburg positioning. With the Xi robot, split leg or lithotomy positioning is not needed. Upon entry and docking of the robot, initial inspection of the abdomen is performed to assess the anatomy.

W. R. Visser · L. J. Hampton (✉)
Virginia Commonwealth University Health System, Richmond, VA, USA
e-mail: william.visser@vcuhealth.org; lance.hampton@vcuhealth.org

Seminal Vesicle Exposure

Initially, lysis of adhesions may need to be undertaken in order to free up the sigmoid colon from the left lateral body wall. This can be vitally important in that if the sigmoid is tethered, cephalad retraction will be difficult and can affect the posterior dissection. Once the sigmoid is free, it is retracted cephalad and the far-left arm (with the Prograsp grasper) is used to hold the sigmoid in place with gentle posterior traction. This maneuver pulls the posterior cul-de-sac taut and will improve visualization. The posterior peritoneum in the cul-de-sac is then incised midway between the bladder "fold" and the reflection of the peritoneum by the rectum. The assistant's suction irrigator is placed in this space and retracted anteriorly (Fig. 9.1).

Seminal Vesicle Dissection Via the Posterior Approach

At this point, using a combination of sharp and blunt dissection the bilateral vasa and seminal vesicle complex is dis-

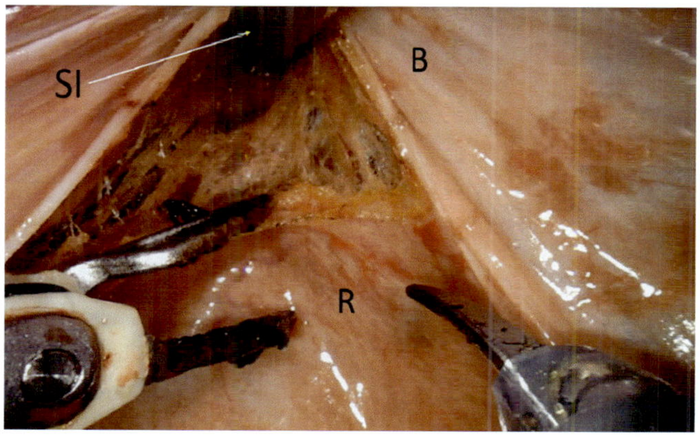

Fig. 9.1 An incision is made in the cul-de-sac of the peritoneum between the bladder (B) and rectum (R) using the curved monopolar scissors. The assistants laparoscopic suction irrigator (SI) can then provide retraction anteriorly to help develop the operative space

S. Ren et al. (eds.), *Robot-Assisted Radical Prostatectomy*, https://doi.org/10.1007/978-3-031-05855-4_9

sected both anteriorly and posteriorly taking care not to dissect the vasa off of the seminal vesicles or from each other in the midline (Fig. 9.2). It is unnecessary to dissect the vasa away from the seminal vesicles and could, theoretically, lead to a positive margin for very high stage disease. It is very important to see both vasa deferentia and seminal vesicles before anything is cut. Patients with ectopic ureters or with extreme "J-Hooking" of the ureters may have an injury in this area if the complex is not dissected carefully (Fig. 9.3).

Once this posterior complex has been freely dissected, the vas on either side is cut as laterally as possible near the tip of the seminal vesicle. This maneuver also keeps as much tissue as possible on the vas/SV complex (Fig. 9.4). Immediately caudal to the vas lies the vasal artery. This can be cauterized easily with either monopolar or bipolar energy. Clips are unnecessary. The seminal vesicles will now be more freely mobile and can be gently pulled medially exposing the lateral surface. Frequently, there are small vessels in this area as well which are easily identifiable and addressed with cauterization. This dissection is carried caudally until the insertion of the vas/SV complex can be seen entering the posterior prostate. The same dissection is performed on the contralateral side typically with the assistant pulling the left vas/SV complex medially. Counter traction should always be performed by pulling the complex towards the midline to avoid the lateral nerve tissue which may be present in this area.

Once the entire vas/SV complex has been freed, the assistant will grab the complex and lift anteriorly. The suction irrigator is placed posterior putting gentle traction in this area. This exposes Denonvillier's fascia. At this point, the surgeon may decide to split the fascia to be as close to the prostate as possible or to purposefully enter Denonvillier's, keeping all posterior fascial tissue on the posterior surface of the prostate (Fig. 9.5). This decision should be based on each patient's individual pathology and preoperative imaging.

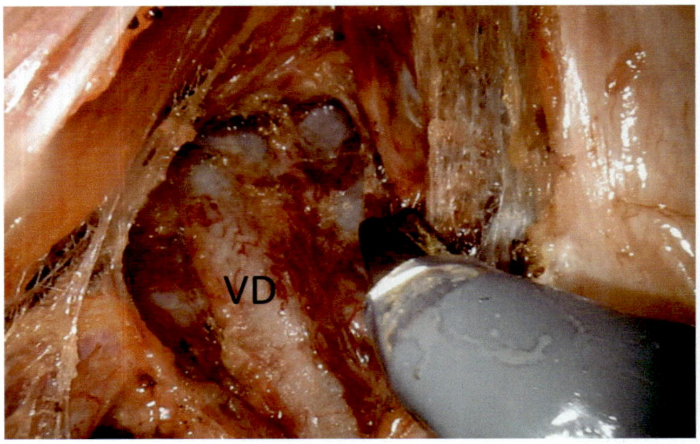

Fig. 9.2 Blunt and electrocautery dissection are used to identify the right vas deferens (VD) on the course towards the right internal inguinal ring

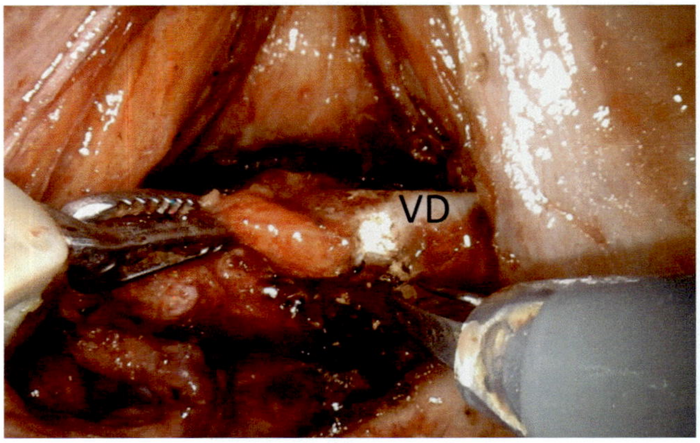

Fig. 9.3 The right vas deferens (VD) is dissected both anteriorly and posteriorly prior to transection. This allows for identification of aberrant or ectopic ureters in this space

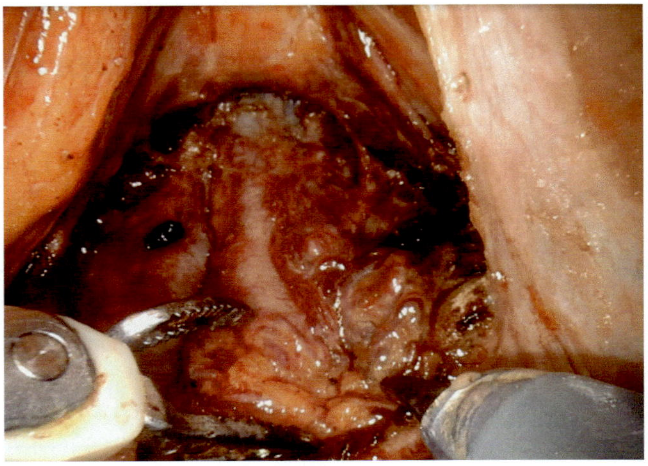

Fig. 9.4 The vas deferens is cut on the right side of the image depicting a lateral transection. The seminal vesicles and vas deferens are not separated from this point on

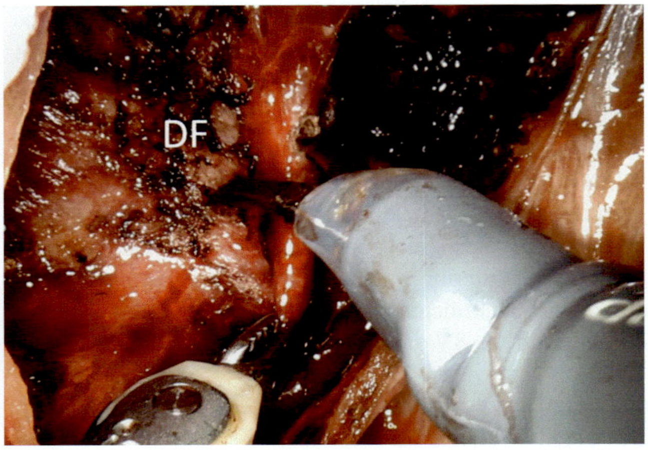

Fig. 9.5 The seminal vesicles have been dissected free and are being lifted anteriorly by the assistant. The surgeon can then enter Denonvillier's fascia (DF) posterior to the prostate

Caudal dissection can then be performed with both sharp and blunt dissection as distal as possible. A 30° up lens can also be used at this point to facilitate this dissection if needed. At this point, the focus of the operation is shifted to the anterior side where the surgeon will start by dropping the bladder.

Advantages

Knowledge of and ability to perform both the anterior and posterior dissection of the SV is crucial for a urologist that plans on performing radical prostatectomies. Each case may require a specific technique based on varying factors. Regardless, the posterior approach consistently offers several key advantages when compared to the anterior dissection. Immediately, the surgeon will notice improved working area and visualization for the SV dissection. By performing the SV dissection first from a posterior approach, the bladder and prostate remain suspended to the anterior abdominal wall, which gives the surgeon improved visualization. Furthermore, the vas deferens can be seen coursing towards its exit through the interior inguinal ring allowing for ease of identification. The second noticeable benefit is decreased pooling of the blood in the rectoprostatic space. Posterior entrance affords improved suctioning by the assistant and a cleaner operative field. If performed first, the posterior dissection will then make for a safe and reliable bladder neck transection into the space created initially [3].

Outcomes

Intraoperative choice of the posterior dissection technique is typically based on surgeon preference. Yasui et al. demonstrated that the approach was safe and efficient in their retrospective analysis of 300 consecutive patients undergoing robot-assisted laparoscopic radical prostatectomy (RALP) with an initial posterior approach. In this study, the researchers found a median operative time 160 min, complication rate of 3.0%, and estimated blood loss, including urine, of 200 mL. At 6 months post-operative follow-up, approximately 82.4% of patients did not use more than one absorbent pad in 24 h [3]. The posterior SV dissection may be most beneficial for patients undergoing RALP who are found to have a large prostatic volume. Maddox et al. enrolled 404 patients in a prospective study comparing anterior and posterior seminal vesicle dissection. Of the patients enrolled, 187 patients underwent a posterior surgical approach and 217 were approached anteriorly. The investigators found no difference in console time, transfusion rate, positive margins, or complication rate. However, when each group was stratified based on prostate volume, the posterior approach was found to have statistically significant shorter operative times for the two highest quartiles of prostate volume (163.8 vs. 145.9 min and 183.8 vs. 166.2 min, $p = 0.02$, $p = 0.04$) [4]. Post-operative quality of life is important to consider in patients undergoing RALP as this procedure can be curative for a large population of men. Maruyama et al. compared 201 patients in a retrospective study where 146 underwent robot-assisted radical prostatectomy with an anterior approach and 55 with a posterior approach. The Expanded Prostate Cancer Index Composite (EPIC) score was used to assess HRQOL 3 months pre-operatively and post-operatively at 2 weeks, 1, 3, 6, and 12 months. There was no difference in HRQOL post-operatively between the anterior and posterior surgical approaches [5]. Surgeons can therefore choose either approach without the fear of a difference in long term quality of life issues and can focus on refining their operative technique.

Conclusion

Performing a posterior SV dissection during RALP is the preferred method for many urologists. This method may be most useful on patients with exceptionally large prostate glands. It is both safe and effective and can assist with visualization and identification of the structures posterior to the prostate. The ability to perform both the anterior and posterior approach is crucial for surgeons performing RALP as variations in pelvic anatomy may be best suited by one or the other depending on several factors.

References

1. Guillonneau B, Vallancien G. Laparoscopic radical prostatectomy: the Montsouris technique. J Urol. 2000;163(6):1643–9.
2. Lee DI, Fagin R. The timing and route of seminal vesicle dissection during robotic prostatectomy. J Robot Surg. 2008;1(4):253–5.
3. Yasui T, Tozawa K, Okada A, Kurokawa S, Kubota H, Mizuno K, et al. Outcomes of robot-assisted laparoscopic prostatectomy with a posterior approach to the seminal vesicle in 300 patients. Int Sch Res Notices. 2014;2014:565737.
4. Maddox M, Elsamra S, Kaplon D, Cone E, Renzulli J, Pareek G. The posterior surgical approach to robot-assisted radical prostatectomy facilitates dissection of large glands. J Endourol. 2013;27(6):740–2.
5. Maruyama Y, Sadahira T, Araki M, Mitsui Y, Wada K, Tanimoto R, et al. Comparison of longitudinal health-related quality-of-life outcomes between anterior and posterior surgical approaches to robot-assisted radical prostatectomy. J Robot Surg. 2020;14(2):255–60.

10 Retrograde Release of Neurovascular Bundles with Preservation of the Dorsal Venous Complex

Jonathan Noël, Marcio Covas Moschovas, Rafael Ferreira Coelho, and Vipul Patel

Introduction

Robotic-assisted laparoscopic radical prostatectomy (RALP) presents opportunities to use magnification and dexterity in a minimal access approach. Compared to open surgery, robotics has allowed delicate dissection of the periprostatic fascia, with significantly less bleeding in the operative field [1], to enhance preservation of the neurovascular bundles (NVBs). However, in some series the return of erectile function can range from 62% to 80% [2, 3]. In an effort to improve rates of potency recovery, refinement in surgical technique along with consideration of the pelvic neuroanatomy can lead to an optimal outcome for the patient.

Prior to the landmark discovery by Walsh and Donker [4], open radical prostatectomy had been a curative procedure for prostate cancer, but carried a high incidence of post-operative impotence and overall morbidity. Surgeons of that time understood that nerves involved in potency, existed within the prostate, and so had to be sacrificed to treat cancer of the gland. Additionally, the venous plexus found anterolaterally on the prostate, would be entered and brisk bleeding hindered the ability to identify key landmarks. This translated to poor outcomes and hesitancy of new patients to undergo surgery. Walsh defined the complex arrangement of the dorsal venous plexus [5], which when controlled, made prostatectomy a safe procedure, with shorter operative times and allowed anatomy to further be explored.

This formed the basis for the collaboration between Walsh and Donker, to define the autonomic innervation of the corpora cavernosa. This was achieved by cadaveric examination of the male fetus, as dissection in the adult was difficult. In the anatomy laboratory of the Netherlands, the connective and adipose tissue was easily dissected away from the neurovascular structures and they were nerves easily identifiable. The pelvic nerve plexus to the bladder, prostate and urethra formed the basis of roadmap that current surgeons use to aid in potency in patients following radical prostatectomy. The posterolateral prostatic margin must be carefully dissected to displace the NVB so it can be preserved. In this chapter, we discuss the anatomical and surgical details that have helped achieve trifecta after RALP.

Pelvic Neuroanatomy

The autonomic innervation of the pelvis starts at its plexus, which is formed by sacral levels S2 to S4 (parasympathetic) and thoracolumbar levels T11 to L2 (sympathetic) nerve fibres. The pelvic (inferior hypogastric) plexus exists as a rectangular structure that is found in the retroperitoneum and pararectally [6] (see Fig. 10.1). It is close to the tip of the seminal vesicles (SV) and inferior vesical artery, the former must be cautiously handled during elevation and placement of a vascular clip inferiorly [7]. The NVB commences from an inferior branch of the plexus, that runs between the rectum and the posterolateral surface of the prostate. Other major branches of the pelvic plexus includes an anterior branch that runs on the SV surface and inferior bladder aspect; and an anteroinferior branch to the prostatovesical junction and lateral prostate surface [6].

The NVB extends laterally to and within the lateral pelvic fascia (LPF). The LPF meets the pararectal fascia, as does the Denonvilliers' fascia (DF) posteriorly. The pararectal fascia continues on the lateral rectal surface and the lateral pelvic fascia lies between the levator ani muscles/fascia and the lateral surface of the prostate. The DF separates the prostate and the rectum and the NVB lies underneath and within it. Maintaining a plane between the prostate and DF is the first step to ensuring an optimal nerve spare RALP is carried out. This is confirmed from the colorectal experience in rectal excision, where potency and urogenital function is opti-

J. Noël · M. C. Moschovas · V. Patel (✉)
Global Robotics Institute, AdventHealth, Celebration, FL, USA
e-mail: jonathan.noel.md@adventhealth.com; marcio.moschovas.md@adventhealth.com; vipul.patel.md@adventhealth.com

R. F. Coelho
Hospital Albert Einstein, Sao Paulo, Brazil

S. Ren et al. (eds.), *Robot-Assisted Radical Prostatectomy*, https://doi.org/10.1007/978-3-031-05855-4_10

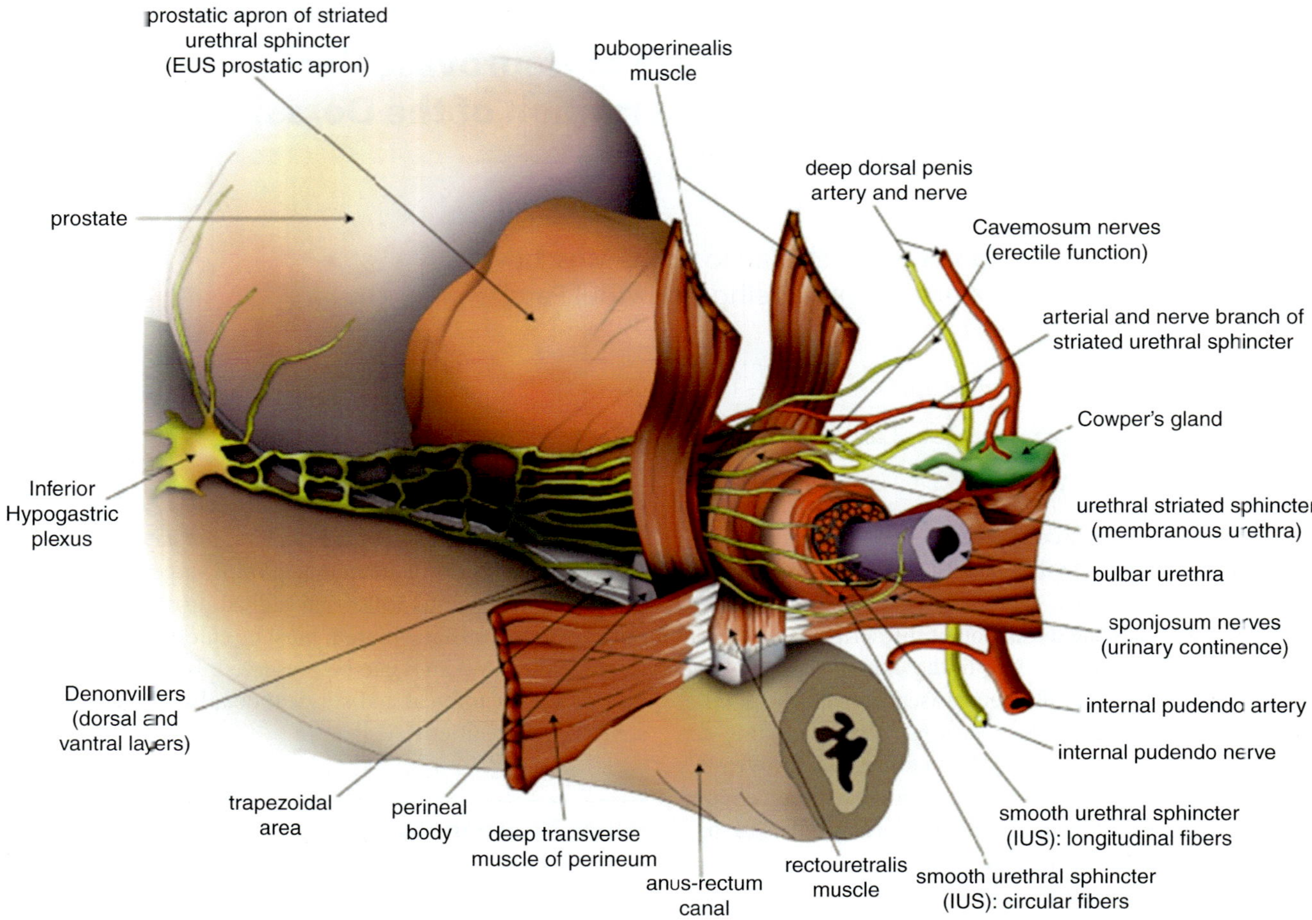

Fig. 10.1 (Permission from Springer Publishing) Laucirica O, Catalá V, Vilanova JC. Anatomy of the prostate. Atlas of Multiparametric Prostate MRI. 2017:23–45. https://doi.org/10.1007/978-3-319-61786-2_2

mised by leaving DF intact [8, 9]. In prostatectomy, to spare the NVB begins with staying superior to DF, medial the lateral pelvic fascia (LPF) and superior to the pararectal fascia: leaving the triangular space intact. This space becomes progressively narrow from the prostate base to the apex. The cavernosum, levator ani and rectal branches of the NVB meet at the mid prostatic level, which is a point where we focus during our lateral incision and plane development for nerve spare (NS) later. Authors have also previously described the importance of maintaining the arterial supply of the pudendal artery and its branches, such as an accessory pudendal artery to enhance postoperative potency [10].

Figure 10.1 shows the cavernosum nerve courses the mid-prostate gland to the prostatic apex. It is recognised that this nerve's position is lateral to capsular vessels and gives nerve branches that travel intraprostatic. Therefore, once the mid-portion of prostate has had the NVB spared by releasing the LPF, it allows a natural plane of retrograde separation for an otherwise difficult identification of the cavernosal nerves at the prostatic base and apex. There is usually no standard functional organization of the neural constituent at the base and apex, the nerves can spread over these areas while enclosed within their fascial planes. Delicate preservation of the cavernosum nerve off the apex, while the pudendal nerve is avoided 3–1.3 mm distal to supply the striated urethral sphincter [11]. This translates to the care in surgical apical dissection to achieve a balance of oncological cure versus functional outcome.

This cavernosal nerve regulates vasomotor tone of the cavernous arteries to be regulated through its autonomic function, by releasing acetylcholine, nitric oxide (NO) and cyclic guanosine monophosphate (cGMP) will decrease calcium intracellularly [12]. The resultant decrease in smooth muscle vessel tone allows inflow of blood into the penis to achieve a rigid corpora (erection).

It is paramount to appreciate the injury of nerves by revisiting definitions. Neurapraxia is the least severe due to intact neural structural elements, but with ischemia and/or demyelination this affects conduction with resolution up to 3 months. Axonotmesis involves disrupted of axons and myelin sheaths but the endoneurium left intact with consequent Wallerian degeneration distal to the level of injury and proximal axon degenerates. An intact endoneurium equates to incomplete recovery in months but may not be complete. Neurotmesis occurs when the endoneurial tubes and connective tissue components are disrupted with fibrosis, axonal regeneration cannot occur, thus inhibiting nerve recovery. Tissue trauma as a result of dissection from surgery will generate inflammation and response and oxidative stress further mitigating neuronal regeneration. The surgical technique chosen and delicacy of carrying out RALP will always dictate the recovery of potency after NVB preservation.

Veil of Aphrodite

The publication from Lunacek et al. [13] showed that cavernous nerves can be displaced further anterolaterally than previously described. To compensate for this, the technique of releasing the lateral pelvic fascia from a high anterior release dissection, could preserve the neurovascular bundle with more surety. It is paramount for the reader to appreciate that the innervation to the pelvis and erectile tissue is complex and varies according to previous published cadaveric work [14]. Eichelberg et al. [15] gathered histology on sections of post RP specimens which found median number of nerve was lower at apex compared to mid and basal part of the prostate gland. This group observed a significant count of nerves above a transverse line through the prostate, with 21.5–28.5% of nerves from apex to base.

Menon et al. would publish this as the "Veil of Aphrodite" technique, in order optimise post prostatectomy functional outcomes [16]. Aphrodite was an ancient Greek goddess of love, beauty and fertility. In the "veil" procedure, a plane between the prostatic capsule and the prostatic fascia is developed cranially, from the base of the seminal vesicles. A plane between the prostatic fascia and the prostate is developed, with careful blunt peeling of the neurovascular bundle. Since this plane can have minimal bleeding up until the anterior segment of the dorsal venous plexus (between the puboprostatic ligaments) a resultant curtain of periprostatic fascia either side is left behind; similar to a veil. In this series published in 2007, of 1142 patients (pre-operative SHIM score of >21) who underwent bilateral NS with at least 1 year follow-up, 70% were able to achieve sexual intercourse after surgery with or without the use of PDF-5 inhibitors. This technique was refined, and a "superveil" approach was adopted to incorporate the puboprostatic ligaments and dorsal venous plexus, leaving a connected veil with a hood of anterior tissue. This did not require control of the dorsal vein with a suture oversew, for the most part [17]. In 85 patients who had the superveil approach to bilateral NS, 94% had erections sufficient for penetration on a median follow-up of 18 months.

Clipless Thermal Antegrade Approach

Chien et al. [18] developed an approach to robotic prostatectomy that continued in standard method of a posterior plane developed between Denonvilliers fascia to elevate the prostate off the rectum. Staying within the posterior plane, a blunt dissection approach to tease as much of the vascular pedicles away from the prostate (medial to lateral) as was feasible. Returning to an anterior vantage point, the vascular pedicle release was continued antegradely until the branching intraprostatic vessels were encountered. These distal small vessels were controlled with bipolar diathermy before division. Once the vascular supply had been controlled, the remaining NVB was sharply released along the line of the periprostatic dissection and prior released vascular pedicle. The release of thick pedicles, with each vessel being addressed individually, allowed the NVBs to be spared from excessive traction forces of an en masse pedicle clip. The authors of this technique managed to avoid monopolar electrocautery and vascular clips during this dissection, but allowed selective bipolar coagulation. This ability to have a clipless approach, and precisely bipolar cauterise the intraprostatic branches of the pedicle, was attributed to the vision afforded by robotics as well as pneumoperitoneal pressure. This technique avoids less optimal methods of overuse of monopolar cauterisation and imprecise bulk clipping of a prostatic pedicle.

To assess the outcome of this technical point, Zorn et al. followed 300 patients over 2 years [19]. Unilateral NS was performed in 79 patients and bilateral NS was performed in.179 patients. In the unilateral NS group, 52% of the patients were potent at the end of 6 months while 62% were potent at the end of 24 months while those with bilateral NS were 53% and 83% respectively.

Clipless Athermal Antegrade Approach

Ahlering et al. utilised an approach to their NS with the application of 30 mm vascular bulldog clamps to the vascular pedicle [20]. Initially posterior dissection is performed to create space between the prostate and the rectum, the pedicle clamp is applied and is followed by ligation for control, with a running 3-0 polyglycolic acid suture. The theory is this would protect the NVBs both from traction force and thermal injury, as the dissection is strictly without the use of monopolar or bipolar cautery. When the clamp is removed, the suture is used to control any remaining pedicle vessels. Once the pedicle is controlled first and divided, the lateral pelvic fascia is dissected to allow the antegrade release of the NVBs down to the urethra. In 2009, Ahlering et al. selected 58 patients aged less than 65 years with an International

Index of Erectile Function (IIEF)-5 score greater than 21. Potency (defined as erections sufficient for penetration with or without oral PDE-5 inhibitors) was 40% at 3 months and 80% at 2 years for those unilateral NS, while for bilateral NS; the rate was 29.3% and 93% respectively [21].

The Retrograde Release of the NVB

This chapter's novel technique is the applicability of lessons from techniques discussed above, with that of the traditional open NS radical retropubic prostatectomy [22]. During the period of laparoscopic radical prostatectomy, Rassweiler et al. [23] published their approach of periprostatic fascia incision at the prostatic apex and the NVB dissected off retrogradely. All vascular branches entering the prostate were controlled by 5-mm titanium clips. The pedicles were controlled with Hem-o-lok clips thereafter. Guillonneau and Vallancien [24] from Montsouris in Paris, France described the periprostatic fascia incision being made after the prostatic pedicles were clipped and divided. Systematic bipolar coagulation of the arteries was utilised. After the pedicle was controlled, antegradely a pericapsular fatty space would be encountered to preserve the NVB. Small arteries are coagulated with bipolar forceps and the plane is extended to the point of posterolateral exit of the nerve, to the periurethra.

In 2021, our technique has been heralded at a Society of Robotic Surgery Conference, by Professor Costello as that of a true anatomic nerve-sparing (NS). As mentioned, this was constructed on the knowledge of Walsh's description of radical prostatectomy [25]. The forces exerted on the NVBs during prostatectomy will result in erectile dysfunction and so to mitigate these, we first must appreciate what the risks are. Excessive traction and thermal application will cause the nerve to be directly damaged during dissection, resulting in neuropathies defined in the introduction: neurapraxia, axonotmesis, and neurotmesis.

Our experience dictates that NVB preservation from the prostate base to the apex (antegrade) or from the apex to the base (retrograde) makes a difference to potency. There is an earlier identification and release of the NVB at the time of posterior dissection and then anteriorly, starting at the mid prostate. This occurs before controlling the prostatic pedicle to optimally limit a misplaced clip, all performed without thermal energy use on intraprostatic branches. We compared antegrade or retrograde approaches on functional recovery after bilateral NS robot-assisted RP (RARP), we published this [26] and the technique is explained as follows.

After the bladder neck is opened, the pelvic plexus close to the tip of the seminal vesicle (SV) is protected, using an athermal reflection of the nerve rich ventral surface of Denonvillier's fascia (DF) off the SV. The blood supply to the SV tip is taken with a clip while limiting traction and elevation of these structures by a sequence of robotic athermal movements published by our Institution [7]. A right sided bedside assistant and robotic auxiliary left arm lift the divided vas deferens and SVs upward, to present the posterior plane.

It is at this point that the commencement of nerve spare begins with careful separation of DF to achieve the appropriate plane between it and the prostatic fascia (intrafasical) or within the multiple leaves of the DF and lateral pelvic fascia (interfascial). The plane both above and within DF is usually avascular; and to further develop this posterolateral dissection, the 30° camera is toggled upwards. It is this manoeuvre that gives the robotic surgeon an optimal vantage point, similar to looking carefully under "the hood" of an automobile. This approach with the robotic camera allows identification and release from medial to lateral, of the leaflet of the respective fascia (PF or DF) but underneath the prostate initially. The camera is placed anteriorly and 30° down, a plane between the prostate and the NVB is created at the level of the mid prostate, which is chosen for the reason of nerve confluence, discussed in the neuroanatomy subsection earlier. The will isolate and protect the NVB completely, when the previously created posterior plane is in view. This method of mid release the NVB (prior to pedicle manipulation and division) minimises traction induced neuropraxia [27].

Prior to anterior mid prostate lateral incision, during a left retrograde release, a right sided bedside assistant will manually grasp the anterior cranial edge of the prostate and rotate it medially. Likewise, the robotic auxiliary left arm will grasp the prostate and rotate it medially, to optimise a right sided retrograde release of NVB. The balance of pedicle control and avoiding the NVB at the base with an overzealous assistant's clip gives little room for error. Costello et al. [6] published work on cadaveric dissection, confirming this point, as the prostatic base and seminal vesicles is where a NVB anterior to posterior distance can be up to 3 cm wide. The hybrid technique of releasing the NVB posteriorly then anteriorly; as well as rotating the prostate prior to clipping the pedicle should create more distance between the NVB and the pedicle base. When divided by NS approach in our comparative study of antegrade versus retrograde NS, the achievement of potency rates were significantly higher in retrograde group: 48.3% versus 64.5% at 3 months ($p = 0.002$), 52.9% versus 70.3% at 6 months ($p = 0.001$), 66.3% versus 83.7% at 9 months $p < 0.001$) and 67.3% versus 86.0% at 12 months ($p < 0.001$) [21].

To further enhance our level of NS ability during posterolateral dissection described above, we investigated the role of a landmark (capsular) artery. This artery runs lateral to the prostate and can aid in preserving the NVB tissue lateral to it. They form a mesh throughout the thickness of the NVB with the most superficial recognized after opening the levator fascia. In the publication by Schatloff et al. [28] 73.3% of

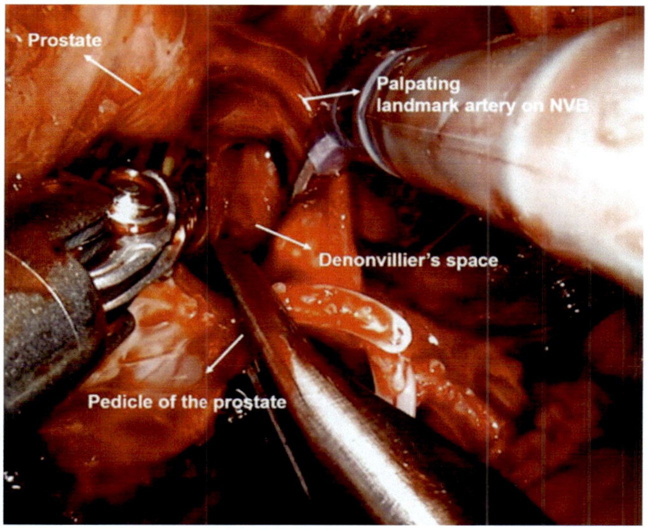

Fig. 10.2 Kang SG, Shim JS, Onol F, Bhat KRS, Patel VR. Lessons learned from 12,000 robotic radical prostatectomies: is the journey as important as the outcome? Investig Clin Urol. 2020;61(1): 1–10. https://doi.org/10.4111/icu.2020.61.1.1

cases the artery was observed and residual nerve tissue on the prostate was measured and compared to NS medial to the landmark artery (LA) and lateral to it. The median (interquartile range) of histological nerve tissue on the specimen was 0 (0–3) mm^2 versus 14 (9–25) mm^2; ($p < 0.001$) respectively.

Utilising this prostate vessel is a routine step in our performance of retrograde release of NVB and the medial border of the LA can consistently result in a complete or near complete NS, whereas performing the NS on its lateral border results in several degrees of incomplete NS (see Fig. 10.2). When the LA is not easily visible due to its embedding in fatty tissue, the NVB fat forms an apron of support to the prostate on the postero-lateral aspects, and this should be identified as a plane of release retrogradely as described above.

Dorsal Venous Complex Preservation

If we consider contemporary studies, a complex neural organization exists around the prostate, which is inclusive of the ventral surface in nearly 25% of patients assessed [29]. Electrophysiological stimulation of the prostate with bipolar electrodes ventrally, evoked increased cavernosal pressures, although it was weaker than the stimulated posterolateral zones [30]. As surgeons and experts in anatomy, we should accept that the direction of cavernosum nerve fibers will vary at times beyond the standard NVB location [31]. A study correlated that patients with no NVB identified on MRI, experienced inferior post-operative outcomes compared to patients with a NVB that was MRI visible. The authors suggested that the nerves spread more anterolaterally in the former case of an MRI revealing lack of a macroscopic NVB [32].

These findings suggest that nerve-sparing (NS) techniques, including sparing the anterior fibres, could contribute to functional recovery after RALP [10]. A landmark study from Costello et al. [33] demonstrated that parasympathetic and sympathetic nerve supply are present in electrophysiological [27] and immunohistochemical [6, 30] (21.5–28.5%) amount at the 9–3 o'clock position of the prostate. To be precise, Costello's group found at the anterolateral base, mid, and apex of the prostate: parasympathetic fibres accounted for 4%, 5% and 6.8% respectively. Whereas, the sympathetic nerves represented 15% of the total number of nerves anterolaterally. It supported the basis for the modified prostate fascia-preserving (veil) nerve sparing or superveil to preserve the dorsal venous complex (DVC) and puboprostatic ligaments. As stated prior, this resulted in a 94% potency recovery rate in their study, using this technique. With all findings above considered, our standard surgical approach of to the DVC of partially preserving and experience with preserving further proximally, will be described in detail.

The DVC lies superior to the prostatic apex and urethral sphincter and so with an anterior approach, prophylactic ligation or incision and oversewing is usually performed. At the time of DVC en bloc suture ligation, the surgeon must take care to not incorporate the striated/external urethral sphincter (seen in Fig. 10.3) which will have obvious impacts on postoperative continence recovery. Ganzer et al. [34] demonstrated that 37% and 30% of the urethral sphincter surface area is covered by the DVC at the apex and 0.5 cm distal to the apex, respectively. Hence, the approach to the DVC, in addition to apical dissection (Fig. 10.3, steps 3–5), will preserve sphincteric function or hinder it.

After performing the retrograde release of NVB, our modified approach to the apical complex of the puboprostatic ligaments and apical endopelvic fascia is to leave these structures intact. We have shown that by avoiding the exaggerated lateral opening of the endopelvic fascia to expose levator ani muscles, these fibres can be left to blend with the rhabdosphincter, where important branches from the pudendal nerve run [35]. Apical dissection is performed by going under the puboprostatic ligaments with the aim of leaving the DVC undisturbed. The result is by avoiding the need for a DVC suspension or oversew suture, it preserves vascularisation of the sphincter complex and apical NVB. This modification to our previous technique of RALP technique also resulted in better potency outcomes. Prior to this modification, a periurethral suspension stitch was placed with a 12-in monofilament polyglytone suture on a CT-1 needle and tied with a mild tension from pubic bone. Moschovas et al. [36] showed that the comparison of the suspension stitch to our

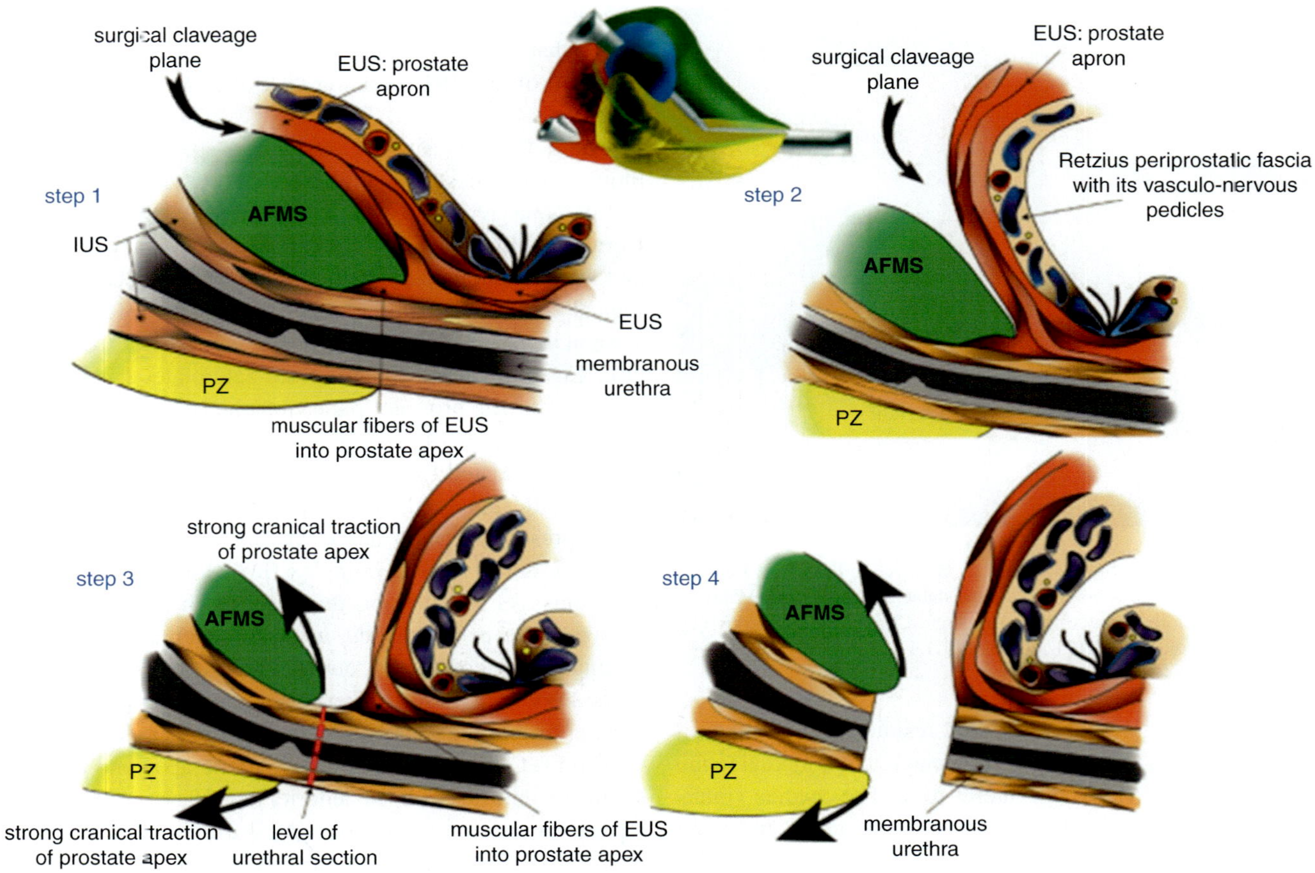

Fig. 10.3 (Permission from Springer Publishing) Laucirica O, Catalá V, Vilanova JC. Anatomy of the prostate. Atlas of Multiparametric Prostate MRI. 2017:23–46. https://doi.org/10.1007/978-3-319-61786-2_2

modification, allowed for a 6 week potency recovery increase from 21% to 44%; a 3 month potency recovery rate increase from 35% to 57%.

A further modification of preserving the DVC is the development of the plane between the prostate and the anterior fascial layer proximally, as described by de Carvalho and Coelho. A plane that may pose risk of entering the prostatic stroma in the early learning curve, and it is accepted that expert level mentoring is recommended. Once the initial incision is made correctly, detrusor apron can be tented up with left hand, while the prostate is manipulated away with the fourth arm or auxiliary left hand. This allows the right hand to advance the plane towards the apex and laterally. The lateral dissection will allow one to fall into the dissected free edge of the medial leaflet (PF or DF) from the previous posterior dissection and NVB release. The NVB is spared and cleared retrogradely to the base, to precisely clip the pedicle (see Fig. 10.4c).

The innovation of this technique is to perform the early retrograde release of the NVBs without opening the endopelvic fascia and without ligating the dorsal venous complex (DVC).

Our technical modification is the release of the NVB starting at the level of the bladder neck, developing an avascular plane underneath the DVC (Fig. 10.1b). This dissection continues laterally respecting the anatomical landmarks of the NVB described by Patel [28]. The prostatic apex is dissected maximizing preservation of the urethral stump; this dissection is carried out underneath the DVC using blunt and sharp dissection, avoiding injury to the anterior vascular structures. Routinely, the periprostatic collar is continuously oversewn as a safety measure, with small bleeding points from the DVC sutured in interrupted fashion.

Impact on Outcomes

Table 10.1 has summarised key papers earlier in the chapter. With the adoption of our retrograde approach to NVB preservation and the addition to proximal sparing of DVC, a case series of 128 consecutive patients from author R.C. was published [38]. It is known that the anterior layer is thicker in smaller prostates, than in BPH, and so the majority of cases (70%), were 20–40 g prostate weight. This is important to

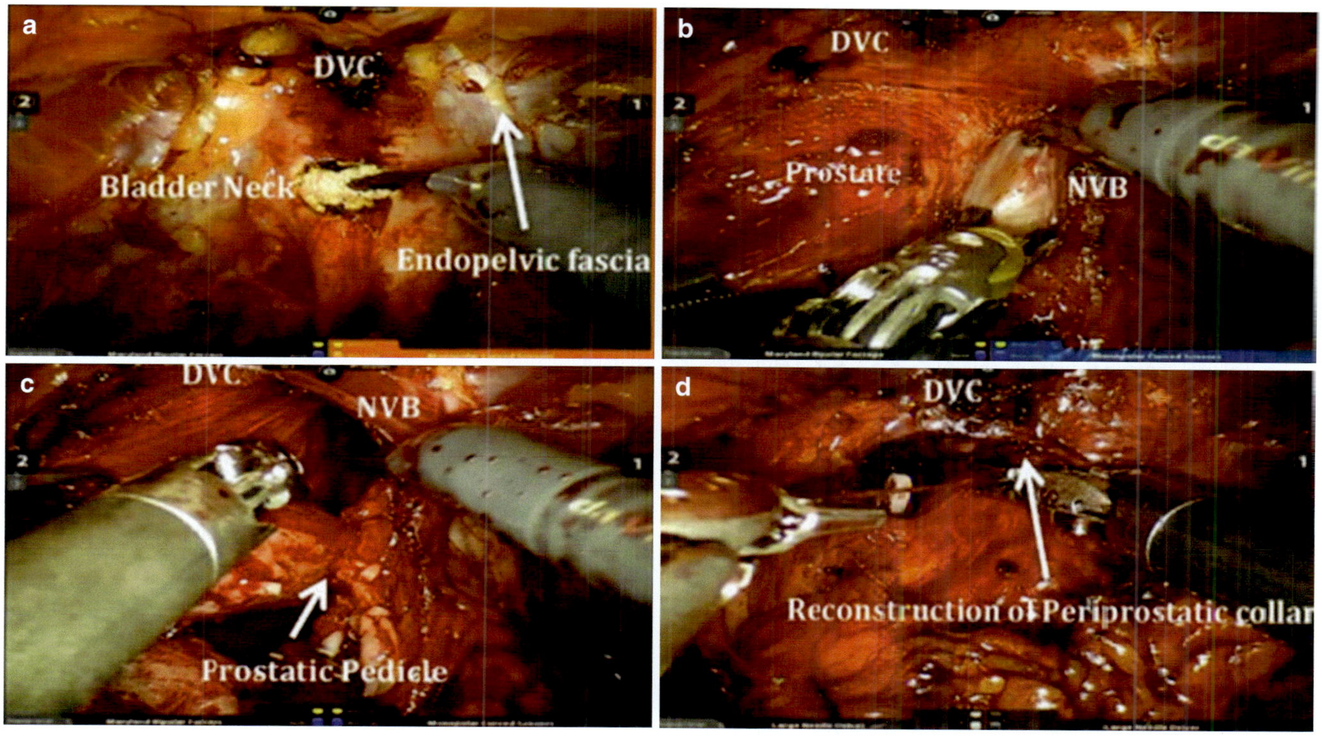

Fig. 10.4 Surgical steps. (**a**) The anterior bladder neck being incised with the endopelvic fascia and the dorsal venous complex preserved. (**b**) Retrograde release of the right neurovascular bundles. (**c**) Dissection of the right neurovascular bundles before ligation of the prostatic pedicle. (**d**) The endopelvic fascia and periprostatic collar are reconstructed with a continuous suture. (From de Carvalho PA, Barbosa JABA, Guglielmetti GB, Cordeiro MD, Rocco B, Nahas WC, Patel V, Coelho RF. Retrograde release of the neurovascular bundle with preservation of dorsal venous complex during robot-assisted radical prostatectomy: optimizing functional outcomes. Eur Urol. 2020;77(5):628–35. https://doi.org/10.1016/j.eururo.2018.07.003. Epub 2018 July 21. PMID: 30041833

Table 10.1 Potency outcomes (adequate for penetration) following RALP

Study	Patient N	Mean age	Follow up months	% Potent unilateral nerve spare	% Potent bilateral nerve spare	% Potent overall
Patel [26]	172	57.8	12	—	—	86
Chien [18]	56	58.9	12	44	50	40
Menon [37]	721	60.2	12	—	79.2	79.2
Ahlering [20]	58	57	3 24	40 80	29.3 93	32.1 89.7
Coelho [38]	128	62.6	3 12	—	—	69 86

note for surgeons developing in their expertise and considering adopting this method: where the margin for error is greater in such patients. The rates of continence immediately was 85%, and 98.4% at 1 year which in itself attests to the impact of preserving endopelvic and levator ani fascia; while the potency was 86% at 1 year with or without PDE5i. The addition of our experience in retrograde release of NVB is objectively superior to an antegrade approach as mentioned earlier [14].

Conclusion

Post RALP potency is dependent on numerous factors including age at surgery, preoperative potency status, co-morbidity (diabetes, hypertension, neurological disorder) and technique/extent of NS. Therefore it is incumbent on us to optimise the factor we can in the operating room: NS.

The reproducibility of outcomes can vary from surgeon to surgeon, such as the skill of an athlete to a rookie, where a similar series of movements will have different end results. Our aim is to share new strategies and combination of movements, with our retrograde NVB preservation. We also incorporated an anterior plane and DVC preservation, made possible with robotic technology. We have shown this helped patients in early recovery of continence and potency [32].

It is the senior authors' collective view that after 15,000 RALPs, the perfect outcome is still elusive but should be realised for patients in the future. Prospective evaluation of outcome data from differing techniques should be continuously reviewed, compared and readers should consider independent and thoughtful replication and development.

References

1. Ficarra V, Novara G, Artibani W, Cestari A, Galfano A, Graefen M, Guazzoni G, Guillonneau B, Menon M, Montorsi F, Patel V, Rassweiler J, Van Poppel H. Retropubic, laparoscopic, and robot-assisted radical prostatectomy: a systematic review and cumulative analysis of comparative studies. Eur Urol. 2009;55(5):1037–63. https://doi.org/10.1016/j.eururo.2009.01.036. Epub 2009 Jan 25. PMID: 19185977.
2. Rocco B, Matei DV, Melegari S, et al. Robotic vs open prostatectomy in a laparoscopically naive centre: a matched-pair analysis. BJU Int. 2009;104:991–5.
3. Porpiglia F, Morra I, Lucci Chiarissi M, et al. Randomised controlled trial comparing laparoscopic and robot-assisted radical prostatectomy. Eur Urol. 2013;63:606–14.
4. Walsh P, Donker P. Impotence following radical prostatectomy: insight into etiology and prevention. J Urol. 1982;128:492–7.
5. Reiner WG, Walsh PC. An anatomical approach to the surgical management of the dorsal vein and Santorini's plexus during radical retropubic surgery. J Urol. 1979;121(2):198–200.
6. Costello AJ, Brooks M, Cole OJ. Anatomical studies of the neurovascular bundle and cavernosal nerves. BJU Int. 2004;94(7):1071–6. PMID: 15541130. https://doi.org/10.1111/j.1464-410X.2004.05106.x.
7. Kalan S, Coughlin G, Palmer KJ, Patel VR. Robot-assisted laparoscopic radical prostatectomy: an athermal anterior approach to the seminal vesicle dissection. J Robot Surg. 2008;2(4):223–6. Epub 2008 Nov 19. PMID: 27637791. https://doi.org/10.1007/s11701-008-0117-3.
8. Fang J, Zheng Z, Wei H. Reconsideration of the anterior surgical plane of total mesorectal excision for rectal cancer. Dis Colon Rectum. 2019;62(5):639–41. PMID: 30964796. https://doi.org/10.1097/DCR.0000000000001358.
9. Lindsey I, Guy RJ, Warren BF, Mortensen NJM. Anatomy of Denonvilliers' fascia and pelvic nerves, impotence, and implications for the colorectal surgeon. Br J Surg. 2000;87(10):1288–99. https://doi.org/10.1046/j.1365-2168.2000.01542.x.
10. Castiglione F, Ralph DJ, Muneer A. Surgical techniques for managing post-prostatectomy erectile dysfunction. Curr Urol Rep. 2017;18(11):90. PMID: 28965315; PMCID: PMC5622908. https://doi.org/10.1007/s11934-017-0735-2.
11. Narayan P, Konety B, Aslam K, Aboseif S, Blumenfeld W, Tanagho E. Neuroanatomy of the external urethral sphincter: implications for urinary continence preservation during radical prostate surgery. J Urol. 1995;153(2):337–41. PMID: 7815577. https://doi.org/10.1097/00005392-199502000-00012.
12. Saenz de Tejada I, Goldstein I, Azadzoi K, et al. Impaired neurogenic and endothelium-mediated relaxation of penile smooth muscle from diabetic men with impotence. N Engl J Med. 1989;320:1025–30.
13. Lunacek A, Schwentner C, Fritsch H, et al. Anatomical radical retropubic prostatectomy 'curtain dissection' of the neurovascular bundle. BJU Int. 2005;95:1226–31.
14. Tewari A, Peabody JO, Fischer M, et al. An operative and anatomic study to help in nerve sparing during laparoscopic and robotic radical prostatectomy. Eur Urol. 2003;43:444–54.
15. Eichelberg C, Erbersdobler A, Michl U, Schlomm T, Salomon G, Graefen M, Huland H. Nerve distribution along the prostatic capsule. Eur Urol. 2006;51(1):105–10; discussion 110–1. PMID: 16814455. https://doi.org/10.1016/j.eururo.2006.05.038.
16. Menon M, Shrivastava A, Kaul S, Badani KK, Fumo M, Bhandari M, Peabody JO. Vattikuti Institute prostatectomy: contemporary technique and analysis of results. Eur Urol. 2007;51(3):648–58. https://doi.org/10.1016/j.eururo.2006.10.055.
17. Menon M, Shrivastava A, Bhandari M, Satyanarayana R, Siva S, Agarwal PK. Vattikuti Institute prostatectomy: technical modifications in 2009. Eur Urol. 2009;56(1):89–96. https://doi.org/10.1016/j.eururo.2009.04.032.
18. Chien GW, Mikhail AA, Orvieto MA, Zagaja GP, Sokoloff MH, Brendler CB, Shalhav AL. Modified clipless antegrade nerve preservation in robotic-assisted laparoscopic radical prostatectomy with validated sexual function evaluation. Urology. 2005;66(2):419–23. https://doi.org/10.1016/j.urology.2005.03.015.
19. Zorn KC, Gofrit ON, Orvieto MA, Mikhail AA, Zagaja GP, Shalhav AL. Robotic-assisted laparoscopic prostatectomy: functional and pathologic outcomes with interfascial nerve preservation. Eur Urol. 2007;51:755–62; discussion 763.
20. Ahlering TE, Eichel L, Chou D, Skarecky DW. Feasibility study for robotic radical prostatectomy cautery-free neurovascular bundle preservation. Urology. 2005;65:994–7.
21. Rodriguez E Jr, Finley DS, Skarecky D, Ahlering TE. Single institution 2-year patient reported validated sexual function outcomes after nerve sparing robot assisted radical prostatectomy. J Urol. 2009;181:259–63.
22. Walsh PC, Lepor H, Eggleston JC. Radical prostatectomy with preservation of sexual function: anatomical and pathological considerations. Prostate. 1983;4:473–85.
23. Rassweiler J, Seemann O, Hatzinger M, Schulze M, Frede T. Technical evolution of laparoscopic radical prostatectomy after 450 cases. J Endourol. 2003;17(3):143–54. https://doi.org/10.1089/089277903321618707.
24. Guillonneau B, Vallancien G. Laparoscopic radical prostatectomy: the montsouris technique. J Urol. 2000;163(6):1643–9. https://doi.org/10.1016/s0022-5347(05)67512-x.
25. Walsh PC. Anatomic radical prostatectomy: evolution of the surgical technique. J Urol. 1998;160:2418–24.
26. Ko YH, Coelho RF, Sivaraman A, Schatloff O, Chauhan S, Abdul-Muhsin HM, et al. Retrograde versus antegrade nerve sparing during robot-assisted radical prostatectomy: which is better for achieving early functional recovery? Eur Urol. 2013;63(1):169–77. https://doi.org/10.1016/j.eururo.2012.09.051.
27. Kowalczyk KJ, Huang AC, Hevelone ND, et al. Stepwise approach for nerve sparing without countertraction during robot-assisted radical prostatectomy: technique and outcomes. Eur Urol. 2011;60:536–47.
28. Schatloff O, Chauhan S, Sivaraman A, Kameh D, Palmer KJ, Patel VR. Anatomic grading of nerve sparing during robot-assisted radical prostatectomy. Eur Urol. 2012;61(4):796–802. https://doi.org/10.1016/j.eururo.2011.12.048.
29. Eichelberg C, Erbersdobler A, Michl U, et al. Nerve distribution along the prostatic capsule. Eur Urol. 2007;51:105–11.
30. Kaiho Y, Nakagawa H, Saito H, et al. Nerves at the ventral prostatic capsule contribute to erectile function: initial electrophysiological assessment in humans. Eur Urol. 2009;55(1):148–54. https://doi.org/10.1016/j.eururo.2008.09.022.
31. Takenaka A, Soga H, Hinata N, et al. Classification of the distribution of cavernous nerve fibers around the prostate by intraoperative electrical stimulation during laparoscopic radical prostatectomy. Int J Impot Res. 2011;23:56–61. https://doi.org/10.1038/ijir.2011.4.
32. Lee SE, Hong SK, Han JH, Han BK, Yu JH, Jeong SJ, et al. Significance of neurovascular bundle formation observed on preoperative magnetic resonance imaging regarding postoperative erectile function after nerve-sparing radical retropubic prostatectomy. Urology. 2007;69:510–4.
33. Costello AJ, Dowdle BW, Namdarian B, Pedersen J, Murphy DG. Immunohistochemical study of the cavernous nerves in the periprostatic region. BJU Int. 2010;107(8):1210–5. https://doi.org/10.1111/j.1464-410x.2010.09711.x.

34. Ganzer R, Stolzenburg JU, Neuhaus J, Weber F, Burger M, Brundl J. Is the striated urethral sphincter at risk by standard suture ligation of the dorsal vascular complex in radical prostatectomy? An anatomic study. Urology. 2014;84:1453–8.
35. Takenaka A, Hara R, Soga H, Murakami G, Fujisawa M. A novel technique for approaching the endopelvic fascia in retropubic radical prostatectomy, based on an anatomical study of fixed and fresh cadavers. BJU Int. 2005;95:766–71.
36. Moschovas MC, Bhat S, Onol FF, Rogers T, Roof S, Mazzone E, et al. Modified apical dissection and lateral prostatic fascia preservation improves early postoperative functional recovery in robotic-assisted laparoscopic radical prostatectomy: results from a propensity score-matched analysis. Eur Urol. 2020;78(6):875–84. https://doi.org/10.1016/j.eururo.2020.05.041.
37. Badani KK, Kaul S, Menon M. Evolution of robotic radical prostatectomy: assessment after 2766 procedures. Cancer. 2007;110:1951–8.
38. de Carvalho PA, Barbosa JABA, Guglielmetti GB, Cordeiro MD, Rocco B, Nahas WC, Patel V, Coelho RF. Retrograde release of the neurovascular bundle with preservation of dorsal venous complex during robot-assisted radical prostatectomy: optimizing functional outcomes. Eur Urol. 2020;77(5):628–35. Epub 2018 July 21. PMID: 30041833. https://doi.org/10.1016/j.eururo.2018.07.003.

The Hood Technique for Robotic-Assisted Radical Prostatectomy: Preserving Vital Structures in the Space of Retzius and the Pouch of Douglas

11

Ash Tewari, Vinayak Wagaskar, Parita Ratnani, Sneha Parekh, Adriana Pedraza, and Bhavya Shukla

Introduction

Robotic-assisted radical prostatectomy (RARP) is the most common treatment for managing localized prostate cancer [1]. The Hood technique for RARP is unique in helping to accomplish three important but competing goals: cancer control, urinary continence, and recovery of sexual function [2]. While cancer control is the primary goal for prostate cancer treatment, preserving and providing better quality of life are equally important. Of the two most significant post-RARP quality-of-life issues, urinary incontinence and sexual dysfunction, the former has had a declining impact on survivorship as, over time, several intra-operative technical modifications have optimized continence after robotic-assisted radical prostatectomy [3]. In this chapter, we describe the novel Hood technique which was developed to help achieve early and better continence outcomes post-RARP.

The Anatomical and Functional Foundations of Continence

Urinary continence in men depends on adequate bladder function and the urethral sphincter complex [4]. After surgery, return of continence is influenced by the optimal angulation and support of the vesicourethral junction; the length of the membranous urethra; and bladder compliance, along with the coordinated muscular contraction of the sphincter complex; and preservation of the neural hammock [5]

A. Tewari (✉) · V. Wagaskar · P. Ratnani · S. Parekh · A. Pedraza
B. Shukla
Department of Urology, Icahn School of Medicine at Mount Sinai Hospital, New York, NY, USA
e-mail: ashtewari@mountsinai.org; parita.ratnani@mountsinai.org; sneha.parekh@mountsinai.org; Adriana.PedrazaBermeo@mountsinai.org; bhavya.shukla@mountsinai.org

Innervation of the Urethral Sphincter

Different neural pathway interactions allow coordinated responses between the bladder and the urinary sphincters. During the storage phase, the bladder maintains lower filling pressure through the activation of potassium channels that stimulate relaxation in response to the distention of the bladder wall. Additionally, the neurotransmitter norepinephrine (NE) is released by sympathetic fibers in the hypogastric nerve. NE acts on B3 adrenergic receptors potentiating relaxation of the detrusor muscle, and at the same time stimulating alpha-1 adrenergic receptors in the urethra to contract its smooth muscle. The pudendal nerve simultaneously releases Ach, which acts on nicotinic receptors to sustain the tonic contraction of the external urethral sphincter (EUS) [6]. Once the mechanoreceptors detect the fullness of the bladder, afferent myelinated Aδ and unmyelinated C-fibers within the pelvic nerve reach the maximal frequency of depolarization and transmit this information to the cortical centers [7]. Next, the pontine micturition center (PMC) triggers the release of ACh by the parasympathetic fibers, which stimulate muscarinic (M3) receptors to contract the detrusor smooth muscle and initiate the micturition process. Meanwhile, nitric oxide (NO) is released to induce bladder neck and urethral relaxation, and the sympathetic system is inhibited [8].

The pelvic plexus is a fan-like structure located in the retroperitoneum between the bladder and the rectum. It is formed by sympathetic fibers from the hypogastric nerve and parasympathetic fibers from the pelvic splanchnic nerve. Somatic fibers originating from cell bodies of the sacral spinal cord (S2–S4) also travel within the pelvic plexus [8]. The exact anatomy of the periprostatic nerves is unknown. However, different studies have shown a complex distribution that is not limited to the posterolateral position. In fact, a trizonal "neural hammock" was described by Tewari and colleagues, to better approach these structures [9]. This ham-

S. Ren et al. (eds.), *Robot-Assisted Radical Prostatectomy*, https://doi.org/10.1007/978-3-031-05855-4_11

mock is composed of the proximal neurovascular plate (PNP) or pelvic plexus, the predominant neurovascular bundle (PNB), and the accessory neural pathways (ANP). Preservation of the periprostatic nerves plays a key role in urinary continence given the autonomic and somatic innervation of the urethral sphincter (US).

Somatic innervation of the US travels through the pudendal nerve or the pelvic plexus. Two pudendal pathways have been described, the extrapelvic and intrapelvic branches. Extrapelvic fibers penetrate the prostatic urethra at 9–12 o'clock and 1–3 o'clock close to the prostatic apex, while the intrapelvic branches of the pudendal nerve penetrate the EUS at 5 and 7 o'clock. Some somatic fibers run with the autonomic nerves mainly in the posterior surface of the bladder and the anterolateral surface of the US [5].

Autonomic innervation of the US travels through the posteromedial aspect of the prostatic apex and through the rectourethral muscle [10]. Careful dissection of this complex "neural hammock" poses a challenge for achieving optimal functional outcomes while balancing the risk of tumoral extracapsular extension.

The Hood technique, however, which allows us to preserve the anterolateral covering structures of the prostate, including the detrusor apron, puboprostatic ligaments, and associated fascia, helps avoid dissection of the majority of the nerves running postero-laterally and which are intermingled between the layers of fascia [2]. Hence, we are able to preserve the antero-lateral structures that have a major anatomic role in and which provide structural support for, the mechanisms of sphincter contraction and relaxation during continence.

Support Structures of the Sphincter Complex

Paraurethral skeletal and fibrous structures support the prostatic musculoligamentous complex, which comprises muscles like the levator ani and puboperinealis. Fibrous structures, including Retzius fibrous attachments, the detrusor apron, the arcus tendineus, the endopelvic fascia, the periprostatic fascia, puboprostatic ligaments, Denonvilliers' fascia, urethropelvic ligaments, and the pelvic bones also play important roles in support of the sphincter complex [11].

The periprostatic fascia is composed mainly of two layers known as the (lateral/parietal) levator ani fascia and the (medial/visceral) prostatic fascia. Anteriorly, the fascia covers the detrusor apron; the dorsal venous complex (DVC) fuses with the anterior fibromuscular stroma (AFMS) in the midline, fuses at the lateral aspect of the bladder and prostate, forms the Arcus tendineus, and posteriorly covers the seminal vesicles closely forming the Denonvilliers' fascia. Posteriorly at the midline, the periprostatic fascia is in close conjunction with the prostate capsule. Posterolaterally, it has no significant adherence. The fascia is a dual/multi-layered entity with the neurovascular bundle (NVB) running between these layers. The parietal layer mainly covers the levator ani muscle forming the levator ani fascia lateral to the NVB and the inner visceral layer/prostatic fascia which is medial to the NVB and covers the underlying prostate capsule [12].

The puboprostatic ligaments are pyramid shaped condensations of the endopelvic fascia extending from the pubic bone and attaching to the prostate, bladder, and membranous urethra leading to urethral stability. They are composed of a pubourethral component which runs deep from the symphysis pubis and attaches to the membranous urethra; a puboprostatic component which merges with the anterior prostatic capsule; a flimsy pubovesical section which travels to the anterior aspect of the bladder in alignment with muscle fibers of the bladder wall and constitutes the so-called detrusor apron; and a curved sickle-shaped extension, which fuses with the arcus tendinous [13].

The arcus tendineus is a lateral fibrous thickening of endopelvic fascia extending from the puboprostatic ligaments to the ischial spine.

The puboperinealis is a paired muscle that originates from the pubis, flanks the prostatic-urethral junction, and terminates at the perineal body, the deep part of the external anal sphincter and bulbospongiosus muscles. The puboperinealis acts as a muscular hammock supporting the urethra posteriorly and serving as a dynamic sling responsible for the quick-stop phenomenon of urination. During surgery, it is important to identify the long pelvic nerve or levator ani nerve, which innervates the puboperinealis muscle [13].

The Denonvilliers' fascia extends posteriorly covering the seminal vesicles and extending distally to the prostatic apex, ending at the prostatic-urethral junction. The Denonvilliers' fascia separates the posterior bladder from the rectum.

The detrusor apron is a dense interwoven network composed of three smooth muscle layers which cover the bladder circumferentially: an inner longitudinal layer, a middle circular layer, and an outer longitudinal layer [14]. Some anterior fibers of the outer longitudinal muscle layer travel anteriorly to the pubic bone covering the prostate anterolaterally to form the detrusor apron which merges with the puboprostatic ligaments, contributing to the sling continence mechanism. Preservation of the detrusor apron in RARP is important for better functional outcome. Additionally, a layer of the detrusor apron contributes to the formation of the anterior fibromuscular stroma and another layer joins the fascial sheath of the dorsal venous complex.

The Urethral Sphincter Complex

The urethral sphincter is a complex of muscles surrounding the urethra and controlling the flow of urine.

The proximal urethral (internal) sphincter or vesical sphincter is ring-shaped muscular tissue under involuntary control and which is compromised during surgery at the vesico-prostatic junction.

The distal urethral (external) sphincter at the prostato-urethral junction is a complex of external rhabdosphincter and inner lissosphincter muscles surrounding the membranous urethra. The external sphincter is under voluntary control and is innervated by somatic pudendal nerves originating from the S2, S3, and S4 sacral nerve roots.

The external rhabdosphincter has outer striated fibers which become sparse posteriorly where the fibrous median raphe (the most anterior part of the perineal body) can be identified. Some of its anterior fibers are known to merge with the supporting fibrous structures that flank the urethra, providing continence through tonic contraction along with the puboperinealis sling through the quick-stop mechanism. Rabdosphincter contractions result in a kind of anterior loop rather than a true circumferential constriction of the urethra. Rabdosphinchter fibers extend up to the prostatic apex with inter-individual variability in the overlap of prostatic tissue that covers the sphincter circumferentially, symmetrically bilaterally, asymmetrically unilaterally, anteriorly only, or posteriorly only, or ending bluntly above the sphincter.

The inner smooth muscle layer (the lissosphincter) consists of outer circular and inner longitudinal muscle fibers extending up to the verumontanum/seminal colliculus making preservation of longer urethral length important for better functional outcome [15].

The membranous urethra, the narrowest part of the urethra, connects the prostatic and bulbar urethra extending from the prostatic apex and piercing the urogenital diaphragm. The membranous and prostatic urethra, together with the bladder neck, form a high-resistance channel. Preserving longer membranous urethral length (MUL) helps achieve early continence post RARP [16].

The Role of the Vesicle Angle in Continence

The vesical angle is also a strong predictor of urinary continence after surgery. A recent study found that bladder neck angle fewer than 100°, measured between the bladder neck and the bilateral margin over the pelvic inlet, is related to poor urinary continence outcomes [17]. It has been hypothesized that a narrow vesical angle may also decrease bladder compliance impacting intravesical pressure. Total anatomic reconstruction to provide anterior and posterior support to the sphincter complex has been described with a finding of better rates of urinary continence recovery at 1, 6, 12, and 24 weeks after surgery [18]. MRI findings in patients before and after surgery have found a positive association between postoperative membranous urethral length and the depth of urethrovesical junction with urinary continence recovery, the latter measured as the craniocaudal distance from the most proximal margin of the symphysis pubis to the level of the urethrovesical junction [19].

The Pathophysiology of Post-Radical Prostatectomy Urinary Incontinence (PPI)

Urinary incontinence following radical prostatectomy is attributed to sphincter and/or bladder dysfunction. Sphincter dysfunction, also known as intrinsic sphincter deficiency, is caused by injury to the sphincter mechanism during surgery. Sphincter dysfunction commonly presents as stress urinary incontinence and is the most common form of post-radical prostatectomy urinary incontinence (PPI) [20]. Bladder mobilization and incision of the arcus tendineus render the urethra hypermobile, descending from the pelvic floor. Shortening or thinning of the membranous urethra during partial excision of the sphincter, or devascularization due to apical tumor location, damage sphincter mechanisms. Additionally, the posterior connections of the puboperinealis sling are disrupted during posterior apical dissection causing weakness in the dynamic sling mechanism resulting in sphincter dysfunction [21]. Detrusor instability and decreased bladder compliance are associated with increases in detrusor pressure in urine storage resulting in bladder dysfunction and PPI. Classically, bladder dysfunction presents as incontinence urgency. Probable mechanisms of bladder dysfunction include disruption of anterior bladder wall fixations resulting in a collapsed bladder, and damage to the bladder nerve supply during bladder neck and seminal vesicle dissection. In addition, loss of retro trigonal support causes weakness at the posterior half of the bladder neck [22].

The "Hood" Concept

The last decade has seen efforts, led by Dr. A. Massimo Bocciardi, to preserve structures in the space of Retzius [23]. This approach preserves the entire space of Retzius and its contents by approaching the prostate and bladder neck through the pouch of Douglas. Convincing data provide support for the impact of this approach on the early return of

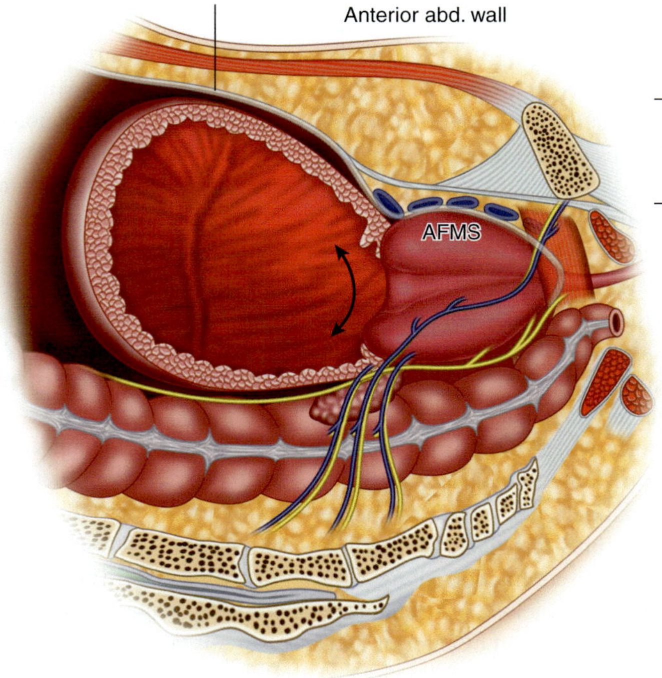

Fig. 11.1 A sketch demonstrating Hood surgical anatomy. Anatomical components of the hood surround and safeguard the membranous urethra and external urethral sphincter. *Abbreviations*: *AFMS* anterior fibromuscular stroma, *DA* detrusor apron, *Pubo P ligament* pubo-perinealis muscle and accompanying ligament, *DVC* deep venous complex, *Plane of tunnel* plane of development of retropubic space

continence, and many surgeons have embraced the space of Retzius preservation technique for robotic-assisted prostatectomy. While there is considerable enthusiasm for this approach, the majority of robotic surgeons continue to perform robotic prostatectomy from the anterior aspect; more than one million such surgeries have been performed. Surgeons who prefer the anterior approach believe it to be a more versatile technique allowing for greater exposure by providing the ability to visualize the interior of the bladder (ureteric orifices and median lobes); perform simultaneous lymph nodal dissection; tailor grades of nerve sparing through access to the peri-prostatic space to place a suprapubic catheter (if chosen) with a direct view without violating the pouch of Douglas where most of the neurovascular tissue travels to the penile and pelvic structures.

To address this concern, our team sought to modify the anterior approach to capture the benefits of space of Retzius preservation while maintaining the advantages of the conventional anterior approach. We made modifications to the technique, defined and characterized the structures that contribute to early continence following the space of Retzius sparing approach, reviewed the results of this modification in 272 cases, and compared these results with our traditional anterior approach. Our novel Hood technique, inspired by the work of Dr. Robert Myers, preserves tissue after prostate removal takes on the appearance of a "hood" comprises of the detrusor apron, arcus tendineus, puboprostatic ligaments, anterior vessels, and some fibers of the detrusor muscle [14]. This hood surrounds and safeguards the membranous urethra, the external sphincter, and supportive structures (Fig. 11.1).

The Hood Surgical Technique

Because the Hood technique involves the anterior supporting structures, we excluded men whose biopsy was positive at the anterior prostate or whose pre-operative multiparametric Magnetic resonance imaging (MRI) showed an anterior prostatic lesion. While not a formal exclusion criterion for the technique, patients who received prior hormonal treatment or radiotherapy for prostate cancer were also excluded from our study on the Hood technique.

Surgical Steps

A four-arm da Vinci Xi System (Intuitive Surgical-ISRG, Sunnyvale, CA, USA) was used to perform the Hood technique for robot-assisted radical prostatectomy.

1. Position and port placement. The patient was placed in the steep Trendelenberg position.

   Pneumoperitoneum was induced by a Veress needle. Six laparoscopic trocars were placed as previously published [13].

2. Development of the retropubic space. Using a 0° optic camera lens, the peritoneum was incised with an inverted U-shaped incision beginning high at the midline median-to-medial umbilical ligaments. We performed blunt and sharp dissection to expose the bladder and anterior prostate without exposing the puboprostatic ligaments (Fig. 11.2).
3. Bladder neck transection. The bladder neck was incised and deepened until the Foley catheter was seen (Fig. 11.3). Visualization of the Foley catheter ensured that the anterior bladder neck had been properly incised. The Foley catheter was grasped by the tip with firm anterior traction. Using the shaft of the catheter as a landmark, the mucosa at the posterior bladder neck was incised precisely. We then developed a plane behind the posterior wall of the bladder neck exposing a consistent fibromuscular layer, known as "the retrotrigonal layer" [24] (Fig. 11.4). Cutting this layer exposed the vasa and the seminal vesicles.
4. Vas deferens and seminal vesicles dissection. The vas deferens were lifted one at time and dissected using an athermal technique to clip and cut the ends. The cut ends were then lifted up by the fourth arm of the robot. Then, we created a plane between the seminal vesicles and the surrounding fascia, which is called "the median avascular plane" (Fig. 11.5). This plane was followed proximally to identify the arteries that enter the seminal vesicles. These vesicles were cut using clips and sharp dissection. Every attempt was made to preserve the neurovascular bundles

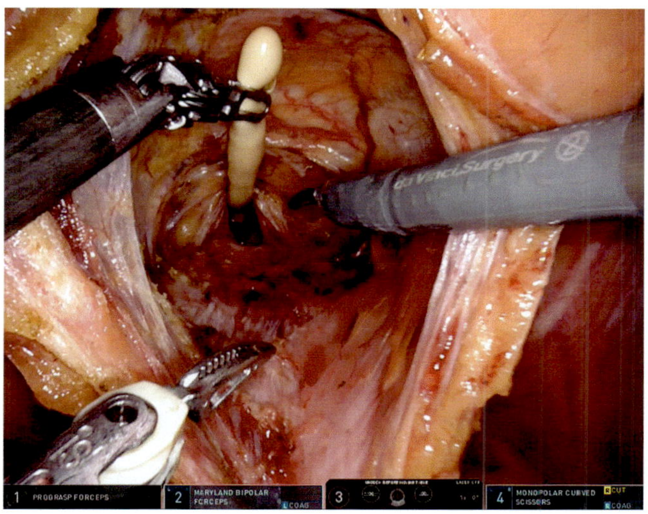

Fig. 11.2 Development of the retropubic space

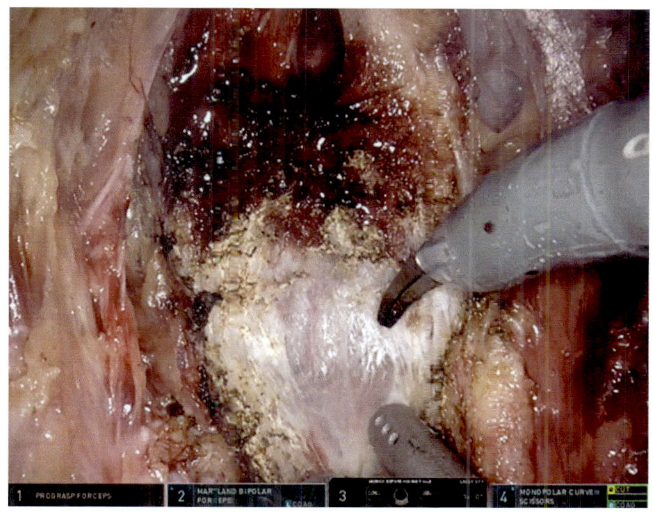

Fig. 11.4 Development of the retro-trigonal layer

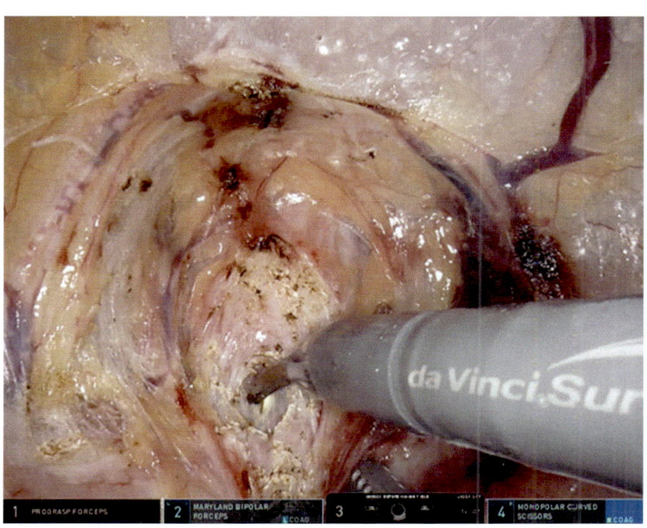

Fig. 11.3 Bladder neck dissection

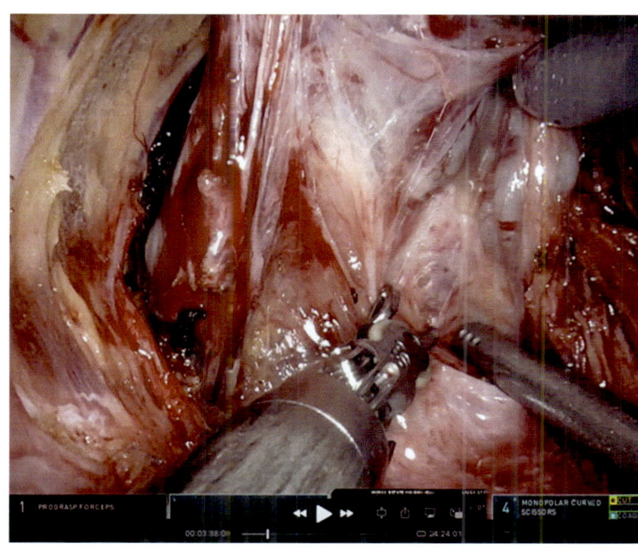

Fig. 11.5 Dissection of seminal vesicles. Development of medial avascular plane

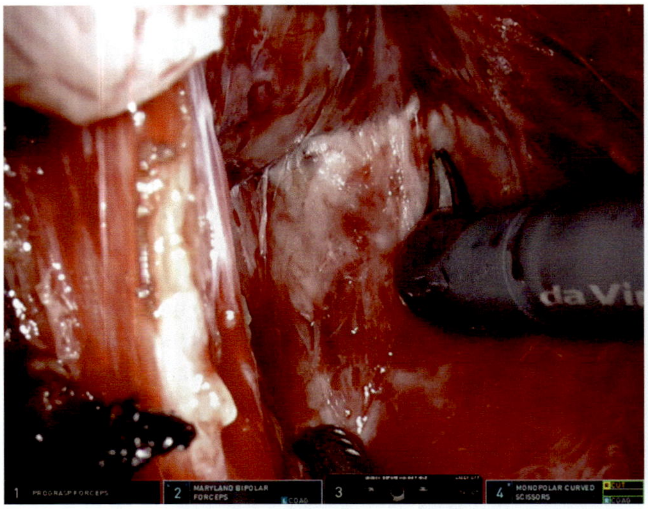

Fig. 11.6 Athermal plane created between prostate capsule and Denonvilliers' fascia

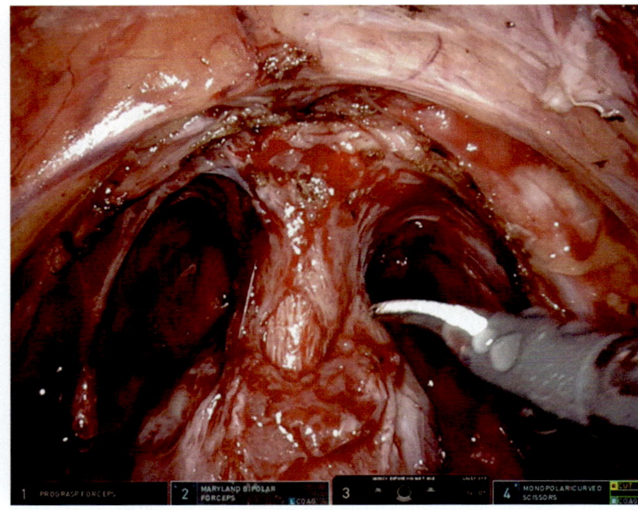

Fig. 11.7 Circumferential apical dissection

which are lateral to the seminal vesicles. Both the seminal vesicles and vas deferens were then pulled upwards.

5. Lateral pedicle control. A plane was created between the prostatic capsule and Denonvilliers' fascia athermally by sharp and blunt dissection, proceeding distally toward the apex and laterally on either side allowing us to access the lateral attachments where the perforating arteries enter the prostatic capsule (Fig. 11.6). We sharply cut these attachments and developed a plane between the capsule and the medial aspect of the pedicular vessels.
6. Circumferential apical dissection. The prostate was lifted anteriorly towards the pubic symphysis. The camera lens was changed to 30° optic with upward direction. Using blunt dissection with monopolar scissors and retracting the apex from the urethra, we were able to gain 1–2 mm of ventral membranous urethral length prior to transection. The camera lens was changed again to 0° optic. The prostate was retracted to one side and anterolateral dissection was performed with the goal of preserving the urethral sphincter (Fig. 11.7). This process was repeated on the contralateral side.
7. Control of the dorsal venous complex. The dorsal venous complex was ligated using a 2-0 Vicryl suture (Fig. 11.8) in continuous fashion followed by urethropexy.
8. Development of "hood" and urethral transection. A plane was developed between the detrusor apron and the anterior fibromuscular layer of prostate. This plane was followed until we reached the prostatic apex. Using blunt dissection, we then mobilized the dorsal membranous urethral length. With a direct view, the anterior urethra was sharply cut and the prostate was freed. The specimen was then sent to Surgical Pathology where the margins were inked and examined under a microscope to assess the extra-capsular extension (Fig. 11.9).

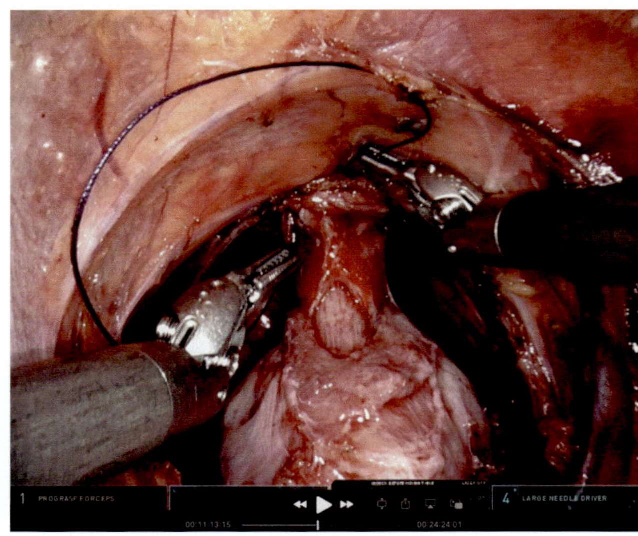

Fig. 11.8 Control of dorsal venous complex

9. Total anatomical reconstruction and anastomosis. The first step in posterior reconstruction was creating a "mattress" for anastomosis using V-lock sutures. This mattress consisted of the Denonvilliers' musculo fascial plate and the posterior bladder neck (Fig. 11.10). Two-layer bladder neck reconstruction was then performed using V-lock sutures. Watertight, tension-free Urethro-vesical anastomosis was performed using barbed sutures (Fig. 11.11). The arcus tendineus was sutured to partial thickness bites of the detrusor muscle which aided in stabilizing and positioning the vesico-urethral junction.

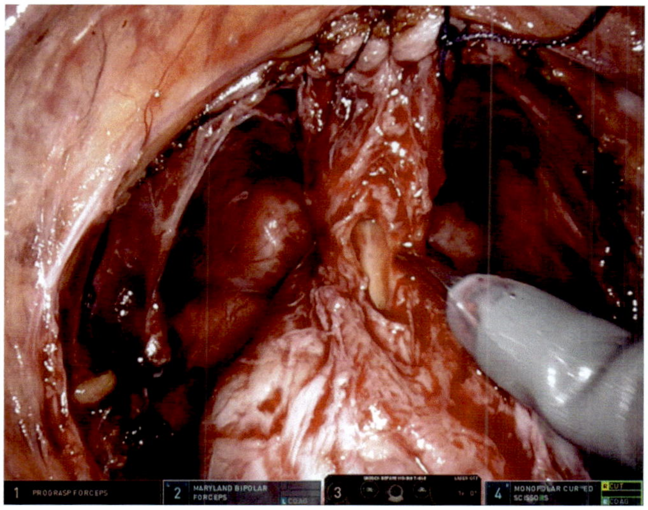

Fig. 11.9 Urethral transection

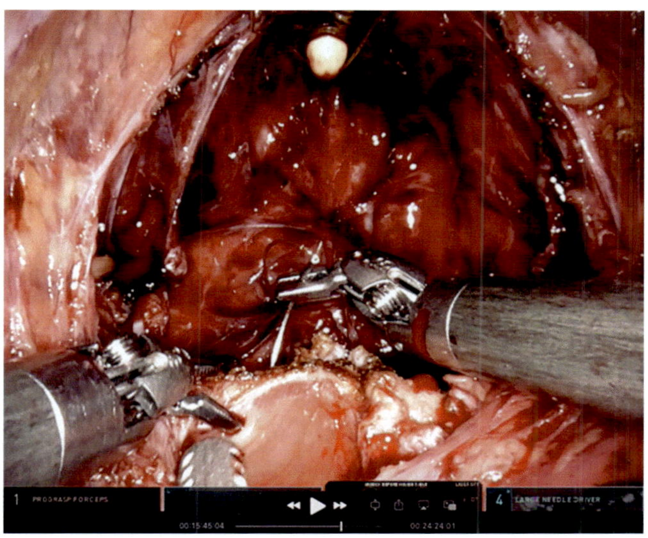

Fig. 11.10 Posterior reconstruction. Consists of the Denonvilliers' musculofascial plate and the posterior bladder neck

Results

We compared our novel "Hood" technique with the "non-Hood" technique for RARP in 330 consecutive patients. The non-Hood technique was performed in patients who were not eligible for the Hood technique (as per the exclusion criteria described above). We did not preserve the "hood" structures in any of the non-Hood technique patients. Of the 330 patients who underwent RARP, 272 patients underwent the Hood technique and 58 patients underwent the non-Hood technique. Preoperative, intraoperative, and oncological outcomes of the study population are summarized in Table 11.1. The median age of the patients was 63 and 67 years for the Hood-technique and

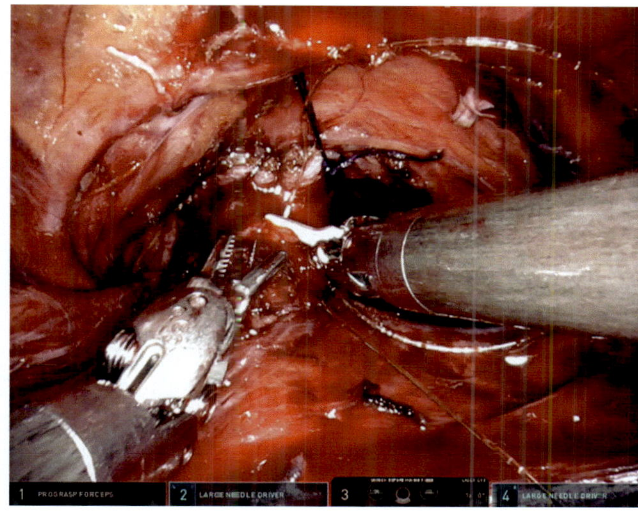

Fig. 11.11 Urethro-vesical anastomosis

Table 11.1 Preoperative and intraoperative parameters and surgical pathology outcomes of the study population

	Overall N = 330 (%)	Non-Hood N = 58 (%)	Hood N = 272 (%)	P value
Median age in years [IQR]	64 (59, 69)	67 (62, 70)	63 (58, 68)	0.001
Median BMI in kg/m² [IQR]	27 (25, 29)	27(24, 29)	27 (25, 29)	0.9
PSA, ng/mL [IQR]	5.8 (4.5, 8.7)	7.5 (5.1, 15.0)	5.7 (4.5, 8.0)	0.001
PSA density [IQR]	0.1 (0.1, 0.2)	0.1 (0.1, 0.3)	0.1 (0.1, 0.2)	0.007
Prostate volume in mL [IQR]	52 (42, 65)	51 (43, 66)	52 (40, 65)	0.6
cT stage, n				0.0004
T1	167 (51)	17 (29)	150 (55)	
T2	163 (49)	41 (71)	122 (45)	
Nerve sparing pattern, n				<0.0001
Bilateral	249 (67)	28 (47)	22[illegible] (71)	
Monolateral	50 (24)	30 (27)	51 (23)	
Non-nerve sparing	31 (9)	15 (26)	16 (6)	
Final pathology ISUP GGG				<0.0001
1	45 (14%)	3 (5%)	42 (15%)	
2	156 (47%)	13 (22%)	143 (53%)	
3	85 (26%)	24 (41%)	61 (22%)	
4	9 (3%)	4 (8%)	5 (2%)	
5	35 (10)	14 (24)	21 (8%)	
pTNM stage, n				0.045
T2N0	252 (76%)	36 (62%)	215 (79%)	
T2N1	4 (1%)	0 (0)	4 (2%)	
T3N0	61 (18%)	17 (29%)	44 (16%)	
T3N1	13 (5%)	5 (9%)	8 (3%)	
Surgical margins				0.004
Negative	313 (95%)	50 (86%)	263 (97%)	
Positive	17 (5%)	8 (14%)	9 (3%)	

IQR interquartile range, *BMI* body mass index, *PSA* prostate specific antigen, *ISUP* International Society on Urologic Pathology Gleason grading group, *pTNM stage* pathological tumor, node and metastases stage

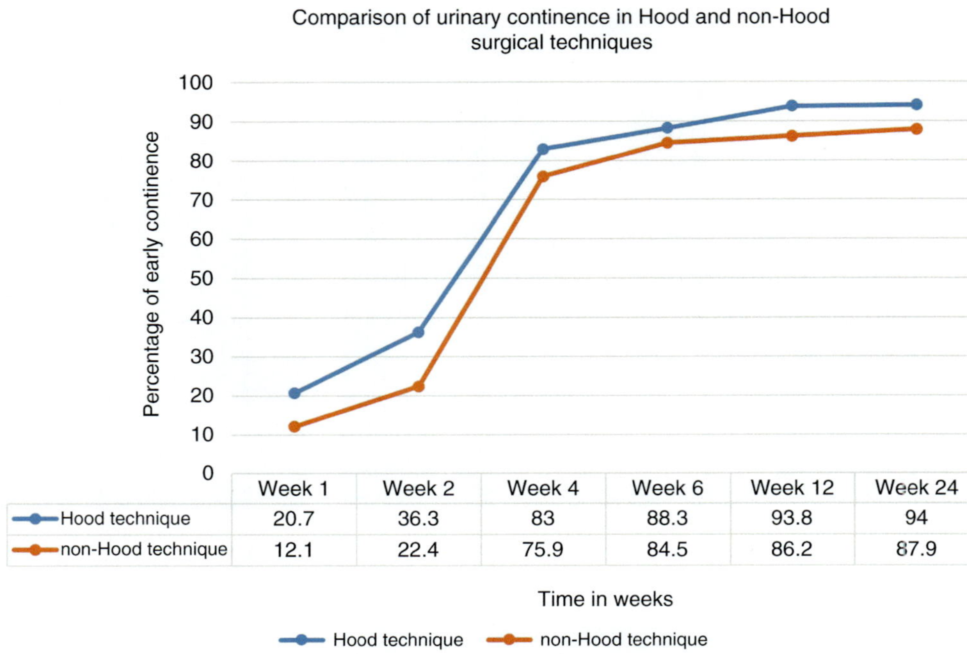

Fig. 11.12 Comparison of urinary continence rates of the hood technique and non-hood technique

non-Hood technique patients, respectively. Median body mass index was 27 for both groups. Median PSA was 5.7 ng/dL and 7.5 ng/dL for Hood-technique and non-Hood technique patients, respectively; median prostate volume was 52 and 51 cc for Hood-technique and non-Hood technique patients, respectively. Bilateral nerve sparing, monolateral nerve sparing, and non-nerve sparing was performed in 71%, 23%, and 6% patients of Hood-technique patients, respectively, and 47%, 27%, and 26% patients of non-Hood technique patients, respectively. Final pathology International Society of Urologic Pathology (ISUP) Gleason grades of 1, 2, 3, 4 and 5 were seen in 15%, 53%, 22%, 2%, and 8% of patients who underwent the Hood technique, while ISUP Gleason grades 1, 2, 3, 4 and 5 were seen in 5%, 22%, 14%, 8%, and 24% patients who underwent the non-Hood technique.

Effect of Technique on Urinary Continence (Fig. 11.12)

Patients were followed up 1, 2, 4, 6 and 12 weeks after catheter removal (which was performed at 1 week) as a part of standard protocol and additional third-party telephone interviews were conducted by urology fellow (V.G.W.). Patients were considered continent if they were pad free for 24 h. Urinary continence data has been verified independently by two other co-authors (U.F. and P.T.).

The continence rates with Hood technique at 1, 2, 4, 6, 12 and 24 weeks after catheter removal were 21%, 36%, 83%, 88%, 93% and 94% while continence rates with non-Hood technique at 1, 2, 4, 6, 12 and 24 weeks after catheter removal were 12%, 22%, 76%, 85%, 86% and 88% at 1, 2, 4, 6, 12 and 24 weeks after catheter removal.

Conclusion

The Hood technique has proven to achieve early return of continence, better functional outcomes, and improved quality of life and survival. The detrusor apron, puboprostatic ligaments, and surrounding fascia are the major components of the "hood," providing attachment along the bladder, prostate, and urethra to the surrounding pelvic muscles and bone. The anatomic and functional roles of all of these "hood" structures have an impact on the mechanism of continence through coordinated bladder and urethral sphincter contractions and relaxation. The Hood technique allows for preservation of these important structures, while providing optimal post-operative cancer-free outcomes, functional outcomes, and better quality of life and survival.

Acknowledgement We thank Ms. Sima Rabinowitz for editorial assistance.

Conflicts of Interest None.

References

1. Sandoval Salinas C, González Rangel AL, Cataño Cataño JG, Fuentes Pachón JC, Castillo Londoño JS. Efficacy of robotic-assisted prostatectomy in localized prostate cancer: a systematic review of clinical trials. Adv Urol. 2013;2013:105651.
2. Wagaskar VG, Mittal A, Sobotka S, Ratnani P, Lantz A, Falagario UG, et al. Hood technique for robotic radical prostatectomy-preserving periurethral anatomical structures in the space of Retzius and sparing the pouch of Douglas, enabling early return of continence without compromising surgical margin rates. Eur Urol. 2021;80(2):213–21.
3. Hwang J, Kim B, Uchio E. Improving urinary continence after radical prostatectomy: review of surgical modifications. Korean J Urol. 2009;50:935–41.
4. Golomb J, Chertin B, Mor Y. Anatomy of urinary continence and neurogenic incontinence. Therapy. 2009;6(2):151–5.
5. Bessede T, Sooriakumaran P, Takenaka A, Tewari A. Neural supply of the male urethral sphincter: comprehensive anatomical review and implications for continence recovery after radical prostatectomy. World J Urol. 2017;35(4):549–6.
6. Ikeda Y. Neurophysiological control of urinary bladder storage and voiding—functional changes through development and pathology. Pediatr Nephrol. 2021;36(5):1041–52.
7. Groat W, Yoshimura N. Afferent nerve regulation of bladder function in health and disease. Handb Exp Pharmacol. 2009;194:91–138.
8. Groat W, Yoshimura N. Anatomy and physiology of the lower urinary tract. Handb Clin Neurol. 2015;130:61–108.
9. Srivastava A, Grover S, Sooriakumaran P, Tan G, Takenaka A, Tewari AK. Neuroanatomic basis for traction-free preservation of the neural hammock during athermal robotic radical prostatectomy. Curr Opin Urol. 2011;21(1):49–59.
10. Nyangoh Timoh K, Moszkowicz D, Creze M, Zaitouna M, Felber M, Lebacle C, et al. The male external urethral sphincter is autonomically innervated. Clin Anat. 2021;34(2):263–71.
11. Reeves F, Everaerts W, Murphy DG, Costello A. Chapter 29: The surgical anatomy of the prostate. In: Mydlo JH, Godec CJ, editors. Prostate cancer. 2nd ed. San Diego: Academic; 2016. p. 253–63.
12. Gandaglia G, Briganti A, Suardi N, Gallina A, Cucchiara V, Vizziello D, et al. Fascial layers in nerve sparing robot-assisted radical prostatectomy. Urol Pract. 2014;1(2):86–91.
13. Takenaka A, Tewari AK. Anatomical basis for carrying out a state-of-the-art radical prostatectomy. Int J Urol. 2012;19(1):7–19.
14. Myers RP. Detrusor apron, associated vascular plexus, and avascular plane: relevance to radical retropubic prostatectomy—anatomic and surgical commentary. Urology. 2002;59(4):472–9.
15. Koraitim MM. The male urethral sphincter complex revisited: an anatomical concept and its physiological correlate. J Urol. 2008;179(5):1683–9.
16. Cho DS, Choo SH, Kim SJ, Shim KH, Park SG, Kim SI. Postoperative membranous urethral length is the single most important surgical factor predicting recovery of postoperative urinary continence. Urol Oncol. 2020;38(12):930.e7–930.e12.
17. Sugi M, Kinoshita H, Yoshida T, Taniguchi H, Mishima T, Yoshida K, et al. The narrow vesicourethral angle measured on postoperative cystography can predict urinary incontinence after robot-assisted laparoscopic radical prostatectomy. Scand J Urol. 2018;52(2):151–6.
18. Tewari A, Jhaveri J, Rao S, Yadav R, Bartsch G, Te A, et al. Total reconstruction of the vesico-urethral junction. BJU Int. 2008;101(7):871–7.
19. Haga N, Ogawa S, Yabe M, Akaihata H, Hata J, Sato Y, et al. Association between postoperative pelvic anatomic features on magnetic resonance imaging and lower tract urinary symptoms after radical prostatectomy. Urology. 2014;84(3):642–9.
20. Kretschmer A, Nitti V. Surgical treatment of male postprostatectomy incontinence: current concepts. Eur Urol Focus 2017;3(4–5):364–76.
21. Shin TY, Lee YS. Detrusorrhaphy during robot-assisted radical prostatectomy: early recovery of urinary continence and surgical technique. Biomed Res Int. 2019;2019:1528142.
22. Chung M, Lee SH, Jung H, Park W, Chung B. Impact of a retrotrigonal layer backup stitch on post-prostatectomy incontinence Korean J Urol. 2011;52:709–14.
23. Galfano A, Ascione A, Grimaldi S, Petralia G, Strada E, Bocciardi AM. A new anatomic approach for robot-assisted laparoscopic prostatectomy: a feasibility study for completely intrafascial surgery. Eur Urol. 2010;58(3):457–61.
24. Tewari A, El-Hakim A, Rao S, Raman JD. Identification of the retrotrigonal layer as a key anatomical landmark during robotically assisted radical prostatectomy. BJU Int. 2006;98(4):829–32.

Apical Dissection During Trans-Peritoneal, Anterior Robot-Assisted Radical Prostatectomy

12

Alexandre Mottrie and Carlo Andrea Bravi

Introduction

The prostatic apex is a common location for tumor involvement and the most common site of positive surgical margins (PSMs) after radical prostatectomy. Considering robot-assisted radical prostatectomy, which nowadays represents the most widely employed approach for PCa surgery in western countries [1], PSMs may be considered as an unsuccessful outcome of prostate cancer surgery, since patients harboring PSMs on final pathology are at higher risk of biochemical recurrence (BCR) [2], and require additional salvage treatments that could impair functional outcomes and quality of life. Moreover, it has been demonstrated that apical PSMs are associated with a higher risk of cancer recurrence [3, 4].

To obviate apical PSMs, the urethra could be transected farther from the prostatic apex, but this might impair urinary continence recovery due to a shortage of the urethra and damage of the urethral sphincter complex (USC). Therefore, apical dissection still remains the "Achilles heel" of PCa surgery [5], since it may affect not only cancer control, but also postoperative urinary continence recovery [6]. Anatomical preservation of each component of USC, including the external rhabdosphincter and the inner lissosphincter, is essential in order to optimize continence recovery [7]. Apical dissection should therefore represent a compromise between cancer control (avoiding apical PSMs) and urinary continence recovery (maximizing the urethral length).

A. Mottrie (✉)
Department of Urology, OLV Ziekenhuis Aalst, Aalst, Belgium

ORSI Academy, Ghent, Belgium

C. A. Bravi
Department of Urology, OLV Ziekenhuis Aalst, Aalst, Belgium

ORSI Academy, Ghent, Belgium

Unit of Urology/Division of Oncology, URI, IRCCS Ospedale San Raffaele, Milan, Italy

Anatomy

The urethral sphincter complex is composed of two morphologically related but functionally unrelated components:

- Inner layer lissosphincter of smooth muscle: it forms a complete cylinder of circular and longitudinal muscle fibers around the urethra.
- Outer layer rhabdosphincter of skeletal muscle: is composed of skeletal muscle fibers from the perineal membrane to the prostatic apex that unite behind the urethra in a central fibrous raphe, while proximally they form a cap on the anterolateral side of the prostate [7, 8].

With high magnification (Fig. 12.1) it is possible to clearly recognize three different layers of musculature at the level of prostate-membranous urethra: the rhabdosphincter (light blue), the circular smooth muscles (dark blue) and the longitudinal smooth muscles (red) which surround the urethral mucosa (yellow) [6].

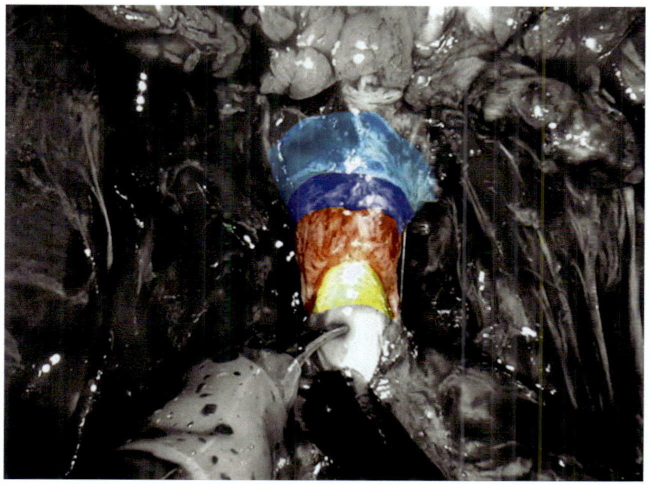

Fig. 12.1 Intraoperative anatomic definition of the three different muscular layers at the level of the urethral sphincter complex

S. Ren et al. (eds.), *Robot-Assisted Radical Prostatectomy*, https://doi.org/10.1007/978-3-031-05855-4_12

The ventral part of the sphincter is covered by the deep venous complex (DVC) and ridges of rudimentary striated muscle fibers; the lateral and posterior aspects are surrounded by the apex and neurovascular tissue [9]. The rhabdosphincter sometimes invades the pseudocapsule of the prostate and the glandular tissues at the level of the apex. Thus, dissection in this area may cause an inadvertent injury of the prostatic apex. In addition, some anatomical considerations are noteworthy during apical dissection, including the lack of a capsule-like structure in the apex, variability of the prostatic apex shape [10], and variation in the structure of the USC [6]. Anatomic and functional studies have shown that an important functional part of the USC is located intraprostatically between the prostatic apex and the colliculus seminalis [9, 11] due to the development of prostate at the onset of puberty. Koraitim clearly showed that continence at rest is primarily a function of the lissosphincter and that a minimal length of 1.5 cm of the USC is essential to maintain continence [7]. All these considerations, therefore, confirm the great importance of preservation of maximal urethral length at the time of radical prostatectomy in order to preserve urinary continence.

Surgical Technique

The visualization of the operative field and the ability to limit bleeding from the deep venous complex facilitate apical prostatic dissection during robot-assisted radical prostatectomy. Up to this point in the operation, antegrade dissection has permitted complete mobilization of the lateral, base, and posterior prostate, leaving division of the DVC and urethra from the prostatic apex for last. It is critical to avoid entry into the anterior prostate during division of the deep DVC because this may result in an iatrogenic positive margin. Although the previously placed DVC stitch may become dislodged or divided during this step, further sutures to secure the deep DVC can be easily placed. Also, bleeding from the deep DVC during attempts at re-suturing can be kept to a minimum by transiently increasing the CO_2 insufflation pressure to 20 mmHg to improve the tamponade effect on venous bleeding. Once the DVC is divided, there should be good visualization of the prostatic apex and its junction with the urethra.

The anatomy of the prostatic apex is variable and should be carefully inspected before division of the urethra. As much urethral length as possible should be maintained, but an overlying anterior lip of prostate must be recognized, as well as posterior extension of prostatic tissue beneath the urethra. Nevertheless, leaving a small rim of urethra along the prostatic apex may be advisable to reduce the incidence of apical positive margins because this does not appear to have an adverse effect on the return of urinary continence [12]. To prevent thermal injury to the external striated sphincter and nearby neurovascular bundles (NVB), sharp dissection with limited use of electrocautery is preferred during the prostatic apical dissection and division of the urethra.

Recently, the EAU Robotic Urology Section (ERUS) Scientific and Educational Working Groups established specific metrics for the assessment of intra-operative skills during robotic radical prostatectomy [13]. These metrics comprise 12 phases and 80 procedural steps that represent a "good practice" in robotic radical prostatectomy. With respect to apical dissection, the panel of experts identified six steps which are described below:

1. Instrument positioning. The additional arm should either be parked in a position that will avoid collision with the other instruments or can be used for traction on the prostate.
2. Preservation of the urethra by releasing the prostate from the urethra. During this phase, rotation of the prostate helps with the dissection and delineation of the apex laterally and posteriorly. Dissect the urethra away from the capsule of the prostate both anteriorly and posteriorly (taking care to optimize the urethral length).
3. Transection of the urethra preserving urethral length and following the anatomy of the prostatic apex. The dissection of the prostatic apex can be carried out with a sharp and direct division of the membranous urethra at the level of the urethra-prostatic junction.
4. Transection of any remnants of tissue attaching the prostate staying close to the capsule of the prostate.
5. Bagging of the prostate (and it may be sent for frozen section).
6. Reduce pneumoperitoneum to look for bleeding. Suction irrigation to visualize NVB and DVC. Control arterial and venous bleeding with combination of ligation of bleeders, point coagulation and/or clips, suturing or use of tissue coagulants.

Collar Technique

A different technique for apical dissection has been described recently as the "collar" technique [14]. It consists in progressively dissecting the three different muscular layers at the level of the urethral sphincter complex (rhabdosphincter, circular smooth muscle, longitudinal smooth muscle, and mucosa) in order to optimize the recovery of urinary continence while not increasing the risk on positive surgical margins.

The technique was describe in a series of 189 consecutive patients receiving robotic radical prostatectomy at a high volume European center [14]. A 0° lens was used for the whole procedure. The DVC was sharply divided without any previous ligation, thus providing optimal visualization of the underlying urethra and preventing inadvertent cutting into the prostatic apex or damage of sphincteric apparatus. After complete transection, the DVC was selectively sutured with a running V-Loc 3-0 barbed suture. At this point, the prostatic apex is fully exposed and the UCS is clearly visualized.

The collar technique for apical dissection consists of the following steps:

1. The USC is circumferentially incised 2–3 mm distally to the prostatic apex, first at the level of the rhabdosphincter and then at the level of the circular smooth muscle, in order to stay farther from the prostatic apex and reduce PSM risk (Fig. A-a).

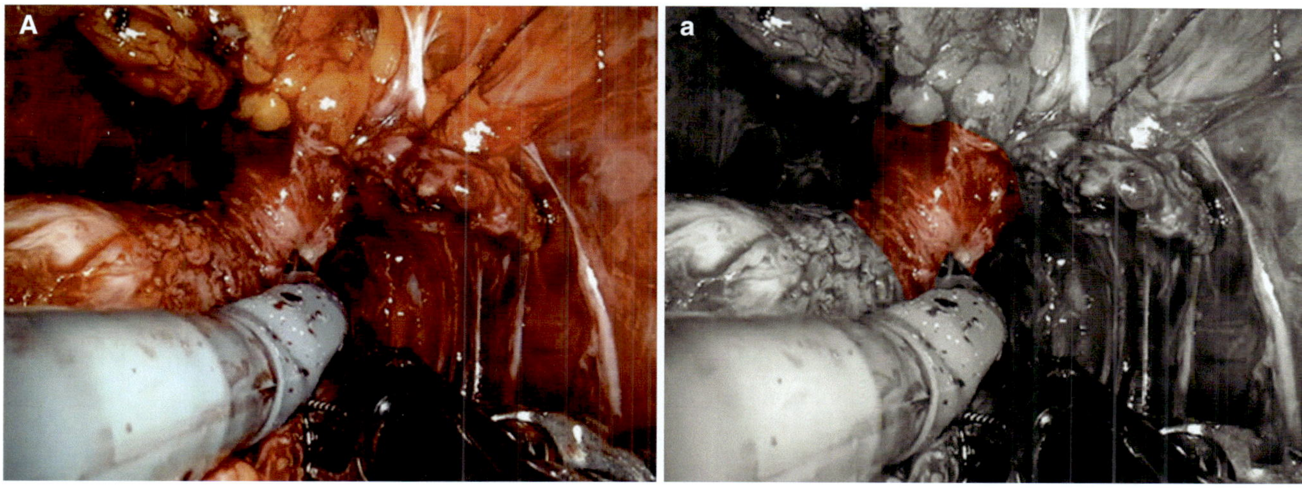

2. The underlying smooth longitudinal muscle is exposed with blunt and sharp dissection (Fig. B-b).

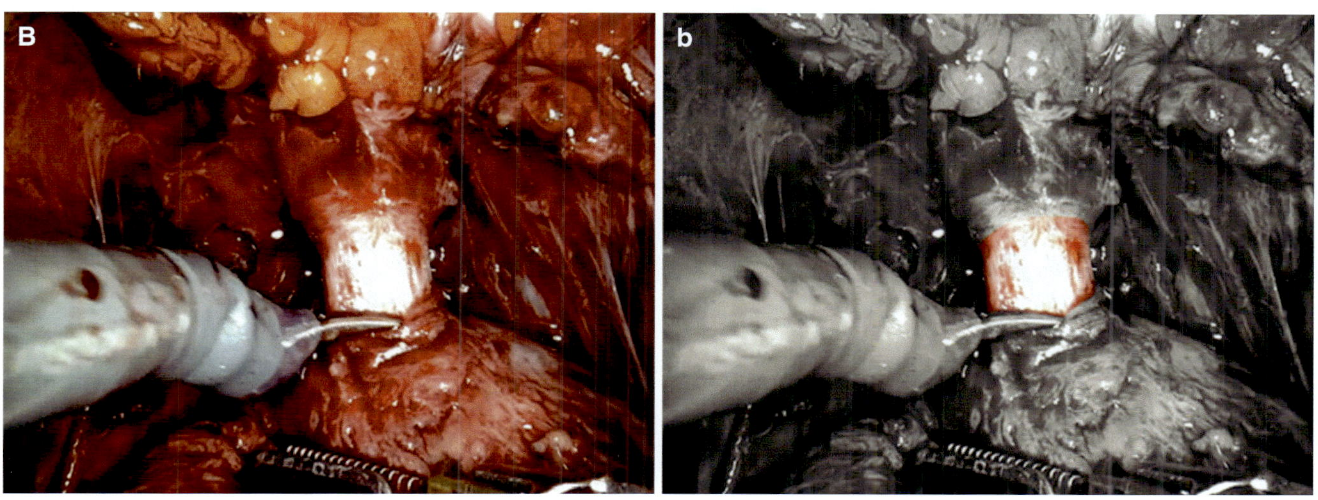

3. Two to three millimeters of the rhabdosphincter and of the circular smooth muscle remain to cover the prostate (Fig. C-c).

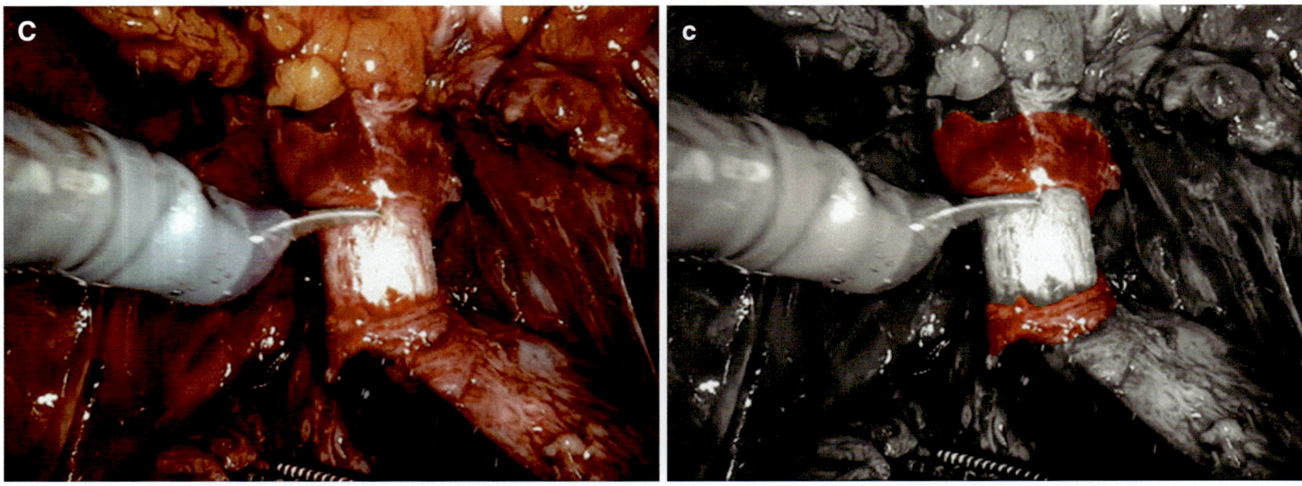

4. The longitudinal smooth muscle is sharply incised close to the prostatic apex in order to achieve maximal length of the functional lissosphincter (Fig. D-d).

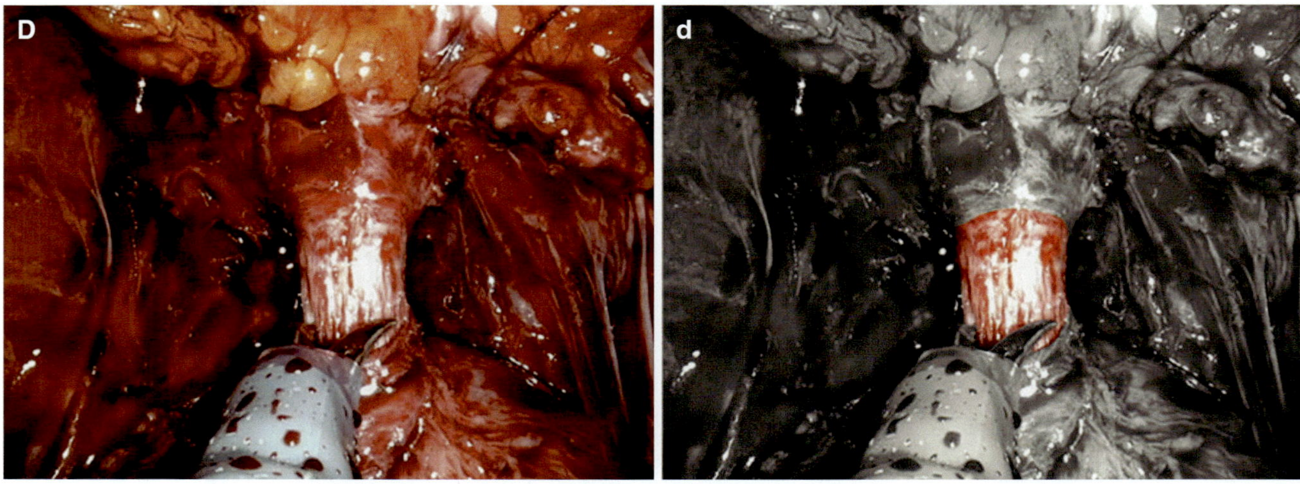

5. The underlying mucosa is exposed, and the catheter is visualized and retracted (Fig. E-e).

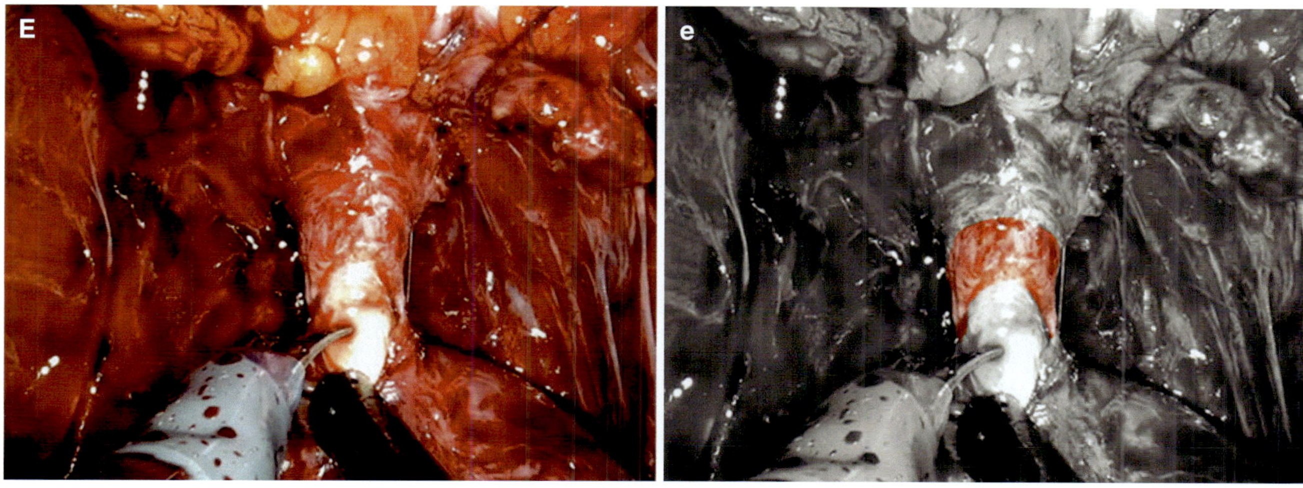

6. The mucosa of the posterior aspect of the urethra is incised just caudally to the colliculus, and the posterior aspect of the longitudinal smooth muscle is exposed (Fig. F-f).

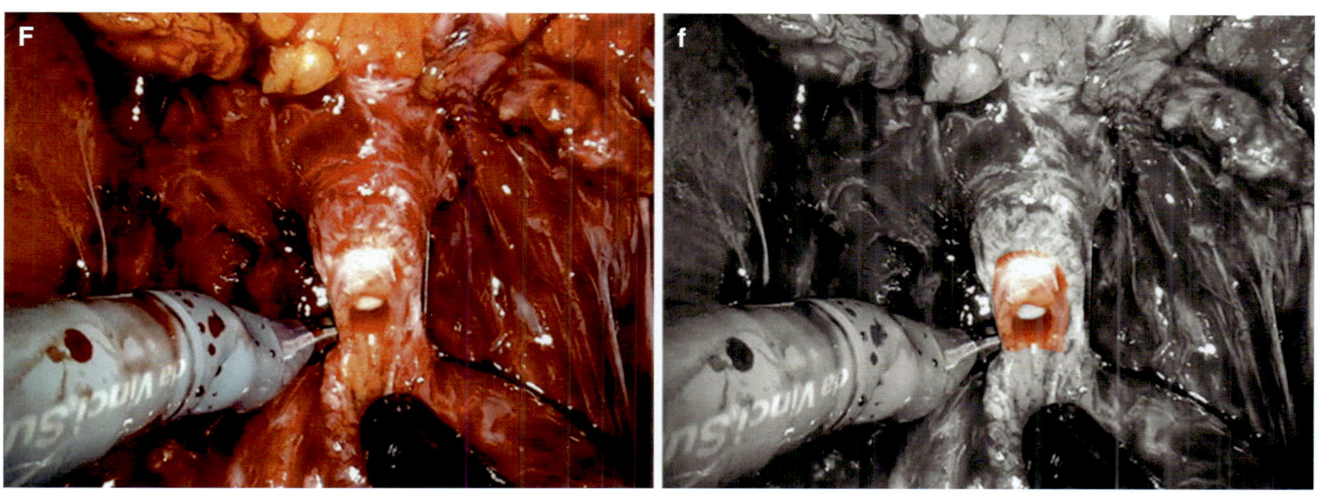

7. The posterior aspect of the longitudinal smooth muscle is sharply incised (Fig. G-g).

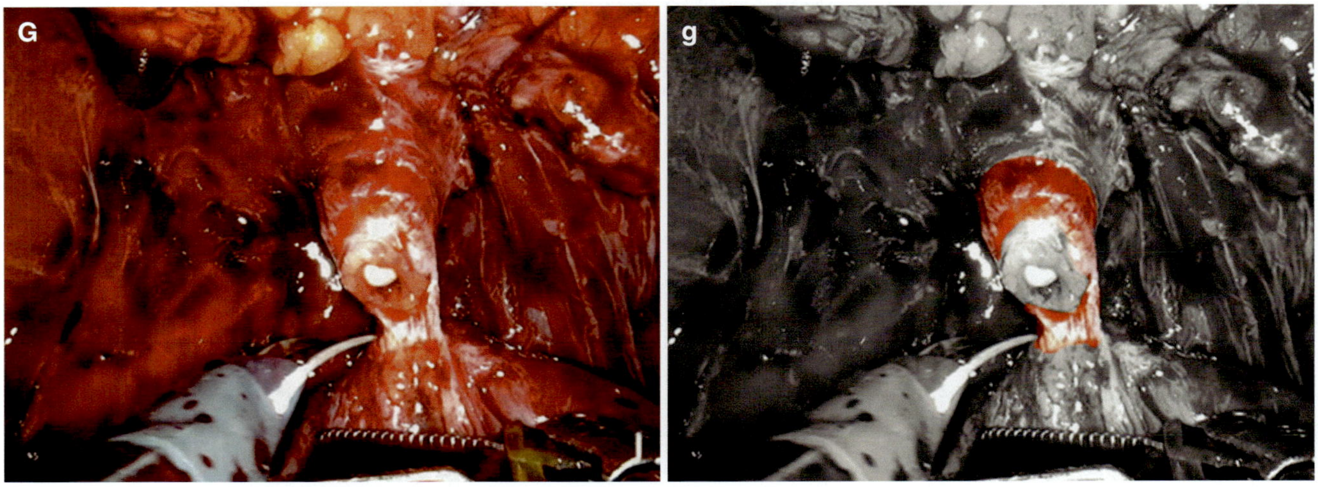

8. At the end of the dissection, lengths of the smooth longitudinal muscle and the mucosa are preserved (Fig. H-h).

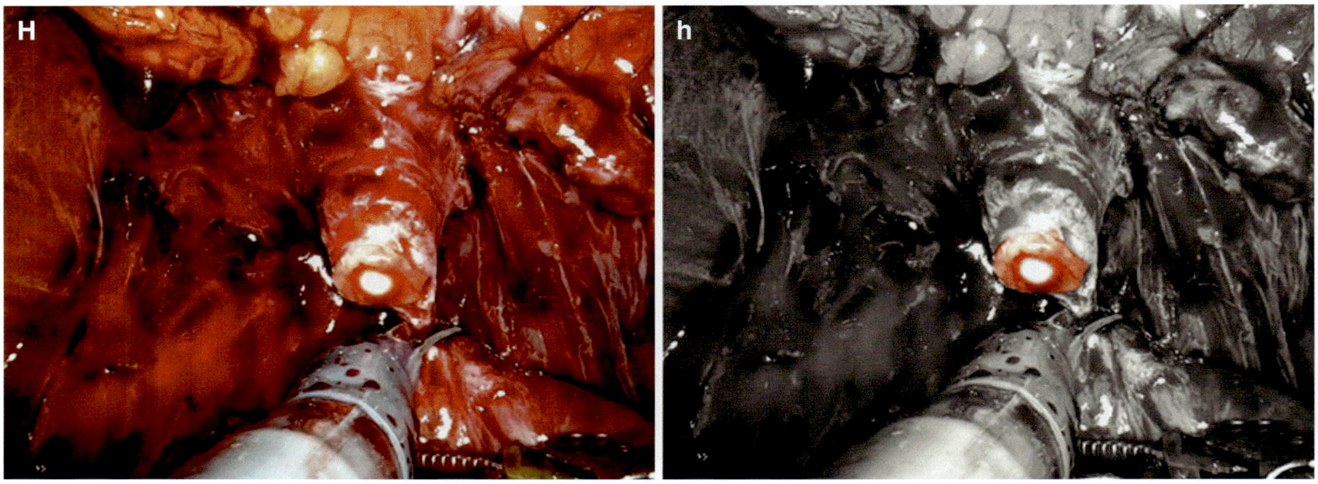

Figure 12.2 shows the collar of peri-urethral tissue covering the prostatic apex in the final specimen; conversely, Fig. 12.3 demonstrates how the apex is not protected in the specimens resulting from standard apical dissection.

To investigate the oncologic and functional outcomes of this new technique, authors compared 108 individuals who received the "collar" technique with patients operated prior to the introduction of this novel technique (81 patients, control group), whose apical dissection was performed by sharp and direct division of membranous urethra at the level of the urethra-prostatic junction without dissection of the single components of the USC.

Overall, 20 out of 189 (10.6%) patients revealed PSMs at final pathology, without a significant difference between the two samples (13.6% in the control group and 8.3% in the collar technique group; $p = 0.2$). The vast majority of PSMs was found to be apical (7.4%), including 5.6% in the collar technique group and 9.9% in the control group ($p = 0.7$). After stratifying PSMs according to pathologic stage, a significant difference was noted between the two groups only when considering patients with pT2 disease (0% in the collar

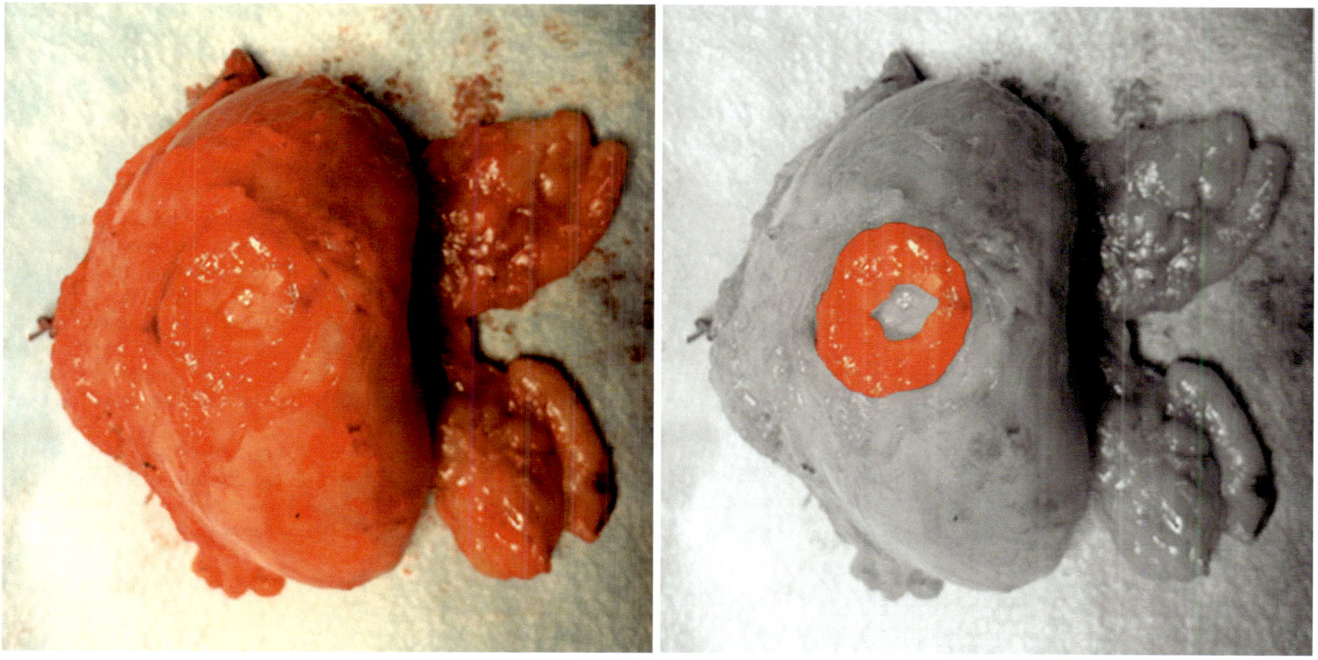

Fig. 12.2 Macroscopic evidence of the collar of peri-urethral tissue covering the prostatic apex in the final specimen

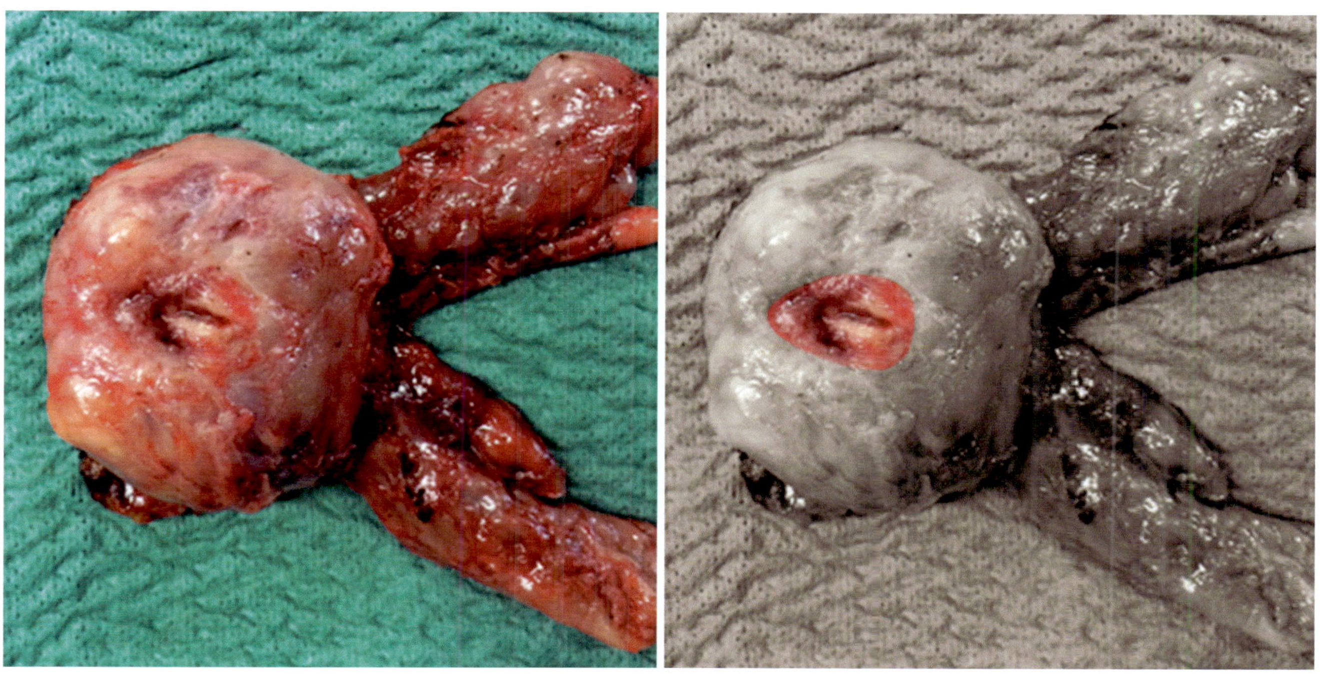

Fig. 12.3 Final specimen of a procedure in which the collar technique was not employed: the apex is not protected by any collar of peri-urethral tissue

technique group vs. 8.9% in the control group; p = 0.01). Similarly, patients treated with the collar technique experienced significantly lower apical surgical margins compared with the control group, when considering individuals with organ-confined disease at final pathology (0% vs. 7.1%; p = 0.03). This was further confirmed on univariate analyses: considering patients with the suspicion of an index tumor located in the apical region at preoperative mpMRI ($n = 43$), men referred to the collar technique had a significantly lower risk of apical PSMs as compared with those who underwent standard apical dissection (OR: 0.05, $p = 0.009$). With regard to intra- and post-operative complications, no significant differences were found between the two groups.

Considering functional outcomes, the urinary continence recovery rates were comparable between the two groups: the rate of patients who utilized zero pads with no leakage of urine in the collar vs. standard technique was, respectively, 42% and 54%, 46% and 60%, 74% and 84%, 94% and 88%, and 99% and 93% on catheter removal and at 1, 3, 6, and 12 months after surgery (all $p \geq 0.052$).

Conclusions/Discussion

Apical dissection represents one of the most challenging steps during robot-assisted radical prostatectomy. Specific precautions have to be taken into consideration to balance the risk of positive surgical margins and the preservation of delicate structures involved in the recovery of urinary continence. In this regard, detailed surgical steps have been described and validated by experts. Moreover, the "collar" technique for apical dissection allows for a reduction of apical positive surgical margins, especially in case of patients with prostate cancer located at the apex.

References

1. Leow JJ, Chang SL, Meyer CP, et al. Robot-assisted versus open radical prostatectomy: a contemporary analysis of an all-payer discharge database. Eur Urol. 2016;70(5):837–45.
2. Boorjian SA, Karnes RJ, Crispen PL, Carlson RE, Rangel LJ, Bergstralh EJ, Blute ML. The impact of positive surgical margins on mortality following radical prostatectomy during the prostate specific antigen era. JURO. 2010;183:1003–9.
3. Novara G, Ficarra V, Mocellin S, et al. Systematic review and meta-analysis of studies reporting oncologic outcome after robot-assisted radical prostatectomy. Eur Urol. 2012;62:382–404.
4. Dev HS, Wiklund P, Patel V, Parashar D, Palmer K, Nyberg T, Skarecky D, Neal DE, Ahlering T, Sooriakumaran P. Surgical margin length and location affect recurrence rates after robotic prostatectomy. Urol Oncol. 2015;33:109.e7–109.e13.
5. Tewari AK, Srivastava A, Mudaliar K, Tan GY, Grover S, El Douaihy Y, Peters D, et al. Anatomical retro-apical technique of synchronous (posterior and anterior) urethral transection: a novel approach for ameliorating apical margin positivity during robotic radical prostatectomy. BJU Int. 2010;106(9):1364–73.
6. Hinata N, Sejima T, Takenaka A. Progress in pelvic anatomy from the viewpoint of radical prostatectomy. Int J Urol. 2013;20(3):260–70.
7. Koraitim MM. The male urethral sphincter complex revisited: an anatomical concept and its physiological correlate. J Urol. 2008;179(5):1683–9.
8. Walz J, Epstein JI, Ganzer R, et al. A critical analysis of the current knowledge of surgical anatomy of the prostate related to optimisation of cancer control and preservation of continence and erection in candidates for radical prostatectomy: an update. Eur Urol. 2016;70:301–11.
9. Schlomm T, Heinzer H, Steuber T, Salomon G, Engel O, Michl U, Haese A, Graefen M, Huland H. Full functional-length urethral sphincter preservation during radical prostatectomy. Eur Urol. 2011;60(2):320–9.
10. Walz J, Burnett AL, Costello AJ, et al. A critical analysis of the current knowledge of surgical anatomy related to optimization of cancer control and preservation of continence and erection in candidates for radical prostatectomy. Eur Urol. 2010;57(2):179–92.
11. Mayers RP. Practical surgical anatomy for radical prostatectomy. Urol Clin North Am. 2001;28(3):473–90.
12. Borin JF, Skarecky DW, Narula N, Ahlering TE. Impact of urethral stump length on continence and positive surgical margins in robot-assisted laparoscopic prostatectomy. Urology. 2007;70(1):173–7.
13. Mottrie A, Mazzone E, Wiklund P, Graefen M, Collins J, De Groote R, Dell'Oglio P, et al. Objective assessment of intra-operative skills for robot-assisted radical prostatectomy (RARP): results from The ERUS Scientific and Educational Working Groups Metrics Initiative. BJU Int. 2020;128(1):103–11.
14. Bianchi L, Turri FM, Larcher A, et al. A novel approach for apical dissection during robot-assisted radical prostatectomy: the "collar" technique. Eur Urol Focus. 2018;4(5):677–85.

Part IV

Intraoperative Assessment of Surgical Margins

Intra-operative Assessment of Surgical Margins: NeuroSAFE

13

Eoin Dinneen and Greg Shaw

Introduction

The aim of all cancer surgery ought to be to cure cancer where it is found and to leave as little evidence as possible of surgical intervention. In the case of radical prostatectomy (RP) for localised prostate cancer, this lofty ambition is often referred to by surgeons and researchers as the trifecta outcome; cancer cure (or freedom from biochemical recurrence (BCR)), urinary continence and recovery of erectile function [1].

All advanced surgical techniques should aim to assist the surgeon during robot-assisted radical prostatectomy (RARP) to achieve these goals, and different surgical techniques will influence surgery and thus, potentially, benefit the patient in different ways. Intra-operative assessment of surgical margins during RP relates to the moments during RP upon which the patient's functional and oncological outcomes may critically depend, i.e. decisions on the planes of dissection and the radicality of surgical resection. In RP, as a consequence of the unique position and relations of the prostate, these decisions and thus intra-operative margin assessment, can have considerable influence on a man's recovery from RP.

Already in this book, there have been chapters on the surgical anatomy of the pelvis, the prostate, and its intimate neighbours such as the neurovascular bundles (NVB). There are a variety of different techniques for applying intra-operative assessment to the surgical of the prostate using frozen section, of which the NeuroSAFE technique is the most well-known. All intra-operative margin assessment techniques (frozen section or other) share in common the aim to assist the surgeon with realtime feedback to optimise the balance between *preservation* and *avoidance* during RARP:

- *Preservation*—of peri-prostatic structures that confer improved post-operative functional recovery.
- *Avoidance*—of positive surgical margins (PSM) by checking for them during RARP.

To understand these simultaneous but sometimes competing surgical goals, it is helpful to briefly consider them separately so that we may appreciate why they are independently advantageous, but also how they can be difficult to balance and achieve in certain patients.

Preservation of the Peri-prostatic Structures

Preservation of all peri-prostatic structures will facilitate improved recovery, but particularly preservation of the NVB by way of "nerve-sparing" (NS) is one of the most important decisions for a man undergoing RARP. Since the original description of these nerves by Walsh et al. in the 1980s [2] many other authors have characterised and improved our understanding of the course of the NVBs using cadaveric studies and, more recently, tensor diffusion tractography MRI [3, 4]. Now it is very well recognised that NS RARP is essential for recovery of erectile function [5, 6]. Some groups have also demonstrated that NS RARP is associated with improved time to recovery of urinary continence [7, 8]. The closer the dissection the plane to the prostate, the more neuronal tissue can be preserved and thus the greater the opportunity for erectile function recovery. Thus, intrafascial NS where the dissection is made just outside the prostatic capsule with the aim to maintain the complete neural hammock is associated with the best opportunity for recovery of erectile function [9].

Elsewhere on the prostate, dissection in close proximity to the prostate may preserve structures that contribute to the recovery of urinary continence such as the bladder neck [10], the maximal functional length of membranous urethra [11], and anterior structures such dorsal venous complex [12]. Again, preservation of these anatomical structures

E. Dinneen · G. Shaw (✉)
Division of Surgery and Interventional Science, University College London, London, UK

Department of Urology, University College Hospital London, London, UK
e-mail: gregshaw@doctors.net.uk

S. Ren et al. (eds.), *Robot-Assisted Radical Prostatectomy*, https://doi.org/10.1007/978-3-031-05855-4_13

requires intimate dissection as close to the prostate as possible without entering the prostate itself or the disease within.

Avoidance of PSM

PSM will reduce the likelihood of cure from surgery and leave a man at increased risk of BCR and as such avoidance of PSM is a surgical imperative [13]. At the postero-lateral margin of the prostate, extra-prostatic extension (EPE) reduces the distance from the tumour to the NVBs [14], and therefore can increase the chance of PSM if the dissection plane is close to the capsule. Even in the absence of EPE, capsular incision into malignant glands giving intra-prostatic PSM seems also increase the risk of BCR [15]. Intuitively, this is more likely to occur when the surgical dissection plane is very close to the prostatic capsule and disease volume is higher, such as in pT2c disease, though evidence to support this in the published literature is lacking.

Historically surgeons have used digital rectal examination (DRE), intra-operative palpation [16], and nomograms to estimate the likelihood of EPE, but these are flawed [17]. More recently, mpMRI has been used to predict EPE and safety of NS, and although use of mpMRI continues to evolve and mature, the updated systematic review on mpMRI for staging by Abrams-Pompe et al. again highlights the great heterogeneity in its performance according to centre [18].

Overall, the conundrum for surgeons planning on "aggressive NS strategy" is that prediction of EPE before surgery is difficult and the detection of PSM during surgery is not currently possible even with the improved magnification and endoscope optics of modern robotic surgery platforms.

Role of Intra-operative Margin Assessment

Given these often-times competing intentions to *preserve* peri-prostatic structures and *avoid* PSM, when the extent each man's tumour burden is different and difficult to accurately predict prior to RARP, the role of realtime intra-operative margin assessment of the prostate has become attractive. Fresh Frozen section is the only widely available technology for the purpose of intra-operative margin assessment during to RARP, though new, interesting, albeit untested, microscopic digital imaging technologies are emerging and will be discussed in this book in the next chapter [19].

In this chapter, we will discuss the merits, the disadvantages, and the currently unanswered questions according to the available evidence with regards to (a) intra-operative frozen section assessment of the prostate margin, (b) the NeuroSAFE technique, which is the most well-known and prominent of the IFS approaches.

Intra-operative Frozen Section (IFS): Quality of Evidence

A recent systematic review of intra-operative margin assessment during RP has been conducted by our group [20]. Ten studies were included (see Table 13.1) that reported on 22 separate outcomes of importance to RP. Detailed analysis of all ten studies included in the review are beyond the remit of this chapter, however, all of these studies were retrospective and the majority of the outcomes reported upon were deemed to be at serious risk of bias according to the RoBINs tool for assessment of reporting in observational studies. There have been some notable additions to the literature since the performance of this review including several studies on the NeuroSAFE technique, however, this summary gives an indication of the generally low-quality evidence which is commonplace in relation to intra-operative margin assessment during RARP.

Moreover, this review and a further review paper by Sighinolfi et al. [21] both identified the considerable heterogeneity in the techniques of frozen section used, the site of the prostate where they are applied, the reasons why IFS is performed, the technique for secondary resection (when PSM identified) and the outcomes reported by the studies identified. To date, there has been only one prospective, randomised study in the field of intra-operative frozen section, the NeuroSAFE PROOF Feasibility Study, which has not reported upon patient-centred oncological nor functional outcomes, however the ongoing, fully powered successor NeuroSAFE PROOF trial will.

Different Approaches to IFS on the Prostate

Directing IFS by Surgeon Discretion

The NeuroSAFE technique is the best-known application of intra-operative frozen section during RP, and this will be described and reviewed in greater detail later in this chapter, however it is not the only application of IFS during RP. Numerous groups have applied IFS directed to evaluate areas that are perceived to be of concern for EPE or PSM. In five studies the area of concern was directed on an "ad lib" basis by the operating surgeon. Of these five studies, two noted an increase in PSM rate in the IFS group, though both were high risk of bias favouring the non-IFS group. Conversely, the other three studies that reported performing

Table 13.1 Characteristics of eligible studies in the systematic review and their baseline characteristics

First author and year	Country	Recruitment period	No. of patients	Type of surgery	Site of IFS	Oncological outcomes	NVB status	EF recovery
Cangiano 1999 [39]	USA	1989–1997	142	Open	Posterolateral only when surgeon concern	Yes	Yes	Yes
Tsuboi 2005 [27]	USA	1998–2002	760	Open	Area of concern by surgeon	No	No	No
Lavery 2010 [40]	USA	2007–2009	970	RARP	"Visual concern" by surgeon	Yes	Yes	Yes
Heinrich 2010 [41]	Germany	2004–2006	287	Open	Posterolateral only when surgeon concern	No	No	No
Schlomm 2012 [29]	Germany	2002–2011	11,069	Open (10,427) RALP (642)	NeuroSAFE technique	Yes	Yes	No
Kakiuchi 2013 [26]	USA	2004–2011	2608	RARP	Surgeon discretion	No	No	No
Petralia 2015 [42]	Italy	2010–2012	268	RARP	MRI-guided EPE concern	No	Yes	No
Obek 2018 [43]	Turkey	2014–2016	170	RARP	Entire prostate margin	No	Yes	No
Mirmilstein 2018 [33]	UK	2008–2017	277	RARP	NeuroSAFE technique	Yes	No[a]	Yes
Preisser 2019 [34]	Germany	2014–2018	346	Open (126) RARP (220)	NeuroSAFE technique	No	Yes	No
Fossa[b] 2019 [36]	Norway/ Germany	2013–2016	307	RARP (183) Open (124)	NeuroSAFE technique	No	No	Yes
van der Slot[b] 2020 [37]	Netherlands	2018–2019	258	RARP	NeuroSAFE technique	No	Yes	No
Dinneen[b] 2020 [44]	UK	2018	50	RARP	NeuroSAFE technique	Yes[c]	Yes	No

[a]NVB status results presented for before and after the introduction of the NeuroSAFE technique to their hospital, but not according to whether IFS/NeuroSAFE was performed
[b]Studies not included in systematic review as published after
[c]Limited oncological outcomes presented for men with PSM on IFS, not the entire trial

intra-operative margin assessment according to surgeon suspicion noted a reduction in PSM rates in favour of the IFS group. The best of these results was achieved by Heinrich et al. demonstrating the most notable reduction in PSM rates (−12.2%) when applying the IFS to the postero-lateral margin of the prostate compare to men who did not have IFS during RP.

Directing IFS by Pre-op MRI Discretion

Also of note, Petralia et al. describe using IFS directed by pre-operative MRI scan to an area of concern for EPE and/or PSM. In a study of 268 patients, they noted that this technique was able to reduce PSM rate by −11.2% (7.5% IFS group vs. 18.7% non-IFS group), though their report did not include mature oncological outcomes.

IFS at Multiple Sites

Some groups have used IFS for multiple areas on the prostate at the same time. Von Bodman and colleagues describe applying IFS to the NVBs, the apex and the base of the prostate simultaneously. In their 2013 report, they note that IFS was positive in 22% of cases, including the NVBs in 56.9%, the apex in 34.5% and the base in 8.6% of cases, though they do not comment on the initial NS strategy opted for by the surgeon when margin was positive at the NVB. They comment that the surgeon was able to convert the frozen section PSM to negative in 92.3%, though again, mature oncological outcomes are awaited from this group.

Pak and colleagues described performing IFS by taking biopsies of the urethra and the bladder neck and performing further tissue resection if these were positive for malignant or atypical cells [22]. Overall, IFS analyses were initially negative in 1799 patients, converted to negative in 139 patients and were persistently positive in 75 patients. Among 1799 patients with initially negative IFS, PSMs at the negative IFS site were found in 49 patients (2.7%). When the results of IFS and permanent specimen analyses were compared, the sensitivity, specificity, negative predictive value and positive predictive value of IFS analysis were 78.1%, 97.8%, 97.3% and 81.8%, respectively. Interestingly, in this study the authors reported an improved 5 year BCR-free survival (BCRFS) in patients who had an initial PSM on IFS converted to NSM by secondary resection. The 5-year BCRFS rates of patients with negative surgical margins (NSM), negative converted surgical margins (NCSM) and PSMs were 89.6%, 85.1% and 57.1%, respectively ($P < 0.001$).

There are, however, other groups who have analysed their single-arm, retrospective surgical series of RP using and concluded that there is limited value to performing IFS based upon underwhelming improvements in oncological outcomes in men who had secondary resection performed. For instance, Gillitzer et al. assessed BCR in 188 patients who underwent RP with IFS [23]. They reported 5 year BCRFS at 94.9%, 75.3%, and 62.5% for patients who had NSM, PSM with negative frozen section and PSM, respectively. Their conclusions were similar to others [24–27], with similar study designs, who found it difficult to improve oncological outcomes significantly with IFS, though the level of evidence in these studies is low. All of these studies were non-comparative, IFS methods were not standardised, and there was no focus on other important elements of recovery after RP such as functional outcomes.

NeuroSAFE Technique

As highlighted in both recent review papers on the topic, the NeuroSAFE technique is the only technical application of IFS during RP that has been disseminated, developed and published upon by multiple groups [20], as such, we will consider this here in greater detail.

NeuroSAFE stands for "neurovascular structure adjacent frozen section examination" of the prostate margin using IFS applied exclusively to the postero-lateral margin of the prostate. The technique was first described in 2008 by Eichelberg et al. [28] from the Martini Klinik, Hamburg, Germany and was followed by two further large, retrospective case-control studies from the same institution [29, 30].

The NeuroSAFE technique is gaining in popularity and consequently the volume of published evidence available from different groups is greater (see Table 13.1). The application of IFS realtime assessment of the posterolateral margin is particularly relevant because of the adjacent NVBs, preservation of which can have profound impact on functional recovery, not just oncological outcomes.

NeuroSAFE Technique: Technical Description

The NeuroSAFE technique involves removal of the prostate from the body as soon as it has been detached from its surrounding structures. In RARP, this entails an enlarged umbilical incision and a bespoke endoscope arm port to enable re-establishment of pneumoperitoneum should be used. Immediately upon removal of the prostate, the postero-lateral neuro-vascular structure adjacent surfaces are painted in theatres by the operating surgeon (Fig. 13.1a). The inked prostate is then transported to the histopathology department where the entire inked margin is cleaved by a straight blade. This inked postero-lateral portion of prostate is further divided by perpendicular cuts at intervals of 5 mm from apex to base. A minimum of four and a maximum of seven pieces from the postero-lateral prostate on each side are submitted for freezing in this manner depending on the size of the prostate. Each piece of prostate tissue is then embedded into optimal cutting temperature (OCT) compound on a cryostamp and frozen (see Fig. 13.1b). The frozen prostate tissue is then transferred to the cryostat for sectioning at a tissue thickness of 5 μm before staining with haematoxylin and eosin (Fig. 13.1c). Slides are examined by a consultant genito-urinary histopathologist and the results are conveyed to the console surgeon in the operating room (OR) (see Fig. 13.2). This process is followed systematically in the same fashion irrespective of any other surgeon or image-based index of concern for EPE or large volume organ-confined disease in the region of the NVBs on either side.

NeuroSAFE Technique: Secondary Resection

If a positive margin is reported on the IFS during the NeuroSAFE technique, then this information is conveyed to the operating console surgeon who according to local protocol may or may not perform a secondary resection depending on the length, grade, and number of PSMs noted on a side (see Fig. 13.2 for schematic cartoon and 13.3 for example images of margin status). When SR is performed all tissue from the cut edge of Denonvilliers' fascia medially, the pararectal fat laterally, the pedicle cranially, and just beyond the urethrovesical anastomosis (including the puboprostatic ligament and Walsh's pillar) caudally is removed en bloc by the surgeon as originally described by the Martini Klinik authors [29] (see Fig. 13.4 for a collage of console images depicting this process). Secondarily resected tissue is sent for routine paraffin embedded histological analysis and is not routinely analysed intra-operatively.

NeuroSAFE Technique: Histological Outcomes

Frozen Section Concordance to Final Pathology

In terms of the diagnostic accuracy of the NeuroSAFE technique compared to the reference standard (final formalin fixed paraffin embedded haematoxylin and eosin stained margin assessment), IFS can be considered in comparison to (a) the final margin status at the posterolateral margin only and (b) the final margin status on a whole gland level.

Four studies have reported on the diagnostic accuracy of the NeuroSAFE technique comparing IFS to final margin assessment at the NVB margin only. Firstly, Schlomm et al. from the Martini Klinik in the report of their experience after 11,069 patients noted sensitivity and specificity of 93.4% and 98.8%, respectively. Mirmilstein et al. reported a UK-based experience of 120 NeuroSAFE RARPs noted sen-

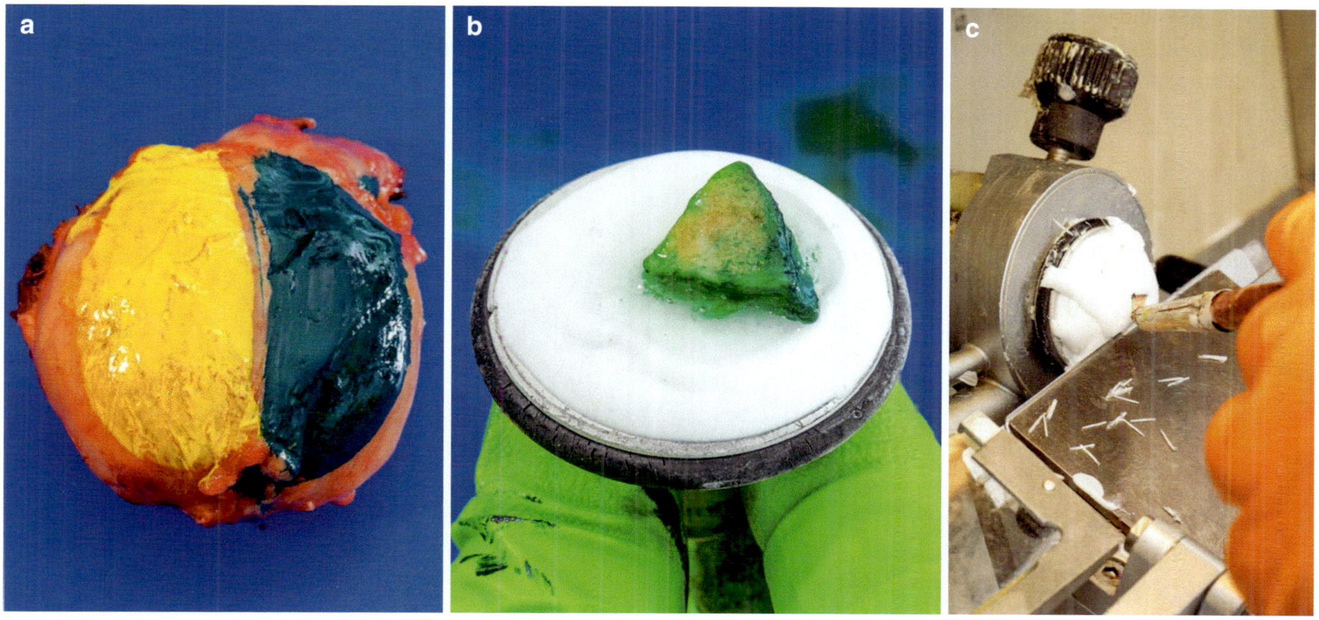

Fig. 13.1 Photos of the NeuroSAFE Technique. (**a**) Ink stains the left (yellow) and right (green) neurovascular structure adjacent prostate margin, respectively. (**b**) After cleaving the right side and slicing perpendicularly a 5 mm piece of prostate tissue sits on the cryostat before freezing. (**c**) Once embedded in OCT and frozen 5 μm sections are prepared on the microtome before staining

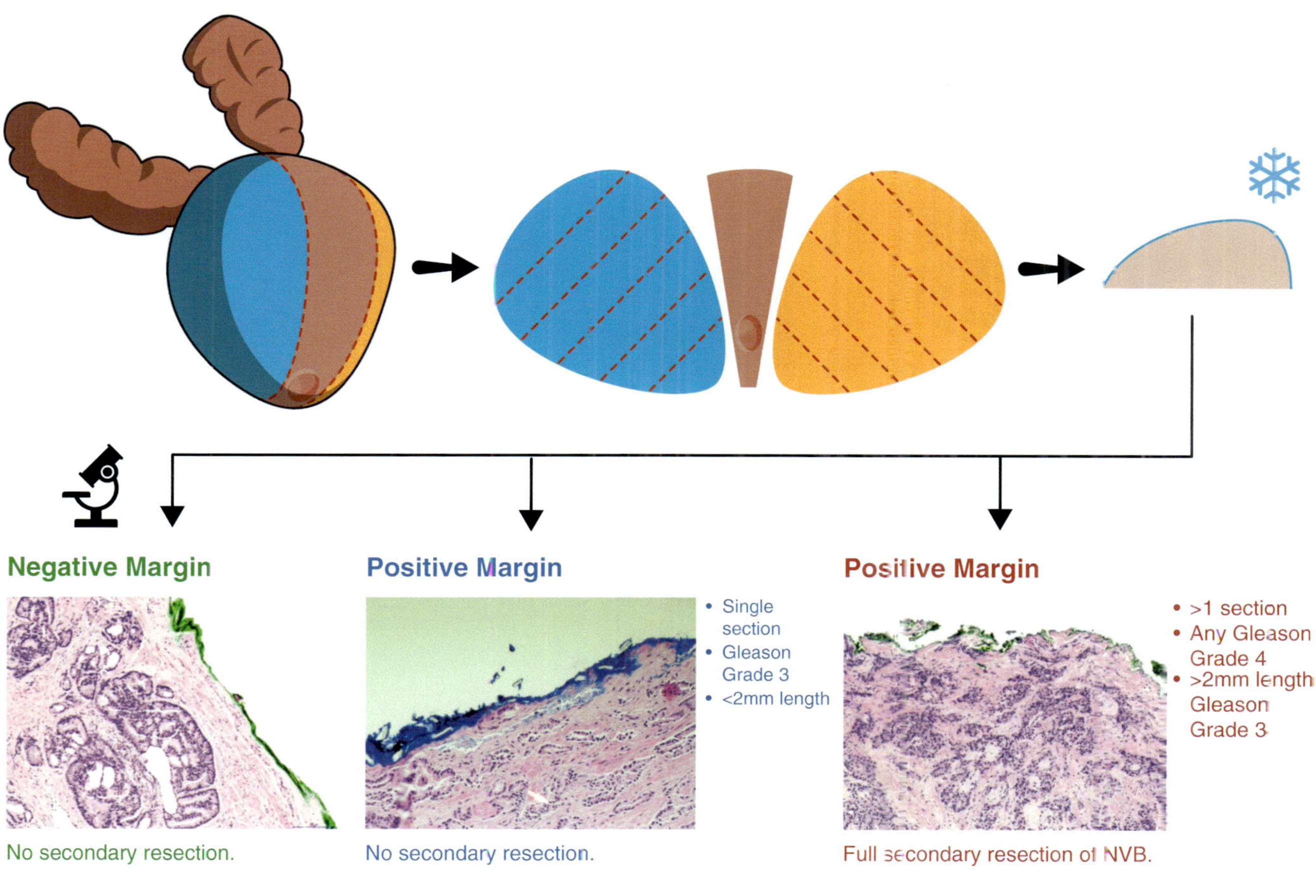

Fig. 13.2 Pictorial representation of the steps involved in the NeuroSAFE Technique during RP

sitivity of 90% and specificity of 97.4%. van der Slot reported upon the pathological outcomes following the introduction of the NeuroSAFE technique at the Erasmus Centre in the Netherlands. Their series included 491 NeuroSAFE procedures in 258 patients, during the introduction of the technique to their centre and reported sensitivity was 76.8% and specificity 97.3%. Lastly, Dinneen et al. reported the diagnostic accuracy of IFS vs. final pathology (see Fig. 13.3

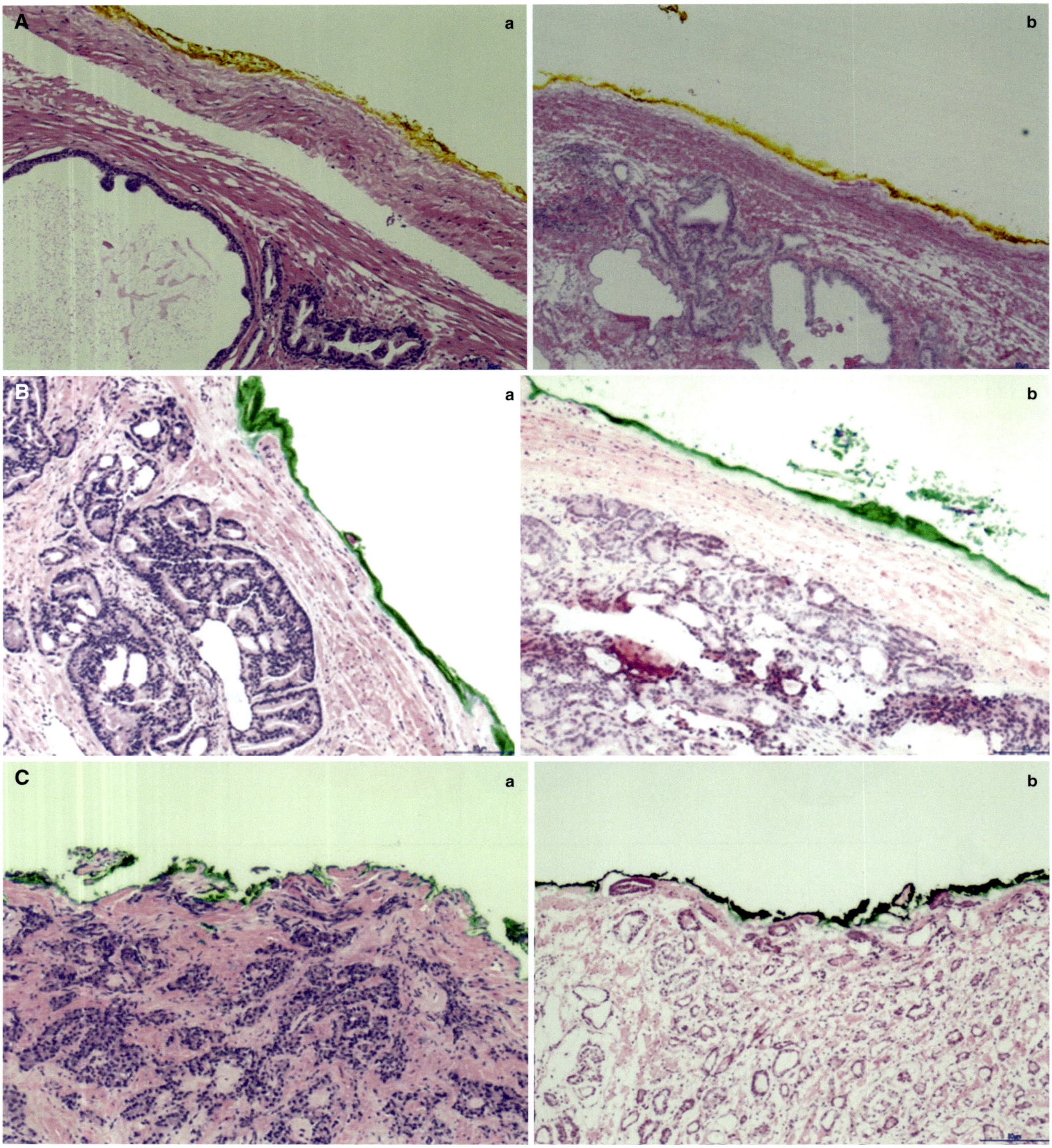

Fig. 13.3 (**A**) (a) Formalin Fixed Paraffin Embedded (final) section of margin CLEAR ×10 magnification. (b) Intra-operative Frozen Section (IFS) of corresponding CLEAR margin section also at ×10 magnification. (**B**) (a) Final section of NARROWLY CLEAR margin ×10 magnification. (b) IFS section of corresponding NARROWLY CLEAR margin section at ×10 magnification. (**C**) (a) Final section of POSITIVE margin ×10 magnification. (b) IFS section of corresponding POSITIVE margin section at ×10 magnification

for illustration of IFS and final margin classifications) at the NVB within the NeuroSAFE PROOF Feasibility RCT and found sensitivity of 100% and specificity 92.7% [31, 32] (Fig. 13.4).

Only one study (Mirmilstein et al.) has reported on the concordance between NVB margin status as per NeuroSAFE IFS and final whole gland RP margin status [33]. As is to be expected given that the NeuroSAFE technique only takes account margin status in a limited section of the overall gland, diagnostic accuracy was inferior compared to at the NVB level alone, with sensitivity and specificity of 82.4% and 91%, respectively.

Interestingly, the study from the Erasmus Centre in the Netherlands included a detailed analysis of IFS margin, final paraffin margin and whether cancer was present in the secondarily resected NVB to inform their NeuroSAFE technique protocol for the future. They performed secondary resection in 61 of 491 NeuroSAFE procedures. In 72.2% of secondary NVB resections prompted by a NeuroSAFE PSM, no tumour was present. These cases more often had a positive surgical margin of ≤1 mm (48.7% vs. 20.0%; $p = 0.001$) and only one positive slide (69.2% vs. 33.3%; $p = 0.008$). None of the nine patients with Gleason pattern 3 at the surgical margin, a positive surgical margin length of ≤1 mm and one positive slide had tumour in the secondary resection. They concluded that secondary resection of the NVB might be omitted in cases with limited amount of low-grade disease at the positive IFS surgical margin.

Similarly, Dinneen et al. analysed the presence of cancer in the secondary resection NVB and included 12-month oncological follow-up for these patients who had PSM on the IFS in their report on the NeuroSAFE PROOF Feasibility Study [31]. In total 11/25 patients had PSM identified by the NeuroSAFE technique. Bilateral PSM was identified in one man. 7/11 patients underwent SR (Table 13.2). Of the seven patients who had SR, four patients underwent partial and three patients full SR of the ipsilateral NVB. Cancer was found in the SR in three out of seven cases on final histological examination (two full SR and one partial SR). Of the four patients who underwent partial SR, one had cancer present in the SR specimen and three had RP failure by 12-months (defined as requiring adjuvant therapy or BCR). Of the three patients who underwent full SR, two out of the three had cancer present in the SR specimen and two went on to have RP failure by 12-months.

Four men (patient 5, 6, 7 and 11 in Table 13.3) had five PSMs on IFS and no SR was performed because of short length and low grade of PSM. In all three cases where PSM was single and up to 1 mm, no RP failure was noted at 12-months follow-up. Moreover, three men (5, 7, and 9 Table 13.3) had single PSM <1 mm in length, all three of which were converted to clear on final section analysis.

Also in the NeuroSAFE PROOF Feasibility study, four men (patients 2, 3, 6 and 8 in Table 13.3) who had multiple section PSMs during IFS all had RP failure regardless of whether they had SR. Of these four men, two had full SR (of which one had cancer within), one man had a partial resection with cancer seen in it, and the last had no SR. Although these numbers are small, these findings were taken into account alongside the results of the Erasmus group, and have helped inform the NeuroSAFE technique secondary resection protocol for the full study (see below).

NeuroSAFE Technique: PSM Evidence and Secondary Resection

With regards to the comparative studies that are available where a NeuroSAFE RARP cohort are compared to a non-NeuroSAFE control cohort there are three studies to date that report. All report a reduction in PSM rate in the NeuroSAFE RP group attributable to the ability to convert a PSM noted during IFS into a final NSM by SR (see Table 13.2). Schlomm et al., Mirmilstein et al. and Preisser et al. note a reduction in rate of PSM by 6.5%, 8.6% and 14.1%, respectively in the NeuroSAFE group compared to the non-NeuroSAFE technique. All of these studies are retrospective case-control studies, though Schlomm and colleagues performed propensity score matched analysis. van der Slot and colleagues report a final PSM rate of 34.5%, but no comparison group is provided where RP was performed without the NeuroSAFE technique for comparison of PSM. The NeuroSAFE PROOF team have not published their surgical margin status results from the feasibility study because the full trial is ongoing.

NeuroSAFE Technique: Oncological Outcomes

Schlomm and colleagues from the Martini Klinik have presented long term oncological outcomes in their retrospective case control of 11,069 men. In summary, according to their propensity score-based model, BCR did not differ significantly according to NeuroSAFE and non-NeuroSAFE patients [29]. In the single surgeon series of 417 patients reported by Mirmilstein and colleagues, though only short-term oncological follow-up was available (median 15.6 NeuroSAFE group and 31.4 non-NeuroSAFE group), BCR occurred in 1.7% and 1.9% of patients, respectively ($p = 0.88$).

NeuroSAFE Technique: NVBs and Functional Recovery

There is an increasing body of evidence to suggest that the NeuroSAFE technique during RARP can increase the pro-

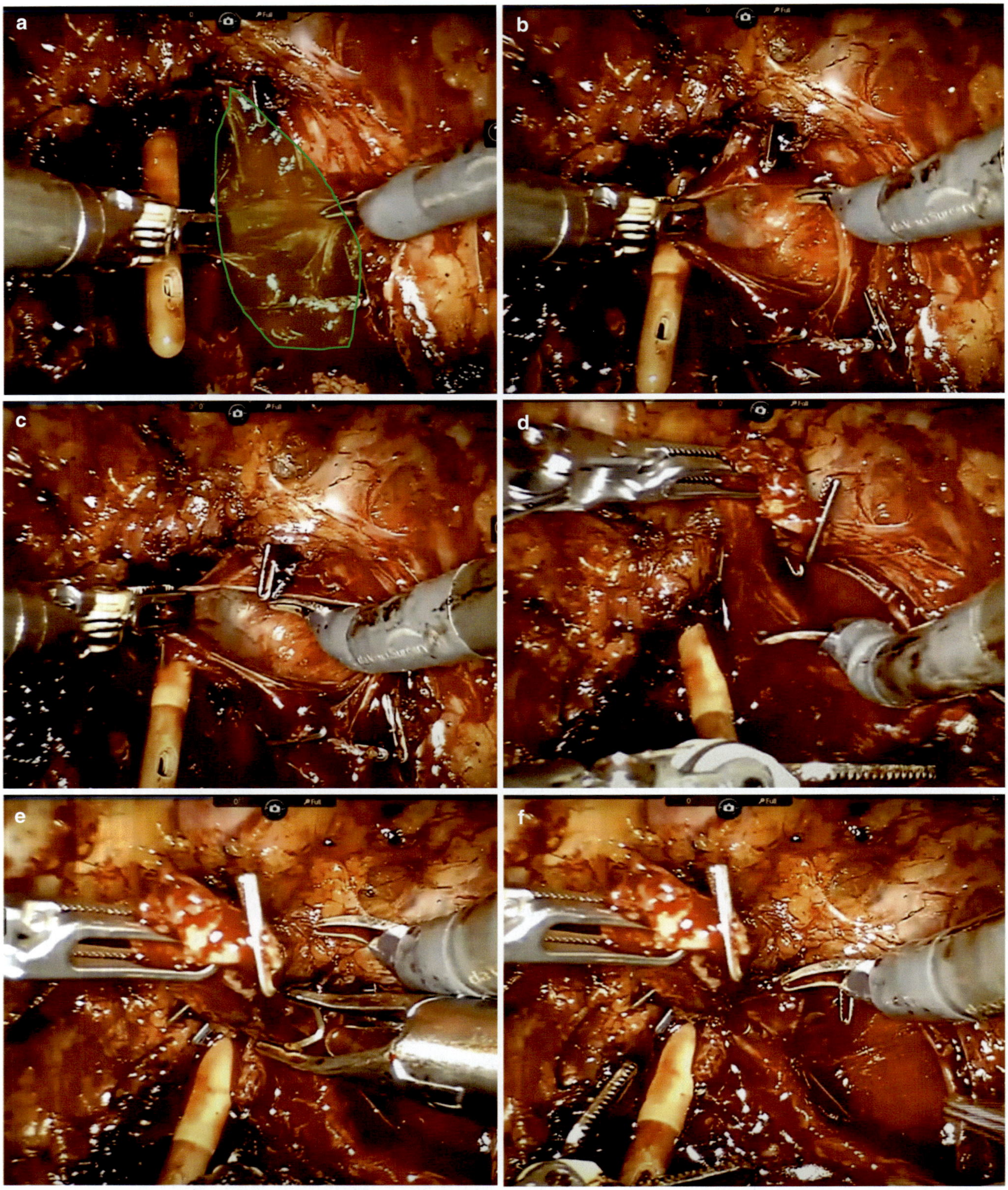

Fig. 13.4 Still images collated to demonstrate the secondary resection of an ipsilateral NVB in response to a positive NeuroSAFE intra-operative frozen section margin. (**a**) The right NVB is distracted medially (**b**) and the overlying fascia incised to develop a plane between NVB and the rectum. (**c**) Dissection plane is extended distally to the insertion of the NVB into the pelvic floor and proximally to its origin at the prostatic pedicle. (**d**) Further dissection of the NVB towards the apical limit for en bloc resection. (**e**) The distal (apical) end of the NVB is clipped and cut. (**f**) The excised NVB is removed and sent for formalin fixation, paraffin embedding final histopathological examination with the rest of the RP specimen. The outer aspect of the secondarily resected NVB can be inked to demonstrate new limit of the surgical margin

Table 13.3 Summary of histological and oncological outcomes for patients in the NeuroSAFE Arm who had a positive margin on IFS

Patient[a]	IFS margin (number, length)	Final margin[b]	SR performed	SR +ve cancer	PSA	Biopsy ISUP	Tumour biopsy	DRE	Path ISUP	pT	pN	RP failure
1	Single, 3 mm	P	Partial	No	5.8	2	Bilateral	T2	2	3a	NX	N
2	Multiple, 7 mm	P	Full	Yes	11	2	Bilateral	T3	2	3a	NX	Y
3	Multiple, 5 mm	P	Full	No	7.1	2	Left	T1	2	2c	NX	Y
4	Single, 2 mm	P	Partial	No	8	2	Bilateral	T2	2	3a	NX	Y
5	Single, <1 mm	C	Nil	n/a	4	2	Bilateral	T1	2	2c	NX	N
5 (other side)	Single, <1 mm	P	Nil	n/a	4	2	Bilateral	T1	2	2c	NX	N
6	Multiple (each only 1 mm) 2 mm	P	Nil	n/a	14.3	3	Bilateral	T3	3	3b	N0	Y
7	Single, 0.5 mm	C	Nil	n/a	1.2	2	Left	T2	2	2a	NX	N
8	Multiple, 4 mm	P	Partial	Yes	7.5	3	Bilateral	T3	2	3a	NX	Y
9	Single, <1 mm	C	Partial	No	8	2	Bilateral	T1	2	3a	NX	Y
10	Single, 1 mm	P	Full	Yes	6.7	2	Left	T2	2	2c	NX	N
11	Single, 1 mm	P	Nil	n/a	9.4	2	Right	T1	2	2c	N0	N

RP failure defined as adjuvant therapy or PSA > 0.2 ng/mL at follow-up of 12 months

[a]Patient numbers arbitrary not chronological in this table to preserve anonymity. *P* positive, *C* clear, *Y* yes, *N* no

[b]Final margin at the corresponding final section only

Table 13.2 PSM rates according to NeuroSAFE PROOF published studies where data is available

Study	IFS (n=)	Non-IFS (n=)	PSM rate IFS	PSM rate non-IFS	δ PSM rate	% IFS positive	Ability convert PSM IFS to NSM RP	% SNR tissue +ve cancer
Schlomm [29]	2567	2567	15.2%	21.7%	−6.5%	27.2%	86.2%	23%
Mirmilstein [33]	120	157	9.2%	17.8%	−8.6%	14.5%	NA	42.4%
Preisser [34]	156	190	15.4%	29.5%	−14.1%	NA	NA	NA

portion of NS RARP performed. Firstly, the original report from the Martini Klink including 2567 propensity score matched men in each group reported an increase in NVB preservation from 80.6% to 96.6% overall, and from 52% to 63.3% for bilateral NS. Preisser and colleagues reported an even more pronounced increase in the proportion of men having NS following the introduction of the NeuroSAFE technique at their institution [34]. In a retrospective unadjusted case-control study with 190 non-NeuroSAFE and 156 NeuroSAFE RP, they noted overall NS increase from 55.3% to 95.5%, and bilateral NS increase 55.3% to 85.3%.

In the NeuroSAFE PROOF Feasibility, 25 men underwent NeuroSAFE RARP and 24 men underwent standard RARP. NS status was prospectively recorded by the operating surgeon immediately after the completion of surgery. Considering each NVB as the denominator 60% of NVB had some degree of NS (intrafascial, interfascial, partial) in the standard arm vs to 89.6% in the NeuroSAFE arm. Considering each participant as the denominator, 33% of men in the standard arm had bilateral intrafascial NS compared to 62.5% of men in the NeuroSAFE arm [35]. Mature functional outcomes are not available for review until the full study has completed recruitment (see below).

In terms of patient-centred functional outcomes, two studies to date have published results. Mirmilstein and colleagues, reported improvement in erectile function recovery [33]. They defined potency as the ability to have penetrative sexual intercourse with or without the assistance of oral medications at 12-months after surgery and was assessed by physician interview unblinded to operation type. At 12-months, 77.3% of men who had NeuroSAFE RARP were potent vs. 50.9% who had standard RARP.

Fossa and colleagues, from Norway, are the only group to date to publish validated patient reported outcome measures (PROM) for men undergoing RP with the NeuroSAFE technique [36]. Their study is limited by retrospective design and confounded by the fact that the NeuroSAFE group were younger and underwent RP at the Martini Klinik, whereas the non-NeuroSAFE group underwent surgery during the same period at Oslo University Hospital, Norway. They compared 95 men in the NeuroSAFE group against 312 men in the Non-NeuroSAFE group in whom bilateral NS was achieved in 79% and 29%, respectively. The Norwegian version of the EPIC-26 was used wherein 66% of men in the NeuroSAFE group reported "No erectile dysfunction" compared to 36% of men in the Non-NeuroSAFE group. After RP with NeuroSAFE technique, 83% of the men reported effective use of pro-erectile aids compared to 50% of men in the non-NeuroSAFE group.

NeuroSAFE Technique: Cost and Resources

Early reports from the Martini Klinik about time required to perform the NeuroSAFE technique suggest that the additional time for IFS can be used to perform the Rocco stitch, urethra-vesical anastomosis, and lymph node dissection; therefore, no additional time, at their centre is spent under general anaesthesia despite the fact that technical laboratory steps takes 35 min [29]. Mirmilstein and colleagues estimated the additional cost of the NeuroSAFE technique at £550 per case in the NHS UK healthcare system [33].

Dinneen et al. showed in their Feasibility RCT that whilst no patients experienced any harm for longer time spent under general anaesthesia, NeuroSAFE RARP took 57 min longer than standard RARP [31]. However, two points were highlighted by the authors to help explain the considerable increase in operation length in the intervention arm; (a) in both sites, the pathology laboratory was located in a different building to the OR therefore transportation time had to be taken into account, and (b) only 22% or men had lymph node dissection, therefore the average length of RARP in the standard arm was shorter than previous reports, which made the difference more pronounced.

Similarly, van der Slot et al. estimated that the additional time required for the NeuroSAFE technique during RARP was 43 min (IQR 39–50 min) but this decreased over time [37]. The median pathology time for the first 100 NeuroSAFE procedures was 46 min (IQR 40–53 min), and that for the last 100 was 41 min (IQR 37–48 min) ($p = 0.004$).

NeuroSAFE PROOF Trial

Despite the advent of robotic surgery technology, many centres have struggled to improve sexual health recovery outcomes for their patients over the last decade [38]. Consequently, surgeons and researchers should be investigating and evaluating new avenues to improve this important part of recovery and achievement of trifecta. The NeuroSAFE PROOF study is part of this endeavour.

Many of the design features of the NeuroSAFE PROOF trial have been developed in order to provide evidence that will be of assistance to health policy makers considering methods and advanced techniques in RARP to improve outcomes, particularly erectile function recovery, for men with localised prostate cancer undergoing surgery. No clinical trial is truly explanatory nor pragmatic, but in many aspects the NeuroSAFE PROOF trial has been based upon decisions to represent real life, or pragmatic conditions as this will help surgeons and policy makers around the world understand whether the technique will be appropriate for their patients. As such, the trial will involve multiple sites, surgeons, pathologists, radiologists and clinicians. Similarly, there will be no standardised penile rehabilitation program after RARP as this is not routine practice where the trial will be conducted.

Conversely, the exclusion of men with poor baseline erectile function (IIEF-5 < 22) represents a step away from usual conditions and thus may reduce external validity compared to all candidates for RARP. However, this decision reflects a desire on the part of the researchers to maximise the conditions for favourable effects from intervention to be apparent if they are present.

The NeuroSAFE PROOF Feasibility Study demonstrated better than expected recruitment and feasibility of the trial intervention in more than one centre in the UK. Moreover, the feasibility study has helped the trial team to stabilise and standardise the trial intervention and follow-up measures so that, as much as possible, treatment effects seen in the outcomes of the study can be attributed to the trial intervention rather than divergent surgical practices, bias or confounding from variations in follow-up regimen. Following the analysis of the men who had PSM on NeuroSAFE technique in the feasibility study, the trial protocol now instructs that only full SR is performed and partial SR has been eliminated. Secondly, the indications for full SR are now: (1) any PSM on multiple sections on a side; (2) any Gleason grade 4 or grade 5 adenocarcinoma at the margin; and (3) any single section PSM >1 mm of Gleason Grade Group 1 (see Fig. 13.2). At the time of writing, the NeuroSAFE PROOF Trial has recruited 330 patients from a total of approximately 400. Covid-19 pandemic has interrupted and delayed recruitment, but the trial is still open to recruitment and performing interventions as per random allocation at five UK sites.

Conclusions

In conclusion, intra-operative margin assessment using frozen section (IFS) has long been an appealing option for surgeons attempting to tailor and optimise surgical dissection for their patients during RP. Realtime microscopic margin status feedback can, certainly in theory, allow the surgeon to get the balance between *preservation* of important periprostatic structures and *avoidance* of PSM correct irrespective of the differences between each man's disease and anatomical characteristics.

With regards to the evidence on IFS, there is some evidence that IFS can reduce PSMs, but this is largely lower quality within the hierarchy and only one single centre series have reported that this can impact beneficially on BCR.

Evidence to suggest IFS can benefit functional outcomes appears generally more promising than exclusively focussing on oncological outcomes by way of altering margin status. Arguably, the area of the prostate where the correct balance between preservation and avoidance is most important and influenced by the surgeon is the posterolateral neurovascular structure adjacent margin. That is one of the reasons why the NeuroSAFE Technique IFS has become prominent in recent years. To summarise the important considerations and evidence to date on the NeuroSAFE technique:

- There is evidence of good to excellent histological concordance from several centres on the use of frozen section for the posterolateral neurovascular structure adjacent margin comparing to final margin status at the same portion of the prostate.
- Increased duration of surgery may or may not occur depending on centre. If surgery is lengthened by the technique, there is no evidence that this causes harm to the patient, though there may be additional costs associated with the technique.
- There is evidence that the NeuroSAFE technique can affect a modest reduction on PSM rates, though the evidence of the long-term oncological outcomes with the NeuroSAFE technique is limited to a single centre, the Martini Klinik.
- There are several studies from numerous centres that note a marked increase in NS during RP when the NeuroSAFE technique is used.
- There is some observational evidence to suggest improved erectile function outcomes when the NeuroSAFE technique is used.
- The NeuroSAFE PROOF randomised controlled trial has been designed to attempt to answer many of the questions not yet answered in this chapter, and will have patient-reported functional outcomes as the primary outcome.

References

1. Eastham JA, Scardino PT, Kattan MW. Predicting an optimal outcome after radical prostatectomy: the trifecta nomogram. J Urol. 2008;179(6):2207–10; discussion 10–1.
2. Walsh PC, Lepor H, Eggleston JC. Radical prostatectomy with preservation of sexual function: anatomical and pathological considerations. Prostate. 1983;4(5):473–85.
3. Costello AJ, Brooks M, Cole OJ. Anatomical studies of the neurovascular bundle and cavernosal nerves. BJU Int. 2004;94(7):1071–6.
4. Sievert KD, Hennenlotter J, Dillenburg T, Toomey P, Wollner J, Zweers P, et al. Extended periprostatic nerve distributions on the prostate surface confirmed using diffusion tensor imaging. BJU Int. 2019;123(6):995–1004.
5. Walz J, Burnett AL, Costello AJ, Eastham JA, Graefen M, Guillonneau B, et al. A critical analysis of the current knowledge of surgical anatomy related to optimization of cancer control and preservation of continence and erection in candidates for radical prostatectomy. Eur Urol. 2010;57(2):179–92.
6. Wang X, Wu Y, Guo J, Chen H, Weng X, Liu X. Intrafascial nerve-sparing radical prostatectomy improves patients' postoperative continence recovery and erectile function: a pooled analysis based on available literatures. Medicine (Baltimore). 2018;97(29):e11297.
7. Michl U, Tennstedt P, Feldmeier L, Mandel P, Oh SJ, Ahyai S, et al. Nerve-sparing surgery technique, not the preservation of the neurovascular bundles, leads to improved long-term continence rates after radical prostatectomy. Eur Urol. 2016;69(4):584–9.
8. Reeves F, Preece P, Kapoor J, Everaerts W, Murphy DG, Corcoran NM, et al. Preservation of the neurovascular bundles is associated with improved time to continence after radical prostatectomy but not long-term continence rates: results of a systematic review and meta-analysis. Eur Urol. 2015;68(4):692–704.
9. Tewari AK, Srivastava A, Huang MW, Robinson BD, Shevchuk MM, Durand M, et al. Anatomical grades of nerve sparing: a risk-stratified approach to neural-hammock sparing during robot-assisted radical prostatectomy (RARP). BJU Int. 2011;108(6 Pt 2):984–92.
10. Ma X, Tang K, Yang C, Wu G, Xu N, Wang M, et al. Bladder neck preservation improves time to continence after radical prostatectomy: a systematic review and meta-analysis. Oncotarget. 2016;7(41):67463–75.
11. Schlomm T, Heinzer H, Steuber T, Salomon G, Engel O, Michl U, et al. Full functional-length urethral sphincter preservation during radical prostatectomy. Eur Urol. 2011;60(2):320–9
12. Lei Y, Alemozaffar M, Williams SB, Hevelone N, Lipsitz SR, Plaster BA, et al. Athermal division and selective suture ligation of the dorsal vein complex during robot-assisted laparoscopic radical prostatectomy: description of technique and outcomes. Eur Urol. 2011;59(2):235–43.
13. Dev HS, Wiklund P, Patel V, Parashar D, Palmer K, Nyberg T, et al. Surgical margin length and location affect recurrence rates after robotic prostatectomy. Urol Oncol. 2015;33(3):109.e7–13.
14. Inoue S, Shiina H, Hiraoka T, Mitsui Y, Sumura M, Urakami S, et al. Retrospective analysis of the distance between the neurovascular bundle and prostate cancer foci in radical prostatectomy specimens: its clinical implication in nerve-sparing surgery. BJU Int. 2009;104(8):1085–90.
15. Philippou Y, Harriss E, Davies L, Jubber I, Leslie T, Bell RW, et al. Prostatic capsular incision during radical prostatectomy has important oncological implications: a systematic review and meta-analysis. BJU Int. 2018. https://doi.org/10.1111/bju.14522.
16. Rapp DE, Orvieto MA, Lucioni A, Gong EM, Shalhav AL, Brendler CB. Intra-operative prostate examination: predictive value and effect on margin status. BJU Int. 2005;95(7):1005–8.
17. Rocco B, Sighinolfi MC, Sandri M, Eissa A, Elsherbiny A, Zoeir A, et al. Is extraprostatic extension of cancer predictable? A review of predictive tools and an external validation based on a large and a single center cohort of prostate cancer patients. Urology. 2019;129:8–20.
18. Abrams-Pompe RS, Fanti S, Schoots IG, Moore CM, Turkbey B, Vickers AJ, et al. The role of magnetic resonance imaging and positron emission tomography/computed tomography in the primary staging of newly diagnosed prostate cancer: a systematic review of the literature. Eur Urol Oncol. 2021;4(3):370–95.
19. Eissa A, Zoeir A, Sighinolfi MC, Puliatti S, Bevilacqua L, Del Prete C, et al. "Real-time" assessment of surgical margins during radical prostatectomy: state-of-the-art. Clin Genitourin Cancer. 2020;18(2):95–104.
20. Dinneen EP, van der Slot M, Adasonla K, Tan J, Grierson J, Haider A, et al. Intraoperative frozen section for margin evaluation during radical prostatectomy: a systematic review. Eur Urol Focus 2020;6(4):664–73.
21. Sighinolfi MC, Eissa A, Spandri V, Puliatti S, Micali S, Reggiani Bonetti L, et al. Positive surgical margin during radical prostatectomy: overview of sampling methods for frozen sections and tech-

niques for the secondary resection of the neurovascular bundles. BJU Int. 2020;125(5):656–63.
22. Pak S, Park S, Kim M, Go H, Cho YM, Ahn H. The impact on oncological outcomes after radical prostatectomy for prostate cancer of converting soft tissue margins at the apex and bladder neck from tumour-positive to -negative. BJU Int. 2019;123(5):811–7.
23. Gillitzer R, Thuroff C, Fandel T, Thomas C, Thuroff JW, Brenner W, et al. Intraoperative peripheral frozen sections do not significantly affect prognosis after nerve-sparing radical prostatectomy for prostate cancer. BJU Int. 2011;107(5):755–9.
24. Nunez AL, Giannico GA, Mukhtar F, Dailey V, El-Galley R, Hameed O. Frozen section evaluation of margins in radical prostatectomy specimens: a contemporary study and literature review. Ann Diagn Pathol. 2016;24:11–8.
25. Dillenburg W, Poulakis V, Witzsch U, de Vries R, Skriapas K, Altmansberger HM, et al. Laparoscopic radical prostatectomy: the value of intraoperative frozen sections. Eur Urol. 2005;48(4):614–21.
26. Kakiuchi Y, Choy B, Gordetsky J, Izumi K, Wu G, Rashid H, et al. Role of frozen section analysis of surgical margins during robot-assisted laparoscopic radical prostatectomy: a 2608-case experience. Hum Pathol. 2013;44(8):1556–62.
27. Tsuboi T, Ohori M, Kuroiwa K, Reuter VE, Kattan MW, Eastham JA, et al. Is intraoperative frozen section analysis an efficient way to reduce positive surgical margins? Urology. 2005;66(6):1287–91.
28. Eichelberg C, Erbersdobler A, Haese A, Schlomm T, Chun FK, Currlin E, et al. Frozen section for the management of intraoperatively detected palpable tumor lesions during nerve-sparing scheduled radical prostatectomy. Eur Urol. 2006;49(6):1011–6. discussion 6–8.
29. Schlomm T, Tennstedt P, Huxhold C, Steuber T, Salomon G, Michl U, et al. Neurovascular structure-adjacent frozen-section examination (NeuroSAFE) increases nerve-sparing frequency and reduces positive surgical margins in open and robot-assisted laparoscopic radical prostatectomy: experience after 11,069 consecutive patients. Eur Urol. 2012;62(2):333–40.
30. Beyer B, Schlomm T, Tennstedt P, Boehm K, Adam M, Schiffmann J, et al. A feasible and time-efficient adaptation of NeuroSAFE for da Vinci robot-assisted radical prostatectomy. Eur Urol. 2014;66(1):138–44.
31. Dinneen E, Haider A, Grierson J, Freeman A, Oxley J, Briggs T, et al. NeuroSAFE frozen section during robot-assisted radical prostatectomy: peri-operative and histopathological outcomes from the NeuroSAFE PROOF feasibility randomized controlled trial. BJU Int. 2021;127(6):676–86.
32. Dinneen E, Haider A, Freeman A, Oxley J, Briggs T, Nathan S, et al. NeuroSAFE PROOF randomised controlled feasibility study: brief report of perioperative outcomes, histological concordance, and feasibility. Eur Urol. 2020;78(3):476–8.
33. Mirmilstein G, Rai BP, Gbolahan O, Srirangam V, Narula A, Agarwal S, et al. The neurovascular structure-adjacent frozen-section examination (NeuroSAFE) approach to nerve sparing in robot-assisted laparoscopic radical prostatectomy in a British setting—a prospective observational comparative study. BJU Int. 2018;121(6):854–62.
34. Preisser F, Theissen L, Wild P, Bartelt K, Kluth L, Kollermann J, et al. Implementation of intraoperative frozen section during radical prostatectomy: short-term results from a German Tertiary-care Center. Eur Urol Focus. 2021;7(1):95–101.
35. Dinneen E, Haider A, Grierson J, Briggs T, Nathan S, Allen C, Heffernan-Ho D, Persad R, Oakley N, Freeman A, Shaw G. The NeuroSAFE RCT feasibility study. Eur Urol Suppl. 2019;18(5):e2548.
36. Fossa SD, Beyer B, Dahl AA, Aas K, Eri LM, Kvan E, et al. Improved patient-reported functional outcomes after nerve-sparing radical prostatectomy by using NeuroSAFE technique. Scand J Urol. 2019;53(6):385–91.
37. van der Slot MA, den Bakker MA, Klaver S, Kliffen M, Busstra MB, Rietbergen JBW, et al. Intraoperative assessment and reporting of radical prostatectomy specimens to guide nerve-sparing surgery in prostate cancer patients (NeuroSAFE). Histopathology. 2020;77(4):539–47.
38. Capogrosso P, Vertosick EA, Benfante NE, Eastham JA, Scardino PJ, Vickers AJ, et al. Are we improving erectile function recovery after radical prostatectomy? Analysis of patients treated over the last decade. Eur Urol. 2019;75(2):221–8.
39. Cangiano TG, Litwin MS, Naitoh J, Dorey F, deKernion JB. Intraoperative frozen section monitoring of nerve sparing radical retropubic prostatectomy. J Urol. 1999;162(3 Pt 1):655–8.
40. Lavery HJ, Xiao GQ, Nabizada-Pace F, Mikulasovich M, Unger P, Samadi DB. 'Mohs surgery of the prostate': the utility of in situ frozen section analysis during robotic prostatectomy. BJU Int. 2011;107(6):975–9.
41. Heinrich E, Schon G, Schiefelbein F, Michel MS, Trojan L. Clinical impact of intraoperative frozen sections during nerve-sparing radical prostatectomy. World J Urol. 2010;28(6):709–13.
42. Petralia G, Musi G, Padhani AR, Summers P, Renne G, Alessi S, et al. Robot-assisted radical prostatectomy: multiparametric MR imaging-directed intraoperative frozen-section analysis to reduce the rate of positive surgical margins. Radiology. 2015;274(2):434–44.
43. Obek C, Saglican Y, Ince U, Argun OB, Tuna MB, Doganca T, et al. Intra-surgical total and re-constructible pathological prostate examination for safer margins and nerve preservation (Istanbul preserve). Ann Diagn Pathol. 2018;33:35–9.
44. Dinneen E, Haider A, Grierson J, Freeman A, Oxley J, Briggs T, et al. NeuroSAFE frozen section during robot-assisted radical prostatectomy (RARP): peri-operative and histopathological outcomes from the NeuroSAFE PROOF feasibility randomised controlled trial. BJU Int. 2021;127(6):676–86.

Ex Vivo Fluorescence Confocal Microscopy

14

Bernardo Rocco, Luca Sarchi, Tommaso Calcagnile, Simone Assumma, Alessandra Cassani, Sofia Maggiorelli, and Maria Chiara Sighinolfi

Introduction

Fluorescence Confocal Microscopy (FCM) is an imaging technique able to generate digital images from fresh tissue in real time, without the need for traditional processing. The appearance of microscopical slides is in hematoxylin-eosin (HE), similar to the conventional images that pathologists are usually dealing with. The FCM analysis on the fresh sample does not affect specimen integrity and does not prevent the samples from undergoing subsequent histopathological examination or supplementary studies (e.g. immunohistochemistry) [1].

Device Technical Features

The confocal microscope outperforms the traditional wide field light microscope in terms of both maximum lateral resolution (0.25 m vs. 0.5 m) and maximum axial resolution (0.7 m vs. 1.6 m). Moreover, the ability of removing "out-of-focus" brightness at various magnifications is a typical feature of FCM [2]. Reflectance (488 nm) and fluorescence (785 nm) can be adjusted depending on the laser wavelength; modern FCM devices are able to provide a combination of the two modalities, characterizing either stromal and subcellular features, simultaneously displaying two color scale mosaics that resemble HE pattern. Fluorescence mode is based on the use of dyes; Acridine Orange, which selectively binds to DNA and allows for clear visualization of the nuclei, is the most commonly used.

Ex vivo FCM has been applied in dermatology field [3–5] and compared with traditional frozen sections analysis for the detection of basal cell carcinoma and cutaneous inflammatory diseases. A prospective study found that FCM has a high degree of accuracy [3]. Analogously, it has shown 95.2% agreement with conventional hematoxylin-eosin (HE) in the interpretation of lung, liver, adrenal gland, kidney, bone, pleura, lymph nodes and soft tissues [6].

FMC has been successfully applied in the urological area for renal tissue analysis. In the context of the renal biopsy procedure, Mir et al. recorded 100% agreement of FMC with HE for the identification of both tumor tissue and normal renal parenchyma. The aim of the study was to find a suitable core sample, and FCM's real-time analysis proved to be effective in reducing the number of non-diagnostic renal mass biopsies [7].

The purpose of this chapter is to present the evidence for FCM's application in prostate tissue analysis and to describe the state of the art for its use in prostate cancer diagnosis and treatment.

FCM Technology: Historical Background

Marvin Minsky developed in 1955 the first model of confocal microscope [8]. This first version consisted of a transmitted light microscope, composed by a light source with a small hole for allowing the passage of a light beam, which was then centered on the biological sample by a lens [9]. After passing through the biological sample, the light beam was focused by a second lens and a second small hole with the same focus as the first: the definition of "confocal" comes from this mechanism. The light passing through the second hole impacted against a detector, creating a signal equal to the brightness of the beam that passed through the hole; however, the light above and below the plane was protected by

B. Rocco (✉)
Department of Urology, ASST Santi Paolo e Carlo—Università degli Studi di Milano, Milan, Italy

Department of Urology, Ospedale Policlinico e Nuovo Ospedale Civile S.Agostino Estense Modena, University of Modena and Reggio Emilia, Modena, Italy

L. Sarchi · T. Calcagnile · S. Assumma · A. Cassani · S. Maggiorelli · M. C. Sighinolfi
Department of Urology, Ospedale Policlinico e Nuovo Ospedale Civile S.Agostino Estense Modena, University of Modena and Reggio Emilia, Modena, Italy
e-mail: 213144@studenti.unimore.it

S. Ren et al. (eds.), *Robot-Assisted Radical Prostatectomy*, https://doi.org/10.1007/978-3-031-05855-4_14

the second hole. The image was produced by shifting the sample manually [2, 9].

The reflected light microscope was another variation of the same microscope: it had a light source and a small hole that generated a light ray, which was reflected by a dichromatic mirror and focused on the biological sample by a lens. The beam was then mirrored by the sample and centered by the same lens as before, passing through the same dichromatic mirror and impacting on the detector through a second hole [2, 9, 10].

Many technological advancements have occurred since these first prototypes, including high resolution monitors, faster computers, laser-based light sources, optimized reflective mirrors and filters, more sensitive and silent photodetectors, more accurate data acquisition techniques, optimized biological sample preparation, more innovative image analysis software and bioinformatics methods [2, 9, 10].

In the late 1980s, the final version of confocal laser microscope which could be considered the prototype of more recent ones, usable for both research and clinical purposes, was developed by a group of researchers in Cambridge. The optical sections created by the microscope were thin enough to examine the items of interest; thickness could be varied by adjusting the diameter of the hole in front of the detector, providing the chance of zooming the image without losing resolution by decreasing the scanned area. Modern confocal microscopes can be categorized based on the biological sample's scanning process, which can be either the movement of the sample (stage scanning) or the movement of the light beam (beam scanning) [2, 9, 10].

Further progress was made in recent decades, as laser stability and power (which was reduced in modern microscopes to avoid photo damage), efficacy of dichromatic mirrors and photo detectors, electronic filters and software systems for digitalization were enhanced. These advancements increase the versatility of confocal microscopes for a variety of current applications.

Current FCM Device Available for Clinical Application on Prostatic Tissue

The Fluorescence Confocal Microscopy (FCM) with VivaScope® 2500 M-G4 (Mavig GmbH, Munich, Germany; Caliber I.D.; Rochester, NY, USA) is an optical imaging instrument which uses two lasers: reflectance (785 nm) and fluorescence (488 nm) modes [1, 11]. FCM has been applied in the prostate setting to evaluate in real time (ex vivo) fresh dissected specimens. Its maximum examination depth consists of 200 μm, its vertical resolution of up to 4 μm, its maximum magnification of ×550 and its maximum scan size of 25 × 25 mm. It should be also remarked that the penetration depth can be improved by adjusting the laser power and/or the specimen's incubation time in the dye. The resulting image is a mosaic of square-shaped images with a resolution of 1024 × 1024 pixels. The laser filter has a ×38, 0.85 numerical aperture water immersion objective lens. VivaScan® (Version 11.0.1140 Mavig GmbH; Caliber I.D.), VivaBlock®, and VivaStack® are software packages which respectively allow for image reconstruction from the sensors, multiple picture acquisition in the X/Y directions within a single plane at a fixed depth, and a survey of multiple frames along the Z axis to visualize deeper tissue [1, 11]. Grayscale fluorescence and reflectance mosaics were mixed after being digitally stained with color. Purple and pink colors are used to enhance correlation respectively with cellular nuclei and non-cellular structures, in order to produce pictures similar to hematoxylin and eosin (HE) and to strengthen the interpretation process performed by the pathologists [11]. Zooming capabilities allow for a more detailed view of cell morphology. The current FCM device is small and compact, making it easy to store in an operating room or an office.

Prostate Tissue Interpretation

Handling and Preparation of the Specimens

The fresh tissue—not formalin-fixed—is dyed separately with acridine orange dye. The dye currently used in clinical practice is Acridine orange (Sigma-Aldrich®), 0.6 mM solution; the sample is first soaked in it for 30 s and then washed in saline solution. The stained specimen is then positioned between two glass slides secured with silicon glue, before being out put on the FCM stage for image capture [1, 12]. The FCM can inspect both sides of the glass slides, allowing for a more precise inspection of the sample. The entire procedure for each specimen, including staining and image acquisition, should not take more than 5 min, depending on sample size: the wider the region to scan is, the longer it would require for picture acquisition. Then, the sample is formalin fixed (immersion in 10% neutral buffered formalin for 24 h) and paraffin embedded, as the standard processing practice requires. If necessary, the specimen is handled, during FCM and HE histopathological examinations, to maintain the correct orientation [1, 13]. FCM inspection of several urological tissues, including renal parenchyma [7], nodes, and urothelium, has proved to be effective using the same procedure (unpresented data, manuscript in submission).

Benign Prostatic Tissue and Benign Prostatic Hyperplasia

Benign prostate tissue appears as round-oval typical glands, consisting in two cell layers: low flat or cuboidal basal cells on the outside and tall columnar mucin-secreting epithelial cells on the inside [1, 12, 14]. The glands are organized in a non-infiltrating pattern of development and a thin connective tissue surrounds them. Corpora amylacea can be easily identified even if small in size [1, 12, 14]. Increased amount of epithelial pale to transparent cytoplasm and enlarged nuclei without atypia (epithelial hyperplasia) and/or stromal cells (stromal hyperplasia) are signs of hyperplastic changes (benign prostatic hyperplasia). Spindle cells and hyalinized matrix can be observed in stromal hyperplasia, which is characterized by fibrovascular and fibromuscular proliferation. Basal cells are clearly visible in hyperplastic glands at FCM (Fig. 14.1).

High-grade prostatic intraepithelial neoplasia is characterized in FCM images by glands with stratified epithelium, cells with pleomorphic nuclei and prominent nucleoli; the basal cell layer is preserved [1, 12, 14].

Acinar Adenocarcinoma

Acinar adenocarcinoma is constituted by tight packages of irregular glands that differ in size and form and are arranged in a back-to-back pattern [1, 12, 14]. The atypical glands are usually separated from one another by a small amount of stroma and they can look compressed in certain conditions. The presence of enlarged, hyperchromatic nuclei and a prominent nucleolus (colored in purple) in FCM is a crucial feature for defining the malignant nature of the glands, associated with the absence of the basal cell layer and the glands' disorganized morphology (Fig. 14.1).

The presence of cribriform glands appears to be noticeable as well, allowing for the differentiation of GG2 and GG3 tumors. PCa is classified as GG4 when undifferentiated cell patterns and poorly formed/fused glands are observed [1, 12, 14].

Periprostatic Components

In cases of extracapsular extension or positive surgical margins, specimens from extra-prostatic soft tissues were examined to distinguish between normal features—such as fatty, connective, and muscular tissues—and the persistence of prostate cancer at this site [1, 15]. The FCM appearance of extra-prostatic features, such as fatty tissues and muscle bundles, was presented in a study of 41 samples from 20 patients; these components were usually seen in a pink-color resem-

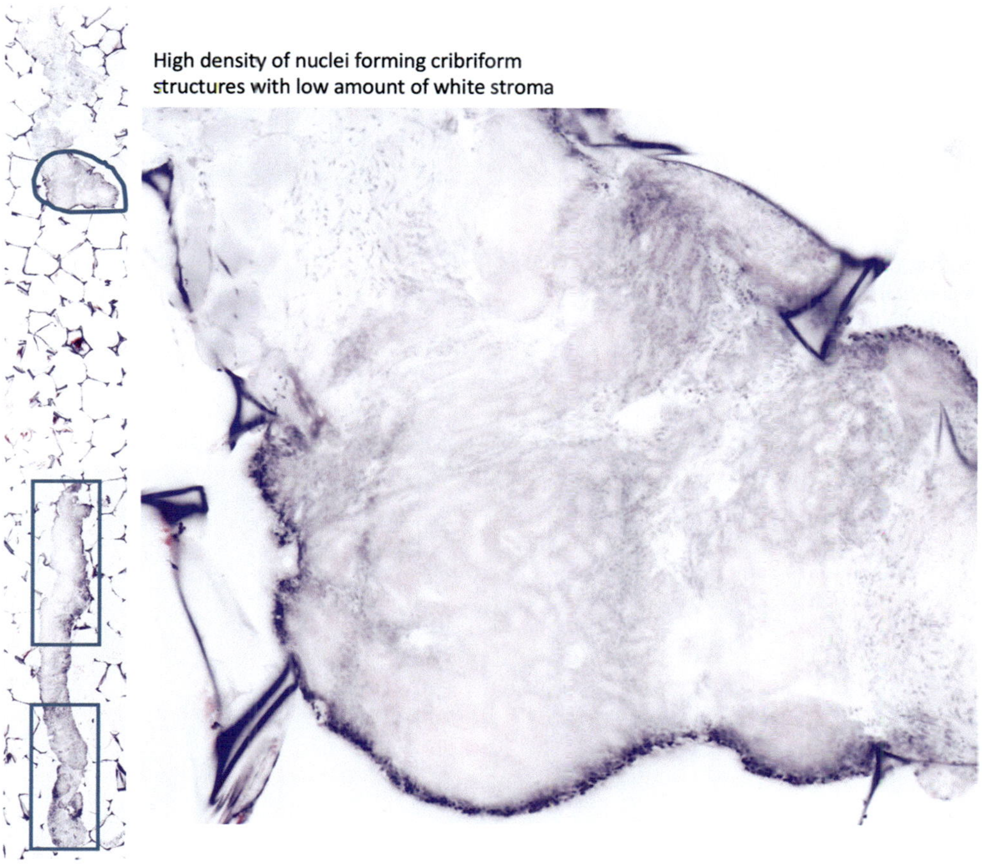

Fig. 14.1 Microscopical details: the presence of enlarged, hyperchromatic nuclei and a prominent nucleolus (purple) in FCM is crucial for defining the malignant nature of the glands, associated with the absence of the basal cell layer and the glands' disorganized morphology

bling eosin staining from the reflectance mode. The prostate glandular parenchyma, on the other hand, is different: it shows a prevalent purple color due to acridine-stained nuclei and given from the fluorescence modality (Fig. 14.2) [1, 15]. According to Rocco et al., there was 97.14% agreement between FCM and HE for muscular, 97.14% for nervous, 97.14% for vascular and 94.2% for fatty tissue [15]. The identification of benign and malignant prostate glands was feasible and consistent between FCM and the gold standard (Figs. 14.3 and 14.4).

Current FCM Fields of Applications

Diagnostic Setting

Prostate biopsy is one of the most common urological procedures, with over one million prostate biopsies performed each year in Europe and the United States, owing to the high prevalence of PCa among adult males [16]. The microscopic pathological examination of prostatic cores is essential for PCa diagnosis. Prostate biopsy may be done either in a sys-

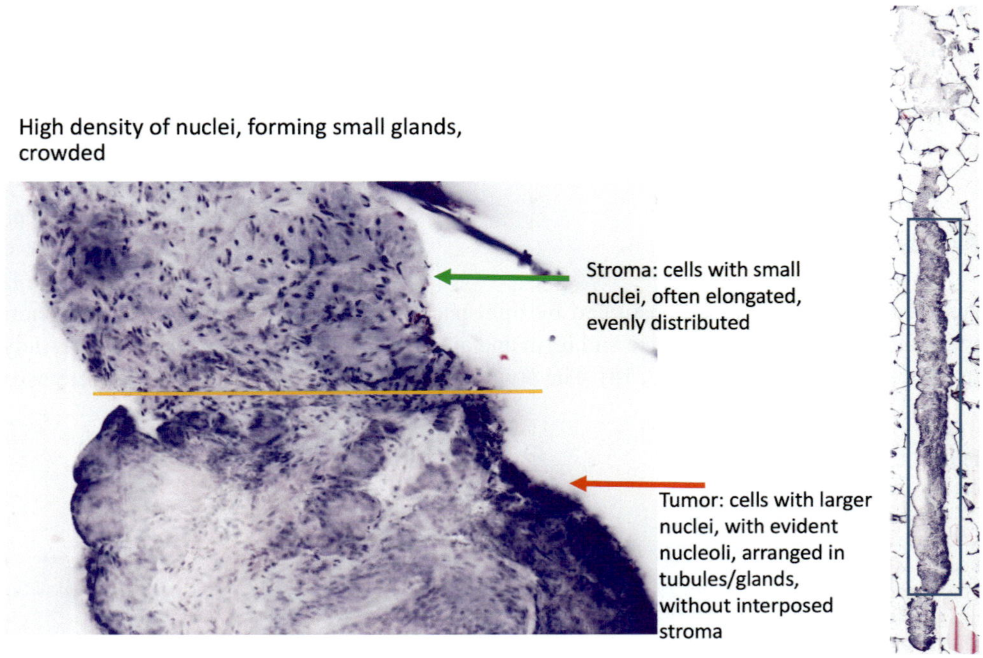

Fig. 14.2 The FCM appearance of extra-prostatic features, such as fatty tissues and muscle bundles, is usually seen in a pink-color resembling eosin staining; the prostate glandular parenchyma, shows a prevalent purple color due to acridine-stained nuclei

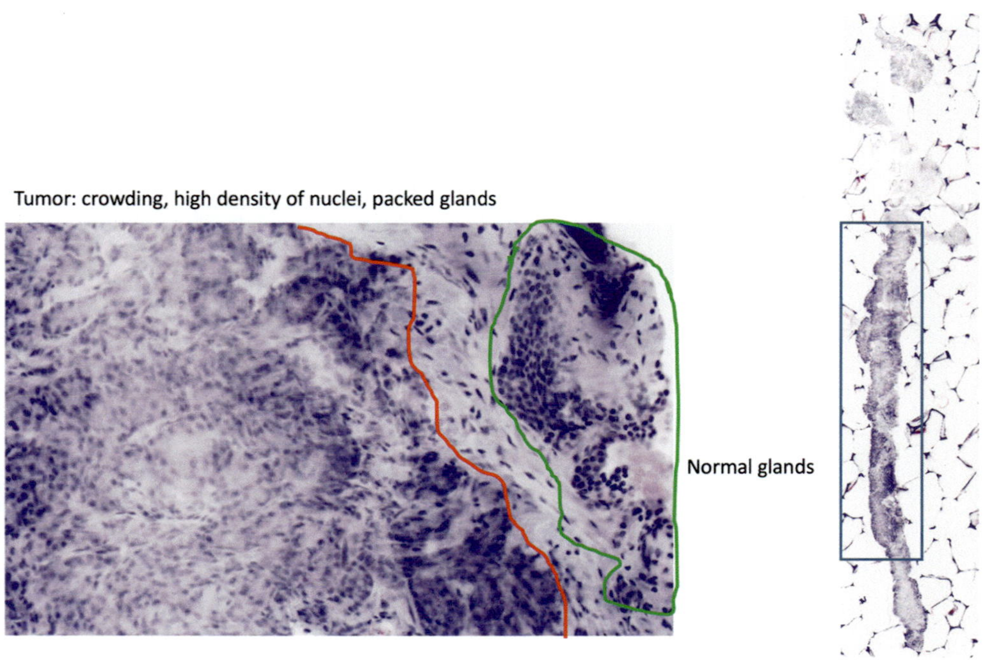

Fig. 14.3 Identification of benign and malignant prostate glands, part 1

Fig. 14.4 Identification of benign and malignant prostate glands, part 2

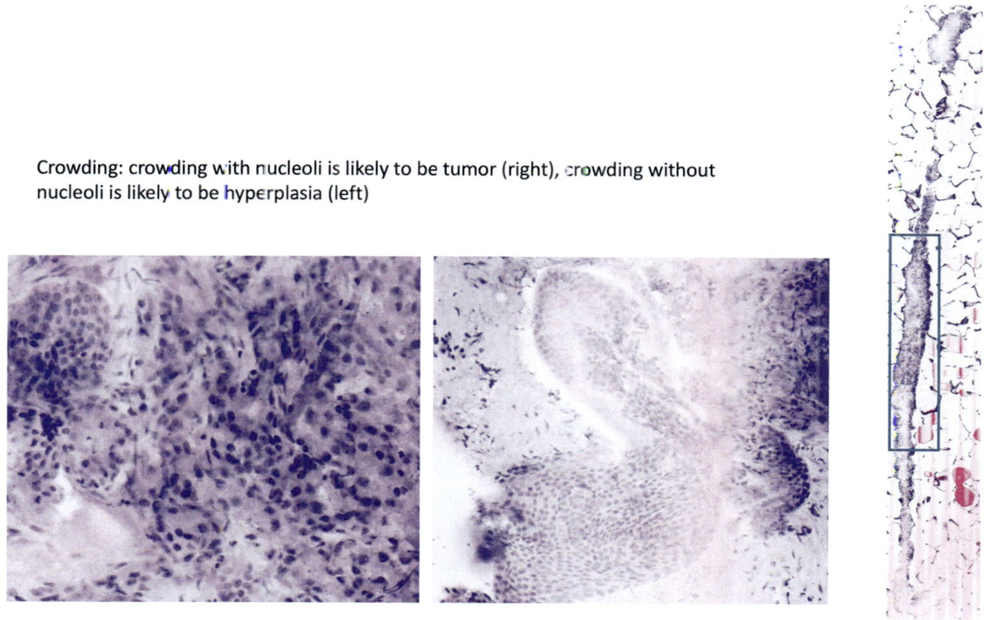

tematic (12 bilateral cores) or target fashion, if suspicious lesions are visible on mpMRI [17]. The best detection rate of clinically relevant PCa appears to be achieved by sampling using the combination of systematic and target method. The traditional histopathological analysis consists of processing, slide preparation, and pathological evaluation after the biopsy cores have been retrieved. Authors report that, in almost 25% of the cases, the average processing time for the pathological result is calculated to be longer than the standard recommended by the College of American Pathologists (CAP) [18]. This can be related to the time needed for the processing of the sample—formalin fixation, paraffin embedding, specimen cut and slide assembly—as well as the operational workload that often affects different pathological divisions in distinct regions of the world.

FCM's capacity to discriminate prostate tissue on bioptic cores in real time was investigated in two prospective clinical trials [14, 19]. The primary endpoint was to assess the concordance between FCM and HE for prostate cancer diagnosis (presence vs. absence of PCa). A prospective study conducted by Rocco et al. [14] included 427 cores from 54 patients, retrieved from either mpMRI targeted or random prostate areas. FCM was used to create and collect digital pictures from all the prostatic cores, that in the end were examined with conventional HE.

Four pathologists from different institutions and diverse backgrounds evaluated the pictures, both the digital biopsy and the corresponding HE digitized slides, in a random fashion. The agreement between FCM and HE in terms of cancer detection (k value, AUC) was the outcome measure, the inter-observer agreement between pathologists was also assessed. Interestingly, diagnosis alignment between FCM and HE for the identification of cancerous tissue was nearly perfect (k = 0.84; range: 0.81–0.88 for four pathologists), with 95.1% of accurate diagnoses obtained (range: 93.9–96.2). With an average AUC of 0.92 (95% CI 0.90–0.94), FCM's discriminative efficiency was outstanding [14].

In parallel, another prospective study by the group of Marenco and Calatrava, focused on target biopsy, was published [19]. A total of 182 cores from 65 regions of interest (ROI) at mpMRI were taken and analyzed with FCM by a single pathologist. Afterward, a second pathologist, who was blinded to the FCM findings, conducted HE analysis and interpreted HE pictures. An agreement between the two pathologic techniques of 0.81 and 0.69 was discovered by the authors at biopsy core and ROI level, high positive predictive value (85% vs. 83.78%) and negative predictive value (95.1% vs. 85.71%) were also demonstrated, respectively.

Marenco et al. did not investigated ISUP scoring attribution, claiming a lack of expertise to adequately apply grading to the FCM cores, suggesting a sort of learning curve effect [19]

Rocco et al., on the other hand, referred at ISUP scoring as a secondary endpoint for inter-observer agreement.

Unfortunately, the gold standard HE pathway's high inter-observer variability found FCM results inconclusive as well [14]; further research on FCM's potential to differentiate between ISUP groups—built and directed to this outcome—are required.

Intra-operative Digital Frozen Sections During Radical Prostatectomy

Radical prostatectomy (RP) represents the treatment of choice in case of low and intermediate risk PCa, while is part of a multimodal approach for high-risk and locally advanced disease [17]. The aim of RP is to remove the entire gland according to the principles of oncological safety, along with the purpose of preserving as much as possible functional outcomes in terms of continence and potency. The preservation of neurovascular bundles (NVB) is critical for erectile function rehabilitation, according to Walsh's preliminary report, but somehow may affect surgical margin status [20].

Authors describe the presence of positive surgical margins (PSM) in 15% of cases according to any pT staging; the estimated PSM rate for pT2 is 9%, while the rate for pT3 status is 37%. PSM can have an effect on biochemical recurrence and, potentially, PCa-related mortality [21–23].

The intra-operative microscopical control of surgical dissection can be the game changer in the trade-off between nerve conservation and reduction of the chance of positive SM. Few papers investigating Cellvizio and confocal laser endomicroscopy attempted to verify in vivo the presence of NVBs in the aim of sparing as much healthy tissue as possible: although, poor results were published in both an experimental [24] and a clinical in vivo study [23] due to a lack of detail, a small FOV, and, most noticeably, a difficult interpretation of Cellvizio black-and-white images that limited an indepth characterization of the prostate capsule [25].

To date, the most common method of controlling surgical dissection in real time is microscopical examination of surgical margin on a fresh specimen (ex vivo). Besides this, the standard method for this is to perform a frozen section sample of the prostate (FSA) [17]. The optimal sampling strategy [26] and the correct sites of FS in reducing positive SM are subject to debate [27].

The use of intra-operative FS concerning postero-lateral margins of the prostate may help to increase the rate of NS procedures while ensuring a negative margin status, as suggested by the study from Schlomm et al. [28], where the authors described a systematical approach aimed to evaluate the bundles. According to the authors, the NeuroSAFE methodology requires a specialized setup, including a fully equipped laboratory with cryostats, dedicated personnel handling and preparing the specimen, and pathologists on-site ready to evaluate it and provide the surgeon with an immediate assessment of the specimen [29]. Significantly, the NeuroSAFE needs to take 35 min to perform in facilities with a good solid setup, making it difficult to be sustained in all pathology centers [29].

The role of FCM digital biopsy in implementing real-time control of surgical dissection has been identified in this scene. Microscopical analysis using FCM has been shown to recognize both random and systematic sampling. Suspicious areas may be observed during prostate dissection, inducing a larger excision if not differently characterized. This is the case often with traumatic neuroma, which is an inflammatory condition caused by prostate biopsy [30]: a thick adhesion of peri-prostatic tissue to the capsule may be misinterpreted by the surgeon as a region of extracapsular extension (ECE), possibly requiring a wider plane of excision. A prospective study run by Rocco et al. [15] investigated this issue, focusing on 41 samples collected intra-operatively during robotic prostatectomy at suspicious areas or from sites corresponding to suspected ECE on preoperative mpMRI. The aim of the study was to see whether FCM could identify prostate glands in extra-prostatic soft tissues, which could indicate ECE or an accidental incision within the prostate capsule [15]. The paper assessed the concordance between FCM and HE for determining each component of the extra-prostatic environment. As a result, the investigators observed a 90% agreement rate for all components, with connective, fatty, and muscular tissues being the easier to interpret; within these tissues, the presence of the prostatic glandular pattern is readily identifiable [15].

Moreover, FCM has been adopted for the en-face examination of the prostatic surface to evaluate for surgical margin status (known as MOHS approach), in addition to the analysis of small samples suspicious of cancer from the peri-prostatic regions. Similar to the case of the NeuroSAFE [28], a study focused on the ability of confocal microscopy to systematically evaluate the postero-lateral aspects of the prostate, which are likely to be at risk of a PSM during a nerve sparing procedure, was carried out recently.

Rocco et al. [13] harvested a slice shaved section of each lobe of the prostate specimen from eight men undergoing radical prostatectomy in a prospective exploratory study (36 samples overall). These slices were made by cutting the glands tangentially from the base to the apex and then flattening them on the confocal microscopy device for en-face tissue evaluation using the lowest thickness optical settings [13]. Depending on prostate thickness, longitudinal slices were occasionally split into two or three sections to match the 2.5 × 2.5 cm scanning field. This procedure differs significantly from the one used with traditional frozen sections (including NeuroSAFE), which focused on circumferential evaluation of the inked margin from a specific number of prostate transverse sections (10–12 per lobe for NeuroSafe). The images were then evaluated by two pathologists and the study definitively demonstrated a perfect concordance between FCM—applied to the flat specimen—and conventional HE analysis—applied to the circumferential margin of the prostate [13]. Within 25 min, FCM was able to provide high-definition digital images of the margins; regarding all of these, one out of eight patients had a PSM in an area of ECE. In the event of a positive margin, the confocal microscope software allows you to measure the distance from a previously positioned reference (for example a clip), in order to track on the operating field the precise site of the PSM and eventually allowing for a focal secondary resection and optimize NVB preservation without compromising oncological safety [13].

Recently, a systematic approach to evaluate surgical margins during RARP with FCM has been described [31]: once the prostate has been removed through a supraumbilical wound retractor, the fresh specimen is sectioned using the Mohs technique (shaving) in three basic slices: one regards the apex, the other two include the right and left posterolateral aspects. Digital images are obtained from the shavings and immediately acquired via FCM and shared with a remote pathologist, that can take over the control of the device and investigate the slides. In case of suspicious areas, a focal secondary resection can be performed owing to the ability of FCM to track a region of interest on the flat sample.

FCM Learning Curve

Evidences describe FCM as a reliable technique able to differentiate between different types of prostatic and periprostatic tissues including benign prostatic glands, benign prostatic hyperplasia, high-grade intraepithelial neoplasm, and prostatic adenocarcinoma. Furthermore, authors demonstrated a short learning curve for the interpretation of FCM images [1]. Bertoni et al. conducted a study regarding 89 FCM digital images obtained from prostate specimen, showing them to two pathologists with different background, blinded to final histopathologic diagnosis; they were asked to detect the presence vs. absence of PCa at a baseline and after 90 days, in a random order. The consensus between FCM and HE improved from a range of 86% to 92% at the baseline, up to 95% in the second interpretation for both pathologists. Interestingly, 10% of specimens needed immunohistochemistry for histopathological diagnosis, which may address the minimal (5%) discrepancy found in the second round [1]. In fact, the region under the receiver operating characteristic (ROC) curve at the first reading was 0.87, suggesting that FCM has outstanding discriminative efficiency since the first reading, that was even better at the second reading with AUC 0.92–0.93. In conclusion, the paper assessed that the learning curve for FCM is short due to HE-like appearance that makes easy the interpretation of prostate tissue [1].

In their prospective study on prostate biopsy, Rocco et al. [14] did not directly mention the learning curve effect; nevertheless, the large rate of agreement for prostate cancer diagnosis among pathologists who had no experience with FCM could imply that this technique has a limited learning curve.

Further researches regarding ISUP score attribution are encouraged to evaluate specific prostate cancer grading assessment with FCM.

Limits

Among the clear advantages of fast and direct digital pictures creation, few technical aspects could improve. One limit is the restricted scanning area, which is ideal for analyzing small specimens [13, 14], such as biopsies but may be not enough when evaluating the postero-lateral aspects of large prostates. To date, currently accessible system (MAVIG VivaScope 2500) has a single field of view (FOV) of 500 × 500 m and can scan areas up to 2.5 × 2.5 cm. The sample is shifted under the objective by a mechanized stage to produce a mosaic image of 2.5 × 2.5 cm, and hundreds of FOVs are fitted together by the microscope software during the acquisition process. A motorized stage, which leads to a higher mobility of the sample under the objective, may be used to increase the overall scanning area.

The amount of time needed to create digital pictures is directly proportional to the size of the specimen [13, 14]: the scanning is processed faster when the sample is smaller. In fact, the amount of FOVs required to generate a mosaic image of a given area determines the duration of the process needed to acquire that area from the specimen. An increased of the FOV would decrease the numbers of FOVs used to produce the mosaic image, lowering specimen acquisition time.

Additionally, there is space for storage programs and reporting tools to be implemented, allowing researchers to transfer pictures, homogenize reporting, and add prospective studies with standardized methods for evaluating outcomes.

Future FCM Fields of Application

Clinical Applications

The potential of detecting PCa in real time with digital biopsy introduces previously unexplored areas of application. Ultimately, focal therapy has been described as a treatment option for localized unilateral PCa. In this scenario, patients may undergo a diagnostic and therapeutic treatment in the same session in this context: FCM can be used to acquire a digital biopsy of cores from an mpMRI region, which can therefore be evaluated in real time by a remote pathologist, and the detection of PCa could trigger concurrent treatment of the cancerous site [14, 19]. Another suggestive hypothesis is represented by the application of FCM to rule out PCa diagnosis in the case of patients affected by lower urinary tract symptoms due to bladder output obstruction and ambiguous PSA level. In this case, FCM technology may potentially avoid the need for a previous prostate biopsy and allow for diagnosis and therapeutic treatment in the same hospitalization regimen, lowering health care costs.

Regarding the intraoperative use of FCM as control of surgical margins during RARP, a tailored surgical dissection is no longer a future development, but rather an emerging scenario whose adoption may lead to improved functional outcomes. According to Rocco et al. proof of concept study [13], FCM essentially allows the accurate mapping of the positive surgical margin on the postero-lateral portion of the prostate specimen, with the potential of tracking the same site on the spared NVB. As a result, the study opens the way for a focal wedge secondary resection of NVB without the need for a complete bundle demolition. In fact, authors describe the presence of cancerous tissue on about 23–42% of the NVBs that were secondarily resected [29]: implementing FCM, a partial wedge resection on NVB may resect cancerous foci while sparing as much healthy functional tissue as possible. Indeed, further research is needed to assess the oncological benefit along with the potential benefit in preserving erectile function in this setting.

Eventually, the almost perfect discrimination between cancerous and benign tissue reported for the prostate may be applied to other malignancies in diagnostic settings, including all histopathology tests done for oncological concern.

Management and External Support Applications

Several healthcare systems in the western countries, such as Canadian and the United Kingdom, have seen a drop in pathologist personnel in past years [32]. According to Metter et al., insufficient manpower affects 97% of departments, which may contribute in diagnostic delays and rising costs as a result of the need to focus on outsourced services or temporary employees [32]. FCM accessibility and quick acquisition of digital images is expected to make the process easier, and it fits in well with the current trend in digitalization, web access, and real-time sharing. Remote access to virtual microscopical images offers the advantage of consulting specialists not physically present, and digital storage may represent a dataset dedicated for training novel pathologists [33–36]. The health system may be able to deliver partial services more efficiently at various global areas, as well as receive responses from subspecialized and/or experts in the field, shortening waiting time prior to diagnosis. To date, pathology, is not particularly prone to the emerging telemedicine prospective: telepathology involves the acquisition of microscopical images from one area to another for diagnostic purposes, and it may be helpful in low-income or developing nations where hospitals practice surgical procedures but lack on-site pathology resources [37–39]. In this light, FCM adoption could have strategic impacts, since it contributes to the dual concerns of workload balance and tele-reporting.

Furthermore, FCM application may find its role regarding the recent pandemic scenario. Lastly, pathologists are worried about the risk of pathogen viability from fresh tissue while treating and harvesting specimen from Covid-19 infected patients [40–43]. A report of COVID-19 detection in numerous types of specimens showed that SARS-CoV-2 RNA could be found in feces and blood [42]. During the pandemic, the routine use of frozen section analysis was discouraged. In this case, FCM's ability to have pathological specimens entirely treated by the surgeon, preventing undue contact to external staff such as technicians and pathologists, may represent a benefit relevant for the actual situation.

Conclusions

FCM was evaluated in the field of prostate tissue interpretation and showed diagnostic results comparable to that of traditional histopathology for cancer diagnosis. To summarize, the following are some of the benefits of FCM:

- Direct digital images creation from fresh specimen
- Quick and easy to handle preparation of the specimen
- No need for dedicated laboratory or specialized technicians
- Acquisition of digital images with HE-like appearance
- High reliability and concordance with conventional pathology
- Tissue integrity preservation for further histopathological examination
- Digital storage of the images allows for web-sharing and remote pathological reporting
- Fast learning curve for image interpretation
- En-face examination of a flattened sample allows to preserve the specimen's proper orientation and map the location of malignant tissue inside of it (measurement provided by FCM ruler)

Oncological implementation of FCM is expected to grow in the coming years, especially regarding prostate cancer; multicentric clinical trials are encouraged to validate the transferability of current evidences, assess FCM evaluation of ISUP scoring, and move on to innovative surgical applications.

References

1. Bertoni L, Puliatti S, Reggiani Bonetti L, Maiorana A, Eissa A, Azzoni P, Bevilacqua L, Spandri V, Kaleci S, Zoeir A, Sighinolfi MC, Micali S, Bianchi G, Pellacani G, Rocco B, Montironi R. Ex vivo fluorescence confocal microscopy: prostatic and periprostatic tissues atlas and evaluation of the learning curve. Virchows Arch. 2020;476(4):511–20. https://doi.org/10.1007/s00428-019-02738-y.
2. Paddock SW, Eliceiri KW. Laser scanning confocal microscopy: history, applications, and related optical sectioning techniques. Methods Mol Biol. 2014;1075:9–47. https://doi.org/10.1007/978-1-60761-847-8_2.
3. Longo C, Pampena R, Bombonato C, et al. Diagnostic accuracy of ex vivo fluorescence confocal microscopy in Mohs surgery of basal cell carcinomas: a prospective study on 753 margins. Br J Dermatol. 2019;180:1473–80.
4. Bertoni L, Azzoni P, Reggiani C, et al. Ex vivo fluorescscence confocal microscopy for intra-operative real-time diagnosis of cutaneous inflammatory diseases: a preliminary study. Exp Dermatol. 2018;27:1152–9.
5. Reggiani C, Pellacani G, Reggiani Bonetti L, et al. An intraoperative study with ex vivo fluorescence confocal microscopy: diagnostic accuracy of the 3 visualization modalities. J Eur Acad Dermatol Venereaol. 2020;35(1):e92–4. https://doi.org/10.1111/jdv.16831.
6. Krishnamurthy S, Sabir S, Ban K, et al. Comparison of real-time fluorescence confocal microscopy with hematoxylin eosin stained sections of core-needle biopsy specimens. JAMA Net Open. 2020;3:e200476.
7. Mir MC, Bancalari B, Calatrava A, Casanova J, Dominguez Escrig JL, Ramirez-Backhaus M, Gomez-Ferrer A, Collado A, Wong A, Iborra I, Sanmarti O, Rubio-Briones J. Ex-vivo confocal fluorescence microscopy for rapid evaluation of renal core biopsy. Minerva Urol Nefrol. 2020;72(1):109–13. Epub 2019 Dec 12. PMID: 31833726. https://doi.org/10.23736/S0393-2249.19.03627-0.
8. Minsky M. Memoir on inventing the confocal scanning microscope. Scanning. 1988;10:128–38.
9. Pawley JB. Handbook of biological confocal microscopy. 3rd ed. NY: Plenum Press; 2006.
10. Amos WB, White JG. How the confocal laser scanning microscope entered biological research. Biol Cell. 2003;95:335–42.
11. MAVIG. Datasheet VivaScope® 2500M-G4. 2018. https://www.vivascope.de/wp-content/uploads/2019/06/DS_VS-2500M-G4_287_0219-ohne-Mohs.pdf. Accessed 4 Jan 2020.
12. Puliatti S, Bertoni L, Pirola GM, Azzoni P, Bevilacqua L, Eissa A, Elsherbiny A, Sighinolfi MC, Chester J, Kaleci S, Rocco B, Micali S, Bagni I, Bonetti LR, Maiorana A, Malvehy J, Longo C, Montironi R, Bianchi G, Pellacani G. Ex vivo fluorescence confocal microscopy: the first application for real-time pathological examination of prostatic tissue. BJU Int. 2019;124(3):469–76. https://doi.org/10.1111/bju.14754.
13. Rocco B, Sighinolfi MC, Cimadamore A, Reggiani Bonetti L, Bertoni L, Puliatti S, Eissa A, Spandri V, Azzoni P, Dinneen E, Shaw G, Nathan S, Micali S, Bianchi G, Maiorana A, Pellacani G, Montironi R. Digital frozen section of the prostate surface during radical prostatectomy: a novel approach to evaluate surgical margins. BJU Int. 2020;126(3):336–8. https://doi.org/10.1111/bju.15108.
14. Rocco B, Sighinolfi MC, Sandri M, et al. Digital biopsy with fluorescence confocal microscopy for effective real time diagnosis of prostate cancer: a prospective, comparative study. Eur Urol Oncol. 2021;4(5):784–91.
15. Rocco B, Sighinolfi MC, Bertoni L, et al. Real-time assessment of surgical margins during radical prostatectomy: a novel approach that uses fluorescence confocal microscopy for the evaluation of peri-prostatic soft tissue. GBJU Int. 2020;125(4):487–9.
16. Cicione A, De Nunzio C, Manno S, et al. An update on prostate biopsy in the era of magnetic resonance imaging. Minerva Urol Nephrol. 2018;70:264–74.
17. Mottet N, Cornford P, van der Bergh RCN et al. EAU-EANM-ESTRO-ESUR-ISUP-SIOG guidelines on prostate cancer. 2019 edn.
18. Alshieban S, Al-Surimi K. Reducing turnaround time of surgical pathology reports in pathology and laboratory medicine departments. BMJ Qual Improv Rep. 2015;4(1):u209223.w3773.
19. Marenco J, Calatrava A, Casanova J, et al. Evaluation of fluorescent confocal microscopy for intraoperative analysis of prostate biopsy core. Eur Urol Focus. 2021;7(6):1254–9.
20. Walsh PC, Donker PJ. Impotence following radical prostatectomy: insight into etiology and prevention. J Urol. 1982;128:492–7.
21. Mauermann J, Fradet V, Lacombe L, et al. The impact of solitary and multiple positive surgical margins on hard clinical end points in 1712 adjuvant treatment-naive pT2-4 N0 radical prostatectomy patients. Eur Urol. 2013;64:19–25.
22. Yossepowitch O, Briganti A, Eastham JA, et al. Positive surgical margins after radical prostatectomy: a systematic review and contemporary update. Eur Urol. 2014;65:303–13.
23. Lopez A, Zlatev DV, Mach KE, et al. Intraoperative optical biopsy during robotic assisted radical prostatectomy using confocal endomicroscopy. J Urol. 2016;195:1110–7.
24. Boyette LB, Reardon MA, Mirelman AJ, et al. Fiberoptic imaging of cavernous nerves in vivo. J Urol. 2007;178:2694–700
25. Jaudlim A, Aydin A, Hebrain F, et al. Imaging modalities aiding nerve sparing during radical prostatectomy. Turk J Urol. 2019;45:325–30.
26. Sighinolfi MC, Rocco B. Re: EAU guidelines: prostate cancer 2019. Eur Urol. 2019 76(6):871.
27. Dinneen EP, Van Der Slot M, Adasonla K, et al. Intraoperative frozen section for margin evaluation during radical prostatectomy: a systematic review. Eur Urol Focus. 2020;6(4):664–73.
28. Schlomm T, Tennstedt P, Huxhold C, et al. Neurovascular structure-adjacent frozen-section examination (NeuroSAFE) increases nerve-sparing frequency and reduces positive surgical margins in open and robot-assisted laparoscopic radical prostatectomy: experience after 11,069 consecutive patients. Eur Urol. 2012;62(2):333–40.
29. Oxley J, Bray A, Rowe E. Could a Mohs technique make NeuroSAFE a viable option? BJU Int. 2018;122(3):358–9.
30. Sighinolfi MC, Rocco B. Reply to Alessia Cimadamore, Marina Scarpelli, Liang Cheng, et al.'s Letter to the Editor. re: Maria Chiara Sighinolfi, Bernardo Rocco's words of wisdom, re: EAU guidelines: prostate cancer 2019. Mottet N, van den Bergh RCN, Briers E, et al. https://uroweb.org/guideline/prostate-Cancer/. Eur Urol. 2019;76:871. Eur Urol. 2020;77(5):e128–9.
31. Rocco B, Sarchi L, Assumma S, et al. Digital frozen sections with fluorescence confocal microscopy during robot-assisted radical prostatectomy: surgical technique. Eur Urol. 2021;80(6):724–9. https://doi.org/10.1016/j.eururo.2021.03.021.
32. Metter DM, Colgan TJ, Leung ST, et al. Trends in the US and Canadian pathologist workforces from 2007 to 2017. JAMA Netw Open. 2019;2:e194337.
33. Bulten W, Pinckaers H, van Boven H, et al. Automated deep-learning system for Gleason grading of prostate cancer using biopsies: a diagnostic study. Lancet Oncol. 2020;21:233–41.
34. Ström P, Kartasalo K, Olsson H, et al. Artificial intelligence for diagnosis and grading of prostate cancer in biopsies: a population-based, diagnostic study. Lancet Oncol. 2020;21:222–32.
35. Nir G, Karimi D, Goldenberg SL, et al. Comparison of artificial intelligence techniques to evaluate performance of a classifier for automatic grading of prostate cancer from digitized histopathologic images. JAMA Netw Open. 2019;2:e190442.

36. Chen PHC, Gadepalli K, MacDonald R, et al. An augmented reality microscope with real-time artificial intelligence integration for cancer diagnosis. Nat Med. 2019;25:1453–7.
37. Huang EY, Knight S, Guetter CR, et al. Telemedicine and telementoring in the surgical specialties: a narrative review. Am J Surg. 2019;218:760–6.
38. Montironi R, Cheng L, Cimadamore A, et al. Uropathologists during the COVID-19 pandemic: what can be learned in terms of social interaction, visibility, and social distance. Eur Urol. 2020;78(3):478–81. Epub 2020 May 11.
39. Cimadamore A, Lopez-Beltran A, Scarpelli M, et al. Digital pathology and COVID-19 and future crises: pathologists can safely diagnose cases from home using a consumer monitor and a mini PC. J Clin Pathol. 2020;73(11):695–6.
40. Comperat E. What does COVID-19 mean for the urology-pathology interaction? Eur Urol. 2020;78(1):e43–4.
41. Wang W, Xu Y, Gao R, et al. Detection of SARS-CoV-2 in different types of clinical specimens. JAMA. 2020;323(18):1843–4.
42. Gerston KF, Blumberg L, Tshabalala VA, Murray J. Viability of mycobacteria in formalin-fixed lungs. Hum Pathol. 2004;35:571–5.
43. Badia JM, Rubio-Pérez I, Arias Díaz J, et al. Protocolo de actuación quirúrgica en casos confirmados o sospechosos de enfermedad por Ébola y otras enfermedades víricas altamente transmisibles. Cir Esp. 2016;94:11–5.

Part V

Reconstruction of Continence Mechanisms

The Single Knot Running Vesico-Urethral Anastomosis

15

Simone Albisinni, Romain Diamand, Massimo Valerio, and Roland van Velthoven

Introduction

The last 20 years have seen an exponential increase in the application of robotic-assisted and laparoscopic surgery to radical prostatectomy. The vesico-urethral anastomosis (VUA) represents the conclusion of this complex operation, remaining a challenging step especially for novice laparoscopic surgeons. The reasons are numerous: first, the anatomic position of the urethra makes the vesico-urethral anastomosis a technically difficult procedure, especially in men with a narrow and/or deep pelvis in whom running the urethral stitches may be extremely challenging. Second, robotic-assisted and laparoscopic radical prostatectomy, especially in the beginning of a surgeon's learning curve, is a long and wearing procedure. Therefore, surgeons face a complex step in the procedure (i.e. the VUA) after several hours of concentration and difficult dissection, boosting the VUA's complexity. Finally, although this applies only to pure laparoscopic surgery, laparoscopic intra-corporeal suturing and knot-tying is one of the most complicated technical gestures that a surgeon must learn during his training. Obviously, the robotic platform has simplified this procedure, yet it remains a fundamental step in the training of young uro-oncologic surgeons.

In 2000, in our center we introduced a single-knot running VUA, today more known as the van Velthoven technique. Its initial series was published in 2003 [1]. This technique requires only one intracorporeal knot, it allows a water-tight approximation of the bladder neck to the urethra, it is reproducible and versatile, as a consequence it is easy to teach. As such, although many variations have been proposed and are currently in use in centers worldwide [2–4], this technique has been widely accepted by many urologists and is frequently used today to perform VUA [5].

S. Albisinni (✉)
Urology Department, University Clinics of Brussels, Hôpital Erasme, Université libre de Bruxelles, Brussels, Belgium
e-mail: simone.albisinni@erasme.ulb.ac.be

R. Diamand
Urology Department, University Clinics of Brussels, Institut Jules Bordet, Université libre de Bruxelles, Brussels, Belgium
e-mail: romain.diamand@bordet.be

M. Valerio · R. van Velthoven
Department of Urology, Centre Hospitalier Universitaire Vaudois, Lausanne, Switzerland
e-mail: massimo.valerio@chuv.ch; Roland.vanvelthoven@chuv.ch

The Single Knot Running Vesico-Urethral Anastomosis Technique

The basic principle of a valid vesico-urethral anastomosis is to align the urethral and bladder mucosae without traction. The mucosa approximation guarantees a water-tight anastomosis, while the absence of traction avoids ischemic complications. A good quality VUA is responsible for preventing urinary leakage and stricture formation. The success of a vesico-urethral anastomosis therefore depends upon meticulous attention to details and the optimization of technical factors that affect anastomotic integrity. The single-knot running vesico-urethral anastomosis respects this principle and has become a commonly used method of reconstruction [1].

After having performed a posterior reconstruction, the technique begins by inspecting the bladder neck with careful attention to ureteral orifices (Fig. 15.1). The degree of bladder neck preservation will dictate the length of the stitch. It varies accordingly between 12 cm and 20 cm The running suture is prepared extracorporeally by tying together the two ends of a twin dyed 6 in. sutures of 3-0 Monocryl RB-1 (Ethicon, USA). The second step is to identify the urethral stump (Fig. 15.1). A 18 French urethral catheter is positioned and suspended anteriorly to expose the dorsal urethral mucosa. At times the urethral stump is short and might retract into the pelvic floor musculature, or is positioned deep underneath the symphysis pubis. In these cases, visualizing and placing the anastomotic sutures in laparoscopy could be difficult. A simple trick to facilitate suturing is to exert an external perineal pressure with a sponge stick at the bulbar urethra during the initial throws of the suture, thus everting

S. Ren et al. (eds.), *Robot-Assisted Radical Prostatectomy*, https://doi.org/10.1007/978-3-031-05855-4_15

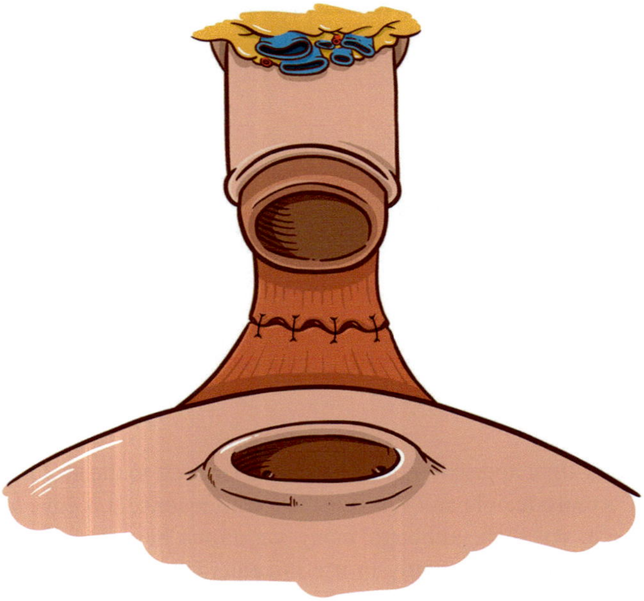

Fig. 15.1 Posterior reconstruction

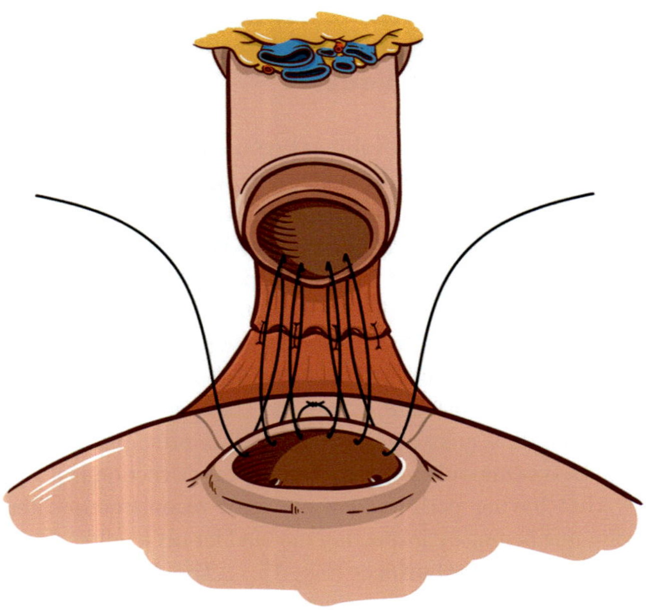

Fig. 15.2 First posterior suture throws, allowing via a pulley system to approximate the bladder neck to the urethra

the urethral stump. The running stitch is initiated by placing both needles outside-in through the bladder neck and inside-out on the urethra, one needle at the 5:30-o'clock position and the other needle at the 6:30-o'clock position. The sutures are run from the 6:30 and 5:30-o'clock positions toward the 9:00 and 3:00-o'clock positions (Fig. 15.2), respectively. After two throws through the urethra and three throws through the bladder are completed, the sutures are cinched down with gentle traction on each thread simultaneously or alternately, bringing the bladder neck as a unit tightly into position with the urethra (Fig. 15.3). This approximation provides a secure posterior wall with no gap visualised between sutures and allows a 18F catheter to be placed into the bladder. A transition suture is completed at the 11:00-o'clock positions, by taking an extra bite on the urethra, going outside in. The transition suture allows the stitch to now exit the bladder on its outer surface (Fig. 15.4). The sutures are continued to the 12:00-o'clock position and tied to each other. This solitary intracorporeal knot now, like the initial extracorporeal knot, rests on the exterior aspect of the bladder (Fig. 15.5). If discrepancy persists between the diameters of the bladder neck and urethra, an anterior retrograde tennis racket-type closure is performed. On the other

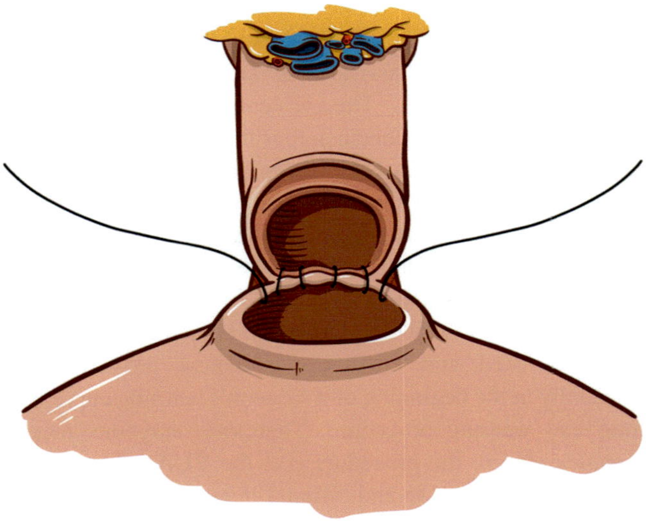

Fig. 15.3 Reduction of the posterior throws, securing the bladder neck to the urethra

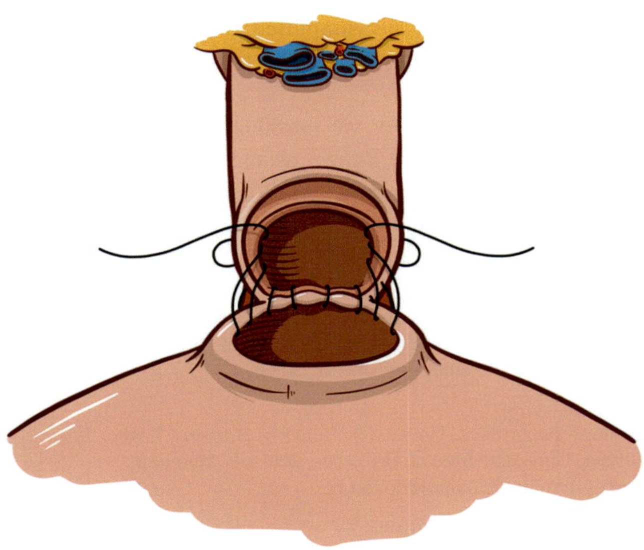

Fig. 15.4 Lateral throws and U-turn to block the running suture

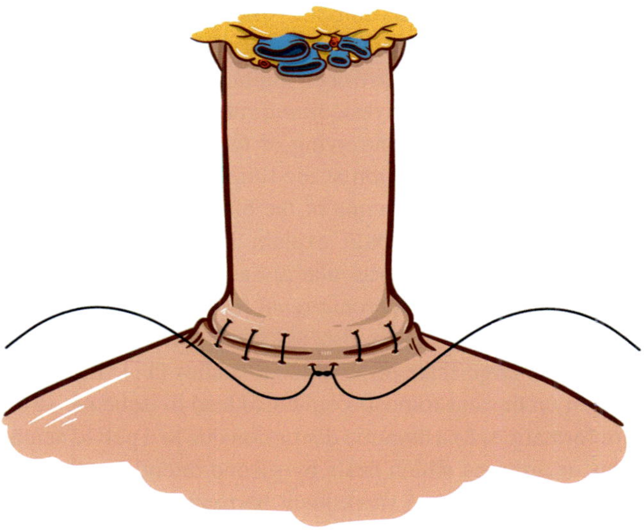

Fig. 15.5 Anterior throws and finalization of the anastomosis

hand, if the ureteral orifices are close, a posterior tennis racket-type closure is advised prior to begin the anastomosis.

A part from the VUA, we strive to maximise the chances of preserving urinary function after prostatectomy by combining an anatomical preservation of key functional structures to a total anatomical reconstruction. Prior to dissecting the bladder neck, we place a suspending stitch in the anterior mid-part of the prostate. Afterwards, by counter-traction on the bladder, the anatomical cleavage plane between the bladder and the prostate is identified, and the dissection is pursued in a funnel-shape fashion in order to preserve as much as possible the bladder neck. At the end of the antegrade dissection, to maximise the urethral length, we initially divide and ligate the DVC in order to achieve a clear visualisation of the urethra, the apex and the rhabdo-sphincter. We release the fibrotic tissue anchoring the urethra and the apex from lateral to medial bilaterally, and finally we sharply divide the urethra close to the apex to preserve its maximal length. We routinely perform a total anatomical reconstruction combining a posterior reconstruction following the technique divulgated by Rocco et al. [6], as well as an anterior reconstruction as proposed by Tewari et al. [7]. We firmly believe the combination of these technique reduce the direct tension on the VUA, mimic the supporting anatomy to the sphincter complex and accelerate the healing process as well as the recovery of urinary continence [8]. The catheter is normally left in place for 3–7 days, as shorter catheter times are associated to non-negligible rates of urinary retention due to oedema, whereas prolonged catheter times are useless and increase pain and infectious complications.

The single knot running anastomosis was associated with a significantly decreased anastomotic time compared to interrupted and modified interrupted technique in an analysis of three different techniques performed by Teber et al. [9]. The median time to perform a single knot running anastomosis laparoscopically was 15.3 min (range 11–31) in their series. Furthermore, the system of symmetric loops acts as a block and pulling mechanism, thereby enabling approximation of the dorsal part of the anastomosis to be carried out without tension or traction.

Complications of the Single-Knot Running VUA

As any surgical step in radical prostatectomy, the vesico-urethral anastomosis is characterized by possible complications. The surgeon must master the technique of VUA to reduce these events, which however remain inevitable, as expected in any surgical procedure.

An anastomotic leak is a short term complication following vesico-urethral anastomosis and is associated with significant morbidity including postoperative ileus, infection, prolonged hospital stay and urinoma formation with potential risk of anastomotic disruption. The long-term relevance of anastomotic leak is controversial in the literature, although it does seem a major risk factor in the development of anastomotic strictures [10]. Surya et al. suggest that prolonged urinary leakage results from an anastomotic gap which heals by second intention, thereby causing scarring and anastomotic stricture. By contrast, other studies have reported no significant increase in anastomotic stricture due to leakage [9, 11, 12]. The reported incidence of anastomotic leak with single knot running sutures has been very variable ranging from 0% to 7.5% [13–15] in series of surgeons using the single-knot running technique. In a study by [16], urine leak was significantly reduced in the group of single knot running sutures compared to the interrupted technique. Teber et al. [9] also demonstrated significantly less dorsal urine leak with the van Velthoven technique than with interrupted sutures.

Treatment of a urinary leakage can be troublesome. First, we recommend that conservative measures should be preferred over operative surgical repair, unless urinary peritonitis is present. We have published our technique to treat with little morbidity the vast majority of anastomotic leakages [17]. A 20F "fenestrated" catheter is prepared by incising two drainage holes proximal to the anchoring balloon. The fenestrated catheter is positioned, eventually under fluoroscopy to verify the correct intravesical position. The two proximal drainage holes will divert urine away from the leakage and into the drainage catheter, thus allowing the fistula to heal in a dry environment. In fact, in the majority of cases, the ureteral orifices are positioned too close to the VUA, with a consequent immediate emission of urine on the suture and the fistula (Fig. 15.6), this supports the leakage

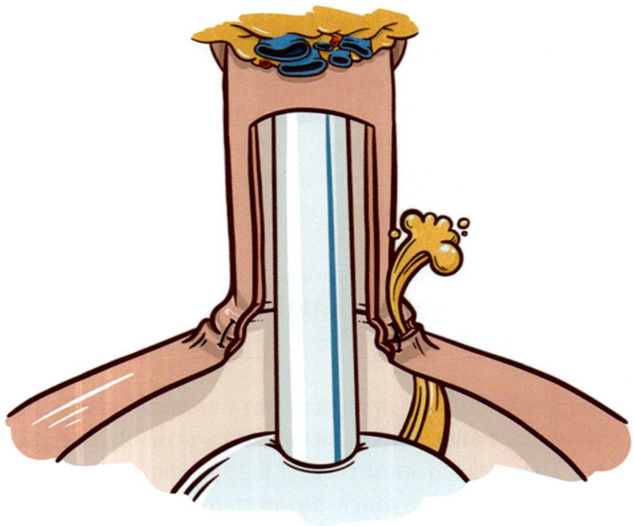

Fig. 15.6 Anastomotic urinary leakage, with urine leaking outside of the bladder

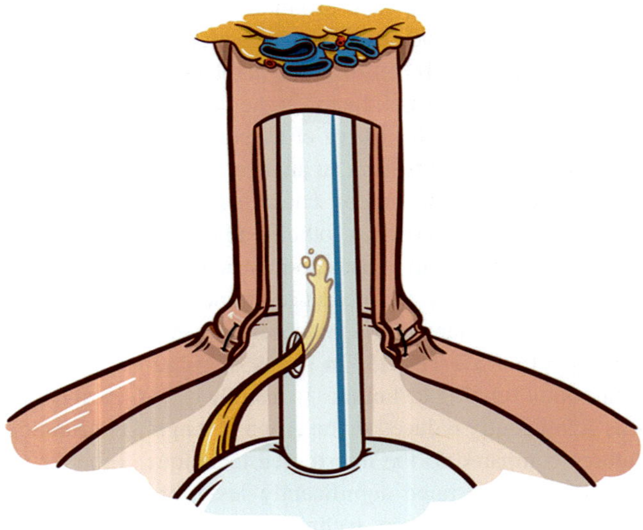

Fig. 15.7 The fenestrated catheter help directing the leakage outside of the bladder and optimizes drainage

and prevents healing. As standard catheters only drain the urine once this is above the balloon, in case of a fistula, urine will more like extravasate than be drained in the catheter. Our fenestrated catheter represents a simple and extremely effective solution in case of anastomotic leakage (Fig. 15.7).

Anastomotic stricture is a late complication which has hopefully become less frequent since the standardisation of laparoscopy and robotic radical prostatectomy. Significant morbidity may be associated with the development of anastomotic stenoses, including infection, urinary retention, the need for additional invasive surgery and further stress incontinence [9]. While several factors have been associated with the development of anastomotic stricture, its exact pathophysiology remains poorly defined. Both technical and patient-related factors have been implicated in their development [10]. The type of vesico-urethral anastomosis plays a major role. Excessive narrowing of the anastomosis and/or lack of mucosal apposition at the time of the procedure are known risk factors. Ischemia of the bladder neck and/or the membranous urethra could explain higher rates in older patients with peripheral vascular disease. Smoking, diabetes, hypertension, obesity, chronic renal insufficiency and coronary artery disease were also associated with anastomotic stricture in large scale observational studies [11]. Too much tension on the anastomosis could also lead to ischemic stricture formation. Anastomotic disruption due to a pelvic hematoma or urinoma which heals by second intention may lead to scar formation and subsequent narrowing. Postoperative radiation is also a well-known cause of anastomotic stricture by inducing ischemia and fibrosis [12]. Technical improvements and surgeon experience may explain lower incidence rates in contemporary series [5]. Clearly robotic-assisted surgery has had a major impact in reducing the occurrence of anastomotic strictures. First, the reduced blood loss and clean field allow the surgeon to perfectly visualize the urethral stump. Second, the improved dexterity deep in the pelvis allows a meticulous placement of the stitches. Finally, the single knot running technique creates a direct wide vesicourethral alignment with an end-to-end mucosal apposition. Ischemia is also reduced by the running "funnelling parachute" anastomosis.

Complex Situations

Minimally invasive radical prostatectomy is often challenging. There are particular situations in which the dissection and the reconstructive phase of the intervention can be particularly complex. Regarding VUA, major challenges can arise when a salvage prostatectomy is performed after another primary prostate cancer treatment (i.e. radiation therapy, HIFU, cryoablation), or after prostate surgery for benign prostatic enlargement. Indeed, these are all situations in which the dissection is very complicated, particularly at the level of the bladder neck, as surgical planes are usually blended together and massive fibrosis is present. Frequently in these situations the bladder neck is excessively opened, with a subsequent mis-match of the bladder neck and the urethra. To face this problem, the bladder neck can be reconstructed with a posterior or anterior tennis-racket. As mentioned above, we advise a posterior racket if the ureteral orifices are too close to the suture. Moreover, if there has been exposure to radiation or thermal energy, tissue healing is usually impaired and the risk of post-operative complications is therefore elevated. This should be kept in mind by the surgeon, especially with regard to urine leakage and anastomotic strictures. An in-depth analysis has been performed by Ouzaid et al., who retrospectively analyzed 2215 patients undergoing LRP or RARP with the Van Velthoven technique. Anastomotic strictures occurred overall in 30 (1.4%), and both previous radiotherapy and previous TURP were significant predictors of such adverse event [18].

Series describing functional outcomes of salvage RARP after primary treatment (radiation, brachytherapy, HIFU) confirm that complications following such procedure are frequent [19, 20]. In the largest contemporary series exploring results of salvage radical prostatectomy, 395 men, of which 186 were operated by an open and 209 by a robotic approach, were analyzed. Robotic salvage radical prostatectomy yielded lower blood loss and a shorter hospital stay (each $p < 0.0001$). Anastomotic stricture was more frequent for open salvage radical prostatectomy group (16.57% vs. 7.66%, $p < 0.01$), yet confirming the major role of previous oncologic treatment on the development of such a complications. Yuh et al., analyzed complications and functional outcomes of salvage RALP in 51 men with recurrent prostate cancer. Complication rate was elevated (25% minor complications; 43% major complications), and regarding anastomosis, 18% of patients experienced an anastomotic leakage and 16% an anastomotic stricture [21]. Salvage radical prostatectomy after focal therapy appears to determine improved outcomes compared to whole gland radiotherapy. Herrera-Caceres et al. reported on 38 patients with a 91.2% continence rate. In their series, 11.8% of patients developed a bladder neck contracture [22].

After BPH surgery, as transurethral resection of the prostate or surgical adenomectomy, RARP can be particularly challenging due to the absence of the bladder neck, requiring unavoidable reconstruction. Porpiglia and colleagues reported results from 40 patients undergoing RARP after BPH surgery [23]. 8/40 (20%) patients experienced Clavien 1 complications, and continence rate at 1, 4, 12, 24, and 52 weeks from catheter removal was 77.5%, 82.5%, 90%, 92.5%, and 95%, respectively. A group from India published a study in which 26 men with previous transurethral resection of the prostate underwent RARP, and compared them to a cohort of 132 men undergoing RARP with no history of prostatic surgery [24]. In their work the authors point out the multiple difficulties associated with RARP in these patients, as the thickening of the bladder wall (a discrepant thickness of walls of the bladder and the urethra may determine difficulties in the VUA), difficult bladder neck dissection, increased periprostatic adhesions, difficulty in individualizing the ureteral orifices with increased risk of injury and poor healing of the vesico-urethral junction. Indeed, they found not only increased per-operative difficulties (which reflected in an increased blood loss and increased conversion to open surgery), but also worst post-operative functional outcomes: a prolonged urine leakage and an anastomotic stricture were found in 11.5% and 14% of men in the post-TURP group, respectively.

Surgeons must keep in mind that patients with prior treatment for prostate cancer or surgery for benign prostatic enlargement represent a true challenge, even for experts in the field of minimally invasive prostatectomy. Regarding the VUA, these patients present difficulties as a consequence of the frequently imperfect bladder neck conformation and local ischemia. We advise a prolonged catheter drainage of 7–21 days in these situations, depending on the local tissue conditions and the quality of bladder neck reconstruction.

Barbed Sutures

In the first description of the single-knot running VUA technique we were using two 3/0 poliglecaprone-25 absorbable monofilament sutures (Monocryl™) tied at their end, and the median time required for performing the anastomosis was 35 min (range 18–80) [1]. Today performing the single-knot VUA has become an easier and faster task, which usually requires about 10 min in expert hands [13, 25, 26]. This improvement is the consequence of different innovations: first, the robotic platform has incredibly eased the throwing of stitches, and second unidirectional and bidirectional barbed sutures are increasingly being used to facilitate the VUA. Barbed sutures are characterized by small barbs which allow the suture to run only in one direction, without losing tension if the sutured is not held during the throw of successive stitches.

V-LOC™ has been commercialized by Covidien and is characterized by a high density of barbs, 20 per cm, and unidirectionality: at the end of the suture is a small loop which serves to lock the suture after the first throw. As such, when used for VUA, two V-LOC™ are used and locked together at their ends. V-LOC is designed such that the first 3 cm of thread after the needle are non-barbed: this allows the surgeon to undo a stitch if it is misplaced. V-LOC™ is available in 1, 0, 2/0, 3/0 and 4/0, with two types of absorbable materials (90 and 180, referring respectively to the average absorption time) and one non-absorbable texture. Quill™ by Angiotech Pharmaceutics, is a barbed suture available either in uni- or bi-directional form: the bi-directional suture has two needles at its ends, with barbs oriented in opposite direction in the two halves of the suture, starting from a transition point at the center. Quill™ sutures have 8 barbs per cm, disposed in a helical pattern to allow equal distribution of strength. The bidirectional Quill™ device is available in absorbable and non-absorbable materials and its sizes range from 4-0 to 2. The equivalence in biocompatibility and strength of barbed sutures compared to standard sutures has been demonstrates in different animal studies [27], making these sutures a very interesting option for VUA. Stratafix™, by Ethicon (JnJ), currently offers a wide variety of barbed sutures applicable for vesico-urethral anastomosis. Both monocryl and PDS materials are available with a wide variety of needles, mounted on uni-or bidirectional sutures. Stratafix features a triclosan coating, reducing the colonization of the suture by Gram positive bacteria.

The advantages of barbed sutures on retaining the traction are evident. This translates into a reduction of surgical time and avoids to loose traction on some throws. Erdogru et al. recently performed a matched pair analysis comparing 70 men in which barbed sutures were used for VUA to 70 in which standard monofilament was employed. Minimal differences were reported in anastomotic time (11.2 vs. 13.2 min, $p < 0.001$) and watertightness (91% vs. 85%, $p < 0.001$). Of note, complication rate was similar across the two groups (25 vs. 20%, $p = 0.89$) [28]. Tewari et al. analyzed 50 men in which VUA was performed with a V-LOC™ and 50 men in which a polyglecaprone suture (Monocryl™) was used. They found that V-LOC significantly reduces anastomotic time by around 5 min; however, the clinical significance of such time saving is questionable [26, 29]. Similarly, Moran et al. tested a bidirectional barbed suture (Quill™), comparing it to Monocryl™, finding minimal differences in time and in surgeon security score [30]: although the Quill™ suture was faster to deploy (17.3 vs. 19.2 min), and the security score by the surgeon was greater, also in this case it is important to keep in mind clinical and not only mathematical differences. Sammon et al., at the Vattikuti Institute in Detroit, performed a randomized controlled trial with 64 men undergoing RARP. When performed with a barbed suture, the VUA was terminated faster, though no difference in leaks or bladder neck contractures were found compared to standard suture [31]. Zorn et al. in a prospective randomized trial, evaluating Monocryl™ vs. V-LOC™ in 70 men, found that barbed sutures reduced reconstruction time (13.1 vs. 20.8 min; $p < 0.01$), and the need to readjust suture tension or to place additional sutures was greater in the standard monofilament group [32]. Moreover, after an average follow-up of 6.2 months, no leakage nor anastomotic stricture was observed in the V-LOC group, and continence rates were similar across the two groups (88 vs. 92%, $p = 0.70$). In a prospective cohort study with 12 months of follow-up, Massoud et al. compared VUA performed with interrupted Vicryl™ stiches to VUA with a continuous V-LOC™ suture [29]: it is of note that after 1 year, no difference in anastomotic stricture rate requiring internal urethrotomy (2.5% in each group) was found across the two groups. Moreover, continence rates at 12 months were comparable in the two arms (97.5% with V-LOC™ vs. 95% with interrupted sutures, $p = 0.368$).

Concerns associated with barbed sutures are costs, the possibility of increased tissue inflammation and a possible more traumatic tissue injury in case of incorrect manipulation of the thread. Regarding costs, indeed barbed sutures are more expensive than standard threads: in Europe, a V-LOC suture costs around 17€, making VUA material cost approximately 34€, compared to 7€, which is roughly the cost of two Monocryl™ 3/0 sutures. Regarding tissue inflammation, there is no evidence that barbed sutures determine its increase [33, 34]. Finally, it should be noted that once a barbed suture has been passed and locked, one cannot reverse the procedure without major tissue tearing. As such, the surgeon must gain full confidence with the needle and suture manipulation before locking a throw.

Indeed, some surgeons may prefer barbed sutures while performing VUA, as they are self-cinching, do not require intracorporeal knot tying and can save time and reduce technical complications. Nonetheless, the method utilized for VUA most frequently remains the one we described 17 years ago [1]: new materials, same technique.

Future Perspectives and Conclusions

Today, surgeons across the world perform VUA in multiple manners. However, many of them have readapted the original single-knot running technique, making minor modifications. In the opinion of many surgeons, continuous sutures seem more appealing than separate stitches [5, 35]. We conducted a worldwide internet survey, asking urologists involved in minimally invasive surgery several questions regarding our technique [36]. Overall, it appeared that our technique has been widely accepted, and many urologists consider it a well-established technique in urology. Although the results of such survey are encouraging, further research will probably lead us to advance and develop better, faster and easier techniques for VUA, which especially in the pure laparoscopic approach, remains a challenging step. In this setting, an interesting research was conducted by Hruby et al.: these investigators in 2007 described a novel tissue apposing device to perform VUA and tested it on a pig model [37]. This device, developed by American Medical Systems (Minnetonka, MN), is similar to a Foley catheter with two sets of opposing retractable nitinol tines which approximate the bladder neck to the urethra, thereby eliminating the need for suturing. In their animal model, this system not only was significantly faster than standard VUA (12 vs. 41 min), but it was also associated with a reduced fibrotic reaction. As it happened with colo-rectal cancer, it is possible that in the near future we will see mechanic transurethral devices that aid in performing VUA, however to date the work of Hruby et al. represents, to our knowledge, the only attempt in such direction.

In conclusion, close to 20 years have passed since the introduction of the single-knot running VUA technique and today it still seems a valid and safe technique for VUA. Though with minor modifications, this method is now widely applied by many surgeons involved in minimally invasive urologic surgery and should be the gold standard against which to compare novel techniques that certainly will be developed in the next future.

References

1. Van Velthoven RF, Ahlering TE, Peltier A, Skarecky DW, Clayman RV. Technique for laparoscopic running urethrovesical anastomosis: the single knot method. Urology. 2003;61(4):699–702.
2. Menon M, Hemal AK, Tewari A, Shrivastava A, Bhandari A. The technique of apical dissection of the prostate and urethrovesical anastomosis in robotic radical prostatectomy. BJU Int. 2004;93(6):715–9.
3. Simone G, Papalia R, Ferriero M, Guaglianone S, Gallucci M. Laparoscopic «single knot-single running» suture vesico-urethral anastomosis with posterior musculofascial reconstruction. World J Urol. 2012;30(5):651–7.
4. Meeks JJ, Zhao LC, Greco KA, Wu SD, Nadler RB. Application of continuous tension to aid in performing the vesicourethral anastomosis for robot-assisted prostatectomy. J Endourol. 2009;23(12):1941–4.
5. Montorsi F, Wilson TG, Rosen RC, Ahlering TE, Artibani W, Carroll PR, et al. Best practices in robot-assisted radical prostatectomy: recommendations of the Pasadena Consensus Panel. Eur Urol. 2012;62(3):368–81.
6. Rocco F, Carmignani L, Acquati P, Gadda F, Dell'Orto P, Rocco B, et al. Restoration of posterior aspect of rhabdosphincter shortens continence time after radical retropubic prostatectomy. J Urol. 2006;175(6):2201–6.
7. Tewari A, Jhaveri J, Rao S, Yadav R, Bartsch G, Te A, et al. Total reconstruction of the vesico-urethral junction. BJU Int. 2008;101(7):871–7.
8. Vis AN, van der Poel HG, Ruiter AEC, Hu JC, Tewari AK, Rocco B, et al. Posterior, anterior, and periurethral surgical reconstruction of urinary continence mechanisms in robot-assisted radical prostatectomy: a description and video compilation of commonly performed surgical techniques. Eur Urol. 2019;76(6):814–22.
9. Teber D, Erdogru T, Cresswell J, Gözen AS, Frede T, Rassweiler JJ. Analysis of three different vesicourethral anastomotic techniques in laparoscopic radical prostatectomy. World J Urol. 2008;26(6):617–22.
10. Surya BV, Provet J, Johanson KE, Brown J. Anastomotic strictures following radical prostatectomy: risk factors and management. J Urol. 1990;143(4):755–8.
11. Schatzl G, Madersbacher S, Hofbauer J, Pycha A, Reiter WJ, Svolba G, et al. The impact of urinary extravasation after radical retropubic prostatectomy on urinary incontinence and anastomotic strictures. Eur Urol. 1999;36(3):187–90.
12. Williams TR, Longoria OJ, Asselmeier S, Menon M. Incidence and imaging appearance of urethrovesical anastomotic urinary leaks following da Vinci robotic prostatectomy. Abdom Imaging. 2008;33(3):367–70.
13. Hemal AK, Agarwal MM, Babbar P. Impact of newer unidirectional and bidirectional barbed suture on vesicourethral anastomosis during robot-assisted radical prostatectomy and its comparison with polyglecaprone-25 suture: an initial experience. Int Urol Nephrol. 2012;44(1):125–32.
14. Hu JC, Nelson RA, Wilson TG, Kawachi MH, Ramin SA, Lau C, et al. Perioperative complications of laparoscopic and robotic assisted laparoscopic radical prostatectomy. J Urol. 2006;175(2):541–6; discussion 546.
15. Rebuck DA, Haywood S, McDermott K, Perry KT, Nadler RB. What is the long-term relevance of clinically detected postoperative anastomotic urine leakage after robotic-assisted laparoscopic prostatectomy? BJU Int. 2011;108(5):733–8.
16. Cohen MS. J Endourol. 2006;20(8):574–9. https://doi.org/10.1089/end.2006.20.574.
17. Diamand R, Al Hajj Obeid W, Accarain A, Limani K, Hawaux E, van Velthoven R, et al. Management of anastomosis leakage post-RALP: a simple trick for a complex situation. Urol Case Rep. 2017;12:28–30.
18. Ouzaid I, Xylinas E, Ploussard G, Hoznek A, Vordos D, Abbou C-C, et al. Anastomotic stricture after minimally invasive radical prostatectomy: what should be expected from the Van Velthoven single-knot running suture? J Endourol. 2012 26(8) 1020–5.
19. Gontero P, Marra G, Alessio P, Filippini C, Oderda M, Munoz F, et al. Salvage radical prostatectomy for recurrent prostate cancer: morbidity and functional outcomes from a large multicenter series of open versus robotic approaches. J Urol. 2019;202(4):725–31.
20. Rocco B, Cozzi G, Spinelli MG, Grasso A, Varisco D, Coelho RF, et al. Current status of salvage robot-assisted laparoscopic prostatectomy for radiorecurrent prostate cancer. Curr Urol Rep. 2012;13(3):195–201.
21. Yuh B, Ruel N, Muldrew S, Mejia R, Novara G, Kawachi M, et al. Complications and outcomes of salvage robot-assisted radical prostatectomy: a single-institution experience. BJU Int. 2014;113(5):769–76.
22. Herrera-Caceres JO, Nason GJ, Salgado-Sanmamed N, Goldberg H, Woon DTS, Chandrasekar T, et al. Salvage radical prostatectomy following focal therapy: functional and oncological outcomes. BJU Int. 2020;125(4):525–30.
23. Campobasso D, Fiori C, Amparore D, Checcucci E, Garrou D, Manfredi M, et al. Total anatomical reconstruction during robot-assisted radical prostatectomy in patients with previous prostate surgery. Minerva Urol Nefrol. 2019;71(6):605–11.
24. Gupta NP, Singh P, Nayyar R. Outcomes of robot-assisted radical prostatectomy in men with previous transurethral resection of prostate. BJU Int. 2011;108(9):1501–5.
25. Dev H, Sharma NL, Dawson SN, Neal DE, Shah N. Detailed analysis of operating time learning curves in robotic prostatectomy by a novice surgeon. BJU Int. 2012;109(7):1074–80.
26. Tewari AK, Srivastava A, Sooriakumaran P, Slevin A, Grover S, Waldman O, et al. Use of a novel absorbable barbed plastic surgical suture enables a «self-cinching» technique of vesicourethral anastomosis during robot-assisted prostatectomy and improves anastomotic times. J Endourol. 2010;24(10):1645–50.
27. Weld KJ, Ames CD, Hruby G, Humphrey PA, Landman J. Evaluation of a novel knotless self-anchoring suture material for urinary tract reconstruction. Urology. 2006;67(6):1133–7.
28. Erdogru T, Celik O, Hladun T, Kazimoglu H, Micoogullari U, Akincioglu E, et al. Comparison of suture material for vesico-urethral anastomosis in robotic radical prostatectomy. Cent Eur J Urol. 2020;73(2):134–9.
29. Massoud W, Thanigasalam R, El Hajj A, Girard F, Théveniaud PE, Chatellier G, et al. Does the use of a barbed polyglyconate absorbable suture have an impact on urethral anastomosis time, urethral stenosis rates, and cost effectiveness during robot-assisted radical prostatectomy? Urology. 2013;82(1):90–4.
30. Moran ME, Marsh C, Perrotti M. Bidirectional-barbed sutured knotless running anastomosis v classic Van Velthoven suturing in a model system. J Endourol. 2007;21(10):1175–8.
31. Sammon J, Kim T-K, Trinh Q-D, Bhandari A, Kaul S, Sukumar S, et al. Anastomosis during robot-assisted radical prostatectomy:

randomized controlled trial comparing barbed and standard monofilament suture. Urology. 2011;78(3):572–9.
32. Zorn KC, Trinh Q-D, Jeldres C, Schmitges J, Widmer H, Lattouf J-B, et al. Prospective randomized trial of barbed polyglyconate suture to facilitate vesico-urethral anastomosis during robot-assisted radical prostatectomy: time reduction and cost benefit. BJU Int. 2012;109(10):1526–32.
33. Murtha AP, Kaplan AL, Paglia MJ, Mills BB, Feldstein ML, Ruff GL. Evaluation of a novel technique for wound closure using a barbed suture. Plast Reconstr Surg. 2006;117(6):1769–80.
34. Warner JP, Gutowski KA. Abdominoplasty with progressive tension closure using a barbed suture technique. Aesthet Surg J. 2009;29(3):221–5.
35. Sengupta S, Ischia J, Webb DR. Single-layer anatomical reconstruction of the vesico-urethral anastomosis during robot-assisted laparoscopic prostatectomy (RALP). BJU Int. 2011;107(2):340–3.
36. Albisinni S, Limani K, Hawaux E, Peltier A, Van Velthoven R. Evaluation of the single-knot running vesicourethral anastomosis 10 years after its introduction: results from an international survey. J Laparoendosc Adv Surg Tech A. 2014;24(9):640–6.
37. Hruby G, Weld KJ, Marruffo F, Collins S, Durak E, Mitchell R, et al. Comparison of novel tissue apposing device and standard anastomotic technique for vesicourethral anastomoses. Urology. 2007;70(1):190–5.

Urethral Suspension

16

Ryoichi Shiroki, Kiyoshi Takahara, Kenji Zennami, Masashi Takenaka, Makoto Sumitomo, and Mamoru Kusaka

Introduction

Urinary incontinence following radical prostatectomy (RP) is still a major source of morbidity and significant concern for patients facing with surgery. Urinary sphincteric complex contains periurethral smooth muscles, rhabdosphincter consisting of omega-shaped loop of striated muscles around the membranous urethra, and further supporting connective tissues. This combined anatomical functionality is aimed to withstand increased abdominal pressure, leading to facilitate urinary continence [1]. Surgical reconstruction of pelvic-floor structures aims to enhance anatomical support, returning to the presurgical state. It is, however, yet unknown which reconstructive techniques add any further to the stabilization of pelvic-floor structures to improve continence recovery post RP.

There have been various different kinds of surgical procedures used in an attempt to make urinary continence recovery earlier post Robot-Assisted Radical Prostatectomy (RARP). Some of the technical variations showed a certain effect on the recovery of urinary continence without compromising the oncologic outcomes. Robotic assistance made it possible to adopt the variety of techniques to improve continence recovery. This situation is thought to be totally different from pure laparoscopic approach which involve technical difficulty for the specific technique such as longitudinal-directed suturing. Urethral suspension during RARP are mainly comprised of stitch suspension with sutures or sling suspension using various materials and combination of these. Table 16.1 gives an overview of the continence rates in time after surgery as reported by the studies of various reconstructive procedures. This chapter illustrates the different kinds of urethral suspension techniques and outcomes of continence recovery after RARP.

R. Shiroki (✉) · K. Takahara · K. Zennami · M. Takenaka · M. Sumitomo · M. Kusaka
Department of Urology, Fujita Health University School of Medicine, Toyoake, Aichi, Japan
e-mail: rshiroki@fujita-hu.ac.jp; kiyoshi@fujita-hu.ac.jp; zenken@fujita-hu.ac.jp; masashi.takenaka@fujita-hu.ac.jp; m-sumi@fujita-hu.ac.jp; mkusaka@fujita-hu.ac.jp

Urethral Stitch Suspension

Urethral stitch suspension is one of the most popular and simple method to deliver during RARP. Because of the robotic articulation, various types of suspension stitches were proposed in an attempt to improve continence post RARP. The concept of urethral suspension is primarily thought to be associated with the stabilization of the vesicourethral anastomosis. The periurethral retropubic suspension stitch has been described by Walsh in an open RP series [2]. Anterior reconstruction might be reserved for techniques that anchor the urethra to the pubic fascia or, alternatively, for fixation of the periurethral tissues to the bladder neck and endopelvic fascia.

In 2009, Patel et al. first introduced this suspension technique in RARP as the anterior reconstruction through anchoring the urethra and urethral supportive structures to the pubic bone [3]. The technique is based on placement of a puboperiurethral suspension stitch after ligation of the dorsal venous complex (DVC). The suture is placed between urethra and DVC, passed through the periosteum of the pubic bone, and back through to the DVC in multiple figure-eight loops. The suspension of the periurethral complex can provide additional anterior support to the striated sphincter, stabilizing the posterior urethra in its anatomical position within the pelvic floor. This stabilization can aid in the preservation of the urethral length during the dissection of the prostatic apex, facilitating the vesicourethral anastomosis. They reported that the suspension technique resulted in significantly better continence rates at 3 months after RARP than a non-suspension technique (92.8% vs. 83.0%, $p = 0.013$). The median/mean interval to recovery of continence was also statistically significantly shorter in the suspension group (median 6 weeks; mean 7.3) than in the non-suspension

S. Ren et al. (eds.), *Robot-Assisted Radical Prostatectomy*, https://doi.org/10.1007/978-3-031-05855-4_16

Table 16.1 Urethral suspension and outcomes of urinary continence after Robotic-Assisted Radical Prostatectomy (RARP)

Surgical type of procedure				Continence rate post RARP			
Authors (year)	Type of study	No. of cases	Surgical technique	1 month (%)	3 months (%)	12 months (%)	Efficacy
Suture suspension							
Patel (2009) [3]	Non-RCT	237	Periurethral suspension	40.0	92.8	97.9	p = 0.013
		94	No suspension	33.0	83.0	95.7	
Kojima (2014) [4]	C	27	Bladder neck suspension	29.6	29.6	ND	p < 0.05
		30	No suspension	10.0	25.9	ND	
Canvasser (2016) [5]	C	36	Posterior urethral suspension	54	64	ND	p < 0.05
		56	No suspension	24	36	ND	
Sling suspension							
Bahler (2016) [7]	RCT	73	Artificial material (Surgisis)	55.2	75.2	94.5	N.S.
		74	No sling	47.1	73.8	86.7	
Cestari (2017) [8]	RCT	60	Six-arm sling (vas deference)	87	ND	ND	p = 0.04
		60	Two-arm sling (vas deference)	70	ND	ND	
Nguyen (2017) [9]	RCT	95	Two-arm sling (vas deference)	45	76	ND	N.S.
		100	No sling	49	75	ND	
Combination							
Kalisvaart (2009) [10]	C	50	Ant and post reconstruction (simple stitch)	ND	90.9	ND	p = 0.014
		50	No reconstruction	ND	48.2	ND	
Sammon (2010) [11]	RCT	59	Ant and post reconstruction	80.0	ND	ND	N.S.
		57	Post reconstruction	82.6	ND	ND	
Tan (2010) [12]	C	1383	Ant and post reconstruction	70.0	91.7	98.0	p < 0.001
		214	No reconstruction	35.2	61.9	82.1	
Hurtes (2012) [13]	RCT	34	Ant and post reconstruction	26.5	45.2	ND	p = 0.047
		28	No reconstruction	7.1	15.4	ND	p = 0.016
Beattie (2013) [14]	C	81	Ant and post reconstruction	20.5	44.3	ND	p = 0.025
		51	Post reconstruction	8.2	26.7	ND	
Han (2015) [15]	C	60	Ant and post reconstruction	25.0	60.0	ND	N.S.
		70	No reconstruction	23.9	57.7	ND	
Karabulut (2020) [16]	C	20	Ant suspension and long urethra	ND	85	100.0	p = 0.031
		20	No reconstruction	ND	50.0	95.0	

C retrospective cohort study, *RCT* randomized clinical trial, *N.S.* not significant

group (median 7 weeks; mean 9.6, $p = 0.02$), suggesting that the suspension stitch resulted in a statistically significantly shorter interval to recovery of continence and higher continence rates at 3 months after the procedure. The effect of continence recovery, however, did not last as the continence rates were similar to those in the long run postoperatively.

Kojima et al. described another technique for suspension stitch [4]. They adopted the sling-type suspension suture to anchor the anastomosis just behind the pubic bone. The percentages of patients with no leakage on the 1-h pad test 4, 12, and 24 weeks after RARP were 29.6%, 29.6%, and 36.7% in the sling group, whereas they were 10.0%, 25.9%, and 33.3% in the non-sling group, respectively. There was a significant difference between two groups at 4 weeks after RARP ($p < 0.05$). The authors concluded that bladder neck sling suspension suture is a simple and feasible procedure and can improve the early return of continence after RARP.

Canvasser et al. reported posterior urethral suspension using preplaced suture into posterior urethral rhabdosphincter connective tissue at the 5 and 7 o'clock positions [5]. After completion of the vesico-urethral anastomosis, each suspension suture is secured to the ipsilateral pubic bone periosteum 3–4 cm from the pubic symphysis using a slipknot technique to suspend the anastomosis. Pad-free rates for this procedure were 37%, 47%, 54%, and 60% compared with controls 15%, 18%, 24%, and 36%, at weeks 1, 2, 4, and 12 after catheter removal, respectively. They concluded this technique resulted in statistically significant improvement in urinary control 4 week post-operation. By 12 weeks, however, the differences in pad-free rates between two groups had resolved.

Urethral Sling Suspension

Some types of the sling suspension of vesicourethral anastomosis were reported to improve early continence recovery using isogenic tissues or artificial materials. Bladder neck sling suspension procedures, which have been used for the management of female stress urinary incontinence (SUI), can support the proximal urethra and bladder neck. As a result, sling provides a direct compressive force on the vesicourethral anastomosis, increasing the functional length of the urethral sphincteric complex, and potentially reestablishing and reinforcing the suburethral tissue used as a backboard for urethral closure.

In open RP, there were some techniques for sling suspension of the vesicourethral anastomosis with a strip harvested from the fascia of the rectus muscle and reported significant effect on continence recovery [6]. The disadvantages of this procedure, however, include the additional morbidity of harvesting the fascia, which seemed to be crucial on endoscopic surgery, and the risk of urinary retention. There were some reports for sling suspension using artificial and autologous materials for anastomosis support.

Bahler et al. applied an artificial strip made from small intestinal submucosal tissue as urethral sling [7]. Soft tissue graft, Surgisis® (Cook Biodesign), was laid posterior to the urethra and bladder neck to suture-fixed to the both sides of Cooper's ligament. While not statistically significant, the continence rate was higher in the sling group than the control group at 1 month (55.2% vs. 47.1%, p = 0.34) and 12 months (94.5% vs. 86.7%, p = 0.15). For those patients who regained continence during the course of the clinical study the median time to return of continence was 90 days for the control group and 77 days for the sling group. This difference was not statistically different either.

Cestari et al. assessed the effectiveness of six-arms sling using autologous vas deferens harvested during RARP [8]. They applied two- or six-arms sling underneath the urethral anastomosis to fix to the symphysis of the pubic bone. The continence rate was higher in the six-arms group than the two-arms group at 1 month (87% vs. 70%, p = 0.04). Compared with two-arms sling, patients submitted to six-arms sling reported higher rate of early urinary continence until 30 days postoperatively.

Nguyen et al. also organized prospective trial using vas deferens as autologous sling materials during RARP [9]. After harvesting the vas deferens, the sling was placed on the rectum underneath the site of the vesicourethral anastomosis and the anastomosis was completed. The sling was then placed around the vesicourethral anastomosis, suspended to the pubic symphysis and tensioned to allow elevation of the vesicourethral anastomosis. Their study failed to demonstrate a benefit of autologous sling placement on early return of continence at 6 months. Continence was related to patient age, not to the sling procedure, in background-adjusted model.

Combination Technique (Anterior Suspension and Posterior Reconstruction)

Some studies tried anterior suspension combined with posterior reconstruction, and showed improvements on the early return of continence.

Kalisvaart et al. compared posterior reconstruction and anterior suspension by single anastomotic suture (PRASS) with no reconstruction [10]. Patients who underwent the PRASS reconstruction had significantly improved urinary control at 3 months compared with the control group; 90.9% of the patients in the PRASS group wore 0–1 pads per day vs. 48.2% in the control group (p = 0.014). They concluded PRASS technique resulted in statistically significant improvement in urinary control 3 months post RARP.

Sammon et al. compared continence recovery between double-layer anastomosis consisted of the reapproximation of Denonvilliers' fascia and the posterior rhabdosphincter, as well as reapproximation of the puboprostatic ligaments to the anterior pubovesical collar [11]. They reported pad usage rates and weights were equivalent between two groups.

Tan et al. proposed another combination technique with posterior reconstruction and anterior suspension which composed of preservation of anterior structures and suspension sutures to the arcus tendineus and puboprostatic ligaments alleviate downward prolapse of the bladder on the anastomosis [12]. They compared recovery of continence and showed the mean time to continence recovery was 19.0, 7.3, and 5.7 weeks in the no reconstruction, anterior suspension alone, and total reconstruction cohorts, respectively (P < 0.001). They concluded total reconstruction, which composed of anterior and posterior reconstruction, was the most significant variable for early continence.

Hurtes et al. conducted a randomized prospective multicenter trial using anterior suspension combined with posterior reconstruction [13]. They reported that the continence rates in combined group (26.5% and 45.2%, respectively) at 1 and 3 months after RARP were significantly higher than with the standard technique (7.1% and 15.4%; p = 0.047 and p = 0.016, respectively).

Beattie et al. introduced bladder neck imbrication suture continued to anterior fixation [14]. Their technique showed significant improvement at all stages of follow-up compared with posterior reconstruction alone, from 8.2% to 20.5%, 26.7% to 44.3%, and 47.7% to 62.3% at 1.5, 3 and 6 months, respectively (p = 0.025).

Some other studies also reported that patients undergoing the combined technique had earlier or even continence recovery than patients undergoing the standard reconstruction [15–18]. From several small studies, it seems that some studies of the combined anterior and posterior or total reconstruction has advantage over the standard technique at 1 or 3 months after RARP, whereas long-term outcomes are unknown and have largely not been supported by RCTs.

It is striking that all described reconstructive techniques show good-to-fair outcomes 1 year after surgery, that is, continence rates between 87% and 98% of cases. Apparently, all reconstructive surgical techniques result in similar short-term continence rates, without significant differences in long-term continence rates as compared with "no reconstruction." The effect of continence recovery, however, did not last as the continence rates were similar to those in the long run postoperatively.

Complications with Urethral Suspension During RARP

Overall, certain procedures of urethral suspension showed some effects on the recovery of urinary continence without compromising the oncologic outcomes. Urethral suspension may, however, cause postoperative urinary tract complications such as increased residual urine, retention or anastomosis stricture. Patel et al. reported no significant postoperative morbidity related to the placement of the suspension stitch, such as pubic osteitis, or no acute urinary retention after catheter removal [3]. Kojima et al. showed no significant difference in MFR and Post-void residual (PVR) between two groups 4, 12, and 24 weeks after RARP by sling suture suspension [4]. Posterior urethral suspension with stitch (PUS) was reported to result in similar postoperative complications rates with control, without grade IV or higher complications [5]. Only two cases of PUS (2.4%) developed urinary retention who had endoscopic-confirmed bladder neck edema treated with extended catheter placement uneventfully, while the other developed a bladder neck contracture that required intraluminal dilation.

For the sling procedure, urinary complication rates seemed to be a little higher than stich suspension [17, 18]. Bahler et al. applied an artificial strip as sling suspension and the total percentage of patients with adverse events was similar between the control and sling groups (10.8% vs. 13.7%, respectively) [7]. They reported that no particular adverse events were related to the sling. Cestari et al. reported that one patient treated with six-arms sling suspension experienced acute urinary retention at the time of catheter removal and treated with longer placement uneventfully [8]. Nguyen et al. also organized prospective trial using vas deferens as autologous sling materials during RARP [9]. They reported that no incidence of urine infection, erosion, bleeding, bladder neck contracture or injury to adjacent structures that was related to sling placement. Urinary obstruction requiring short-term catheterization developed in 12 patients (6%) and did not differ between the groups. The number of cases with PVR volume greater than 150 mL did not differ significantly between groups (three in the non-sling and one in the sling group). No patients experienced with anastomotic stricture in both the groups. In summary, there seemed no particular complications or elevated rates related to the different types of suspension procedures.

Conclusions/Discussion

The concept of urethral suspension is mainly associated with the stabilization of the vesicourethral anastomosis. Because of the robotic articulation, urethral stitch suspension is one of the most popular and simple method to deliver during RARP. Almost all reconstructive surgical techniques result in similar short-term continence rates and excellent outcomes 1 year after surgery. There are only a few randomized clinical trials comparing a reconstructive technique with "no reconstruction" or a different reconstructive technique, and outcomes are conflicting. Although many of the procedures reported a benefit with respect to early continence, benefits seem to diminish with longer follow-up. Whether any of the reconstructive techniques is superior to another is a matter of study.

Further improvement of urinary continence through further advancement and modification of the procedure during RARP are expected.Financial or Material SupportNone.

Conflict of Interest The authors have no conflicts of interest to declare.

References

1. Burnett AL, Mostwin JL. In situ anatomical study of the male urethral sphincteric complex: relevance to continence preservation following major pelvic surgery. J Urol. 1998;160:1301–6.
2. Walsh PC. Anatomical radical prostatectomy: evolution of the surgical technique. J Urol. 1998;160:2418–24.
3. Patel VR, Coelho RF, Palmer KJ, Rocco B. Periurethral suspension stitch during robot-assisted laparoscopic radical prostatectomy: description of the technique and continence outcomes. Eur Urol. 2009;56:472–8.
4. Kojima Y, Hamakawa T, Kubota Y, Ogawa S, Haga N, Tozawa K, Sasaki S, Hayashi Y, Kohri K. Bladder neck sling suspension during robot-assisted radical prostatectomy to improve early return of urinary continence: a comparative analysis. Urology. 2014;83:632–9.
5. Canvasser NE, Lay AH, Koseoglu E, Morgan MS, Cadeddu JA. Posterior urethral suspension during robot-assisted radical prostatectomy improves early urinary control: a prospective cohort study. J Endourol. 2016;30:1089–94.
6. Jorion JL. Rectus fascial sling suspension of the vesicourethral anastomosis after radical prostatectomy. J Urol. 1997;157:926–8.
7. Bahler CD, Sundaram CP, Kella N, Lucas SM, Boger MA, Gardner TA, Koch MO. A parallel randomized clinical trial examining the

return of urinary continence after robot-assisted radical prostatectomy with or without a small intestinal submucosa bladder neck sling. J Urol. 2016;196:179–84.
8. Cestari A, Ferrari M, Sangalli M, Zanoni M, Ghezzi M, Fabbri F, Sozzi F, Lolli C, Dell'Acqua V, Rigatti P. Simple vs six-branches autologous suburethral sling during robot-assisted radical prostatectomy to improve early urinary continence recovery: prospective randomized study. J Robot Surg. 2017;11:415–21.
9. Nguyen HG, Punnen S, Cowan JE, Leapman M, Cary C, Welty C, Weinberg V, Cooperberg MR, Meng MV, Greene KL, Garcia M, Carroll PR. A randomized study of intraoperative autologous retropubic urethral sling on urinary control after robotic assisted radical prostatectomy. J Urol. 2017;197:369–75.
10. Kalisvaart JF, Osann KE, Finley DS, Ornstein DK. Posterior reconstruction and anterior suspension with single anastomotic suture in robot-assisted laparoscopic radical prostatectomy: a simple method to improve early return of continence. J Robot Surg. 2009;3:149–53.
11. Sammon JD, Muhletaler F, Peabody JO, Diaz-Insua M, Satyanaryana R, Menon M. Long-term functional urinary outcomes comparing single- vs double-layer urethrovesical anastomosis: two-year follow-up of a two-group parallel randomized controlled trial. Urology. 2010;76:1102–7.
12. Tan G, Srivastava A, Grover S, Peters D, Dorsey P Jr, Scott A, Jhaveri J, Tilki D, Te A, Tewari A. Optimizing vesicourethral anastomosis healing after robot-assisted laparoscopic radical prostatectomy: lessons learned from three techniques in 1900 patients. J Endourol. 2010;24:1975–83.
13. Hurtes X, Rouprêt M, Vaessen C, Pereira H, Faivre d'Arcier B, Cormier L, Bruyère F. Anterior suspension combined with posterior reconstruction during robot-assisted laparoscopic prostatectomy improves early return of urinary continence a prospective randomized multicentre trial. BJU Int. 2012;110:875–83.
14. Beattie K, Symons J, Chopra S, Yuen C, Savdie R, Thanigasalam R, Haynes AM, Matthews J, Brenner PC, Rasiah K, Sutherland RL, Stricker PD. A novel method of bladder neck imbrication to improve early urinary continence following robotic-assisted radical prostatectomy. J Robot Surg. 2013;7:193–9.
15. Han KS, Kim CS. Effect of pubovesical complex reconstruction during robot-assisted laparoscopic prostatectomy on the recovery of urinary continence. J Laparoendosc Adv Surg Tech A. 2015;25:814–20.
16. Karabulut I, Yilmazel FK, Yilmaz AH, Celik EC, Ceylan O, Ozkaya F, Adanur S, Polat O. Effect of reconstructive techniques on continence in robot-assisted laparoscopic prostatectomy: novel combination of long urethral stump and anterior suspension suture. Eurasian J Med. 2020;52:57–60.
17. Vis AN, van der Poel HG, Ruiter AEC, Hu JC, Tewari AK, Rocco B, Patel VR, Razdan S, Nieuwenhuijzen JA. Posterior, anterior, and periurethral surgical reconstruction of urinary continence mechanisms in robot-assisted radical prostatectomy: a description and video compilation of commonly performed surgical techniques. Eur Urol. 2019;76:814–22.
18. Vora AA, Dajani D, Lynch JH, Kowalczyk KJ. Anatomic and technical considerations for optimizing recovery of urinary function during robotic-assisted radical prostatectomy. Curr Opin Urol. 2013;23:78–87.

Posterior Reconstruction

17

Jonathan Noël, Bernardo Rocco, Maria Chiara Sighinolfi, Simone Assumma, and Vipul Patel

Introduction

Post prostatectomy urinary incontinence is a potential side effect of surgical treatment of prostate cancer [1]. However the majority of patients will recover in several months after radical prostatectomy (RP). To improve quality of life after prostatectomy, we must adopt techniques that not only limit this side effect, but minimize the recovery period for patients. After all, post RP urinary incontinence is the most troublesome side effect when compared to erectile dysfunction.

It is recognized that there are a wide range of definitions for continence; the majority being the use of a daily safety pad or no pads at all. The rate can range anywhere from 2% to 47% [2] and this is likely due to the non-uniformity of continence as a definition and the assessor (whether it is indirectly by the surgical team or directly from the patient). For non-persistent incontinence, the cause is frequently down to stress incontinence from weakness in the striated urethral sphincter and pelvic floor. Published urodynamic studies of persistent post RP incontinence reveal it is caused by intrinsic sphincter deficiency [3] while recognizing that decreased urethral and/or detrusor compliance, and detrusor overactivity will contribute in some cases. This supports evidence that urethral closure pressure, bladder stability and functional urethral length all contribute to achieving continence post-surgery [4]. An appreciation of the urethral sphincter complex anatomy and the closely related structures is key to the reader appreciating the aims of this chapter's technique.

Anatomical Disruption of Prostatectomy

The rhabdosphincter (RS) surrounds the urethra in a cylindrical fashion, starting from the perineal membrane to the bladder base. It is mostly made up of skeletal muscle fibres that originate in the perineal membrane to insert into the prostate apex with anterior extension towards the detrusor apron. It has a horse shoe appearance axially, and contracts the skeletal muscles anterolaterally to close the urethral lumen by a "fulcrum" action on the fixed posterior wall. This posterior wall of the RS is a rigid and fibrous connective tissue as opposed to striated muscle [5, 6], and it becomes contiguous with the posterior median raphe (PMR). Therefore, the posterior suspension system of the male pelvis is the posterior portion of the RS, PMR, the prostatic fascia and Denonvilliers' fascia (DF).

During a radical prostatectomy, this continuous posterior suspension system is disrupted. In our centres, the bladder is dropped by division of the urachus, to access the space of retzius. The rectovesical pouch will change in position as a result, and this may contribute to a change of the orientation in cranial insertions of the posterior suspension system, since the DF is related directly to this pouch.

After the bladder neck is opened, we perform a series of manoeuvres to optimise visualisation of the seminal vesicles (SV) athermally, with blunt sweeping off of the ventral layer of DF before a Hem-o-Lok clip is applied to blood vessels. The absence of cautery near the tip of the SV is paramount to spare the pelvic plexus from electrical current nearby [7, 8]. Once the SVs are elevated, the DF is sharply dissected to create a plane between the rectum and the prostate, which is then extended laterally to an pre-planned grade of neurovascular bundle (NVB) sparing that is appropriate for the patient [9].

Our technique has always evolved to optimise functional outcomes. In the past, once the prostate is fully mobilised cranially, the puboprostatic ligaments and deep venous complex (DVC) were suture ligated and fixed to the pubic bone with the urethra [10]. Moschovas et al. [11] published our modified approach to the endopelvic fascia and apical dis-

J. Noël · V. Patel (✉)
Global Robotics Institute, AdventHealth, Celebration, FL, USA
e-mail: jonathan.noel.md@adventhealth.com; vipul.patel.md@adventhealth.com

B. Rocco
Department of Urology, ASST SANTI Paolo e Carlo—Università degli Studi di Milano, Milan, Italy

M. C. Sighinolfi · S. Assumma
Department of Urology, Ospedale Policlinico e Nuovo Ospedale Civile S.Agostino Estense Modena, University of Modena and Reggio Emilia, Modena, Italy

S. Ren et al. (eds.), *Robot-Assisted Radical Prostatectomy*, https://doi.org/10.1007/978-3-031-05855-4_17

section, by opening the endopelvic fascia while conscientiously preserving levator ani fascia on the muscle. A plane medial to the lateral prostatic fascia is then made, with a communicating window to the previous posterior nerve spare plane, which allows a retrograde NVBs sparing technique with minimal traction [12, 13]. The apical complex of the puboprostatic ligaments and apical endopelvic fascia are left intact, keeping the anatomy of the apex undisturbed and avoiding a deep venous complex (DVC) stitch. This allows the sphincteric complex anteriorly to remain attached to the pubis, to have an optimal craniocaudal length. The anterolateral walls of the RS are carefully teased off the prostate apex and at the point of the anterior urethra, a cold cut with scissors is performed until the foley catheter is in view and subsequently retracted.

Other centres have advocated a more proximal approach to sparing the anterior fascia of the prostate, to enhance the preservation of the puboprostatic ligaments and DVC complex. These results have been published with a rate of potency and continence recovery at 1 year of follow up (86% and 98.4% respectively [14]).

A contemporary technique of avoiding to drop the bladder and leave the space of retzius intact (retzius sparing RALP) has been employed by centres worldwide, and the results show significantly increased rates of immediate recovery of continence. A randomised trial revealed median time to continence of 21 days for retropubic RALP and 1 day for retzius sparing RALP [15], with further comparative studies confirming this advantage in their respective series [16]. However, there is an association of patients undergoing retzius sparing RALP to have positive surgical margins (PSM) and in tandem their long term biochemical recurrence (BCR) remains to be determined, according to a Cochrane Database systematic review [17].

The posterior wall of the urethra is then cold cut divided; the prostatic fascia and PMR is encountered and bipolar diathermy applied to control associated vessels before it is dissociated. This is the final step in the disruption of the entire posterior suspension system: DF at the beginning of posterior plane development and the apical dissection.

After the prostate specimen is placed in an endocatch bag, hemostatic selective suturing and bladder neck reconstruction is performed as our standard practise. Our preference is to perform lateral plication bladder neck reconstruction. Bladder neck sparing is not performed in our centre to limit the risk of positive surgical margins on pathological assessment, as confirmed in a systematic review by Bellangino et al. [18].

The important functional consequences of disruption of the posterior musculofascial suspensory system are:

- The urethral sphincteric complex will not be continuous with the prostatic apex and Denonvilliers' fascia, and so the fixed framework to close the urethra is compromised.
- The urethral sphincteric complex shortens due to being withdrawn into the pelvic floor from the remaining longitudinal muscles, making the RS similarly shortened.
- The perineum can also prolapse, especially if there is a weak pelvic floor, and so this further adds to the caudal displacement of the urethral sphincteric complex.

Posterior Reconstruction Description and Evolution

The posterior musculofascial reconstruction has been born out of the following objectives:

- Suturing the posterior median raphe to the cut edge of Denonvilliers' fascia, thereby re-establishing the posterior suspensory support system post prostatectomy.
- Fixing this to the bladder.
- The retracted urethral sphincteric complex is restored closer to its normal anatomical position.

The overall goal being to facilitate improved recovery of post prostatectomy urinary continence, and so this reconstruction has evolved over years. The technique was first described by F. Rocco et al. in 2006 [19], during open radical prostatectomy where it shortened the time to continence recovery in patients. The restoration of the posterior support system is by reconstruction of the PMR to the residual layers of DF, followed by suspending the urethral sphincteric complex to the posterior bladder. In detail, the PMR is marked with two sutures before dissecting the prostatic apex, being careful to separate it from the NVB (see Fig. 17.1).

The PMR is fixed to the residual Denonvilliers fascia using the two stay sutures and then attached to the posterior bladder wall with two sutures about 1–2 cm cranial: to suspend and lengthen the urethral sphincter complex in reference to the bladder neck. An interrupted vesicourethral anastomosis is then performed in a separate plane and create a tension less approximation. This was described as a modification of Walsh's open RP, and it was compared to patients who did not have this reconstructive step. The continence of posterior reconstruction vs. non reconstruction was at discharge (62.4% vs. 14%), 1 month (74% vs. 30%) and at 3 months (85.2% vs. 46%).

B. Rocco described his experience using a laparoscopic transperitoneal approach [20]. The original technique by F. Rocco, used two (pre urethral incision) placed sutures in

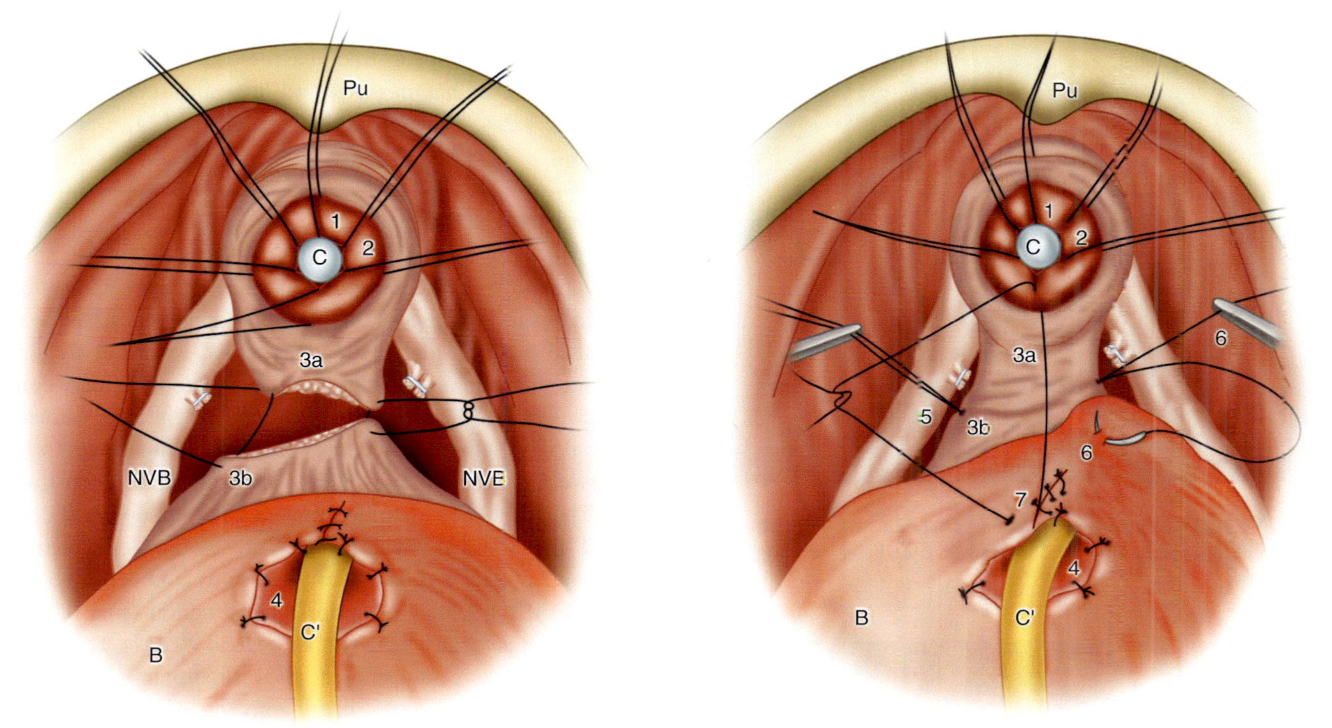

Fig. 17.1 *Left*: Suturing the RS and median fibrous raphe to the Denonvilliers fascia. *Pu* pubis, *C* urethral catheter, *C′* bladder catheter, *B* bladder, *NVB* neurovascular bundle, *1* membranous urethra, *2* anterolateral wall of RS, *3a* sectioned posterior wall of RS and MFR, *3b* sectioned Denonvilliers fascia, *4* bladder-neck eversion. *Right*: Fixation of the RS and DV (5) to the posterior wall of the bladder 2 cm dorsocephalad to the bladder neck (6). *Pu* pubis, *C* membranous urethral catheter, *C′* bladder catheter, *B* bladder, *1* membranous urethra, *2* anterolateral wall of RS, *3a* sectioned posterior wall of RS and MFR, *3b* sectioned Denonvilliers fascia, *4* bladder-neck eversion, *7* posterior urethrovesical anastomosis. (Permission from Springer Publishing, Robotic Urologic Surgery, V. Patel, 2nd edn. 2012)

the PMR, so as to avoiding the urethra entirely. The trocars are placed as follows:

- 12-mm umbilical port
- 12-mm paramedian right port
- 5-mm paramedian left port
- 5-mm pararectal ports (two)

After the urethra is divided, the PMR was incised proximal to the urethral transection, obviating the placement of two stay sutures initially. The open approach described sutures being placed in all the structures and tied in one step. To overcome initial challenges of tissue tearing due to imbalanced tension during the laparoscopic approach, the PMR and RS with DF was tied first followed by the RS-DF complex to the bladder. This controlled tension to a more reproducible standard, with gentle pressure in the perineum externally where necessary. The study compared 62 patients who underwent laparoscopic RP, and 31 underwent posterior reconstruction and other 31 did not. The results of reconstruction vs. no reconstruction were documented at catheter removal (74.2% vs. 25%), 1 month (83.8% vs. 32.3%) and 3 months (92.3% vs. 76.9%) post-surgery.

Posterior reconstruction was first described by our group in a robotic approach [21]; by utilising a double armed 2-0 poliglecaprone RB-1 needle suture or 2-0 monocryl. As previously described, the free edge of the remaining Denonvilliers' fascia is identified and approximated to the RS with one arm of the suture (Fig. 17.2).

The second layer we initially described was performed with the second arm of the suture including 2 cm of proximal posterior bladder in relation to the bladder neck, and then the first layer of reconstruction. After this is secured, then it was incorporated to a Van Velthoven vesicourethral anastomosis [22]. The early continence rate (0–1 pad per day) was 72%. The accuracy of finding the exact anatomy without placing a safety suture in the PMR prior to urethral transection (as described in the open approach) is made up for with the robotic camera endoscope's magnification. Precise identification of the relevant anatomy, particularly in placing the distal sutures in the PMR and RS, is the challenging aspect for a new adoption of this technique.

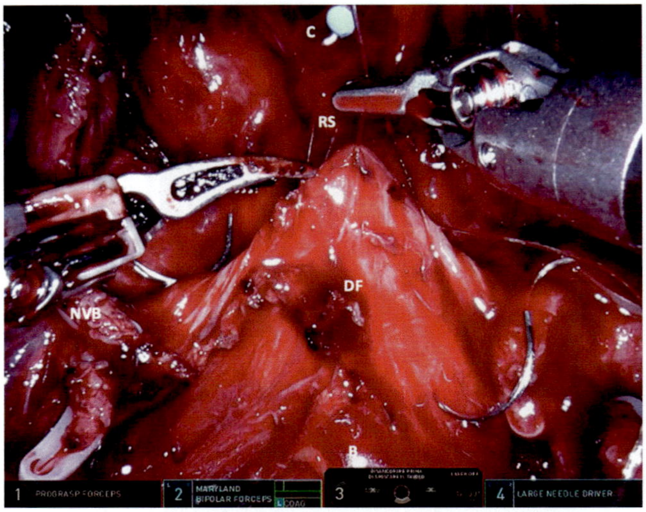

Fig. 17.2 First layer of robotic posterior reconstruction. *DF* Denonvilliers fascia, *RS* rhabdosphincter, *C* catheter. (Photographs by B. Rocco)

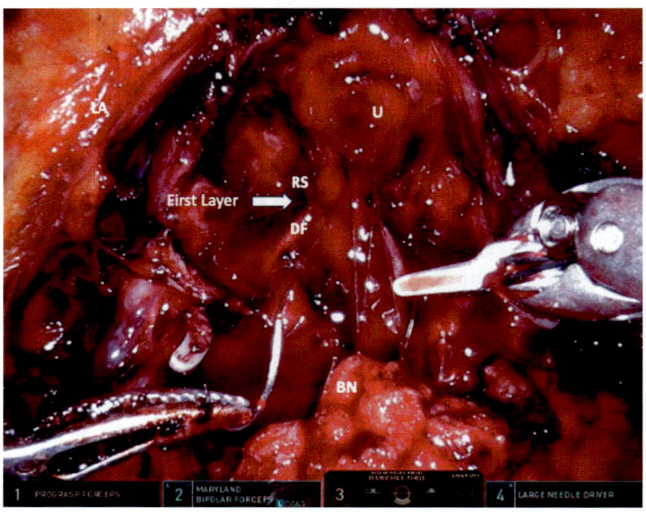

Fig. 17.3 Second layer of robotic posterior reconstruction. DF: Denonvilliers fascia is already reconstructed to the RS: rhabdosphincter (first layer). The posterior U = urethra is taken with the first layer, and then the posterior BN = bladder neck. (Photographs by B. Rocco)

A further modification to the second layer of RALP by Patel [23] (which is used in current practise at our Institution) was to utilise the posterior bladder neck and the vesicoprostatic muscle followed by the posterior urethral edge. This was incorporated into the first reconstructed layer of RS-PMR and DF and all performed with a double armed suture (Fig. 17.3).

One of the key steps for an appropriate reconstruction is the preservation of the DF when dissecting the posterior plane between the prostate and the rectal wall. In addition, the connective tissue of the PMR of the prostate apex, is a usable surgical plane that can be preserved and allow reconstructive advantages of the retracted posterior RS fibres. The more DF and RS spared, the more robust the reconstructive layers can be. A tension free anastomosis follows, with the added benefit of haemostasis and less anastomosis associated urine leaks, as evaluated by cystograms [24].

Impact on Outcomes

A systematic review of posterior musculofascial reconstruction only in open, laparoscopic and robotic approaches has been published and considered for this chapter. Rocco et al. [25] explored the main outcome of post prostatectomy urinary continence at 3–7, 30–45, 90, 180 days and 1 year after catheter removal. The authors included studies comparing cohorts who underwent prostatectomy with or without posterior reconstruction. The 11 studies identified included two randomised controlled trials (RCTs) which revealed no significant difference; comparative studies showed early return of continence within the first 30 days after posterior reconstruction ($p = 0.004$), while continence rates were similar beyond 90 days. This similarity after 90 days maybe due to the difficulty in isolating the effect of a posterior reconstruction only; as bladder neck sparing, nerve spare and anterior structure preservation will all have impacts on continence recovery. These could not be controlled for as is the heterogeneity among surgical skill, per the study by Vickers et al. [26] ($p < 0.001$ for outcomes). Employing the posterior RS reconstruction did not result in a statistically significant difference in positive surgical margin (PSM) rates nor bladder neck stricture (BNS).

With the continued wide scale adoption of this technique, a meta-analysis was carried out in 2016; where 21 studies that employed this technique with comparison to cases without, in all surgical approaches [27]. Once again, it confirmed no statistical significant difference in postoperative complications or positive surgical margin profile with patients undergoing posterior reconstruction. The main advantage was seen in post prostatectomy urinary continence, where an advantage at 3–7, 30, 90 days after catheter removal was observed in open, laparoscopic and robotic modalities. A less but noteworthy statistically significant advantage was seen at 180 days after catheter removal in this study across all surgical approaches. The limitations of this study were similar to the 2012 systematic review, in respect to surgeon heterogeneity, the modifications used in posterior reconstruction as opposed to the first description by F Rocco in 2006. The premise of the original description being that besides the restoration of the posterior musculofascial support, elongation of the dorsal wall of the urethral sphincteric complex occurred by the 2 cm cranial anchoring suture to the dorsal bladder. Table 17.1 summarises a select profile of publications that compared this technique to the absence of its utilisation in RALP.

Table 17.1 Continence at time points after RALP with and without posterior reconstruction

Author	Type of study	Number of patients		Continence at catheter removal (3–7 days)		Continence at 30 days		Continence at 45–75 days		Continence at 90 days		Continence at 180 days		Continence at 1 year	
		PR	No PR	PR	No PR	PR	No PR	PR	No PR	PR	No PR	PR	No PR	PR	No PR
Tewari A et al. 2008	Retrospective	182	214	38.37% ($p < 0.01$)	13.5%	82.56% ($p < 0.01$)	35.21%			91.30% ($p < 0.01$)	50.23%	97.14% ($p < 0.01$)	61.97%		
Menon M et al.2008	Randomized trial	59	57	1 Day 34.0% 2 Days 46.0% 7 Days 54.0% ($p < 0.01$)	1 Day 26.0% 2 Days 49.0% 7 Days 51.0%	80.0% ($p < 0.01$)	74.0%								
Nguyen MM et al. 2008	Retrospective	32	30	34.0% ($p = 0.007$)	3.0%	56.0% ($p = 0.006$)	17.0%								
Krane LS et al. 2009	Retrospective	34	37					85.0%	86.0%						
Kim IY et al. 2010	Retrospective	25	25	19.0% ($p = 0.306$)	38.1%	72.6% ($p = 1$)	71.4%			88.0% ($p = 0.718$)	80.0%	96.0%	96.0%		
Joshi N et al. 2010	Prospective	53	54							75.0% ($p = 0.391$)	69.0%	51.0% ($p = 0.686$)	43.0%		
Coelho RF et al. 2010	Prospective	473	330	28.7% ($p = 0.045$)	22.7%	51.6% ($p = 0.016$)	42.7%			91.1% ($p = 0.908$)	91.8%	97.0% ($p = 0.741$)	96.3%		
Sutherland DE et al. 2011	Randomized trial	47	47							63% ($p = 0.007$)	81%				
Brien JC et al. 2011	Retrospective	31	58							64.0% ($p = 0.05$)	50.0%	69.0% ($p = 0.27$)	62.0%		
Atug F et al. 2012	Retrospective	125	120	71.2% ($p < 0.0001$)	23.33%	72.8% ($p < 0.0002$)	49.1%			80.8% ($p < 0.5176$)	76.6%	84.8% ($p < 0.5088$)	80.8%	91.2% ($p < 0.5956$)	88.33%
Hurtes X et al. 2012	Randomized trial	39	33			26.5% ($p = 0.047$)	7.1%			45.2% ($p = 0.016$)	15.4%	65.4% ($p > 0.5$)	57.9%		
Gondo T et al. 2012	Retrospective	160	39	48.7%	15.4%	75.0%	20.5%	86.9%	53.9%	91.2%	71.8%	95.6%	79.5%	96.3%	87.2%
You YC et al. 2012	Retrospective	28	31			57.2%	35.5%			89.2%	71%	92.8%	87.5%	94.5%	92.1%

Permission from Springer Publishing, Robotic-assisted radical prostatectomy. J.W. Davis, 2016

The European Association of Urology Robotic Urology Section (ERUS) carried out a survey in 2013 [28], and reported that posterior reconstruction was performed by 51.7% as a standard step for surgeons carrying out RALP; and "sometimes" by 19.8% of them. This would imply that in Europe, it is being utilised in practise widely and a contemporary survey would be anticipated.

Conclusion

Regaining early post prostatectomy continence is challenging, even after technical adaptions, but with further anatomical restoration and innovation to techniques, there will be more patient benefits to gain. It is known that the definition and assessment of continence is largely responsible for globally published outcome variability. Nonetheless, recent meta-analysis [29] have concluded that posterior reconstruction of musculofascial plate offers early continence recovery.

The reproducibility of outcomes is dependent on the skill of the surgeon, but the inherent advantage of robotic technology as a platform, along with mentorship and collaboration will make this attainable. The authors' collective experience of more than 15,000 RALPs, would dictate that the "Rocco" posterior reconstruction be a standard adjunct to any RP approach.

References

1. Litwin MS, Hays RD, Fink A, Ganz PA, Leake B, Leach GE, et al. Quality-of-life outcomes in men treated for localized prostate cancer. JAMA. 1995;273:129.
2. Catalona WJ, Carvalhal GF, Mager DE, Smith DS. Potency, continence and complication rates in 1,870 consecutive radical retropubic prostatectomies. J Urol. 1999;162:433.
3. Groutz A, Blaivas JG, Chaikin DC, et al. The pathophysiology of post-radical prostatectomy incontinence: a clinical and video urodynamic study. J Urol. 2000;163:1767–70.
4. Hammerer P, Huland H. Urodynamic evaluation of changes in urinary control after radical retropubic prostatectomy. J Urol. 1997;157(1):233–6. PMID: 8976260.
5. Myers RP. Male urethral sphincteric anatomy and radical prostatectomy. Urol Clin North Am. 1991;18:211.
6. Burnett AL, Mostwin JL. In situ anatomical study of the male urethral sphincteric complex: relevance to continence preservation following major pelvic surgery. J Urol. 1998;160:1301.
7. Kalan S, Coughlin G, Palmer KJ, Patel VR. Robot-assisted laparoscopic radical prostatectomy: an athermal anterior approach to the seminal vesicle dissection. J Robot Surg. 2008;2(4):223–6. Epub 2008 Nov 19. PMID: 27637791. https://doi.org/10.1007/s11701-008-0117-3.
8. Orvieto MA, Patel VR. Evolution of robot-assisted radical prostatectomy. Scand J Surg. 2009;98:76–88.
9. Schatloff O, Chauhan S, Sivaraman A, Kameh D, Palmer KJ, Patel VR. Anatomic grading of nerve sparing during robot-assisted radical prostatectomy. Eur Urol. 2012;61(4):796–802. https://doi.org/10.1016/j.eururo.2011.12.048.
10. Patel VR, Shah KK, Thaly RK, Lavery H. Robotic-assisted laparoscopic radical prostatectomy: the Ohio State University technique. J Robot Surg. 2007;1(1):51–9. https://doi.org/10.1007/s11701-007-0018-x.
11. Moschovas MC, Bhat S, Onol FF, Rogers T, Roof S, Mazzone E, Mottrie A, Patel V. Modified apical dissection and lateral prostatic fascia preservation improves early postoperative functional recovery in robotic-assisted laparoscopic radical prostatectomy: results from a propensity score-matched analysis. Eur Urol. 2020;78(6):875–84. Epub 2020 June 24. PMID: 32593529. https://doi.org/10.1016/j.eururo.2020.05.041.
12. Coughlin G, Dangle PP, Palmer KJ, et al. Athermal early retrograde release of the neurovascular bundle during nerve-sparing robotic-assisted laparoscopic radical prostatectomy. J Robot Surg. 2009;3:13–7. https://doi.org/10.1007/s11701-009-0127-9.
13. Ko YH, Coelho RF, Sivaraman A, Schatloff O, Chauhan S, Abdul-Muhsin HM, Carrion RJ, Palmer KJ, Cheon J, Patel VR. Retrograde versus antegrade nerve sparing during robot-assisted radical prostatectomy: which is better for achieving early functional recovery? Eur Urol. 2013;63(1):169–77. Epub 2012 Sep 28. PMID: 23092543. https://doi.org/10.1016/j.eururo.2012.09.051.
14. de Carvalho PA, Barbosa JABA, Guglielmetti GB, Cordeiro MD, Rocco B, Nahas WC, Patel V, Coelho RF. Retrograde release of the neurovascular bundle with preservation of dorsal venous complex during robot-assisted radical prostatectomy: optimizing functional outcomes. Eur Urol. 2020;77(5):628–35. Epub 2018 July 21. PMID: 30041833. https://doi.org/10.1016/j.eururo.2018.07.003.
15. Asimakopoulos AD, Topazio L, De Angelis M, et al. Retzius-sparing versus standard robot-assisted radical prostatectomy: a prospective randomized comparison on immediate continence rates. Surg Endosc. 2019;33:2187–96. https://doi.org/10.1007/s00464-018-6499-z.
16. Umari P, Eden C, Cahill D, Rizzo M, Eden D, Sooriakumaran P. Retzius-sparing versus standard robot-assisted radical prostatectomy: a comparative prospective study of nearly 500 patients. J Urol. 2021;205(3):780–90. Epub 2020 Oct 20. PMID: 33086025. https://doi.org/10.1097/JU.0000000000001435.
17. Rosenberg JE, Jung JH, Edgerton Z, Lee H, Lee S, Bakker CJ, Dahm P. Retzius-sparing versus standard robotic-assisted laparoscopic prostatectomy for the treatment of clinically localized prostate cancer. Cochrane Database Syst Rev. 2020;(8):CD013641. https://doi.org/10.1002/14651858.CD013641.pub2.
18. Bellangino M, Verrill C, Leslie T, et al. Systematic review of studies reporting positive surgical margins after bladder neck sparing radical prostatectomy. Curr Urol Rep. 2017;18(12):99. https://doi.org/10.1007/s11934-017-0745-0.
19. Rocco F, Carmignani L, Acquati P, Gadda F, Dell'Orto P, Rocco B, et al. Restoration of posterior aspect of rhabdosphincter shortens continence time after radical retropubic prostatectomy. J Urol. 2006;175(6):2201–6. https://doi.org/10.1016/s0022-5347(06)00262-x.
20. Rocco B, Gregori A, Stener S, et al. Posterior reconstruction of the rhabdosphincter allows a rapid recovery of continence after transperitoneal videolaparoscopic radical prostatectomy. Eur Urol. 2007;51(4):996–1003. https://doi.org/10.1016/j.eururo.2006.10.014.
21. Coughlin G, Dangle PP, Patil NN, et al. Surgery illustrated—focus on details. Modified posterior reconstruction of the rhabdosphincter: application to roboticassisted laparoscopic prostatectomy. BJU Int. 2008;102:1482–5.
22. Van Velthoven RF, Ahlering TE, Peltier A, Skarecky DW, Clayman RV. Technique for laparoscopic running urethrovesical anastomosis: the single knot method. Urology. 2003;61(4):699–702. PMID: 12670546. https://doi.org/10.1016/s0090-4295(02)02543-8.
23. Coelho RF, Chauhan S, Orvieto MA, Sivaraman A, Palmer KJ, Coughlin G, Patel VR. Influence of modified posterior recon-

struction of the rhabdosphincter on early recovery of continence and anastomotic leakage rates after robot-assisted radical prostatectomy. Eur Urol. 2011;59(1):72–80. https://doi.org/10.1016/j.eururo.2010.08.025.

24. Menon M, Muhletaler F, Campos M, Peabody JO. Assessment of early continence after reconstruction of the periprostatic tissues in patients undergoing computer assisted (robotic) prostatectomy: results of a 2 group parallel randomized controlled trial. J Urol. 2008;180:1018–23.
25. Rocco B, Cozzi G, Spinelli MG, Coelho RF, Patel VR, Tewari A, et al. Posterior musculofascial reconstruction after radical prostatectomy: a systematic review of the literature. Eur Urol. 2012;62(5):779–90. https://doi.org/10.1016/j.eururo.2012.05.041.
26. Vickers A, Savage C, Bianco F, et al. Cancer control and functional outcomes after radical prostatectomy as markers of surgical quality: analysis of heterogeneity between surgeons at a single cancer center. Eur Urol. 2011;59:317–22.
27. Grasso AAC, Mistretta FA, Sandri M, Cozzi G, De Lorenzis E, Rosso M, et al. Posterior musculofascial reconstruction after radical prostatectomy: an updated systematic review and a meta-analysis. BJU Int. 2016;118(1):20–34. https://doi.org/10.1111/bju.13480.
28. Ficarra V, Wiklund PN, Rochat CH, et al. The European Association of Urology Robotic Urology Section (ERUS) survey of robot-assisted radical prostatectomy (RARP). BJU Int. 2013;4:596–603.
29. Grasso AA, Mistretta FA, Sandri M, Cozzi G, De Lorenzis E, Rosso M, et al. Posterior musculofascial reconstruction after radical prostatectomy: an updated systematic review and a meta-analysis. BJU Int. 2016;118(1):20–34. https://doi.org/10.1111/bju.13480.

18

CORPUS: Complete Posterior Reconstruction to Improve Continence After Robotic Prostatectomy

Alessandro Morlacco, Valeria Lami, Nicola Zanovello, and Fabrizio Dal Moro

Introduction

Urinary incontinence (UI) after radical prostatectomy is a frequent event and remains a frustrating side effect significantly impairing patients' quality of life. Prospective data indicate that continence improves up to at least 24 months after surgery [1].

In 2001, a technique for restoration of the posterior aspect of the rhabdomyosphincter was developed by Rocco et al. [2]. This technique is based on the principle of providing a fixation point for the posteriorly deficient urethral rhabdomyosphincter using a musculofascial plate. Several technical modifications have been proposed, such as adding a pubo-periurethral suspension [3]. However, despite several surgical solutions have been proposed, complete resolution of the problem of postoperative UI after RP has still not been achieved. AdVance retrourethral transobturator male sling (AMS), based on the hypothesis that relocation of the posterior urethra to a more proximal position plays an important role in regaining continence [4], has shown high effectiveness in post-RP stress urinary incontinence (SUI) [5]. Therefore, starting from anatomic and radiologic evidence [6] of the efficacy of the relocation of the posterior urethra and of intraoperative posterior reconstruction of the musculofascial plate, we designed and tested a novel intraoperative technique for the COmplete Reconstruction of the Posterior Urethral Support (CORPUS).

Surgical Technique

After radical prostatectomy, CORPUS reconstruction was performed [7]. A 2-0 monofilament running suture was used, passing through the fibers of the right portion of the pubo-perinealis muscle, the medial portion of the levator ani, close to the urethra, through the rectourethralis muscle, and then through the fibers of the left portion of the pubo-perinealis muscle, close to the urethra, the suture was passed through Denonvilliers' fascia and then tied (Figs. 18.1 and 18.2). After ligation (without cutting), the same suture was first passed through the perivesical tissue close to the bladder neck, then through the couple of pleated fibers of the pubo-perinealis muscle and tied again (Fig. 18.3). This double pas-

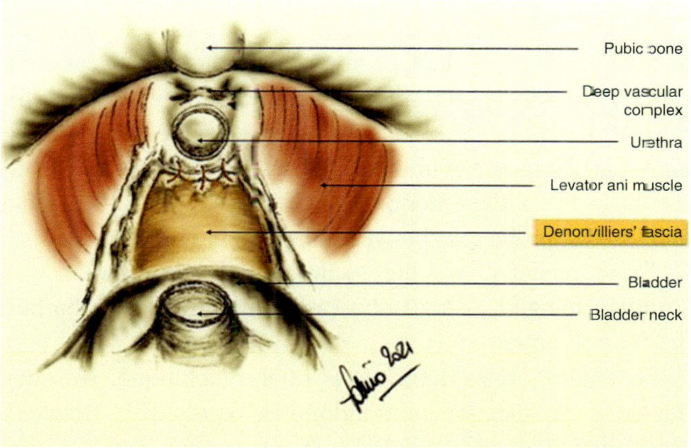

Fig. 18.1

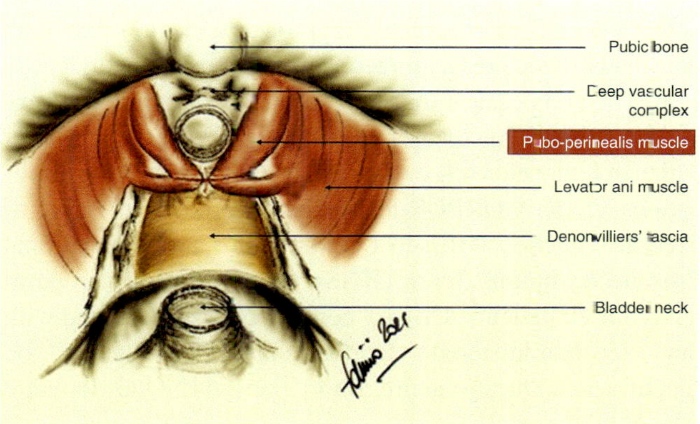

Fig. 18.2

A. Morlacco · V. Lami · N. Zanovello · F. Dal Moro (✉)
Department of Surgery, Oncology and Gastroenterology, Urology Clinic, University of Padova, Padova, Italy
e-mail: alessandro.morlacco@unipd.it; fabrizio.dalmoro@unipd.it

S. Ren et al. (eds.), *Robot-Assisted Radical Prostatectomy*, https://doi.org/10.1007/978-3-031-05855-4_18

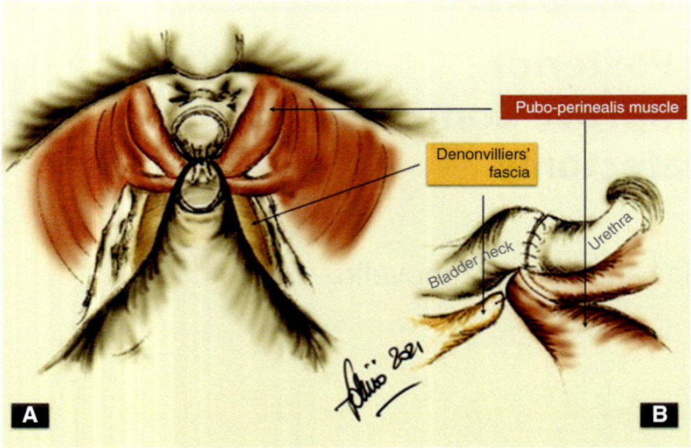

Fig. 18.3

sage and double ligation of the crossing sutures allowed posterior fixation of the dorsal wall of the urethra to the rhabdomyosphincter. The fibers of the pubo-perinealis muscle were carefully arranged as a posterior/lateral hammock, more supportive than the standard posterior reconstruction of the musculofascial plate. After the reconstruction, the anastomosis was performed in a standard fashion using all cases, with 2-0 monofilament stitches at the 6 o'clock position and a double 2-0 monofilament running suture was then emplaced and tied at the 12-o'clock position, over a Foley 18F catheter. After anastomosis, two stitches were bilaterally placed to fix the lateral wall of the bladder to the endopelvic fascia. At the end of anastomosis in both groups, a single stitch was placed medially, to fix the anterior wall of the bladder to the pubis and thus align the axis between bladder and urethra.

More recently, we the technique of anastomosis was slightly changed, using only a running suture with barbed 3/0 monofilament.

To analyze the effectiveness of the technique, we conducted a prospective nonrandomized study [7]. Between November 2012 and June 2013, 36 consecutive patients suitable for non nerve-sparing RARP and pelvic lymphadenectomy for clinically localized prostate cancer were alternatively assigned to two groups: one treated with the new CORPUS reconstructive approach and the other with the standardized posterior reconstruction according to Rocco et al. The end point of the study was comparison of the very early continence recovery rate in the two RARP groups after catheter removal, with evaluation of the short-term complications of the CORPUS technique. International Index of Erectile Function (IIEF-5) Questionnaire and International Prostate Symptom Score (IPSS) were collected preoperatively for all patients. Urinary continence was evaluated with the self-administered International Consultation on Incontinence Questionnaire, Short Form 642 Questionnaire (ICIQ-SF) [8] preoperatively, 24 h after catheter removal after RARP (answers #1 and #2 to the first question were not considered to be applicable) and then repeated 30 days later. To collect homogeneous data, inclusion criteria comprised patients with diagnoses of clinically localized prostate cancer but not eligible for nerve-sparing RARP (Gleason score $\geq$ 8, preoperative erectile dysfunction documented with IIEF-5 questionnaire). Patients with large median lobes or large prostate volume, traditionally considered as potentially affecting continence recovery, were also included in our analyses, because of the limited role they play in patients undergoing RARP, as demonstrated by Coelho et al. [9] in a recent series. In all cases, transperitoneal extrafascial non nerve-sparing RARP was performed.

Results: Preliminary Study

Patients' demographic and clinical characteristics were comparable in both the groups. There were no intraoperative complications during RARP. Two patients in the CORPUS group had postoperative complications: one patient developed ileus, treated conservatively, and another developed a lymphocele, which was treated with percutaneous drainage. Cystography 6 days after surgery revealed only one case of urinary leakage (CORPUS group). A further check after 7 days was normal.

The mean ICIQ-SF score 24 h after catheter removal was 7.05 (SD 2.4; range, 3–12) in the CORPUS group and 9.1 (SD 2.9; range, 4–16) in controls, with a statistically significant difference (P ¼ .015). Mean ICIQ-SF at day 30 was 4.5 (SD 1.9; range, 1–8) in the CORPUS group and 6.7 (SD 2.9; range, 0–14) in controls, with a statistically significant difference (P ¼ .0058). 50% of patients were continent immediately after catheter removal in the CORPUS group, and 83% after 30 days. In the control group, the percentages were 16% and 61%, respectively. The differences were statistically significant in both cases. No patient underwent any specific "rehabilitation" until day 30, but only basic Kegel exercises (not standardized) were prescribed, not to mask the real effects of the reconstruction. No patient reported perineal pain during the postoperative period. No patient has developed acute urinary retention or lower urinary tract symptoms in the follow-up period until the present, as demonstrated by the results of IPSS at 30 days in both the groups. Comparing urinary patterns 1 month after RARP in both groups, no difference was found in the IPSS score (P = .0837). Despite the CORPUS reconstruction, no patients developed clinically evident urethral and/or anastomotic strictures during follow-up, nor did any patients in the control group.

Comment

SUI after radical prostatectomy can be treated in various ways, but one of the most interesting and promising is the use of sub urethral suspension, providing posterior support to the membranous urethra after removal of the prostate gland. The efficacy of placing an AdVance sling 8–10 mm retrourethrally and/or suburethrally is not because of direct compressive effect on the urethral wall and lumen, as confirmed by two studies showing that urodynamic variables were unchanged after sling emplacement [10, 11]. In fact, the sling supports the distal sphincteric urethra, creating a sort of hammock during moments of increased abdominal pressure during stress and physical activity. Another element examined was the efficacy of the intervention of posterior reconstruction of the musculofascial plate as initially described by Rocco et al. In particular, the aforementioned authors noted that the dorsal aspect of the prostate, with Denonvilliers' fascia and the posterior median raphe with the connected dorsal wall of the rhabdomyosphincter, constitute an important support structure, appearing to serve as a fixation point for the muscle fibers of the rhabdosphincter [12]. In addition, as reported in several anatomic studies on cadavers, Denonvilliers' fascia ends at the rectourethralis muscle, which consequently provides a posterior attachment for the rhabdomyosphincter [13]. We reached the concept of CORPUS by examining the rationale of these two aspects and combining the anatomic principles of both techniques. In particular, we postulate that there are six main anatomo-functional effects of our approach: (1) CORPUS provides a hemi-circumferential dynamic support for the urethral sphincter complex, similar to the effects of an AdVance sling; (2) it creates a fixation point for the fibers of the rhabdomyosphincter through the reconstructed musculofascial plate; (3) it avoids bladder prolapse (as the space previously occupied by the prostate is filled) and also reduces the pressure of the bladder on the anastomosis during micturition; (4) the final stitch from the anterior wall of the bladder to the pubis allows the bladder-anastomosis-urethra axis to be properly aligned; and (5) the complete reconstruction provides a dynamic suspensory system for the membranous urethra, allowing pubo-perinealis muscle contractions to increase urethral pressure (6) the inclusion of the pubo-perinealis fibers into the reconstruction creates a fixation point for the perineal body, which tends to become more mobile after removal of the prostate and the surrounding tissues. Regarding this last point, the continence effects of the CORPUS technique might be enhanced with Kegel exercises (perineal contraction), owing to the active participation of the fibers of the pubo-perinealis muscle. These combined elements are a distinctive of the present technique. Our results demonstrate that the previously mentioned technique can further increase the efficacy of the philosophy of Rocco's technique, enhancing very early recovery of urinary continence.

In this preliminary experience study, continence rates were affected by both careful patient selection and the non nerve-sparing technique. To limit possible confounding factors, we restricted selection of patients only to cases suitable for non nerve-sparing RARP, bearing in mind two aspects: how the preservation of neuro-vascular bundles can increase continence rates [14–16] and how difficult it is to define a correct nerve-sparing procedure, although standardization of the procedure might be achieved [17].

Conclusion

We presented the CORPUS technique as a novel alternative approach for early continence recovery after RARP. Extension of the inclusion criteria, to comprise patients treated with nerve-sparing RARP, and standardization of rehabilitation programs are needed to evaluate the impact of the new technique in a more heterogeneous group, better reflecting real clinical practice.

References

1. Wei JT, Dunn RL, Marcovich R, Montie JE, Sanda MG. Prospective assessment of patient reported urinary continence after radical prostatectomy. J Urol. 2000;164:744–8. https://doi.org/10.1016/s0022-5347(05)67294-1.
2. Rocco F, Gadda F, Acquati P, Carmignani L, Favini P, Dell'Orto P, et al. Personal research: reconstruction of the urethral striated sphincter. Arch Ital Urol Androl. 2001;73:127–37.
3. Patel VR, Coelho RF, Palmer KJ, Rocco B. Periurethral suspension stitch during robot-assisted laparoscopic radical prostatectomy: description of the technique and continence outcomes. Eur Urol. 2009;56:472–8. https://doi.org/10.1016/j.eururo.2009.06.007.
4. Rehder P, Gozzi C. Transobturator sling suspension for male urinary incontinence including post-radical prostatectomy. Eur Urol. 2007;52:860–7. https://doi.org/10.1016/j.eururo.2007.01.110.
5. Novara G, Ficarra V. AdVance sling in postprostatectomy urinary incontinence: more data available and some questions still open. Eur Urol. 2012;62:146–7. https://doi.org/10.1016/j.eururo.2012.03.054.
6. Papin G, Tissot V, Le Penndu H, Nonent M, Fournier G. Évaluation du positionnement de la bandelette rétro-urétrale transobturatrice par IRM pelvienne statique et dynamique. Prog Urol. 2012;22:602–9. https://doi.org/10.1016/j.purol.2012.03.001.
7. Dal Moro F, Crestani A, Valotto C, Zattoni F. CORPUS—Novel COmplete reconstruction of the posterior urethral support after robotic radical prostatectomy: preliminary data of very early continence recovery. Urology. 2014;83:641–7. https://doi.org/10.1016/j.urology.2013.12.010.
8. Avery K, Donovan J, Peters TJ, Shaw C, Gotoh M, Abrams P. ICIQ: a brief and robust measure for evaluating the symptoms and impact of urinary incontinence. Neurourol Urodyn. 2004;23:322–30. https://doi.org/10.1002/nau.20041.
9. Coelho RF, Chauhan S, Guglielmetti GB, Orvieto MA, Sivaraman A, Palmer KJ, et al. Does the presence of median lobe affect out-

comes of robot-assisted laparoscopic radical prostatectomy? J Endourol. 2012;26:264–70. https://doi.org/10.1089/end.2011.0132.
10. Rehder P, Mitterberger MJ, Pichler R, Kerschbaumer A, Glodny B. The 1 year outcome of the transobturator retroluminal repositioning sling in the treatment of male stress urinary incontinence. BJU Int. 2010;106:1668–72. https://doi.org/10.1111/j.1464-410X.2010.09400.x.
11. Bauer RM, Soljanik I, Füllhase C, Karl A, Becker A, Stief CG, et al. Mid-term results for the retroluminar transobturator sling suspension for stress urinary incontinence after prostatectomy. BJU Int. 2011;108:94–8. https://doi.org/10.1111/j.1464-410X.2010.09729.x.
12. Rocco F, Carmignani L, Acquati P, Gadda F, Dell'Orto P, Rocco B, et al. Restoration of posterior aspect of rhabdosphincter shortens continence time after radical retropubic prostatectomy. J Urol. 2006;175:2201–6. https://doi.org/10.1016/S0022-5347(06)00262-X.
13. Uchimoto K, Murakami G, Kinugasa Y, Arakawa T, Matsubara A, Nakajima Y. Rectourethralis muscle and pitfalls of anterior perineal dissection in abdominoperineal resection and intersphincteric resection for rectal cancer. Anat Sci Int. 2007;82:8–15. https://doi.org/10.1111/j.1447-073X.2006.00161.x.
14. Suardi N, Moschini M, Gallina A, Gandaglia G, Abdollah F, Capitanio U, et al. Nerve-sparing approach during radical prostatectomy is strongly associated with the rate of postoperative urinary continence recovery. BJU Int. 2013;111:717–22. https://doi.org/10.1111/j.1464-410X.2012.11315.x.
15. Nandipati KC, Raina R, Agarwal A, Zippe CD. Nerve-sparing surgery significantly affects long-term continence after radical prostatectomy. Urology. 2007;70:1127–30. https://doi.org/10.1016/j.urology.2007.07.042.
16. Choi WW, Freire MP, Soukup JR, Yin L, Lipsitz SR, Carvas F, et al. Nerve-sparing technique and urinary control after robot-assisted laparoscopic prostatectomy. World J Urol. 2011;29:21–7. https://doi.org/10.1007/s00345-010-0601-z.
17. Schatloff O, Kameh D, Giedelman C, Samavedi S, Abdul-Muhsin H, Coelho RF, et al. Proposal of a method to assess and report the extent of residual neurovascular tissue present in radical prostatectomy specimens. BJU Int. 2013;112:E301–6. https://doi.org/10.1111/bju.12038.

Total Anatomical Reconstruction

19

Francesco Porpiglia, Paolo Verri, Stefano Granato, Michele Sica, Daniele Amparore, Cristian Fiori, and Enrico Checcucci

Introduction

Urinary incontinence represents the most feared functional complication after robot-assisted radical prostatectomy (RARP), since it can deeply impact the patient's quality of life [1].

The achievement of the so called "pentafecta", as described by some authors [2] by the concurrent presence of urinary continence, sexual potency, absence of positive surgical margins, early complications and biochemical recurrence, cannot prescind, as previously said, from satisfying urinary continence. These factors together, describe the perfect results after radical prostatectomy and represent the goal of every surgeon facing prostate cancer.

The introduction of robotic surgery revolutionized prostate cancer surgery, since it offered the surgeon greater image magnification and definition, microsurgical instruments with a wide range of movements and the minimization of physiological hands' shaking. Robotic surgery, thanks to the aforementioned technical characteristics, stated its superiority as a surgical technique, allowing to reach better results in terms of oncological and functional outcomes [3].

During RARP, one of the most challenging and delicate passage of the surgical act is represented by the urethrovesical anastomosis, which constitutes the crucial step in order to reach perfect continence. In the last decades, as also reported in the previous chapters of this book, different techniques have been proposed and validated.

In the following chapter, we describe the Total Anatomical Reconstruction performed during robot-assisted radical prostatectomy, as introduced by Professor Francesco Porpiglia and collaborators in 2015.

F. Porpiglia (✉) · P. Verri · S. Granato · M. Sica · D. Amparore
C. Fiori · E. Checcucci
Division of Urology, Department of Oncology, School of Medicine, San Luigi Gonzaga Hospital, University of Turin, Turin, Italy
e-mail: daniele.amparore@unito.it; cristian.fiori@unito.it

Technical Specifications

Before explaining in detail the total anatomical reconstruction (TAR) surgical technique, it is important to outline some anatomical and technical aspects, which need to be considered in order to fully comprehend the milestone of TAR technique.

Dorsal Venous Complex (DVC)

Also known as Santorini plexus, this vascular structure is intimately in contact with rabdosphincter fibers, with the pubo-prostatic ligaments and with the ventral side of the prostate before merging with the prostatic veins. As a consequence, during the suturing maneuvers, if the suture is placed too deeply, a damage to the sphincter and the underlying nervous structures may be caused. An anatomical landmark, whose knowledge is important in order to avoid damage to sphincter fibers, is represented by the avascular plane located at the level of the prostatic-urethral junction, which represents the ideal location for DVC hemostasis. As described by several authors [4, 5], after dissecting the fibers of levator ani muscle, separating them from the urethra and prostate, a selective ligation of the DVC can be performed. This maneuver avoids the damage to surrounding structures (i.e., levator ani, sphincter) and is related to higher early urinary continence recovery rates

Pubo-Prostatic Ligaments

Arising from the visceral layer of the endopelvic fascia, they insert inferiorly to the prostate, stabilizing the prostate-bladder-urethra complex. Thanks to their stiffness, these ligaments determine an angle at the level of the membranous urethra, which is important in the mechanism of urinary continence [6]. As proved by Stolzenburg et al. [7], the safeguarding of this anatomical structure allows to preserve the

S. Ren et al. (eds.), *Robot-Assisted Radical Prostatectomy*, https://doi.org/10.1007/978-3-031-05855-4_19

maximal urethral length and its anterior support, allowing to reach better function results in terms of urinary continence after radical prostatectomy.

Endopelvic Fascia

Thanks to the intimacy of its visceral layer with the pelvic organs (i.e., rectum, bladder, prostate) and to its merging with the fibromuscular stroma on the ventral side of the prostate. This complex interweaving of fascial layers constitutes an anatomical scaffold which gives solidity to the pelvic organs. For this reason, the preservation of this fascia determines higher stability of the urethra-vesical anastomosis, conferring better functional outcomes [8, 9].

Bladder Neck

The bladder neck corresponds to the urethro-vesical junction and is formed by muscular fibres, variably oriented, coming from the bladder trigone, the detrusor muscle and the urethra itself. Its function is essential in the micturition process and, consequently, in providing urinary continence. The careful dissection of this structure is fundamental in order to guarantee better functional outcomes after RARP. The preservation of the detrusor fibers (arranged into a longitudinal, middle circular and outer longitudinal layer) and of the internal sphincter is the key-point to reach optimal results. Notwithstanding the approach to the bladder neck dissection (e.g., anterior, lateral, anterolateral), it is fundamental to reach the bladder neck preservation in order to achieve the best functional outcomes, as outlined in a systematic review and meta-analysis [10].

Urinary Sphincter and Urethral Length

The urethral sphincter complex is located distally to the prostate apex, close to the levator ani muscle (*pars puboperinealis*) and is formed by two muscular layers: the outer striated muscle and the inner smooth muscle layer. The shape, the extension and the relationship of these muscular layers with the urethra and prostate apex can slightly vary, representing a variable during the apex dissection. For this reason, it is important to preserve the sphincter and urethra as much as possible. In a work of Schlomm et al. [11] it is clearly stated that a full-length urethral preservation together with the urinary sphincter preservation leads to an improvement of early urinary continence. In addition, the urethral length, volume and an anatomically close relationship between the levator ani muscle and membranous urethra are associated with a better recovery of urinary continence [12].

Prostate Apex and Neurovascular Bundles

The prostate apex presents a wide variety in terms of shape and volume between the individuals, making the apex dissection a challenging phase during radical prostatectomy. In addition, the prostate apex is intimately close to part of the periprostatic nerves which, after arising from the hypogastric plexus (i.e., pelvic plexus) surround laterally the bladder neck, the prostate base and the seminal vesicles. These nerves, located posterolaterally and anterolaterally with respect to the apex [13], are immersed in a fibrofatty tissue, which also surrounds arterial and venous vasa. This tissue plate surrounding the aforementioned pelvic organs is called the Neuro Vascular Bundle (NVB). As described by Tewari et al. [14] the NVBs can be divided into three longitudinal compartments: the proximal neurovascular place, the predominant NVB and the accessory neuronal pathways. Other authors, instead, divided the NVBs based on their position with respect to the levator ani muscle [15]. The interindividual variants of the nervous structures and the variable characteristics of the malignancy don't allow the reproduction of a specific and standardized surgical approach for every patient. On the other hand, the multilayered character of the periprostatic fascia allows to perform a modulable approach, including more or less periprostatic tissue and, consequently, periprostatic nervous fibers of the NVBs. These approaches (i.e., intrafascial, interfascial and extrafascial) have been widely described and discussed [16] and it has been demonstrated that the preservation of NVBs together with the careful dissection of the prostate apex is associated with better functional outcomes [17, 18]. Robotic surgical equipment, thanks to its advantages in terms of precision, allows the surgeon to perform a careful dissection of these delicate structures, leading to optimal and never reached before oncological and functional results.

Bladder Neck and Posterior Reconstruction

The bladder neck reconstruction consists in the restoration of the bladder neck orifice, after the dissection of the bladder neck itself. The dedicated suturing of the bladder orifice allows to reduce the diameter of the bladder neck, allowing a better realignment with the resected urethra. Several surgical variants have been described [19, 20], showing improved results after meticulous and precise bladder neck reconstruction.

The posterior reconstruction technique, firstly developed by Rocco et al. [21] has been object of discussion during the years, and several variants of the initial technique have been proposed [22, 23], including (in 2016) the TAR technique. The rationale of this technique is that the posterior musculofascial plate (i.e., posterior median raphe, rabdosphincter and dorsal aspect of Denonvilliers' fascia) covers a role of utmost importance in supporting dynamically the preserved urethra. This supporting structure is extended from the peritoneum (i.e., Douglas pouch) to the perineal membrane and median raphe [24]. During the years, the posterior reconstruction during RARP and its role in the urinary continence preservation and in the diminishing of postoperative complications has been extensively validated, having become at all effects a fundamental step in the reconstructive phase of radical prostatectomy [25].

Anterior Reconstruction

The rationale of anterior reconstruction is to restore the anatomical position of the pubo-prostatic ligaments, providing support to the rabdosphincter by positioning a monofilament suspension suture between the DVC, the urethra and pubic bone periosteum. After its first development in 1998 by Walsh [4], this technique was furtherly studied and validated [26], demonstrating its important role in the urinary continence recovery. The functional results of this technique were furtherly improved by its association with posterior reconstruction [27, 28].

The two aforementioned types of reconstructions represent an important step in the TAR technique. In the following paragraphs, the various steps of the reconstructing process will be explained in detail.

Total Anatomical Reconstruction: Surgical Technique

Demolitive Phase

The demolitive phase is standardized and in line with the most popular surgical approaches to perform robot-assisted radical prostatectomy. The description of this first phase of the surgical procedure allows to describe and highlight the anatomical structures which will be later essential to perform the total anatomical reconstruction.

Patient Positioning and Preliminary Time

After positioning the patient in the classical fashion for performing RARP (supine, legs slightly spread, Trendelenburg position) and after inducing pneumoperitoneum, the abdominal cavity can be explored. Subsequently, the parietal peritoneum can be incised, accessing the retropubic space. The endopelvic fascia, exposed after dissecting the periprostatic fatty tissue, is carefully incised in order to preserve the pubo-prostatic ligaments. At this point, the prostatic apex is identified.

Suture of Deep Venous Complex (DVC) and Bladder Neck Incision

The deep venous complex, in order to avoid excessive bleeding, is sutured using separated 2/0 monofilament sutures, with attention to pubeprostatic ligaments' preservation. At this point, after slicing cranially the visceral layer of the endopelvic fascia, the bladder neck is incised and dissected. Thanks to the robotic fourth arm, the catheter is pulled cranially, allowing to identify the dorsal portion of the vesical trigone. Following a vertical course and continuing the incision posteriorly, at the level of the circumference ridge, the muscular fibers attaching the prostatic base to the bladder are dissected. In order to access the retrotrigonal space, the posterior aspect of the bladder neck, a small lingula of muscular tissue known as the "retrotrigonal fascia", is dissected. At this point, by incising the anterior layer of Denonvilliers' fascia, the seminal vesicles are identified and dissected.

Incision of Posterior Denonvilliers' Fascia and Dissection of Prostatic Apex

Performing a U-shaped incision, the posterior layer of Denonvilliers' fascia is incised, creating an access to the perirectal space. At this point, the visceral layer of the endopelvic fascia and the apron, laying underneath and covering the anterior face of the prostate, are incised while sparing the pubo-prostatic ligaments. Thanks to the robotic miniaturized instruments, it is possible to perform a blunt and sharp microdissection of the smooth muscular fibers arising from the peri-urethral structures towards the prostatic apex. It is important to underline that, in this particular phase, a minimal use of electrocauterization is recommended, in order to avoid damages to the anatomical structures. At the end of the dissecting phase, the prostatic apex is completely isolated and the urethra can be incised at the level of the prostatic ridge. The surgical field, after removing the prostate and seminal vesicles is shown in Fig. 19.1.

Reconstructive Phase

Now that the demolitive phase has been completed and the pivotal anatomical structures have been dissected and spared variably, we can get to the heart of the TAR technique.

Posterior Reconstruction

Firstly, the posterior reconstruction is performed by using 3/0 barbed sutures, creating three distinct layers. The first layer is created by approaching the previously sectioned Denonvilliers' fascia and the median raphe, suturing them together from right to left (Fig. 19.2). The second layer is created by suturing, from left to right, the retrotrigonal fascia and the median raphe (Fig. 19.3). The third and last layer

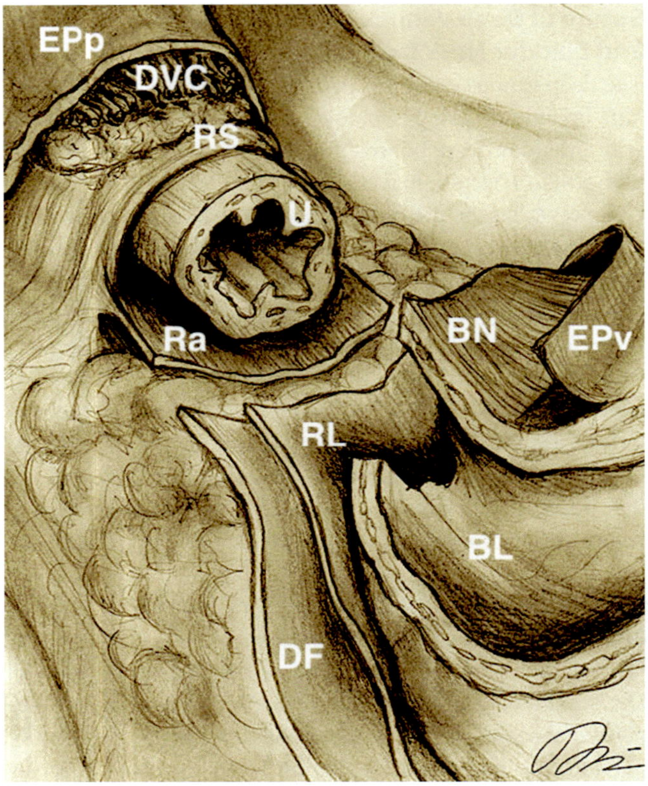

Fig. 19.1 Operative field at the end of the demolitive phase. *EPp* Endopelvic fascia, parietal layer, *DVC* deep venous complex, *RS* rabdosphincter, *U* urethra, *Ra* median raphe, *RL* retrotrigonal layer, *BN* bladder neck, *EPv* endopelvic fascia, visceral layer, *BL* bladder lumen, *DF* Denonvilliers' fascia. (Courtesy of Dr. Amparore—SCDU Urologia, San Luigi Gonzaga Hospital, Orbassano (TO), Italy)

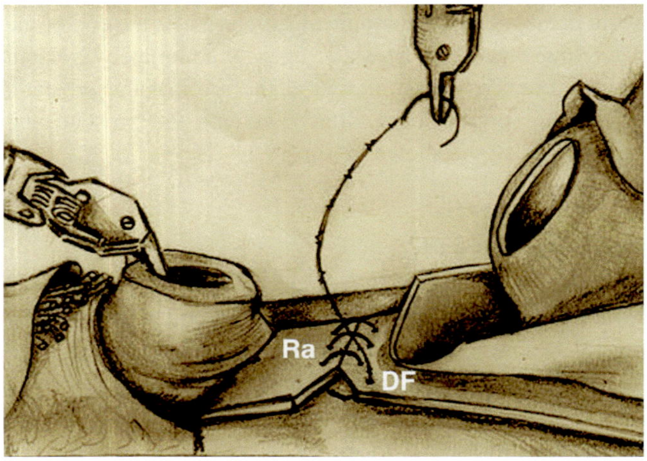

Fig. 19.2 Lateral view. First layer of posterior reconstruction. *Ra* median raphe, *DF* Denonvilliers' fascia. (Courtesy of Dr. Amparore—SCDU Urologia, San Luigi Gonzaga Hospital, Orbassano (TO), Italy)

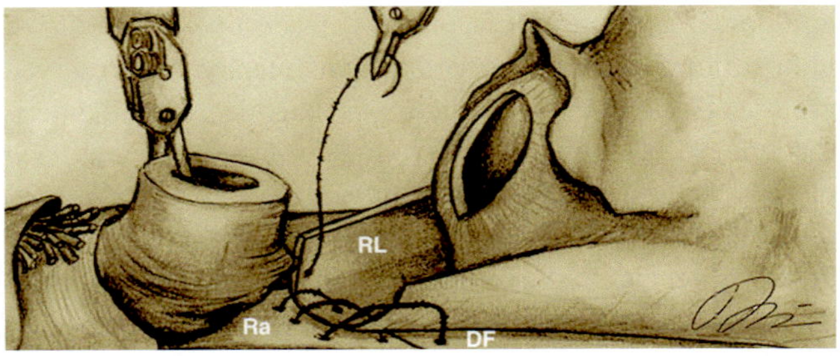

Fig. 19.3 Lateral view. The second layer involves the retrotrigonal fascia and the median raphe moving from left to right. *Ra* Median Raphe, *DF* Denonvilliers' fascia, *RL* retrotrigonal layer. (Courtesy of Dr. Amparore—SCDU Urologia, San Luigi Gonzaga Hospital, Orbassano (TO), Italy)

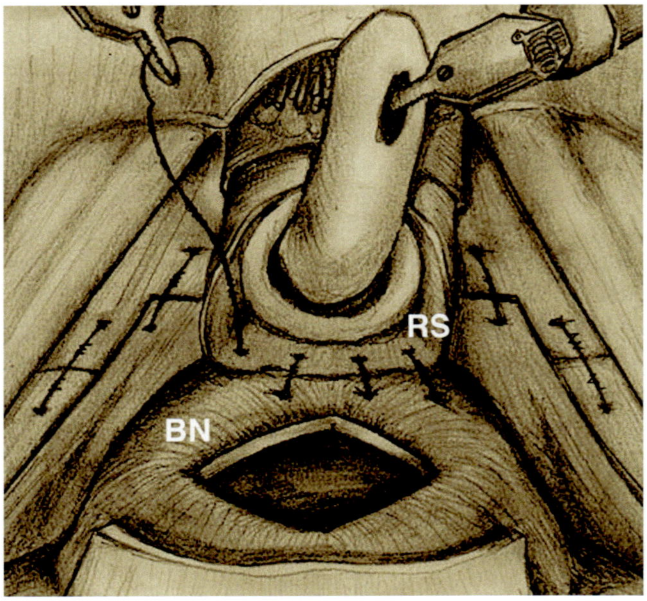

Fig. 19.4 Frontal view. The third layer involves the bladder neck (excluding the mucosa of the bladder) and the posterior aspect of the rabdosphincter again moving from right to left. *BN* bladder neck, extramucosal, *RS* rabdosphincter. (Courtesy of Dr. Amparore—SCDU Urologia, San Luigi Gonzaga Hospital, Orbassano (TO), Italy)

includes the bladder neck, avoiding the vesical mucosa, and the posterior edge of the rabdosphincter, which are sutured together from right to left (Fig. 19.4).

Urethro-Vesical Anastomosis

For this phase, the use of a 3/0 barbed suture is recommended. Starting at 4 o'clock and proceeding clockwise, a running suture is performed, including the urethra and bladder at full thickness (Fig. 19.5). When needed, in order to reinforce the anastomosis, the surgeon may add a single stitch. When operating on patients with large bladder neck, the anastomosis' creation is "split" and performed separately, performing two hemi-running sutures. On the anterior side, eventually, single stitches of reabsorbable monofilament 3/0 sutures may be added.

Anterior Reconstruction

The vesical muscular fibers are sutured to the dissected peri-urethral tissue, located between the urethra and the DVC, using a 3/0 barbed running suture, similarly to the previous procedural step. The suture begins from the right side and is carried on towards the left side, anti-clockwise (Fig. 19.6). This suture has a double aim: firstly, it allows to restore the preoperative anatomy, reallocating the muscular fibers towards the abdominal cavity; secondly, to reinforce the anastomosis. Using the same suture and heading towards the starting point, the visceral layer of the endopelvic fascia and the apron, covering the anterior surface of the bladder, are sutured to the endopelvic fascia at the level of the DVC. It is important, while performing this suture, to include the pubo-prostatic ligaments which, it could be speculated, at this point become "pubo-vesical" ligaments. In order to secure the end of the newly performed running suture, a single 3/0 monofilament stitch can be added. At the end of the reconstructive phase the anastomosis is actually covered and protected by three posterior layers and two anterior layers which, together, determine the full restoration of the preoperative peri-urethral anatomy (Fig. 19.7)

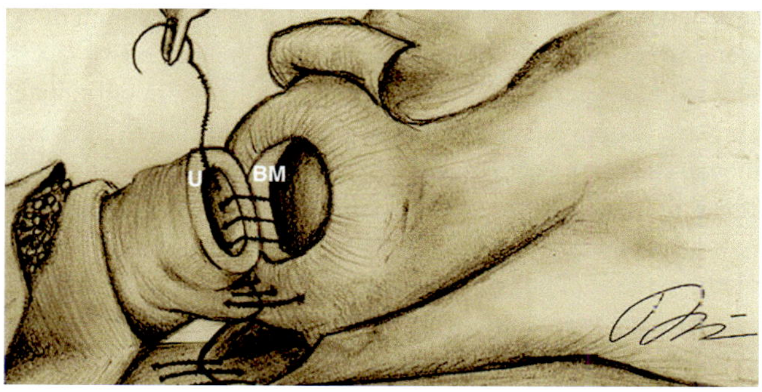

Fig. 19.5 Lateral view. The urethro-vesical anastomosis performed by a 3/0 "barbed" running suture, starting at 4 o'clock on the urethra and proceeding clockwise. The suture involves the full thickness of either the bladder or the urethra. *U* urethra, *BM* bladder mucosa. (Courtesy of Dr. Amparore—SCDU Urologia, San Luigi Gonzaga Hospital, Orbassano (TO), Italy)

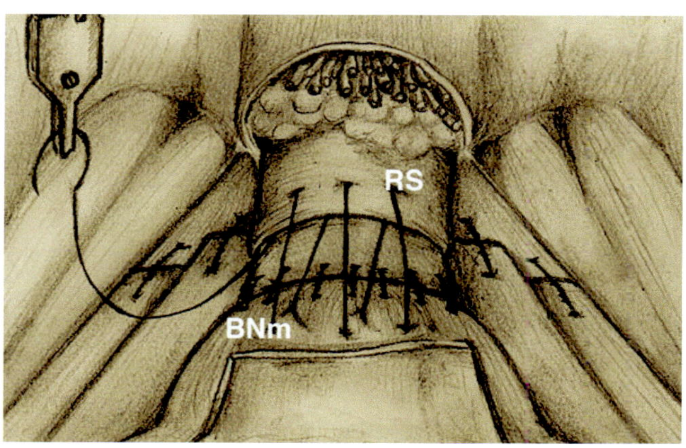

Fig. 19.6 Frontal view. Beginning from the right side and moving to the left, the muscular fibers of the bladder are 3/0 "barbed" running sutured to the previously dissected peri-urethral tissue located between the urethra and the deep venous complex. *RS* rabdosphincter; *BNm* bladder neck, muscular fibers. (Courtesy of Dr. Amparore—SCDU Urologia, San Luigi Gonzaga Hospital, Orbassano (TO), Italy)

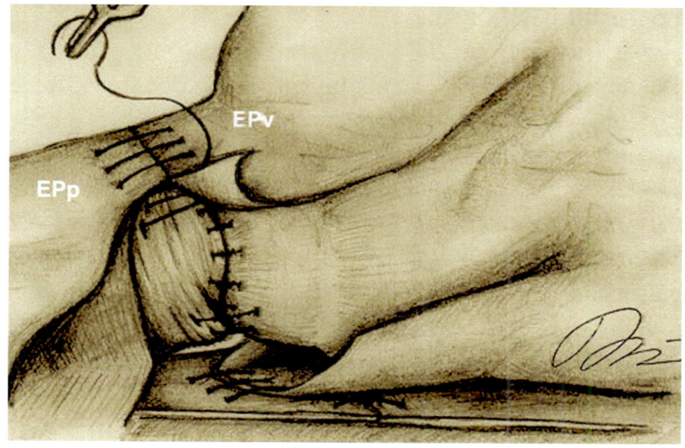

Fig. 19.7 Lateral view. Moving from left to right, the visceral layer of the endopelvic fascia and the underlying apron, still covering the anterior surface of the bladder, are sutured to the portion of the endopelvic fascia while involving the pubo-prostatic ligaments, renamed "pubo-vescical" ligaments. *EPp* endopelvic fascia, parietal layer, *EPv* endopelvic fascia, visceral layer. (Courtesy of Dr. Amparore—SCDU Urologia, San Luigi Gonzaga Hospital, Orbassano (TO), Italy)

Hemostasis, Peritoneal Reconstruction, Drainage, Specimen Extraction

A perfect control of the hemostasis, performed by using bipolar forceps and hemostatic agents, is fundamental to guarantee a perfect seal at the level of the anastomosis. To avoid the formation of suprapubic hematomas, which may push and dislocate the anastomosis, a small drainage is placed through a small suprapubic incision. The peritoneal sac is reconstructed using a 3/0 barbed suture, fixed with Hem-o-lok. The peritoneal reconstruction involves the ventral peritoneum, located medially respect to the umbilical ligament. In this manner, the incision (lateral to the ligament) remains opened on both sides, preventing the communication between the retropubic space and the intraperitoneal cavity.

Postoperative Care

For at least the first 24 h after the surgical procedure, the patients are invited to remain in bed. Gradually, they can be seated on the bad and, after approximately 48 h from the surgical procedure, they can stand and start to walk. Depending by the volume and quality of the drained fluid, the drainages can be removed after 48 h from the surgical procedure. Catheter is usually removed on 5th POD, after performing a pelvic ultrasound or a retrograde cystography.

Outcomes and Functional Results

As previously stated, the superiority of robot-assisted surgery in terms of oncological and functional outcomes has already been extensively proven [29, 30]. In the majority of studies, Authors and expert surgeons highlight the importance of the preservation of anatomical structures and integrity, considering it a pivotal factor in order to maintain postoperative urinary continence. During the years, several authors have experimented technical procedural (i.e., bladder neck preservation, intussusception of bladder neck …) and instrumental (i.e., types of suspension sutures) variations, in order to obtain the best postoperative results. The majority of authors have particularly stressed the importance of urethral support, which was provided by performing different reconstructive strategies in order to maximize urethral length and restore the urethral stabilization [31].

The previously described total anatomical reconstruction (TAR) technique aims to create a tension-free anastomosis, providing the best support to the sphincter. The key points of the TAR technique, which makes it unique in the scenario of urethro-vesical anastomosis, are the following:

- Preservation of pubo-prostatic ligaments: the incision of the endopelvic fascia together with the preservation of these ligamentous structures allows for a precise apex dissection. Even when suturing the DVC, the surgeon must pay attention to the ligaments' preservation.
- Bladder neck incision: this phase must be performed in a bloodless operative field, in order to easily identify the retrotrigonal fascia and preserve it, since it will be important in the posterior reconstruction's phase.
- Incision of posterior Denonvilliers' fascia: the previously cited U-shape incision allows for a more effective reconstruction.
- Management of prostatic apex: the surgeon should pay major attention in the apical dissection, trying to avoid the use of electrocauterization as much as possible. The dissection should always be performed remembering the high anatomical variability and the goal to obtain negative surgical margins.
- Multi-layer reconstruction: the creation of a double anterior and a triple posterior layer allows the creation of a tension-free anastomosis, providing optimal tissue vascularization, and helping the healing process.

The results of this technique are encouraging. In the study by Porpiglia et al. [32], which represent the first study describing the TAR technique, 252 patients were included. The median IPSS-score was 7 and 85% of patients were affected by intermediate or low risk prostate cancer, as classified accordingly to the D'Amico Score. Among the patients, a percentage of 77.8%, 89.3%, 89.3%, 94,4% and 98% of patients were continent at 1, 4, 12 and 24 weeks after the surgical procedure, respectively. Five cases of postoperative urinary incontinence were recorded: in one case, urodynamic study revealed the presence of detrusor hyperactivity causing severe incontinence; in the latter four patients, of which three were affected by mild incontinence, the postoperative stress was pointed out as the causing factor of the incontinence. Univariate analysis found a significative correlation between the nerve sparing (NS) approach and the functional outcome, being the full NS approach associated with the best results. After performing a multivariate analysis, the low and intermediate malignancies, as classified by the D'Amico classification, were associated with the best functional results. After 1000 procedures, the results were slightly adjusted. The continence rates at 24 h and after 1, 4, 12, 24 and 48 weeks after the removal of the catheter were 61.6%, 58.93%, 79.66%, 90.48% and 94.84% respectively. In this population of patients, an analysis of the potency outcomes was also performed. Overall, 102 patients underwent a full NS bilateral procedure whilst 18 patients reported an andrological drop-out. After considering this data, the overall. Potency recovery rate was 24.82%, 38.20%, 58.10%, 67.74% and 74.90% at 1, 3, 6 and 12 months respectively. The main factors influencing the preservation of urinary continence after RARP with TAR, as proven by multivariate analysis, were the nerve sparing approach, the D'Amico risk group, the execution of ePLND and the prostatic volume [33]. The impact of the aforementioned factors on postoperative results may be in relationship with two reasons: the need to perform a more demolishing surgical approach during the procedure and potential involvement of the sacral plexus.

RARP with TAR in Previously Treated Prostate

As it is widely known, the prostate and the surrounding tissues are altered by the surgical maneuvers, since the inflammation caused by capsular perforation and fluid absorption during the endoscopic procedure determines tissue alteration. In particular, it is more challenging to find and dissect anatomical planes, making nerve sparing procedures very difficult to fulfill; in addition, the bladder neck reconstruction phase is characterized, in the postoperative period, by higher rates of urinary leak and urethro-vesical anastomosis' stricture [34, 35].

In a dedicated study [36] a sub-cohort of patients, who underwent previous prostate endoscopic surgery for BPH, was analyzed. A total of 40 patients underwent RARP with TAR after previous surgery for BPH: specifically, 36 patients underwent TURP, one Greenlight photo vaporization of the prostate, one open adenomectomy (Millin technique) and two open transvesical adenomectomy. There was no intraoperative conversion to open surgery nor complication and, in all patients, it was possible to execute a nerve sparing approach. In ten cases, it was necessary to perform a bladder neck reconstruction: in this subgroup, the catheter was maintained for 7 day after the procedure and, before the removal, a retrograde cystography was executed, revealing urine leak in seven patients. This Clavien 1 complication was treated in all cases with further maintenance of the catheter for a minimum of 3 days. There were no cases of urethra-vesical anastomosis' stricture and, after bilateral NS procedure, 73.9% of patients had sexual intercourse. Continence rate at 1, 4, 12, 24 and 52 weeks from the procedure was 77.5%, 82.50%, 90%, 92.5% and 95% respectively. In 20% of the patients, positive surgical margins were found at the pathological examination: in 75% of the cases, the malignancy was locally infiltrating (≥pT3). At 90 days after RARP, eight complications (Clavien I) were reported. The results showed that the functional results of this specific group of patients was not affected by a history of previous prostate surgery. Nonetheless, is important to underline that all procedures in the reported series were performed by a single expert laparoscopic surgeon (F.P.) in a high-volume tertiary referral center, confirming that the surgeon's experience plays a crucial role in the management.

Conclusions

The robot-assisted radical prostatectomy, after decades of surgical evolution, still represents one of the most fascinating and challenging procedures in the urological field. The impact of this surgical act on the patient's quality of life has become object of major interest, given the great and largely proven oncological results. During the years, many surgeons have given their contribution, with the aim to find the best surgical technique to reach the best functional results in terms of urinary continence and potency preservation. In this scenario, the TAR technique has proven to be feasible, safe and effective, giving the chance to obtain, in experienced hands, optimal results and to offer a satisfying postoperative quality of life to patients.

References

1. Ficarra V, Novara G, Rosen RC, Artibani W, Carroll PR, Costello A, Menon M, Montorsi F, Patel VR, Stolzenburg JU, Van der Poel H, Wilson TG, Zattoni F, Mottrie A. Systematic review and meta-analysis of studies reporting urinary continence recovery after robot-assisted radical prostatectomy. Eur Urol. 2012;62(3):405–17. Epub 2012 June 1. PMID: 22749852. https://doi.org/10.1016/j.eururo.2012.05.045.
2. Patel VR, Abdul-Muhsin HM, Schatloff O, Coelho RF, Valero R, Ko YH, Sivaraman A, Palmer KJ, Chauhan S. Critical review of 'pentafecta' outcomes after robot-assisted laparoscopic prostatectomy in high-volume centres. BJU Int. 2011;108(6 Pt 2):1007–17. PMID: 21917104. https://doi.org/10.1111/j.1464-410X.2011.10521.
3. Ficarra V, Novara G, Fracalanza S, D'Elia C, Secco S, Iafrate M, Cavalleri S, Artibani W. A prospective, non-randomized trial comparing robot-assisted laparoscopic and retropubic radical prostatectomy in one European institution. BJU Int. 2009;104(4):534–9. Epub 2009 Mar 5. PMID: 19281468. https://doi.org/10.1111/j.1464-410X.2009.08419.
4. Walsh PC. Anatomic radical prostatectomy: evolution of the surgical technique. J Urol. 1998;160(6 Pt 2):2418–24. PMID: 9817395. https://doi.org/10.1097/00005392-199812020-00010.
5. Porpiglia F, Fiori C, Grande S, Morra I, Scarpa RM. Selective versus standard ligature of the deep venous complex during laparoscopic radical prostatectomy: effects on continence, blood loss, and margin status. Eur Urol. 2009;55(6):1377–83. Epub 2009 Feb 14. PMID: 19243886. https://doi.org/10.1016/j.eururo.2009.02.009.
6. Soljanik I, Bauer RM, Becker AJ, Stief CG, Gozzi C, Solyanik O, Brocker KA, Kirchhoff SM. Is a wider angle of the membranous urethra associated with incontinence after radical prostatectomy? World J Urol. 2014;32(6):1375–83. Epub 2014 Jan 23. PMID: 24452450. https://doi.org/10.1007/s00345-014-1241-5.
7. Stolzenburg JU, Liatsikos EN, Rabenalt R, Do M, Sakelaropoulos G, Horn LC, Truss MC. Nerve sparing endoscopic extraperitoneal radical prostatectomy—effect of puboprostatic ligament preservation on early continence and positive margins. Eur Urol. 2006;49(1):103–11; discussion 111–2. Epub 2005 Nov 2. PMID: 16314031. https://doi.org/10.1016/j.eururo.2005.10.002.
8. van der Poel HG, de Blok W, Joshi N, van Muilekom E. Preservation of lateral prostatic fascia is associated with urine continence after robotic-assisted prostatectomy. Eur Urol. 2009;55(4):892–900. Epub 2009 Jan 21. PMID: 19171418. https://doi.org/10.1016/j.eururo.2009.01.021.
9. Kwon SY, Lee JN, Kim HT, Kim TH, Kim BW, Choi GS, Kwon TG. Endopelvic fascia preservation during robot-assisted laparoscopic radical prostatectomy: does it affect urinary incontinence? Scand J Urol. 2014;48(6):506–12. Epub 2014 July 10. PMID: 25008957. https://doi.org/10.3109/21681805.2014.913259.
10. Ma X, Tang K, Yang C, Wu G, Xu N, Wang M, Zeng X, Hu Z, Song R, Yuh B, Wang Z, Ye Z. Bladder neck preservation improves time to continence after radical prostatectomy: a systematic review and meta-analysis. Oncotarget. 2016;7(41):67463–75. PMID: 27634899; PMCID: PMC5341889. https://doi.org/10.18632/oncotarget.11997.
11. Schlomm T, Heinzer H, Steuber T, Salomon G, Engel O, Michl U, Haese A, Graefen M, Huland H. Full functional-length urethral sphincter preservation during radical prostatectomy. Eur Urol. 2011;60(2):320–9. Epub 2011 Mar 22. PMID: 21458913. https://doi.org/10.1016/j.eururo.2011.02.040.
12. von Bodman C, Matsushita K, Savage C, Matikainen MP, Eastham JA, Scardino PT, Rabbani F, Akin O, Sandhu JS. Recovery of urinary function after radical prostatectomy: predictors of urinary function on preoperative prostate magnetic resonance imaging. J Urol. 2012;187(3):945–50. Epub 2012 Jan 20. PMID: 22264458; PMCID: PMC4768862. https://doi.org/10.1016/j.juro.2011.10.143.

13. Ganzer R, Blana A, Gaumann A, Stolzenburg JU, Rabenalt R, Bach T, Wieland WF, Denzinger S. Topographical anatomy of periprostatic and capsular nerves: quantification and computerised planimetry. Eur Urol. 2008;54(2):353–60. Epub 2008 Apr 15. PMID: 18436370. https://doi.org/10.1016/j.eururo.2008.04.018.
14. Tewari A, Takenaka A, Mtui E, Horninger W, Peschel R, Bartsch G, Vaughan ED. The proximal neurovascular plate and the trizonal neural architecture around the prostate gland: importance in the athermal robotic technique of nerve-sparing prostatectomy. BJU Int. 2006;98(2):314–23. PMID: 16879671. https://doi.org/10.1111/j.1464-410X.2006.06266.x.
15. Costello AJ, Brooks M, Cole OJ. Anatomical studies of the neurovascular bundle and cavernosal nerves. BJU Int. 2004;94(7):1071–6. PMID: 15541130. https://doi.org/10.1111/j.1464-410X.2004.05106.x.
16. Walz J, Epstein JI, Ganzer R, Graefen M, Guazzoni G, Kaouk J, Menon M, Mottrie A, Myers RP, Patel V, Tewari A, Villers A, Artibani W. A critical analysis of the current knowledge of surgical anatomy of the prostate related to optimisation of cancer control and preservation of continence and erection in candidates for radical prostatectomy: an update. Eur Urol. 2016;70(2):301–11. Epub 2016 Feb 2. PMID: 26850969. https://doi.org/10.1016/j.eururo.2016.01.026.
17. Michl U, Tennstedt P, Feldmeier L, Mandel P, Oh SJ, Ahyai S, Budäus L, Chun FKH, Haese A, Heinzer H, Salomon G, Schlomm T, Steuber T, Huland H, Graefen M, Tilki D. Nerve-sparing surgery technique, not the preservation of the neurovascular bundles, leads to improved long-term continence rates after radical prostatectomy. Eur Urol. 2016;69(4):584–9. Epub 2015 Aug 12. PMID: 26277303. https://doi.org/10.1016/j.eururo.2015.07.037.
18. Reeves F, Preece P, Kapoor J, Everaerts W, Murphy DG, Corcoran NM, Costello AJ. Preservation of the neurovascular bundles is associated with improved time to continence after radical prostatectomy but not long-term continence rates: results of a systematic review and meta-analysis. Eur Urol. 2015;68(4):692–704. Epub 2014 Oct 29. PMID: 25454614. https://doi.org/10.1016/j.eururo.2014.10.020.
19. Seaman EK, Benson MC. Improved continence with tubularized bladder neck reconstruction following radical retropubic prostatectomy. Urology. 1996;47(4):532–5. PMID: 8638363. https://doi.org/10.1016/S0090-4295(99)80490-7.
20. Lin VC, Coughlin G, Savamedi S, Palmer KJ, Coelho RF, Patel VR. Modified transverse plication for bladder neck reconstruction during robotic-assisted laparoscopic prostatectomy. BJU Int. 2009;104(6):878–81. PMID: 19706036. https://doi.org/10.1111/j.1464-410X.2009.08784.x.
21. Rocco F, Gadda F, Acquati P, Carmignani L, Favini P, Dell'Orto P, Ferruti M, Avogadro A, Casellato S, Grisotto M. Ricerca personale: la ricostruzione dello sfintere striato uretrale [Personal research: reconstruction of the urethral striated sphincter]. Arch Ital Urol Androl. 2001;73(3):127–37. Italian. PMID: 11822054.
22. Dal Moro F, Crestani A, Valotto C, Zattoni F. CORPUS—novel COmplete Reconstruction of the Posterior Urethral Support after robotic radical prostatectomy: preliminary data of very early continence recovery. Urology. 2014;83(3):641–7. PMID: 24581526. https://doi.org/10.1016/j.urology.2013.12.010.
23. Ogawa S, Hoshi S, Koguchi T, Hata J, Sato Y, Akaihata H, Kataoka M, Haga N, Kojima Y. Three-layer two-step posterior reconstruction using peritoneum during robot-assisted radical prostatectomy to improve recovery of urinary continence: a prospective comparative study. J Endourol. 2017;31(12):1251–7. Epub 2017 Nov 20. PMID: 29061068. https://doi.org/10.1089/end.2017.0410.
24. Burnett AL, Mostwin JL. In situ anatomical study of the male urethral sphincteric complex: relevance to continence preservation following major pelvic surgery. J Urol. 1998;160(4):1301–6. PMID: 9751340.
25. Wilson TG, Guru K, Rosen RC, Wiklund P, Annerstedt M, Bochner BH, Chan KG, Montorsi F, Mottrie A, Murphy D, Novara G, Peabody JO, Palou Redorta J, Skinner EC, Thalmann G, Stenzl A, Yuh B, Catto J, Pasadena Consensus Panel. Best practices in robot-assisted radical cystectomy and urinary reconstruction: recommendations of the Pasadena Consensus Panel. Eur Urol. 2015;67(3):363–75. Epub 2015 Jan 9. PMID: 25582930. https://doi.org/10.1016/j.eururo.2014.12.009.
26. Patel VR, Coelho RF, Palmer KJ, Rocco B. Periurethral suspension stitch during robot-assisted laparoscopic radical prostatectomy: description of the technique and continence outcomes. Eur Urol. 2009;56(3):472–8. Epub 2009 June 16. PMID: 19560260. https://doi.org/10.1016/j.eururo.2009.06.007.
27. Hurtes X, Rouprêt M, Vaessen C, Pereira H, Faivre d'Arcier B, Cormier L, Bruyère F. Anterior suspension combined with posterior reconstruction during robot-assisted laparoscopic prostatectomy improves early return of urinary continence: a prospective randomized multicentre trial. BJU Int. 2012;110(6):875–83. Epub 2012 Jan 19. PMID: 22260307. https://doi.org/10.1111/j.1464-410X.2011.10849.x.
28. Koliakos N, Mottrie A, Buffi N, De Naeyer G, Willemsen P, Fonteyne E. Posterior and anterior fixation of the urethra during robotic prostatectomy improves early continence rates. Scand J Urol Nephrol. 2010;44(1):5–10. PMID: 19958072. https://doi.org/10.3109/00365590903413627.
29. Porpiglia F, Morra I, Lucci Chiarissi M, Manfredi M, Mele F, Grande S, Ragni F, Poggio M, Fiori C. Randomised controlled trial comparing laparoscopic and robot-assisted radical prostatectomy. Eur Urol. 2013;63(4):606–14. Epub 2012 July 20. PMID: 22840353. https://doi.org/10.1016/j.eururo.2012.07.007.
30. Di Pierro GB, Baumeister P, Stucki P, Beatrice J, Danuser H, Mattei A. A prospective trial comparing consecutive series of open retropubic and robot-assisted laparoscopic radical prostatectomy in a centre with a limited caseload. Eur Urol. 2011;59(1):1–6. Epub 2010 Oct 21. PMID: 21035248. https://doi.org/10.1016/j.eururo.2010.10.026.
31. Manfredi M, Fiori C, Amparore D, Checcucci E, Porpiglia F. Technical details to achieve perfect early continence after radical prostatectomy. Minerva Chir. 2019;74(1):63–77. Epub 2018 July 23. PMID: 30037176. https://doi.org/10.23736/S0026-4733.18.07761-1.
32. Porpiglia F, Bertolo R, Manfredi M, De Luca S, Checcucci E, Morra I, Passera R, Fiori C. Total anatomical reconstruction during robot-assisted radical prostatectomy: implications on early recovery of urinary continence. Eur Urol. 2016;69(3):485–95. Epub 2015 Aug 19. PMID: 26297603. https://doi.org/10.1016/j.eururo.2015.08.005.
33. Manfredi M, Checcucci E, Fiori C, Garrou D, Aimar R, Amparore D, De Luca S, Bombaci S, Stura I, Migliaretti G, Porpiglia F. Total anatomical reconstruction during robot-assisted radical prostatectomy: focus on urinary continence recovery and related complications after 1000 procedures. BJU Int. 2019;124(3):477–86. Epub 2019 Mar 15. PMID: 30801887. https://doi.org/10.1111/bju.14716.
34. Yazici S, Inci K, Yuksel S, Bilen CY, Ozen H. Radical prostatectomy after previous prostate surgery: effects on surgical difficulty and pathologic outcomes. Urology. 2009;73(4):856–9. Epub 2008 Nov 20. PMID: 19022487. https://doi.org/10.1016/j.urology.2008.09.024.

35. Menard J, de la Taille A, Hoznek A, Allory Y, Vordos D, Yiou R, Abbou CC, Salomon L. Laparoscopic radical prostatectomy after transurethral resection of the prostate: surgical and functional outcomes. Urology. 2008;72(3):593–7. https://doi.org/10.1016/j.urology.2008.03.019. PMID: 18762050.

36. Campobasso D, Fiori C, Amparore D, Checcucci E, Garrou D, Manfredi M, Porpiglia F. Total anatomical reconstruction during robot-assisted radical prostatectomy in patients with previous prostate surgery. Minerva Urol Nefrol. 2019;71(6):605–11. https://doi.org/10.23736/S0393-2249.19.03446-5. Epub 2019 July 8. PMID: 31287254.

Part VI

Transperitoneal RALP Retzius-Sparing Approach

Transperitoneal RALP Retzius-Sparing Approach: Bocciardi Technique

20

Aldo Massimo Bocciardi, Stefano Tappero, Mattia Longoni, Paolo Dell'Oglio, and Antonio Galfano

Introduction

In developed countries prostate cancer (PCa) represents the most common solid organ malignancy of the male population [1]. Robot-assisted radical prostatectomy (RARP) is the gold standard for surgical removal of the prostate according to the European Association of Urology (EAU) [2] and the American Urological Association (AUA) guidelines [3].

The goal of a RARP is to achieve complete cancer control while preserving urinary and sexual faculties. Several variations of the original standard retropubic template have been designed and standardized, aiming to make the most of the potentiality of the robotic technology and minimize the inner comorbidities and *sequaele* of the prostate removal [4, 5].

Retzius-sparing robot assisted radical prostatectomy (RS-RARP) was conceived by Aldo Massimo Bocciardi at Niguarda Hospital of Milan in 2010 [6]. As the Montsouris technique, the RS-RARP starts with the incision of the retrovesical pouch [7], but subsequently the whole prostatectomy is exclusively carried out through the Douglas space.

The rationale of this approach stems on the preservation of all the structures thought to play a role in continence and potency preservation:

- The pubo-prostatic ligaments stabilize the prostate, the urethra and the bladder to the pubic bone and are considered an important part of the suspensory system of the continence mechanism [8, 9]. The preservation of these ligaments may improve early recovery of urinary continence as well as the preservation of the endopelvic fascia, whose parietal component covers the medial aspects of the levator ani muscle while the visceral component covers the pelvic organs, including prostate, bladder and rectum.
- The prostate artery terminates in two main pedicles: a posterior pedicle surrounding seminal vesicles and deferential ducts reaching the prostate base and an anterior pedicle running to the prostate apex as an anterior capsular branch. The anterior pedicle, when preserved, might relate with postoperative erectile function and penile integrity because it may be responsible for the ancillary penile blood flow [10, 11].
- The network of vascular and nervous fibers surrounding the lateral aspect of the bladder neck, the proximal prostate, and the seminal vesicles in a cage-like fashion is known as neuro-vascular bundle and it is responsible for the mechanisms of urinary continence, erection and ejaculation [8]. Since one-third of the periprostatic nerves course anteriorly and anterolaterally [12], proceeding through the posterior path most of them are spared.

  Lack of identification of these structures during radical prostatectomy may potentially result in inferior oncologic results as well as in a higher risk of incontinence or erectile dysfunction [3].

Thus, the bladder is not detached, the surgical trauma is minimized, and the normal pelvic anatomy is maximally preserved, leading to an enhanced urinary continence recovery (UCR) [4]; this is crucial since incontinence is one of the most feared and, perhaps, under-reported complications of RARP, which strongly affects the quality of life (QoL) of the patient [13].

After more than 2000 of cases performed at the Niguarda Hospital in a decade and several thousands throughout the World, in 2020, the EAU guidelines included RS-RARP among the available surgical treatments for prostate cancer [2].

A. M. Bocciardi · S. Tappero (✉) · M. Longoni · P. Dell'Oglio · A. Galfano
Urology Unit, Niguarda Hospital, Milan, Italy
e-mail: m.longoni@campus.unimib.it

S. Ren et al. (eds.), *Robot-Assisted Radical Prostatectomy*, https://doi.org/10.1007/978-3-031-05855-4_20

Surgical Technique

The patient is placed in a steep Trendelemburg position (25–30°) and pneumoperitoneum is induced either by an open Hasson technique, preferred in case of suspect of intra-abdominal adhesions, or using a Veress needle.

A front and a side docking of the patient cart are required for the Da Vinci Si and Xi platforms, respectively.

Transperitoneal port placement is performed under direct vision in the same fashion displayed in Fig. 20.1. The 30° lens camera is accommodated through the latero-umbilical 12-mm trocar, downwards oriented during the first phase of the procedure and upwards after the dissection of the seminal vesicles. The main operative arms are placed in 8-mm trocars with the monopolar scissor on the right, in the midline between the umbilicus and the right anterior superior iliac spine (ASIS), and the bipolar Maryland forceps on the left, at least two fingerbreadths medially and cranially to the left ASIS. A third 8-mm trocar for a grasper instrument (usually a Cadiere forceps) is placed on the left, at two-thirds along the line connecting the camera and the Maryland ports and 2–3 fingerbreadths cranially to the umbilicus. A 12-mm and a 5-mm ports are positioned for the assistant on the right, with the first one connected to the Airseal insufflation system when recommended. The 12-mm assistant port is placed directly between the two right-sided robotic ports approximately 3 cm superior to a line drawn between the two trocars and the 5-mm assistant port is placed at least two fingerbreadths superomedial to the right ASIS.

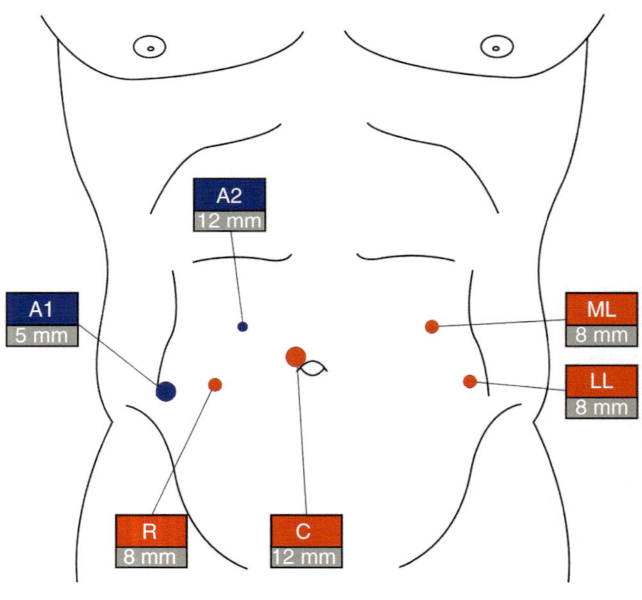

Fig. 20.1 Port positioning. *C* camera, *R* right robotic arm, *ML* medial left robotic arm, *LL* lateral left robotic arm, *A1* right assistant arm, *A2* left assistant arm

Especially in obese patients or in case of narrow and small pelvis, the release of the adhesions of the left colon may be key in expanding the operatory field and displacing the bowel cranially. The so-called *Pansadoro stitch* may further help retracting the colon backwards; this suture (Ethilon 2-0, straight needle) passes through the 5-mm assistant port and gently retracts the sigma stretching its epiploic appendixes (Fig. 20.2).

A horizontal semicircular incision is made at the level of the vas deferens, identified as an arch anterior to the rectum, about 1 cm over the reflection of the Douglas space (Fig. 20.3). Vas deferens and seminal vesicles are isolated and incised, possibly avoiding cautery (Fig. 20.4). Once the seminal vesicles are completely dissected down to the prostatic base, two transabdominal suprapubic stitches (Ethilon 2-0, straight needle) can be passed to lift the bladder and retract the seminal vesicles, with a significant widening of the surgical space (Fig. 20.5a–c).

Depending on the clinical assessment of the malignancy and the preoperatory functional conditions of the patients the nerve-sparing plane is chosen. Hence, the 30° camera is turned upwards and the dissection of the posterior aspect of the prostate begins with the incision of the Denonvillier's

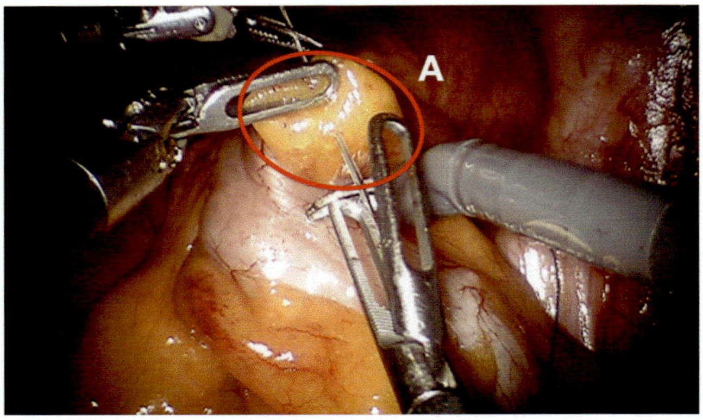

Fig. 20.2 Pansadoro stitch (*A* epiploic appendix of the sigma)

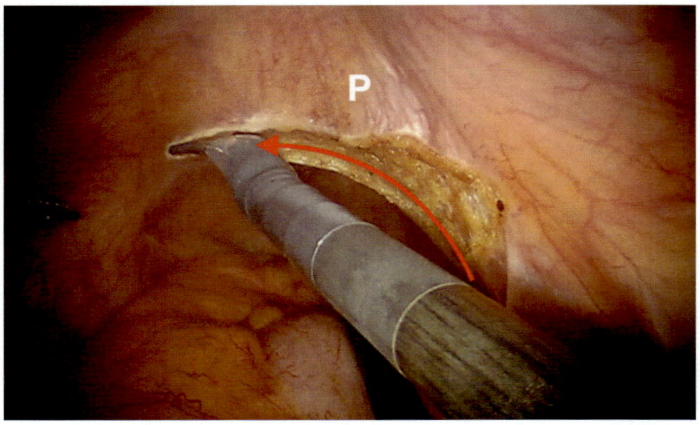

Fig. 20.3 Incision of the peritoneum (P)

fascia from the midline where the slightly less dense vascularization usually offers a clearer plane. The dissection proceeds towards the prostatic capsule reaching an inter- or intrafascial plane.

The upwards oriented traction offered by the Cadiere grasper is crucial while bluntly dissecting the postero-lateral surface of the prostate from the Denonvillier's fascia anterogradely down to the prostate apex. Approaching the apex along the midline and proceeding laterally to the bundles yields a harmless isolation of the prostatic pedicles (Fig. 20.6). Thus, the lateral prostatic pedicles are sectioned and the neurovascular bundles are fully/partially spared or sacrificed according to the planned surgical strategy

Once dissected the postero-lateral aspects of the prostate, the bladder neck is identified pushing downwards the seminal vesicles with the Cadiere forceps. The vesico-prostatic junction is reached from its posterior surface through a blunt dissection of the vesico-prostatic muscle (or posterior detrusor apron) [14] which lays over the circular fibers of the detrusor (Fig. 20.7).

The bladder neck isolation is complete when the anterior surface of the vesico-prostatic junction can be surrounded by

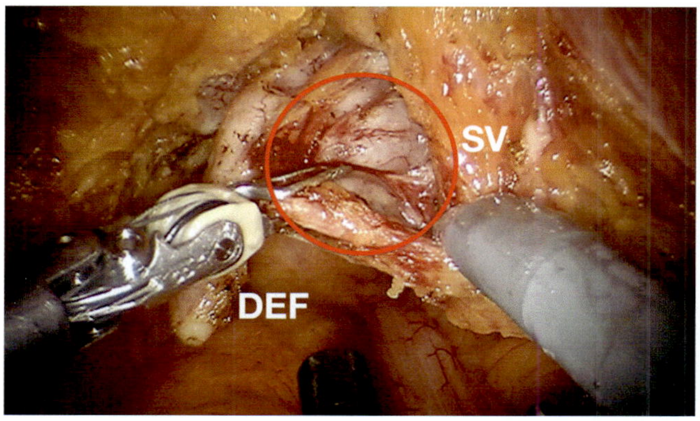

Fig. 20.4 Vas deferens (DEF) and seminal vesicle (SV) isolation

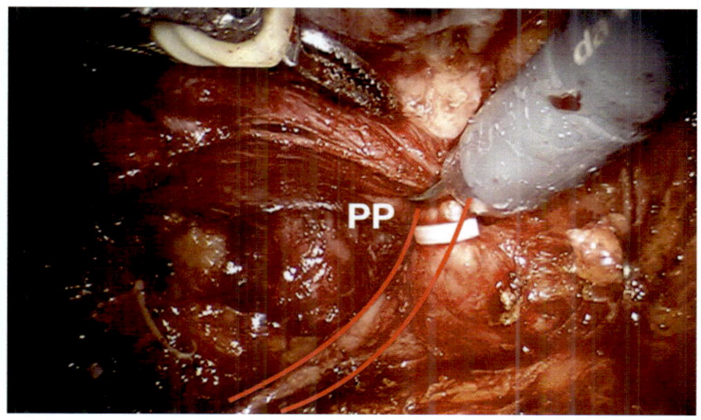

Fig. 20.6 Isolation of the prostatic pedicle (PP)

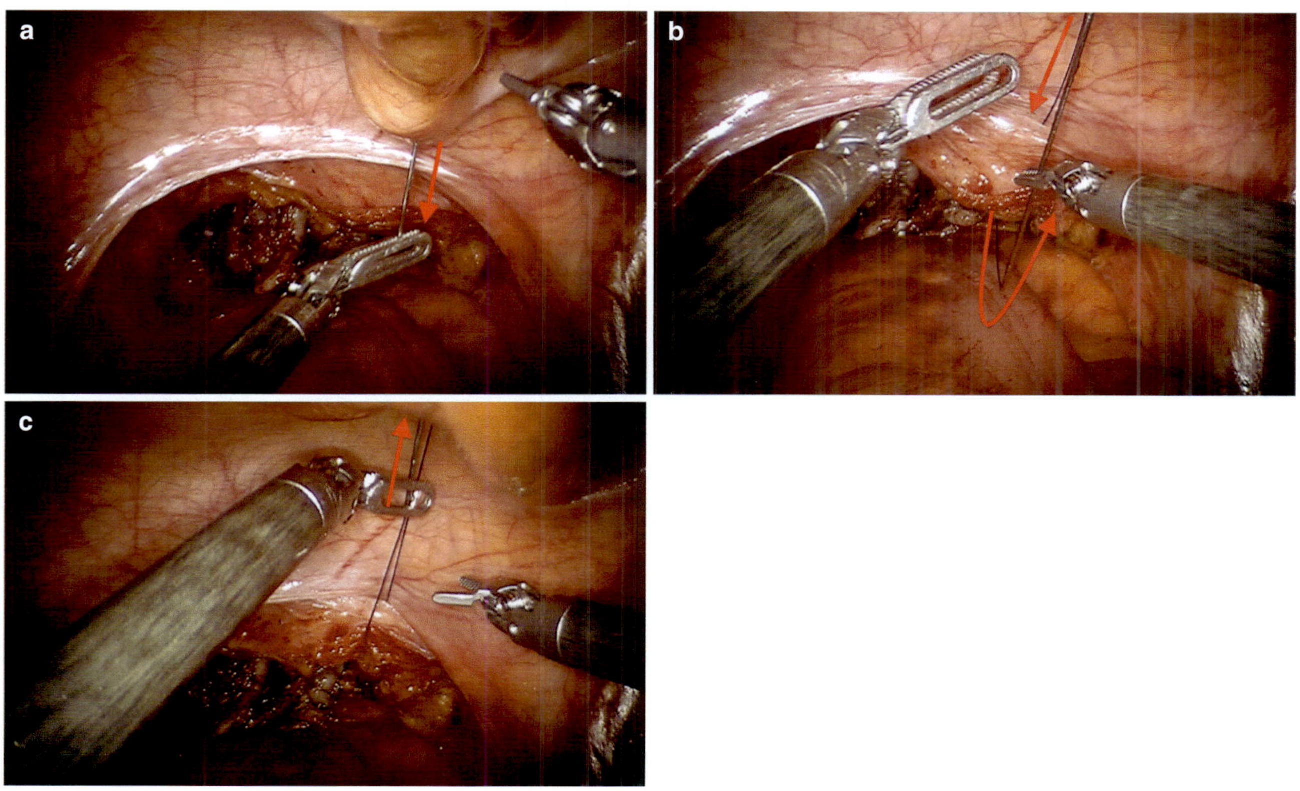

Fig. 20.5 (**a**–**c**) Sequence of positioning of the suprapubic stitch and retraction of the seminal vesicle

the Maryland forceps. At this point, two quickly absorbable stay stitches (Vycril rapide 3-0, curve needle) at 6 and 12 o'clock in the bladder neck help fixing the mucosa and recognizing both starting and ending points of the following anastomosis. This maneuver also helps keeping the bladder neck closed during the dissection and avoids urine spillage against the camera.

The isolation bluntly advances on the anterior surface of the prostate, carefully avoiding opening the Dorsal Vascular Complex (DVC, the Santorini plexus), whenever technically feasible.

Since more than one-third of the striated urethral sphincter's surface area is located ventrally to the DVC [15], sparing the DVC reduces the damage to the urethral sphincter and may allow an earlier recovery of the continence [14].

In case of locally advanced anterior prostate cancer, an extra-fascial dissection usually implies a partial or complete resection of the Santorini plexus.

When the apex is circumferentially isolated (Fig. 20.8), the urethra can be resected and the prostate removed from the pelvis into an endobag.

A modified Van Velthoven anastomosis with two separate 15-cm barbed sutures (V-Loc 3-0, 5/8 needle) is performed as follows: left anterior quadrant (12 o'clock–9 o'clock); right half circle (12 o'clock–6 o'clock); left posterior quadrant (9 o'clock–6 o'clock). The length and the number of the sutures may vary depending on the width of the bladder neck (Fig. 20.9a, b).

If the anastomosis proves to be watertight (200–300 cc) the transurethral catheter can be removed and a supra-pubic tube (SPT) positioned under direct vision by the table assistant. The SPT is commonly better tolerated and thereby it is meant to reduce the patient discomfort and faster the discharge at home. The SPT is also safer than the transurethral catheter as its involuntary tractions are less likely related to anastomosis damages or urethral strictures.

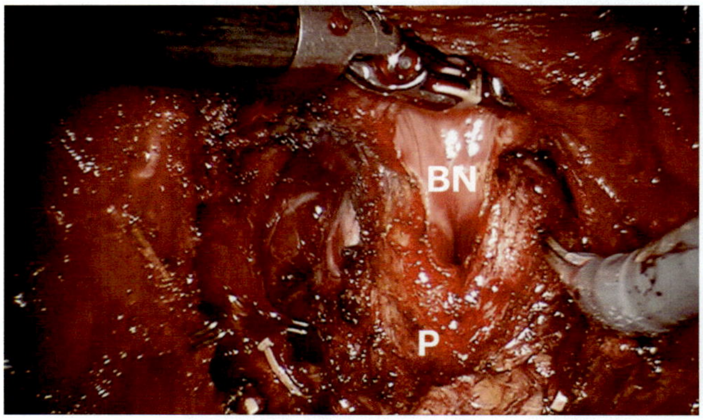

Fig. 20.7 Bladder neck (BN) dissection (*P* prostate)

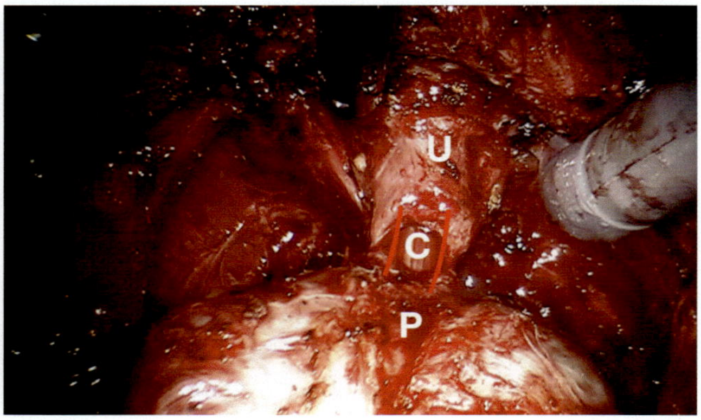

Fig. 20.8 Dissection of the urethra (U) (*C* bladder catheter, *P* prostate apex)

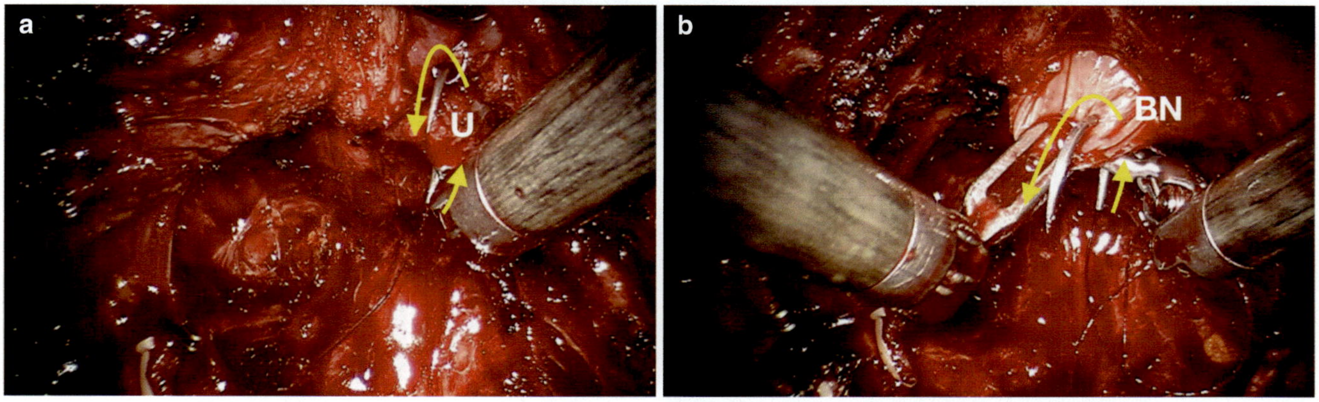

Fig. 20.9 (**a**, **b**) Beginning of the anastomosis from 12 o'clock position; (**a**) on the urethra (from outside to inside); (**b**) on the bladder neck (from inside to outside)

Outcomes

The available literature regarding RS-RARP is gradually growing as several institutions worldwide adopted the posterior technique as routinary approach for radical prostatectomy and began publishing their comparative results [16].

As the surgeons become more familiar to the Retzius-sparing technique, a noteworthy improvement of the oncologic and functional outcomes is recorded, although a reasonable expertise cut-off between novice and skilled operators still has not been properly stated [5, 16, 17].

A consistent lack of evidence regarding the reliability of the RS-RARP in the specific setting of high-risk patients still needs to be filled since currently the available published RCTs only focused on low and intermediate PCa patients.

Positive Surgical Margins (PSMs)

Several retrospective and prospective cohort studies reported variable PSM rates predominantly due to the different inclusion criteria the patients were selected with, and to the surgeon's expertise in RS-RARP (Table 20.1). A systematic review of the literature found RS-RARP prone to a higher rate of PSMs, especially in case of anterior tumours [18] but ought to be disclosed how in the considered studies the surgeons had extensive expertise for S-RARP and initial expertise for RS-RARP.

When the comparison concerned two large cohorts of standard and Retzius-sparing prostatectomies performed by a single surgeon extensively proficient in both techniques, the PSM rates did not significantly differ [19, 20].

Table 20.1 The Bocciardi Approach around the World

Author, year	Country	Patients (n)	Surgeon's expertise in RS-RARP	PSMs (%)
Lim, 2014 [5]	South Korea	50 No risk group classification	Initial	14
Dalela, 2017 [22]	USA	60 Only low-intermediate grade PCa	50 cases	25
Sayyid, 2017 [27]	USA	100 27% high risk PCa	Initial	≤T2: 16.7 >T3: 47.1
Chang, 2018 [23]	Taiwan	30 No risk group classification	Initial	23.3
Eden, 2018 [28]	UK	40	Initial	T2: 16.7 T3: 31.8
Menon, 2018 [29]	USA	60 Only low-intermediate grade PCa	60 cases	Focal: 13.3 Non-focal: 11.7
Asimakopoulos, 2019 [21]	Italy	45 Only low-intermediate grade PCa	Initial	T2: 19 T3: 41.2
Lee, 2020 [19]	South Korea	609	Advanced (including initial)	T2: 11 T3: 36
Egan, 2020 [24]	USA	70 No risk group classification	Initial	Focal: 27.1 Non-focal: 7.1
Umari, 2021 [20]	UK, Italy	282 37.2% high risk PCa	Advanced (including initial)	15.6

Urinary Continence (UC)

The posterior approach yields a faster and higher recovery of continence as its aforementioned anatomical rationale let foresee. A significative advantage in terms of immediate continence recovery rate was assessed by several single surgeon series studies [20–22], and moreover it was found to be related to a minor bladder neck descent at postoperative cystography [23].

A recent meta-analysis and systematic review by Checcucci and colleagues registered a statistically significant and persistently improved continence at 1, 3, 6, and 12 months, without increased risk of complications [18]. The quality of life (QoL) after prostatectomy as banner outcome of the prostatic surgery was specifically evaluated by Egan in 2020, who emphasized how overall QoL was significantly better in men undergoing RS-RARP rather than S-RARP at any time along the 12-month follow-up period [24].

Erectile Function (EF)

Potency recovery is clearly dependent on the oncological feasibility of an anatomically conservative surgery. Up-to-date, potency remains a secondary and mostly under-reported outcome of the available literature. The last metanalysis regarding the argument did not find any differences in terms of return to intercourses after surgery between anterior and posterior techniques [25].

Selecting from the Niguarda Hospital series the <65 years old preoperatively potent patients, undergone fully intra-fascial nerve-sparing surgery, the 38% reported a complete sexual intercourse within 1 month from surgery, rising to 65%, 77% and 81% at 3, 6 and 12 months respectively, with a median time to erectile function recovery of 48 days.

Besides, the 12-months sexual recovery rate was 43% when considering high-risk patients submitted to mono- or bilateral nerve sparing RS-RARP.

Complications

Rosemberg performed a metanalysis of 5 RCTs, overall including 502 patients, and did not highlight disparities in adverse events between standard and posterior RARP, although with a very low-certainty level of evidence [25]. Likewise, both Phukan [26] and Checcucci [18], considering retrospective and prospective series comparative studies, did not encountered RS-RARP being related to higher overall and major complication rates.

Unpublished data of the Niguarda Hospital series mirror the current literature evidence in terms of RS-RARP complications rate. Overall, the major intraoperative adverse events are mainly associated to the trocars positioning and the lymph nodes dissection, being the injuries of the external iliac vessels the most common complications (0.48%). The most common post-operatory Clavien ≥ 3 complication was the infection of lymphocele needing for percutaneous drainage (3%).

Conclusions

This chapter provides an overview of the key steps of the Retzius-sparing RARP with its anatomical landmarks. RS-RARP enhances early urinary continence recovery without compromising oncologic safety. Current literature mainly considers low and intermediate risk prostate cancer patients, thereby prospective multicentric data regarding high-risk patients will be crucial in widening the indication and elucidating strength points and pitfalls of this approach.

References

1. Siegel RL, et al. Cancer statistics, 2016. CA Cancer J Clin. 2016;66:7–30.
2. Mottet N, et al. EAU-EANM-ESTRO-ESUR-SIOG Guidelines on Prostate Cancer—2020 Update. Part 1: Screening Diagnosis and Local Treatment with Curative Intent. Eur Urol. 2021;79(2):243–62.
3. American Urologic Association, Oncology Guidelines, Prostate Cancer. https://www.auanet.org/guidelines/guidelines/prostate-cancer-clinically-localized-guideline.
4. Asimakopoulos AD, et al. Retzius-sparing robot-assisted laparoscopic radical prostatectomy: critical appraisal of the anatomic landmarks for a complete intrafascial approach. Clin Anat. 2015;28:896–902.
5. Lim SK, et al. Retzius-sparing robot-assisted laparoscopic radical prostatectomy: combining the best of retropubic and perineal approaches. BJU Int. 2014;114(2):236–44.
6. Galfano A, et al. A new anatomic approach for robot-assisted laparoscopic prostatectomy: a feasibility study for completely intrafascial surgery. Eur Urol. 2010;58(3):457–61.
7. Guillonneau B, et al. Laparoscopic radical prostatectomy: the Montsouris technique. J Urol. 2000;163(6):1643–9.
8. Walz J, et al. A critical analysis of the current knowledge of surgical anatomy related to optimization of cancer control and preservation of continence and erection in candidates for radical prostatectomy. Eur Urol. 2010;57(2):179–92.
9. Steiner MS. The puboprostatic ligament and the male urethral suspensory mechanism: an anatomic study. Urology. 1994;44:530–4.
10. Patel VR, et al. The role of the prostatic vasculature as a landmark for nerve sparing during robot-assisted radical prostatectomy. Eur Urol. 2012;61:571–6.
11. Secin FP, et al. Anatomy and preservation of accessory pudendal arteries in laparoscopic radical prostatectomy. Eur Urol. 2007;51:1229–35.
12. Alsaid B, et al. Division of autonomic nerves within the neurovascular bundles distally into corpora cavernosa and corpus spongiosum components: immunohistochemical confirmation with three-dimensional reconstruction. Eur Urol. 2011;59:902–9.
13. Liss MA, et al. Continence definition after radical prostatectomy using urinary quality of life: evaluation of patient reported validated questionnaires. J Urol. 2010;183:1464–8.
14. Walz J, et al. A critical analysis of the current knowledge of surgical anatomy of the prostate related to optimisation of cancer control and preservation of continence and erection in candidates for radical prostatectomy: an update. Eur Urol. 2016;70:301–11.
15. Ganzer R, et al. Is the striated urethral sphincter at risk by standard suture ligation of the dorsal vascular complex in radical prostatectomy? An anatomic study. Urology. 2014;84:1453–60.
16. Galfano A, et al. Retzius-sparing robot-assisted laparoscopic radical prostatectomy: an international survey on surgical details and worldwide diffusion. Eur Urol Focus. 2020;6:1021–3.
17. Galfano A, et al. Beyond the learning curve of the Retzius-sparing approach for robot-assisted laparoscopic radical prostatectomy: oncologic and functional results of the first 200 patients with ≥ 1 year of follow-up. Eur Urol. 2013;64(6):974–80.
18. Checcucci E, et al. Retzius-sparing robot-assisted radical prostatectomy vs the standard approach: a systematic review and analysis of comparative outcomes. BJU Int. 2020;125:8–16.
19. Lee J, et al. Retzius sparing robot-assisted radical prostatectomy conveys early regain of continence over conventional robot-assisted radical prostatectomy: a propensity score matched analysis of 1,863 patients. J Urol. 2020;203(1):137–44.
20. Umari P, et al. Retzius sparing versus standard robot-assisted radical prostatectomy: a comparative prospective study of nearly 500 patients. J Urol. 2021;205(3):780–90.
21. Asimakopoulos AD, et al. Retzius-sparing versus standard robot-assisted radical prostatectomy: a prospective randomized comparison on immediate continence rates. Surg Endosc. 2019;33(7):2187–96.
22. Dalela D, et al. A pragmatic randomized controlled trial examining the impact of the Retzius-sparing approach on early urinary continence recovery after robot-assisted radical prostatectomy. Eur Urol. 2017;72(5):677–85.

23. Chang LW, et al. Retzius-sparing robotic-assisted radical prostatectomy associated with less bladder neck descent and better early continence outcome. Anticancer Res. 2018;38(1):345–51.
24. Egan J, et al. Retzius-sparing robot-assisted radical prostatectomy leads to durable improvement in urinary function and quality of life versus standard robot-assisted radical prostatectomy without compromise on oncologic efficacy: single-surgeon series and step-by-step guide. Eur Urol. 2021;79(6):839–57.
25. Rosenberg JE, et al. Retzius-sparing versus standard robotic assisted laparoscopic prostatectomy for the treatment of clinically localized prostate cancer. BJU Int. 2021;128(1):12–20.
26. Phukan C, et al. Retzius sparing robotic assisted radical prostatectomy vs. conventional robotic assisted radical prostatectomy: a systematic review and meta-analysis. World J Urol. 2020;38(5):1123–34.
27. Sayyd RK., et al. Retzius-Sparing Robotic-Assisted Laparoscopic Radical Prostatectomy: A Safe Surgical Technique with Superior Continence Outcomes. J Endourol. 2017;31(12):1244–50.
28. Eden CG., et al. Urinary continence four weeks following Retzius-sparing robotic radical prostatectomy: The UK experience. J Clin Urol. 2018;11(1):15–20.
29. Menon M., et al. Functional Recovery, Oncologic Outcomes and Postoperative Complications after Robot-Assisted Radical Prostatectomy: An Evidence-Based Analysis Comparing the Retzius Sparing and Standard Approaches. J Urol. 2018;199(5):1210–17.

Transperitoneal Robot-Assisted Laparoscopic Radical Prostatectomy Retzius-Sparing Approach: Yonsei Technique

21

Sylvia L. Alip, Periklis Koukourikis, and Koon Ho Rha

Introduction

The past decade has seen an exponential growth in robot-assisted prostatectomy cases potentially unmatched by any other shifting trend in urology in recent times. It is arguably one of game changers of the field, with its increasing accessibility, attractive learning curve (compared to most minimally-invasive approaches), and rigorous industry-driven support. In the United States alone, the shift to robotic from traditional laparoscopic and open surgery has seen a 376% rise in a decade [1]. It is no surprise that an explosion of modifications, variations, and nuances for the approach have been explored. Major areas of contention include: single port versus multi-port, extraperitoneal versus transperitoneal, anterior versus posterior approaches, retropubic versus perineal, all of which are addressed in various segments in this book.

As with previous pioneering Retzius-sparing modifications discussed elsewhere in the text, the theoretical basis of the authors' technique is the preservation of the neurovascular bundles (NVBs) and Aphrodite veil, puboprostatic ligaments, accessory pudendal arteries and Santorini plexus, which all help to preserve potency and continence [2–4]. The Retzius-sparing approach affords the advantages of both the perineal approach and retropubic approach in the minimally-invasive setting.

This theoretical advantage has translated into multiple retrospective [5–7] and prospective randomized controlled trials [8] comparing the anterior and posterior approaches, emphasizing an earlier return to continence in most studies, but with similar long-term outcomes in functional recovery and quality of life.

S. L. Alip
Department of Urology, Urological Science Institute, Yonsei University College of Medicine, Seoul, South Korea

Division of Urology, University of the Philippines—Philippine General Hospital, Manila, Philippines
e-mail: slalip@up.edu.ph; slalip@alum.up.edu.ph

P. Koukourikis · K. H. Rha (✉)
Department of Urology, Urological Science Institute, Yonsei University College of Medicine, Seoul, South Korea
e-mail: khrha@yuhs.ac

Pre-operative Evaluation and Post-operative Medical Management

In the author's institution, each patient comes in with a prostate specific antigen (PSA) measurement, a prostate MRI, and a prostate biopsy. Biopsies are usually done using magnetic resonance imaging (MRI)-fusion transperineally or traditional transrectal ultrasound-guided double sextant biopsies. Biopsies done in an outside institution are routinely reviewed by the institution's in-house pathologist. An MRI is performed nearing the patient's admission or on the day of admission. A bone scan is done for high risk and intermediate risk disease. The patient is admitted a day before the surgery, during which baseline data for continence, potency and sexual health, lower urinary tract symptoms and bladder function are assessed with validated questionnaires. Blood tests include a basic electrolyte and kidney function panel, a complete blood count, a urinalysis and urine culture.

The authors employ wide patient selection and all radical prostatectomies are performed with this approach. Both localized prostate cancer and locally-advanced disease are candidates for the procedure. Decision making for oligometastatic disease is shared with the patient, and all therapies are offered and discussed. Metastatic disease is treated hormonally.

Pre-operative preparation does not routinely entail enemas or rigid diet restriction. Prophylactic antibiotics are similar to most guidelines employing a first generation cephalosporin or an extended Beta-lactam/Inhibitor combination [9]. The urine is ensured sterile prior to the operation.

The length of stay in our institution averages 5 days. The pelvic drain is removed on the second day post-operatively. Patients are sent home with a urethral catheter. The first outpatient follow-up visit is on Day 8–10 after the operation,

S. Ren et al. (eds.), *Robot-Assisted Radical Prostatectomy*, https://doi.org/10.1007/978-3-031-05855-4_21

where the catheter is removed and voiding is observed immediately post catheter removal; a uroflowmetry is also done at this time. The first serum PSA determination is 6 weeks post-operatively. After which it is measured on months 3, 6, and 9, then q6–12 months thereafter, congruent with multi-institutional guidelines [10–12].

Patient Positioning, Trocar Insertion and Peritoneal Access

Da Vinci Si Template

The patient is initially positioned in a low lithotomy position in YellowFins stirrups (Allen Medical, MA, USA) with the knees at >90° of flexion, and the hips at 45° of flexion. All pressure points are padded and the patient is strapped to the operating table. Povidone iodine preparation and draping are done. An initial 1 cm incision is done in the supraumbilical area to ensure a snug fit of the optical trocar. The 12 mm vision port is placed using a Veress needle approach and secured to the skin with a single suture; the pneumoperitoneum is set at 12 mmHg. The 0° endoscope is inserted and an initial survey of the intraperitoneal area is done to check for adhesions and overt pathologies or abnormalities. Robotic and assistant ports are then inserted as in Fig. 21.1, along a line 15 cm from the upper border of symphysis pubis, with an 8 cm distance between ports. If adhesions are encountered, it is the authors' preference that all ports that may be placed safely are inserted and the robot is docked with lysis of adhesions performed robotically prior to completion of port insertion. If only the assistant ports are initially deemed safe for insertion, laparoscopic adhesiolysis is performed prior to docking the robot. After all ports are inserted, the patient is repositioned to a 30° Trendelenburg and the robot is docked in between the patient's legs.

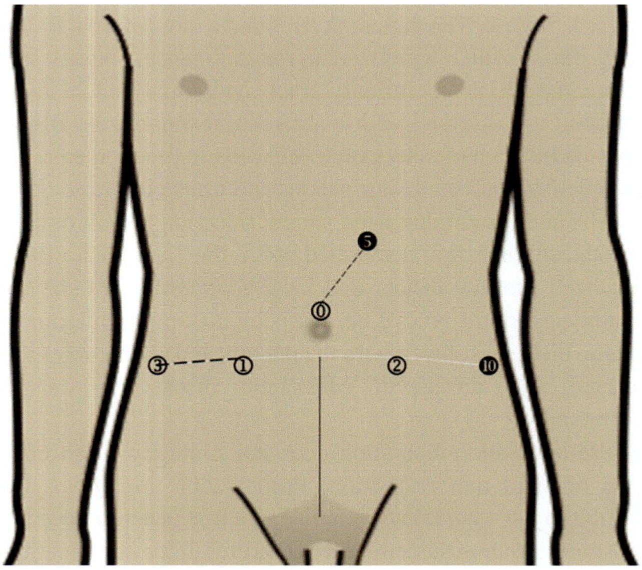

Fig. 21.1 Clear numbered circles *0–3*, *0* being the vision port, and *1–3* being robotic arms *1–3*. Dark numbered circles 5, 10 are the assistant ports, 5 and 10 mm. Dark vertical line is a 15 cm distance from the superior border of the pubic symphysis to a line bisecting all ports. The dashed lines are an 8 cm distance between all ports

It is noteworthy that the Yonsei technique departs from earlier Retzius-sparing techniques [13] in that the 12 and 5 mm assistant ports (and consequently, the bedside surgeon assist) are on the patient's left. This configuration is easily adapted by left and right-handed surgeons alike in the authors' institution.

The EndoWrist Maryland bipolar forceps is inserted into Arm 2 in the left side, the Endowrist monopolar curved scissors is inserted into Arm 1 in the right side, and the Endowrist Prograsp forceps (all Intuitive Surgical, CA, USA) is inserted into Arm 3 in the right side. The 12 mm assist port is for titanium, Weck Hem-o-lok (Teleflex, NC, USA), Lapra-Ty (Ethicon, Somerville NJ, USA) clip appliers, insertion and removal of surgical sutures, and introduction of the specimen bag. The 5 mm assist port is for the suction apparatus and drain placement.

Da Vinci Xi Key Differences

Two new features introduced by the Da Vinci Xi that are relevant to technique modifications are the Port-hopping technology, which enables any of the four robotic arms to carry the endoscope, and the 8 mm diameter endoscope [14], which allows for smaller incisions. In the Xi set-up, trocar placement is the same as in Si. Instruments maintain their relative positions. Arm designations are from the patient's left to right, Arm 1–4, with Arm 2 carrying the endoscope. The 0° camera is used. An additional feature of the Xi is the ability to change the direction of the 30° endoscope with the press of a button, the authors do not switch angles during different parts of the surgery as the 0° endoscope is used throughout the procedure; however, this may be done when preferred. The assistant ports are the same as in Si.

Da Vinci SP Key Differences

The authors perform a pure single port Retzius sparing robot-assisted laparoscopic radical prostatectomy (SP-RSRARP) using the Da Vinci SP. The incision is a single supraumbilical incision measuring 3.5–4 cm that is fitted with an Alexis O wound protector/retractor (Applied Medical, Rancho Santa Margarita, CA, USA). The Da Vinci SP cannula with a 2.5 cm inner diameter is fitted into the GelPOINT Access

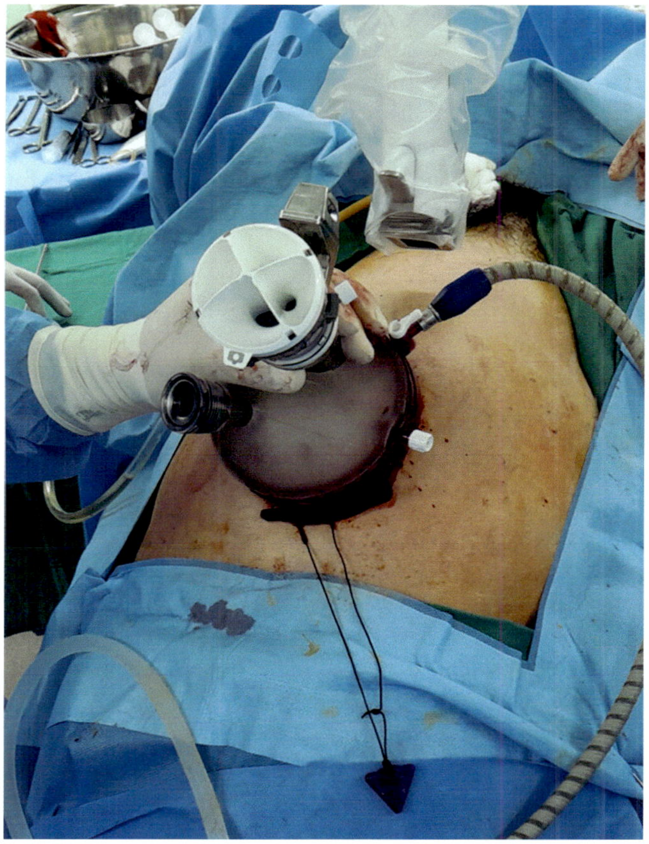

Fig. 21.2 Da Vinci SP single port configuration; the camera appears below in the intraoperative field, the "camera down" position

Platform (Applied Medical, Rancho Santa Margarita, CA, USA) at the caudad 6 o'clock position and a 1.2 cm cannula in the 2 o'clock position as the single assistant port, as in Fig. 21.2. The Da Vinci SP cannula can be rotated to position the camera at each of the four quadrants (with the boom rotating and docking to match the camera position): authors prefer the "camera down" position, which places the camera at the craniad 12 o'clock position, and as the inferior-most arm in the intraoperative view. The three instrument arms' positions are the same as for the Si. A single assistant port is used for all tasks of the bedside surgeon.

Revo-I Key Differences

The Revo-i (Meerecompany Inc., Seongnam, Republic of Korea) is a Korean-developed robot that functions much like the Da Vinci Si, with a surgeon console, a robotic patient cart with four arms, and a vision cart (Fig. 21.3). Multiple published studies have described the feasibility and ease of use of the Revo-i in urologic operations [16] and in other surgical fields [17–20]. The Revo-i has been increasingly used in the authors' institution for RSRARP since its Ministry of Food and Drug Safety approval for commercial use in 2018 [15]. The initial peritoneal access, trocar positions and instrument positions (albeit using Revo-i compatible robotic bipolar forceps, grasping forceps, and monopolar shears) are the same as those described for the Si.

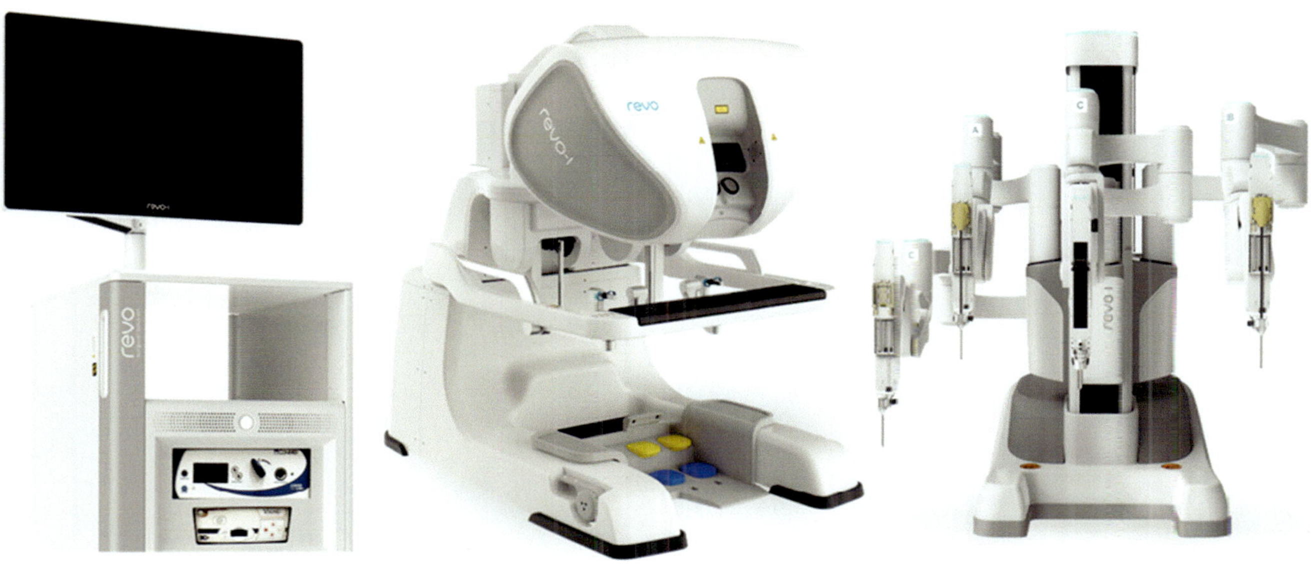

Fig. 21.3 The Revo-i vision cart, surgeon console and patient cart [15]

Surgical Technique

Radical Prostatectomy

Lysis of attachments of the cecum and sigmoid is important in allowing the bowel to fall back into the abdomen by gravity, emptying the pouch of Douglas. In the authors' institution, this is done for sigmoid colon, and the ileocecal area, if needed. The proximal extent of the dissection is indicated as the attachments surrounding the 12 mm assistant port are reached (Fig. 21.4).

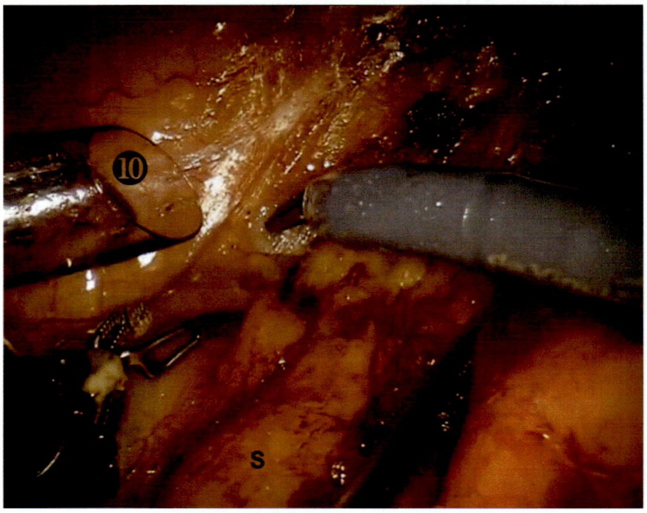

Fig. 21.4 Proximal extent of dissection in the sigmoid mesentery; *10–10 mm assistant port. S—Sigmoid mesentery*

The Prograsp forceps lifts up the peritoneum covering the bladder. The peritoneum is incised 5 cm above the reflection of the Douglas space, midway between the impression of the seminal vesicles and the transverse vesical fold (Fig. 21.5a). This is higher than traditionally described by Bocciardi and Galfano [13]. The authors have found that this has allows for a larger working space posterior to the prostate and prevents collapse of the posterior bladder wall obstructing the field, without the need for bladder stay sutures. Dissection is continued leaving a thin peritoneal fold posteriorly, locating the vas and seminal vesicles. Efficient traction of the Prograsp forceps, adequately tenting the field of dissection over the posterior bladder wall is important in avoiding bladder injury. The vasa are clipped and ligated at their take-off laterally (Fig. 21.5b). Upon freeing each vas, the forceps is repositioned to exert traction on the vas in an upward and contralateral direction; the seminal vesicles are freed off the surrounding tissue, using a combination of titanium clips, and sharp dissection. The authors find it helpful to decompress the seminal vesicle by incising its substance and suctioning the contents. This facilitates ease of handling and more efficient Prograsp traction.

The Denonvillier fascia is peeled off from the posterolateral surface of the prostate in a gentle sweeping motion and dissection proceeds in an antegrade fashion. The role of the assistant is to exert controlled counter-traction in pushing down the Denonvillier's fascia (Fig. 21.6). Proper exposure of dissection planes is invaluable in avoiding rectal injury. Diathermy is avoided as posterior dissection proceeds towards the apex of the prostate.

Attention is brought to the lateral prostate maintaining athermic dissection in the intrafascial or interfascial plane,

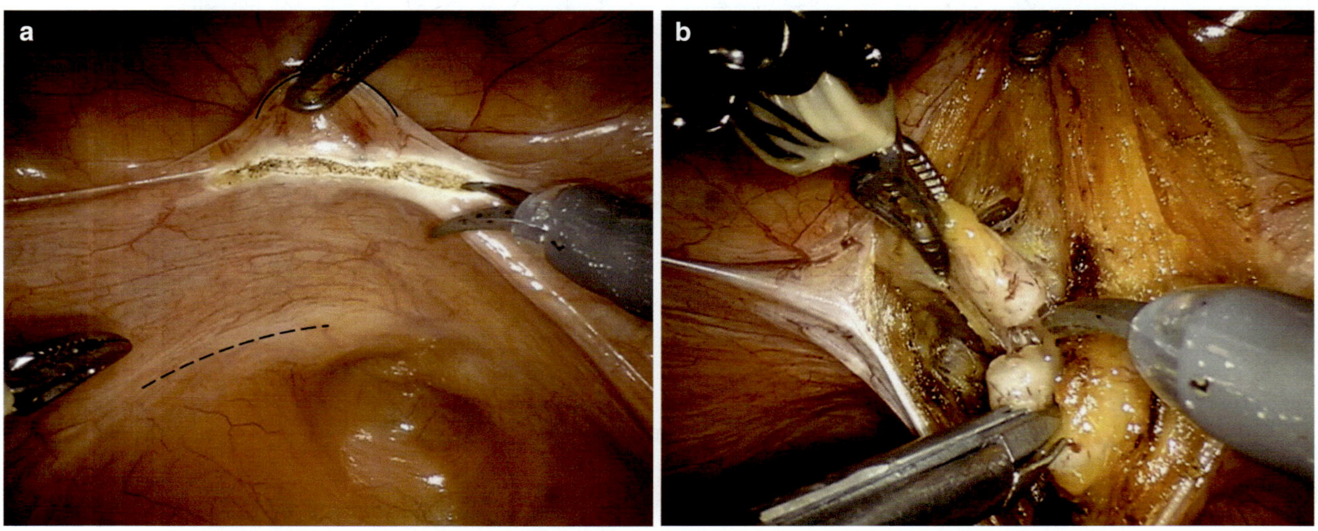

Fig. 21.5 (**a**) Initial incision showing the position of the three arms, (**b**) transection of the right vas deference showing the lower most instrument as the titanium clip applier controlled by the surgeon assistant from the 10 mm port (doubling as a counter-traction instrument); *solid line—transverse vesical fold, dashed line—impression made by the vas deferens*

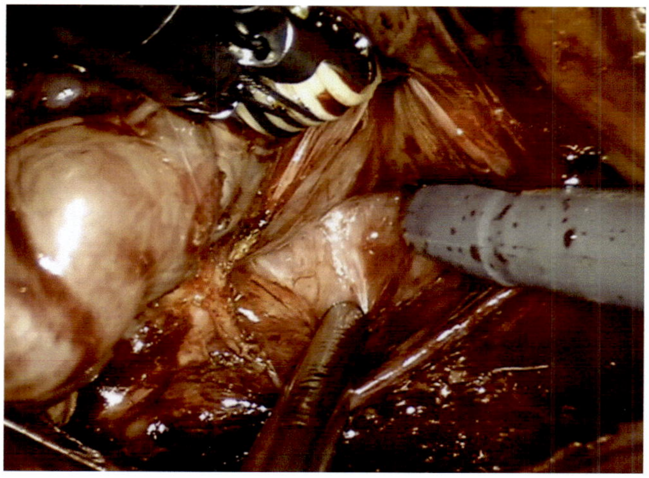

Fig. 21.6 Posterior dissection at the Denonvillier fascia. The lowermost instrument is the assistant suction from the 5 mm port. The Denonvillier fascia is the thick white structure in the middle of the field. A seminal vesicle is shown in the left of the field

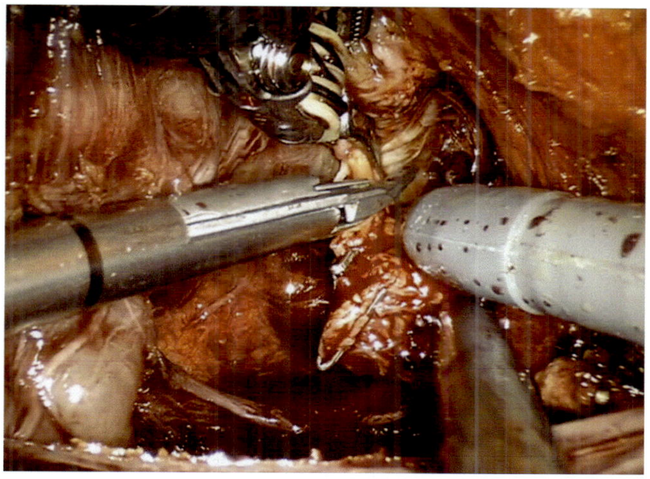

Fig. 21.7 Lateral dissection in the area of the right neurovascular bundle (NVB). The right NVB is the clipped structure in the middle of the field. The Prograsp forceps is lifting the prostate upwards and contralaterally

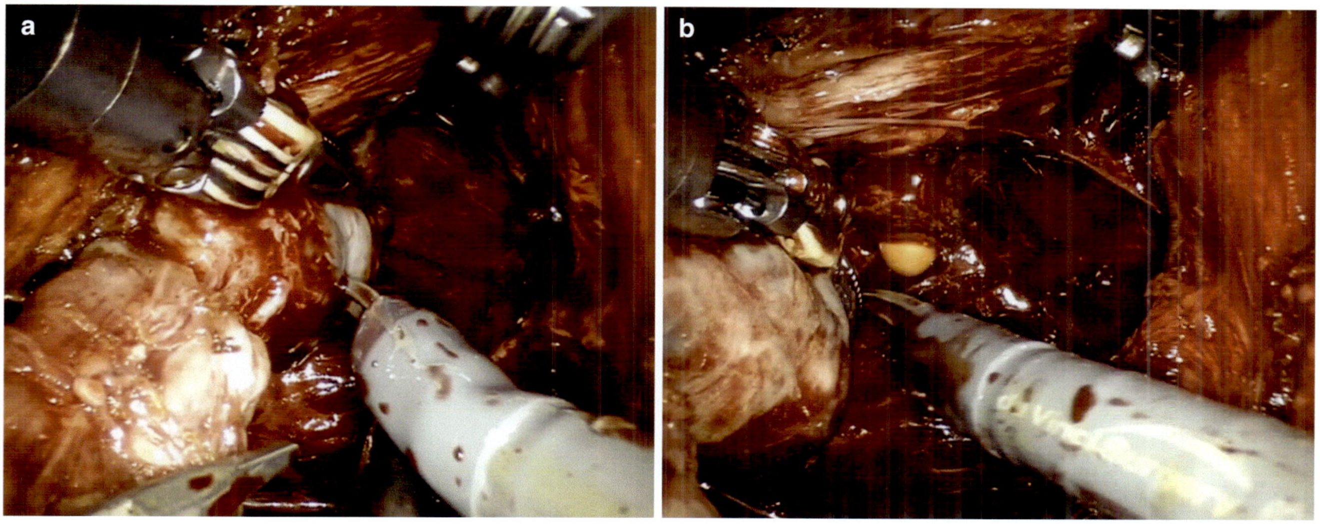

Fig. 21.8 (**a**) Dissection at the apex and urethra. The prostate is the white structure at the center of the field. The seminal vesicles are partly seen at the lower left of the field. (**b**) The catheter is retracted and the urethral transection is completed

until the apex of the prostate is reached. At this point in the dissection, the Prograsp forceps is reapplied to lift the prostate upwards towards the pubic symphysis and contralaterally, away from the neurovascular bundle (NVB), which runs posterior to the former. Care is taken to preserve bilateral NVBs without compromising surgical margins. The authors use titanium clips and cold shears in approaching the NVB (Fig. 21.7).

After meticulous posterior and lateral dissection, the Prograsp forceps is repositioned to exert traction on the right pelvic side wall, as the prostate is pulled contralaterally by the surgeon's left hand, aided by the assistant (Fig. 21.8a). The urethra will then come into view. The transection of the urethra is done, and the Foley catheter identified and retracted. Urethral transection is completed using sharp dissection (Fig. 21.8b).

The vesicoprostatic junction is identified. The starting point of this dissection is the anterior surface and base of the seminal vesicles. The Prograsp forceps is repositioned to hold the bladder up, the left Maryland exerts downward traction on the prostate and seminal vesicles, while dissection continues on their anterior surface peeling them off the posterior bladder serosa and bladder neck. The bladder is entered, and the Foley catheter identified, ensuring grossly adequate surgical margins (Fig. 21.9).

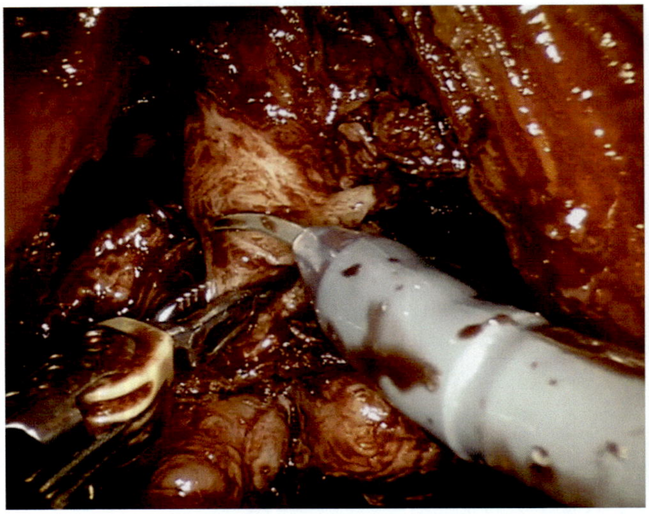

Fig. 21.9 The vesicoprostatic junction and entry into the bladder lumen

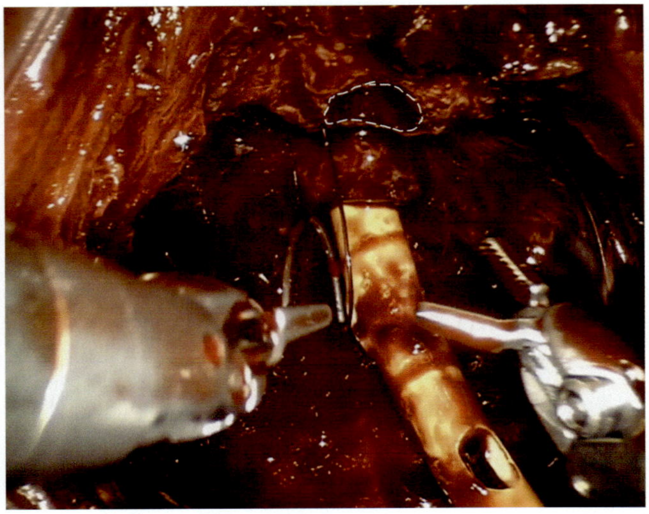

Fig. 21.10 Placement of anterior sutures. The left suture is shown. The catheter marks the urethral lumen, while the *white dashed line* encircles the entry into the bladder lumen

The prostate is now expected to be mobile with few remaining attachments, most commonly to the posterior Denonvillier fascia. The prostate is rolled off the prostatic fossa combining effective traction and sharp dissection. The specimen bag is inserted and the prostate secured within. Diligent hemostasis of the prostatic fossa is accomplished prior to creation of the anastomosis.

The authors use a polydioxanone barbed 2-0 suture with triangular stopper for a knotless first bite, Monofix PDO (Polydioxanone; Samyang Biopharmaceuticals Corp, Seoul, South Korea) for the urethrovesical anastomosis. The anastomosis is done anteriorly in a single-layer running fashion with two threads (one running from 12 o'clock to 6 o'clock from the right, and one in the left), first securing the anterior bladder to the anterior urethra (Fig. 21.10). After the anterior sutures are in place, the catheter is inserted all the way up to the bladder to serve as a guide in keeping the lumen open for the posterior stitches, after which the posterior sutures are completed. (This is in contrast with conventional anterior RARP, in which the posterior sutures are accomplished first.) (Fig. 21.11) The Yonsei technique again departs from the Galfano technique with posterior urethrovesical sutures all placed in an inside-to-outside fashion to avoid inadvertent injury to the catheter (Fig. 21.12); the catheter is also manipulated periodically to make sure it is untethered. After the bites are placed circumferentially, the working catheter is replaced with a 14-Fr silicone catheter and a leak test is done with 150 mL of saline. The anastomosis is secured with a Lapra-Ty clip on each suture end, or knotting both ends together. The peritoneal incision is closed in a running fashion with a single layer of a barbed absorbable suture.

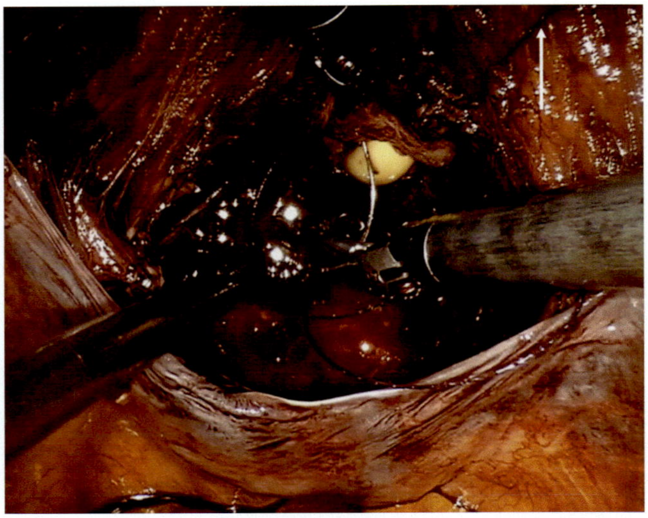

Fig. 21.11 Placement of posterior sutures after the catheter is inserted into the bladder. The left suture is being handled by the instruments. The right suture is anchored taut into the right abdominal fat and is indicated by a *white arrow*

Pelvic Lymph Node Dissection

Several templates of pelvic lymph node dissection (PLND) are noted in literature, the classification by Ploussard is used here [21]. A more extensive discussion of this is available in the succeeding chapters. The standard template (sPLND) excises the lymph nodes in the external iliac, obturator, and hypogastric packets. The extended template (ePLND) includes all packets in the sPLND and

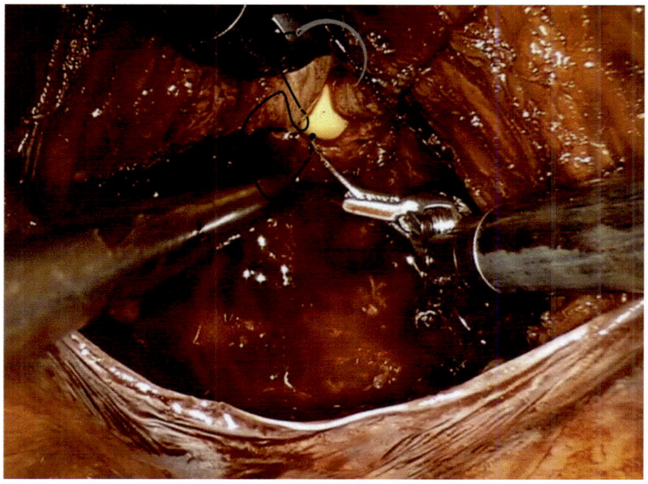

Fig. 21.12 The inside-to-outside Yonsei technique of suturing the posterior anastomosis to avoid catheter injury. *Dashed lines are impressions of sutures under the tissue*

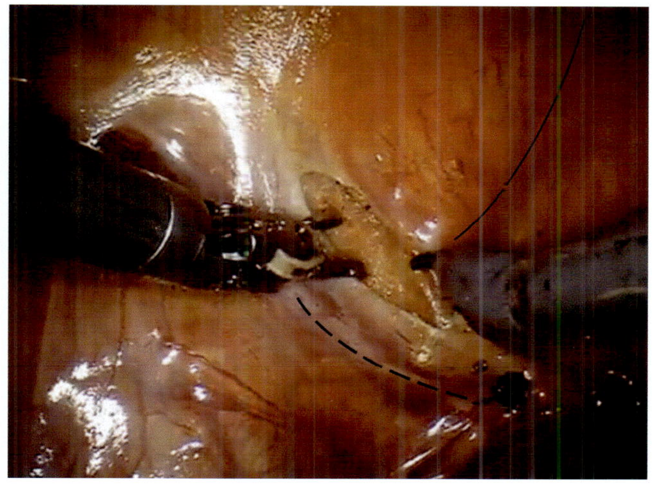

Fig. 21.13 The Yonsei incision for a left pelvic lymph node dissection. The *dashed line indicates the left vas impression, the solid line indicates the left medial umbilical ligament*, the end of the peritoneal closure after the prostatectomy is indicated by the Lapra-Ty clip in the lower right of the field

the proximal common iliac nodes. The limited template which has fallen out of favor and is considered to be inadequate [21, 22]. Guidelines are in agreement that, although positive nodes are detected at an increased rate in the extended template, this has not translated into a survival benefit [11, 23]. The authors' technique is to routinely remove nodes in the standard template for patients with ≥2% risk of nodal metastases [12, 24, 25], and to use the extended template if grossly enlarged lymph nodes are noted intraoperatively, or as a shared decision with younger patients. An alternative is to use a risk cut-off of over 5% to identify candidates for ePLND [10]; some advocate performing an ePLND routinely in all patients in lieu of sPLND [12].

Briefly, the Yonsei standard template dissection begins with a diagonal incision paralleling the vas, continuing proximally towards the bifurcation of the common iliac. This exposes an area bordered by the external iliac vein laterally, the obturator vessels internally, and the medial umbilical ligament as the medial border of the incision in the peritoneal fold (Fig. 21.13). The incision is typically 2–3 cm. The traction of the assistant surgeon maximizes exposure despite the smaller incision that ensures that the Retzius space is truly preserved. The node of Cloquet indicates the distal extent of the dissection, while the bifurcation indicates the proximal extent. The authors' prefer ligation of the vas segment contained in the field above. Muscular perforators are controlled using bipolar cautery, and a cut-and-roll motion over the anterior surface of vessels and nerves helps facilitate complete nodal excision.

Specimen Extraction and Surgical Closure

A drain is inserted into the 5 mm assistant port and guided by the surgeon into the pelvis. The instruments are removed, and the robot is undocked. The midline incision is enlarged to approximately 3–5 cm, depending on the estimated prostate size, the specimen is removed. The fascia of the midline wound is repaired in an interrupted fashion using absorbable braided sutures; the fascia of the 12 mm assistant port is closed with a figure of eight stitch; the rest of the incisions are closed subcutaneously with absorbable subcuticular sutures.

Outcomes, Pitfalls, and Addressing Complications

Single surgeon outcomes for the authors' technique have been published in peer-reviewed journals. The largest study is on 713 RS-RARP patients operated on from 2013–2018 [6]. The RS-RARP group showed significantly shorter operative time than the conventional RARP group (mean ± SD 149 ± 41 vs. 194 ± 44 min), and this reached clinical significance. Clavien-Dindo major complications, blood loss, and transfusion rate were the same between the groups. Additional reconstructive procedures were performed at a markedly higher rate in conventional RARP (69% vs. 8%). As regards oncologic outcomes, positive surgical margins for organ-confined disease is pegged at 11%, and 36% for pT3 or greater. This is consistent with most studies of RS-RARP and C-RARP.

As regards functional outcomes, at month 1 postoperatively the continence recovery rate in cRARP and RS-RARP cases was 9.0% and 45%, respectively. By month 6 postoperatively continence was recovered in 77% and 98% of the patients in the cRARP and RS-RARP groups, respectively. Statistical significance was reached for both points [6]. An earlier recovery of continence has been consistent across several trials with varying techniques of RS-RALP [26–28].

Prostate Size

This technique has been attempted at the authors' institution for various prostate sizes, the largest operated on was 165 ml and no complications were incurred. Difficulty in exposure was encountered, due to a decreased maneuverability expected with a larger organ. This was addressed by a wider initial peritoneal incision and maximizing traction-countertraction maneuvers of the third arm and the surgeon assistant. The surgeon assistant's role in widening the field-of-view is invaluable in these cases, the use of both right and left-hand surgeon instruments as retractors in spreading the incision open is crucial.

Organ Injury

The authors prefer immediate repair once an organ injury is identified. Bowel is repaired with a figure-of-eight suture for pinpoint burns or lacerations less than 1 cm in length, or a running single-layer approximation for longer defects. Absorbable braided sutures are used. Rectal injuries are repaired in a double-layer fashion, with fat interposition. Debridement of any nonviable edges is done prior to repair. The repair is done without the need for a diverting stoma. Air tightness of the repair is ensured with an insufflation test. Copious irrigation of the pelvis with saline is done post-repair.

Ureteral injury is rare in our series [6]. Because the bladder is viewed from below, the ureteral orifices are not visualized. Injury is avoided by meticulous dissection of the prostate base that the bladder neck is identified in its entirety prior to incising. Moreover, incising from the lateral may be done and as the bladder lumen is encountered, a clearer picture of the bladder neck configuration may be ascertained.

Bleeding

The authors occasionally use Surgicel (J&J Medical Devices, IN, USA) absorbable hemostat and Greenplast (GreenCross, Yongin, Republic of Korea) fibrin sealant on the raw areas in the prostatic fossa and lymph node packets post-lymphadenectomy. More important than any of these implements, however, is meticulous field inspection. Pinpoint bleeding may be addressed by monopolar or bipolar coagulation. Persistent bleeding from pelvic muscle perforators or the prostatic pedicle may be controlled by a figure-of-eight hemostatic suture. Bleeding from the Santorini plexus is rare in the Retzius-sparing procedure as this complex is undisturbed. Suspicious bleeding, however, especially during apical and urethral transection should be explored further. For the venous plexus, transient compression is usually sufficient.

Conclusion

Retzius-sparing robot-assisted laparoscopic radical prostatectomy is a safe and efficient way of primary treatment for both localized and locally-advanced prostate cancer. The highly standardized Yonsei method facilitates satisfactory oncologic outcomes, and superb continence outcomes that are sustained in the long-term. Future randomized controlled trials are appropriate to ascertain technique modifications and definitive advantages of this method.

References

1. Oberlin DT, Flum AS, Lai JD, Meeks JJ. The effect of minimally invasive prostatectomy on practice patterns of American urologists. Urol Oncol Semin Orig Investig. 2016;34:255.e1–5. https://doi.org/10.1016/j.urolonc.2016.01.008.
2. Walz J, Burnett AL, Costello AJ, et al. A critical analysis of the current knowledge of surgical anatomy related to optimization of cancer control and preservation of continence and erection in candidates for radical prostatectomy. Eur Urol. 2010;57:179–92. https://doi.org/10.1016/j.eururo.2009.11.009.
3. Rogers CG, Trock BP, Walsh PC. Preservation of accessory pudendal arteries during radical retropubic prostatectomy: surgical technique and results. Urology. 2004;64:148–51. https://doi.org/10.1016/j.urology.2004.02.035.
4. Stolzenburg JU, Schwalenberg T, Horn LC, et al. Anatomical landmarks of radical prostatecomy. Eur Urol. 2007;51:629–39. https://doi.org/10.1016/j.eururo.2006.11.012.
5. Umari P, Eden C, Cahill D, et al. Retzius-sparing versus standard robot-assisted radical prostatectomy: a comparative prospective study of nearly 500 patients. J Urol. 2021;205:780–90. https://doi.org/10.1097/JU.0000000000001435.
6. Lee J, Kim HY, Goh HJ, et al. Retzius sparing robot-assisted radical prostatectomy conveys early regain of continence over conventional robot-assisted radical prostatectomy: a propensity score matched analysis of 1,863 patients. J Urol. 2020;203(1):137–44. https://doi.org/10.1097/JU.0000000000000461.
7. Martini A, Falagario UG, Villers A, et al. Contemporary techniques of prostate dissection for robot-assisted prostatectomy. Eur Urol. 2020;78:583–91. https://doi.org/10.1016/j.eururo.2020.07.017.
8. Rosenberg JE, Jung JH, Edgerton Z, et al. Retzius-sparing versus standard robotic-assisted laparoscopic prostatectomy for the treatment of clinically localized prostate cancer. Cochrane Database Syst Rev. 2020;(8):CD013641. https://doi.org/10.1002/14651858.CD013641.pub2.

9. Lightner DJ, Wymer K, Sanchez J, et al. Best practice statement on urologic procedures and antimicrobial prophylaxis. J Urol. 2020;203:351.
10. Mottet N, Bellmunt J, Briers E, Bolla M, Bourke L, Cornford P, De Santis M, Henry A, Joniau S, Lam T, Mason MD, Van den Poel H, Van den Kwast TH, Rouvière O, Wiegel T. members of the EAU—ESTRO—ESUR—SIOG Prostate Cancer Guidelines Panel. EAU— ESTRO—ESUR—SIOG Guidelines on Prostate Cancer. Edn. presented at the EAU Annual Congress Milan. Arnhem: EAU Guidelines Office; 2021.
11. Sanda MG, Cadeddu JA, Kirkby E, et al. Clinically localized prostate cancer: AUA/ASTRO/SUO guideline. Part I: Risk stratification, shared decision making, and care options. J Urol. 2018;199(3):683–90. https://doi.org/10.1016/j.juro.2017.11.095.
12. National Comprehensive Cancer Network. Prostate cancer (version 2.2021). 2021. http://www.nccn.org/professionals/physician_gls/pdf/prostate.pdf. Accessed 17 Apr 2021.
13. Galfano A, Di Trapani D, Sozzi F, et al. Beyond the learning curve of the Retzius-sparing approach for robot-assisted laparoscopic radical prostatectomy: Oncologic and functional results of the first 200 patients with ≥1 year of follow-up. Eur Urol. 2013;64:974–80. https://doi.org/10.1016/j.eururo.2013.06.046.
14. Da Vinci Xi System User Manual (551400-11). California: Intuitive Surgical; 2018.
15. Revo Surgical Solution. 2021. http://revosurgical.com. Accessed 20 Apr 2021.
16. Chang KD, Abdel Raheem A, Choi YD, et al. Retzius-sparing robot-assisted radical prostatectomy using the Revo-i robotic surgical system: surgical technique and results of the first human trial. BJU Int. 2018;122:441–8. https://doi.org/10.1111/bju.14245.
17. Abdel Raheem A, Troya IS, Kim DK, et al. Robot-assisted Fallopian tube transection and anastomosis using the new REVO-I robotic surgical system: feasibility in a chronic porcine model. BJU Int. 2016;118:604–9. https://doi.org/10.1111/bju.13517.
18. Kang CM, Chong JU, Lim JH, et al. Robotic cholecystectomy using the newly developed Korean robotic surgical system, Revo-i: a preclinical experiment in a porcine model. Yonsei Med J. 2017;58:1075–7. https://doi.org/10.3349/ymj.2017.58.5.1075.
19. Kang I, Hwang HK, Lee WJ, Kang CM. First experience of pancreaticoduodenectomy using Revo-i in a patient with insulinoma. Ann Hepatobiliary Pancreat Surg. 2020;24:104. https://doi.org/10.14701/ahbps.2020.24.1.104.
20. Lim JH, Lee WJ, Park DW, et al. Robotic cholecystectomy using Revo-i Model MSR-5000, the newly developed Korean robotic surgical system: a preclinical study. Surg Endosc. 2017;31:3391–7. https://doi.org/10.1007/s00464-016-5357-0.
21. Ploussard G, Briganti A, De La Taille A, et al. Pelvic lymph node dissection during robot-assisted radical prostatectomy: Efficacy, limitations, and complications—a systematic review of the literature. Eur Urol. 2014;65:7–16. https://doi.org/10.1016/j.eururo.2013.03.057.
22. Smith JA, Howards SS, Preminger GM, et al., editors. Hinman's atlas of urologic surgery. 4th ed. Philadelphia: Elsevier; 2018.
23. Fossati N, Willemse PPM, Van den Broeck T, et al. The benefits and harms of different extents of lymph node dissection during radical prostatectomy for prostate cancer: a systematic review. Eur Urol. 2017;72:84–109. https://doi.org/10.1016/j.eururo.2016.12.003.
24. Briganti A, Larcher A, Abdollah F, et al. Updated nomogram predicting lymph node invasion in patients with prostate cancer undergoing extended pelvic lymph node dissection: the essential importance of percentage of positive cores. Eur Urol. 2012;61:480–7. https://doi.org/10.1016/j.eururo.2011.10.044.
25. Cimino S, Reale G, Castelli T, et al. Comparison between Briganti, Partin and MSKCC tools in predicting positive lymph nodes in prostate cancer: a systematic review and meta-analysis. Scand J Urol. 2017;51:345–50. https://doi.org/10.1080/21681805.2017.1332680.
26. Dalela D, Jeong W, Prasad MA, et al. A pragmatic randomized controlled trial examining the impact of the retzius-sparing approach on early urinary continence recovery after robot-assisted radical prostatectomy. Eur Urol. 2017;72:677–85. https://doi.org/10.1016/j.eururo.2017.04.029.
27. Asimakopoulos AD, Topazio L, De Angelis M, et al. Retzius-sparing versus standard robot-assisted radical prostatectomy: a prospective randomized comparison on immediate continence rates. Surg Endosc. 2019;33:2187–96. https://doi.org/10.1007/s00464-018-6499-z.
28. Menon M, Dalela D, Jamil M, et al. Functional recovery, oncologic outcomes and postoperative complications after robot-assisted radical prostatectomy: an evidence-based analysis comparing the Retzius sparing and standard approaches. J Urol. 2018;199:1210–7. https://doi.org/10.1016/j.juro.2017.11.115.

Retzius Sparing Robot-Assisted Radical Prostatectomy: Evolution, Technique and Outcomes

22

Deepansh Dalela, Wooju Jeong, Mani Menon, and Firas Abdollah

Introduction and History

Radical prostatectomy (RP) continues to be one of the most common definitive treatment approaches for men diagnosed with clinically localized prostate cancer, with over 80% of RPs (as of 2015) in the US being done via the robotic approach [1]. Along with ensuring perioperative safety, the trifecta (urinary continence, erectile function and surgical margins) have long served as aspirational benchmarks for a successful robot-assisted RP (RARP). Ever since the inception of RARP and its initial reports by Menon and colleagues [2], myriad technical modifications have attempted to minimize urinary incontinence and improve urinary function-associated quality of life (QoL). Sparing the space of Retzius (Retzius sparing RARP, or posterior RARP) is one of the few approaches to optimize UC that is supported by Level 1 evidence [3–7].

The idea of sparing the space of Retzius during a radical prostatectomy is by itself not new: indeed, the initial descriptions of perineal radical prostatectomy by Hugh Hampton Young centered around approaching the prostate transperineally without dropping the bladder or disrupting the anterior pelvic support. This approach, however, became less popular after the description of radical retropubic prostatectomy in late 1940s, despite reports describing continence rates of nearly 90–95% with perineal prostatectomy. Kavoussi's group attempted performing a Retzius sparing laparoscopic radical prostatectomy in the 1990s [8]. In their series of nine patients, the operating time was almost 9 h, blood loss ranged from 500–800 mL, and around 33% patients had serious complications. Even in the hands of one of the world's leading laparoscopic surgeons, the authors concluded that minimally invasive radical prostatectomy did not offer any significant benefits. Yet, somewhat remarkably, 6/9 (66%) were completely continent, with an additional 2 (22%) requiring one pad/day. Regardless, laparoscopic radical prostatectomy did not achieve much popularity in the US, until Menon's path breaking descriptions for RARP (that recapitulated open retropubic prostatectomy) revolutionized minimally invasive surgery [9].

Ten years later, Aldo Bocciardi and colleagues renewed interest in Retzius-sparing robotic prostatectomy in a small published series of three patients, noting a continence of 66% [10]. This was followed by a more formal evaluation in 200 patients, with a continence rate of 90% (defined as no pad/one safety liner) 1 week after catheter removal, and approximately 75% were potent 1 year after surgery [11]. Halfway across the world, Rha's group [12] and our own unpublished data showed similar results with Retzius-sparing prostatectomy: ~90% were either dry or using one safety liner 1 month postoperatively. Encouraged by these findings, we conducted the first randomized controlled trial comparing the standard (anterior) approach to Retzius-sparing (posterior) approach [5]. The results convincingly were in favor of Retzius sparing RARP.

Anatomical Basis for Retzius-Sparing Prostatectomy

The standard (anterior) RARP approach starts off with incising across the median and medial umbilical ligaments that hold up the bladder to the anterior abdominal wall and developing the space of Retzius (Fig. 22.1). In contrast, RS-RARP entails accessing the prostate from the rectovesical space by incising the pouch of Douglas. Theoretic rationale for expediting continence recovery through this approach are

1. Sparing the anterior pelvic support structures (dorsal venous complex, accessory pudendal arteries if any, pubovesical and puboprostatic ligaments, detrusor apron and the endopelvic fascia) and potentially allowing a more thorough Intrafascial dissection [11, 13]. Indeed,

D. Dalela · W. Jeong · M. Menon · F. Abdollah (✉)
VUI Center for Outcomes Research Analytics and Evaluation, Vattikuti Urology Institute, Henry Ford Hospital, Detroit, MI, USA
e-mail: ddalela1@hfhs.org; wjeong1@hfhs.org; mmenon1@hfhs.org

S. Ren et al. (eds.), *Robot-Assisted Radical Prostatectomy*, https://doi.org/10.1007/978-3-031-05855-4_22

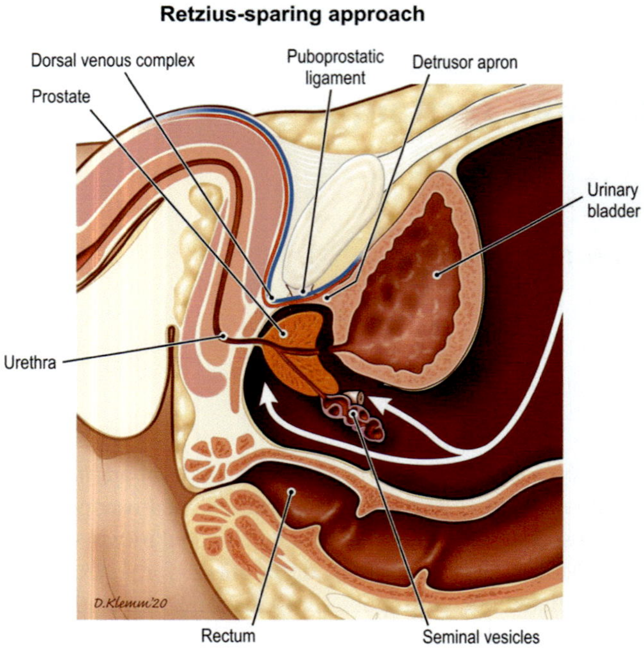

Fig. 22.1 White arrows illustrate the access for Retzius-sparing robot-assisted radical prostatectomy. (Borrowed, with permission, from Davis et al. [16])

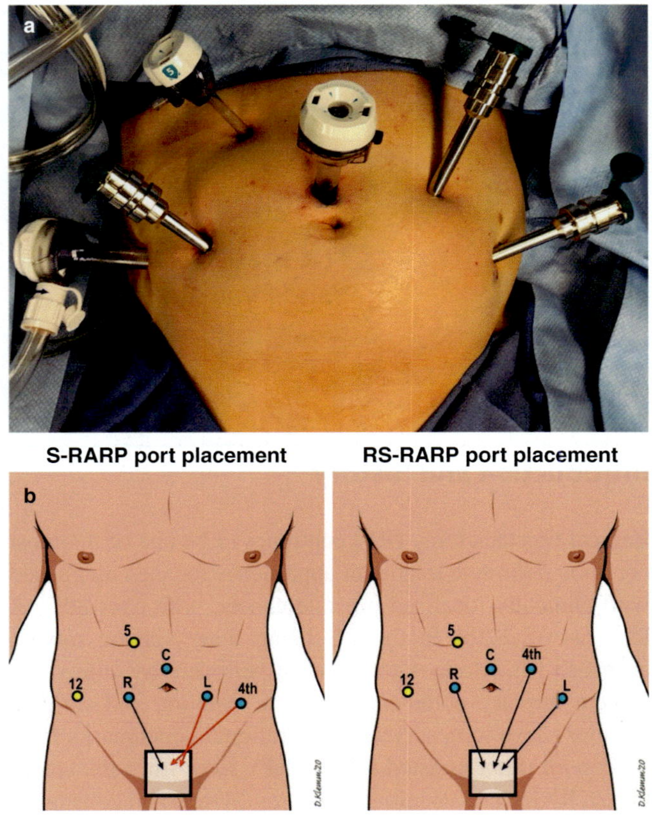

Fig. 22.2 Actual (**a**) and schematic (**b**) Schematic of port placement for both RS-RARP and S-RARP. Some groups place the Prograsp forceps is placed in the left medial robotic port and in a more caudal position, as this minimizes instrument clashing in the small operative space. *RS-RARP* Retzius-sparing robot-assisted radical prostatectomy, *S-RARP* standard robot-assisted radical prostatectomy. (Borrowed, with permission, from Egan et al. [17])

Chang and colleagues [14] showed that RS-RARP was associated with lesser bladder neck descent (calculated as bladder neck to pubic symphysis ratio on postoperative cystogram) compared to standard RARP, and the degree of descent was independently associated urinary continence recovery (HR 0.048, p = 0.006). Alternatively, RS-RARP may allow preservation of a longer membranous urethra (>12.1 mm on MRI imaging based on a recent study), which translated into faster continence recovery [15].

2. Decreasing or obviating the need for ligation of dorsal venous complex (DVC), which can have variable degree of overlap with the external urethral sphincter, especially at the level of the apex (up to 37%) [13, 16].

Current Technique for RSP

Port placement for RSP is slightly different from anterior RARP, and further needs to be modified based on patient's habitus, co-existing abdominal pathologies/prior surgeries, and comparatively smaller working space with the Retzius sparing approach. In our group, we have used the similar port placement to the conventional port placement, since some of the attempted RSP converted to anterior RARP due to body habitus. The camera port is placed below the umbilicus and 30°-up lens is used for the entire dissection of the prostate gland and the anastomosis. Alternatively, the camera port can be placed above the umbilicus and 0° lens can be used. Egan and colleagues [17] suggested a modified port placement: swapping the left arm (with the Maryland bipolar) and the fourth arm (with the Prograsp forceps) such that the fourth arm is medial and left arm is more lateral (Fig. 22.2).

Once the abdominal cavity is entered into and the sigmoid colon is mobilized out of the way, the sacrogenital fold (semilunar fold of parietal peritoneum between the bladder anteriorly and the rectum posteriorly) is grasped and incised for about 5–7 cm just above the level of vas deferens (VD) (Fig. 22.3).

In contrast to other practices, our technique starts with posterior dissection prior to the VD and SV dissection. Posterior dissection involves creating the posterior plane by incising into the leaves of the Denonvilliers' fascia, which is then carried down towards the apex and laterally towards the neurovascular bundles at the apex and the mid-gland of the prostate as intra-, inter- or extra-fascial nerve sparing, depending upon the intended degree of nerve sparing and visual approximation of tumor extent (Fig. 22.4). The

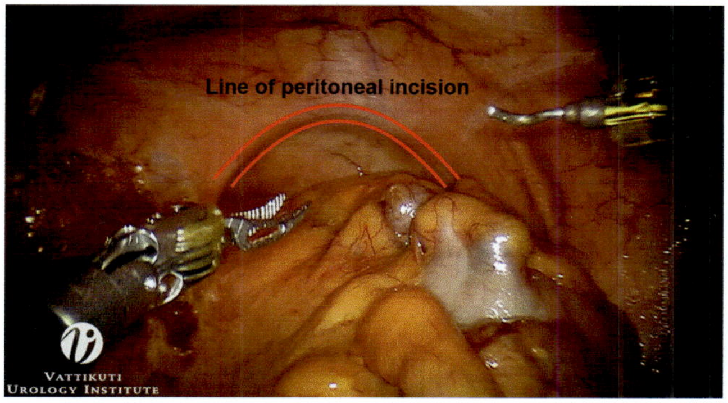

Fig. 22.3 Initial incision is made through the pouch of Douglas. (Borrowed, with permission, from Dalela et al. [5])

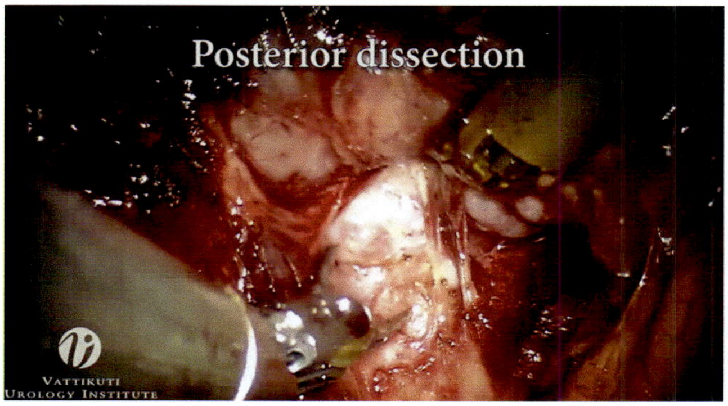

Fig. 22.4 Dissection through Denonvilliers' fascia to create a posterior plane. (Borrowed with permission, from Dalela et al. [5])

Prograsp (and suction by the bedside assistant) can be vital in providing countertraction, since working space can be limited. This posterior dissection prior to SV and VD dissection might eliminate the special need for suspension stitch to pull up the SV and VD during the posterior dissection.

Alternatively, VD/SV dissection can be performed prior to posterior dissection. The VD is dissected and followed towards the ampulla and seminal vesicles, which is freed from the posterior aspect of the bladder anteriorly and the Denonvilliers' fascia posteriorly. The VD is transected. The Prograsp forceps (or the assistant grasper) provide countertraction by retracting the ipsilateral ampulla of vas/SV contralaterally.

- Some authors may leave a 1-cm remnant of tip of the SV (SV-sparing), in an effort to maximize preservation of neuronal cage surrounding it that may contribute to recovery of erectile function [3].
- Others [10, 17] use a suspension stitch (such as a 3-0 prolene) on a Keith needle that goes through the anterior abdominal wall, cut edge of the sacrogenital fold of peritoneum, looping behind the SV and VD, and back out to the abdominal wall where they are secured with clamps. This frees the Prograsp for retraction for the remaining posterior and lateral dissection.

The ipsilateral SV/cut end of VD are retracted anteromedially, and the posterolateral plane is developed using a combination of blunt and sharp dissection.

Following adequate creation of a posterior plane, small individual vessels penetrating the prostate are clipped (using 5 mm clips) or cauterized (using bipolar grasper). Dissection at the base of the prostate continues until the plane cooperate with the dissected plane at the mid-gland and the apex. The authors start the bladder neck dissection prior to the circumferential dissection of the prostate gland as described by another group. The key point for the bladder neck dissection is that the posterior bladder and the trigone cover the base of the prostate like an apron and the posterior bladder wall needs to be peeled off from the base of the prostate to identify the posterior bladder neck. The lateral dissection of the prostate might be helpful to identify the bladder neck.

Once the lateral plane is developed, dissection curves anteriorly, where the anterior detrusor apron is gently swept away from the anterior surface of the prostate (Fig. 22.5). The left hand can provide upward traction on the bladder, with the Prograsp maintaining posterior retraction on the prostate. The prostate has now been freed circumferentially, remaining attached at the apex caudally and bladder neck cranially. The latter is then identified and circumferentially dissected, and then transected posteriorly. This exposes the Foley catheter, which is withdrawn, and Bladder neck dissection continues anteriorly. After anterior bladder neck is transected, the dissection is advanced to the anterior surface of the prostate (Fig. 22 6). The Prograsp is again repositioned to provide downward traction, and the previously dissected anterolateral plane can be followed to remain underneath the detrusor apron and dorsal venous complex (DVC) using blunt and bipolar dissection. The apex is freed of any attachments, and the urethra is divided sharply just distal to it, maximizing the length of preserved membranous urethral stump.

Urethrovesical anastomosis (UVA) presents some unique challenges with the Retzius-sparing approach, given the opposite orientation of bladder and prostate in standard vs. Retzius-sparing approach. We perform our UVA using two single 6 or 9 in. 3-0 V-loc on CV-23 needle. Anastomosis begins at the 1 o'clock position, outside-in on the anterior bladder neck, and inside-out bite at the 1 o'clock of the anterior urethra. After the second bite at the 11 o'clock of the anterior bladder neck, the stitch is cinched down tight enough to approximate the anterior anastomosis. The anastomosis is then sequentially carried out anticlockwise from the 11 o'clock to the 8 o'clock position (Fig. 22.7a–c).

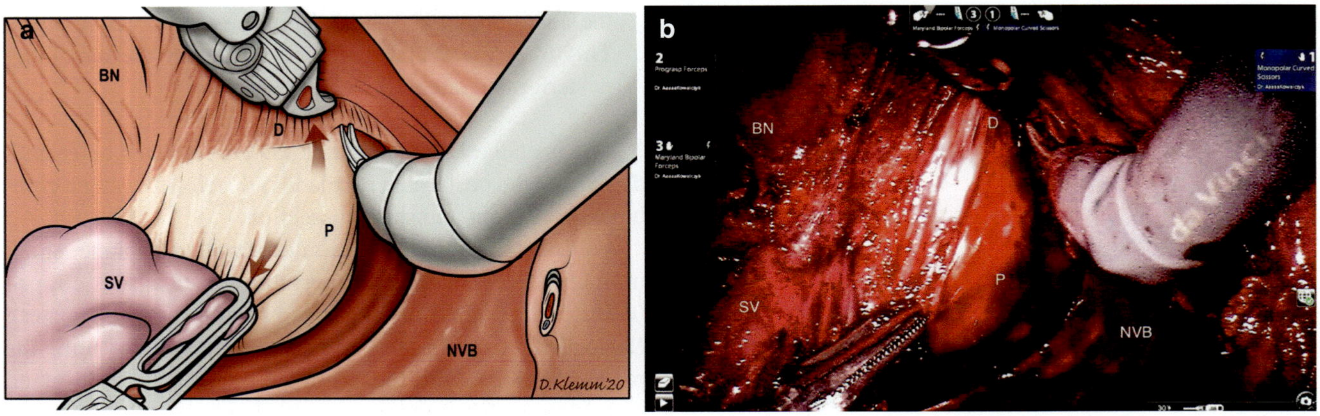

Fig. 22.5 Showing the development of the anterior plane, schematic (**a**) and intraoperative (**b**) description. The anterolateral surface and apex of the prostate are further developed prior to dissecting the bladder neck. Continuous upward traction on the bladder with the left hand along with posterior retraction with the Prograsp will often reveal the interface between the detrusor fibers and prostate, and this is developed from the apex to the medial bladder neck utilizing gentle monopolar and blunt dissection. *BN* bladder neck, *D* detrusor, *NVB* neurovascular bundle, *P* prostate, *SV* seminal vesicle. (Borrowed, with permission, from Egan et al. [17])

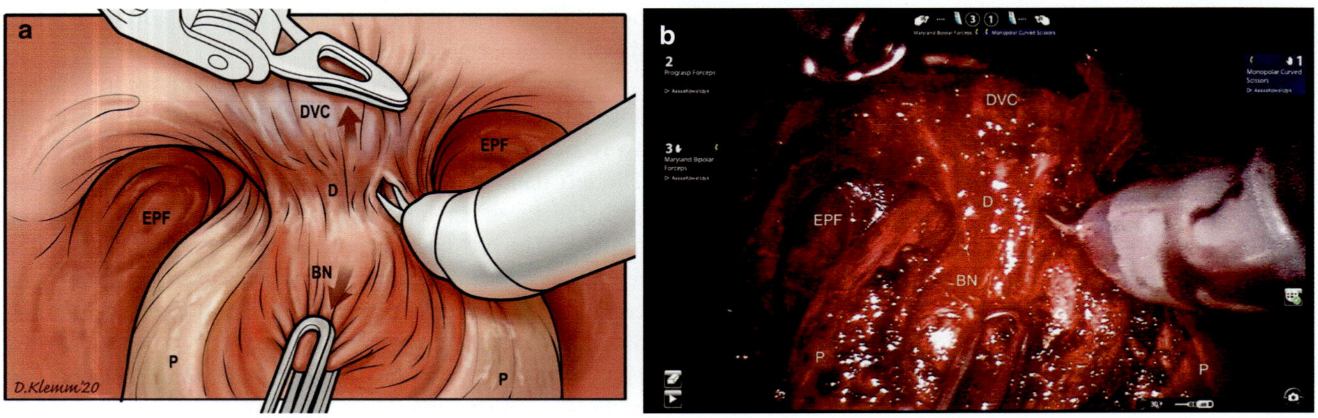

Fig. 22.6 After transection of the bladder neck, the plane between the anterior prostate and the dorsal venous complex is developed (schematic (**a**) and intraoperative (**b**) images). Blunt and bipolar dissection allows maintaining the correct plan, and the apex is used as a visual guide during dissection. If necessary, the posterior portion of the DVC can be entered if the plane is difficult to establish or in men with anterior lesions. *BN* bladder neck, *D* detrusor, *DVC* dorsal venous complex, *EPF* endopelvic fascia, *P* prostate. (Borrowed with permission, from Egan et al. [17])

A second V-loc suture is then introduced, and the anastomosis starts at the 2 o'clock position on the bladder neck from the outside to the inside. Same as the first stitch, the stitch is cinched down after 3 o'clock bladder bite (Fig. 22.7d). The anastomosis is then continued clockwise up to the 5 o'clock position. The 7 o'clock and 6 o'clock stitches are then placed using the initial and the second V-loc sutures respectively. Additional bites may be taken to reinforce the anastomoses, and the anastomosis is completed by burying in or tying off. If the size of the bladder neck is wider than what was planned, the second stitch may start in between the 1- and 11-o'clock stitches, so called anterior bladder neck reconstruction. Alternatively, bladder neck reconstruction at 3- and 9-o'clock of the bladder neck can be done using extra sutures prior to UVA.

Closing off the pouch of Douglas is optional based on surgeon's preference and 3-0 V-Loc can be used to close it. At our institution, the pouch of Douglas is not necessarily closed.

Pelvic lymph node dissection (PLND) is performed by making a longitudinal peritoneal incision at the junction of the VD and external iliac artery. The external iliac vessels are identified, and the obturator lymph nodes are dissected off the lateral surface of the bladder. Care should be taken to identify some critical structures such as the obturator nerve and the ureter during PLND. The anterior packet is well cauterized or clipped with 10 mm Hem-o-Lok clips, and the posterior packet is dissected away from the iliac bifurcation. Above steps are repeated for the contralateral side. Peritoneal incisions are left open to avoid lymphocele.

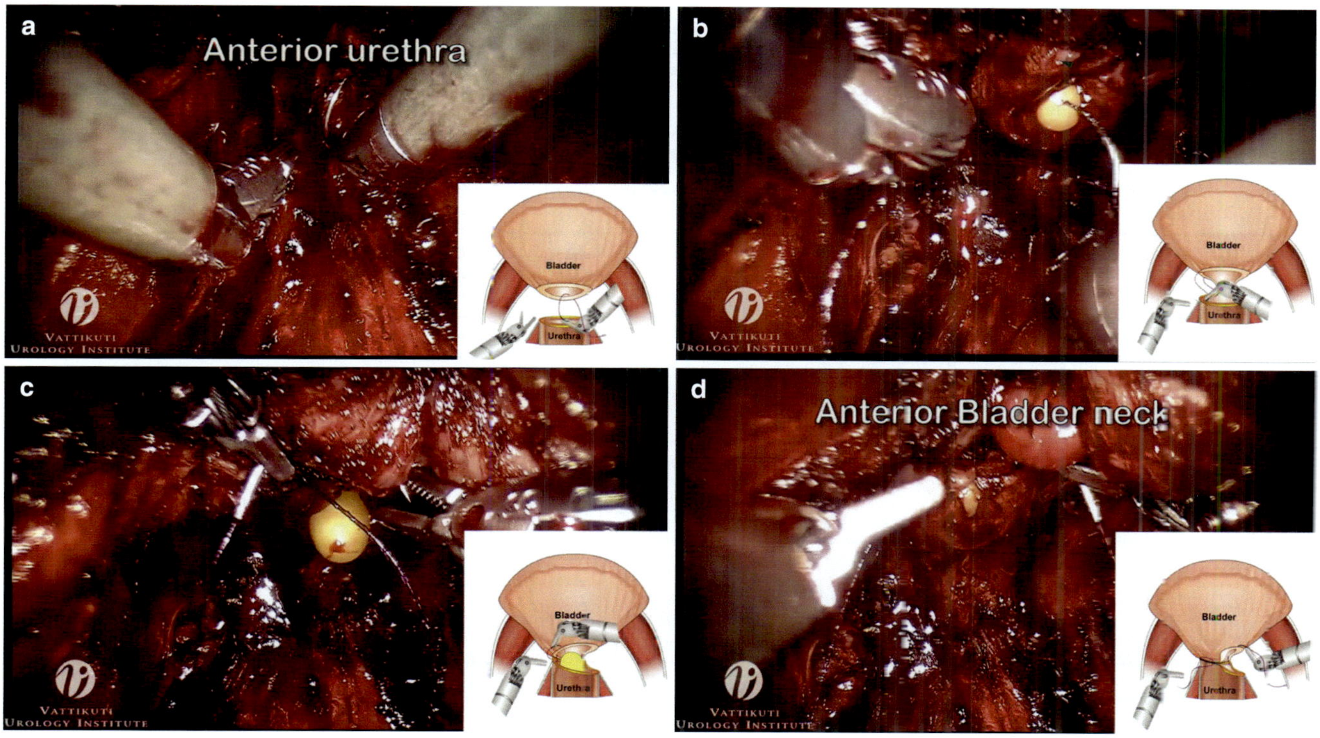

Fig. 22.7 (**a**–**d**) Steps of the urethro-vesical anastomosis. (Borrowed, with permission, from Dalela et al. [5])

Current Evidence: Summary of Outcomes for Retzius-Sparing Radical Prostatectomy

These have been summarized in multiple meta-analyses, and one Cochrane review [18] (Fig. 22.8, Tables 22.1 and 22.2). Overall, perhaps no other technical modification of robotic radical prostatectomy has been so extensively studied in a Level 1 fashion.

Functional Outcomes

Urinary Continence

As can be assessed from Tables 22.1 and 22.2, the major benefits of the Retzius sparing approach are realized in terms of functional outcomes, specifically expediting recovery of urinary continence. As of May 31, 2021, five randomized controlled trials comparing RS-RARP to standard RARP have been reported, all conducted in different countries and all consistently showing faster recovery of continence with Retzius sparing approach [3–7]. Another trial is ongoing at Heidelberg University, Germany (NCT03787823), results of which should be forthcoming shortly.

Continence rates (measured as no pads or use of one safety pad/day) following catheter removal have approached ~50–70% [3, 5, 6] rising to ~70–90% a month postoperatively and ~90–95% 3 months after surgery [3–7], significantly better compared to standard RARP at those time points. This was further confirmed in our detailed analyses including pad weights. Similar results have been seen from non-randomized retrospective comparisons between the two approaches. Of note, Level 1 evidence so far has focused on early continence (<3–6 months postoperatively) as their primary end point. Longer term follow up of our trial [19] showed that the incremental continence benefit of RS-RARP approach was muted at 1-year follow up, with 98% continence rate (0–1 pad/day) compared to 93% with standard approach (log rank $p = 0.09$), and while a statistically higher proportion of men were using 1 pad/day with the standard approach, there was no difference in pad weights compared to RS-RARP. Non-randomized data from other institutions have suggested sustained continence benefit with the RS approach 1 year after surgery [17], although this may be related to lower continence rates in the standard RARP arm (81.4% vs. 97.6% for RS-RARP).

More importantly, only one trial [7] included patients with clinically high risk disease (n = 36, ~33% of study population): twice as many (~58%) men with D'Amico high risk disease were continent 1 week post catheter removal with RS-RARP compared to standard (29%), although the smaller sample size precluded statistical significance ($p = 0.08$). While a recently reported prospective non-randomized comparison between RS and standard RARP included 37%

Study	Age (years)	Clinical stage	Surgeon experience	No participants per arm	No participants receiving nerve sparing	Continence definition (pads/day)	Primary outcome	Secondary outcomes	Duration of follow-up (months)
Asimakopoulos 2019	RS: 66 Standard: 65	cT1-cT2, Gleason score ≤ 7, PSA ≤10 ng/mL	< 50 cases each technique	RS: 45 Standard: 57	RS: 39 (86.7%) Standard: 44 (77.1%)	0	Continence rates at catheter removal	PSM	6
Bhat 2020	N/A	T1 or T disease	> 400 cases	N/A	N/A	0	BCR, urinary continence return, erectile function	Operative time, blood loss, PSMs	12
Dalela 2017	RS: 60 Standard: 60	Low-intermediate risk (NCCN)	"varying levels of expertise" including residents and fellows	RS: 59 Standard: 60	RS: 37 (62.7%) Standard: 39 (65%)	0–1	Continence rates within 1 week of catheter removal	PSM, BCR, adverse events	12
Kolontarev 2016	Median age: 67.4	Not reported	N/A	RS: 39 Standard: 40	Not reported	0–1	Urinary continence within 1 week of catheter removal	Urinary bother symptoms	3
Qiu 2020	RS: 68 Standard: 67	low, intermediate, and high risk (EAU)	> 200 RS approach > 300 standard approach	RS: 55 Standard: 55	RS: 36 (65.5%) Standard: 38 (69.1%)	0	Urinary continence within 1 week of catheter removal	PSM, BCR, adverse events	12

BCR: biochemical recurrence; cT: clinical stage; EAU: European Association of Urology; PSA: prostate-specific antigen; PSM: positive surgical margin; N/A: not applicable; NCCN: National Comprehensive Cancer Network; RALP: robotic-assisted laparoscopic prostatectomy; RS: Retzius-sparing.

Fig. 22.8 Summary table showing the characteristics of randomized controlled trials comparing Retzius-sparing robot-assisted radical prostatectomy (RARP) with standard RARP

patients with clinically high risk disease, their outcomes were not separately analyzed. Nyarangi-Dix et al. [20] operated upon 50 men with clinically high risk PCa: 3-month continence rates after RS-RARP were 82% (0–1 pad; 50% 0 pad) and increased to 98% (72% with 0 pad/day) at 12 months, despite 34% undergoing adjuvant radiotherapy.

In line with aforementioned data, a recent Cochrane review concluded that RS-RARP probably improves continence 1 week after catheter removal (moderate certainty, relative risk [RR] 1.74), may improve continence 3 months after surgery (low certainty, RR 1.33) and probably results in little to no difference in continence at 12 months postoperatively (moderate certainty, RR 1.01) [18].

Sexual Function

Although preservation of DVC and pudendal arteries may theoretically impact recovery of sexual function, we [19] and others [17] have not noted a statistically significant improvement with RS-RARP. A year after surgery, about 44% of preoperatively potent men had s Sexual Health Inventory for Men score ≥17 with either approach, and 86% men undergoing RS-RARP (vs. 69% with S-RARP) were able to have intercourse ($p = 0.5$). The Cochrane review [18] therefore concluded that there is uncertainty about the effect of RS-RARP on potency 12 months after surgery (RR 0.98).

Oncological Outcomes

As referenced earlier, most of the evidence for RS-RARP has been limited to low-intermediate risk disease, with only one randomized trial (~33% [7]) and prospective non-randomized series (~37% [21]) including a sizeable proportion of men with clinically high risk prostate cancer. Interestingly, despite our cohort of predominantly clinically intermediate risk, 45% of RS-RARP cohort eventually harbored pT3 disease [5, 19] which was the same proportion noted in the Qiu trial comprising 33% clinically high risk PCa. In contrast, Nyarangi-Dix retrospectively reviewed the outcomes of 50 men with exclusively clinically high-risk PCa [20].

Postoperatively, one of the criticisms of RS-RARP approach has been the higher risk of positive surgical margins (PSM): the Cochrane review [18] states with low certainty that RS-RARP may increase positive surgical margin (RR 1.95). Data from RCTs show a PSM rate of 25–30% in RS-RARP (compared to ~15% in S-RARP). While these differences were not statistically significant, and the proportion of non-focal PSM (defined as PSM ≥2 mm) was much lower in both groups, they were (non-significantly) accentuated in men with pT3 disease (35–40% with RS-RARP vs. ~20–25% with S-RARP) . Further, as expected, PSMs were more likely to occur anteriorly or at the apex with RS-RARP [7, 11, 17, 19], with some authors advocating partial DVC

Table 22.1 Summary of findings from published randomized controlled trials comparing standard robot-assisted radical prostatectomy (S-RARP) with Retzius-sparing RARP

Author, year, (region)	Primary time point for continence	Continence definition	Continence outcomes	Potency	Pertinent histopathology	Positive surgical margins	BCR-free survival
Dalela et al. 2017 (USA) [5]	1 week after catheter removal	0–1 ppd 0 ppd Median Pad weights	48% vs. 71%* 15% vs. 42%* 1 week: 25 vs. 5 g* 2 week: 12 vs. 0 g* 1 month: 5 vs. 0 g*	n/a	75% clinically intermediate risk pT3 disease: 23% vs. 45%*	Overall: 13.3% vs. 25% pT3 disease: 21.4% vs. 37%	0.91 vs. 0.91
Asimakopoulos et al. 2019 (Italy) [3]	Immediately after catheter removal		30% vs. 51.3%* At 6 months: 64% vs. 90%* Median TTC: 21 vs. 1 day*	n/a	70% biopsy GG1, 33% pT3	Overall: 10% vs. 28% pT3: 22.2% vs. 41.2%	n/a
Kolontarev et al. 2016 (Russia)[a] [6]	1 week after surgery (? Immediately after catheter removal)	0–1 ppd	25% vs. 46.1%* At 3 months 82.5% vs. 94.8%	n/a	n/a	n/a	n/a
Qiu et al. 2020 (China) [7]	1 week after catheter removal	0 ppd	Overall: 30.9% vs. 69.1%* At 6 months 90% vs. 93% HR 1.56 (RS vs. S-RARP)* Clinically high risk patients: 29.4% vs. 57.9% (p = 0.08) At 6 months: 100% vs. 95% (HR 1.26, p = 0.1)	n/a	~33% overall had clinically high risk disease, with 20% ≥ GG4 ~45% overall with pT3 disease	Overall: 14.5% vs. 23.6% Clinically high risk: 23.5% vs. 36.8% pT3 disease 25.9% vs. 36.4% PSM location: Apex (37.5%) and lateral (50%) vs. lateral (38.5%) and anterior (30.8%)	At 12 months: 95% vs. 90% (p = 0.1)
Bhat et al. 2020 (India)[a] [4]	1 month post-op	0 ppd	23% vs. 80%* At 6 months: 86% vs. 96%*	n/a	n/a	n/a	n/a
Menon et al. 2018[b] (USA) [19]	6–12 months postop	0–1 ppd 0 ppd	93% vs. 98% 74% vs. 92% (6 months)* 88% vs. 96% (12 months)	ESI at 12 months: 86% vs. 69% SHIM ≥ 17 at 12 months: 44.6% vs. 44.1%	75% clinically intermediate risk pT3 disease: 23% vs. 45%*	Overall: 13.3% vs. 25% pT3 disease: 21.4% vs. 37%	At 18 months: 92.7% vs. 83.8%

ppd pads per day, *SHIM* Sexual Health Inventory for Men, *ESI* erection for intercourse
*$p < 0.05$
[a]Only abstract forms available
[b]One-year follow up of Dalela et al. study

resection anteriorly to potentially decrease PSMs at this location [12]. More recent studies have however, allayed some of these concerns, especially with wider acceptance of the RS approach and overcoming the learning curve [22]. Recent prospective comparative series have shown similar rates of overall and nonfocal PSMs in RS-RARP vs. S-RARP [17, 21], and more importantly, no difference in biochemical recurrence free survival at 1–1.5 year follow up (long term data pending). Even amongst 50 men with clinically high risk PCa undergoing RS-RARP (84% with ≥pT3 disease) and >50% of those undergoing adjuvant therapy, 1-year recurrence-free survival was 96% [20].

Challenges, Limitations and Opportunities

Certain surgical scenarios such as very large prostates/median lobes, post-TURP, kidney transplant recipients and salvage prostatectomies may present increased complexities and technical challenges, however do not preclude performance of RS-RARP, especially with adequate experience with the technique. One of the stated challenges with the Retzius sparing approach is men with large prostates or median lobes, given the smaller working space to start off with. However, studies from high volume center have shown

Table 22.2 Summary of findings from published non-randomized controlled trials comparing standard RARP (S-RARP) with Retzius-sparing RARP (RS-RARP)

Author, year (country)	Continence definition	Continence outcomes	Potency	Pertinent histopathology	Positive surgical margins	BCR-free survival
Lim et al. 2014 (South Korea) [12] S-RARP n = 50 RS-RARP N = 50	0–1 ppd 0 ppd	1-month post op: 74% vs. 92%* 50% vs. 70%*	n/a	Biopsy Gleason 8–10: ~18% in either arm pT3: ~18% in either arm	Overall: 14% vs. 14% pT3 disease: 24% vs. 18%	n/a
Sayyid et al. 2017 (USA) [36] S-RARP n = 100 RS-RARP n = 100 (Prospective study)	Mean pad number	3-month post op: 3.2 vs. 1.5* 6-month post op: 2.3 vs. 0.9*	n/a	Clinically high risk: ~25% either arm pT3 disease: 23% vs. 34%	Overall: 13% vs. 17%. pT3 disease: 47.1 vs. 47.8%	n/a
Eden et al. 2018 (UK) [37] S-RARP n = 40 RS-RARP n = 40	0 ppd 0–1 ppd	1-month post op: 37.5% vs. 90% 70% vs. 97.5%	n/a	n/a	pT2 disease: 7.7 vs. 16.7% pT3 disease: 14.3% vs. 31.8%	n/a
Lee et al. 2020 (South Korea) [38] S-RARP n = 609 RS-RARP n = 609 (Propensity score matched cohort)	<1 safety liner/day	1-month post op: 9% vs. 45%* 6-month post op: 77% vs. 98%*	n/a	Biopsy Gleason 8–10: 29 vs. 26% Clinical high risk: ~50% in either arm pT3 disease: 43% vs. 39%	pT2 disease: 15% vs. 11% pT3 disease: 32% vs. 36%	n/a
Egan et al. 2021 (USA) [17] S-RARP n = 70 RS-RARP n = 70	EPIC-CP urinary incontinence scores 0–1 ppd	6 weeks post op: 4.4 vs. 3.2* 6 month: 2.4 vs. 1.7* 12-month: 81.4% vs. 97.6%*	12-month ESI: 62.9% vs. 65.7%	Clinical high risk: ~10% in either arm pT3 disease: ~33% in either arm	Overall: 30% vs. 34% Location: posterior (70.6%) vs. anterior (52%)	1-year: 82% vs. 87%
Umari et al. 2021 (UK) [21] S-RARP n = 201 RS-RARP n = 282 (Prospective study)	0–1 ppd	58.1% vs. 70.4%* No difference in overall urinary scores	Mean IIEF scores at 12-months: 10.5 vs. 8.9 (p = 0.2)	37% D'Amico high risk RS-RARP 30% pT3 disease	Overall: 13.9% vs. 15.6% pT3 disease: 20.3% vs. 33.7% (p = 0.2)	1-year: 93% vs. 98.6%*

EPIC-CP Expanded Prostate Cancer Index Composite for Clinical Practice, *IIEF* International Index for Erectile function, *ESI* erection sufficient for intercourse, *ppd* pad per day
*$p < 0.05$

that although larger prostates (>60–80 mL) may be associated with more blood loss and longer console time, immediate and 3-month urinary continence rates (~80% and 90%, respectively) were comparable to smaller ones [23, 24]. Similarly, even in men with enlarged median lobes >10 mm (longitudinal distance from the bladder neck to the highest portion of the median lobe of the prostate as measured on preoperative MRI), RS-RARP expedited continence recovery (HR 1.83, p = 0.002) without compromising perioperative outcomes, blood loss or BCRFS [25]. Rha and colleagues recently published a short case series of 17 patients undergoing RS-RARP with a history of prior transurethral resection of prostate, with no significantly inferior outcomes [26].

Other concerns with the Retzius sparing approach entail the higher risk of positive surgical margins, especially in the anterior or apical location. While studies so far have not conclusively proven this association, patients with anterior tumors, clinical T3 disease or body mass index may nonetheless demand higher technical expertise coupled with continuous evolution and adaptation of surgical technique. Perioperative complications have been comparable, and once again, likely to improve with the learning curve as with all new approaches (including standard RARP). One notable complication has been the potential for higher incidence of postoperative lymphoceles: one series noted a symptomatic lymphocele rate of 18% (most of which required percutaneous drainage) [9], although this was not noted in our experience (7–8% with both standard and RS-RARP) since lateral peritoneal incisions for pelvic lymphadenectomy remain open with either approach.

Like with all new surgical techniques, there is a likely element of learning curve. A multi-institutional analysis of 14 surgeons showed that console time, continence and rate of Clavien-Dindo ≥2 complications improved over the first 50 cases, while reducing rate of PSMs may take longer [11, 22]. However, no appreciable learning curve phenomenon was seen in other high volume centers [27], including ours [5], suggesting that the impact of learning curve can be safely mitigated by expert proctoring and prior experience with robotic prostatectomy platform. Specifically, given the predilection of anterior PSMs, patients with high risk anterior or transitional zone tumors on preoperative MRI may be offered S-RARP [28], or a wider dissection with partial DVC resection may be performed anteriorly in experienced hands and appropriately counseled patients [12].

Potentially Beneficial Scenarios

On the other hand, RS-RARP can be a valuable tool in the armamentarium in patients who have had prior inguinal hernia/extraperitoneal mesh surgeries, by virtue of avoiding that space entirely [29]. Similarly, patients with kidney transplant in-situ may be good candidates for RS approach [29, 30]. Interestingly, Chang et al. noted that RS-RARP was associated with a lower risk of postoperative inguinal hernia over a 3-year follow up: of the 6.3% patients (53 out of 839) who had an inguinal hernia, 79% had undergone standard RARP [31]. The authors postulate that this is likely due to maintaining the attachment between the bladder and anterior abdominal wall structures, preserving the myopectineal orifice ("shutter mechanism") and preventing medialization and dilation of internal ring.

Modifications of the Retzius-Sparing Approach

Lastly, given the documented superiority of RS-RARP in expediting continence recovery, different groups have proposed modifications of the Retzius sparing approach in an effort to make it more reproducible. Ash Tewari's group in New York [32] proposed a "hood" technique for performing RARP (Figs. 22.9 and 22.10), whereby the surgery proceeds in the usual S-RARP fashion after developing the space of Retzius, going through the anterior/posterior bladder neck to the retrotrigonal layer posteriorly, and developing the plane between detrusor apron and anterior fibromuscular stroma anteriorly, such that a hood of tissue remains behind (including puboprostatic ligaments, arcus tendineus, puboperinealis muscle, retrotrigonal layer and Denonvilliers' fascia for posterior musculofascial reconstruction). The authors reported urinary continence rates similar to RS-RARP (83% 1 month after catheter removal), without adversely affecting complication rate or positive surgical margin (6%), although the majority of patients had pT2 disease (81%) and patients with high risk disease or anterior tumors were excluded. Zhou and colleagues in China discussed a transvesical, Retzius-sparing approach, where a cystotomy is made on the postero-superior aspect of the bladder and the prostate is accessed through a circumferential incision around the internal urethral meatus/bladder

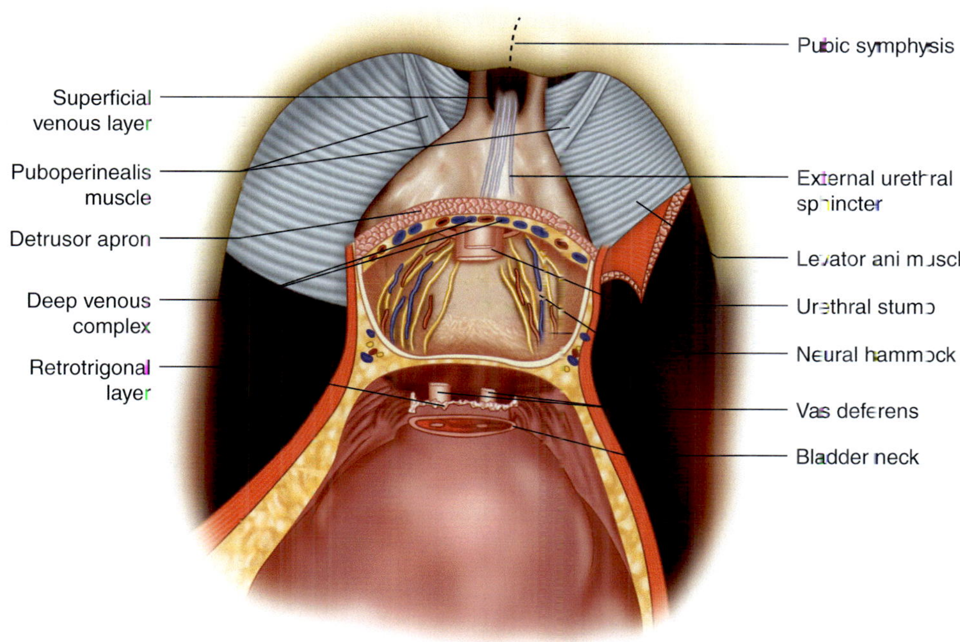

Fig. 22.9 Sketch demonstrating hood surgical anatomy. Anatomical components of the hood surround and safeguard the membranous urethra and the external urethral sphincter, and thereby urethrovesical anastomosis. 1 = pubic symphysis; 2 = external urethral sphincter; 3 = superficial venous layer; 4 = puboperinealis muscle; 5 = levator ani muscle; 6 = detrusor apron; 7 = urethral stump; 8 = deep venous complex; 9 = neural hammock; 10 = vas deferens; 11 = retrotrigonal layer; 12 = bladder neck. (Borrowed, with permission, from Wagaskar et al. [32])

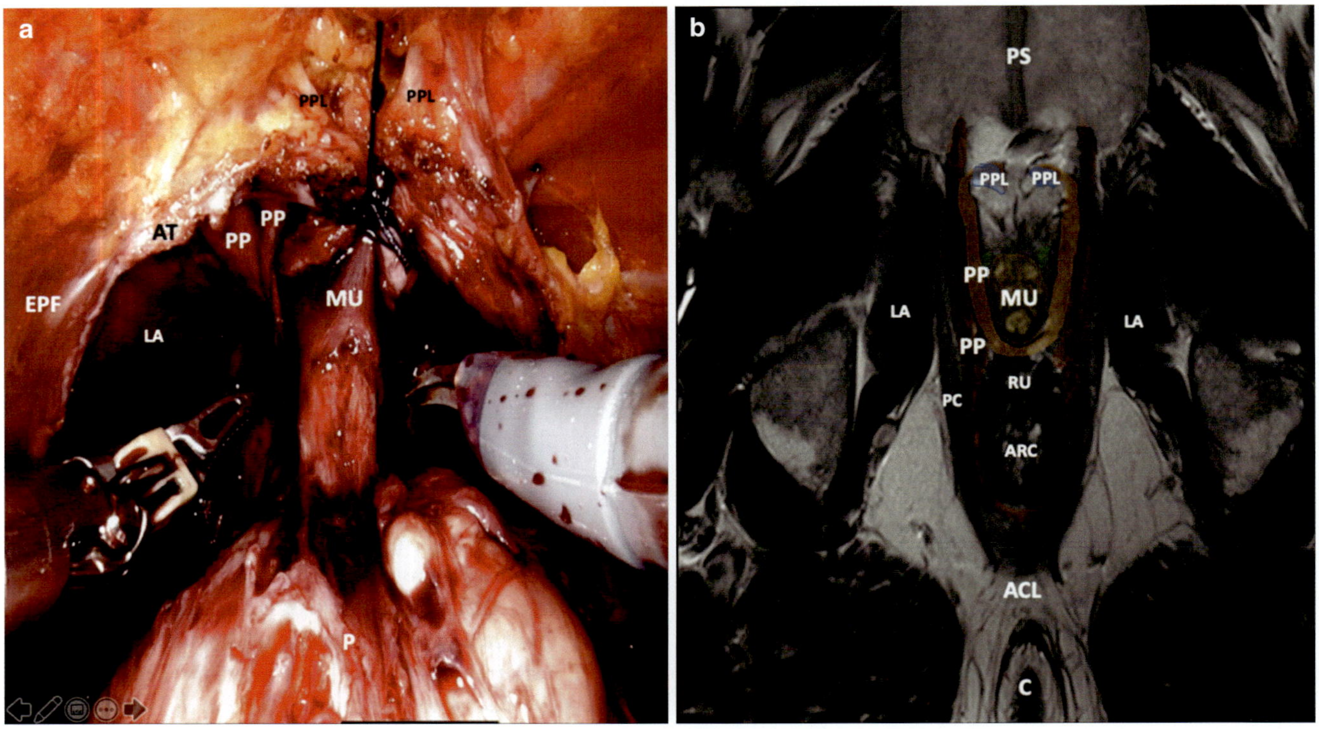

Fig. 22.10 MRI and intraoperative images corresponding to section **b**. (**a**) Intraoperative image showing the membranous urethra and muscles surrounding the urethral sphincter. (**b**) MRI of the pelvis (cross section) corresponding to the intraoperative image. *ACL* anococcygeal ligament, *ARC* anorectal canal, *AT* arcus tendineus, *C* coccyx, *EPF* endopelvic fascia, *LA* levator ani, *MRI* magnetic resonance imaging, *MU* membranous urethra, *PC* prostatic capsule, *PP* puboperinealis muscle, *PPL* puboprostatic ligaments, *PS* pubic symphysis, *RU* rectourethralis muscle. (Borrowed, with permission, from Wagaskar et al. [32])

neck [33]. Continence outcomes (0–1 ppd) were comparable to RS-RARP performed through the posterior (pouch of Douglas) approach (91% 1 week after catheter removal) with a PSM rate of 11.4%, although their series did not include clinically high risk, anterior tumor or pathological T3 disease [34]. Kaouk and colleagues adapted the transvesical Retzius-sparing approach to the single-port RARP platform (making a 2-cm vertical cystotomy extracorporeally through a 4 cm vertical midline incision and a "floating" single port with Gelpoint mini docked inside the bladder, with 75% (15/20) continent immediately post catheter removal, 30% harboring ≥pT3a disease and 15% with PSMs [35].

References

1. Preisser F, Nazzani S, Mazzone E, et al. Regional differences in total hospital charges between open and robotically assisted radical prostatectomy in the United States. World J Urol. 2019;37:1305.
2. Menon M, Tewari A, Baize B, et al. Prospective comparison of radical retropubic prostatectomy and robot-assisted anatomic prostatectomy: the Vattikuti Urology Institute experience. Urology. 2002;60:864.
3. Asimakopoulos AD, Topazio L, De Angelis M, et al. Retzius-sparing versus standard robot-assisted radical prostatectomy: a prospective randomized comparison on immediate continence rates. Surg Endosc. 2019;33:2187.
4. Bhat S, Sharma H, Gregory P, et al. Retzius sparing versus non Retzius sparing prostatectomy—a randomised control trial. Indian J Urol. 2020;36(5 Suppl):1–56.
5. Dalela D, Jeong W, Prasad MA, et al. A pragmatic randomized controlled trial examining the impact of the Retzius-sparing approach on early urinary continence recovery after robot-assisted radical prostatectomy. Eur Urol. 2017;72:677.
6. Kolontarev K, Govorov A, Rasner P, et al. Retzius-sparing robot-assisted radical prostatectomy: a randomized study evaluating urinary continence recovery. Eur Urol Suppl. 2016;15:282.
7. Qiu X, Li Y, Chen M, et al. Retzius-sparing robot-assisted radical prostatectomy improves early recovery of urinary continence: a randomized, controlled, single-blind trial with a 1-year follow-up. BJU Int. 2020;126:633.
8. Schuessler WW, Schulam PG, Clayman RV, et al. Laparoscopic radical prostatectomy: initial short-term experience. Urology. 1997;50:854.
9. Menon M, Tewari A, Peabody J. Vattikuti Institute prostatectomy: technique. J Urol. 2003;169:2289.
10. Galfano A, Ascione A, Grimaldi S, et al. A new anatomic approach for robot-assisted laparoscopic prostatectomy: a feasibility study for completely intrafascial surgery. Eur Urol. 2010;58:457.
11. Galfano A, Di Trapani D, Sozzi F, et al. Beyond the learning curve of the Retzius-sparing approach for robot-assisted laparoscopic radical prostatectomy: oncologic and functional results of the first 200 patients with ≥1 year of follow-up. Eur Urol. 2013;64:974.

12. Lim SK, Kim KH, Shin TY, et al. Retzius-sparing robot-assisted laparoscopic radical prostatectomy: combining the best of retropubic and perineal approaches. BJU Int. 2014;114:236.
13. Walz J, Epstein JI, Ganzer R, et al. A critical analysis of the current knowledge of surgical anatomy of the prostate related to optimisation of cancer control and preservation of continence and erection in candidates for radical prostatectomy: an update. Eur Urol. 2016;70:301.
14. Chang LW, Hung SC, Hu JC, et al. Retzius-sparing robotic-assisted radical prostatectomy associated with less bladder neck descent and better early continence outcome. Anticancer Res. 2018;38:345.
15. Ota Y, Hamamoto S, Matsuyama N, et al. Pelvic anatomical features after Retzius-sparing robot-assisted radical prostatectomy intended for early recovery of urinary symptoms. J Endourol. 2021;35:296.
16. Davis M, Egan J, Marhamati S, et al. Retzius-sparing robot-assisted robotic prostatectomy: past, present, and future. Urol Clin North Am. 2021;48:11.
17. Egan J, Marhamati S, Carvalho FLF, et al. Retzius-sparing robot-assisted radical prostatectomy leads to durable improvement in urinary function and quality of life versus standard robot-assisted radical prostatectomy without compromise on oncologic efficacy: single-surgeon series and step-by-step guide. Eur Urol. 2021;79:839.
18. Rosenberg JE, Jung JH, Edgerton Z, et al. Retzius-sparing versus standard robotic-assisted laparoscopic prostatectomy for the treatment of clinically localized prostate cancer. Cochrane Database Syst Rev. 2020;8:CD013641.
19. Menon M, Dalela D, Jamil M, et al. Functional recovery, oncologic outcomes and postoperative complications after robot-assisted radical prostatectomy: an evidence-based analysis comparing the Retzius sparing and standard approaches. J Urol. 2018;199:1210.
20. Nyarangi-Dix JN, Görtz M, Gradinarov G, et al. Retzius-sparing robot-assisted laparoscopic radical prostatectomy: functional and early oncologic results in aggressive and locally advanced prostate cancer. BMC Urol. 2019;19:113.
21. Umari P, Eden C, Cahill D, et al. Retzius-sparing versus standard robot-assisted radical prostatectomy: a comparative prospective study of nearly 500 patients. J Urol. 2021;205:780.
22. Galfano A, Secco S, Dell'Oglio P, et al. Retzius-sparing robot-assisted radical prostatectomy: early learning curve experience in three continents. BJU Int. 2021;127:412.
23. Galfano A, Panarello D, Secco S, et al. Does prostate volume have an impact on the functional and oncological results of Retzius-sparing robot-assisted radical prostatectomy? Minerva Urol Nefrol. 2018;70:408.
24. Santok GD, Abdel Raheem A, Kim LH, et al. Perioperative and short-term outcomes of Retzius-sparing robot-assisted laparoscopic radical prostatectomy stratified by gland size. BJU Int. 2017;119:135.
25. Qian J, Fu Y, Wu X, et al. Impact of protruded median lobe on perioperative, urinary continence and oncological outcomes of Retzius-sparing robot-assisted radical prostatectomy. Transl Androl Urol. 2021;10:538.
26. Kim LHC, Santok GD, Raheem AA, et al. Retzius-sparing robot-assisted radical prostatectomy is safe for patients with prior transurethral prostate surgery. Int Braz J Urol. 2018;44:342.
27. Olivero A, Galfano A, Piccinelli M, et al. Retzius-sparing robotic radical prostatectomy for surgeons in the learning curve: a propensity score-matching analysis. Eur Urol Focus. 2021;7(4):772–8.
28. Li Y, Fu Y, Li W, et al. Tumour location determined by preoperative MRI is an independent predictor for positive surgical margin status after Retzius-sparing robot-assisted radical prostatectomy. BJU Int. 2020;126:152.
29. Sayyid RK, Madi R. The untold advantages of Retzius-sparing robotic radical prostatectomy. J Endourol. 2018;32:671.
30. Mistretta FA, Galfano A, Di Trapani E, et al. Robot assisted radical prostatectomy in kidney transplant recipients: surgical, oncological and functional outcomes of two different robotic approaches. Int Braz J Urol. 2019;45:262.
31. Chang KD, Abdel Raheem A, Santok GDR, et al. Anatomical Retzius-space preservation is associated with lower incidence of postoperative inguinal hernia development after robot-assisted radical prostatectomy. Hernia. 2017;21:555.
32. Wagaskar VG, Mittal A, Sobotka S, et al. Hood technique for robotic radical prostatectomy-preserving periurethral anatomical structures in the space of Retzius and sparing the pouch of Douglas, enabling early return of continence without compromising surgical margin rates. Eur Urol. 2021;80(2):213–21.
33. Zhou X, Fu B, Zhang C, et al. Transvesical robot-assisted radical prostatectomy: initial experience and surgical outcomes. BJU Int. 2020;126:300.
34. Deng W, Zhang C, Jiang H, et al. Transvesical versus posterior approach to Retzius-sparing robot-assisted radical prostatectomy: a retrospective comparison with a 12-month follow-up. Front Oncol. 2021;11:641887.
35. Kaouk J, Beksac AT, Zeinab MA, et al. Single port transvesical robotic radical prostatectomy: initial clinical experience and description of technique. Urology. 2021;155:130–7.
36. Sayyid RK, Simpson WG, Lu C, et al. Retzius-sparing robotic-assisted laparoscopic radical prostatectomy: a safe surgical technique with superior continence outcomes. J Endourol. 2017;31:1244.
37. Eden CG, Moschonas D, Soares R. Urinary continence four weeks following Retzius-sparing robotic radical prostatectomy: the UK experience. J Clin Urol. 2018;11:15.
38. Lee J, Kim HY, Goh HJ, et al. Retzius sparing robot-assisted radical prostatectomy conveys early regain of continence over conventional robot-assisted radical prostatectomy: a propensity score matched analysis of 1,863 patients. J Urol. 2020;203:137.

UCL Technique

23

Tushar Aditya Narain and Prasanna Sooriakumaran

Introduction

Robot assisted radical prostatectomy was first performed in 2000 by Binder in Germany, following which it become the preferred surgical approach for radical prostatectomies since 2001 when surgeons at the Vattikutti Urology Institute started performing all radical prostatectomies using robotic assistance [1]. The functional outcomes improved dramatically with this approach, owing to the highly magnified three-dimesional vision and the dexterity the robotic arms provided, resulting in better nerve spare and more meticulous reconstruction. The robotic approach to radical prostatectomy soon became the gold standard and was accepted the world over. Centers and surgeons in different parts of the world adopted this technique and published their own style of performing the surgery, the common denominator being that all these approaches involved going into the space of Retzius and bringing the bladder down. However, the functional outcomes for all these variant approaches were still far from ideal, and surgeons have been in a continuous pursuit to improve urinary incontinence following the surgery, the bane of all robot assisted radical prostatectomies.

Endeavors to achieve the trifecta outcomes following RARP, which became the holy grail since its proposal in 2005, resulted in various modifications being introduced such as the Rocco's stitch suggested by Bernado Rocco, total anatomical reconstruction by Ash Tewari or the use of suprapubic catheters; or the initial access to the seminal vesicles through the pouch of Douglas (Montsouris approach) to improve functional outcomes [2–6]. All of these innovations independently did improve the outcome measures, but rates of urinary incontinence following this surgery were still far from what was desirable.

Galfano and team in 2010 presented a novel approach to radical prostatectomy which preserved all the anterior supports of bladder, endopelvic fascia, puboprostatic and pubovesical ligaments besides the Dorsal venous complex. This was popularized as the Retzius sparing approach to radical prostatectomy where the prostate was removed without violating the space anterior to the bladder, the space of Retzius. The preservation of anterior supports aimed at improving urinary continence following the surgery. The authors even proposed that preservation of Veil of Aphrodite circumferentially improved greatly the potency rates, for the anterior approaches which preserves the Veil of Aphrodite, requires the Veil to be incised anteriorly. Preservation of the Sartorini's plexus also aimed to reduce the blood loss and preserved the blood supply to the striated sphincter and the Corpora Cavernosa, which might have some bearing on the proposed improved outcomes. This team from Milan soon published their experience of first 200 cases and demonstrated very high early continence rates (92%) in the Retzius sparing group with a low 1 year biochemical recurrence rates, establishing the oncological safety of this procedure [7]. However, this was a single arm study with no comparison of outcomes with the Standard RALP, and Koon Rha's group from Korea in 2014 published the results from a matched comparison study comparing 50 patients undergoing RS-RALP with >500 patients how underwent S-RALP. This team also reported excellent immediate functional outcomes with 70% of patients being dry at 1 month (70% vs. 50%), although in their series, the continence rates decreased if the patients had lymph node dissection [8]. Both these initial experiences published were not randomized and the outcomes were reported subjectively. Dalela et al. from Vattikuti Urology Institute, Detroit published the first randomized control trial comparing the outcomes between the two groups. A multivariate regression analysis revealed a 71% 1 week continence rates in the Retzius arm vs. 48% in the

T. A. Narain
Robotic Pelvic Uro-Oncology, University College London Hospital NHS Foundation Trust, London, UK

P. Sooriakumaran (✉)
University College London Hospital NHS Foundation Trust, London, UK

Lead for Urology and Consultant Urological Surgeon, Cleveland Clinic, London, UK
e-mail: psoori@santishealth.org; prasanna.sooriakumaran@nds.ox.ac.uk

S. Ren et al. (eds.), *Robot-Assisted Radical Prostatectomy*, https://doi.org/10.1007/978-3-031-05855-4_23

standard arm (p = 0.01). Incidence of post-operative complications (18% Retzius vs. 12% standard) and probability of BCRF survival (0.91 vs. 0.91) were comparable in the two groups [9]. Our group recently published a comparative prospective study of 500 patients comparing Retzius sparing and the standard approach. We found immediate urinary continence to be better in RS-RARP group (70.4% vs. 58.1%, p = 0.02), with less nocturnal enuresis prevalence (p = 0.011) and bother (p = 0.009) with no significant differences afterwards. A better QOL (p = 0.004) was reported 1 week after surgery with no other differences in functional or QOL outcomes, perioperative parameters, complications, or margin rates [10].

Retzius sparing robot assisted radical prostatectomy has been on the horizon for just over a decade and modifications have constantly been introduced to improve the functional outcomes. Few surgeons across the globe have traversed their learning curves while most surgeons are still in the process of mastering this approach. We present a step by step approach of the "UCL technique of Retzius Sparing Robot Assisted Radical Prostatectomy".

UCL Technique of Retzius Sparing Robot Assisted Radical Prostatectomy

Positioning and Port Placement

The patient is placed under general anesthesia in a steep Trendelenburg position. Initial access to the peritoneum is obtained via the open Hasson's technique where the first 8 mm camera port goes in, just above the umbilicus. We administer the Transverse Abdominis Plane (TAP) block under direct vision in between the transverse abdominis muscle and the fascial layer superficial to it. This aims at anaesthetizing the nerves supplying the anterior abdominal wall (T6 to L1) and reducing the pain post operatively. Three additional 8 mm robotic ports, a 5 and 12 mm additional assistant ports are placed. The robotic ports are placed at the level of the umbilicus, the 5 mm port between the camera and the right robotic port and the 12 mm port two finger breadths above the right anterior superior iliac spine. We use Air Seal device for all our cases, which is connected to the special 12 mm assistant port. The right robotic arm mounts the monopolar curved scissors, while the two left robotic arms use the Maryland bipolar forceps and the Prograsp forceps from medial to lateral.

Posterior Access

The surgery begins with dividing any adhesions of the sigmoid colon if present. The peritoneum is divided posterior to the bladder and access is gained posterior to the bladder (Fig. 23.1). The first structures to be encountered are the vas deferens. Bilateral vas deferens are identified by dividing the overlying fat, and once both the vas have been identified meeting in the center, the right vas is divided (Fig. 23.2). This ensures avoidance of any iatrogenic injuries to the ureter and confusing the ureter for the vas. The assistant holds the divided vas with a retractor inserted from the 12 mm port and retracts it to the opposite side. This exposes the right seminal vesicle situated posterolateral to the vas. The right seminal vesicle is mobilized with blunt dissections medially in the avascular plane between the vesicles and the Denonvilliers fascia posteriorly. Having mobilized medially, the pedicles of the vesicles are dissected laterally, clipped and divided. Care is taken not to use electrocautery near the tips of the vesicles as the caver-

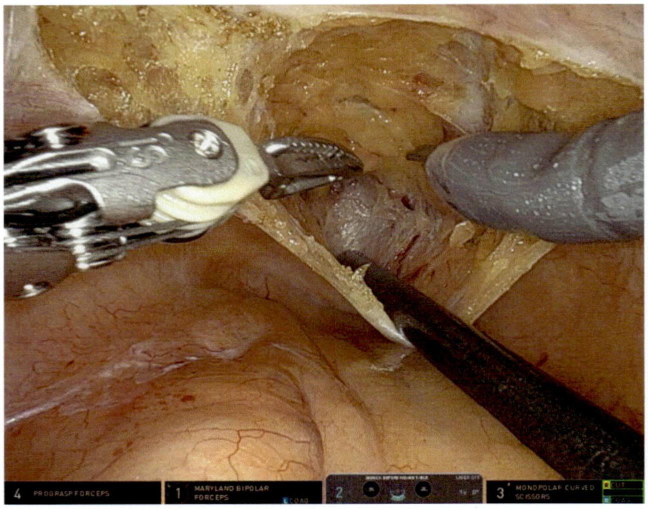

Fig. 23.1 Incision of the posterior peritoneum

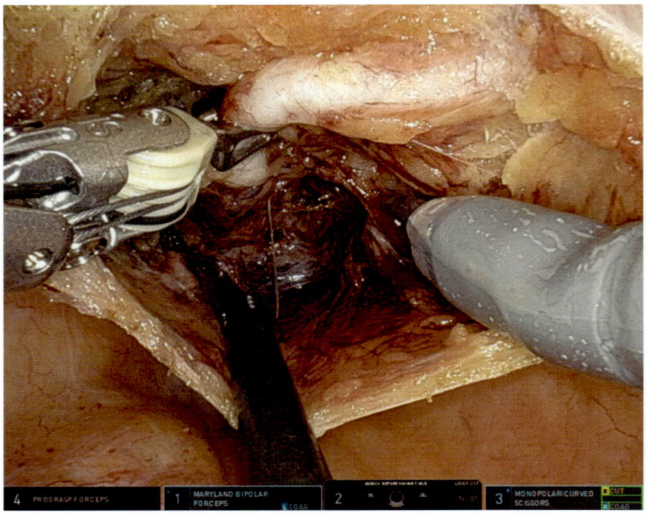

Fig. 23.2 Isolation of the right vas deferens

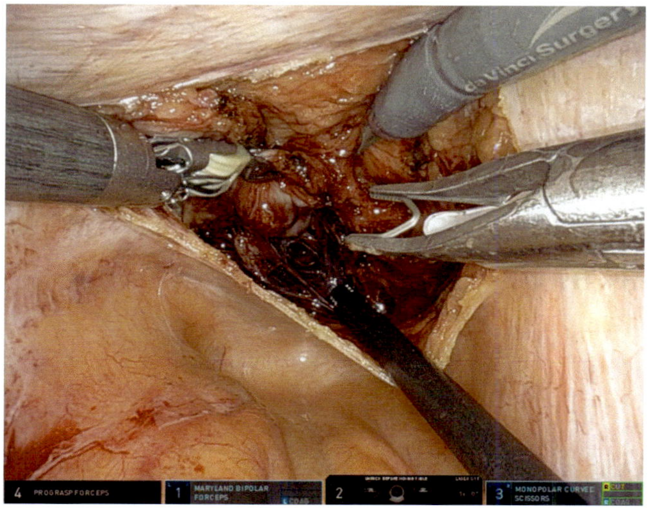

Fig. 23.3 Dissection of the right seminal vesicle tip and clipping of pedicles to seminal vesicle

nosal nerves traverse very close (Fig. 23.3). Having clipped all the vessels laterally and dividing them cold, the right vas and vesicle are completely mobilized off the Denonvilliers fascia posteriorly and the attachments laterally. The left vas and seminal vesicles are dissected and mobilized in a similar fashion.

Dissection Posterior to the Prostate

Depending on the level of nerve spare, dissection is carried further caudally behind the seminal vesicles by sharply dividing the Denonvilliers fascia. Extrafascial dissection proceeds between the Denonvilliers fascia anteriorly and the pre rectal fat posteriorly. Interfascial dissection proceeds between the prostatic fascia and the Denonvilliers fascia, with the assistant retracting the tough Denonvilliers fascia posteriorly with the sucker inserted through the 5 mm port, the left hand Maryland retracting the prostate anteriorly. Dissection is carried on till the apex of the prostate caudally (Fig. 23.4).

Prostatic Pedicles and Lateral Dissection

The prostatic pedicles are dissected out next and clipped with Hem-o-lok clips and divided cold (Figs. 23.5 and 23.6). The Prograsp forceps retracts the prostate medially, Maryland retracts the bladder up and the scissors dissects the prostate laterally preserving the neurovascular bundles. The bladder is slowly dissected off the prostate. Dissection proceeds from lateral to medial, with the bladder being dissected off the lateral and anterior surface of prostate (Figs. 23.7 and 23.8).

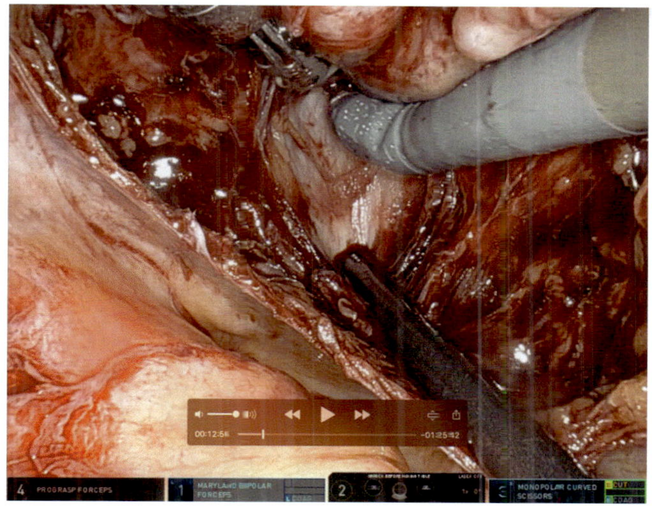

Fig. 23.4 Dissection of the posterior plane

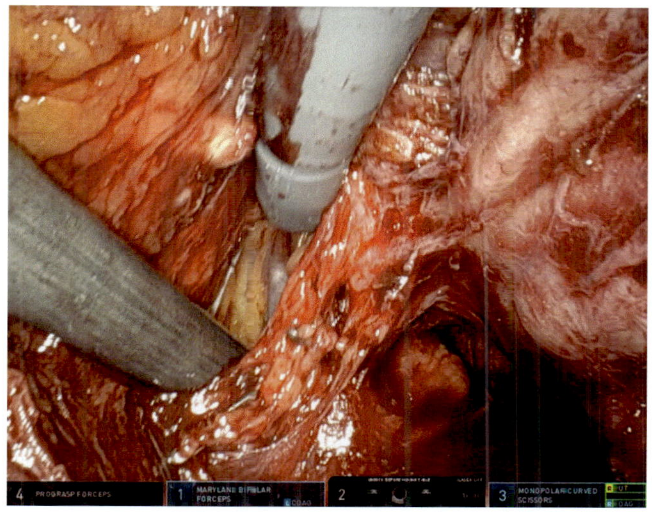

Fig. 23.5 Wide dissection of the left pedicle

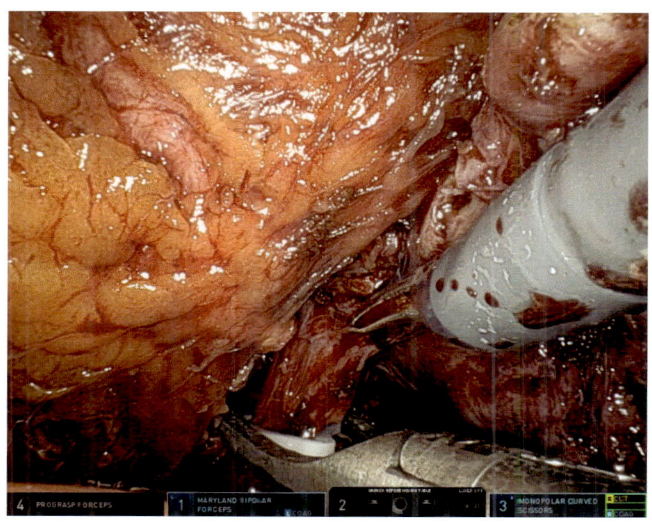

Fig. 23.6 Wide excision of the left pedicle using Hem-o-lok clips

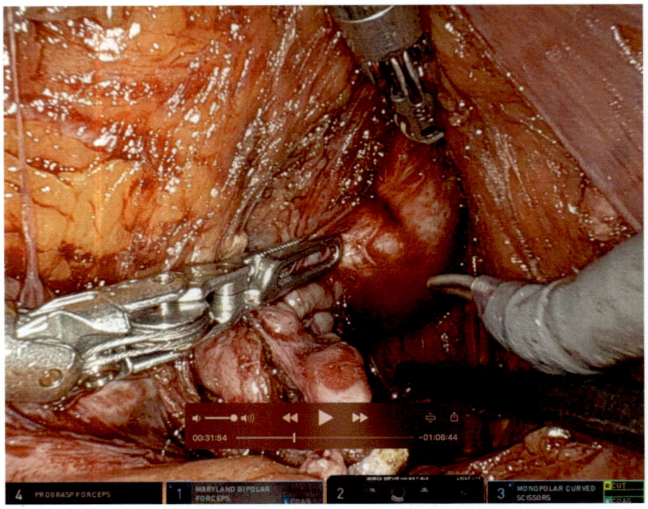

Fig. 23.7 Nerve-sparing dissection on the right side

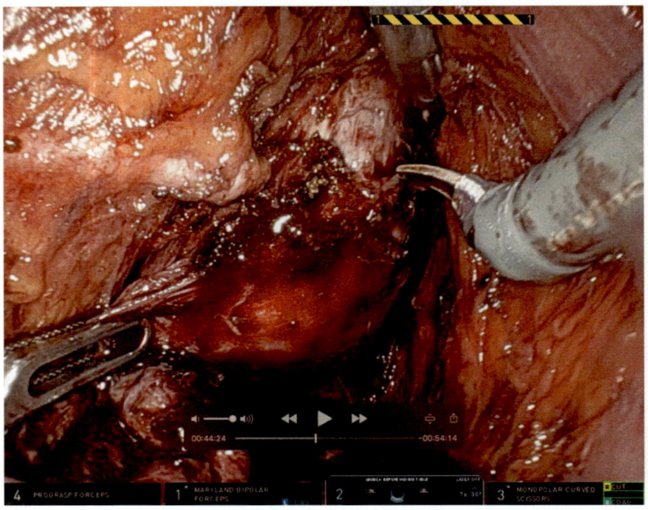

Fig. 23.8 Circumferential dissection completed laterally on the right side

Bladder Neck and Anterior Dissection

Having completed the lateral dissection, the prostatovesical junction is next approached. The urethra is slowly delineated by dividing the detrusor slips between the bladder and the prostate in the midline (Fig. 23.9). Most of the time, it is fairly easy to preserve the bladder neck if the urethra has been delineated well. Urethra is divided using electrocautery and the catheter is pulled back to reveal the anterior prostatovesical junction (Fig. 23.10). Having divided the bladder neck, the dissection proceeds anteriorly between the bladder and the anterior surface of the prostate till the apex of the prostate.

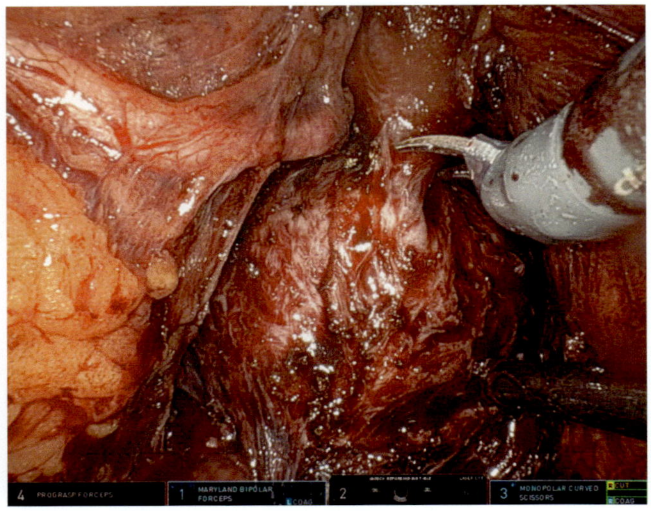

Fig. 23.9 Bladder neck sparing dissection

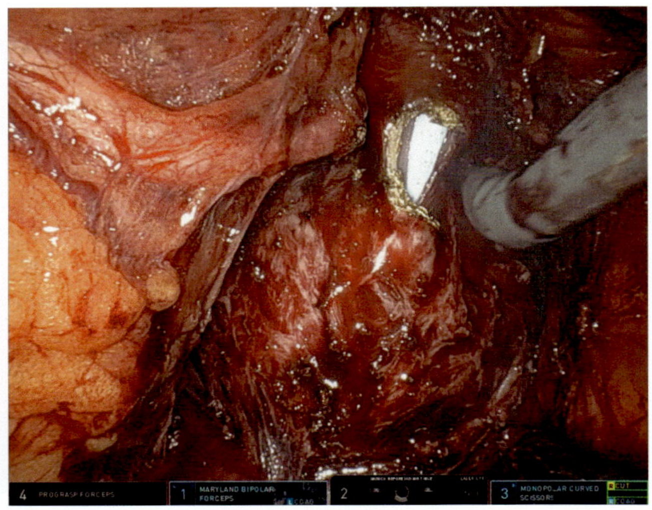

Fig. 23.10 Urethral dissection

Apex and Urethra

The dorsal venous complex (DVC) hugs the apex of the prostate closely. It is possible altogether to avoid dividing the DVC and go beneath the veins while approaching the apex. The prostate is moved side to side and the apex is approached laterally to avoid cutting through the prostate or a possible rectal injury. The urethra is dissected out and the apex is divided cold to avoid any thermal injuries to the sphincter (Figs. 23.11 and 23.12). Any posterior attachments remaining are divided and the prostate along with the seminal vesicles and vas is excised as one specimen and bagged.

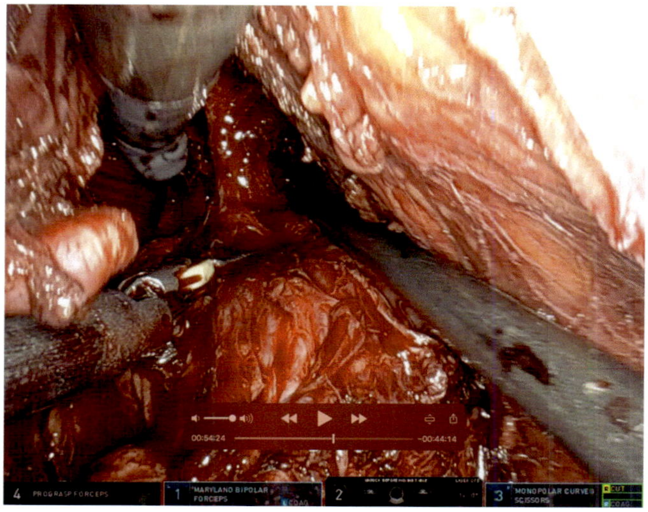

Fig. 23.11 Dorsal venous complex dissection

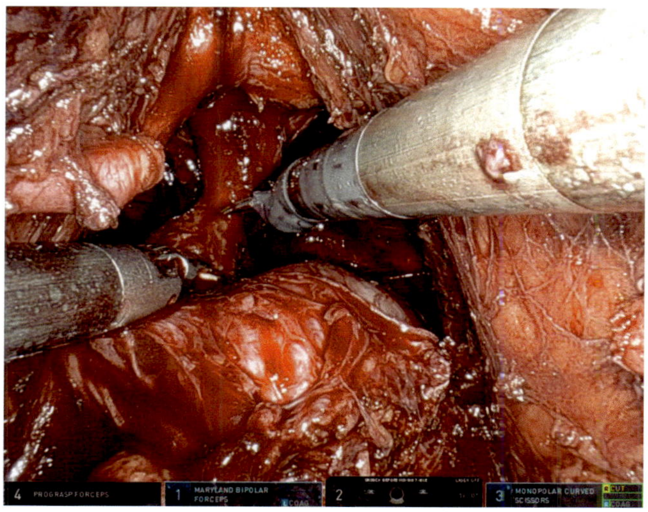

Fig. 23.12 Apical dissection

Vesicourethral Anastomosis

Anastomosis starts at 12 o'clock position outside in on the bladder, ensuring full thickness of the bladder wall along with the mucosa being incorporated in the stitch. We generally use the 3-0 gold V-Loc sutures with a 17 mm 3/8 needle, four of which are required in the complete anastomosis (Fig. 23.13). The direction of the sutures are changed at 3 and 9 o'clock position to inside out on the bladder to facilitate the ease of suturing. The urethral catheter is used to show the lumen of the urethra and to ensure the urethral mucosa is incorporated in the stitches. A final 16 Fr catheter is placed once the anastomosis is completed and the integrity of the sutures are tested by filling up the bladder with 300 ml of saline.

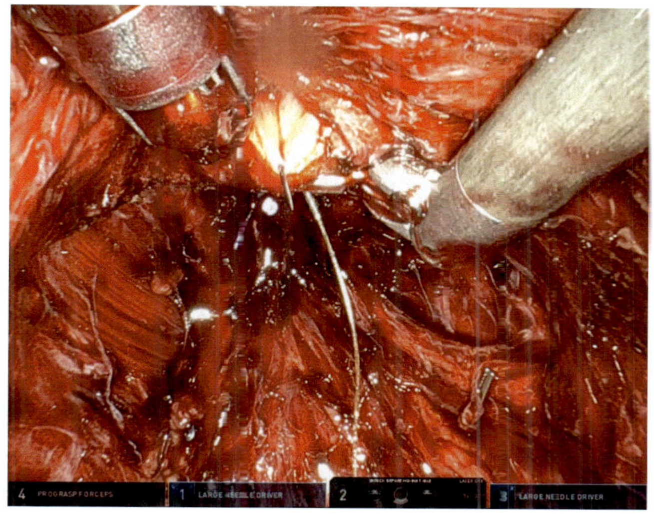

Fig. 23.13 Start of the vesico-urethral anastomosis

Conclusion

The Retzius sparing approach to robot assisted radical prostatectomy is an oncologically safe and technically feasible approach which offers excellent immediate functional outcomes, based on preservation of the anterior supports of the bladder and the urethra.

References

1. Binder J, Kramer W. Robotically-assisted laparoscopic radical prostatectomy. BJU Int. 2001;87(4):408–10.
2. Bianco FJ Jr, Scardino PT, Eastham JA. Radical prostatectomy: long-term cancer control and recovery of sexual and urinary function ("trifecta"). Urology. 2005;66(5):83–94.
3. Patel VR, Coelho RF, Palmer KJ, Rocco B. Periurethral suspension stitch during robot-assisted laparoscopic radical prostatectomy: description of the technique and continence outcomes. Eur Urol. 2009;56(3):472–8.
4. Menon M, Shrivastava A, Bhandari M, Satyanarayana R, Siva S, Agarwal PK. Vattikuti Institute prostatectomy: technical modifications in 2009. Eur Urol. 2009;56(1):89–96.
5. Pasticier G, Rietbergen JB, Guillonneau B, Fromont G, Menon M, Vallancien G. Robotically assisted laparoscopic radical prostatectomy: feasibility study in men. Eur Urol. 2001;40(1):70–4.
6. Menon M, Hemal AK, VIP Team. Vattikuti Institute prostatectomy: a technique of robotic radical prostatectomy: experience in more than 1000 cases. J Endourol. 2004;18(7):611–9.
7. Galfano A, Di Trapani D, Sozzi F, Strada E, Petralia G, Bramerio M, Ascione A, Gambacorta M, Bocciardi AM. Beyond the learning curve of the Retzius-sparing approach for robot-assisted laparoscopic radical prostatectomy: oncologic and functional results of the first 200 patients with ≥1 year of follow-up. Eur Urol. 2013;64(6):974–80.
8. Lim SK, Kim KH, Shin TY, Han WK, Chung BH, Hong SJ, Choi YD, Rha KH. Retzius-sparing robot-assisted laparoscopic radical prostatectomy: combining the best of retropubic and perineal approaches. BJU Int. 2014;114(2):236–44.

9. Dalela D, Jeong W, Prasad MA, Sood A, Abdollah F, Diaz M, Karabon P, Sammon J, Jamil M, Baize B, Simone A. A pragmatic randomized controlled trial examining the impact of the Retzius-sparing approach on early urinary continence recovery after robot-assisted radical prostatectomy. Eur Urol. 2017;72(5):677–85.
10. Umari P, Eden C, Cahill D, Rizzo M, Eden D, Sooriakumaran P. Retzius-sparing versus standard robot-assisted radical prostatectomy: a comparative prospective study of nearly 500 patients. J Urol. 2021;205(3):780–90.

Part VII

Extraperitoneal RALP

Robot-Assisted Radical Prostatectomy: The Extraperitoneal Approach and the Future with Single Port

24

Thomas L. Osinski and Jean V. Joseph

Introduction

The wide adoption of robot-assisted radical prostatectomy (RARP) has made surgical prostatectomies safe and effective with short hospital stays [1]. Furthermore, RARP has been associated with decreased complications when compared to other surgical approaches [2]. This has led to RARP becoming the standard of care in the surgical management of localized prostate cancer at a number of centers. To date, hundreds of thousands of radical prostatectomies have been performed since the approval of the first-generation robot in 2000. There have been several generations of robots used to perform radical prostatectomies aimed at improving outcomes, while decreasing the associated invasiveness of open radical prostatectomies.

While open radical prostatectomy, the previously accepted standard surgical approach, was performed using an extraperitoneal (EP) approach, RARP is most often performed using a transperitoneal approach. The learning curve associated with the creation of the EP space laparoscopically and port placement difficulty have been cited as reasons for its decreased popularity [3]. Multiport EP surgery requires lateral dissection of the EP space to allow lateral robotic and assistant ports placement. The Single-Port (SP) robot however, only requires placement of a midline port in the space of Retzius. Several centers including our own have embarked on SP RARP with encouraging results [4].

In this chapter we review the EP approach to the RARP, which has been our preferred route, in the surgical management of organ confined prostate cancer. Our institution has been performing EP RARP with every robot generation available. The latest da Vinci SP system lends itself to the EP technique, and will potentially lead to increased adoption of the EP approach. Herein, we describe our experience at the University of Rochester Medical Center (URMC) with the EP approach to RARP on the multiport, and the alterations required to perform the procedure using the SP platform. We also review key differences between the multiport and SP RARP experience.

The URMC EP Approach to the RARP

Preoperative and Perioperative Considerations

All patients undergo pre-surgical screening by our anesthesia colleagues to ensure that anesthesia can be administered safely.

We do not have patients undergo bowel prep prior to RARP, except in patients undergoing salvage procedures. Just prior to being brought to the operating room 5000 U of low molecular weight heparin is injected subcutaneously. If the patient has a positive urine culture prior to surgery, culture specific antibiotic therapy is started several days prior to surgery, which is continued throughout the perioperative period. For routine antibiotic surgical prophylaxis, we prefer to give a cephalosporin antibiotic if there is not an allergy to prohibit administration. We ask our anesthesia colleagues to give less than 1.5–2 L of intravenous fluids until the vesicourethral anastomosis (VUA) is completed to avoid saturating the surgical field with urine. With the bladder neck transected, the field can be flooded with urine, which can slow down the procedure, particularly the anastomosis.

Operative Procedure

The following section outlines our technique of the EP RARP with caveats noted when the technique is altered to accommodate the SP platform. We currently use the da Vinci Xi and da Vinci SP surgical systems.

T. L. Osinski · J. V. Joseph (✉)
Department of Urology, University of Rochester Medical Center, Rochester, NY, USA
e-mail: thomas_osinski@urmc.rochester.edu; jean_joseph@urmc.rochester.edu

S. Ren et al. (eds.), *Robot-Assisted Radical Prostatectomy*, https://doi.org/10.1007/978-3-031-05855-4_24

Patient Positioning and Set Up

Patient positioning is critical as improper positioning may contribute to postoperative morbidity. Patients are placed in the supine position over a bean bag. Sequential compression devices (SCDs) are placed on the patient's calves upon arrival to the operating room. General anesthesia is administered and placement of additional intravenous access is performed as necessary. Egg crate protective foam is placed under bony prominences in contact with the surgical bed to prevent pressure injuries. The patient's arms are tucked. A rectal examination is performed to ensure adequate clinical staging, and proper surgical planning with respect to extent of nerve sparing. The abdomen is shaved. Using a vacuum, the beanbag is activated while wrapping the beanbag over the patient's shoulders to prevent sliding when the patient is placed in the Trendelenburg position. We clean and prep the patient with a chlorhexidine scrub from just below the patient's ribs down to the upper thighs with the genitals prepped in the operative field. We drape the patient with the penis in the operative field. A 16 F Foley catheter is placed, the bladder is emptied, and 10 cc of water is placed in the Foley balloon. The patient is placed in a mild (10–15°) Trendelenburg position.

EP Access and Trocar Placement

A Hasson "cut-down" technique is used to gain access to the EP space. Just inferior to the umbilicus, an approximately 3 cm vertical incision is made. We use a combination of blunt dissection and electrocautery until we reach the anterior rectus sheath (Fig. 24.1). The anterior rectus sheath is incised sharply (Fig. 24.2) by making a 1 cm incision and then placing a stay suture. The stay suture is used for retraction to aid in identifying the posterior rectus sheath. Bluntly, the rectus muscle is partially freed from the posterior rectus sheath to facilitate passage of a balloon dilator trocar (Fig. 24.3). This trocar is passed under direct visualization using a 0° laparoscope (a laparoscope is used at this time as the robotic camera can be difficult to manipulate due to the length and weight of the scope). The balloon is inflated under direct vision to create the EP space. Placing a fist over the left lower quadrant during inflation of the balloon can help ensure creation of a symmetric space by varying pressure on the left lower quadrant as the balloon expands. Over inflation should be avoided to lessen the risk of bleeding from the iliac or epigastric vessels, or creating a compromising peritoneal rent. After creating the EP space the external iliacs, the pubic bone and the epigastric arteries should be easily visible.

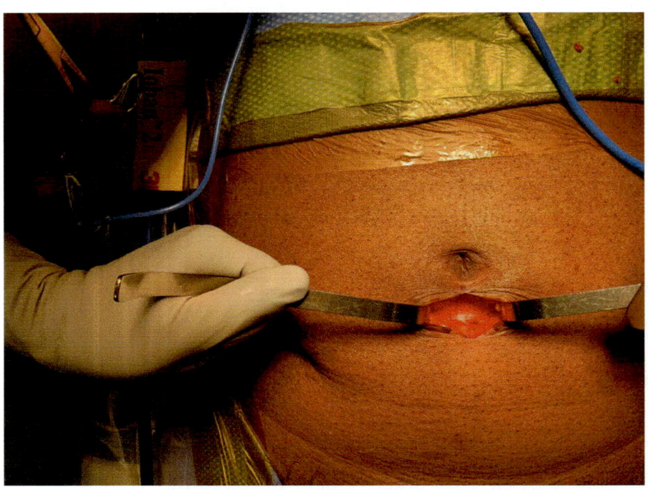

Fig. 24.1 An incision is made just inferior to the umbilicus and the dissection is carried to the anterior rectus sheath as visualized in this image (this patient is status post open appendectomy)

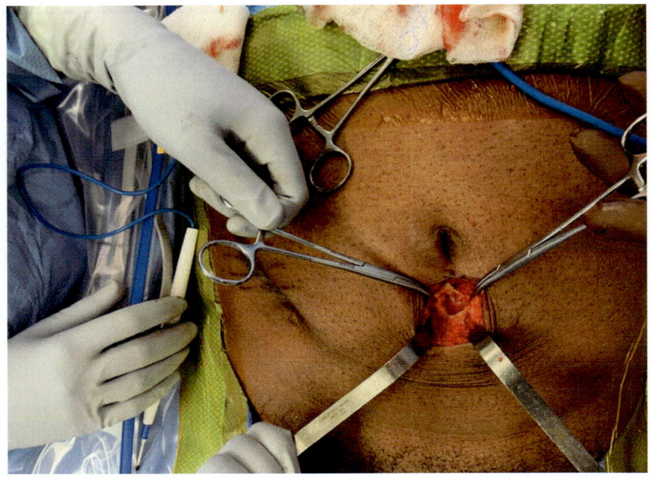

Fig. 24.2 The anterior rectus sheath is incised so a balloon dilator can be placed into the space of Retzius. It is critical to only incise the anterior rectus sheath as incising the posterior rectus sheath will result in entry into the peritoneal space

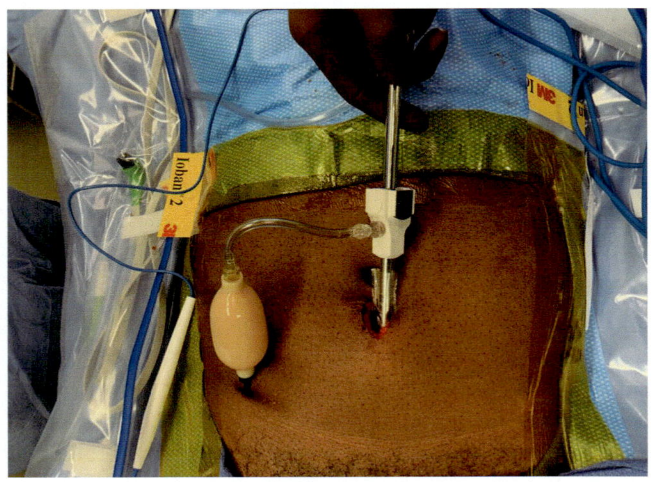

Fig. 24.3 The balloon dilator trocar is passed through the anterior rectus sheath incision into the space of Retzius. The laparoscope is being held by the surgeon's right hand. The balloon dilator is insufflated by hand using the pump connected to the balloon dilator trocar

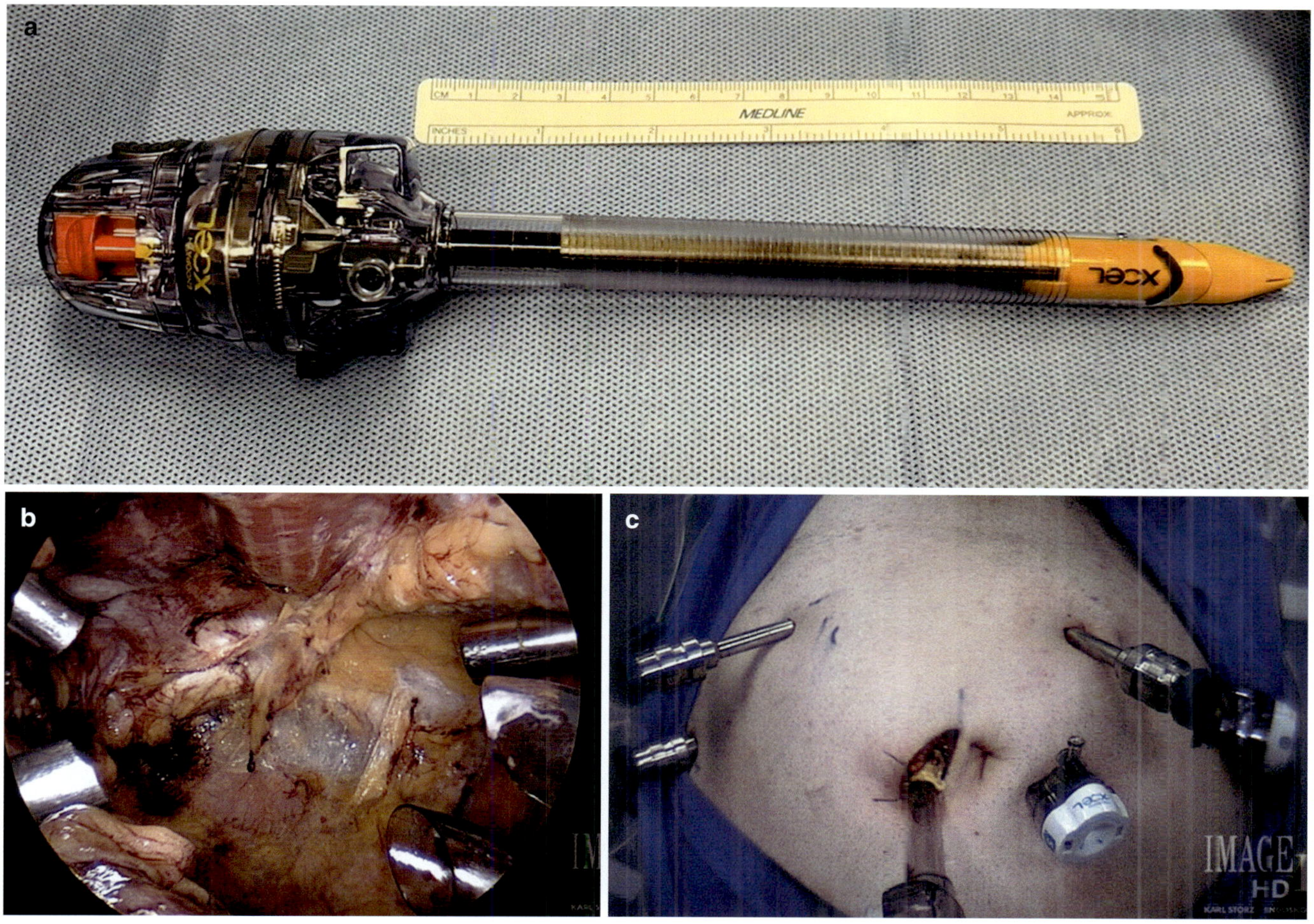

Fig. 24.4 When using multiport robotic platforms the EP space must be maximized for optimal placement of the robotic trocars and assistant ports to minimize collision of the robotic arms. The 10/12 mm 512 XD Ethicon trocar is used to dissect the extraperitoneal space laterally (**a**). Internal (**b**) and external (**c**) view of port placement configured for Si robot. (For Xi robot, the midline trocar is replaced by a 12 mm stapler cannula to accommodate robotic arm used for camera)

If performing surgery with the Xi system, a 10/12 long smooth trocar (Fig. 24.4a) with a bevel is placed in the EP space and insufflation with CO_2 is maintained at a pressure of 15 mmHg. With the multiport robot it is necessary to expand the extraperitoneal space laterally to accommodate the robotic and the assistant trocars (Fig. 24.4b, c). The smooth trocar is critical as it allows us to further develop the EP space by using the beveled edge of the smooth trocar to free the peritoneum cephalad from the transversalis fascia with care taken to avoid inadvertent entry into the peritoneal space. Developing the EP space further as described allows for trocar placement with appropriate distance between each robotic arm and assistant ports while only remaining in EP space. Creating this space is essential when using a multiport robot as appropriate spacing between the robotic ports prevents collision of the robotic arms while maintaining an adequate working space.

The first trocar is placed while the balloon dilator is still in place (Fig. 24.5).

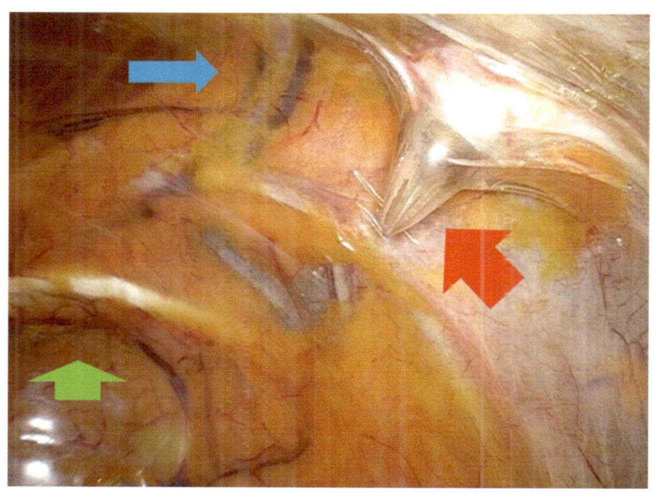

Fig. 24.5 The assistant trocar is being placed while the balloon dilator remains inflated in the EP space. The red arrow is pointing to the assistant trocar being placed the blue arrow is highlighting the epigastric vessels, and the green arrow is pointing to the pubic bone

Each subsequent trocar is placed under direct vision. A 12 mm assistant trocar is inserted in the left or right lower quadrant approximately 2 cm anteromedial to the anterior superior iliac spine (ASIS). We use a hypodermic needle to identify the inferior epigastric vessels so that the left and right 8 mm robotic trocars can be inserted while avoiding injury to these vessels. We place these 8 mm ports 8–10 cm from the camera port on a line between the umbilicus and ASIS. The fourth 8 mm robotic trocar is placed approximately 2 cm anteromedial to the ASIS, opposite to the assistant. Lastly, a 5 mm trocar is placed between the camera port and the most medial port on the same side as the assistant port, to serve as an additional assistant port. To prevent CO_2 leakage at the midline trocar or camera entry site, and maintain insufflation, we use a 12 mm stapler cannula given the larger fascial opening. Additionally, a xeroform gauze is placed around the camera trocar. A suture is used to narrow the fascial opening around the trocar. In older robot generations, the same trocar used to dissect the extraperitoneal space is used for the camera as noted in the external view configuration below.

If performing surgery with the SP system, we enter the retropubic space in the midline approximately 5 cm from the umbilicus. The balloon dilator is used as described above to develop the EP space. However, the lateral dissection required when using the multiport robot is not needed as all the robotic arms are deployed from the single port site. The port is "air docked" to provide adequate working space and deploy the robotic arms with elbows. We use either the Gel Point mini, or the da Vinci SP Access Port. The associated wound protector is inserted in the space of Retzius after extending the fascial incision to 3–4 cm. When the GelPoint Mini is used, a 2.5 cm metal trocar is placed through the Gel Point along with other accessory ports. Instruments such as a suction cannula can be inserted directly through the gel without a trocar. We routinely "air dock" when using the Gel Point to facilitate internal triangulation of the robotic arms. When using the da Vinci SP Access Port, floating of the wound protector, or "air docking" is not necessary (Fig. 24.6). The Access Port is designed to float and allows for easy visualization of the robotic arms upon their entry through the instrument guide. Furthermore, the SP Access Port allows easy removal of the specimen from the working space without losing insufflation. If a "plus one" approach is used, an 8- or 12-mm port is placed medial to the epigastric vessels. We routinely insert this trocar directly into the inflated balloon as previously demonstrated.

Next, we dock the da Vinci patient cart to the trocars. We use a da Vinci camera (0° if using the Xi system or EndoWrist SP camera with COBRA action if using the SP system). We also use monopolar scissors, a bipolar grasper, and the cardiere forceps.

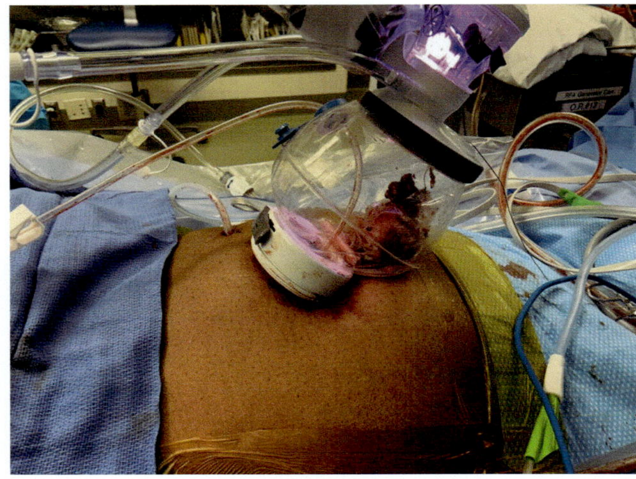

Fig. 24.6 The da Vinci SP Access Port with prostatectomy specimen. The drain in this photo was placed through the "plus one" port site

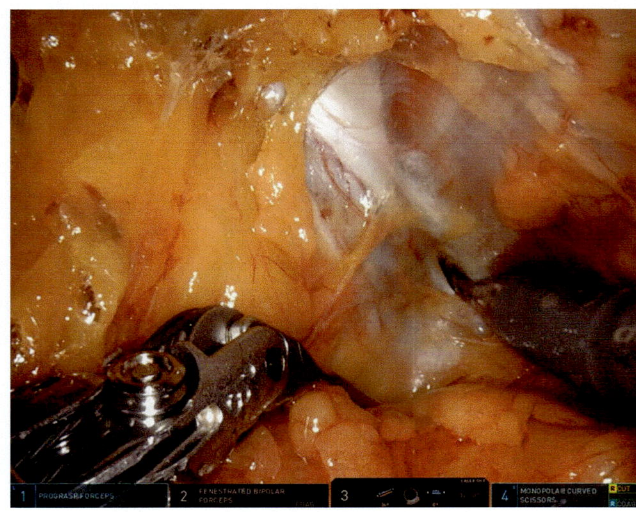

Fig. 24.7 The endopelvic fascia on the right side of the prostate is being incised just lateral to the prostate. The levator ani is seen lateral to the tips to the scissors

Subsequent operative steps of RARP are common to both the multiport and SP platforms. Of note, the EP RARP is performed via an anterior approach whereby the seminal vesicle dissection is performed after bladder neck dissection. The posterior approach to the seminal vesicles cannot be performed as the EP RARP is completed without entering the peritoneum.

Endopelvic Fascia Dissection

Lateral to the prostate, the endopelvic fascia should be easily visible. At times fatty connective tissue needs to be removed in order to visualize the fascia adequately. Just lateral to the prostate, the endopelvic fascia is incised (Fig. 24.7). A sweeping motion is used to push the levator ani muscle off the prostate. Occasionally, sharp dissection or electrocautery is needed to aid dissection as prostatic inflammation can cause the pelvic floor muscles to adhere to the prostatic capsule. Care should be taken to avoid violation of the prostate capsule laterally, or Santorini's plexus anteriorly (which can also be associated with bleeding). This dissection is brought caudally to a "notch" between the urethra and dorsal venous complex (DVC). The puboprostatic ligaments are cut close to the prostate to keep some of their pelvic floor support but facilitate suture ligation of the DVC.

Dorsal Vessel Complex Ligation

A barbed 2/0 V-Lok™ suture with a SH needle is passed through the "notch" between the DVC and urethra in a figure of eight fashion by suspending the stitch to the periosteum of the pubic bone. The DVC suture is secured with surgical clip (Fig. 24.8). Excess suture is left so the suture can be tightened if the suture slips. It is important to pass the figure of eight suture as distal to the apex as possible to ensure negative apical margins and to facilitate apical dissection.

Bladder Neck Dissection

Care with the bladder neck dissection is critical as too large of a bladder neck can be associated with postoperative incontinence, while following a bad plane can lead to positive margins on final pathology. We identify the initial dissection plane by tugging on the Foley and pressing on the bladder on each side of the prostate to identify the plane between prostate and bladder (Fig. 24.9). We then use a "burn and push" technique to develop the plane on either side carrying it to the midline. The "burn and push" technique allows us to follow a plane between the prostate and bladder and the visualization afforded by this technique gives us considerable control of the entire dissection. The anterior bladder neck is incised in the midline at which point the Foley catheter can be observed. The Foley can be retracted toward the pubic bone to facilitate further dissection. Once we transect the posterior bladder neck, the anterior layer of Denonvillier's fascia is now exposed. Incising Denonvillier's fascia should expose the vas deferens and the seminal vesicles.

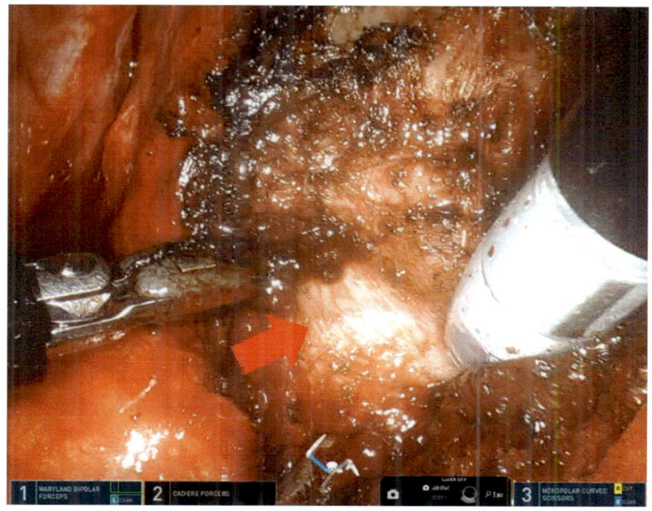

Fig. 24.9 The "burn and push" technique is being utilized to facilitate the bladder neck dissection. The red arrow is showing the bladder neck dissection plane

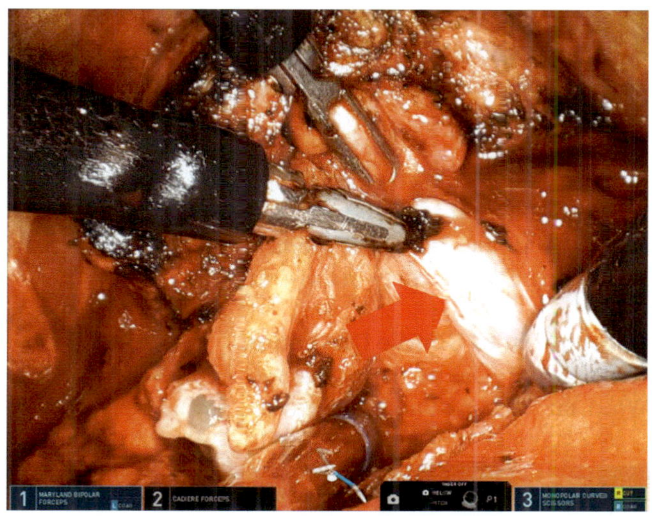

Fig. 24.10 The red arrow in this photo is the medial portion of a partially skeletonized seminal vesicle. The vas and seminal vesicle are being retracted anterior and cranially while the scissors dissect laterally to create a vascular pedicle that will be clipped

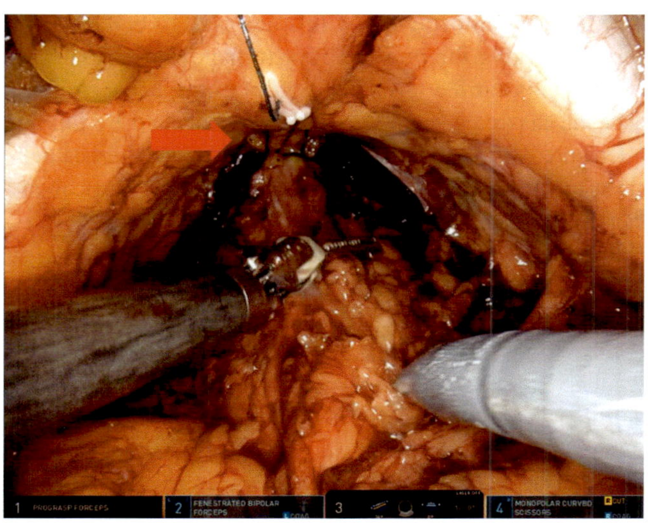

Fig. 24.8 Red arrow pointing towards figure of eight DVC suture suspended to the pubic bone

Vas Deferens and Seminal Vesicle Dissection

This is a challenging part of the dissection as it occurs essentially in a hole and electrocautery should be avoided to prevent damage to the laterally coursing neurovascular bundles, thus retraction is essential. First the vas deferens is dissected distal to the ampulla. The vas deferens are divided between Hem-o-Lok clips. Next, we skeletonize the seminal vesicles, freeing it from the overlying blood vessels (Fig. 24.10).

The grasping forceps are used to retract the seminal vesicle towards the contralateral shoulder (anterior and cranially). For example, the left seminal vesicle should be retracted toward the right shoulder. The dissection starts from the medial aspect of the seminal vesicle and carried laterally as the medial portion of the seminal vesicles is avascular which allows for creation of vascular pedicles. The vascular pedicles that are created can then be easily clipped laterally with Hem-o-lok clips and then sharply divided. Done well, each seminal vesicle will require about three clips for vascular control.

Incision of Denonvillier's Fascia and Posterior Dissection

Once the seminal vesicles are dissected free, the grasping forceps are used to retract the vas deferens and seminal vesicles anteriorly to facilitate dissection (Fig. 24.11). We incise the posterior layer of Denonvillier's fascia starting in the midline close to the prostate to avoid rectal injuries. A plane is then developed between the prostate anteriorly and the rectum posteriorly. We develop this plane mostly bluntly while pushing the rectum down and minimizing electrocautery to avoid rectal injuries. The dissection is carried distally toward the apex.

Securing the Prostatic Pedicle

We control the prostate pedicles with Hem-o-lok clips. To avoid inadvertent damage to the neurovascular bundles we avoid using electrocautery in this area.

Neurovascular Bundle Dissection

The ultimate goal of the procedure is cancer eradication. When the cancer parameters, and the prostate exam under

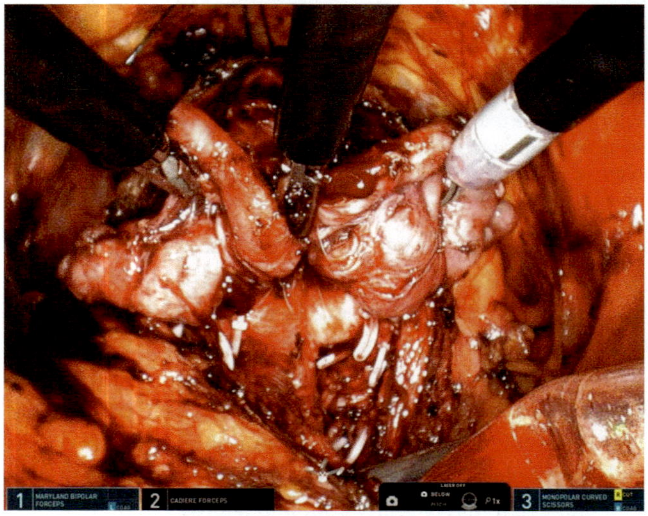

Fig. 24.11 Retraction of the vas deferens and seminal vesicles anteriorly which will help with visualization and facilitate the posterior dissection

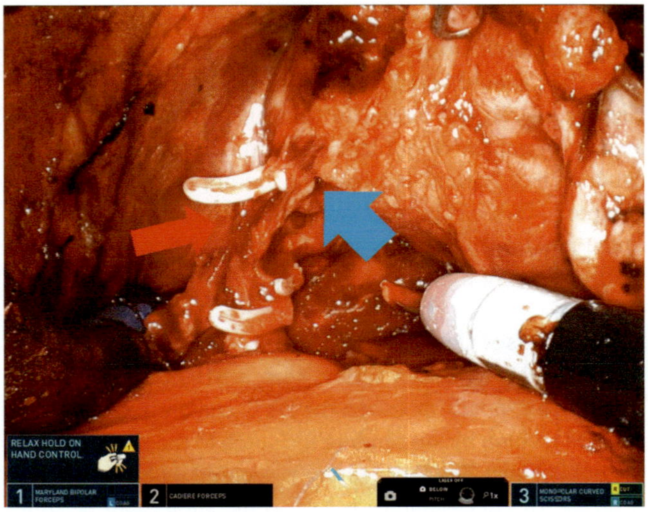

Fig. 24.12 The red arrow is pointing to the left neurovascular bundle that has been dissected free of the prostatic capsule. The blue arrow shows the dissection place between the neurovascular bundle and periprostatic fascia. Note the prostate being retracted anteriorly and slightly to the right to facilitate dissection

anesthesia suggest a low likelihood of extraprostatic disease, we routinely perform a nerve sparing approach. When aggressive cancer is present, we avoid sparing the neurovascular bundle. We often send frozen sections from the periprostatic tissues near the neurovascular bundles to ensure a cancer free dissection plane. When the bundles are spared, the prostate pedicles are selectively clipped while avoiding injury to the adjacent bundles. The prograsp is used to retract the prostate anteriorly, and opposite to the side being dissected (Fig. 24.12). We prefer a combination of antegrade and retrograde dissection. The latter is used to facilitate appropriate visualization and dissection of the bundles coursings posterolaterally. We use scissors to incise the lateral prostatic fascia. The neurovascular bundle is gently dissected from the prostatic capsule. Clips are used to control large vessels entering the prostate prior to their transection. This dissection is carried to the apex. If bleeding is encountered over the dissected bundles, it can be controlled by placing Interrupted 4-0 Vicryl sutures. We avoid using electrocautery close to the neurovascular bundles to prevent electrical and thermal injuries.

Apical Dissection

The previously secured DVC is incised using electrocautery. A plane between the prostatic apex and urethra is created. We then expose and sharply incise the anterior urethra a few millimeters from the prostatic apex. Care should be taken to avoid injuring the neurovascular bundle near the prostatic apex as the neurovascular bundles course anterolaterally to the apex. Once the posterior urethral wall and rectourethralis muscle are dissected, the specimen is completely freed. We then examine the specimen with careful attention to the resection margins. Additional frozen sections may be sent from the specimen if there are concerning areas.

Lymph Node Dissection (LND)

It is possible to perform a LND with the EP approach using either the da Vinci multiport or SP platforms. The difficulty of the dissection is due to the shorter working distance of the robotic arms limiting the range of motion of the robotic arms and ability to obtain optimal angles when performing the LND. Furthermore, compared to transperitoneal approaches, the assistant port is slightly more inferior and medial which also limits the ability of the assistant to place clips and retract. Despite the difficulty in performing LND with the EP approach, there does not seem to be increased rates of symptomatic lymphoceles [5]. Our dissection starts at the node of Cloquet and is carried proximally to the bifurcation of the common iliac vein. The lateral margin is over the external iliac vein and medially to the node packet below the obturator nerve and vessels. Clips and bipolar energy are used to prevent lymphatic leakage. We clip the left lymphatic packet so we can identify which side each lymphatic packet came from for pathologic analysis.

Once the LND is complete, the lymph node packets and prostate specimen are placed in a specimen retrieval bag.

Posterior Reconstruction

The posterior reconstruction is performed as there is some evidence that performing a posterior reconstruction can improve early continence after RARP [6]. Furthermore, performing the posterior reconstruction is helpful as it makes the VUA somewhat simpler as the posterior reconstruction approximates the bladder neck and urethra. This approximation also likely takes tension off the anastomosis. The posterior reconstruction is performed with two separate 3/0 9-in. V-Loc™ sutures. The first suture throw is a good bite through the posterior rhabdosphincter. The suture is then used to pull the rhabdosphincter into the pelvic cavity so that a second suture throw can be made through the posterior rhabdosphincter slightly lateral without incorporating mucosa. The suture from the first throw is then completely removed. Next, the suture is passed through Denonvillier's fascia and the posterior bladder. The suture is then placed through the loop at the end of the V-Loc™ suture. A second throw of the suture is then made more lateral to the first stitch and again incorporates the posterior rhabdosphincter, Denonvillier's fascia and the posterior bladder (Fig. 24.13). We repeat these steps with the second V-Loc™ suture starting on the opposite side of the posterior rhabdosphincter. We then cinch these sutures to approximate the bladder neck to urethra. We eventually suspend these sutures Cooper's ligament after cinching the aforementioned sutures (Fig. 24.14). Suspending these sutures to Cooper's ligament is a technical modification which helps to restore the intrapelvic position of the membranous urethra. This also may be associated with improved early return of urinary continence as the suspension provides a sling-like effect on the bladder neck which prevents the anastomosis from descending through the pelvic diaphragm.

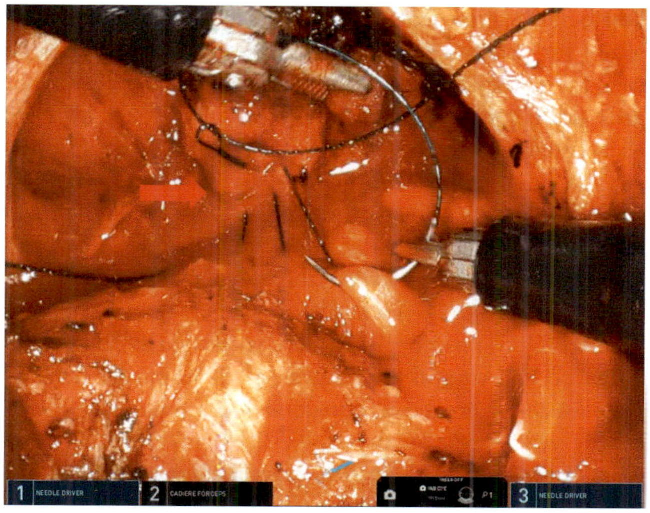

Fig. 24.13 The posterior reconstruction with the posterior rhabdosphincter being highlighted with the red arrow. The needle is currently being driven through Denonvillier's fascia prior to being incorporated into the posterior bladder

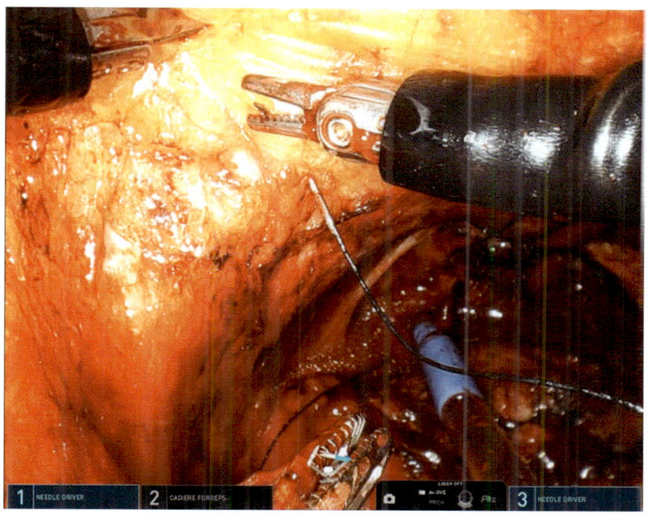

Fig. 24.14 The posterior reconstruction suture being thrown through Cooper's ligament. In this image one can appreciate the placement of the suture in relation to the endopelvic fascia and DVC suture. Note the posterior reconstruction sutures have been cinched as well to approximate the bladder to the rhabdosphincter

Vesicourethral Anastomosis

A watertight anastomosis with good approximation of the urethral and bladder mucosa is important as these measures likely help reduce the risk of bladder neck contractures [7].

Furthermore, urine leaks are a source of post-operative morbidity for patients as a urine leak may lead to prolonged need for a Foley catheter and drain. The urethra and bladder neck are approximated by running two separate 2-0 9-in. Vicryl sutures on RB-1 needles. The first throw is placed at the 5 o'clock position starting on the inside of the urethra and then placed through the bladder ending through the bladder mucosa (Fig. 24.15). The suture is then tied. We then run the suture clockwise from the 5 to 11 o'clock position. Next, we run the second suture anticlockwise from the 4 to 10 o'clock position. The suture is cinched as each suture is placed and careful attention is given to ensure there is good mucosa-to-mucosa apposition. Each suture is tied separately which provides two suture lines and avoids reliance on a single knot. If there is a large bladder neck we close some of the bladder neck by suturing bladder mucosa to bladder mucosa in the anterior midline prior to completing the VUA creating a tennis racket closure. A new 20 F 2-way Foley catheter is placed. The integrity of the anastomosis is evaluated by observing the anastomosis for leaks while the bladder is filled with 180 cc of saline. If a leak is demonstrated, additional sutures are placed to ensure its resolution. Once we are satisfied with the VUA, 15 cc of water is placed in the Foley balloon.

Drain Placement

A 19 F Blake drain is inserted through the most lateral 8 mm trocar site when performing surgery with the multiport robot. During SP "plus one" cases the 8 or 12 mm assistant port is used to place the drain. No fascial closure is absolutely necessary at the assistant port site, given its EP nature of the procedure. The drain is positioned so it is not directly over the anastomosis which may result in a urine leak.

At this point the robot is undocked after removal of instruments.

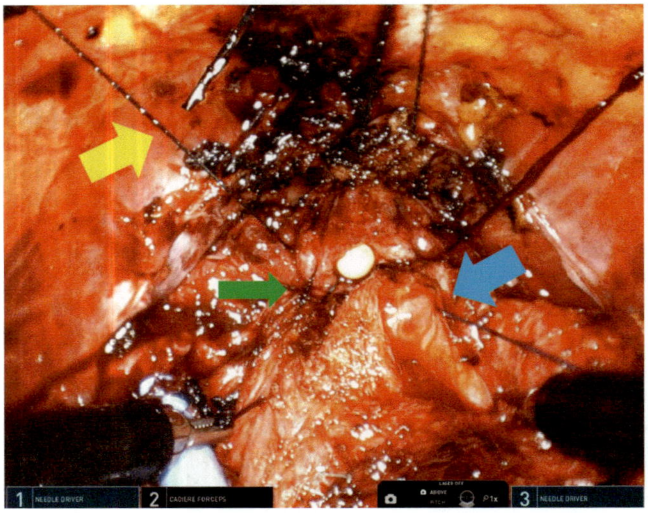

Fig. 24.15 Start of the VUA. The yellow arrow highlights the left posterior reconstruction suspension suture, the green arrow highlights the posterior reconstruction sutures, and the blue arrow is displaying placement of the first suture for the VUA. Note the approximation of the rhabdosphincter to the bladder neck with the posterior reconstruction

Specimen Extraction and Wound Closure

The patient is taken out of Trendelenburg position. With the multiport setup, the specimen bag string is transferred from the assistant's 12 mm port to the robotic 8 mm camera port. The umbilical incision is extended as needed and the specimen is extracted. With the SP setup, the specimen can often be easily removed through the robotic port site as it is approximately 3–4 cm in length. Occasionally the fascial incision needs to be extended to remove the specimen. All additional ports are taken out under direct vision to ensure there is not any significant bleeding.

Once the specimen is removed, we close the fascia with 3–4 interrupted figure of 8's using 0-polyglactin suture.

Skin incisions are closed with 4/0 Monocryl sutures (Fig. 24.16). A 3-0 silk tie is used to secure the drain to the skin. Steri strips and dressings are applied over the incision and local anesthetic is infiltrated prior to the reversal of anesthesia.

Post-operative Care

The patient is recovered in our PACU. Clear liquid diet is administered initially and diet is advanced as tolerated. Patients are ambulated the same day. If there is no significant concern for bleeding, prophylactic chemical thromboembolic prophylaxis is given with intermittent pneumatic compression with SCDs while the patient is in the hospital. We only obtain post-operative labs for clinical concerns. The morning after surgery the drain is removed if there is <100 cc of output in an 8-h shift. Almost all patients are discharged within 24 h of surgery. For straight forward cases, the Foley catheter is removed approximately 7–10 days after surgery. Patients with significant thromboembolic risks are discharged with a course of 10 days of anticoagulation.

Discussion

EP RARP remains an underutilized approach. This route avoids insufflation of the intraperitoneal space. Diaphragmatic splinting, which can cause respiratory compromise, is eliminated. Severe Trendelenburg which is often required with the transperitoneal approach is also avoided. The peritoneum serves as a natural barrier, keeping intraabdominal contents out of the operative field. Furthermore, no lysis of adhesions is necessary in patients with prior abdominal surgeries [8].

The potential advantages of the SP RARP are fewer incisions and possibly better postoperative pain control. We

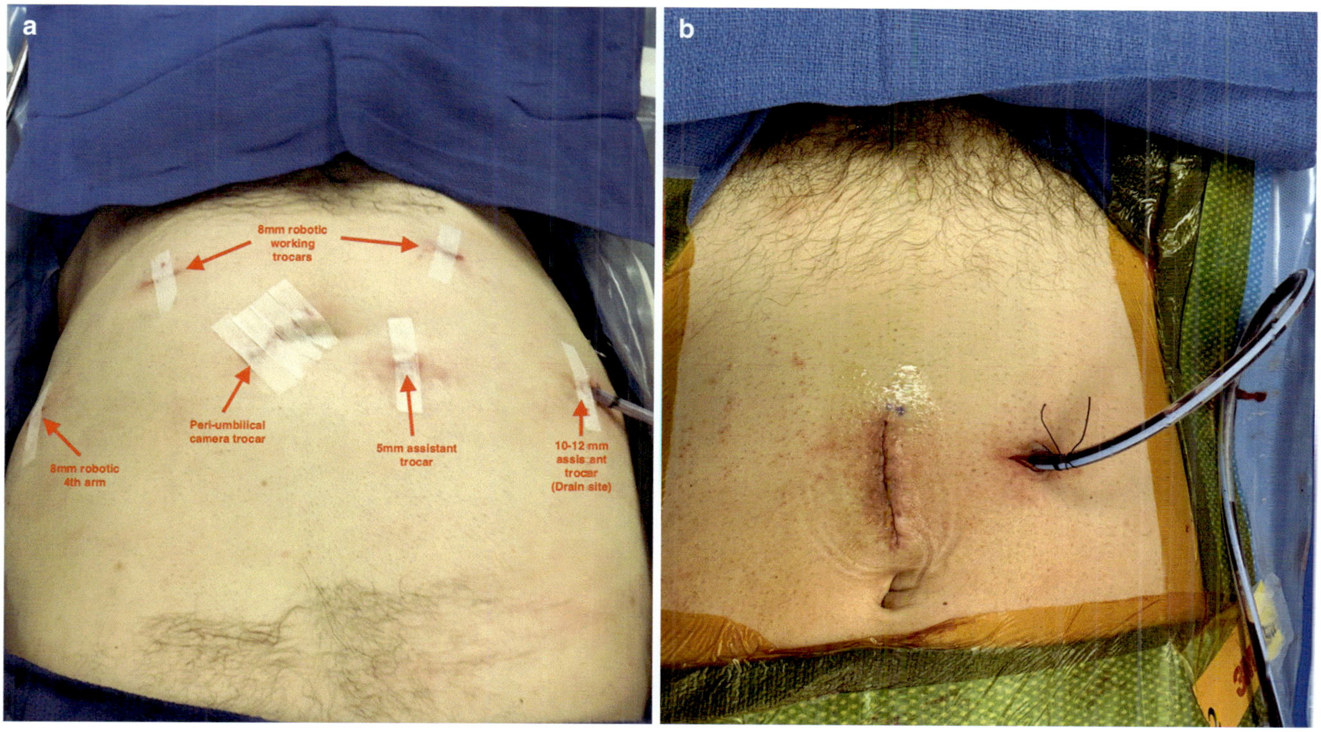

Fig. 24.16 Post-operative views post multiport (**a**) and SP "plus one" (**b**) EP RARP

expect improvement in operative times once the surgical techniques become established and there is better familiarity with the maneuverability of the SP robotic instruments. The camera does have a cobra head allowing better maneuverability, however using this capability to ease the operative procedure is not clearly evident. There are some that will use a 0° scope for the majority of a RARP and switch to a 30° down scope during the bladder neck and seminal vesicle dissections. Thus, for those who use two scopes during RARP the cobra head function of the camera could help save them time and money by providing optimal visualization without needing to change robotic scopes during the case. However, there are currently significant disadvantages of the SP system. Training is an issue for two reasons: currently training consoles are not widely available and the primary surgeon is often still working out the surgical technique and maneuverability of the robot for themselves. Furthermore, maneuverability of the robotic arms with the SP system is an issue. The instruments have an articulating elbow 2–3 cm from the wrists of the robotic instruments which allow the instruments to enter the surgical space and then move out of the view of the camera. Due to the articulating elbows, the range of motion of the instruments are reduced when compared to the multiport robot. Creation of new instruments for the SP robot may help with optimizing the surgical experience while minimizing postoperative complications.

We show in this chapter that the EP approach can be used to perform RARP using both a multiport and a SP robot. However, the EP RARP has not been widely adopted with the multiport robot. This is mainly due to the learning curve associated with the extraperitoneal space expansion laterally. This often challenging EP dissection is no longer necessary with the SP robotic system given the space created in the midline with a finger manually or with a balloon dilator is sufficient to deploy the SP. A lot of progress is on the way to further minimize invasiveness of our surgical approach to RARP. The SP access kit which has only become available in the last year is one such example. With further technological improvement, adoption of the SP robot to perform RARP will undoubtedly continue.

References

1. Yaxley JW, Coughlin GD, Chambers SK, et al. Robot-assisted laparoscopic prostatectomy versus open radical retropubic prostatectomy: early outcomes from a randomised controlled phase 3 study [published correction appears in Lancet. 2017;389(10077):e5]. Lancet. 2016;388(10049):1057–66.
2. Novara G, Ficarra V, Rosen RC, et al. Systematic review and meta-analysis of perioperative outcomes and complications after robot-assisted radical prostatectomy. Eur Urol. 2012;62(3):431–52.
3. Davis JW, Achim M, Munsell M, Matin S. Effectiveness of postgraduate training for learning extraperitoneal access for robot-assisted radical prostatectomy. J Endourol. 2011;25(8):1363–9.
4. Kaouk J, Valero R, Sawczyn G, Garisto J. Extraperitoneal single-port robot-assisted radical prostatectomy: initial experience and description of technique. BJU Int. 2020;125(1):182–9. https://doi.org/10.1111/bju.14885.

5. Horovitz D, Lu X, Feng C, Messing EM, Joseph JV. Rate of symptomatic lymphocele formation after extraperitoneal vs transperitoneal robot-assisted radical prostatectomy and bilateral pelvic lymphadenectomy. J Endourol. 2017;31(10):1037–43.
6. Rocco B, Gregori A, Stener S, Santoro L, Bozzola A, Galli S, Knez R, Scieri F, Scaburri A, Gaboardi F. Posterior reconstruction of the rhabdosphincter allows a rapid recovery of continence after transperitoneal videolaparoscopic radical prostatectomy. Eur Urol. 2007;51(4):996–1003.
7. Webb DR, Sethi K, Gee K. An analysis of the causes of bladder neck contracture after open and robot-assisted laparoscopic radical prostatectomy. BJU Int. 2009;103(7):957–63.
8. Liu S, Hemal A. Techniques of robotic radical prostatectomy for the management of prostate cancer: which one, when and why. Transl Androl Urol. 2020;9(2):906–18.

The CUF Technique: Extraperitoneal Robot-Assisted Radical Prostatectomy

25

António Pinheiro, Pedro Bargão Santos, and Estevao Lima

Introduction

Extraperitoneal approach was described for the first time in laparoscopic approach by Raboy in 1997 [1], although it was with Bollens that this technique became popular [2]. The first report of a robot assisted extraperitoneal radical prostatectomy was made by Gettman and Abbou in 2003 [3].

This approach has advantage of non-entrance in the peritoneal cavity and therefore reduces the risk of intra-abdominal organ lesions, as well as postoperative ileus. In obese patients, as this technique allows less angulation of Trendelenburg position, it might also be advantageous [4].

Technique

To the accomplishment of this surgery, a fourth arm *da Xi DaVinci® Robot system* is used.

The patient is put on dorsal supine position with its legs slightly apart or in classical *Trendelenburg* position. The operating table is with 20° on head-down tilt, to ensure better viewing of the operating, however less angulation might be used 10–20° (Fig. 25.1). The robot is on left side of the patient, lateral to its legs. The assistant is on the right side of the patient and the scrub nurse is on the left side.

After a 16Ch-*Folley* bladder drainage is in place, the surgery's first step is to create the preperitoneal space and the placement of the first trocar. An 8 mm incision is made 2 cm inferiorly and 2 cm laterally to the right of the umbilicus. A blunt dissection is preformed until the identification of the anterior rectus sheath. A horizontal incision on the anterior rectus sheath is then made and enlarged trough blunt dissection. The rectus muscle fibers are identified below and are dissected until identification of the posterior rectus sheath. Afterwards, a gentle fingertip dissection is made in the space between the rectus muscle and the posterior rectus sheath.

A balloon trocar is placed through this space, superiorly to the posterior rectus sheath, up to the pubic bone. Insufflation is done under vision control of the 3D camera system. The pubic bone and the epigastric vessels are important landmarks. After the creation of the preperitoneal space, the balloon trocar is removed and an 8 mm robot trocar is placed. Afterwards the insufflation starts and we proceed to the placement of the other trocars.

The camera is placed on the paraumbilical port and can be used to swipe of peritoneal adhesions laterally and superiorly to facilitate the other port placement.

Two pararectal robot trocars of 8 mm are placed on each side of the patient. The other 8 mm robot trocar is placed anteromedial to the left anterior iliac crest. The AirSeal® 12 mm trocar is placed anteromedial to the right anterior iliac crest (Fig. 25.2).

The robot arms are connected and the instruments are inserted under direct vision. On the right arm a round-tip scissor is placed with monopolar energy connected, on the left pararectal arm a bipolar forceps and on the lateral left arm a standard forceps is placed.

An operating urologist that is not sterile, on the remote console, controlling the camera and the three robot arms, performs the entire surgery.

The assistant uses the right lateral trocar with an aspirator, or a grasper, scissor or a clip of *Hemolock®* applier.

The first step is to proceed with a dissection of the all Retzius space from the pubic symphysis to prostate. Ensure that the bladder is completely drained. The fatty and the areolar tissue overlying the anterior prostatic surface and the

A. Pinheiro · P. B. Santos
CUF Hospitals, Lisbon, Portugal
e-mail: pedro.b.santos@cuf.pt

E. Lima (✉)
CUF Hospitals, Lisbon, Portugal

School of Medicine, University of Minho, Braga, Portugal

Hydrumedical, Avepark—Parque de Ciência e Tecnologia, Zona Industrial da Gandra, Barco, Guimarães, Portugal
e-mail: estevaolima@med.uminho.pt; estevao.lima@CUF.pt; info@hydrustent.com; http://www.icvs.uminho.pt/research-scientists/surgical-sciences/people/estevaolima; https://hydrustent.com/about/#team

S. Ren et al. (eds.), *Robot-Assisted Radical Prostatectomy*, https://doi.org/10.1007/978-3-031-05855-4_25

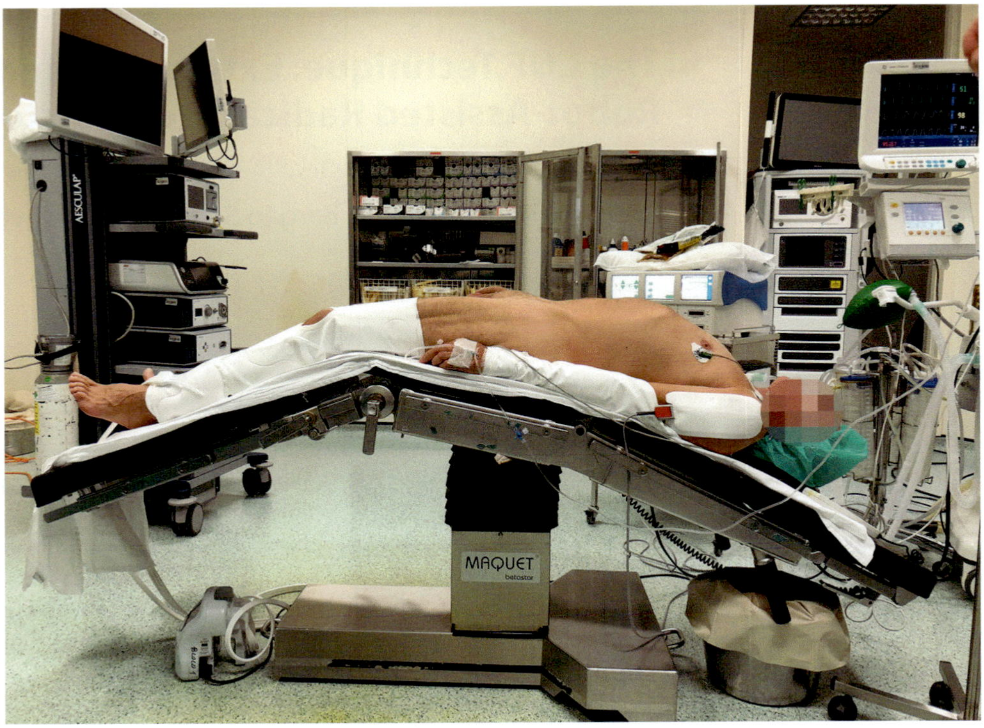

Fig. 25.1 Patient positioning

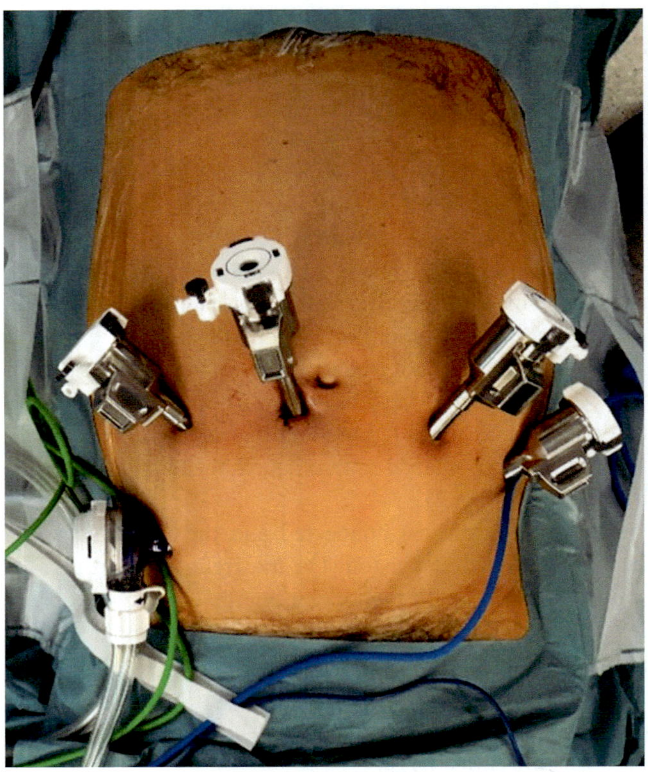

Fig. 25.2 Port placement

endopelvic fascia are gently swept away. The superficial branch of the dorsal vein may be visible and if so is coagulated and sectioned (Fig. 25.3).

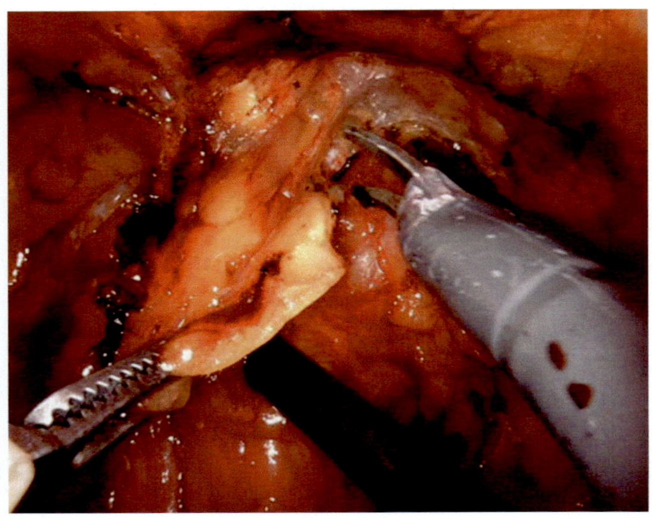

Fig. 25.3 Retzius space dissection

The endopelvic fascia is incised bilaterally. Blunt dissection is made from the prostatovesical junction to puboprostatic/vesical ligaments, until the lateral aspect of the prostate is completely visible and isolated. Sharp dissection may be needed near the prostate apex in case of adhesions (Fig. 25.4).

The next step is bladder neck incision. If it is not easily identifiable use repeated traction on the catheter with the balloon inflated. Then put it completely inside the bladder, at the dome. An incision is made at 12 o'clock and sharp incision from 10 to 2 o'clock is made. The incision extends later-

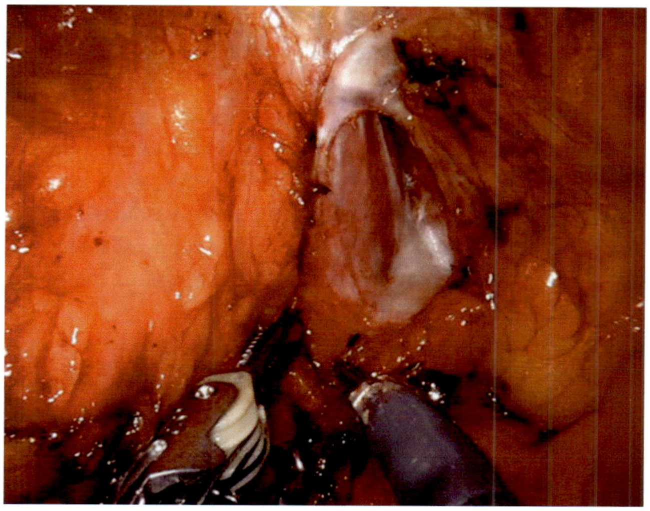

Fig. 25.4 Endopelvic fascia incision

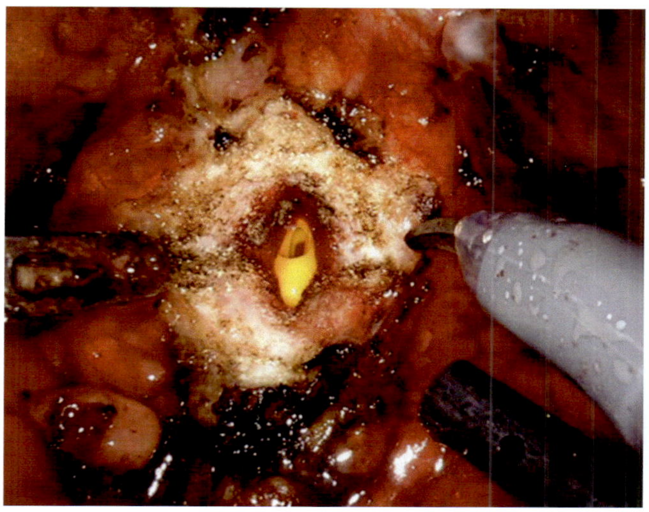

Fig. 25.5 Anterior bladder neck incision

ally only on the superficial layers, to remove adhesions from the bladder to the prostate.

The bladder neck is then incised on its ventral aspect in a descending way, until the prostatic urethra is identified. The prostate is separated from the bladder neck through sharp dissection. The bladder neck should be incise as much distally as possible to allow as much preservation as possible. However, caution must be taken to avoid entrance on the prostate and therefore positive surgical margins (Fig. 25.5).

As soon as the urethra is incised the catheter is grasped and lifted upwards, in order to enhance the dorsal visualization of structures. The dissection continues laterally and then posteriorly always identifying the bladder mucosa.

The dorsal bladder neck is incised, ensure the incision is made on natural groove between the bladder and prostate. In case of middle lobe, the ureteral orifices are close to the plane of dissection, caution must be taken or double pigtail stenting prior to surgery (Fig. 25.6).

The dissection plane continues perpendicularly and posteriorly until the longitudinal seminal-bladder, muscular fibers are identified and sharply dissected (Fig. 25.7). The vas deferens are then dissected, isolated and sectioned bilaterally. In first place, the right vas deferent and seminal vesicle, and afterwards, the left vas deferent and seminal vesicles. On the right side, the surgeon grasps the vesicle. On the left side, the assistant grasps the seminal vesical cranially and medially to facilitate its dissection. Caution must be taken in careful hemostasis of the seminal artery and too much pressure should not be applied on the tip of the vesicle, in order to avoid damage to the neurovascular bundle (Fig. 25.8).

The left deferent is pulled up and to the left by the robot standard forceps and the right deferent to the counter side by

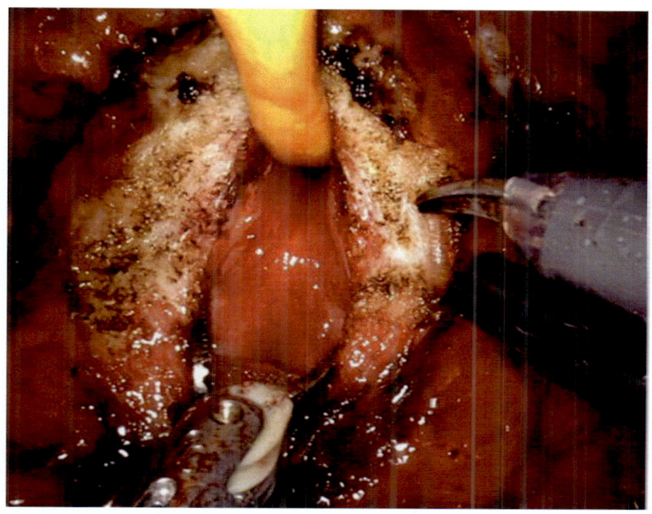

Fig. 25.6 Posterior bladder neck incision

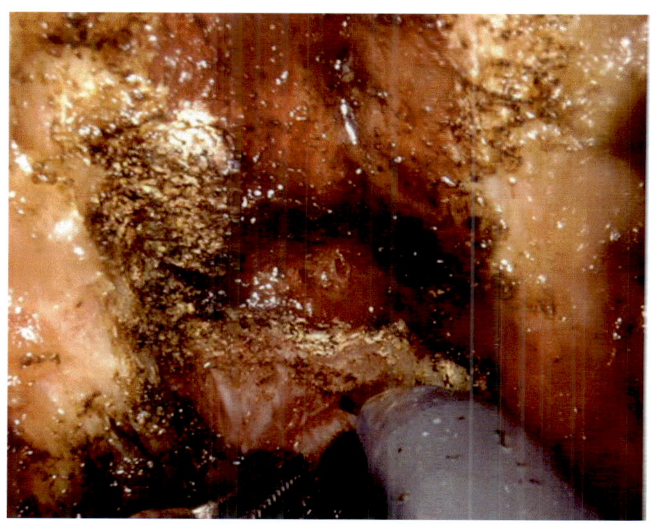

Fig. 25.7 Posterior plane incision

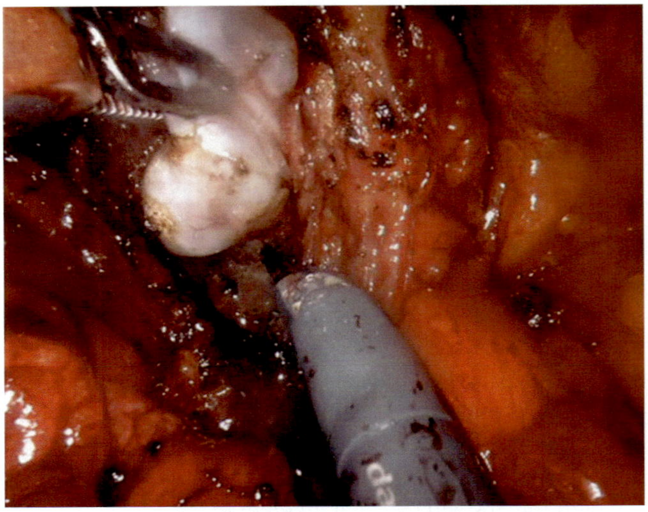

Fig. 25.8 Seminal vesical dissection

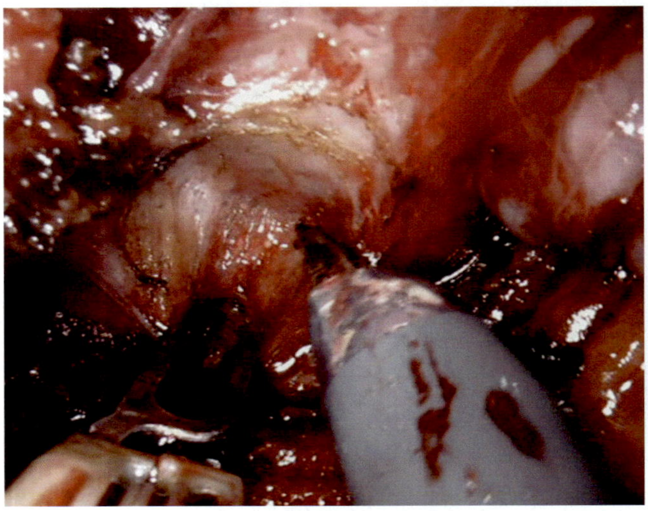

Fig. 25.9 Posterior plane dissection

the assistant grasper. The anterior layer of the *Denonvilliers* fascia is gentle pulled down and opened below the insertion plane of seminal vesical and vas deferens (Fig. 25.9). The prostatic capsule is dissected from the perirectal fat, pushing the rectum inferiorly to avoid its lesion. The dissection continues as far as possible until the apex, on the midline and bilaterally.

Then the attention moves laterally to the neurovascular bundles and the prostatic lateral pedicles.

If nerve-sparing technique is applied, it starts at the right side of the prostate. The right seminal vesicle is pulled to the left side, by the robot standard forceps, to expose the right neurovascular bundle. An incision of the prostate superficial fascia from the lateral ends of the bladder neck to the apex is made. A plane is sharp and bluntly developed, laterally, between the superficial prostatic/periprostatic fascia and the prostate, until the identification of the prostatic pedicles and neurovascular bundle. The same is done on the left side of the prostate (Fig. 25.10).

At this point, *Hemolock*® clips are applied anterogradely, and transversally on the vessels, very close to the prostate capsule. Small distances should be covered with cuts, in order to avoid in advert lesion of the neurovascular bundle. This dissection continues until the prostate apex. Cautery use must be reduced to ensure minimum damage to the nerve bundle (Fig. 25.11).

If nerve sparing is not adequate due to tumor oncological characteristics, the prostate is lifted upwards and contralateral and the rectum is pushed down. The dissection starts posteriorly near the prostatovesical junction and *Hemolock*® clips are applied transversally on the vessels

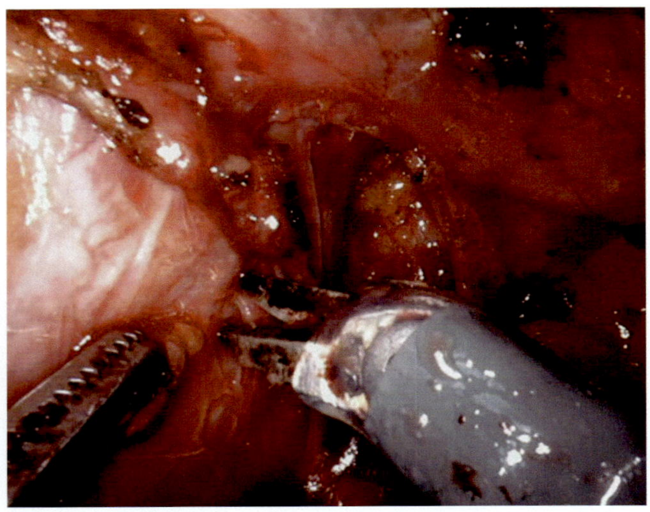

Fig. 25.10 Dissection of the prostate superficial fascia from the prostate capsule

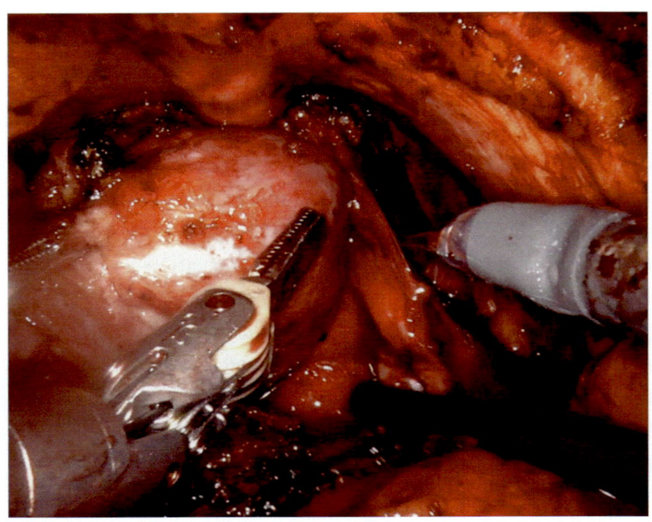

Fig. 25.11 Neurovascular bundle dissection

that travel to the prostate and sharp cut is applied superiorly. Safe margins should be applied to ensure negative surgical margins.

Then attention moves to the anterior surface of the prostate. The plane is developed under the dorsal vein complex, between it and the anterior surface of the prostate. Coagulation of vessels is done with extreme care to avoid large blood loss. Irrigation by the assistant is very important at this time. The puboprostatic ligaments are not divided in this approach. They are detached from the prostate with the dorsal vein complex (Fig. 25.12).

The apex of the prostate and the urethra are isolated by this dissection and the urethra sharply sectioned on the anterior surface. The catheter is removed, the prostate is rotated laterally to the left side and then to the right side, to complete the posterior urethra cut. Caution must be taken to avoid lesion of the neurovascular bundle at this step. Cold scissors should be used on this step.

The prostate is removed and placed inside a specimen retrieval bag.

The posterior musculofascial reconstruction and urethrovesical anastomosis are the next steps. The first starts with a 3-0 5/8 *V-LOC*® suturing—three runs from the anterior *Denonvilliers'* fascia that was cut to the rectourethral muscle also cut (Fig. 25.13). This stich moves the bladder closer to the urethra and reduces tension on the anastomosis. Then with the same stich starts the urethrovesical anastomosis at 5–7 o'clock on the posterior bladder neck (Fig. 25.14). It goes from dorsal to ventral and it is completed with another 3-0 5/8 *V-LOC*® suture starting at 5 o'clock. The sutures are outside-in on the bladder and inside-out on the urethra. Caution on the lateral stitches to avoid lesion on the neurovascular bundle.

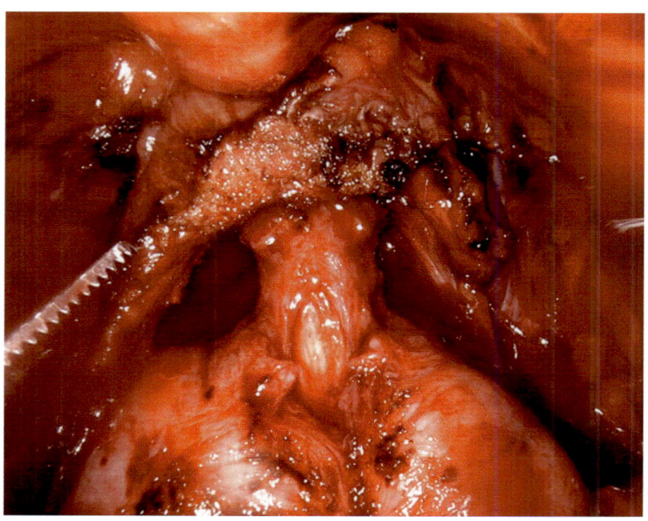

Fig. 25.12 Anterior plane development

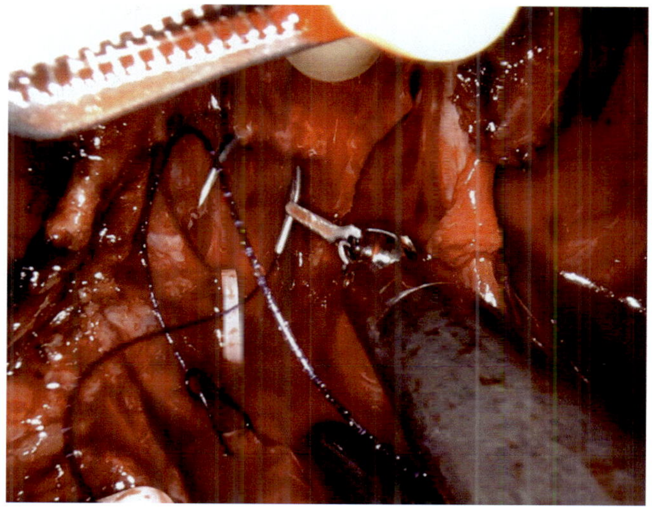

Fig. 25.13 Posterior reconstruction suture

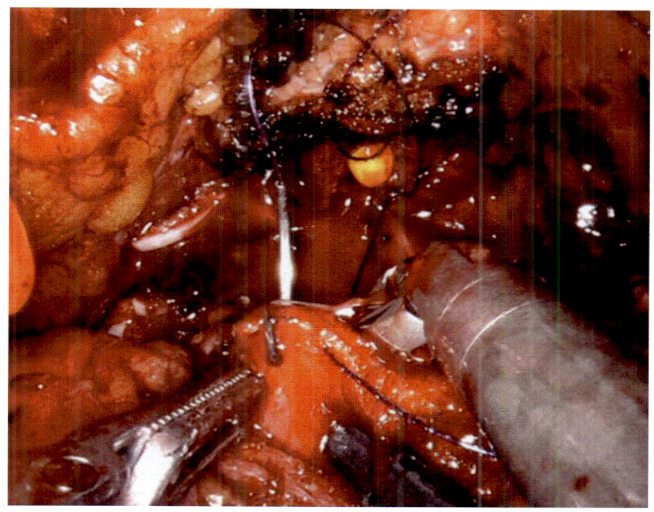

Fig. 25.14 Anastomosis

The same stiches are used to make the anterior reconstruction. They are placed from the anastomosis to the Santorin plexus and then to the bladder, to ensure stabilization of the anastomosis (Fig. 25.15).

After the anastomosis is finished the new sylatic 18Ch bladder catheter is passed. The bladder is filled with 150 mL of saline to ensure watertightness.

A surgical drain is placed through the left lateral port and should remain near although not adjacent to the anastomosis.

The surgical specimen is extracted after enlarging the right lateral port.

The air of the pre and intraperitoneal spaces is removed, the trocars are removed under vision. The incisions are closed in two layers.

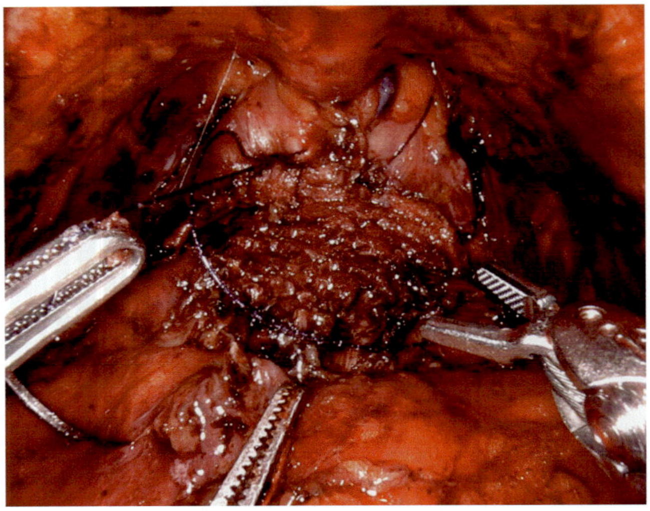

Fig. 25.15 Anterior reconstruction

References

1. Raboy A, Ferlzi G, Albert P. Initial experience with extaperitoneal endoscopic retropubic radical prostatectomy. Urology. 1997;50:849–53.
2. Bollens R, Vanden Bossche M, Roumeguere T. Extraperitoneal laparoscopic radical prostatectomy. Results after 50 cases. Eur Urol. 2001;40:65–9.
3. Gettman MT, Hoznek A, Salomon L, Katz R, Borkowski T, Antiphon P, Lobontiu A, Abbou CC. Laparoscopic radical prostatectomy: description of the extraperitoneal approach using the da Vinci robotic system. J Urol. 2003;170:416–9.
4. Semerjian A, Pavlovich CP. Extraperitoneal robot-assisted radical prostatectomy: indications, technique and outcomes. Curr Urol Rep. 2017;18(6):42.

Part VIII

Pelvic Lymph Node Dissection

Predictive Models in Prostate Cancer

26

Elio Mazzone, Giorgio Gandaglia, Vito Cucchiara, and Alberto Briganti

Introduction

The decision-making process in the field of prostate cancer (PCa) requires the clinician to balance clinical benefits, life expectancy, comorbidities and potential treatment related side effects that could ultimately influence the outcome of patients. Considering the complexity of this phase, the use of predictive tools that can integrate multiple clinical information for each individual patient allows to provide an individualized approach [1]. In consequence, several preoperative and postoperative tools have been developed during the last two decades to assist patients and physicians across the steps of the diagnosis, staging and treatment decision. Those models have been presented in the forms of look-up tables, regression trees, risk-class stratification tools, nomograms and artificial neuronal network [2–6]. Of those, nomograms represent undoubtedly the most frequently proposed tool. Nonetheless, there is a large disparity between the number of developed nomograms and those who are routinely adopted in clinical practice. A possible explanation for the low adoption rate is that a non-negligible proportion of available nomograms share similar endpoints. In consequence, the choice of one nomogram instead of another may be hampered by the large number of alternatives, which may ultimately discourage the end user. Second, the low adoption rate may be related to the intrinsic complexity of the nomogram. Indeed, most of the available nomograms require an elevated number of variables, which may not be always available in routine clinical practice. In consequence, despite an available nomogram showed promising results and high predictive accuracy, its complexity may limit its use. Therefore, risk stratification in few classes have also been proposed as alternatives to more complex nomograms with the goal of providing a user-friendly tool assisting preoperative patient counselling.

The predictive ability of available tools may be improved by the implementation of additional parameters which derive from genomic analyses or radiological parameters. In this context, in the last decade, multiparametric magnetic resonance imaging (MRI) has gained momentum and, to date, it is widely accepted as a key tool in the diagnostic pathway of PCa [1, 7]. However, while this widespread use of upfront MRI, some limitations should be still carefully considered, particularly regarding the risk of missing clinically significant PCa [8]. As a matter of fact, the use of MRI as a component of a model and not as a single tool might indeed mitigate this risk [9–11]. At the same time, the inclusion of MRI parameters in preoperative tools to improve risk classification and local staging have been recently explored [9].

In the current chapter, we aimed to describe the available published predictive tools for PCa, with the intent to discuss the advantages and potential pitfalls related to their use. Particularly, we explored currently available tool predicting: (1) presence of PCa at biopsy; (2) adverse pathological features at final surgical specimen; (3) oncological outcomes after radical treatment.

Main Body of the Chapter

Models Predicting the Presence of PCa at Biopsy

The first step during the PCa decision-making process is the identification of patients who are at higher risk of PCa and who should, therefore receive a prostate biopsy. In this context, several strategies have been developed to optimize the use of prostate biopsies detecting men at higher risk of significant disease (Table 26.1A). Prostatic specific antigen (PSA) alone or free/total (F/T) PSA are widely used and accepted to stratify pre-biopsy PCa risk [12]. In order to

E. Mazzone (✉) · G. Gandaglia · V. Cucchiara · A. Briganti
Division of Oncology/Unit of Urology, URI, IRCCS Ospedale San Raffaele, Milan, Italy

Vita-Salute San Raffaele University, Milan, Italy
e-mail: mazzone.elio@hsr.it; Gandaglia.giorgio@hsr.it; Cucchiara.vito@hsr.it; Briganti.alberto@hsr.it

S. Ren et al. (eds.), *Robot-Assisted Radical Prostatectomy*, https://doi.org/10.1007/978-3-031-05855-4_26

Table 26.1 Relevant predictive models in prostate cancer

Study	Year	Number of patients	Cohort	Covariates	Endpoint	Accuracy (%)
(A) Models predicting presence of PCa at biopsy						
Radtke et al. [23]	2017	1159	Patients with suspected PCa and candidate to prostate biopsy	PSA, prostate volume, DRE and PIRADS	csPCa	83
Truong et al. [27]	2017	285	Patients with suspected PCa and candidate to prostate biopsy	PSA, prostate volume, age, PIRADS	Prediction of absence of PCa	82.5
van Leeuwen et al. [25]	2017	393 + 198	Patients with suspected PCa and candidate to prostate biopsy	Age, PSA, DRE, previous prostate biopsy, prostate volume and PIRADS	csPCa	88
Bjurlin et al. [20]	2019	2063	Patients with suspected PCa and candidate to prostate biopsy	PSA, prostate volume, age, PIRADS	Prediction of absence of PCa	79
(B) Models predicting adverse pathological features at final specimen						
Cagiannos et al. [30]	2003	7014	Candidates to RP and LND	PSA, biopsy Gleason score and clinical stage	LNI	78
Godoy et al. [31]	2011	4176	Candidates to RP and LND	PSA, biopsy Gleason score and clinical stage	LNI	86
Briganti et al. [33]	2012	588	Candidates to RP and LND	PSA, clinical stage and primary and secondary Gleason score	LNI	88
Gandaglia et al. [32]	2017	681	Candidates to RP and LND	Clinical T stage, PSA, biopsy Gleason score, percentage of positive cores with highest and lowest Gleason score	LNI	91
Porpiglia et al. [40]	2018	310	Candidates to RP and LND with estimated risk of LNI <5%	Radiological stage at MRI and predominant Gleason pattern 4 at MRI	LNI	—
Briganti et al. [41]	2012	1366	Candidates to RP and LND	PSA, age, clinical stage, and biopsy Gleason sum	Organ confined disease at final specimen	72
Martini et al. [45]	2018	561	Candidates to RP and LND	PSA, ipsilateral biopsy Gleason grade, ipsilateral percentage of core involvement and ECE at MRI	ECE at final specimen	82
Lebacle et al. [22]	2017	1743	Candidates to RP and LND	PSA, clinical stage, Gleason score, prostate volume and MRI	ECE at final specimen	74
Nyarangi-Dix et al. [46]	2020	264	Candidates to RP and LND	Gleason grade, ESUR criteria, PSA, clinical stage, prostate volume, and capsule contact length at MRI	ECE at final pathology	87
Lantz et al. [47]	2020	1284	Candidates to RP and LND	Age, PSA, PIRADS, MRI prostate volume, systematic and target biopsy grade group and ECE at MRI	Adverse pathology (defined as non-organ-confined disease and/or lymph node invasion and/or pathological grade group ≥3 at RP)	71
Soeterik et al. [48]	2021	1870	Candidates to RP and LND	PSA density, Gleason grade, and mpMRI T stage	ECE at final specimen	78
(C) Models predicting oncological outcomes before RP (preoperative setting)						
Kattan et al. [4]	1998	983	Candidates to RP	PSA, biopsy Gleason score and clinical stage	Treatment failure (defined as clinical evidence of disease recurrence, a rising serum PSA level or initiation of adjuvant therapy)	79
D'Amico et al. [6]	1998	1872	Candidates to RP or RT	PSA, biopsy Gleason score and clinical stage	5-Year BCR	—
Cooperberg et al. [3]	2005	1439	Candidates to RP	PSA, biopsy Gleason score, clinical T stage and age	5-Year BCR	66

Table 26.1 (continued)

Study	Year	Number of patients	Cohort	Covariates	Endpoint	Accuracy (%)
Eastham et al. [49]	2008	2906	Candidates to RP	Preoperative PSA, clinical T stage	Trifecta (i.e. cancer-free status with recovery of continence and potency)	77
Dalela et al. [58]	2017	512	Candidates to RP	pT stage, pathological Gleason score, lymph node invasion, Decipher (genomic classifier)	5- and 10-year CR	85
Lalonde et al. [60]	2017	563	Candidates to RP	31-Locus genomic classifiers, clinical T stage, PSA and biopsy Gleason score	BCR and CR	91, 87
Gandaglia et al. [9]	2020	804	Candidates to RP with preoperative MRI	PSA, PIRADS, SVI at MRI, diameter of index lesion, Gleason grade at target biopsy and presence of csPCa at systematic biopsy	3-Year BCR	77
(D) Models predicting oncological outcomes after RP (postoperative setting)						
Stephenson et al. [50]	2005	1881	Candidates to RP	Preoperative PSA, pathological Gleason score, surgical margins, ECE, SVI, LNI and adjuvant RT	10-Year progression free survival	81
Cooperberg et al. [51]	2011	3837	Patients treated with RP	Preoperative PSA, pathological Gleason score, surgical margins, ECE, SVI and LNI	5-Year Progression-free survival	77
Den et al. [54]	2015	198	Patients treated with ART or SRT for BCR after RP	Expression values for the 22 prespecified biomarkers	Distant metastases at 5-year	83
Stephenson et al. [61]	2007	1540	Patients treated with SRT for BCR after RP	PSA at SRT, pathological Gleason score, surgical margins, PSA doubling time, ADT during SRT and LNI	6-Year progression-free survival	69
Tendulkar et al. [62]	2016	2460	Patients treated with SRT for BCR after RP	Pre-SRT PSA, Gleason score, ECE, SVI, surgical margins, ADT use, and SRT dose	BCR-free survival and distant metastases	68, 74
Briganti et al. [63]	2014	472	Patients treated with eSRT for BCR after RP	pT stage, pathological Gleason score and surgical margins	5-Year BCR after eSRT	74

LNI lymph node invasion, *RP* radical prostatectomy, *MRI* magnetic resonance imaging, *PSA* prostate specific antigen, *ECE* extracapsular extension, *SVI* seminal vesicles invasion, *BCR* biochemical recurrence, *CR* clinical recurrence, *RT* radiation therapy, *DRE* digital rectal examination, *LND* lymph node dissection, *PCa* prostate cancer, *csPCa* clinically significant prostate cancer, *PIRADS* Prostate Imaging Reporting and Data System, *ART* adjuvant salvage radiotherapy, *SRT* salvage radiotherapy, *eSRT* early salvage radiotherapy, *ADT* androgen deprivation therapy

improve the diagnostic performance of PSA, prostate health index (PHI) combines three forms of PSA: total PSA, free PSA and the isoform [−2] proPSA, and it can outperform total and free PSA for PCa detection on biopsy and have an association with aggressive forms of PCa [13–15]. PHI can also be combined with prostate volume to obtain PHI density, improving its diagnostic yield [16], or even with MRI with good results [17]. Since there is increasing evidence that PCa risk is multifactorial and not precisely assessed by a single marker, risk calculators have been developed to estimate individual risk of PCa based on multiple factors. Among these, the European Randomized Study of Screening for Prostate Cancer (ERSPC) calculator is available in different versions and allow to estimate the baseline PCa risk according to different baseline parameters [18]. Another similar tool is the Prostate Cancer Prevention Trial (PCPT) risk calculator, which includes PSA, family history, digital rectal examination and history of prior biopsy. Notably, a head-to-head comparison has shown that ERSPC outperforms PCPT in the prediction of any PCa and clinically significant PCa. It is important to note that these calculators have not been assessed in prospective randomized studies and their potential role in reducing PCa mortality remains unknown. For these reasons, all these calculators are not routinely recommended by the European Association of Urology (EAU) or National Comprehensive Cancer Network (NCCN) guidelines to decide whether prostate biopsy is indicated [1, 7].

To date, the introduction of MRI has contributed to increase the likelihood of identifying significant PCa in men referred to the urologist due to elevated PSA levels. However, systematic reviews and meta-analyses have demonstrated that the MRI might be characterized by a suboptimal sensitivity for the diagnosis of PCa [8]. Thus, investigators attempted to develop nomograms that combined the information derived from the MRI with clinical data [19–25], with the intent of facilitating the clinical decision. For instance, van Leeuwen et al. [25] developed a nomogram integrating prostate MRI and clinical features to predict clinically significant PCa. The performance of the nomogram was greatly improved by the inclusion of MRI features: the application of the model would reduce 28% of prostate biopsies, while missing only 2.6% of clinically significant PCa. Recently, Bjurlin et al. showed that PSA density, age and MRI suspicion category can predict PCa at combined MRI-targeted and systematic biopsy and, as a consequence, developed a nomogram including these data [20] with an estimated accuracy for overall and clinically significant PCa detection of, respectively, 78% and 84% in biopsy naïve men. Similarly, Radtke et al. [23] have recently published a nomogram combining the Prostate Imaging Reporting and Data System (PIRADS) score with clinical variables such as PSA, prostate volume, age and digital rectal exploration findings to identify significant PCa (ISUP grade group ≥2). Of note, the authors included only patients aged 35–80 years, who are potential candidates to radical treatments and in which, therefore, the indication to perform or not a prostate biopsy is crucial. Moreover, they included patients with PSA value between 1 and 40 ng/mL and with a prostate volume between 5 and 100 cc, which represents the majority of PCa patients. Nevertheless, this nomogram lacks external validation, which is mandatory before being considered in daily clinical practice. Another example of MRI-based pre-biopsy nomogram is the tool developed by Truong et al. [26, 27]. The authors developed and validated a nomogram for prediction of negative biopsy results in patients with previously negative prostate biopsy and in whom a second biopsy was required due to persistently elevated or increased PSA. Here, as for the nomogram developed by Radtke et al., clinical variables and MRI-based PIRADS score were combined to develop the model. The Truong nomogram showed high accuracy (82.5%), optimal calibration and elevated clinical benefit in decision curve analyses, in either internal or external validations. One possible limitation of this study is the inclusion of patients with PIRADS 5 (43%) and patients with PSA more than 40 ng/mL [26, 27]. Of note, both these subgroups have elevated likelihood of harboring significant PCa regardless other covariates and may, therefore, overestimate the clinical utility of this model. In consequence, the validity of the nomogram in these patient subgroups would be marginal, if present.

Models Predicting Adverse Pathological Features at Final Surgical Specimen

The use of preoperative predictive tools to assess the risk of having adverse pathological features at pathology in patients undergoing radical prostatectomy (RP) is well-established in routine clinical practice and can guide treatment decision. During the last two decades, several preoperative tools have been developed with the aim to predict lymph node invasion (LNI), positive surgical margins and extracapsular extension at definitive pathology [5] (Table 26.1B). The issue of lymph nodes is particularly relevant because with an accurate definition of LNI risk a significant proportion of patients could avoid lymph node dissection (LND) and the associated morbidity. Based on clinical and biopsy variables, several nomograms have been developed [28]. Historically, well-known pre-RP nomograms such as the Partin Tables [29] and the Memorial Sloan Kettering Cancer Center (MSKCC) score, along with the Godoy, the Cagiannos and the Briganti nomograms [30–33], have been routinely integrated in the clinical practice. Since their introduction, these nomograms have repeatedly proved their validity and accuracy [34–39]. All relied on clinical variables such as baseline PSA value, clinical T stage and biopsy ISUP grade group, but only the Briganti and the MSKCC nomograms included the percentage of positive cores. In the more recent version of the Briganti nomogram, the percentage of positive cores was subdivided into two categories (percentage of higher and lower grade cores/total cores) and showed a 90.8% accuracy in predicting LNI. Using a 7% cut-off, this model would allow sparing almost 70% of pelvic LND with a risk of missing only 1.5% of patients with positive nodes. When a head-to-head comparison between these nomograms was performed, the Cagiannos model and the 2012-Briganti showed the best calibration characteristics and net clinical benefit at the decision-curve analysis. On the other hand, the ability to avoid unnecessary LND was virtually the same for all the nomograms tested in this comparative study (Cagiannos, 2012-Briganti, Godoy and MSKCC) [37].

Some authors have also suggested that MRI could have a role in risk stratification in the setting of patients with Briganti's calculated LNI risk <5%. Specifically, Porpiglia et al. reported the MRI may be crucial in this specific subgroup of patients, where the presence of extracapsular extension (ECE) or seminal vesicle invasion at MRI were independent predictors of LNI at final pathology [40]. In the same direction, Gandaglia et al. developed a nomogram specifically aimed to predict LNI in MRI-diagnosed PCa. Indeed, the Briganti 2012, Briganti 2017 and MSKCC nomograms showed suboptimal performances in this subset of patients with positive MRI and PCa detected at targeted prostate biopsy. The authors developed a new model including PSA, clinical T stage, maximum diameter of the index lesion on MRI, ISUP grade group on MRI-guided biopsy and the presence of clinically significant PCa on concomitant systematic biopsy which was externally validated in a multi-institutional European cohort and showed a Receiving-Operator Characteristics (ROC) derived Area Under the Curve (AUC) of 86% in predicting the presence of LNI at final pathology [10]. This increased accuracy would directly translate into a higher number of unnecessary LND spared and lower risk of missing positive LNI compared to the existing models applied in patients receiving preoperative MRI.

Another frequent clinical question is how to select men with high-risk PCa who will benefit the most from RP by identifying those patients with favourable pathological features at the final specimen. Historically, Briganti et al. developed a model specifically aimed to the identification of men with adverse pathological features [41], identifying 40% of patients with high-risk PCa who have a specimen-confined disease at RP and improving the preoperative selection of RP candidates. In this context, several reports have shown that MRI-derived information may have an incremental role when compared to clinical nomograms alone, although with some controversies [42–44]. Notably, most of the studies showed optimal performance of MRI for local staging (i.e. ECE, seminal vesicle invasion), while the role of MRI for nodal staging was limited, thus confirming the sub-optimal accuracy of MRI along with the good performance of nomograms in regards of this outcome. Based on these evidences, Martini et al. recently published a MRI-based nomogram predicting side-specific ECE of prostate cancer on a model including PSA highest ipsilateral biopsy ISUP grade group, highest ipsilateral percentage core involvement and extracapsular invasion on MRI. After internal validation, the model AUC was 82.11%, with excellent calibration, particularly when compared with MRI prediction of ECE alone. Unfortunately, at external validation, this model reached an AUC of 67.6% with suboptimal calibration characteristics. Moreover, the added value of MRI parameters compared to the other clinical variables was not statistically significant [45]. Several models based on similar integration have been presented in the last few years [22, 46], although most of these nomograms lack an external validation and a formal comparison between these tools has not been performed yet. Among these, the risk tool developed by Lantz et al. [47] was specifically aimed to detect adverse pathology at final specimen and, consequently, to identify those patients who may benefit the most from active surveillance instead of radical treatment. Lastly, a novel nomogram to predict side specific ECE has been recently proposed by Soeterik et al. The model includes PSA density, highest ipsilateral ISUP grade, side-specific percentage of positive cores on systematic biopsy and ipsilateral clinical stage assessed by both digital rectal examination and MRI. Notably, the use of MRI information significantly increased the AUC, while the model based on PSA density, ISUP grade and MRI stage was superior in terms of calibration [48].

Models Predicting Oncological Outcomes of Candidates to Radical Treatment (Preoperative Setting)

The management of candidates to RP with high risk of cancer progression represents one other critical step for urologists in clinical practice. Here, major concerns are related to the use of adjuvant or salvage treatments, which should be considered in the light of potential benefits and related side effects. In this regard, numerous prognostic models have been developed for helping physicians to measure the optimal balance between oncological benefit and adverse events (Table 26.1C). Of note, the ability to assess biochemical recurrence (BCR)-free survival improves pre-treatment counseling of patients and the definition of appropriate therapy, as well as the identification of those patients with more advanced disease who are candidates for novel clinical trials. Historical disease progression predictive tools, such as the D'Amico classification [6], Cancer of the Prostate Risk Assessment (CAPRA) [3], the Kattan nomogram [4] and the TRIFECTA [49] represent examples of prognostic tools that are frequently adopted in clinical practice in the preoperative setting. The Kattan nomogram was one of the first tool developed to predict disease recurrence after local therapy [4]. In this model, as well as in other pre-treatment nomograms, clinical stage, biopsy ISUP grade, and pre-treatment serum PSA level are incorporated to predict the continuous risk of disease progression after definitive local therapy. Regarding patients treated with RP, nearly 1000 patients with clinically localized disease were included; as such, this model is not applicable for those men with evidence of seminal vesicle involvement or regional lymph nodal involvement. Despite providing an accurate estimate of individual patient risk, the use of nomograms in clinical practice is limited by their complex format which limits a straightforward clinical application in the context of preoperative patient counselling. Therefore, to simplify risk stratification, men with prostate cancer can be grouped into fewer categories without compromising the ability to predict disease behavior and response to intervention. D'Amico et al. [6] defined patients at low, intermediate, and high risk for biochemical failure based on pre-treatment disease characteristics (i.e., clinical T stage, PSA value and ISUP grade group). Other versions of simplified risk stratification have been developed and validated, with inclusion of features such as age and pathologic findings [3, 50]. The CAPRA score, ranging from 0 to 10, provides another method to assess risk, with each 2-point increase in score doubling the risk for recurrence after prostatectomy. It is easily calculated from PSA, T stage, patient age, ISUP grade and volume and it has been validated in several populations. Moreover, this score allows to predict disease-specific and overall mortality [51].

Although men with low-risk disease generally have low probability of experiencing biochemical recurrence during follow-up, patients in the intermediate- and high-risk groups may have widely discrepant outcomes. Therefore, men in these groups benefit from more modern and accurate risk prediction models and nomograms [52]. Overall, all these tools relied on clinical and/or pathological variables such as T stage, Gleason score, PSA and surgical margin status to predict the risk of recurrence or progression after radical treatments. Despite the large number of variables involved and the advanced statistical methodology, these tools remain imperfect. To improve the ability to accurately assess the risk of PCa progression, genomic classifiers have been proposed to improve prediction of oncological outcomes after RP or radiation therapy in PCa patients [53–57]. They are based on the identification of predefined biomarkers that the tumor cells may or may not express. Based on the number and on the types of these expressed biomarkers, the genomic classifiers are able to predict the biological behavior of PCa, as well as the risk of BCR and cancer progression. In the light of this evidence, clinical-based nomograms have been implemented with genomic classifiers to increase the predictive accuracy of the original models. For instance, Dalela et al. [58] have developed a genomic classifier-based nomogram for predicting the risk of meta- static progression after RP in order to identify those patients who might benefit the most from adjuvant therapies. The nomogram was generated combining pathological variables such as pathological T stage, ISUP grade and lymph node status with a genomic classifier, which was based on 22 prespecified biomarkers [59]. The resulting nomogram showed high accuracy (85% vs. 79% for the clinicopathologic model only) and elevated ability to identify patients who might benefit from adjuvant radiation therapy. Similarly, Lalonde et al. [60] developed a genomic classifier-based nomogram for prediction of BCR and metastases in patients who underwent RP. Their nomogram combined clinical variables such as clinical T stage, PSA and biopsy ISUP grade with a 100-genes based genomic classifier. The combined model showed higher accuracy compared to the model based on clinical variables alone for prediction of either BCR (91% vs. 87%), or metastases (71% vs. 64%). Taken together, the Lalonde and Dalela nomograms represent new interesting options in clinical decision-making process, where classical clinical variables were combined with genomic variables to predict PCa progression. These encouraging results should prompt the utilization of genomic biomarkers throughout the entire decision-making process in PCa patients. On the other hand, the elevated cost and the scarce availability of these new biomarkers, as well as the lack of external validation studies on large patient sample, may represent initial barriers toward large-scale use of these genomic classifier-based nomograms in clinical practice.

In the same direction, MRI-derived parameters have been proposed to improve the ability to identify patients at higher risk of PCa relapse or progression after radical treatment. Of note, a recent analysis by Gandaglia et al. [9] aimed at introducing MRI features in predicting BCR after treatment. They developed a novel nomogram which depicted superior discrimination (c-index: 77% vs. 62% vs. 60%) and net benefit at decision curve analysis as compared with the CAPRA score and the D'Amico risk groups when predicting BCR at 3-year after surgery. Remarkably, MRI based parameters, such as maximum diameter of the index lesion or tumor stage at MRI, resulted as independent strong predictors of BCR.

Model Predicting Oncological Outcomes After Radical Prostatectomy (Postoperative Setting)

Several tools based on pathological data have been proposed to assess the risk of progression after RP (Table 26.1D). This step is particularly important in order to define the need for additional treatments. Indeed, an accurate selection of patients more likely to benefit from RP vs. those who can be safely managed with observation may allow sparing a relevant proportion treatments-related side effect. Among these, the CAPRA-S [51] and the Stephenson nomogram [50] represent historical risk tools there are still used in clinical practice. The CAPRA-S score [51] is a scoring system based on PSA, pathological Gleason score, ECE and LNI (1 point each), positive surgical margins and SVI. The Stephenson nomograms [50] used similar variables and outperformed the CAPRA-S score in predicting oncological outcomes after RP (c-index 81% vs. 77%). However, despite having lower accuracy, the scoring system represents a user-friendly tool which may be preferred given its simple and straightforward format when compared to the nomogram. Despite the overall good accuracy achieved by these postoperative predictive tools, their predictive role in stratifying patients for additional therapies is still controversial.

After a patient is treated with salvage radiotherapy (RT) for BCR after RP, few nomograms have been developed to predict the survival of patients at long term follow-up. The first model was developed by Stephenson et al. [61], where PSA doubling time and ADT use were added as covariates to pathological data and played a crucial role in predicting risk of further disease recurrence after salvage RT. Recently, the nomogram proposed by Stephenson was updated by Tendulkar et al. [62]. Here the authors also included the dose of RT and achieved higher accuracy when compared to the original model in predicting progression-free survival (c-index 69 vs. 74). In the same context, Briganti et al. proposed a simple model including only pathological variables and, differently from the models previously developed, they included only node-negative patients [63].

In order to further improve the ability to predict long-term oncological outcomes, in the last decade genomic-based biomarkers have been developed to predict both recurrence risk and adjuvant/salvage RT benefit. In this context, Den et al. evaluated a cohort of 188 PCa patients at 10-year follow-up after adjuvant or salvage RT for high-risk features. Genomic classifier score (Decipher®) outperformed conventional risk-assessment tools. Moreover, men with low genomic classifier scores could safely undergo salvage RT in case of PCa recurrence, while patients with a high genomic classifier score are more likely to benefit from adjuvant RT [54]. The same tool was then integrated into a clinical nomogram, which combines pathological variables with the genomic classifier results. The results were provided as a sum of risk factors including pT3b/T4 stage, Gleason score 8–10, LNI and Decipher score >0.6. Here, patients with two or more risk factors where those who benefited the most from receiving adjuvant RT, while those with only one risk factor had similar outcomes when compared to patients managed with observation. Unfortunately, given the high cost and limited availability, the use of biomarkers in the context of PCa is still limited. However, with new evidence supporting and validating the role of genomic-based biomarkers, it is likely that the use of combined clinical and molecular predictive models during the post-RP decision-making process will increase in the next future.

Conclusion

Several prediction models have been developed in the last two decades in the context of PCa, with a specific focus on the ability to predict the presence of PCa at a screening level, the presence of adverse pathological findings at final pathology and oncological outcomes after radical treatment. Most of these tools exhibited elevated accuracy, good calibration characteristics and promising clinical net benefit, when they were internally validated. However, the majority still require external validation to confirm their applicability in routine clinical practice. To date, only few tools have met these criteria. Of note, in the upcoming years, the integration of the clinical tools with information derived from genomic classifiers or MRI results will substantially improve their predictive ability. In consequence, they could represent the gold standard in clinical practice but need proof of their benefits in well-designed validation studies.

Acknowledgements *Disclosure*: The authors declare no conflict of interest.

Formatting of Funding Sources This research did not receive any specific grant from funding agencies in the public, commercial, or not-for-profit sectors.

Financial Disclosures Elio Mazzone certifies that all conflicts of interest, including specific financial interests and relationships and affiliations relevant to the subject matter or materials discussed in the manuscript (e.g., employment/affiliation, grants or funding, consultancies, honoraria, stock ownership or options, expert testimony, royalties, or patents filed, received, or pending), are the following: None.

References

1. Mottet N, van den Bergh RCN, Briers E, et al. EAU-EANM-ESTRO-ESUR-SIOG guidelines on prostate cancer—2020 update. Part 1: Screening, diagnosis, and local treatment with curative intent. Eur Urol. 2021;79:243–62.
2. Preisser F, Cooperberg MR, Crook J, et al. Intermediate-risk prostate cancer: stratification and management. Eur Urol Oncol. 2020;3:270–80.
3. Cooperberg MR, Pasta DJ, Elkin EP, et al. The University of California, San Francisco cancer of the prostate risk assessment score: a straightforward and reliable preoperative predictor of disease recurrence after radical prostatectomy. J Urol. 2005;173:1938–42.
4. Kattan MW, Eastham JA, Stapleton AM, Wheeler TM, Scardino PT. A preoperative nomogram for disease recurrence following radical prostatectomy for prostate cancer. J Natl Cancer Inst. 1998;90:766–71.
5. Bandini M, Fossati N, Briganti A. Nomograms in urologic oncology, advantages and disadvantages. Curr Opin Urol. 2019;29:42–51.
6. D'Amico AV, Whittington R, Bruce Malkowicz S, et al. Biochemical outcome after radical prostatectomy, external beam radiation therapy, or interstitial radiation therapy for clinically localized prostate cancer. J Am Med Assoc. 1998;280:969–74.
7. Schaeffer E, Srinivas S, Antonarakis ES, et al. NCCN guidelines insights: prostate cancer, version 1.2021. J Natl Compr Cancer Netw. 2021;19:134–43.
8. Mazzone E, Stabile A, Pellegrino F, et al. Positive predictive value of prostate imaging reporting and data system version 2 for the detection of clinically significant prostate cancer: a systematic review and meta-analysis. Eur Urol Oncol. 2021;4(5):697–713.
9. Gandaglia G, Ploussard G, Valerio M, et al. Prognostic implications of multiparametric magnetic resonance imaging and concomitant systematic biopsy in predicting biochemical recurrence after radical prostatectomy in prostate cancer patients diagnosed with magnetic resonance imaging-targeted biopsy. Eur Urol Oncol. 2020;3:739–47.
10. Gandaglia G, Ploussard G, Valerio M, et al. A novel nomogram to identify candidates for extended pelvic lymph node dissection among patients with clinically localized prostate cancer diagnosed with magnetic resonance imaging-targeted and systematic biopsies. Eur Urol. 2019;75(3):506–14.
11. Gandaglia G, Ploussard G, Valerio M, et al. The key combined value of multiparametric magnetic resonance imaging, and magnetic resonance imaging–targeted and concomitant systematic biopsies for the prediction of adverse pathological features in prostate cancer patients undergoing radical prostatect. Eur Urol. 2020;77:733–41.
12. Partin AW, Brawer MK, Subong ENP, et al. Prospective evaluation of percent free-PSA and complexed-PSA for early detection of prostate cancer. Prostate Cancer Prostatic Dis. 1998;1:197–203.
13. Catalona WJ, Partin AW, Sanda MG, et al. A multicenter study of [−2]pro-prostate specific antigen combined with prostate specific antigen and free prostate specific antigen for prostate cancer detection in the 2.0 to 10.0 ng/ml prostate specific antigen range. J Urol. 2011;185:1650–5.

14. Tosoian JJ, Druskin SC, Andreas D, et al. Use of the Prostate Health Index for detection of prostate cancer: results from a large academic practice. Prostate Cancer Prostatic Dis. 2017;20:228–33.
15. Giovanni L, Massimo L, Alessandro L, et al. Development and internal validation of a prostate health index based nomogram for predicting prostate cancer at extended biopsy. J Urol. 2012;188:1144–50.
16. Tosoian JJ, Druskin SC, Andreas D, et al. Prostate Health Index density improves detection of clinically significant prostate cancer. BJU Int. 2017;120:793–8.
17. Gnanapragasam VJ, Burling K, George A, et al. The Prostate Health Index adds predictive value to multi-parametric MRI in detecting significant prostate cancers in a repeat biopsy population. Sci Rep. 2016;6:35364.
18. Steyerberg EW, Roobol MJ, Kattan MW, et al. Prediction of indolent prostate cancer: validation and updating of a prognostic nomogram. J Urol. 2007;177:107–12.
19. Distler FA, Radtke JP, Bonekamp D, et al. The value of PSA density in combination with PI-RADS™ for the accuracy of prostate cancer prediction. J Urol. 2017;198:575–82.
20. Bjurlin MA, Rosenkrantz AB, Sarkar S, et al. Prediction of prostate cancer risk among men undergoing combined MRI-targeted and systematic biopsy using novel pre-biopsy nomograms that incorporate MRI findings. Urology. 2018;112:112–20.
21. Lai WS, Gordetsky JB, Thomas JV, Nix JW, Rais-Bahrami S. Factors predicting prostate cancer upgrading on magnetic resonance imaging-targeted biopsy in an active surveillance population. Cancer. 2017;123:1941–8.
22. Lebacle C, Roudot-Thoraval F, Moktefi A, et al. Integration of MRI to clinical nomogram for predicting pathological stage before radical prostatectomy. World J Urol. 2017;35:1409–15.
23. Radtke JP, Wiesenfarth M, Kesch C, et al. Combined clinical parameters and multiparametric magnetic resonance imaging for advanced risk modeling of prostate cancer—patient-tailored risk stratification can reduce unnecessary biopsies. Eur Urol. 2017;72:888–96.
24. Reisæter LAR, Fütterer JJ, Losnegård A, et al. Optimising preoperative risk stratification tools for prostate cancer using mpMRI. Eur Radiol. 2018;28:1016–26.
25. van Leeuwen PJ, Hayen A, Thompson JE, et al. A multiparametric magnetic resonance imaging-based risk model to determine the risk of significant prostate cancer prior to biopsy. BJU Int. 2017;120:774–81.
26. Bjurlin MA, Renson A, Rais-Bahrami S, et al. Predicting benign prostate pathology on magnetic resonance imaging/ultrasound fusion biopsy in men with a prior negative 12-core systematic biopsy: external validation of a prognostic nomogram. Eur Urol Focus. 2019;5:815–22.
27. Truong M, Wang B, Gordetsky JB, et al. Multi-institutional nomogram predicting benign prostate pathology on magnetic resonance/ultrasound fusion biopsy in men with a prior negative 12-core systematic biopsy. Cancer. 2018;124:278–85.
28. Bandini M, Marchioni M, Preisser F, et al. A head-to-head comparison of four prognostic models for prediction of lymph node invasion in African American and Caucasian individuals. Eur Urol Focus. 2019;5:449–56.
29. Eifler JB, Feng Z, Lin BM. An updated prostate cancer staging nomogram (Partin tables) based on cases from 2006 to 2011. BJU Int. 2013;111:22.
30. Cagiannos I, Karakiewicz P, Eastham JA, et al. A preoperative nomogram identifying decreased risk of positive pelvic lymph nodes in patients with prostate cancer. J Urol. 2003;170:1798–803.
31. Godoy G, Chong KT, Cronin A, et al. Extent of pelvic lymph node dissection and the impact of standard template dissection on nomogram prediction of lymph node involvement. Eur Urol. 2011;60:195–201.
32. Gandaglia G, Fossati N, Zaffuto E, et al. Development and internal validation of a novel model to identify the candidates for extended pelvic lymph node dissection in prostate cancer. Eur Urol. 2017;72:632–40.
33. Briganti A, Larcher A, Abdollah F, et al. Updated nomogram predicting lymph node invasion in patients with prostate cancer undergoing extended pelvic lymph node dissection: the essential importance of percentage of positive cores. Eur Urol. 2012;61:480–7.
34. Grivas N, Wit E, Tillier C, et al. Validation and head-to-head comparison of three nomograms predicting probability of lymph node invasion of prostate cancer in patients undergoing extended and/ or sentinel lymph node dissection. Eur J Nucl Med Mol Imaging. 2017;44:2213–26.
35. Hansen J, Rink M, Bianchi M, et al. External validation of the updated Briganti nomogram to predict lymph node invasion in prostate cancer patients undergoing extended lymph node dissection. Prostate. 2013;73:211–8.
36. Walz J, Bladou F, Rousseau B, et al. Head to head comparison of nomograms predicting probability of lymph node invasion of prostate cancer in patients undergoing extended pelvic lymph node dissection. Urology. 2012;79:546–51.
37. Bandini M, Marchioni M, Pompe RS, et al. First North American validation and head-to-head comparison of four preoperative nomograms for prediction of lymph node invasion before radical prostatectomy. BJU Int. 2018;121:592–9.
38. Abdollah F, Schmitges J, Sun M, et al. Head-to-head comparison of three commonly used preoperative tools for prediction of lymph node invasion at radical prostatectomy. Urology. 2011;78:1363–7.
39. Gandaglia G, Martini A, Ploussard G, et al. External validation of the 2019 Briganti nomogram for the identification of prostate cancer patients who should be considered for an extended pelvic lymph node dissection. Eur Urol. 2020;78:138–42.
40. Porpiglia F, Manfredi M, Mele F, et al. Indication to pelvic lymph nodes dissection for prostate cancer: the role of multiparametric magnetic resonance imaging when the risk of lymph nodes invasion according to Briganti updated nomogram is <5. Prostate Cancer Prostatic Dis. 2018;21:85–91.
41. Briganti A, Joniau S, Gontero P, et al. Identifying the best candidate for radical prostatectomy among patients with high-risk prostate cancer. Eur Urol. 2012;61:584–92.
42. Jansen BHE, Nieuwenhuijzen JA, Oprea-Lager DE, et al. Adding multiparametric MRI to the MSKCC and Partin nomograms for primary prostate cancer: improving local tumor staging? Urol Oncol. 2019;37:181.e1–6.
43. Rayn KN, Bloom JB, Gold SA, et al. Added value of multiparametric magnetic resonance imaging to clinical nomograms for predicting adverse pathology in prostate cancer. J Urol. 2018;200:1041–7.
44. Weaver JK, Kim EH, Vetter JM, et al. Prostate magnetic resonance imaging provides limited incremental value over the memorial sloan kettering cancer center preradical prostatectomy nomogram. Urology. 2018;113:119–28.
45. Martini A, Gupta A, Lewis SC, et al. Development and internal validation of a side-specific, multiparametric magnetic resonance imaging-based nomogram for the prediction of extracapsular extension of prostate cancer. BJU Int. 2018;122:1025–33.
46. Nyarangi-Dix J, Wiesenfarth M, Bonekamp D, et al. Combined clinical parameters and multiparametric magnetic resonance imaging for the prediction of extraprostatic disease—a risk model for patient-tailored risk stratification when planning radical prostatectomy. Eur Urol Focus. 2020;6:1205–12.
47. Lantz A, Falagario UG, Ratnani P, et al. Expanding active surveillance inclusion criteria: a novel nomogram including preoperative clinical parameters and magnetic resonance imaging

findings. Eur Urol Oncol. 2020;5:187–94. https://doi.org/10.1016/j.euo.2020.08.001.
48. Soeterik TFW, van Melick HHE, Dijksman LM, et al. Development and external validation of a novel nomogram to predict side-specific extraprostatic extension in patients with prostate cancer undergoing radical prostatectomy. Eur Urol Oncol. 2020. https://doi.org/10.1016/j.euo.2020.08.008.
49. Eastham JA, Scardino PT, Kattan MW. Predicting an optimal outcome after radical prostatectomy: the trifecta nomogram. J Urol. 2008;179:2201–7.
50. Stephenson AJ, Scardino PT, Eastham JA, et al. Postoperative nomogram predicting the 10-year probability of prostate cancer recurrence after radical prostatectomy. J Clin Oncol. 2005; 23:7005–12.
51. Cooperberg MR, Hilton JF, Carroll PR. The CAPRA-S score: a straightforward tool for improved prediction of outcomes after radical prostatectomy. Cancer. 2011;117:5039–46.
52. Mitchell JA, Cooperberg MR, Elkin EP, et al. Ability of 2 pretreatment risk assessment methods to predict prostate cancer recurrence after radical prostatectomy: data from CaPSURE. J Urol. 2005;173:1126–31.
53. Cooperberg MR, Davicioni E, Crisan A, et al. Combined value of validated clinical and genomic risk stratification tools for predicting prostate cancer mortality in a high-risk prostatectomy cohort. Eur Urol. 2015;67:326–33.
54. Den RB, Yousefi K, Trabulsi EJ, et al. Genomic classifier identifies men with adverse pathology after radical prostatectomy who benefit from adjuvant radiation therapy. J Clin Oncol. 2015;33:944–51.
55. Feng FY, Huang H-C, Spratt DE, et al. Validation of a 22-gene genomic classifier in patients with recurrent prostate cancer: an ancillary study of the NRG/RTOG 9601 randomized clinical trial. JAMA Oncol. 2021;7:544–52.
56. Nguyen PL, Haddad Z, Ross AE, et al. Ability of a genomic classifier to predict metastasis and prostate cancer-specific mortality after radiation or surgery based on needle biopsy specimens. Eur Urol. 2017;72:845–52.
57. Van Den Eeden SK, Lu R, Zhang N, et al. A biopsy-based 17-gene genomic prostate score as a predictor of metastases and prostate cancer death in surgically treated men with clinically localized disease. Eur Urol. 2018;73:129–38.
58. Dalela D, Santiago-Jiménez M, Yousefi K, et al. Genomic classifier augments the role of pathological features in identifying optimal candidates for adjuvant radiation therapy in patients with prostate cancer: development and internal validation of a multivariable prognostic model. J Clin Oncol. 2017;35:1982–90.
59. Erho N, Crisan A, Vergara IA, et al. Discovery and validation of a prostate cancer genomic classifier that predicts early metastasis following radical prostatectomy. PLoS One. 2013;8:e66855.
60. Lalonde E, Alkallas R, Chua MLK, et al. Translating a prognostic DNA genomic classifier into the clinic: retrospective validation in 563 localized prostate tumors. Eur Urol. 2017;72:22–31.
61. Stephenson AJ, Scardino PT, Kattan MW, et al. Predicting the outcome of salvage radiation therapy for recurrent prostate cancer after radical prostatectomy. J Clin Oncol. 2007;25:2035–41.
62. Tendulkar RD, Agrawal S, Gao T, et al. Contemporary update of a multi-institutional predictive nomogram for salvage radiotherapy after radical prostatectomy. J Clin Oncol. 2016;34:3648–54.
63. Briganti A, Karnes RJ, Joniau S, et al. Prediction of outcome following early salvage radiotherapy among patients with biochemical recurrence after radical prostatectomy. Eur Urol. 2014;66:479–86.

Extended Lymphadenectomy Technique 27

John W. Davis and Ahmet Urkmez

Introduction

Extended pelvic lymph node dissection (ePLND) is the most reliable method of detecting lymph node metastases (LNM) of prostate cancer (PCa). ePLND also allows for a better understanding of the prognostic risk group a patient is in, guiding the details of the post-operative follow-up protocol, and determining the need for adjuvant or salvage therapy [1]. A decrease in the rate of pelvic lymph node dissection (PLND) performed during radical prostatectomy was noted in the previous studies, possibly due to diagnosis of PCa at early stages and increased application of minimally invasive treatment approaches [2]. Although studies have demonstrated the technical feasibility of PLND during robot-assisted radical prostatectomy (RARP), the concomitant PLND rate was higher in patients who underwent open radical prostatectomy than in those who underwent RARP [3–5]. However, a very recent study assessing the contemporary national trend in PLND during RARP in 115,355 patients with intermediate- to high-risk PCa showed that the PLND rate increased significantly from 2010 to 2016 [6].

Patient Selection

Pre-operative nomograms such as the Briganti nomogram [7] and the Memorial Sloan Kettering Cancer Center (MSKCC) nomogram [8], allow for the identification of PCa patients who would benefit from ePLND. Recently, an external validation study including 12,009 patients who underwent radical prostatectomy with ePLND at eight European centers showed no significant differences in the performance or limitations of the MSKCC nomogram; 2012, 2017, 2019 Briganti nomograms; 2016 Partin nomogram; or Yale model, but it did show a clear benefit for all six of them. The MSKCC and 2012 Briganti nomograms were superior to the other nomograms in the prediction of LNM in PCa patients with only systematic biopsy [9]. The National Comprehensive Cancer Network guidelines for PCa treatment recommend performing an ePLND if the nomogram-predicted LNM probability is 2% or greater [10], whereas the European Association of Urology guidelines set this cut-off at 5% [1].

Over the past decade, the introduction of Gallium-68 (^{68}Ga)- and Fluorine-18 (^{18}F)- prostate-specific membrane antigen (PSMA) positron emission tomography/computed tomography (PET/CT) has provided improved detection of localization of PCa with higher sensitivity and specificity when compared with other imaging modalities (e.g., bone scintigraphy, magnetic resonance imaging, CT, and choline PET/CT) for both primary and recurrent tumors [11–13]. Preoperative ^{68}Ga-PSMA PET/CT was more sensitive in identifying pathological pelvic LNM than was 3 T multiparametric magnetic resonance imaging [14]. Additionally, the risk of LNM was lower in patients with ^{68}Ga-PSMA PET/CT negative for LNM than the risk predicted by Cancer of the Prostate Risk Assessment scores or the MSKCC and Briganti nomograms [14]. A recent study suggested that ePLND could be omitted in patients with intermediate-risk PCa and a radiological T stage less than rT3 according to multiparametric magnetic resonance imaging when PSMA PET/CT shows no LNM (negative predictive value 98.1%). However, ePLND remains the gold-standard staging tool in PCa patients with high-risk disease as LNM are frequently missed in those with PSMA PET/CT negative for LNM [15]. Additionally, in a literature review consisting of eight retrospective studies, the positive predictive value of ^{68}Ga-PSMA PET/CT in detecting pelvic LNM ranged from 70% to 100% in patients with biochemical recurrence (BCR) after initial curative treatment who underwent salvage PLND afterward [13]. Similarly, in a prospective multicenter study, ^{18}F-PSMA PET/CT had a high specificity rate (94%) but a low to moderate sensitivity rate (41%) in the identification of pelvic LNM in patients with primary PCa [16]. In conclusion, although both ^{68}Ga- and ^{18}F-PSMA PET/CT have very high

J. W. Davis · A. Urkmez (✉)
Division of Surgery, Department of Urology, The University of Texas MD Anderson Cancer Center, Houston, TX, USA
e-mail: johndavis@mdanderson.org

S. Ren et al. (eds.), *Robot-Assisted Radical Prostatectomy*, https://doi.org/10.1007/978-3-031-05855-4_27

specificity in detecting pelvic LNM, their sensitivity is only moderate, and small LNM can be missed. Therefore, ePLND cannot be replaced by ^{68}Ga- or ^{18}F-PSMA PET/CT in excluding LNM [13, 16]. The reason ePLND still represents the gold standard for nodal staging is mostly due to the relatively poor diagnostic yield of imaging modalities in the detection of nodal metastases especially those less than 5 mm in diameter [17–19]. PET imaging currently has great utility for recurrent disease management.

Figure 27.1 illustrating a case of recurrent disease after brachytherapy with PET avid lymph node disease with the Axumin tracer.

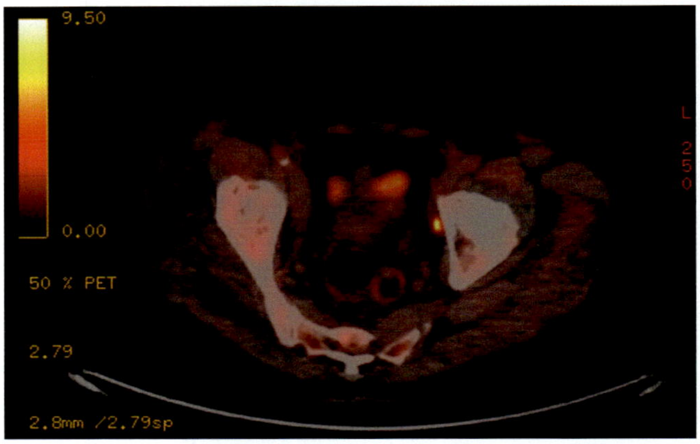

Fig. 27.1 This patient was referred for consideration of salvage prostatectomy for biochemical progression after brachytherapy. However, an Axumin PET showed uptake in the left obturator fossa as well as the prostate. Given his age/co-morbidity he was recommended a trial of androgen deprivation which resulted in resolution of PET uptake 6 months later—consistent with lymph node positive disease

Extent of PLND

As shown in many studies, the number of positive lymph nodes increases proportionally with the extent of the dissection [2, 20]. However, the question of how extensive a PLND should be remains debatable. This is mainly due to the various lymphatic drainage patterns demonstrated in previous studies [21, 22]. The American Urological Association and European Association of Urology guidelines for PCa treatment recommend avoiding PLND in men with low-risk disease because the harm may outweigh the benefits. However, for those with intermediate- or high-risk disease, PLND is suggested, and an extended PLND template should be followed [1, 23].

Researchers have recommended standardization of PLND terminology to better determine the extent of anatomical dissection and more accurately compare the outcomes of studies. The most commonly used terminology with regard to PLND is; limited, standard, extended, and super-extended PLND [2]. In limited PLND, the region between the obturator nerve and external iliac vein is described. In standard PLND, in addition to the region in limited PLND, the area under the obturator nerve and around the internal iliac vessels is described. In extended PLND, in addition to the region in standard PLND, the area around the proximal common iliac artery and vein up to the ureteral crossing is targeted. Finally, in super-extended PLND, in addition to the region in extended PLND, the common iliac vessels up to the aortic and caval bifurcation and the presacral region are included in the dissection field. Figure 27.2a, b show our published diagrams on extended PLND zones by their dissection steps and correlation to standard nomenclature [24].

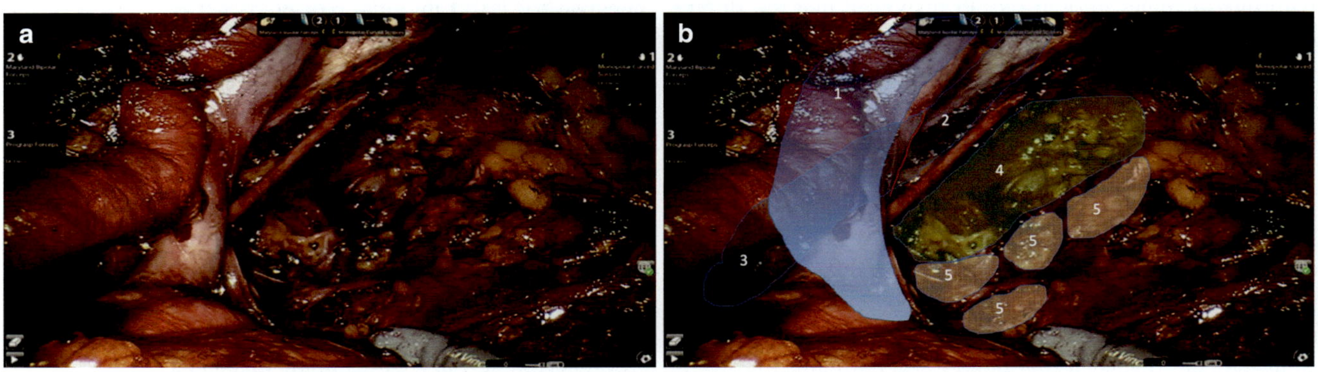

Fig. 27.2 (**a**, **b**) The extent of PLND dissection can be described with blood vessel mapped nomenclature (limited, standard, extended, super-extended) but also thought of in terms of dissection zones and anatomy needed to manipulate. Figure (**a**) shows a completed extended template on the left. Figure (**b**) shows five different dissection zones: 1 = The typical external iliac artery/vein from ureter crossing to node of Cloquet; 2 = The typical obturator fossa space up to the red line where the vein lies naturally; 3 = The continuation of the obturator fossa beneath the external iliac vein—tissue that can be removed by retracting the vein up or for a more complete access dissecting in the triangular space between external iliac artery and vein; 4 = The continuation of obturator fossa beneath the obturator nerve—this space becomes the lateral aspect of the hypogastric artery zone; and 5 = the medial hypogastric lymphatic tissue that often must be dissected out separately between branches of the hypogastric artery. The distal aspect of zone 5 then takes the dissection into the peri-rectal fat adjacent to the prostate endopelvic fascia. For standard nomenclature: limited = zone 2; standard = zones 1–2; extended = zones 1–5; super-extended (not shown) = zones 1–5 plus pre-sacral and more common iliac (Images with permission from Williams SB et al. BJU Int. 2016;117:192–8)

Consensus regarding the optimal number of lymph nodes that should be removed for adequate PCa staging is lacking. Moreover, some surgeons advocated determining PLND adequacy by the borders of anatomical dissection rather than the number of lymph nodes removed. Therefore, it is recommended that the excised lymph nodes be named according to the region they belong to and sent for pathological analysis in separate containers [1]. In our experience, the median lymph node count with extended template was >20—slightly higher with more packets sent but positive yield not affected by number of packets sent [25].

Therapeutic Efficacy of ePLND

Although the benefits of ePLND in PCa staging and consequent guiding of or omitting adjuvant treatment are proven, the therapeutic efficacy of ePLND remains unclear. Several retrospective studies showed that extensive PLND in node-positive PCa patients was associated with improvement of cancer-specific survival [26, 27]. In contrast, the therapeutic role of ePLND was challenged in several other studies. For example, in a recent systematic review including mostly retrospective studies and lacking standardization with regard to definition of the extent of PLND, authors found no significant differences in oncological outcomes favoring any form of PLND over no PLND for BCR, distant metastasis, or survival [28]. Additionally, comparison of ePLND with limited PLND revealed no significant differences in BCR in 11 out of 13 studies. Two studies showed a benefit of ePLND in only specific subgroups of PCa patients: those with intermediate-risk cancer and pN1 disease with less than 15% lymph node invasion [28]. A very recent randomized controlled trial compared the early oncological outcomes of limited PLND (obturator nodes) with those of ePLND (obturator, external iliac, internal iliac, common iliac, and presacral nodes) in 300 PCa patients [29]. Although ePLND significantly improved pathological staging, the study did not show a significant benefit of it over limited PLND in terms of BCR- and metastasis-free survival [29]. However, a few points about therapeutic efficacy of ePLND should be considered. First, PLND may be curative in some patients whose involved lymph nodes are completely removed. For now, though, only limited retrospective evidence supports a possible curative effect of PLND [26, 27, 30]. Second, ePLND, which is accepted as the most accurate staging tool for detecting LNM, may improve survival by identifying patients who would benefit from adjuvant treatments and by omitting adjuvant treatment in those who do not need it. Third, even ePLND can miss 25% of all lymphatic landing sites for PCa metastases [21, 28]. Therefore, including all of the potential lymphatic landing sites with imaging guidance and new techniques may improve the oncological outcomes.

A multicenter study assessing the effect of ePLND on oncological outcomes revealed no significant differences in BCR, cancer-specific mortality, or metastasis-free survival rate 5 years after radical prostatectomy in patients with D'Amico intermediate- or high-risk PCa in whom PLND was or was not performed [31]. Similarly, in a very recent study, we evaluated the data on 1026 PCa patients who underwent RARP from 2006 to 2012 at The University of Texas MD Anderson Cancer Center to show the therapeutic consequences of omitting PLND in patients with biopsy Gleason score $\leq 3 + 4$ and cT1-T2 disease [32]. Our results revealed that low- and intermediate-risk patients who did not undergo PLND and whose PCa was subsequently upgraded or upstaged according to RARP pathology had 5-year BCR-free survival rates similar to those of a propensity score-matched cohort of patients who did undergo PLND [32].

Technical Aspects of ePLND

Placing additional ports is generally not necessary for performing a successful PLND. However, especially for extended and super-extended PLND, a surgeon may consider using a forth robot arm or inserting an additional assistance port. Placing the ports more cranially may help better demonstrate the iliac bifurcation and presacral region in ePLND.

Pelvic lymphadenectomy can be performed either before prostatectomy or after prostatectomy and vesicourethral anastomosis. No related oncological or functional outcomes highlight that any of these options as more advantageous than the other. The main factor here is the surgeon's preference. Surgeons should decide on the method that they believe is most comfortable and effective.

During PLND, an accessory obturator vessel arising from or draining into the external iliac circulatory system may be encountered. Similarly, small perforating vessels may run from the muscle layers in the pelvic sidewall to the pelvic lymph nodes. Paying attention to these vessels is important because they may lead to bleeding that significantly deteriorates the vision in the operative field. Additionally, clipping off relatively large lymphatic vessels will reduce the possibility of prolonged lymph drainage and/or lymphocele development, although advanced energy technologies such as vessel sealer or bipolar may be suitable methods and possibly faster.

Mattei et al. described a standardized ten-step procedure for robot-assisted ePLND to acquire a single tissue monoblock from both sides that includes all lymph nodes within the ePLND template (median number of lymph nodes, 14 [IQR, 11–19]) [33]. Additionally, they suggested a further five-step procedure that includes the super-extended PLND template for patients with at least a 30% risk of lymph node invasion calculated using the 2017 Briganti nomogram (median number of lymph nodes, 23 [IQR, 19–29]) [34].

Sentinel Node Biopsy

Although ePLND is the best available staging method for assessing the presence of LNM in patients with PCa, it can still miss aberrant dissemination pathways to about 25% of lymph nodes located outside the ePLND template [21]. For predicting the routes of lymphatic spread and improving the accuracy of ePLND, fluorescence-supported lymphography and sentinel node biopsy (SNB) have been proposed [1, 35, 36]. Researchers have shown that Indocyanine green-guided ePLND improves the identification of lymphatic drainage and increases the median number of retrieved nodes (22 vs. 14) [37]. Moreover, in vivo guidance of a DROP-IN gamma probe during RARP with ePLND has improved sentinel node yield when compared with a traditional laparoscopic gamma probe and fluorescence imaging (100.0% vs. 76.0% vs. 91.3%), likely owing to its more advanced maneuverability [38]. In a systematic review, SNB exhibited high sensitivity and negative predictive value, and it appeared to increase nodal yield by detecting more positive nodes when combined with ePLND than ePLND alone. However, it infrequently detected positive nodes outside the ePLND template, raising concerns that SNB may not add value to ePLND [39]. Eventually, SNB and fluorescence-supported lymphography are still considered experimental procedures [1].

Multi-Port vs. Single-Port Robotic Surgery Platform

Kaouk and colleagues described a step-by-step technique of single-port (SP) robotic perineal prostatectomy with PLND and reported the results of a comparative analysis of their initial series' perioperative and postoperative outcomes of SP robotic perineal prostatectomy with multiport transperitoneal RARP [40]. After propensity score matching, they included 26 patients in both groups. All of the patients in the multi-port group underwent PLND whereas 16 patients in the SP group underwent PLND. They found that the median lymph node count was lower in the SP group than in the multi-port group (3 [IQR, 1.5–5.5] vs. 6 [IQR, 4–8]; $p = 0.01$) [40]. The same authors also compared the outcomes in patients who underwent SP extraperitoneal RARP and those who underwent multi-port transperitoneal RARP. Ninety-one patients in the SP group and 101 patients in the multi-port group underwent bilateral obturator lymph node dissection. The authors did not observe a significant difference in lymph node yield between the two groups (median, 5 [IQR, 3–7] in the SP group vs. 6 [IQR, 4–7] in the multi-port group) [41]. A very recent pooled analysis of a series of PCa patients who underwent SP RARP ($n = 208$) showed removal of fewer lymph nodes in patients undergoing SP RARP than in those undergoing standard RARP (median, 5.5 vs. 9.0) [42].

Salvage ePLND

The indications for, extent of, and oncological outcome of salvage lymphadenectomy following radical prostatectomy have not been well studied, as only data from retrospective studies of more than 500 patients are reported [43]. ^{68}Ga- and ^{18}F-PSMA PET/CT are generally the preferred imaging studies for identifying patients with potential LNM after RARP [43, 44]. Abreu et al. defined a technique for performing robot-assisted high-extended salvage retroperitoneal and pelvic lymphadenectomy for node-only recurrent PCa [43]. The outcomes of their initial series of ten patients demonstrated that robot-assisted salvage retroperitoneal and pelvic lymphadenectomy is feasible, with a likely increased lymph node yield and decreased morbidity [43]. Similarly, Montorsi et al. presented results from their initial series of 16 patients who underwent robot-assisted salvage lymphadenectomy and showed that the technique is feasible [45]. They also performed retroperitoneal lymph node dissection (the area between the aortic bifurcation and renal vessels) in 81% of patients. In another study including 35 patients at two centers, robot-assisted salvage lymphadenectomy appeared to be feasible and safe, with only Clavien-Dindo grade I or II complications [46].

MD Anderson Experience and Technique

At our center, we started performing ePLND in 2007. Our comparative analysis of standard PLND (obturator fossa) and ePLND showed that ePLND significantly increased the lymph node yield from 8–10 to 14–20 nodes and the node-positive yield from 2.2–6.2% to 17.4–18.4% (both $p < 0.001$) [25]. Also, the median operation times with standard PLND and ePLND were 20 and 37 min, respectively. We did not observe a significant difference in PLND-related complications between the standard PLND and ePLND cohorts [25]. In 2019, we adopted the SP robotic surgery system for RARP along with multi-port robotic surgery systems at MD Anderson [47]. After successful adoption of the new platform, outcomes in our initial series of 17 patients who underwent SP RARP with ePLND demonstrated operative times, complication rates, lymph node yield (median, 14 [IQR, 9–18]), and node-positive yield (15%) similar to those in patients who underwent multi-port RARP with ePLND [47].

Impact of ePLND on Perioperative and Postoperative Morbidity

The technical challenges and potential complications of PLND, especially ePLND, warrant careful consideration when recommending the procedure [48]. A systematic review in which researchers analyzed pooled data from 176 studies of 77,303 PCa patients revealed that those who underwent radical prostatectomy with limited or standard PLND experienced significantly fewer intraoperative (risk ratio, 0.55; $P = 0.01$) and postoperative (risk ratio, 0.46; $P < 0.001$) complications, specifically lymphocele formation and thromboembolic events, than did patients who underwent radical prostatectomy with extended or super-extended PLND [49]. Eighty-four of the 176 studies (28,428 patients) demonstrated that 1.8% of the patients experienced at least one intraoperative complication. In these patients, obturator nerve (52%) and iliac artery (22%) injury were the most commonly observed PLND-related intraoperative complications [49]. Obturator nerve injury is very rare, and researchers observed no long-term complications associated with obturator nerve functions (e.g., adductor function) or neurological deficiency after simultaneous repair of obturator nerve injury with 6-0 polypropylene during RARP [50]. Additionally, a study showed greater risk of hospital readmission in patients who underwent RARP with ePLND than in those who underwent RARP alone (4.4% vs. 0.8%) [51].

Surgical Strategies for Lymphocele Prevention

Lymphocele is the most frequent complication after PLND. Although its real incidence is not known because most of lymphoceles are asymptomatic, 0–8% of PLND patients experience symptomatic lymphocele (SL) after RARP [2]. Previous studies comparing the SL rate for the limited and standard PLND templates with that for the extended PLND template did not show a significant difference [52, 53]. However, a prospective study demonstrated a 5% increase in the risk of SL for every lymph node removed [54]. Additionally, the extent of PLND was an independent predictor of lymphocele formation (risk ratio, 1.77; $P < 0.001$) in a recent meta-analysis of 176 studies [49]. The predictors for SL formation were use of prophylactic low-molecular-weight heparin, an increased number of positive lymph nodes, and extracapsular extension [49]. Similarly, studies comparing lymphocele incidence in PCa patients with extraperitoneal and transperitoneal approaches had controversial results [55]. Authors had reported a higher incidence of SL with the extraperitoneal approach than with the transperitoneal approach [56, 57], whereas a more recent study showed similar SL rates with both approaches [58].

Most SLs can be managed via percutaneous drainage or with conservative treatments; rare cases require surgical marsupialization. Various strategies have been proposed to prevent SL development after RARP, such as peritoneal interposition flap [59], bilateral peritoneal fenestration [60], P.L.E.A.T. (Preventing Lymphocele Ensuring Absorption Transperitoneally) [61], 4PPFF (Four-Point Peritoneal Flap Fixation) [62], placement of pelvic drain [63], and use of hemostatic agents [64, 65], sealing techniques and sealing agents [66]. Randomized controlled trials showed no significant differences in SL development rate after RARP with PLND in comparing non-drainage with pelvic drainage [67], titanium clips with bipolar energy [66], TachoSil (a hemostatic sponge) with control [65], and Arista AH (a hemostatic powder) with control [64]. In a systematic review that included five retrospective studies of 1308 patients, authors found the peritoneal interposition flap to be effective in preventing SL development after RARP with PLND (1.3% vs. 5.7%) [68]. However, a recent randomized controlled trial showed no benefit of the peritoneal interposition flap in reducing the rate of postoperative lymphocele, either asymptomatic or symptomatic [69]. Consequently, increasing lymphatic reabsorption by maximizing the peritoneal surface seems to be a rapid and cost-effective option in preventing or reducing SL development. The use of specific agents and sealing techniques is not supported in the literature, though [55].

References

1. Mottet N, et al. EAU-EANM-ESTRO-ESUR-SIOG guidelines on prostate cancer—2020 update. Part 1: Screening, diagnosis, and local treatment with curative intent. Eur Urol. 2021;79:243–62.
2. Ploussard G, et al. Pelvic lymph node dissection during robot assisted radical prostatectomy: efficacy, limitations, and complications—a systematic review of the literature. Eur Urol. 2014;65:7–16.
3. Canda AE. Re: Is robot-assisted radical prostatectomy safe in men with high-risk prostate cancer? Assessment of perioperative outcomes, positive surgical margins, and use of additional cancer treatments. Eur Urol. 2015;67:347.
4. Davis JW, Shah JB, Achim M. Robot-assisted extended pelvic lymph node dissection (PLND) at the time of radical prostatectomy (RP): a video-based illustration of technique, results, and unmet patient selection needs. BJU Int. 2011;108:993–8.
5. Cooperberg MR, Kane CJ, Cowan JE, Carroll PR. Adequacy of lymphadenectomy among men undergoing robot-assisted laparoscopic radical prostatectomy. BJU Int. 2010;105:88–92.
6. Xia L, et al. Contemporary national trends and variations of pelvic lymph node dissection in patients undergoing robot-assisted radical prostatectomy. Clin Genitourin Cancer. 2021 19(4) 309–15. https://doi.org/10.1016/j.clgc.2021.01.005.
7. Briganti A, et al. Updated nomogram predicting lymph node invasion in patients with prostate cancer undergoing extended pelvic lymph node dissection: the essential importance of percentage of positive cores. Eur Urol. 2012;61:480–7.
8. Memorial Sloan Kettering Institute; Prostate cancer nomograms: pre-radical prostatectomy. Memorial Sloan Kettering Cancer Center. 2020. https://www.mskcc.org/nomograms/prostate/pre_op.
9. Oderda M, et al. Indications for and complications of pelvic lymph node dissection in prostate cancer: accuracy of available nomograms for the prediction of lymph node invasion. BJU Int. 2021;127:318–25.
10. Mohler JL, et al. Prostate cancer, version 2.2019, NCCN clinical practice guidelines in oncology. J Natl Compr Canc Netw. 2019;17:479–505.

11. Perera M, et al. Gallium-68 prostate-specific membrane antigen positron emission tomography in advanced prostate cancer-updated diagnostic utility, sensitivity, specificity, and distribution of prostate-specific membrane antigen-avid lesions: a systematic review and meta-analysis. Eur Urol. 2020;77:403–17.
12. Hofman MS, et al. Prostate-specific membrane antigen PET-CT in patients with high-risk prostate cancer before curative-intent surgery or radiotherapy (proPSMA): a prospective, randomised, multicentre study. Lancet. 2020;395:1208–16.
13. Luiting HB, et al. Use of gallium-68 prostate-specific membrane antigen positron-emission tomography for detecting lymph node metastases in primary and recurrent prostate cancer and location of recurrence after radical prostatectomy: an overview of the current literature. BJU Int. 2020;125:206–14.
14. Franklin A, et al. Histological comparison between predictive value of preoperative 3-T multiparametric MRI and ^{68}Ga-PSMA PET/CT scan for pathological outcomes at radical prostatectomy and pelvic lymph node dissection for prostate cancer. BJU Int. 2021;127:71–9.
15. Meijer D, et al. The predictive value of preoperative negative prostate specific membrane antigen positron emission tomography imaging for lymph node metastatic prostate cancer. J Urol. 2021;205(6):1655–62. https://doi.org/10.1097/JU.0000000000001592.
16. Jansen BHE, et al. Pelvic lymph-node staging with ^{18}F-DCFPyL PET/CT prior to extended pelvic lymph-node dissection in primary prostate cancer—the SALT trial. Eur J Nucl Med Mol Imaging. 2021;48:509–20.
17. O'Shea A, Kilcoyne A, Hedgire SS, Harisinghani MG. Pelvic lymph nodes and pathways of disease spread in male pelvic malignancies. Abdom Radiol (NY). 2020;45:2198–212.
18. Grivas N, et al. Pelvic lymph node distribution and metastases of prostate and bladder cancer: a systematic literature review and template proposal. World J Urol. 2021;39:751–9.
19. Öbek C, et al. Members of Urooncology Association, Turkey. The accuracy of ^{68}Ga-PSMA PET/CT in primary lymph node staging in high-risk prostate cancer. Eur J Nucl Med Mol Imaging. 2017;44:1806–12.
20. Heidenreich A, Ohlmann CH, Polyakov S. Anatomical extent of pelvic lymphadenectomy in patients undergoing radical prostatectomy. Eur Urol. 2007;52:29–37.
21. Mattei A, et al. The template of the primary lymphatic landing sites of the prostate should be revisited: results of a multimodality mapping study. Eur Urol. 2008;53:118–25.
22. Heesakkers RA, et al. Prostate cancer: detection of lymph node metastases outside the routine surgical area with ferumoxtran-10-enhanced MR imaging. Radiology. 2009;251:408–14.
23. Sanda MG, et al. Clinically localized prostate cancer: AUA/ASTRO/SUO guideline. Part II: Recommended approaches and details of specific care options. J Urol. 2018;199:990–7.
24. Williams SB, Bozkurt Y, Achim M, Achim G, Davis JW. Sequencing robot-assisted extended pelvic lymph node dissection prior to radical prostatectomy: a step-by-step guide to exposure and efficiency. BJU Int. 2016;117:192–8.
25. Altok M, et al. Surgeon-led prostate cancer lymph node staging: pathological outcomes stratified by robot-assisted dissection templates and patient selection. BJU Int. 2018;122:66–75.
26. Moschini M, et al. Determinants of long-term survival of patients with locally advanced prostate cancer: the role of extensive pelvic lymph node dissection. Prostate Cancer Prostatic Dis. 2016;19:63–7.
27. Abdollah F, et al. More extensive pelvic lymph node dissection improves survival in patients with node-positive prostate cancer. Eur Urol. 2015;67:212–9.
28. Fossati N, et al. The benefits and harms of different extents of lymph node dissection during radical prostatectomy for prostate cancer: a systematic review. Eur Urol. 2017;72:84–109.
29. Lestingi JFP, et al. Extended versus limited pelvic lymph node dissection during radical prostatectomy for intermediate- and high-risk prostate cancer: early oncological outcomes from a randomized phase 3 trial. Eur Urol. 2020;79(5):595–604. https://doi.org/10.1016/j.eururo.2020.11.040.
30. Seiler R, Studer UE, Tschan K, Bader P, Burkhard FC. Removal of limited nodal disease in patients undergoing radical prostatectomy: long-term results confirm a chance for cure. J Urol. 2014;191:1280–5.
31. Preisser F, et al. Effect of extended pelvic lymph node dissection on oncologic outcomes in patients with D'Amico intermediate and high risk prostate cancer treated with radical prostatectomy: a multi-institutional study. J Urol. 2020;203:338–43.
32. Altok M, Chapin BF, Matin SF, Achim MF, Gregg JR, Davis JW. Therapeutic consequences of omitting a pelvic lymph node dissection at radical prostatectomy when grade and/or stage increase. Urology. 2021;155:144–51. https://doi.org/10.1016/j.urology.2021.01.064.
33. Mattei A, Di Pierro GB, Grande P, Beutler J, Danuser H. Standardized and simplified extended pelvic lymph node dissection during robot-assisted radical prostatectomy: the monoblock technique. Urology. 2013;81:446–50.
34. Mattei A, et al. Standardized and simplified robot-assisted superextended pelvic lymph node dissection for prostate cancer: the monoblock technique. Eur Urol. 2020;78:424–31.
35. Mazzone E, et al. Diagnostic value, oncological outcomes and safety profile of image-guided surgery technologies during robot-assisted lymph node dissection with sentinel node biopsy for prostate cancer. J Nucl Med. 2021;62(10):1363–71. https://doi.org/10.2967/jnumed.120.259788.
36. Harke NN, et al. Fluorescence-supported lymphography and extended pelvic lymph node dissection in robot-assisted radical prostatectomy: a prospective, randomized trial. World J Urol. 2018;36:1817–23.
37. Claps F, et al. Indocyanine green guidance improves the efficiency of extended pelvic lymph node dissection during laparoscopic radical prostatectomy. Int J Urol. 2021;28(5):566–72. https://doi.org/10.1111/iju.14513.
38. Dell'Oglio P, et al. A DROP-IN gamma probe for robot-assisted radioguided surgery of lymph nodes during radical prostatectomy. Eur Urol. 2021;79:124–32.
39. Wit EMK, et al. Sentinel node procedure in prostate cancer: a systematic review to assess diagnostic accuracy. Eur Urol. 2017;71:596–605.
40. Lenfant L, et al. Robot-assisted radical prostatectomy using single-port perineal approach: technique and single-surgeon matched-paired comparative outcomes. Eur Urol. 2021;79:384–92.
41. Lenfant L, et al. Pure single-site robot-assisted radical prostatectomy using single-port versus multiport robotic radical prostatectomy: a single-institution comparative study. Eur Urol Focus. 2020;7(5):964–72. https://doi.org/10.1016/j.euf.2020.10.006.
42. Huang MM, et al. Comparison of perioperative and pathologic outcomes between single-port and standard robot-assisted radical prostatectomy: an analysis of a high-volume center and the pooled world experience. Urology. 2021;147:223–9.
43. Abreu A, et al. Robotic salvage retroperitoneal and pelvic lymph node dissection for 'node-only' recurrent prostate cancer: technique and initial series. BJU Int. 2017;120:401–8.
44. Heidenreich A, Rieke M, Mahjoub S, Pfister D. Management of positive lymph nodes following radical prostatectomy. Arch Esp Urol. 2019;72:182–91.
45. Montorsi F, et al. Robot-assisted salvage lymph node dissection for clinically recurrent prostate cancer. Eur Urol. 2017;72:432–8.
46. Siriwardana A, et al. Initial multicentre experience of ^{68}gallium-PSMA PET/CT guided robot-assisted salvage lymphadenectomy:

acceptable safety profile but oncological benefit appears limited. BJU Int. 2017;120:673–81.
47. Abaza R, Martinez O, Murphy C, Urkmez A, Davis J. Adoption of single-port robotic prostatectomy: two alternative strategies. J Endourol. 2020;34:1230–4.
48. Clark T, et al. Randomized prospective evaluation of extended versus limited lymph node dissection in patients with clinically localized prostate cancer. J Urol. 2003;169:145–8.
49. Cacciamani GE, et al. Impact of pelvic lymph node dissection and its extent on perioperative morbidity in patients undergoing radical prostatectomy for prostate cancer: a comprehensive systematic review and meta-analysis. Eur Urol Oncol. 2021;4(2):134–49. https://doi.org/10.1016/j.euo.2021.02.001.
50. Gözen AS, Aktoz T, Akin Y, Klein J, Rieker P, Rassweiler J. Is it possible to draw a risk map for obturator nerve injury during pelvic lymph node dissection? The Heilbronn experience and a review of the literature. J Laparoendosc Adv Surg Tech A. 2015;25:826–32.
51. Sebben M, et al. The impact of extended pelvic lymph node dissection on the risk of hospital readmission within 180 days after robot assisted radical prostatectomy. World J Urol. 2020;38:2799–809.
52. Liss MA, Palazzi K, Stroup SP, Jabaji R, Raheem OA, Kane CJ. Outcomes and complications of pelvic lymph node dissection during robotic-assisted radical prostatectomy. World J Urol. 2013;31:481–8.
53. Yuh BE, Ruel NH, Mejia R, Novara G, Wilson TG. Standardized comparison of robot-assisted limited and extended pelvic lymphadenectomy for prostate cancer. BJU Int. 2013;112:81–8.
54. Capitanio U, et al. How can we predict lymphorrhoea and clinically significant lymphocoeles after radical prostatectomy and pelvic lymphadenectomy? Clinical implications. BJU Int. 2011;107:1095–101.
55. Motterle G, et al. Surgical strategies for lymphocele prevention in minimally invasive radical prostatectomy and lymph node dissection: a systematic review. J Endourol. 2020;34:113–20.
56. Chung JS, et al. Comparison of oncological results, functional outcomes, and complications for transperitoneal versus extraperitoneal robot-assisted radical prostatectomy: a single surgeon's experience. J Endourol. 2011;25:787–92.
57. Porpiglia F, et al. Transperitoneal versus extraperitoneal laparoscopic radical prostatectomy: experience of a single center. Urology. 2006;68:376–80.
58. Horovitz D, Lu X, Feng C, Messing EM, Joseph JV. Rate of symptomatic lymphocele formation after extraperitoneal vs transperitoneal robot-assisted radical prostatectomy and bilateral pelvic lymphadenectomy. J Endourol. 2017;31:1037–43.
59. Lebeis C, Canes D, Sorcini A, Moinzadeh A. Novel technique prevents lymphoceles after transperitoneal robotic-assisted pelvic lymph node dissection: peritoneal flap interposition. Urology. 2015;85:1505–9.
60. Stolzenburg JU, et al. Reduction in incidence of lymphocele following extraperitoneal radical prostatectomy and pelvic lymph node dissection by bilateral peritoneal fenestration. World J Urol. 2008;26:581–6.
61. Dal Moro F, Zattoni F. P.L.E.A.T.—Preventing Lymphocele Ensuring Absorption Transperitoneally: a robotic technique. Urology. 2017;110:244–7.
62. Stolzenburg JU, et al. Four-point peritoneal flap fixation in preventing lymphocele formation following radical prostatectomy. Eur Urol Oncol. 2018;1:443–8.
63. Danuser H, Di Pierro GB, Stucki P, Mattei A. Extended pelvic lymphadenectomy and various radical prostatectomy techniques: is pelvic drainage necessary? BJU Int. 2013;111:963–9.
64. Gilbert DR, Angell J, Abaza R. Evaluation of absorbable hemostatic powder for prevention of lymphoceles following robotic prostatectomy with lymphadenectomy. Urology. 2016;98:75–80.
65. Buelens S, Van Praet C, Poelaert F, Van Huele A, Decaestecker K, Lumen N. Prospective randomized controlled trial exploring the effect of TachoSil on lymphocele formation after extended pelvic lymph node dissection in prostate cancer. Urology. 2018;118:134–40.
66. Grande P, et al. Prospective randomized trial comparing titanium clips to bipolar coagulation in sealing lymphatic vessels during pelvic lymph node dissection at the time of robot-assisted radical prostatectomy. Eur Urol. 2017;71:155–8.
67. Chenam A, et al. Prospective randomised non-inferiority trial of pelvic drain placement vs no pelvic drain placement after robot-assisted radical prostatectomy. BJU Int. 2018;121:357–64.
68. Deutsch S, Hadaschik B, Lebentrau S, Ubrig B, Burger M, May M. Clinical importance of a peritoneal interposition flap to prevent symptomatic lymphoceles after robot-assisted radical prostatectomy and pelvic lymph node dissection: a systematic review and meta-analysis. Urol Int. 2021;10:1–7.
69. Bründl J, et al. Peritoneal flap in robot-assisted radical prostatectomy. Dtsch Arztebl Int. 2020;117:243–50.

Fluorescence Guided Node Dissection

28

A. C. Berrens, O. Özman, T. Maurer, F. W. B. Van Leeuwen, and H. G. van der Poel

Introduction

Because of limited ability to visually discriminate targeted tissue from surrounding tissue the demand for new image guided surgery has increased. New ways to provide real-time guidance have developed rapidly. In this chapter we provide the insight into the physics of fluorescence and the clinical application of fluorescence during lymph node dissection in prostate cancer.

History of Fluorescence

Fluorescence was observed by the Aztecs. They observed a peculiar blue-light emission when water was added to a diuretic type of wood. A phenomenon later called "lignum nephriticum", meaning "kidney wood" in Latin (Fig. 28.1). When the Europeans arrived it was not the medical use but the color effects used to distinguish this rare and expensive wood from counterfeits that attracted attention; wooden cups made from lignum nephriticum were even given as gifts to royalty [1].

In 1565 a Spanish physician and botanist, Nicolas Monardes, first reported the fluorescence phenomenon [2]. A century later Robert Boyle, a famous chemist, also mentions his observation about fluorescence in his notes; *"If you make an infusion of Lignum Nephriticum in spring water it will appear of a deep color; like that of an orange, when you place*

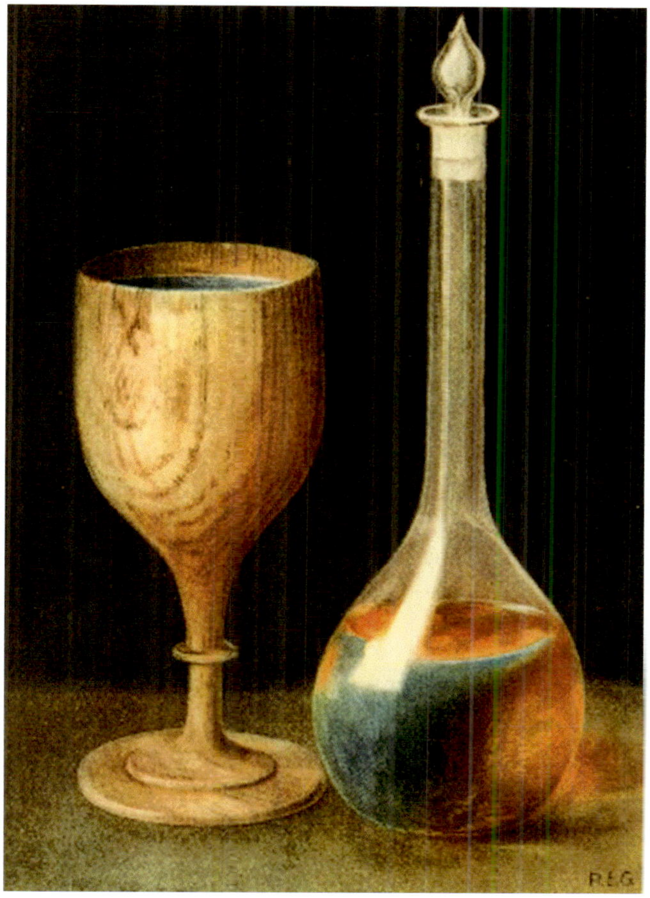

Fig. 28.1 "Lignum nephriticum". The color effect of adding water to a special type of wood

A. C. Berrens · O. Özman
Department of Urology, Netherlands Cancer Institute, Antoni van Leeuwenhoek Hospital, Amsterdam, The Netherlands
e-mail: a.berrens@nki.nl

T. Maurer
Department of Urology, University Hospital Hamburg-Eppendorf, Hamburg, Germany

Martini-Klinik Prostate Cancer Center, University Hospital Hamburg-Eppendorf, Hamburg, Germany
e-mail: t.maurer@uke.de

F. W. B. Van Leeuwen
Interventional Molecular Imaging Laboratory, Department of Radiology, Leiden University Medical Center, Leiden, The Netherlands
e-mail: f.w.b.van_leeuwen@lumc.nl

H. G. van der Poel (✉)
Department of Urology, Amsterdam University Medical Center, Location VUmc, Amsterdam, The Netherlands
e-mail: h.vd.poel@nki.nl

S. Ren et al. (eds.), *Robot-Assisted Radical Prostatectomy*, https://doi.org/10.1007/978-3-031-05855-4_28

the vial between the window and your eye; and of a fine deep blue when you look on it with your eye placed between it and the window" [3]. Later, it was discovered that the UV components in sunlight excited a small fluorescent molecule called formononetin, yielding the blue fluorescent emission [4].

British scientist Sir George G. Stokes, discovered the concept of excitation and emission spectra and introduced the term fluorescence. It was, however, not until 1929 that the mechanism of fluorescence on molecular level was described; *the mechanism of excited substances passing through an intermediate state before emission* [5]. Since then fluorescent compound also made their way to diagnostic medical applications. Two prime examples being fluorescein and indocyanine green (ICG). Fluorescein, when emitted with ultraviolet (UV)-light emits a bright yellow green ($\lambda = 488–515$ nm) and was first used as a tracer for intra operative differentiation of normal and malignant tissues in the 1940s [6].

ICG was developed in the second world war as a dye in photography. It is nontoxic and non-radioactive. Its ability to provide near-infrared fluorescence imaging got it into clinical use and it has been approved for intravenous administration by the U.S. Food and Drug Administration (FDA) since the 1950s for a broad range of surgical indications [7, 8].

Physics of Fluorescence

Fluorescence is part of the broader concept of luminescence. Essentially, the focus of luminescence-based imaging is the detection of light that is emitted from a particular area. The emission spectrum of luminescent tracers intended for medical use encompasses UV-light (400 nm), visible light (400–650 nm), far-red light (650–780 nm), and near-infrared range of 780–2000 nm [9].

Fluorescence is the spontaneous emission of light radiation from a substance that is electronically excited by a light source. Meaning that light needs to go in first and a light-sensitive camera is required to detect the emitted light. Dyes that have fluorescent properties are named fluorophores or fluorescent dyes. The light absorbance and emission aspects of fluorescent dye are dictated by the size and shape of conjugated system in their molecular structure, meaning each specific molecule has a unique absorption maximum ($\lambda_{ex\ max}$). When a fluorescent dye is excited in its "fingerprint" absorption spectrum, the molecule can convert to an unstable excited energy state. The energy that is lost by the decay back to the stable state, as seen in the Jablonski diagram (Fig. 28.2), converts it into light of a longer wavelength which provides the emitted fluorescent light. Again, the (maximum) emission wavelength ($\lambda_{em\ max}$) is unique for each fluorescent dye as it also depends on the specific conjugation system in a molecule. The strength (also called brightness) of a fluorescence emission is a combination of a couple of factors a.o.: the concentration of the dye (please note that in some cases e.g. for ICG the fluorescence drops at concentration over 5×10^{-5} M) [10]. The intensity of the excitation light source (assuming it is matched to the absorption maximum), the efficiency by which the excitation light is absorbed by the molecule (called extinction coefficient) and the conversion of the absorbed energy into a fluorescent emission (called quantum yield) [11].

$$Brightness = Extinction\ Coefficient(\varepsilon) \times Fluorescence\ Quantum\ Yield(\Phi)$$

Clinical use has been reported for a wide range of fluorescent dyes with greatly varying molecular structures and properties. Non structurally related dyes are fluorescein ($\lambda_{em\ max}$ 515 nm; brightness in aqueous solutions $\approx 10^5$) [11] which has been used in non-conjugated [6] and conjugated form [12], methylene blue (MB (λ_{em} 686 nm; brightness $\approx 10^3$) [13] and the metabolically formed dye PpIX ($\lambda_{em\ max}$ 515 nm; quantum yield 0.06 and extinction coefficient 4866 $M^{-1}\ cm^{-1}$) [14, 15]. Apart from these structures most medical applications make use of structurally related cyanine dyes, e.g. conjugated Cy5 (λ_{em} 651 nm; brightness = 5×10^4) [16, 17], IRDye 800CW (λ_{em} 800 nm; quantum yield of 9% with an extinction coefficient of $2.42 \times 10^5\ M^{-1}\ cm^{-1}$ [18] and non-conjugated ICG (λ_{em} 820 nm; brightness = $\approx 10^3$) [19]. Based on this list the dye application can be separated on their wavelength and on non-conjugated (dye only) and conjugated (dye attached to a vector).

Fluorescein is a non-conjugated dye in its purest form. When administered intravenously fluorescein can be used to measure extravasation from blood vessels and renal clearance [20]. Local administrations have seen application in lymphangiography [21].

ICG, although not having a specific moiety for chemical conjugation, has the tendency to non-covalently bind to proteins such as human serum albumin. In fact the binding to serum proteins is so efficient (80%) that dyes are protein bound when in vivo [22]. As a result intravenously administered ICG does not extravasate from blood vessels and remains intravascular for up to 20–30 min, after which it is hepatically cleared via bile [7, 23]. These properties have driven its used during (retinal) angiography [24] and cholangiography [23]. Following local injections ICG, bound to serum proteins, provides an effective lymphangiographic agent [21].

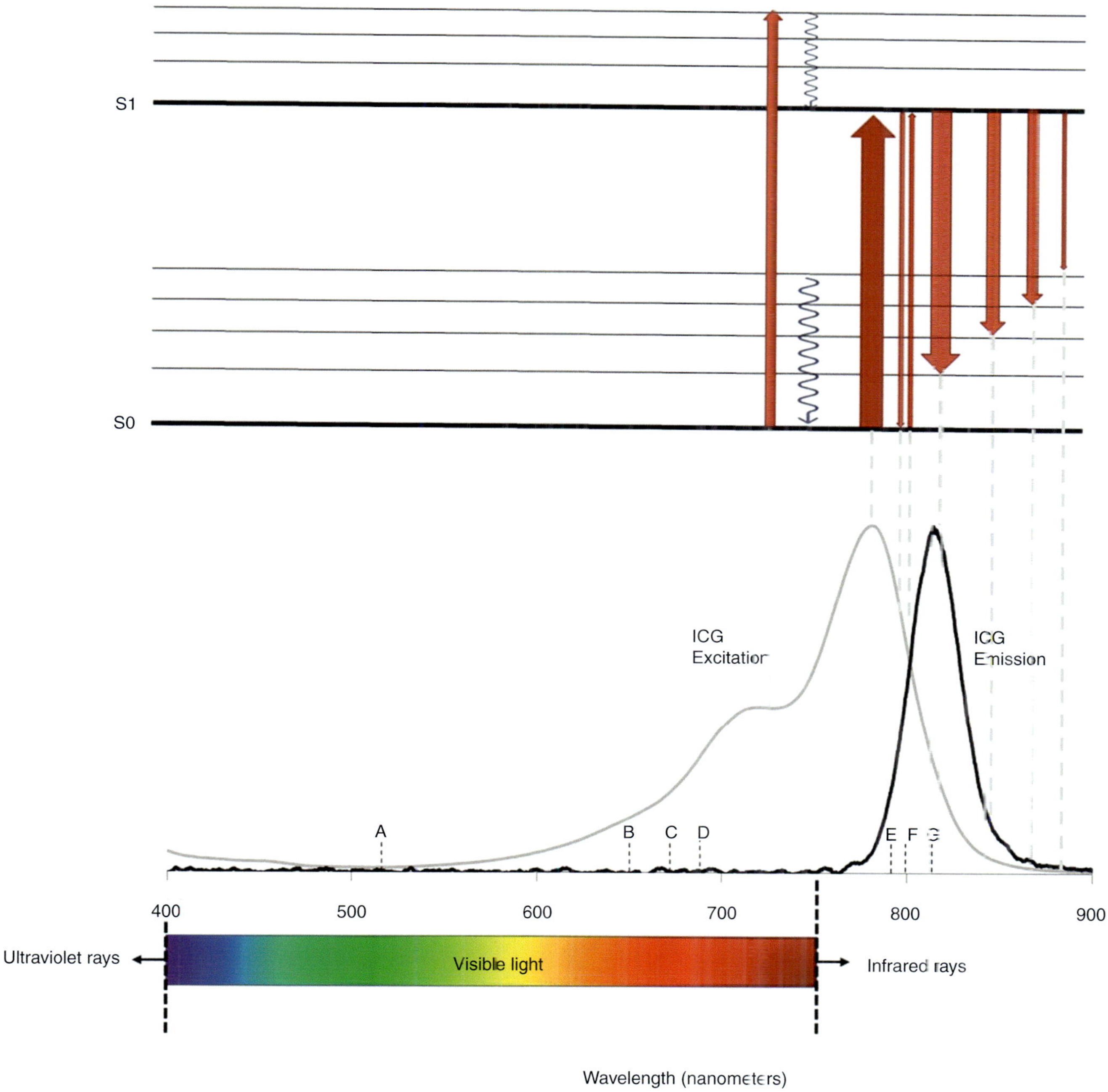

Fig. 28.2 Simplified Jablonski diagram with electromagnetic spectrum of visible light. Example of excitation and emission shown for ICG. Emission wavelengths for mentioned dyes: (**a**) EC17, fluorescein and PpIX (λ_{em} 515 nm). (**b**) Cy5 (λ_{em} 651 nm). (**c**) EMI-137 (λ_{em} 670 nm). (**d**) MB (λ_{em} 686 nm). (**e**) IRDye 800CW (λ_{em} 800 nm). (**f**) IR800 IAB2M and OTL38 (λ_{em} 738 nm), OTL78 (λ_{em} 793 nm). (**g**) ICG (λ_{em} 820 nm)

Non-covalently bound ICG has also been successfully applied to locate the draining lymph nodes for different cancers such as those of the uterus [25–27], breast cancer, melanoma, squamous cell carcinoma of the oral cavity [28], gastric cancer [29, 30] and colon carcinoma [31] but the less specific accumulation of non-bound ICG in the sentinel nodes make it less suitable for sentinel node biopsy (SNB). The definition of sentinel node in prostate cancer remains under debate (Table 23.1).

To more specifically targeted the sentinel node and have ICG retained in it the non-covalent interactions between ICG and albumin have been exploited to create ICG-complexes with nano-particles that are based on albumin aggregates viz. nanocolloid. A feature that helps drive the nodal uptake fol-

Table 28.1 Selection of literature on fluorescence guidance in sentinel node procedures

Article	Pts (n)	Risk group	Operating technique	Template	Tracer	Most important results	Conclusion	Future
Jeschke (2005)	71	All	Laparoscopic	sPLND	^{99m}Tc-Senti-Scint	Radioactivity was detected on two sides in 70.4%, one side in 26.7 and zero in 2,8%. In 54.7% SNs were exclusively outside of the obturator fossa. Histopathological examination showed LNM in SNs in 12.9%. 72.7% of all LNM were outside of the obturator fossa. LNM were exclusively found in Tc containing LNs	Lap. SN procedure is feasible and detects micrometastases outside of the obturator fossa. A gamma probe with a 90° window and the transperitoneal approach were the most important factors for success	On SN NR. The lower threshold of super paramagnetic nanoparticles in conjunction with high resolution MR must be clearly defined in the future
Jeschke (2008)	140	All	Laparoscopic	sPLND	^{99m}Tc-Senti-Scint	SNs were identified on two sides in 68.1% and one side in 25.7%. No SNs were found in 5.7%. In 48.2% of the pelvic sidewalls, SNs were exclusively outside the obturator fossa. Histopathological examination showed LNM in SNs 13.5% of patients; 71.4% of the LNM were outside the current standard LND template	Confirmation of lap. LND + SN in staging PC. Significant amount of LNM were outside of the routine LND template. Small sized metastases are still undetectable by currently available preoperative imaging modalities	SN technique is in need of standardization and more comparative studies
van der Poel (2011)	11	Intermediate/high	Robot assisted laparoscopic	ePLND	ICG-^{99m}TC-nanocolloid	SNs were identified by SPECT/CT preoperatively. The multimodal nature of the imaging agent also enabled via fluorescence imaging intraoperatively. Surgical guidance improved by fluorescence particularly in areas with radioactive background signal. A strong correlation was revealed ex vivo in excised LNs between the radioactive and fluorescent content. Fluorescence guidance was limited by tissue attenuation of the signal	Multimodal ICG-^{99m}Tc-NanoColloid, combined with a laparoscopic fluorescence camera, can be used for SN biopsy during RALP	Further improvement of accuracy is expected when it will be integrated into the robotic system to guide the tip of the laparoscope toward the region of interest
Jeschke (2012)	26	Intermediate/high	Laparoscopic	ePLND + SN	^{99m}Tc-Senti-Scint and ICG	Two drainage patterns were identified as characteristic: along medial umbilical ligament and the internal iliac region. In 11.5% direct connection was found with para-aortic LNs. Additional fluorescence guided LNs demonstrated 120 extra LNs, not identified with radio guidance	Using the described technique of fluorescence navigation, not only lymph nodes but also lymphatic vessels are visualized in real time. The technique appears to be as effective as sentinel LND but easier to apply	Investigate whether fluorescence guided surgery can replace radioguided surgery

Kleinjan (2014)	40	Intermediate/high	Robot assisted laparoscopic	ePLND	ICG-^{99m}Tc-NC	Mean fluorescence-based SN identification improved from 63.7% (gamma-probe + FI and old tracer) to 85.2% and 93.5% for groups 2 (gamma-probe + FI and new tracer) and 3 (FI only), respectively ($p = 0.012$). BCR occurred in three patients (pN0). No differences in postoperative complications were found	Optimisation of the hybrid tracer and imaging systems led to a significant improvement in fluorescence-guided identification of SNs. Preoperative SPECT-CT remained essential for intraoperative guidance	NR
Manny (2014)	50	All	Robot assisted laparoscopic	ePLND	ICG	Robotic-guided ICG injection intraprostatic proved superior to cystoscope or transrectal delivery. Tissue marking was achieved in all patients, positively identifying the prostate with uniform fluorescence relative to surrounding structures at a mean of 10 min postinjection. At a mean of 30 min postinjection SNs were identified in 76% of patient and had 100% sensitivity, 75.4% specificity, 14.6% PPV, and 100% NPV for the detection of nodal metastasis	Robotic-guided injection intraprostatic is safe, feasible, and allows for reliable prostate tissue marking and identification of SNs. ICG SNs are highly sensitive but relatively nonspecific for the detection of nodal metastasis	Reproduction of results in bigger cohort is needed
Yuen (2015)	66	All	Open	ePLND	ICG	SN identification was successful in 97%. A median of 4 SNs per patient was detected. Three lymphatic pathways were identified, the paravesical, internal and lateral routes. Pathological examination revealed LNM in SNs in 9%. 100% was detected as SNs using this imaging	Intraoperative fluorescence imaging with ICG aids with the detection of lymphatic vessels and SNs with high SSY. This method is technically feasible, safe and easy to apply	Further studies are needed to determine the suitable area for SN examination and to evaluate this application of fluorescent imaging
Backhaus (2016)	84	Intermediate/high	Laparoscopic	ePLND	ICG	Median of seven ICG stained LNs. LNM was identified 29.7% of patients, in 27% disease was properly classified by ICG guided LND. Pathological examination revealed 82 positive LNs, of which 60% with ICG	ICG staged 97% correctly. Cannot replace ePLND	Future could allow to avoid ePLND if accurate intraoperative lymph fluorescent analysis is done

(continued)

Table 28.1 (continued)

Article	Pts (n)	Risk group	Operating technique	Template	Tracer	Most important results	Conclusion	Future
Miki (2016)	28	Intermediate/ high	Laparoscopic	ePLND	ICG	SNs were identified in 96.4% with a median of 4.9 SNs per patient. The incidence of LNM was 10.7% (15 LNs: SNs and 9 no-SNs). In two patients, the SN was the only LNM. These two were found in internal iliac and obturator region. On a per-patient basis, the SSY of the SN biopsy was 100%. Three characteristic lymphatic pathway patterns were also identified, the predominant one being along the medial umbilical ligament and laterally to internal iliac, obturator, and external iliac. No complications occurred	Intraoperative fluorescence imaging is safe and feasible with ICG during RP. Real-time visualization being a great advantage. LNs along the internal iliac and obturator should be invariably dissected for accurate pathological staging especially in low-volume patients	NR
Nguyen (2016)	12	Intermediate/ high	NR	ePLND	ICG	It was found that (1) majority of SNs are along external and internal iliac regions, (2) that common iliac regions contain up to 22% of all SNs, (3) that drainage to the contralateral group of pelvic LNs is possible, and (4) that the significant drainage goes through the fossa of Marcille. Among the patients with systematic ICG injections, 42% had a total of 29 LNM. Of these, 16 were ICG positive: SSY of 55%	The drainage pattern is very complex and the SN technique is not able to replace ePLND (yet)	NR
Aoun (2018)	Systematic review of ten clinical trials	NR	All	PLND	ICG	The pooled patient detection rates were 0.88 (0.82–0.92) and 0.92 (0.84–0.96), respectively. The pooled node detection rates were 0.71 (95% CI: 0.68–0.74). Significant heterogeneity existed among studies for patients and for nodes. In patient detection rate ($P < 0.001$) and in nodes detection rate ($P < 0.001$) significant publication bias was found	SN mapping in bladder and prostate cancer has a high detection rate, although SPY to predict LNM remains poor	Large trials are needed to assess the impact of ICG-fluorescence guided sentinel LND

Miki (2018)	50	Intermediate/high	Laparoscopic	ePLND	ICG	In 94% SNs were successfully identified, with median of 4 per patient. LNM were found in 12%, all of whom had positive SNs. 91% of the positive SNs were located along two of three characteristic lymphatic pathways for PC. The first site located at the junction between internal and external iliac vessels. The others located along the inferior vesical artery	Over 90% of positive SNs nodes located at two predominant sites. The removal of the SNs closer to the prostate should be prioritized in PLND. To reduce the chance of overlooking LNM, particular attention should be paid to identifying these nodes	A randomized study with a larger cohort is required to further confirm these findings
Meershoek (2020)	25	Briganti >5%	Robot assisted laparoscopic	ePLND	(ICG)-^{99m}Tc-NC, ^{99m}Tc-NC + free ICG	No differences were seen in the SN identification rate between ICG-^{99m}Tc-nanocolloid and ^{99m}Tc-nanocolloid. Fluorescence guidance allowed intraoperative removal of all SNs in 20% in the free-ICG group and only in 40% of the hybrid-tracer group. 51.8% of the SNs in the free-ICG group were removed solely under fluorescence guidance and 75.9% in hybrid-tracer group. After unmasking, 18 remaining SNs were identified. In the free-ICG group, ex vivo evaluation revealed that 14 SNs removed had radioactivity but no fluorescence	The hybrid tracer outperformed free ICG. The preoperative imaging with SPECT/CT enhanced the detection of prostate SNs. Fluorescence-guided PLND underestimated the number of SNs in 60–80% of patients.	Data from future randomized studies that apply tumor-specific tracers will be needed to confirm if preoperative imaging is indispensable

(continued)

Table 28.1 (continued)

Article	Pts (n)	Risk group	Operating technique	Template	Tracer	Most important results	Conclusion	Future
Aras (2021)	10	All	NR	ePLND	[18F]-BF3-Cy3-ACUPA	Absorbed doses by organs were similar to 68Ga-PSMA-11 imaging. The physiologic radiotracer accumulation and urinary/biliary excretion closely resembled the distribution of other published PSMA specific tracers. Tracer was retained in PSMA+ cancer for at least 24 h, allowing for intraoperative fluorescence assessment. The majority of contrast had decayed or cleared from the blood pool after 24 h. Preoperative and intraoperative findings were confirmed with final histopathology and multiphoton microscopy	In two patients it was demonstrated that [18F]-BF3-Cy3-ACUPA is both safe and useful in humans intraoperatively	Larger trials are needed to further define the clinical role of this tracer in the management of PSMA+ tumors
Claps (2021)	214	Briganti >5%	Laparoscopic	ePLND	ICG	The median number of retrieved nodes was significantly higher in ICG guided group 22 vs. 14. LNM was also higher in this group 65.9% vs. 34.1%. Increasing the yield of LND was independently and negatively correlated with the BCR in both overall and pN-positive patients. The 5-year BCR-free survival rates were 75.8% vs. 65.9% in overall cohort	ICG guided ePLND improves identification of lymphatic drainage. More LNs and LNM are identified. This allows more accurate local staging and a prolonged BCR-free survival	NR

SN sentinel node, *LNM* lymph node metastases, *LND* lymph node dissection, *FI* fluorescent imaging, *BCR* biochemical recurrence, *PPV* positive predictive value, *NNV* negative predictive value, *SSY* sensitivity lowing lymphatic drainage [32]. Bound ICG to albumin has shown only limited efficacy in bladder cancer patients [33]. Currently intravenous injection of free ICG is approved by FDA, but local administration in to the prostate not yet. Conjugated (bound) dyes are still only used in clinical research.

These variants can be attached, “targeted”. With conjugated dyes, the dye basically needs to contain a reactive moiety for commonly used amino acid conjugation strategies e.g. a carboxylic acid group that allows conjugation to a primary amine on a peptide or protein. As such the dye functions as a label for disease specific vector. Clinical literature examples contain, but are not limited to the targets: folate-receptor [34], C-Met [17], GE137. It goes without saying that essentially the targeting vectors can be labeled with different dyes, a concept that has been demonstrated for folate which can be targeted by (e.g.) EC17 by binding to folate receptors which are overexpressed on the surface of tumor cells including renal and ovarian cancer cells [34–38]. Important herein is the influence that the dye structure has on the affinity and pharma kinetics of the imaging agent as a whole. This effect is widely studied in the preclinical setting [22, 39–41] but as far as we know there is but one clinical report mentioning such an evaluation [42]. Currently, studies are ongoing for nearly 40 new image guided surgery tracer candidates (Table 28.2) [43].

Tumor Specific Fluorescent Tracers

Currently, most clinically used fluorescent tracers act in the NIR spectrum of light but other optical spectra have been evaluated. Early studies evaluated the role of 5-aminominolevulinic acid (5-ALA) for intraoperative detection of cancer cells [12]. When taken orally, it is converted into protoporphyrin IX (PpIX) which, because of reduced ferrochelatase activity in cancer cells, might accumulate in malignant tissue [45]. The PpIX within the tumor emits red fluorescence under a violet-blue light [46]. 5-ALA is an FDA-approved tracer for image guided surgery based on PpIX 5-ALA is specific for tumor tissue but not tumor type and is therefore widely used in different clinical disciplines. It is used in neurosurgery, especially malignant gliomas, and has found its use in bladder and kidney cancer surgery [47, 48]. The first application of 5-ALA in prostate cancer surgery was as a photodynamic diagnostic tool for evaluation of the surgical margins in radical prostatectomy [49]. Despite relatively promising results in surgical margin evaluation the sensitivity and specificity lacked and has therefore yet been abandoned. There is no study on the use of 5-ALA in pelvic lymph node dissection. In breast cancer studies, the fluorescence of metastatic axillary sentinel lymph nodes was found higher than non-metastatic sentinel lymph nodes after administration of oral 5-ALA [50]. It is thought that a lower depth of penetration of blue light into the abundant connective tissue of lymph nodes limits its use [51].

Prostate Cancer Specific (Fluorescent) Tracers

Prostate specific membrane antigen (PSMA) is a type II transmembrane glycoprotein which is expressed on cells of the prostate gland and overexpressed on prostate cancer cells in >90% [52, 53]. It has therefore gained interest as a tumor-specific target molecule for prostate cancer and has altered the approach of tumor specific imaging and radio guided surgery by adding an exogenous radioisotope [53, 54].

Table 28.2 Selection of fluorescent tracers and their application[a]

Name tracer	Tracer type	Application	Excitation/emission Wavelength (nm)
ICG	Non-conjugated Fluorescent dye	Lymphangiography Sentinel node imaging	807/820
Fluorescein	Non-conjugated Fluorescent dye	Ureter visualization Lymphangiography	488/515
Methylene blue	Non-conjugated Fluorescent dye	Ureter visualization	665/688
EC17 (Folate-FITC)	Folate-targeting small molecule	Ovarian carcinoma Renal cell carcinoma	488/515
OTL38 (Folate-800CW)	Folate-targeting small molecule	Ovarian carcinoma Endometrial cancer	774/788
EMI-137 (GE137)	C-Met targeting peptide	Penile cancer	650/670
IR800 IAB2M	PSMA-targeting minibody	Prostate cancer	774/788

ICG indocyanine green, *Folate-FITC* folate conjugated with fluorescein isothiocyanate. *EMI137* water-soluble compound composed of a 26-amino acid cyclic peptide, *C-Met* hepatocyte growth factor receptor, *IR800 IAB2M* ^{89}Zirconium-desferrioxamine-IAB2M

[a]Edited from van Beurden et al. [44]

PSMA-targeted fluorescent tracers might meet the desire of high resolution visual feedback intraoperatively. These tracers can be classified according to the emitting wavelength of the fluorophores; visible, far-red and NIR preferably combined with a radioactive component to the tracer for preoperative imaging and intraoperative navigation, comparable to the developed SNB tracers [39]. The first small molecule PSMA-NIR fluorophore tracers were produced in 2005 by conjugating the PSMA inhibitor GPI to IRDye78 to create GPI-78 [55]. After this, many more passed through research facilities all over the world. An example of a PSMA-specific fluorophore that did meet most of the conditions is OTL78 and is now in first in man trials [56]. The research for tracers targeting prostate cancer is not limited to PSMA. Infrared fluorophore conjugated anti-Prostate Stem Cell Antigen (PSCA) is an emerging tracer offering real-time intraoperative fluorescent imaging [57].

A problem with many of the conjugated fluorophores was that the physicochemical properties could drastically alter characteristics of the PSMA-targeting molecule [55, 58, 59]. Some never even made it to in vivo trials in mice [41, 60]. Also, large variations in dosage makes it difficult to compare clinical effectiveness of different tracers.

Combining Fluorescent Tracers and Radioactive Tracers

Combined fluorophores have also been applied to image lymphatic drainage patterns. van den Berg et al. used both ICG and fluorescein as fluorescent tracers to identify lymph nodes and lymphatic ducts simultaneously [61]. Similarly, using multispectral fluorescent camera systems ICG was successfully combined with fluorescein and Cy5 [62].

A limitation of fluorescence guided surgery is the tissue penetration. E.g. ICG and Cy5 can be seen from approximately 15 mm distance to the source emitting the signal. Tissue penetration is influenced by many things like the type of tissue (e.g. more fatty tissue, or more blood containing tissue) which has effect on the absorption and scattering of the signal. For ICG the tissue penetration was comparable in different types of tissue but it outperformed Cy5 in tissue with high blood content. Furthermore, the type of imaging camera used and the height of the background signal can play an important role. Practically, this means that for the use of NIR imaging it is important to get close to the tissue to be able to tell if the surgical margins are tumor free and if any fluorescent tissue is left behind [63]. This still prevents fluorescence guided surgery from being ideal for lymphatic road mapping for deep lymph nodes and vessels.

Combining a fluorescent tracer with a radioactive tracer emerged as a promising solution. Like with fluorescence there was already significant experience with solely radioactive tracers.

Currently, lymph node involvement is evaluated by radiological and radionuclide imaging methods in preoperative assessments of prostate cancer. PSMA PET/CT is a suitable alternative for conventional imaging methods, providing high diagnostic accuracy [64].

Radioisotopes such as beta and gamma-emitting PSMA-targeted tracers like ^{99m}Tc-PSMA-I&S (imaging and surgery) were introduced to give acoustic guidance during pelvic lymph node dissection [39]. Early studies have shown the feasibility of developing fluorescent PSMA targeting tracer and clinical trials are [41, 56, 65].

Again, combining a radioactive and fluorescent tracers may emerge as a promising next step comparable to the SNB tracers [66].

Fluorescence Guided Urological Surgery

First with the use of PpIX and fluorescein fluorescence was of aid in the spectrum visible to the human eye (white light). Because of the unique properties of certain dyes outside of the visible spectrum, however, the conventional white light sources were not enough. This required the NIR technology to integrate with daily practice inside the operating room. First open cameras and later laparoscopic handheld cameras were introduced. In 2011 the first lymphangiography with ICG using a fluorescence laparoscope was described in prostate cancer [67]. A camera to image fluorophores at different wavelengths was integrated with the da Vinci Si surgical robotic system®[1] when robot assisted surgery made his advance [10]. Now surgeons are able to control the images real-time directly from the surgical console, facilitating routine use of this camera.

In the field of urology fluorescence guided surgery has been used to unravel vascular perfusion during partial nephrectomy, to aid with ureteral reconstructions and in clinical trials to investigate minimalizing positive surgical margins of the primary tumor and sentinel node procedures in penile and prostate cancer [17]. The results from an extended pelvic lymph node dissection (ePLND) are still being considered the "gold standard" for nodal staging. However, ePLND has limitations. Research showed that 31% of tumor containing lymph nodes are missed by the standard ePLND template [68, 69].

When attached to nanocolloid the ICG is "trapped" in the first lymphnode making it suitable for identifying sentinel nodes. A potential benefit of SNB is the detection of tumor containing lymph nodes outside the ePLND template. In a systematic review 4.9% of sentinel nodes were documented

[1] Firefly; Intuitive Surgical, Sunnyvale, CA, USA.

outside the ePLND template [70]. Recently, a randomized control trial (RCT) showed higher detection rate of positive nodes using ICG nodal tracing and in recent literature a successful sentinel node detection rate of 86–100% is described when using ICG [26, 71, 72]. However, no difference in biochemical recurrence (BCR) was observed [73]. In the latest EAU guidelines sentinel node detection in intermediate/high-risk prostate cancer is still considered experimental. Also, the role of sentinel node detection in low-risk prostate cancer remains unclear [74].

During those first interventions with fluorescence some disadvantages were revealed. By intraoperative dissection of the lymphatic network leakage of the fluorescent tracer may occur leading to "contamination" of the surgical field. It also has to be taken into account that when tracers are injected intravenously excretion in bile and/or in urine can occur, and are therefore likely to give interfering background signal during prostatectomy. Currently, the best window for injecting the different fluorescent tracers is still under investigation. The way of administering the tracer has been researched by Korne et al. in 2019 concluding that intratumoral tracer deposition increased the chance of visualizing nodal metastases in comparison to intraprostatic (extra tumoral) tracer deposition [32, 75].

For use of hybrid tracers preoperatively a SPECT/CT is done as a control for tracer activity. During surgery it is possible to navigate on this SPECT/CT using acoustic guidance. Simultaneously, simplifying resection and visualization of the surgical margins with fluorescence guidance. Another benefit is when ICG is used in the hybrid tracer it is covalently bound to the nanocolloid particle. This approach provides a more specific nodal targeting and less nonspecific leakage of tracer compared to the use of free-ICG [76].

In comparison to only ICG, adding SN biopsy to ePLND during prostatectomy using a hybrid tracer Mazzone et al. (2021) showed increased detection of nodal metastases and a trend to improved BCR-free survival compared to ePLND only [77]. This benefit was obtained without an increased risk of procedure related complications.

The hybrid tracer ^{99m}Tc-ICG-nanocolloid was successfully applied in a variety of cancers including prostate cancer [77–80]. This raises the question what the additional value of preoperative SPECT/CT tracing is compared to intraoperative fluorescence imaging. In a study where surgeons were blinded for the preoperative SPECT/CT images, detection of all fluorescent nodes became difficult due to the low penetration of the fluorescent signal and additional nodes were found in at least 10% of cases after SPECT/CT unblinding [78]. This was confirmed in a recent retrospective analysis that showed a benefit for the hybrid tracer but not free-ICG for BCR after prostatectomy (Mazzone et al., Eur Urol, 2021) [77].

Furthermore, in 70% of patients with a BCR after local treatment metastases are found in a lymph node [81]. Recent literature already proves that radio guided salvage surgery is feasible and may results in early biochemical responses in recurrent prostate cancer but data on longer term outcome are to be awaited [82]. Suggesting that in the future there is a place for hybrid tracer guided salvage surgery as is already been done for the sentinel node group.

Summarizing, free fluorescent dyes are used in lymphatic mapping and in sentinel node biopsies when combined with human serum albumin Tumor specific (conjugated) dyes are of aid in preoperative imaging and intraoperative judgement of surgical margins. and salvage lymph node dissection. Especially when (tumor-specific) fluorescent tracers and radioactive tracers are combined into a hybrid tracer. In the future more of these hybrid tracers will be developed and eventually implemented in daily practice in robot assisted surgery.

Conclusions

Fluorescence-guided lymph node surgery in prostate cancer was shown to provide anatomical details of lymphatic drainage that can be used to the tailor lymphadenectomy and early data suggest improved outcome. Novel hybrid tracers allow both preoperative imaging and intraoperative tracing. Experience gained from SNB tracer development will aid in the further development of tumor specific tracers, such as those targeting PSMA that hold great promise.

References

1. Garrison FH. An introduction to the history of medicine. Philadelphia: WB Saunders: 1917. p. 283, 285.
2. Acuña AU, Amat-Guerri F. Early history of solution fluorescence: the lignum nephriticum of nicolás monardes. In: Fluorescence of supermolecules, polymers, and nanosystems. Springer series on fluorescence, vol. 4. Berlin, Heidelberg: Springer; 2007.
3. Benham CE. Fluorescence of lignum nephriticum. Nature. 1909;80:159.
4. Muyskens M. The fluorescence of Lignum nephriticum: a flash back to the past and a simple demonstration of natural substance fluorescence. J Chem Educ. 2006;83:765.
5. Valeur B, Berberan-Santos MN. A brief history of fluorescence and phosphorescence before the emergence of quantum theory. J Chem Educ. 2011;88:731.
6. Moore GE. Fluorescein as an agent in the differentiation of normal and malignant tissues. Science. 1947;106:130.
7. Cacciamani GE, Shakir A, Tafuri A, et al. Best practices in near-infrared fluorescence imaging with indocyanine green (NIRF/ICG)-guided robotic urologic surgery: a systematic review-based expert consensus. World J Urol. 2020;38:883.
8. Alander JT, Kaartinen I, Laakso A, et al. A review of indocyanine green fluorescent imaging in surgery. Int J Biomed Imaging. 2012;2012:940585.

9. Sheppard N, Willis HA, Rigg JC. Names, symbols, definitions and units of quantities in optical spectroscopy. Pure Appl Chem. 1985;57:105.
10. Meershoek P, KleinJan GH, van Willigen DM, et al. Multi-wavelength fluorescence imaging with a da Vinci Firefly—a technical look behind the scenes. J Robot Surg. 2020;15:751.
11. Tian Y, Halle J, Wojdyr M, Sahoo D, Scheblykin IG. Quantitative measurement of fluorescence brightness of single molecules. Methods Appl Fluoresc. 2014;2(3):035003.
12. Tatsuta M, Iishi H, Ichii M, et al. Diagnosis of gastric cancers with fluorescein-labeled monoclonal antibodies to carcinoembryonic antigen. Lasers Surg Med. 1989;9(4):422–6.
13. Chin PTK, Welling MM, Meskers SCJ, Valdes Olmos RA, Tanke H, Van Leeuwen FWB. Optical imaging as an expansion of nuclear medicine: Cerenkov-based luminescence vs fluorescence-based luminescence. Eur J Nucl Med Mol Imaging. 2013;40(8):1283–91.
14. Roberts DW, Olson JD, Evans LT, et al. Red-light excitation of protoporphyrin IX fluorescence for subsurface tumor detection. J Neurosurg. 2018;128(6):1690–7.
15. Flynn BP, DSouza AV, Kanick SC, Davis SC, Pogue BW. White light-informed optical properties improve ultrasound-guided fluorescence tomography of photoactive protoporphyrin IX. J Biomed Opt. 2013;18(4):046008.
16. Dell'Oglio P, de Vries HM, Mazzone E, et al. Hybrid indocyanine green- ^{99m}Tc-nanocolloid for single-photon emission computed tomography and combined radio- and fluorescence-guided sentinel node biopsy in penile cancer: results of 740 inguinal basins assessed at a single institution. Eur Urol. 2020;78(6):865–72.
17. de Vries H-M, van Oosterom MN, Karakullukcu M, et al. c-MET receptor-targeted fluorescence-guided surgery—first experience in penile squamous cell carcinoma patients, a phase IIa study. J Nucl Med. 2021;63:51–6.
18. Prince AC, Jani A, Korb M, et al. Characterizing the detection threshold for optical imaging in surgical oncology. J Surg Oncol. 2017;116:898–906.
19. Leung K. IRDye 800CW-Human serum albumin. Molecular Imaging and Contrast Agent Database (MICAD).
20. Desmettre T, Devoisselle JM, Mordon S. Fluorescence properties and metabolic features of indocyanine green (ICG) as related to angiography. Surv Ophthalmol. 2000;45:15–27.
21. Manny TB, Patel M, Hemal AK. Fluorescence-enhanced robotic radical prostatectomy using real-time lymphangiography and tissue marking with percutaneous injection of unconjugated indocyanine green: the initial clinical experience in 50 patients. Eur Urol. 2014;65(6):1162–8.
22. Bunschoten A, Buckle T, Kuil J, et al. Targeted non-covalent self-assembled nanoparticles based on human serum albumin. Biomaterials. 2012;33:867.
23. Dip F, LoMenzo E, Sarotto L, et al. Randomized trial of near-infrared incisionless fluorescent cholangiography. Ann Surg. 2019;270:992.
24. Nagaya T, Nakamura YA, Choyke PL, Kobayashi H. Fluorescence-guided surgery. Front Oncol. 2017;7:314.
25. Göppner D, Nekwasil S, Jellestad A, Sachse A, Schönborn K, Gollnick H. Indocyanine green-assisted sentinel lymph node biopsy in melanoma using the "FOVIS" system. J Dtsch Dermatol Ges. 2017;15:169.
26. Eoh KJ, Lee YJ, Kim HS, et al. Two-step sentinel lymph node mapping strategy in endometrial cancer staging using fluorescent imaging: a novel sentinel lymph node tracer injection procedure. Surg Oncol. 2018;27:514.
27. Lin H, Ding Z, Kota VG, Zhang X, Zhou J. Sentinel lymph node mapping in endometrial cancer: a systematic review and meta-analysis. Oncotarget. 2017;8:46601.
28. Kågedal Å, Margolin G, Held C, et al. A novel sentinel lymph node approach in oral squamous cell carcinoma. Curr Pharm Des. 2020;26:3834.
29. Baiocchi GL, Molfino S, Molteni B, et al. Fluorescence-guided lymphadenectomy in gastric cancer: a prospective western series. Updates Surg. 2020;72:761.
30. Chen QY, Xie JW, Zhong Q, et al. Safety and efficacy of indocyanine green tracer-guided lymph node dissection during laparoscopic radical gastrectomy in patients with gastric cancer: a randomized clinical trial. JAMA Surg. 2020;155:300.
31. Petz W, Bertani E, Borin S, Fiori G, Ribero D, Spinoglio G. Fluorescence-guided D3 lymphadenectomy in robotic right colectomy with complete mesocolic excision. Int J Med Robot Comput Assist Surg. 2020;17:e2217.
32. de Korne CM, Wit EM, de Jong J, et al. Anatomical localization of radiocolloid tracer deposition affects outcome of sentinel node procedures in prostate cancer. Eur J Nucl Med Mol Imaging. 2019;46:2558.
33. Schaafsma BE, Verbeek FPR, Elzevier HW, et al. Optimization of sentinel lymph node mapping in bladder cancer using near-infrared fluorescence imaging. J Surg Oncol. 2014;110:845.
34. Van Dam GM, Themelis G, Crane LMA, et al. Intraoperative tumor-specific fluorescence imaging in ovarian cancer by folate receptor-α targeting: first in-human results. Nat Med. 2011;17:1315.
35. Amato RJ, Shetty A, Lu Y, Ellis R, Low PS. A phase I study of Folate immune therapy (EC90 vaccine administered with GPI-0100 adjuvant followed by EC17) in patients with renal cell carcinoma. J Immunother. 2013;36:268.
36. Boogerd LSF, Hoogstins CES, Gaarenstroom KN, et al. Folate receptor-α targeted near-infrared fluorescence imaging in high-risk endometrial cancer patients: a tissue microarray and clinical feasibility study. Oncotarget. 2018;9:791.
37. de Valk KS, Deken MM, Schaap DP, et al. Dose-finding study of a CEA-targeting agent, SGM-101, for intraoperative fluorescence imaging of colorectal cancer. Ann Surg Oncol. 2021;28:1832.
38. Boogerd LSF, Hoogstins CES, Schaap DP, et al. Safety and effectiveness of SGM-101, a fluorescent antibody targeting carcinoembryonic antigen, for intraoperative detection of colorectal cancer: a dose-escalation pilot study. Lancet Gastroenterol Hepatol. 2018;3:181.
39. Hensbergen AW, Van Willigen DM, Van Beurden F, et al. Image-guided surgery: are we getting the most out of small-molecule prostate-specific-membrane-antigen-targeted tracers? Bioconjug Chem. 2020;31(2):375–95.
40. Buckle T, Van Willigen DM, Spa SJ, et al. Tracers for fluorescence-guided surgery: how elongation of the polymethine chain in cyanine dyes alters the pharmacokinetics of a dual-modality c[RGDyK] tracer. J Nucl Med. 2018;59:986.
41. Schottelius M, Wurzer A, Wissmiller K, et al. Synthesis and preclinical characterization of the PSMA-targeted hybrid tracer PSMA-I&F for nuclear and fluorescence imaging of prostate cancer. J Nucl Med. 2019;60:71.
42. Burggraaf J, Kamerling IMC, Gordon PB, et al. Detection of colorectal polyps in humans using an intravenously administered fluorescent peptide targeted against c-Met. Nat Med. 2015;21:955.
43. Barth CW, Gibbs S. Fluorescence image-guided surgery: a perspective on contrast agent development. Proc SPIE Int Soc Opt Eng. 2020;11222:112220J. https://doi.org/10.1117/12.2545292.
44. van Beurden F, van Willigen DM, Vojnovic B, et al. Multi-wavelength fluorescence in image-guided surgery, clinical feasibility and future perspectives. Mol Imaging. 2020;19:1536012120962333.
45. Steinbach P, Wedmgandt H, Baumgartner R, Kriegmair M, Hofstädter F, Knüchel R. Cellular fluorescence of the endogenous photosensitizer protoporphyrin ix following exposure to 5-aminolevulinic acid. Photochem Photobiol. 1995;62:887.

46. Yoon K, Kim E, Kim K, Lee S, Yoo H. A multi-detection fluorescence dye with 5-ALA and ICG using modified light emitting diodes. Curr Opt Photonics. 2019;3:256.
47. Hadjipanayis CG, Stummer W. 5-ALA and FDA approval for glioma surgery. J Neurooncol. 2019;141:479.
48. Stummer W, Pichlmeier U, Meinel T, Wiestler OD, Zanella F, Reulen HJ. Fluorescence-guided surgery with 5-aminolevulinic acid for resection of malignant glioma: a randomised controlled multicentre phase III trial. Lancet Oncol. 2006;7:392.
49. Zaak D, Sroka R, Khoder W, et al. Photodynamic diagnosis of prostate cancer using 5-aminolevulinic acid-first clinical experiences. Urology. 2008;72:345.
50. Frei KA, Bonel HM, Frick H, Walt H, Steiner RA. Photodynamic detection of diseased axillary sentinel lymph node after oral application of aminolevulinic acid in patients with breast cancer. Br J Cancer. 2004;90:805.
51. Casas A. Clinical uses of 5-aminolaevulinic acid in photodynamic treatment and photodetection of cancer: a review. Cancer Lett. 2020;490:165.
52. Hernot S, van Manen L, Debie P, JSD M, Vahrmeijer AL. Latest developments in molecular tracers for fluorescence image-guided cancer surgery. Lancet Oncol. 2019;20:e354.
53. Han S, Woo S, Kim YJ, Suh CH. Impact of 68Ga-PSMA PET on the management of patients with prostate cancer: a systematic review and meta-analysis. Eur Urol. 2018;74(2):179–90.
54. Maurer T, Eiber M, Schwaiger M, Gschwend JE. Current use of PSMA-PET in prostate cancer management. Nat Rev Urol. 2016;13(4):226–35.
55. Humblet V, Lapidus R, Williams LR, et al. High-affinity near-infrared fluorescent small-molecule contrast agents for in vivo imaging of prostate-specific membrane antigen. Mol Imaging. 2005;4:448.
56. Kularatne SA, Thomas M, Myers CH, et al. Evaluation of novel prostate-specific membrane antigen-targeted near-infrared imaging agent for fluorescence-guided surgery of prostate cancer. Clin Cancer Res. 2019;25:177.
57. Zhang M, Kobayashi N, Zettlitz KA, et al. Near-infrared dye-labeled anti-prostate stem cell antigen minibody enables real-time fluorescence imaging and targeted surgery in translational mouse models. Clin Cancer Res. 2019;25:188.
58. Bao K, Lee JH, Kang H, Park GK, El Fakhri G, Choi HS. PSMA-targeted contrast agents for intraoperative imaging of prostate cancer. Chem Commun. 2017;53:1611.
59. Wang X, Huang SS, Heston WDW, Guo H, Wang BC, Basilion JP. Development of targeted near-infrared imaging agents for prostate cancer. Mol Cancer Ther. 2014;13:2595.
60. Derks YHW, Löwik DWPM, Sedelaar JPM, et al. PSMA-targeting agents for radio- and fluorescenceguided prostate cancer surgery. Theranostics. 2019;9:6824.
61. van den Berg NS, Buckle T, KleinJan GH, van der Poel HG, van Leeuwen FWB. Multispectral fluorescence imaging during robot-assisted laparoscopic sentinel node biopsy: a first step towards a fluorescence-based anatomic roadmap. Eur Urol. 2017;72:110.
62. van Willigen DM, van den Berg NS, Buckle T, et al. Multispectral fluorescence guided surgery: a feasibility study in a phantom using a clinical-grade laparoscopic camera system. Am J Nucl Med Mol Imaging. 2017;7:138.
63. Chin PT, Beekman CA, Buckle T, Josephson L, van Leeuwen FW. Multispectral visualization of surgical safety-margins using fluorescent marker seeds. Am J Nucl Med Mol Imaging. 2012;2:151.
64. Hofman MS, Lawrentschuk N, Francis RJ, et al. Prostate-specific membrane antigen PET-CT in patients with high-risk prostate cancer before curative-intent surgery or radiotherapy (proPSMA): a prospective, randomised, multicentre study. Lancet. 2020;395(10231):1208–16.
65. EudraCT Number: 2019-002393-31. https://www.clinicaltrialsregister.eu/ctr-search/trial/2019-002393-31/NL
66. van Leeuwen FWB, Winter A, van Der Poel HG, et al. Technologies for image-guided surgery for managing lymphatic metastases in prostate cancer. Nat Rev Urol. 2019;16:159.
67. Inoue S, Shiina H, Arichi N, et al. Identification of lymphatic pathway involved in the spreading of prostate cancer by fluorescence navigation approach with intraoperatively injected indocyanine green. J Can Urol Assoc. 2011;5(4):254–9.
68. Joniau S, Van Den Bergh L, Lerut E, et al. Mapping of pelvic lymph node metastases in prostate cancer. Eur Urol. 2013;63(3):450–8.
69. Meinhardt W, van der Poel HG, Valdés Olmos RA, Bex A, Brouwer OR, Horenblas S. Laparoscopic sentinel lymph node biopsy for prostate cancer: the relevance of locations outside the extended dissection area. Prostate Cancer. 2012;2012:751753.
70. Wit EMK, Acar C, Grivas N, et al. Sentinel node procedure in prostate cancer: a systematic review to assess diagnostic accuracy. Eur Urol. 2017;71(4):596–605.
71. Togami S, Kawamura T, Fukuda M, Yanazume S, Kamio M, Kobayashi H. Prospective study of sentinel lymph node mapping for endometrial cancer. Int J Gynecol Obstet. 2018;143:313.
72. Bacalbasa N, Balescu I, Diaconu C, et al. Utility of indocyanine green injection in patients with cervical cancer besides the identification of sentinel lymph node (review). Exp Ther Med. 2020;20:3523.
73. Harke NN, Godes M, Wagner C, et al. Fluorescence-supported lymphography and extended pelvic lymph node dissection in robot-assisted radical prostatectomy: a prospective, randomized trial. World J Urol. 2018;36(11):1817–23.
74. van der Poel HG, Wit E, van den Berg N, et al. Sentinel node biopsy: report from a consensus panel meeting. BJU Int. 2017;120:204.
75. Wit EMK, van Beurden F, Kleinjan GH, Grivas N, de Korne CM, Buckle T, Donswijk ML, Bekers EM, van Leeuwen FWB, van der Poel HG. The impact of drainage pathways on the detection of nodal metastases in prostate cancer: a phase II randomized comparison of intratumoral vs intraprostatic tracer injection for sentinel node detection. Eur J Nucl Med Mol Imaging. 2022;49(5):1743–53.
76. van Leeuwen AC, Buckle T, Bendle G, et al. Tracer-cocktail injections for combined pre- and intraoperative multimodal imaging of lymph nodes in a spontaneous mouse prostate tumor model. J Biomed Opt. 2011;16:016004.
77. Mazzone E, Dell'Oglio P, Grivas N, et al. Diagnostic value, oncological outcomes and safety profile of image-guided surgery technologies during robot-assisted lymph node dissection with sentinel node biopsy for prostate cancer. J Nucl Med. 2021;62:1363.
78. Meershoek P, Buckle T, van Oosterom MN, KleinJan GH, van der Poel HG, van Leeuwen FWB. Can intraoperative fluorescence imaging identify all lesions while the road map created by preoperative nuclear imaging is masked? J Nucl Med. 2020;61:834.
79. Rietbergen DDD, Meershoek P, Kleinjan GH, et al. Head-to-head comparison of the hybrid tracer indocyanine green-^{99m}Tc-nanocolloid with ^{99m}Tc-Senti-Scint using sentinel node lymphoscintigraphy and single-photon emission computed tomography combined with computer tomography in melanoma. Nucl Med Commun. 2020;41:1010.
80. Van Den Berg NS, Brouwer OR, Klop WMC, et al. Concomitant radio- and fluorescence-guided sentinel lymph node biopsy in squamous cell carcinoma of the oral cavity using ICG-^{99m}Tc- nanocolloid. Eur J Nucl Med Mol Imaging. 2012;39:1128.
81. Luiting HB, van Leeuwen PJ, Busstra MB, et al. Use of gallium-68 prostate-specific membrane antigen positron-emission tomography for detecting lymph node metastases in primary and recurrent prostate cancer and location of recurrence after radical prostatectomy: an overview of the current literature. BJU Int. 2020;125(2):206–14
82. Knipper S, Tilki D, Mansholt J, et al. Metastases-yield and prostate-specific antigen kinetics following salvage lymph node dissection for prostate cancer: a comparison between conventional surgical approach and prostate-specific membrane antigen-radioguided surgery. Eur Urol Focus. 2019;5(1):50–3.

Radioguided Surgery in Recurrent Prostate Cancer

29

Sophie Knipper and Tobias Maurer

Abbreviations

CT	Computed tomography
MRI	Magnetic resonance imaging
PET	Positron emission tomography
PLND	Pelvic lymph node dissection
PSA	Prostate-specific antigen
PSMA	Prostate-specific membrane antigen
SLND	Salvage lymph node dissection
SPECT	Single-photon emission computed tomography

Introduction

In recent years imaging of recurrent prostate cancer lesions has evolved in an almost revolutionizing way. Especially positron emission tomography (PET) imaging with ligands directed against the prostate specific membrane antigen (PSMA) [1], a type II transmembrane glycoprotein with overexpression on most prostate cancer cells, has substantially changed the diagnostic pathway. While expression on soft fatty tissue and especially lymph nodes is negligible, prostate cancer lesions within lymph nodes or soft tissue show significant tracer uptake and can be visualized already at only several millimeters in diameter [2–4]. Even at low PSA-levels at biochemical recurrence metastatic sites can be detected with PSMA PET imaging [5, 6]. Based on these superb detection rates PSMA PET became the routine imaging modality for biochemical recurrent prostate cancer within the last few years and is increasingly acknowledged in guidelines as imaging modality of choice [7].

Traditionally, in biochemically recurrent prostate cancer with evidence of lymph node involvement, watchful waiting or initiation of systemic treatment such as androgen deprivation therapy upon further progression or symptomatic disease is recommended [7]. However, the above described evolution in imaging fueled the desire for local targeted treatment approaches such as targeted salvage radiotherapy or salvage lymph node dissection (SLND). Although, to date these treatments are considered experimental by guidelines further systemic palliative treatment and associated toxicity may hopefully be delayed and long-lasting PSA-responses might be initiated.

In this context, results from SLND series have been reported already prior to the PSMA PET era. After initial encouraging reports [8–12], more recently rather critical views have been published. In these, oncological long-term outcomes were either unclear or favourable outcomes were only observed in a minority of men [13–15]. However, several limitations of these earlier series have to be acknowledged that might be responsible for the sobering results. First, the indication for salvage surgery was mainly based on the results of choline-based PET or conventional imaging. Secondly, these series also included advanced patients who presented with several lesions on imaging, retroperitoneal disease or who did receive systemic androgen deprivation therapy prior to SLND. And thirdly, in about 20% of patients, pathological examination revealed no metastatic prostate cancer tissue within the removed tissue specimens. This last finding might be due to unspecific imaging or the fact that recurrent tumor lesions were not readily detectable intraoperatively. Previous lymph node dissection at the time of radical prostatectomy or radiation treatment might furthermore hinder successful removal.

S. Knipper
Martini-Klinik Prostate Cancer Center, University Hospital Hamburg-Eppendorf, Hamburg, Germany
e-mail: a.knipper@uke.de

T. Maurer (✉)
Martini-Klinik Prostate Cancer Center, University Hospital Hamburg-Eppendorf, Hamburg, Germany

Department of Urology, University Hospital Hamburg-Eppendorf, Hamburg, Germany
e-mail: t.maurer@uke.de; http://www.martini-klinik.de; http://www.martini-klinik.de/dr-maurer

S. Ren et al. (eds.), *Robot-Assisted Radical Prostatectomy*, https://doi.org/10.1007/978-3-031-05855-4_29

PSMA PET Refines Indication for SLND

The advancement of molecular imaging and especially the recent introduction of PSMA PET for imaging in biochemical recurrence of prostate cancer, fueled the interest for targeted salvage therapies such as SLND. PSMA PET/CT or PET/MRI allows better identification of patients with minimal and localized recurrent disease, provides a detailed anatomical localization and thus creates the opportunity to more accurately apply local therapies. Results from PSMA PET in combination with clinical parameters [14], help to identify patients that might profit from SLND. Thus, the indication for SLND can be refined by the addition of PSMA PET results.

However, intraoperatively, reliable identification and removal of metastatic lymph nodes or soft tissue lesions is challenging as they might be small in size, atypically located and/or morphologically unrecognizable (Fig. 29.1a). Thus, in a subset of patients, postoperative histology might still be negative even if SLND procedures were based on PSMA PET imaging [16]. As PSMA PET shows a high specificity for lymph node staging, false positive findings are not observed commonly. Instead, in the majority of cases with negative histology lymph node metastases are probably missed by surgical resection. Thus, intraoperative real-time guidance for localization of prostate cancer lesions incorporating the idea of precision surgery to ensure successful removal are needed.

Tracers for PSMA-Radioguided Surgery

Here, based on the high specificity of PSMA tracers used for PET imaging labelling with gamma-emitting radiopharmaceuticals could be established that enable SPECT imaging as well as radioguided surgery [17, 18]. Historically, radioguided surgery is known from sentinel surgical procedures where the lymphatic drainage and first draining lymph node can be detected. However, radioguided surgery with PSMA specific tracers enables direct molecular detection of prostate cancer lesions [19, 20]. Several compounds have been developed that can be used for single-photon emission computed tomography (SPECT) and potentially also radioguided surgery: ^{111}In-PSMA-I&T [18], ^{99m}Tc-PSMA-I&S [17], ^{111}In-PSMA-617 [21], ^{99m}Tc-PSMA-1404 [22]. Of these, the most investigated in PSMA radioguided surgery are ^{111}In-PSMA-I&T and ^{99m}Tc-PSMA-I&S. Both agents have been proven to perform well for both, preoperative SPECT imaging and intraoperative surgical guidance using conventional gamma probes [23, 24]. However, major limitations of ^{111}In-labelled tracers are the associated higher costs, higher radiation exposure and restricted availability restraining broad acceptance and every day's usability. ^{99m}Tc for labelling PSMA tracers on the other hand is available in virtually all nuclear medicine departments as it represents the most widely used radionuclide in nuclear medicine.

Preoperative Work-Flow

Patients who are subjected to SLND for early lymphonodular oligorecurrent prostate cancer based on the results of PSMA PET imaging receive an intravenous injection of ^{99m}Tc-PSMA-I&S (mean activity published in literature: 571 MBq, range: 221–857 MBq), ^{111}In-PSMA-I&T (mean activity published in literature: 150 MBq, range: 86–298 MBq) or ^{111}In-PSMA-617 (mean activity published in literature: 110 ± 10 MBq) 1 or 2 days prior to salvage surgery (mean time prior to surgery published for ^{99m}Tc-PSMA-I&S: 19.7 h, range 15.8–24.9 h, for ^{111}In-PSMA-I&T: 22.9 h, range 16.7–28.0 h, for ^{111}In-PSMA-617: 44 h ± 10 h) [23–25]. It has to be noted that the difference in half-life (^{99m}Tc: 6.0 h; ^{111}In: 2.8 days) allows to perform ^{111}In-PSMA based radioguided surgery 1 or 2 days after injection while ^{99m}Tc-PSMA based radioguided surgery is usually performed the day after injection. Initially, unspecific background precludes intraoperative specific targeting and sufficient tracer accumulation within the prostate cancer lesions have to be awaited. However, due to radioactive decay and possible wash-out radioactive signals from the lesions, after a longer period of time, cannot be reliably detected anymore. Thus, ^{99m}Tc-PSMA based radioguided surgery is usually performed within 24 h after injection.

After PSMA tracer administration usually SPECT/CT imaging is performed to cross-validate findings of the previous PSMA PET and document positive tracer uptake within the lesions (Fig. 29.1b). This also serves as quality control for correct tracer injection and distribution. It has to be noted, however, that due to the difference in sensitivity and spatial resolution, PSMA based SPECT imaging tends to miss small lesions that were detectable on PSMA PET [24, 26].

Description of Surgical Technique

The surgical procedure using PSMA radioguidance is generally similar to the conventional open salvage surgery approach. Patients are placed in a supine position and a urinary catheter is inserted. This allows removal of radioactive urine from the bladder which otherwise may impair gamma probe measurements within the close proximity. Additionally, more space for the surgical procedure is created. After preparing the surgical field, a transperitoneal mid-line incision is performed. Adhesiolysis of the bowel to

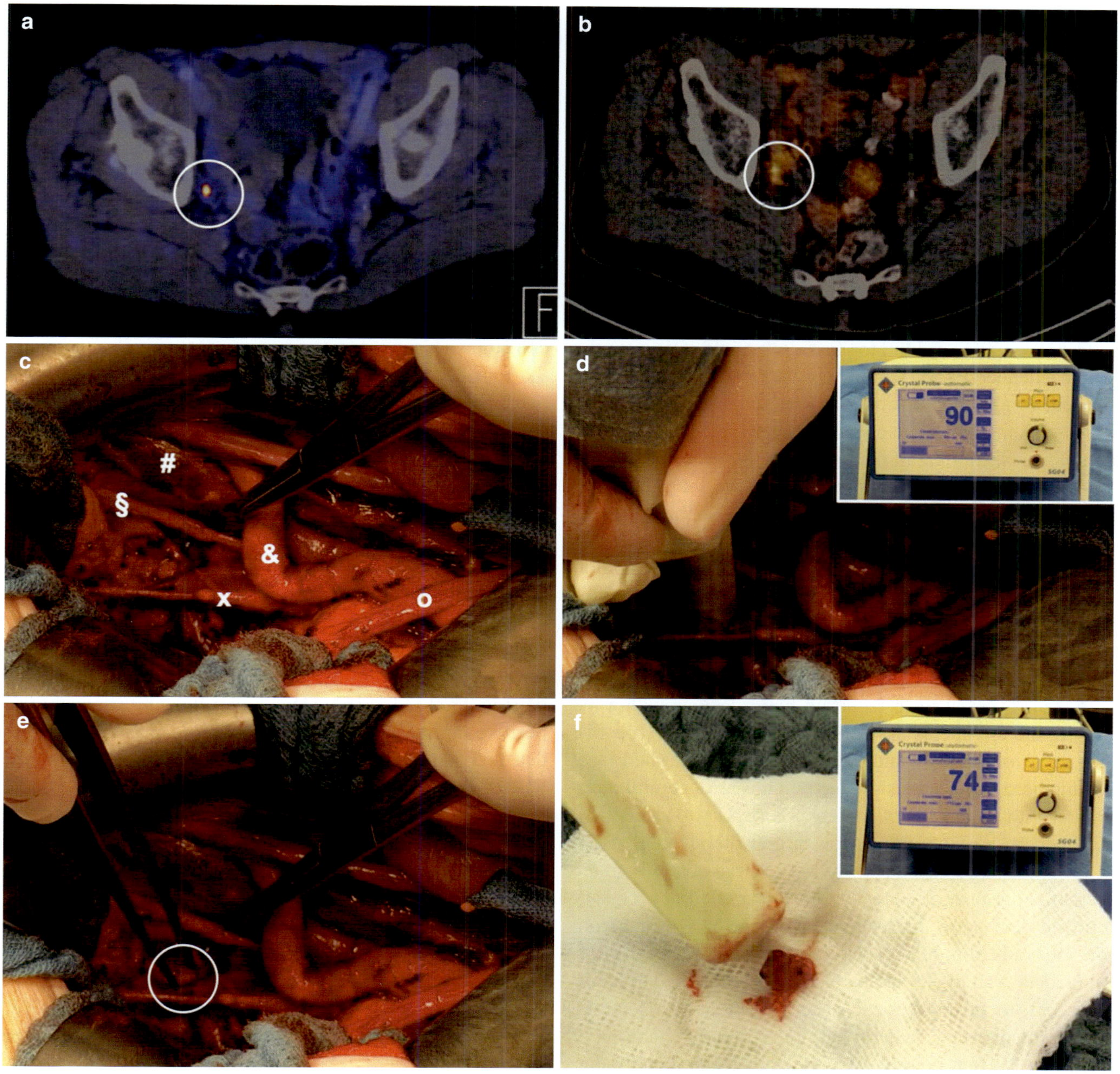

Fig. 29.1 Case of a patient with biochemical recurrent prostate cancer and positive lymph node on PSMA PET suspicious for prostate cancer metastasis: ^{18}F-PSMA-1007 PET/CT fusion imaging shows distinct tracer accumulation within an approximately 5 mm right pelvic lymph node suspicious for prostate cancer metastasis (**a**), that also shows tracer accumulation on ^{99m}Tc-PSMA-I&S SPECT/CT fusion imaging (**b**). Intraoperative view of the right pelvis after almost complete dissection of lymphatic and fatty tissue (& external iliac artery, # external iliac vein, x internal iliac artery, o ureter crossing the common iliac artery, § obturator nerve) (**c**). Intraoperative gamma probe measurement shows distinct localized radioactivity of 90 counts per second (**d**) and aids intraoperative detection of the PSMA PET positive lymph node (white circle, **e**). Ex vivo gamma probe measurement confirms successful removal (**f**). (Image reproduction from Maurer et al., Der Nuklearmediziner, 2020 [33], © Georg Thieme Verlag KG)

the pelvic wall is performed, if necessary. Thereafter, the bowel is retracted cranially. This approach allows immediate access to the lower aorta, inferior vena cava, the bifurcation, the iliac vessels and the ureters as well as the pararectal and presacral area.

During surgery, a sterile draped gamma probe is used for in vivo measurements to facilitate localizing the metastatic lymph nodes and to aid the surgical resection (Fig. 29.1c–f). After excision, ex vivo gamma measurements are performed to immediately confirm the successful removal of the metastatic radioactive lesion(s) on the operation room table or to prompt further search in case of a missing signal. In case of positive identification, defined as measurements exceeding at least twice the background level of the patient's non-cancerous fatty tissue, intraoperative frozen section histopathological analysis to confirm successful resection of a PET positive lesion is usually dispensable. After removal of all metastatic lesions seen on preoperative PSMA PET intraoperative in vivo gamma probe measurements are conducted to exclude additional lesions.

In case of recurrent tumor within the extended PLND template encompassing the external, internal, common iliac field as well as the obturator fossa resection of at least the whole extended PLND template of the respective side is performed. If additional lesions are detected, the planned field of dissection might be extended to increase the probability of complete resection of all tumor-bearing tissue.

Currently, there is no consensus if in the salvage setting and unilateral PSMA PET positive lesions also the contralateral template field should be dissected [27]. For suspicious lesions located elsewhere (pararectal, presacral) a resection of the corresponding region with surrounding tissue is additionally performed. In case of retroperitoneal lesions, the template of dissection usually follows the templates for LND in testicular cancer.

For retrovesical local recurrent tumor lesions within the fatty tissue the ductus deferens and ureter of the respective side serve as landmark and should be clearly identified early during the surgical procedure [28]. In this area, careful preparation with limited use of cautery is necessary to avoid damage or necrosis of the ureter. After careful lateral mobilization of the bladder, an incision of the peritoneum ventrally to the rectum is performed. Here, careful preparation is necessary to avoid damage to the rectum that might be affected from previous radiation. In some cases, a ventral stitch of the dorsal bladder wall to elevate the bladder is performed to facilitate access to the retrovesical space. The use of gamma probe measurements is particularly helpful as fibrotic alteration of the tissue is often present after previous surgery and radiation. Moreover, the distal margin of the recurrent tumor lesion may be identified.

Complications of SLND

As SLND currently is considered an experimental treatment approach risks and benefits need to be carefully considered. In general, salvage surgery procedures seem to be safe [15]. Lymphedema, symptomatic lymphoceles requiring drainage, fever or wound complications are the most frequent reported complications. Most complications are of low grade. In a systematic review, Clavien Dindo grade I and II complications ranged from 0% to 62.5% (mean 21%) and 0% to 37.5% (mean 11%), respectively [15]. Grade 3 complications are reported in less than 10% of cases with varying percentages between series. This is not substantially different for SLND using PSMA radioguided surgery. Of note, no complications associated with PSMA tracer injection are reported to date. The currently largest series on PSMA radioguided SLND encompassing 121 patients reports 24% of Clavien grade I/II and 9% of Clavien grade III complications. Additionally, one death due to pulmonary embolism 6 days after surgery and discharge from hospital was reported [3]. Eleven patients with Clavien grade III complications were affected by hydronephrosis due to ureteral strictures (seven patients), rectal lesions with the need for temporary colostomy (two patients) and urosepsis and osteomyelitis in the foot due to lymphedema (one patient). Although most patients recover well from SLND, these reports highlight that SLND should be only performed in centers with sufficient experience. Moreover, the indication for SLND should be carefully discussed with each patient considering the individual clinical situation.

Outcomes of PSMA Radioguided SLND

In contemporary SLND series postoperative histology did not reveal cancerous tissue in approximately 9–31% of patients [8, 13, 14, 16]. Thus, either imaging showed false positive findings or the prostate cancer lesions could not be detected and removed during SLND. In comparison, in 91–100% of patients undergoing SLND using PSMA radioguidance for PSMA PET positive recurrent lymph nodes showed prostate cancer tissue on final pathology [3, 16, 23–25]. In a small comparative series of patients undergoing SLND for PSMA PET proven lymph node recurrence it could be shown that a PSMA radioguided approach enabled detection of metastatic lymph nodes in all of 13 patients while in 9 (31%) of 29 patients without PSMA radioguidance no metastatic tissue could be removed [16]. This also translated in superior PSA response rates for patients who were treated with SLND utilizing PSMA radioguidance.

It has to be noted, however, that microscopic spread to neighboring lymph nodes cannot be detected using either PSMA PET or PSMA radioguided surgery. Using in vivo and ex vivo gamma probe measurements during PSMA radioguided surgery only metastatic prostate cancer lesions greater than 3 mm can be detected. Smaller microscopic tumor lesions are usually missed. Compared to postoperative histology, accuracy, sensitivity and specificity of gamma probe measurements are 93%, 83.6% and 100%, respectively [24]. Thus, treating only the suspicious lymph node on PSMA PET is not advisable. Conversely, although the extent of SLND is currently under discussion it should at least comprise a clean dissection of the respective side of PSMA PET positive findings.

Currently, oncological outcome data after PSMA radioguided SLND are very limited. In the largest series of 121 patients a complete biochemical response (postoperative PSA <0.2 ng/ml) without any additional prostate cancer treatment (i.e. androgen deprivation therapy or radiotherapy) could be observed in 66% of patients. Not surprisingly, low PSA and single lesion on PSMA PET were associated with higher likelihood of complete biochemical response (84%) and longer median biochemical recurrence-free survival without any additional therapy (14 months) [3]. Compared to conventional SLND series, achieved rates of complete biochemical response seem to be greater, but different baseline characteristics of patients as well as different reported oncological outcome data impede direct comparisons. Thus, the added value is currently hard to establish, while superior removal of affected lymph nodes and a more pronounced postoperative PSA decline might favor the use of PSMA radioguidance compared to conventional SLND. Main limitations of reported series are the retrospective design, short follow-up and lack of a control group.

Future Developments

Noteworthy developments might impact PSMA radioguided SLND in the near future. First, novel development of DROP-IN gamma probes enables minimal-invasive robotic surgery and thus might reduce surgery-associated morbidity [29, 30]. After insertion in the abdominal cavity this device may be handled with more flexibility during robot-assisted laparoscopic surgery than conventional rigid laparoscopic gamma probes. This may be particularly helpful in lesions with retrovesical localizations that could be easily accessed by a robotic approach in a similar fashion like during retrovesical (Retzius-sparing) robotic-assisted radical prostatectomy [31].

Secondly, novel fluorescent or even hybrid (radioactive and fluorescent) PSMA tracers are currently under development and preclinical investigation. These may complement the process of radioguidance by direct optical feed-back using real-time fluorescence imaging [20, 32]. Additionally, the fluorescent probes are partly detectable by currently implemented cameras within the da Vinci™ robotic system and partly by novel dual-imaging camera systems that are still under development.

Conclusion/Discussion

With the recent advancements in molecular imaging and especially with the introduction of PSMA PET a markedly increased interest for targeted salvage therapies such as SLND is observed. The use of PSMA tracers for intraoperative guidance enables successful detection and removal of almost all PSMA PET positive lymph nodes. However, SLND procedures are currently still considered experimental and are not (yet) recommended by guidelines.

Thus, benefits and harms must be critically weighed and discussed in detail with the patients. Identifying optimal candidates for SLND is crucial. Several predictors for beneficial outcomes, such as lower preoperative PSA, absence of retroperitoneal localisation of lymph node involvement and lower number of positive lesions on PET imaging have been established [3, 14]. In the future, additionally blood-borne biomarkers might support the decision for or against a targeted approach.

Furthermore, the boundaries and extent of SLND need to be defined clearly. Currently, the SLND mainly follows the proposed templates for an extended PLND. However, recurrences at different anatomical areas like the presacral or pararectal area might require consideration of alternate lymphatic drainage patterns.

In general, SLND should be performed in specialized centers to ensure highest quality with low complication rates as previous pelvic surgery or radiation treatment might pose challenging situations. In addition, patients should be followed within trials or at least prospective maintained clinical registries to determine the outcomes of this individual treatment approach and to compare the results to current standard treatment consisting of watchful waiting or initiation of systemic androgen deprivation.

References

1. Maurer T, Eiber M, Schwaiger M, Gschwend JE. Current use of PSMA-PET in prostate cancer management. Nat Rev Urol. 2016;13:226–35. https://doi.org/10.1038/nrurol.2016.26.
2. Jilg CA, et al. Diagnostic accuracy of Ga-68-HBED-CC-PSMA-ligand-PET/CT before salvage lymph node dissection for recurrent prostate cancer. Theranostics. 2017;7:1770–80. https://doi.org/10.7150/thno.18421.
3. Horn T, et al. Single lesion on prostate-specific membrane antigen-ligand positron emission tomography and low prostate-specific antigen are prognostic factors for a favorable biochemical response to prostate-specific membrane antigen-targeted radioguided surgery in recurrent prostate cancer. Eur Urol. 2019;76:517–23. https://doi.org/10.1016/j.eururo.2019.03.045.
4. Jilg CA, et al. Detection rate of (18)F-choline PET/CT and (68)Ga-PSMA-HBED-CC PET/CT for prostate cancer lymph node metastases with direct link from PET to histopathology: dependence on the size of tumor deposits in lymph nodes. J Nucl Med. 2019;60:971–7. https://doi.org/10.2967/jnumed.118.220541.
5. Rauscher I, et al. Efficacy, predictive factors, and prediction nomograms for (68)Ga-labeled prostate-specific membrane antigen-ligand positron-emission tomography/computed tomography in early biochemical recurrent prostate cancer after radical prostatectomy. Eur Urol. 2018;73:656–61. https://doi.org/10.1016/j.eururo.2018.01.006.

6. Perera M, et al. Gallium-68 prostate-specific membrane antigen positron emission tomography in advanced prostate cancer-updated diagnostic utility, sensitivity, specificity, and distribution of prostate-specific membrane antigen-avid lesions: a systematic review and meta-analysis. Eur Urol. 2020;77:403–17. https://doi.org/10.1016/j.eururo.2019.01.049.
7. Mottet N, et al. EAU—ESTRO—ESUR—SIOG Guidelines on prostate cancer. 2020. https://uroweb.org/guideline/prostate-cancer/. abgerufen am 10 July 2020.
8. Suardi N, et al. Long-term outcomes of salvage lymph node dissection for clinically recurrent prostate cancer: results of a single-institution series with a minimum follow-up of 5 years. Eur Urol. 2015;67:299–309. https://doi.org/10.1016/j.eururo.2014.02.011.
9. Bandini M, Fossati N, Briganti A. Salvage surgery for nodal recurrent prostate cancer. Curr Opin Urol. 2017;27:604–11. https://doi.org/10.1097/mou.0000000000000437.
10. Steuber T, et al. Standard of care versus metastases-directed therapy for PET-detected nodal oligorecurrent prostate cancer following multimodality treatment: a multi-institutional case-control study. Eur Urol Focus. 2019;5:1007–13. https://doi.org/10.1016/j.euf.2018.02.015.
11. Karnes RJ, et al. Salvage lymph node dissection for prostate cancer nodal recurrence detected by 11C-choline positron emission tomography/computerized tomography. J Urol. 2015;193:111–6. https://doi.org/10.1016/j.juro.2014.08.082.
12. Porres D, et al. The role of salvage extended lymph node dissection in patients with rising PSA and PET/CT scan detected nodal recurrence of prostate cancer. Prostate Cancer Prostatic Dis. 2017;20:85–92. https://doi.org/10.1038/pcan.2016.54.
13. Bravi CA, et al. Long-term outcomes of salvage lymph node dissection for nodal recurrence of prostate cancer after radical prostatectomy: not as good as previously thought. Eur Urol. 2020;78:661–9. https://doi.org/10.1016/j.eururo.2020.06.043.
14. Fossati N, et al. Identifying the optimal candidate for salvage lymph node dissection for nodal recurrence of prostate cancer: results from a large, multi-institutional analysis. Eur Urol. 2019;75:176–83. https://doi.org/10.1016/j.eururo.2018.09.009.
15. Ploussard G, et al. Salvage lymph node dissection for nodal recurrent prostate cancer: a systematic review. Eur Urol. 2019;76:493–504. https://doi.org/10.1016/j.eururo.2018.10.041.
16. Knipper S, et al. Metastases-yield and prostate-specific antigen kinetics following salvage lymph node dissection for prostate cancer: a comparison between conventional surgical approach and prostate-specific membrane antigen-radioguided surgery. Eur Urol Focus. 2019;5:50–3. https://doi.org/10.1016/j.euf.2018.09.014.
17. Robu S, et al. Preclinical evaluation and first patient application of 99mTc-PSMA-I&S for SPECT imaging and radioguided surgery in prostate cancer. J Nucl Med. 2017;58:235–42. https://doi.org/10.2967/jnumed.116.178939.
18. Schottelius M, Wirtz M, Eiber M, Maurer T, Wester HJ. [(111)In]PSMA-I&T: expanding the spectrum of PSMA-I&T applications towards SPECT and radioguided surgery. EJNMMI Res. 2015;5:68. https://doi.org/10.1186/s13550-015-0147-6.
19. Maurer T, et al. Prostate-specific membrane antigen-radioguided surgery for metastatic lymph nodes in prostate cancer. Eur Urol. 2015;68:530–4. https://doi.org/10.1016/j.eururo.2015.04.034.
20. Maurer T, et al. Prostate-specific membrane antigen-guided surgery. J Nucl Med. 2020;61:6–12. https://doi.org/10.2967/jnumed.119.232330.
21. Mix M, et al. Performance of (111)In-labelled PSMA ligand in patients with nodal metastatic prostate cancer: correlation between tracer uptake and histopathology from lymphadenectomy. Eur J Nucl Med Mol Imaging. 2018;45:2062–70. https://doi.org/10.1007/s00259-018-4094-0.
22. Vallabhajosula S, et al. 99mTc-labeled small-molecule inhibitors of prostate-specific membrane antigen: pharmacokinetics and biodistribution studies in healthy subjects and patients with metastatic prostate cancer. J Nucl Med. 2014;55:1791–8. https://doi.org/10.2967/jnumed.114.140426.
23. Rauscher I, et al. Value of (111) In-prostate-specific membrane antigen (PSMA)-radioguided surgery for salvage lymphadenectomy in recurrent prostate cancer: correlation with histopathology and clinical follow-up. BJU Int. 2017;120:40–7. https://doi.org/10.1111/bju.13713.
24. Maurer T, et al. (99m)Technetium-based prostate-specific membrane antigen-radioguided surgery in recurrent prostate cancer. Eur Urol. 2019;75:659–66. https://doi.org/10.1016/j.eururo.2018.03.013.
25. Jilg CA, et al. Results from extended lymphadenectomies with [(111)In]PSMA-617 for intraoperative detection of PSMA-PET/CT-positive nodal metastatic prostate cancer. EJNMMI Res. 2020;10:17. https://doi.org/10.1186/s13550-020-0598-2.
26. Rauscher I, et al. Intrapatient comparison of 111In-PSMA I&T SPECT/CT and hybrid 68Ga-HBED-CC PSMA PET in patients with early recurrent prostate cancer. Clin Nucl Med. 2016;41:e397–402. https://doi.org/10.1097/RLU.0000000000001273.
27. Bravi CA, et al. Assessing the best surgical template at salvage pelvic lymph node dissection for nodal recurrence of prostate cancer after radical prostatectomy: when can bilateral dissection be omitted? Results from a multi-institutional series. Eur Urol. 2020;78:779–82. https://doi.org/10.1016/j.eururo.2020.06.047.
28. Knipper S, et al. Salvage surgery in patients with local recurrence after radical prostatectomy. Eur Urol. 2021;79:537–44. https://doi.org/10.1016/j.eururo.2020.11.012.
29. Dell'Oglio P, et al. A DROP-IN gamma probe for robot-assisted radioguided surgery of lymph nodes during radical prostatectomy. Eur Urol. 2021;79:124–32. https://doi.org/10.1016/j.eururo.2020.10.031.
30. van Leeuwen FWB, et al. Minimal-invasive robot-assisted image-guided resection of prostate-specific membrane antigen-positive lymph nodes in recurrent prostate cancer. Clin Nucl Med. 2019;44:580–1. https://doi.org/10.1097/rlu.0000000000002600.
31. Galfano A, et al. Beyond the learning curve of the Retzius-sparing approach for robot-assisted laparoscopic radical prostatectomy: oncologic and functional results of the first 200 patients with ≥1 year of follow-up. Eur Urol. 2013;64:974–80. https://doi.org/10.1016/j.eururo.2013.06.046.
32. Hensbergen AW, et al. Hybrid tracers based on cyanine backbones targeting prostate-specific membrane antigen: tuning pharmacokinetic properties and exploring dye-protein interaction. J Nucl Med. 2020;61:234–41. https://doi.org/10.2967/jnumed.119.233064.
33. Maurer T, et al. 99mTc-PSMA-I&S: application for radioguided surgery in recurrent prostate cancer. Der Nuklearmediziner. 2020;43:309–15. https://doi.org/10.1055/a-1105-8039.

Part IX

Techniques to Prevent Lymphocele Formation in RALP

Four Point Peritoneal Flap Fixation

30

Jens-Uwe Stolzenburg
and Vinodh-Kumar-Adithyaa Arthanareeswaran

Introduction

Extended pelvic lymph node dissection (ePLND) is indicated in patients with intermediate and high-risk prostate cancer and with an estimated risk of lymph node metastasis of >5% [1]. This procedure performed during radical prostatectomy (RP) disrupts the lymphatic drainage channels and may sometimes result in accumulation of lymphatic fluid within the pelvis. Although these fluid collections are spontaneously absorbed in the majority of cases, few patients may develop lymph collections or lymphoceles. Although most lymphoceles are asymptomatic, some may lead to symptoms which are either mild causing pelvic pain, voiding issues or severe, causing deep vein thrombosis and even sepsis when infected that may require invasive management.

Lymphocele Following Radical Prostatectomy

Lee et al. hypothesize that the peri-vesical fat scars over the lymphadenectomy bed following ePLND and traps lymphatic fluid leading to lymphoceles formation [2]. Lymphoceles are usually detected using ultrasound or CT scan postoperatively. The incidence of lymphocele following RP ranges between 27% to 61% [3–5] with 0% to 8% being symptomatic [6]. Symptomatic lymphoceles have significant impact on postoperative morbidity resulting in increased risk of thrombo-embolism and infection with potential for abscess formation thereby requiring surgical intervention and longer hospital stay.

Prevention of Lymphoceles

Although a wealth of preventive strategies has been tested [7, 8], urologists still face lymphocele formation as an inevitable consequence of PLND without being able to provide reliable measures to avoid it. Extensive clipping using titanium clips to secure pelvic lymphatic channels resulted in 0–0.5% symptomatic lymphoceles following ePLND [9, 10]. However, a recent prospective study by Grande et al. [11] demonstrated high incidence of lymphocele (46%) with no difference following usage of titanium clips and bipolar coagulation.

Peritoneal Flap Interposition

Lebeis et al. [12] performed a peritoneal flap interposition (PIF) technique in which the peritoneum was advanced around the lateral surface of the bladder after transperitoneal robot-assisted ePLND. The authors hypothesise that this procedure prevents the trapping of lymphatic fluid within the pelvis and allows drainage into the peritoneal cavity. The study revealed 0% lymphocele formation among 77 patients compared to 11.6% in patients operated by conventional technique. Lee et al. further validated the utilization of this technique in preventing symptomatic lymphocele formation They reported that the PIF had a lower incidence of symptomatic lymphocele than the control group (0.0% vs. 6.0%, $p = 0.007$).

Four-Point Peritoneal Flap Fixation

Stolzenburg et al. [13] recently described a technical modification to the PIF called the four-point peritoneal flap fixation (4PPFF). The 4PPFF involves mobilizing peri-vesical and pre-peritoneal fat peritoneum to prevent the bladder from scarring over the lymph node dissection bed and create a pathway for lymphatic fluid to drain into the peritoneal cav-

J.-U. Stolzenburg (✉) · V.-K.-A. Arthanareeswaran
Department of Urology, University of Leipzig, Leipzig, Germany
e-mail: jens-uwe.stolzenburg@medizin.uni-leipzig.de

S. Ren et al. (eds.), *Robot-Assisted Radical Prostatectomy*, https://doi.org/10.1007/978-3-031-05855-4_30

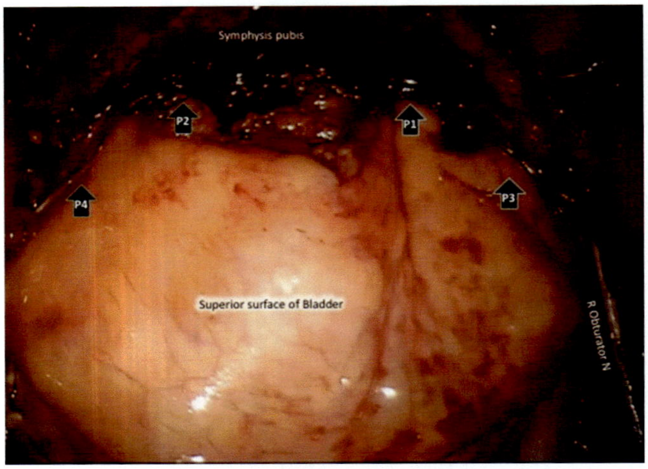

Fig. 30.1 Status following completed Four-Point Peritoneal Flap Fixation (P1, P2, P3, P4). The Obturator nerves on both sides can be visualised. (Credit: Stolzenburg et al. [13])

ity. It also provides direct contact of the peritoneal surface to the lymphatic bed thereby increasing lymph resorption. Asymptomatic lymphoceles were diagnosed by ultrasound examination in only 4 (2.07%) patients with 4PPFF compared to 16 (8.3%) in the other group without 4PPFF. The difference was statistically significant with p = 0.0058. The authors found that patients undergoing the 4PPFF had a lower incidence of symptomatic lymphocele formation after RARP and PLND compared to patients not undergoing the 4PPFF (1.0% vs. 4.6%; p = 0.032).

Surgical Principle

In contrast to the PIF, the 4PPFF requires fixation of the peritoneum to the lateral pelvic wall rather than directly onto the bladder. This was performed by suturing the cut end of the ventral parietal peritoneum at four points (to anterior and lateral pelvic side wall on both sides) following ePLND such that the peritoneal surface is exposed to the iliac vessels and obturator fossa as shown in Fig. 30.1. At the end of the procedure, a 16-F Robinson drainage catheter was placed into the retropubic space in all the patients with and without 4PPFF. As a standard, the drainage catheter was removed on the first postoperative day in all patients.

Conclusions

4PPFF is a safe and effective procedure in preventing lymphocele formation in patients undergoing RP with PLND. The direct contact between lymphatic bed after removal of lymph nodes and the peritoneum following 4PPFF may aid in increased absorption of the accumulating lymph fluid thereby preventing lymphoceles.Conflicts of InterestAuthors have no conflict of interest to declare.

References

1. Mottet N, Bellmunt J, Bolla M, Briers E, Cumberbatch MG, De Santis M, et al. Eau-Estro-Siog Guidelines on prostate cancer. Part 1: Screening, diagnosis, and local treatment with curative intent. Eur Urol. 2017;71(4):618–29.
2. Lee M, Lee Z, Eun DD. Utilization of a peritoneal interposition flap to prevent symptomatic lymphoceles after robotic radical prostatectomy and bilateral pelvic lymph node dissection. J Endourol. 2020;34(8):821–7. Epub 2020 May 13. PMID: 32303137. https://doi.org/10.1089/End.2020.0073.
3. Zorn KC, Katz MH, Bernstein A, Shikanov SA, Brendler CB, Zagaja GP, et al. Pelvic lymphadenectomy during robot-assisted radical prostatectomy: assessing nodal yield, perioperative outcomes, and complications. Urology. 2009;74(2):296–302.
4. Solberg A, Angelsen A, Bergan U, Haugen OA, Viset T, Klepp O. Frequency of lymphoceles after open and laparoscopic pelvic lymph node dissection in patients with prostate cancer. Scand J Urol Nephrol. 2003;37(3):218–21.
5. Spring D, Schroeder D, Babu S, Agee R, Gooding GA. Ultrasonic evaluation of lymphocele formation after staging lymphadenectomy for prostatic carcinoma. Radiology. 1981;141(2):479–83.
6. Ploussard G, Briganti A, De La Taille A, Haese A, Heidenreich A, Menon M, et al. Pelvic lymph node dissection during robot-assisted radical prostatectomy: efficacy, limitations, and complications—a systematic review of the literature. Eur Urol. 2014;65(1):7–16.
7. Karsch JJ, Berthold M, Breul J. Evaluation of lymphorrhea and incidence of lymphoceles: 4dryfield(R) Ph in radical retropubic prostatectomy. Adv Urol. 2016;2016:2367432.
8. Kim WT, Ham WS, Koo KC, Choi YD. Efficacy of octreotide for management of lymphorrhea after pelvic lymph node dissection in radical prostatectomy. Urology. 2010;76(2):398–401.
9. Davis JW, Shah JB, Achim M. Robot-assisted extended pelvic lymph node dissection (Plnd) at the time of radical prostatectomy (Rp): a video-based illustration of technique, results, and unmet patient selection needs. BJU Int. 2011;108(6b):993–8.
10. Eden CG, Zacharakis E, Dundee PE, Hutton AC. Incidence of lymphoceles after robot-assisted pelvic lymph node dissection. BJU Int. 2012;109(5):E14.
11. Grande P, Di Pierro GB, Mordasini L, Ferrari M, Wurnschimmel C, Danuser H, et al. Prospective randomized trial comparing titanium clips to bipolar coagulation in sealing lymphatic vessels during pelvic lymph node dissection at the time of robot-assisted radical prostatectomy. Eur Urol. 2017;71(2):155–8.
12. Lebeis C, Canes D, Sorcini A, Moinzadeh A. Novel technique prevents lymphoceles after transperitoneal robotic-assisted pelvic lymph node dissection: peritoneal flap interposition. Urology. 2015;85(6):1505–9.
13. Stolzenburg JU, Arthanareeswaran VKA, Dietel A, Franz T, Liatsikos E, Kyriazis I, Ganzer R, Yaney K, Do HM. Four-point peritoneal flap fixation in preventing lymphocele formation following radical prostatectomy. Eur Urol Oncol. 2018;1(5):443–8. Epub 2018 May 15. PMID: 31158086. https://doi.org/10.1016/J.Euo.2018.03.004.

PLEAT: A New Technique for Preventing Lymphoceles After Robotic Prostatectomy and Pelvic Lymph Node Dissection

31

Alessandro Morlacco, Valeria Lami, and Fabrizio Dal Moro

Introduction

Pelvic lymphoceles are a common complication of robotic pelvic lymph node dissection (PLND). While the incidence reaches 30%, most cases are asymptomatic and are often an incidental finding during follow-up [1, 2]. If symptoms are present, they are typically related to compression of surrounding structures (pelvic pain, leg oedema, deep vein thrombosis). The incidence of symptomatic lymphoceles (Grade $\geq$ 3, according to the Clavien Dindo Classification [3]) after robotic PLND is 0–8% [4]. Lymphocele, even when asymptomatic, might also affect radiation therapy planning.

Injury to the lymphatic vessels is the main causative factor in the formation of a lymphocele. Potential risk factors have been reviewed by Lee and Kane [5]: many them are not indeed modifiable elements such as patient age, comorbidities, surgeon experience and lymph node involvement.

The current literature strongly supports the idea that the extent of LND should not be guided by the aim of preventing lymphocele formation but rather by the purpose of improving oncologic outcomes. However, this is also supported by results from studies comparing lymphocele incidence in extended vs. standard templates that showed somewhat controversial results [6].

Similar considerations can be made regarding the role of prophylactic anticoagulation (LMWH, low molecular weight heparin) where guidelines already defined its role in the setting of minimally invasive radical prostatectomy and the expected benefits in TVP/PE reduction should outweigh the potential increase risk of lymphocele risk.

A lower incidence of lymphocele has been shown after transperitoneal robotic radical prostatectomy (RARP) with PLND, when compared to traditional open or extraperitoneal approaches. Initial peritoneal incision is probably the main reason for the decreased incidence of lymphocele formation during transperitoneal PLND, allowing free drainage of lymphatic fluid and reabsorption through the peritoneum instead of accumulation in a closed space. Nevertheless, the incidence of lymphocele is also higher than anticipated, in view of the believed protective effect of the transperitoneal approach [7, 8]. However, evidence from retrospective, non-randomized studies, showed significant benefit in terms of symptomatic lymphocele from peritoneal reconfiguration (OR 0.14, 95% CI 0.05–0.44) in comparison to when peritoneum is simply left open or closed completely after the surgical procedure [9].

P.L.E.A.T. technique (acronym: Preventing Lymphocele Ensuring Absorption Transperitoneally) aims to reconfigurate the peritoneum at the end of the surgical procedure thus ensuring a constant drainage of the lymphatic fluid out of the pelvis and into the peritoneal cavity where it can be absorbed.

Description of the Technique

At the beginning of the procedure, after transperitoneal trocar placement and robot docking, the peritoneum is incised starting lateral to umbilical ligament on each side and widely opened on the midline to access the Retzius' space (Figs. 31.1 and 31.2). After performing the surgical procedure, the peritoneum is "pleated" along its midline and fixed to the fibres of the *rectus abdominis* muscles, near the pubis (Fig. 31.3). The P.L.E.A.T. technique, leaving two lateral openings, allows lymphatic fluid to drain away from the pelvis and into the abdomen (Fig. 31.4).

Comparative Study [10]

To test the capability of this technique to prevent symptomatic lymphoceles, we collected series of PLNDs during RARP performed by a single surgeon, comparing 195

A. Morlacco · V. Lami · F. Dal Moro (✉)
Department of Surgery, Oncology and Gastroenterology, Urology Clinic, University of Padova, Padova, Italy
e-mail: alessandro.morlacco@unipd.it; fabrizio.dalmoro@unipd.it

S. Ren et al. (eds.), *Robot-Assisted Radical Prostatectomy*, https://doi.org/10.1007/978-3-031-05855-4_31

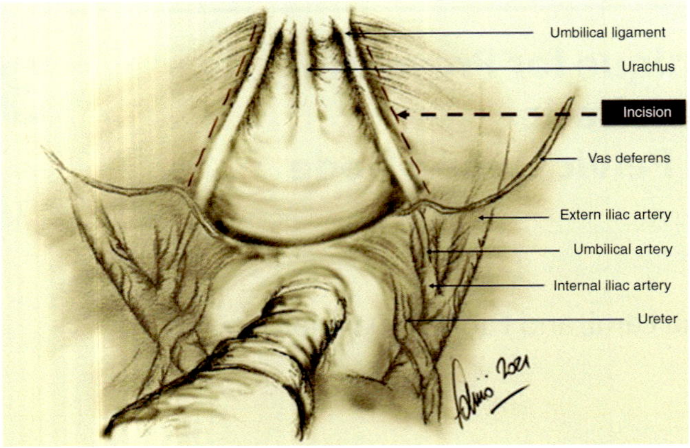

Fig. 31.1 Peritoneal incision at the beginning of the procedure

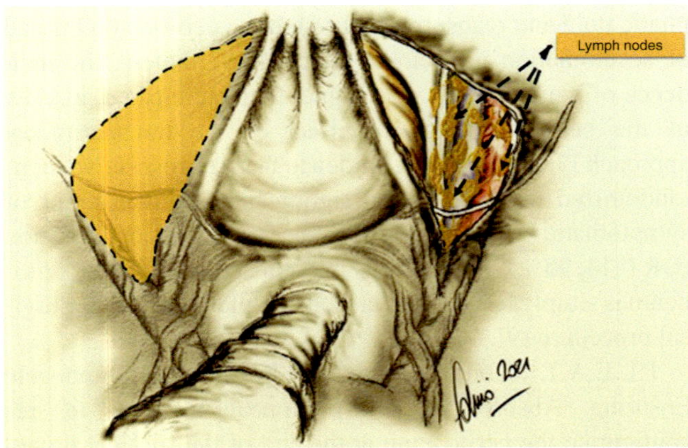

Fig. 31.2 Peritoneal openings for the lymph node dissection

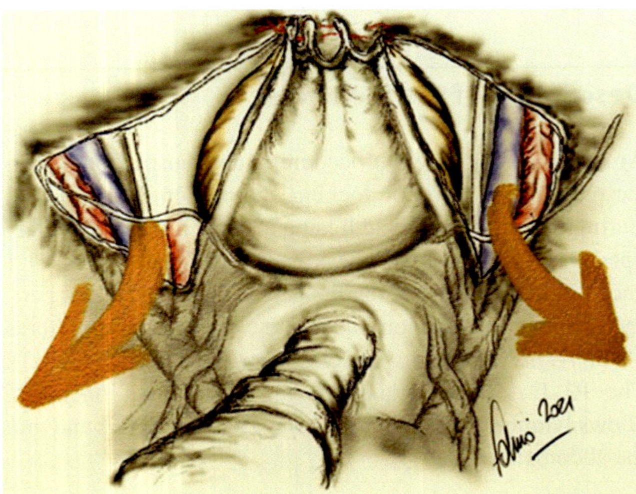

Fig. 31.3 Lymphatic fluid drainage through the peritoneal incisions

"standard" PLNDs (in which the peritoneum was "re-approximated" or left completely open) with 176 cases, in which a "partial" closure of the peritoneum according to

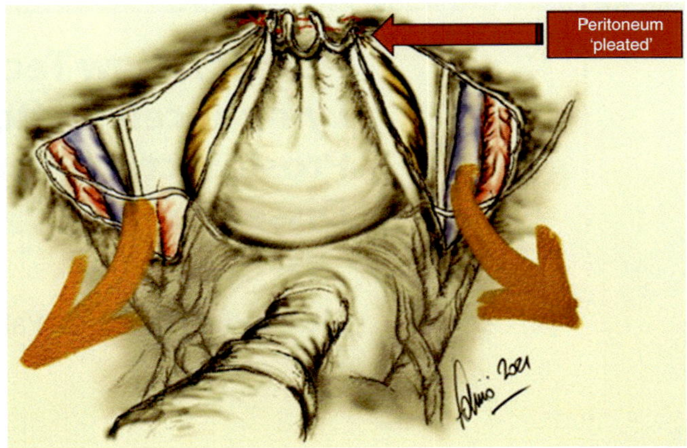

Fig. 31.4 "PLEAT" procedure to ensure continuous drainage through peritoneal incisions

the PLEAT technique was performed. All patients were managed similarly in the perioperative period, particularly, the same time of transurethral catheter (POD 6 with negative cystogram) and pelvic drain removal (POD 1). As Deep Vein Thrombosis (DVP) prophylaxis, we treated all patients with subcutaneous low molecular weight heparin (Enoxaparin) at a dosage of 4000 UI/day (modified according to specific risk, renal function, body mass index) and graduated compression stockings, the DVP prophylaxis was continued for 28 days after discharge as recommended by current guidelines.

We defined "symptomatic" lymphocele any case of pelvic symptoms such as pelvic fullness, fever, or lower abdominal pain, even if slight, with an evidence of lymphocele at ultrasound/CT/MRI, according to Kim's criteria [11].

In suspicious cases of leg DVT (pain, swelling, or discoloration of the affected extremity), the diagnosis was confirmed with Doppler/compression ultrasonography.

Results [10]

The demographic and clinical characteristics of patients in both groups were comparable, as was lymph nodes status ($p > 0.05$), while were statistically significant differences in the pathological staging of cancers ($p < 0.05$), and the median number of lymph nodes removed (5 vs. 10 in standard and P.L.E.A.T. groups, respectively; $p < 0.00001$) were present.

The cases of extended PLND (25 vs. 35, in standard and P.L.E.A.T. groups, respectively) were not statistically different ($p = 0.064$). In the 195 PLNDs without P.L.E.A.T. reconstruction, we found symptomatic lymphocele (Grade ≥ 3, according to the Clavien Dindo Classification) in 8 cases (4.1%). Only one P.L.E.A.T. patient complained of symptoms due to a bilateral lymphocele, requiring percutaneous drainage ($p = 0.039$).

The first 50 cases of PLND performed by the surgeon were excluded: in these cases, four symptomatic lymphoceles were present, but given the limitation linked with the cooperation with other surgeons and the non-standardized PLEAT technique, we decided to exclude these cases to avoid any bias due to the initial learning curve. Although including the first 50 cases would have allowed us to increase the level of significance of the study (p value from 0.038 to 0.01), it would not have been methodologically correct.

Comment

The problem of preventing lymphocele after PLND remains an interesting challenge, particularly in cases of extended PLND. Various solutions have been proposed to limit the risk, such as the use of new energy sources, or collagen patches coated with human coagulation factors which provide rapid and reliable haemostasis by creating a robust fibrin clot adhering to the tissue surface [12].

Peritoneal fenestration has been proposed to prevent the above-mentioned complications: this concept has been extensively studied to prevent lymphocele development in renal transplantation and confirmed in a recent review [13].

In fact, during open radical prostatectomy or extraperitoneal RARP, the occurrence of lymphocele was significantly lower if peritoneal fenestration is performed, and the formation of symptomatic lymphocele requiring surgical intervention was de facto eliminated, without an increase in postoperative morbidity, as documented by Stolzenburg et al. [14].

Nevertheless, although transperitoneal PLND has shown a lower incidence of lymphocele, it still remains significant [15] this may be due to spontaneous "re-approximation" of the edges of the peritoneum, incised laterally to the medial umbilical ligaments. In many cases, after release of the pneumoperitoneum after a RARP with PLND, even though the bladder is left "dropped", perivesical fat may adhere to the PLND bed, creating a closed space in which lymphatic fluid can accumulate. As reported by Lebeis et al., the bladder often forms the medial wall of the lymphocele cavity [16].

In addition, when the peritoneum is completely "re-approximated", the result is similar to an extraperitoneal open/laparoscopic radical prostatectomy.

Some authors have proposed the insertion of a peritoneal flap, thus forming a "window" which should prevents scarring to the bladder over the PLND area, allowing lymphatic fluid to drain into the peritoneal cavity and thus be reabsorbed [15]. As reported by the authors, this peritonealization of the lateral aspect of the bladder with an interposed flap is effective in preventing post-operative lymphoceles. However, this technique fixes the bladder inferiorly.

Starting from these considerations, we devised and applied the P.L.E.A.T. surgical technique. The unique nature of this strategy is that the two lateral "openings" do not collapse when the pneumoperitoneum is removed, because while we fix the bladder into a more natural position) we also pull the peritoneum medially, thereby avoiding any possible spontaneous re-approximation.

The results demonstrated the significant protective effect of this technique in preventing symptomatic lymphocele, compared with the widespread standard approach.

Other published works reported about similar techniques. In particular, Lebeis and colleagues proposed the use of a peritoneal interposition flap ("created by rotating and advancing the peritoneum around the lateral surface of the ipsilateral bladder to the dependent portion of the pelvis and fixing it to the bladder itself"). The rates of lymphocele detection on 77 consecutive patients who underwent this intervention were compared retrospectively to 77 who underwent standard procedure. No lymphocele was observed in the patients with peritoneal flap while 9 (11.6%) symptomatic cases were present in the comparison group [16].

On the other hand, Stolzenburg et al. in 2018 reported US diagnosis of both symptomatic and asymptomatic lymphocele at 8, 28 and 90 days in 193 patients who underwent a reconfiguration through a four-point peritoneal flap fixation (4PPFF) compared to matched controls who did not undergo the procedure. They found a significant difference in the incidence symptomatic lymphocele: two patients (1.03%) in the 4PPFF group vs. nine patients (4.6%) without 4PPFF ($p = 0.0322$). Asymptomatic lymphocele incidence was also lower in the 4PPFF group ($p = 0.0058$).

Meta-analysis results from these studies, including the PLEAT series, showed a significant benefit in terms of symptomatic lymphocele from peritoneal reconfiguration after transperitoneal PNLD (OR 0.14, 95% CI 0.05–0.44) vs. no reconfiguration [17].

Our preliminary analysis confirms that the P.L.E.A.T. technique is a fast, economic, easy-to-perform and safe method for reducing the risk of symptomatic lymphocele after transperitoneal robotic PLND [9].

References

1. Rassweiler J, Hruza M, Teber D, Su LM. Laparoscopic and robotic assisted radical prostatectomy—critical analysis of the results. Eur Urol. 2006;49:612–24. https://doi.org/10.1016/j.eururo.2005.12.054.
2. Orvieto MA, Coelho RF, Chauhan S, Palmer KJ, Rocco B, Patel VR. Incidence of lymphoceles after robot-assisted pelvic lymph node dissection. BJU Int. 2011;108:1185–9. https://doi.org/10.1111/j.1464-410X.2011.10094.x.
3. Dindo D, Demartines N, Clavien P-A. Classification of surgical complications: a new proposal with evaluation in a cohort of 6336 patients and results of a survey. Ann Surg. 2004;240:205–13.

4. Ploussard G, Briganti A, De La Taille A, Haese A, Heidenreich A, Menon M, et al. Pelvic lymph node dissection during robot-assisted radical prostatectomy: efficacy, limitations, and complications—a systematic review of the literature. Eur Urol. 2014;65:7–16. https://doi.org/10.1016/j.eururo.2013.03.057.
5. Lee HJ, Kane CJ. How to minimize lymphoceles and treat clinically symptomatic lymphoceles after radical prostatectomy topical collection on urosurgery. Curr Urol Rep. 2014;15:445. https://doi.org/10.1007/s11934-014-0445-y.
6. Yuh BE, Ruel NH, Mejia R, Novara G, Wilson TG. Standardized comparison of robot-assisted limited and extended pelvic lymphadenectomy for prostate cancer. BJU Int. 2013;112:81–8. https://doi.org/10.1111/j.1464-410X.2012.11788.x.
7. Chung JS, Kim WT, Ham WS, Yu HS, Chae Y, Chung SH, et al. Comparison of oncological results, functional outcomes, and complications for transperitoneal versus extraperitoneal robot-assisted radical prostatectomy: a single surgeon's experience. J Endourol. 2011;25:787–92. https://doi.org/10.1089/end.2010.0222.
8. Solberg A, Angelsen A, Bergan U, Haugen OA, Viset T, Klepp O. Frequency of lymphoceles after open and laparoscopic pelvic lymph node dissection in patients with prostate cancer. Scand J Urol Nephrol. 2003;37:218–21. https://doi.org/10.1080/00365590310008082.
9. Motterle G, Morlacco A, Zanovello N, Ahmed ME, Zattoni F, Karnes RJ, et al. Surgical strategies for lymphocele prevention in minimally invasive radical prostatectomy and lymph node dissection: a systematic review. J Endourol. 2020;34:113–20. https://doi.org/10.1089/end.2019.0716.
10. Dal Moro F, Zattoni F. P.L.E.A.T.—Preventing Lymphocele Ensuring Absorption Transperitoneally: a robotic technique. Urology. 2017;110:244–7. https://doi.org/10.1016/j.urology.2017.05.031.
11. Kim JK, Jeong YY, Kim YH, Kim YC, Kang HK, Choi HS. Postoperative pelvic lymphocele: treatment with simple percutaneous catheter drainage. Radiology. 1999;212:390–4. https://doi.org/10.1148/radiology.212.2.r99au12390.
12. Grande P, Di Pierro GB, Mordasini L, Ferrari M, Würnschimmel C, Danuser H, et al. Prospective randomized trial comparing titanium clips to bipolar coagulation in sealing lymphatic vessels during pelvic lymph node dissection at the time of robot-assisted radical prostatectomy. Eur Urol. 2017;71:155–8. https://doi.org/10.1016/j.eururo.2016.08.006.
13. Mihaljevic AL, Heger P, Abbasi Dezfouli S, Golriz M, Mehrabi A. Prophylaxis of lymphocele formation after kidney transplantation via peritoneal fenestration: a systematic review. Transpl Int. 2017;30:543–55. https://doi.org/10.1111/tri.12952.
14. Stolzenburg JU, Wasserscheid J, Rabenalt R, Do M, Schwalenberg T, McNeill A, et al. Reduction in incidence of lymphocele following extraperitoneal radical prostatectomy and pelvic lymph node dissection by bilateral peritoneal fenestration. World J Urol. 2008;26:581–6. https://doi.org/10.1007/s00345-008-0327-3.
15. Zorn KC, Katz MH, Bernstein A, Shikanov SA, Brendler CB, Zagaja GP, et al. Pelvic lymphadenectomy during robot-assisted radical prostatectomy: assessing nodal yield, perioperative outcomes, and complications. Urology. 2009;74:296–302. https://doi.org/10.1016/j.urology.2009.01.077.
16. Lebeis C, Canes D, Sorcini A, Moinzadeh A. Novel technique prevents lymphoceles after transperitoneal robotic-assisted pelvic lymph node dissection: peritoneal flap interposition. Urology. 2015;85:1505–9. https://doi.org/10.1016/j.urology.2015.02.034.
17. Giovanni M, Alessandro M, Nicola Z, Mohamed A, Filiberto Z, Jeffrey KR, et al. Surgical strategies for lymphocele prevention in minimally invasive radical prostatectomy and lymph-node dissection: a systematic review. J Endourol. 2020;34(2):113–20. https://doi.org/10.1089/end.2019.0716.

Part X

Perineal RALP

32 Tugcu Bakirkoy Technique

Selcuk Sahin and Volkan Tugcu

Introduction/Historical Background

Radical perineal prostatectomy (RPP) was first described by Young in 1905 [1]. Belt later modified this technique by approaching the prostate subsphincterically [2]. Millin developed the radical retropubic prostatectomy (RRP) in 1947 [3]. After, Walsh redefined the anatomical retropubic approach in the early 1980s. The perineal approach became less favored as most urologists preferred the retropubic approach due to its familiar and less complex anatomy [4]. In the minimally invasive era, the robotic transperitoneal approach has become the most popular technique [5, 6].

Nowadays, radical prostatectomy is the most used treatment option for localized prostate cancer [7]. It is used for open retropubic, perineal, laparoscopic and robotic techniques, which are among those used to perform radical prostatectomy. However, there is no evidence to show whether one surgical technique is superior to the others in terms of complications or oncologic and functional outcomes [8–11]. Each of the available techniques has its advantages and disadvantages. The advantages of robotic surgery are well documented. The application of this surgery with robotic arms with multi-directional mobility under a three-dimensional and high-resolution image provides great comfort and advantage to the patients. Robot-assisted radical prostatectomy is frequently performed transperitoneal due to advantages including a large working space and familiar anatomy [12]. However, complications related to patient position, abdominal wall and intraperitoneal structures may occur in cases where this approach is applied [13, 14]. In addition, patients who have had previous abdominal surgery require dissection of visible adhesions [15].

RPP provides relatively easy anatomic access to the prostate through a small incision. However, the deep location of the prostate in the pelvis, the surgeon's narrow operative vision, and the ergonomic issues affecting the operating surgeon are challenging aspects of the perineal approach that make it difficult to use [16]. Kaouk et al. described robot-assisted radical perineal prostatectomy (r-RPP) and reported that it is a safe, reliable and effective surgical technique for selected patients [17]. In a case series consisting of our first 15 cases and then 95 cases, we confirmed that both oncological and functional results of this method were successful [18, 19]. Theoretical advantages of the robotic perineal approach include the small concealed incision, avoidance of the intraperitoneal area, and preservation of the dorsal venous complex. The application of the robotic system to RPP helped in overcoming the above-listed hurdles in conventional RPP [20–22].

We compared the outcomes of robotic-assisted radical perineal prostatectomy (r-PRP) versus robotic-assisted transperitoneal laparoscopic radical prostatectomy (RARP) [23]. In our experience, r-PRP has acceptable morbidity, excellent surgical and oncological outcomes, and satisfactory functional results compared to RARP. The biggest difference between the two techniques is that r-PRP is performed via a different anatomical approach, and this is what strictly distinguishes it from RARP. There is no need to dissect bowel adhesions in patients who have history of major abdominal surgery. In this way, it is possible to preserve the anatomy and physiology of the prostate cancer patients who have previously undergone major abdominal surgery, or those who have received abdominal radiotherapy. Postoperative ileus is caused by many factors, the most important of which is the preferred surgical approach. In our study, ileus was not observed in the r-PRP group. However, spontaneously regressing ileus was detected in 10% of the RARP group. This is an important factors that affects length of hospital stay and recovery.

Until recently, one of the major disadvantages attributed to perineal radical prostatectomy was that patients requiring

S. Sahin (✉)
Department of Urology, Bakirkoy Training and Research Hospital, Istanbul, Turkey

V. Tugcu
Department of Urology, Liv Hospital Vadistanbul, Istanbul, Turkey

S. Ren et al. (eds.), *Robot-Assisted Radical Prostatectomy*, https://doi.org/10.1007/978-3-031-05855-4_32

bilateral pelvic lymph node dissection (BPLND) needed to have it performed through separate access, usually via laparoscopy. Saito and Murakami, however, described a technique for BPLND through the same perineal incision, using several retractors for direct view or laparoscopic assistance. They obtained BPLND via the perineum in 20 patients who underwent RPP [24]. Keller et al. subsequently reported an extended BPLND through the same perineal incision in 90 patients undergoing RPP [25]. After the prostate removal, they performed the extended BPLND under direct vision using a self-retaining system, retracting the bladder medially. Their technique provided sufficient lymph node removal with a reasonable average operative time. Lymphocele developed in seven patients (7.8%), four of whom (3.3%) required treatment. Ramirez et al. described r-RPP and PLND through the same incision in cadavers [26]. We demonstrated that a new The Tugcu Bakirkoy robotic perineal radical prostatectomy and BPLND technique which was previously tested in a cadaveric model can be safely applied for the first time in vivo, and presented our results [27].

Indications and Contraindications

Patient Selection

Patient selection is generally similar to robotic-assisted transperitoneal laparoscopic radical prostatectomy. We do not prefer this approach for patients with locally advanced disease and patients who are not suitable for the exaggerated lithotomy position due to hip arthrosis, ankylosis and/or severe coxarthrosis. We don't recommend selecting patients with large prostates and median lobes, a history of external beam radiotherapy at the beginning of the learning curve.

Surgical Technique

Preoperative Care

After the prostate biopsy, we prefer to wait at least 1 month and perform the surgery. If possible, anticoagulants and antiagregans should be discontinued at least 7 days before the operation. Because of the proximity of the incision to the rectum, antibiotic prophylaxis is indicated. A prophylactic dose of second generation sephalosporin is administered intravenously on call to the operating room and twice postoperatively. The day before the procedure, the patient is given an oral mechanical bowel preparation (e.g., Phospho-soda, a 1.5-oz. dose of which is taken at 9:00 a.m. and 12:00 p.m.). The patient is on a clear liquid diet that day. On the morning of surgery, after arrival at the hospital, the patient is given a 1% neomycin enema. Bowel preparation is very important in this operation. Because a sterile glove is placed in the rectum for further digital rectal examination and rectal damage may happen during the surgery.

Surgical Instruments, Devices, Materials

For open perineal access, scalpel, tissue forceps, Metzenbaum scissors, Allis and right angle forceps, as well as Richardson retractors were used. A GelPOINTMini Advanced Access Platform (Applied Medical, Rancho Santa Margarita, CA) was used, including an Alexis wound retractor and a GelSeal Cap (Applied Medical). The da Vinci Si system (Intuitive Surgical, Sunnyvale, CA) was used in a three-arm configuration. One 8-mm trocar (robotic scope), one 10-mm trocar (assistant), and two 8-mm robotic trocars were inserted through the GelSeal Cap in a diamond-shape configuration, with the 10-mm trocar at the bottom and the camera trocar at the top. Using three 8-mm robotic trocars, and monopolar curved scissors, and when required, a large needle driver was placed on the right side, fenestrated bipolar forceps were placed on the left side and a 30° up scope was placed at the 12 o'clock position.

Patients' Position

The patient is laid in the exaggerated lithotomy and 15° Trendelenburg position. All pressure points are padded, and the upper extremities are maintained in neutral positions (Fig. 32.1). A urethral catheter is placed and the bladder is emptied.

Steps

The operation consists of four stages:

Stage 1; open perineal dissection and Gel point placement
Stage 2; r-RPP

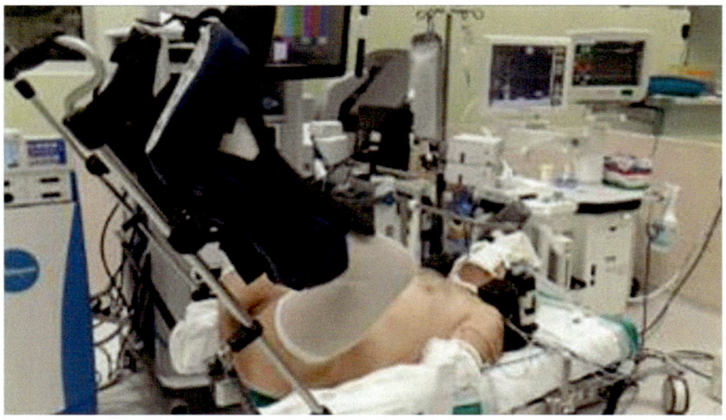

Fig. 32.1 The exaggerated lithotomy position with 15° Trendelenburg

Stage 3; robotic PLND
Stage 4; vesicourethral anastomosis.

Step I: Initial Perineal Dissection and Single Port Placement

A sterile glove is placed in the rectum and the sides of the glove are stitched to the perineal skin (Fig. 32.2). Thus, we aim to avoid rectal damage by using digital rectal examination during perineal dissections. A 6 cm semilunar incision is made between both tuberosity ischiadicum (Fig. 32.3). After the division of the subcutaneous tissue, the perineal body, or central tendon, had to be identified and transected. The perineal dissection is terminated when the dissection margin reaches the membraneous urethra and the apex of the prostate is seen. The subcutaneous tissue lying below the incision margins must be adequately dissected over the superficial perineal fascia to deploy GelPOINT® (Applied Medical, Rancho Santa Margarita, CA, USA).

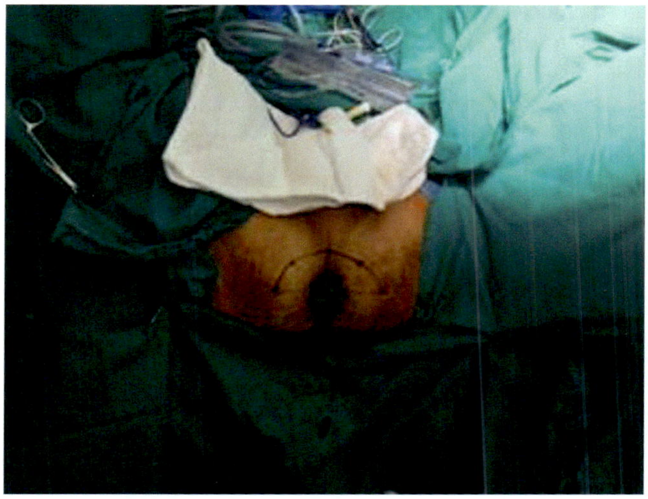

Fig. 32.2 Placing a sterile glove on the rectum

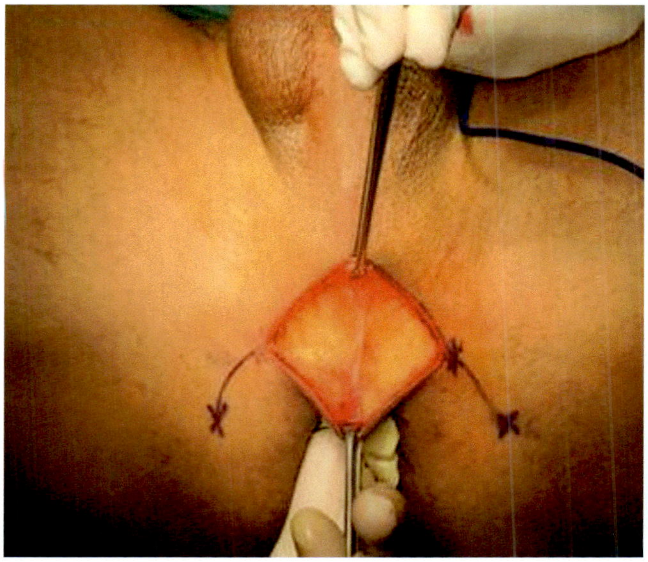

Fig. 32.3 Perineal incision

Step II: Robotic Perineal Radical Prostatectomy

Once the robotic system is docked (Fig. 32.4), dissection is started from the prostate apex (Fig. 32.5) and extended to the lateral sides of the prostate (Fig. 32.6), and then deepened inferiorly to reveal the Denonvilliers' fascia covering the seminal vesicles. Once the Denonvilliers' fascia is incised bilateral vas deferences are revealed, dissected, and cut. Seminal vesicles are completely dissected and freed. Then the membranous urethra is dissected and cut. A Hem-o-lock clip (Weck Closure Systems, Research Triangle Park, NC, USA) is then placed on the urethral catheter to keep the balloon inflated, the catheter can then be used as a handle to aid dissection and manipulation of the prostate (Fig. 32.7). The lateral prostatic pedicles are dissected and hemostatic control is achieved using Hem-o-Lock® Clips (Fig. 32.8). After completing the lateral dissections of the prostate bilaterally, the bladder neck is identified and incised with monopolar scissors. Once the bladder neck dissection is completed, the robotic arms are undocked and the prostate is removed from the surgical field.

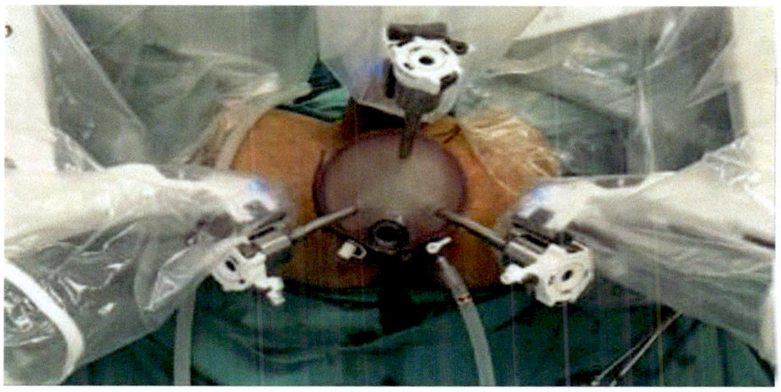

Fig. 32.4 The docking of the three robotic arms

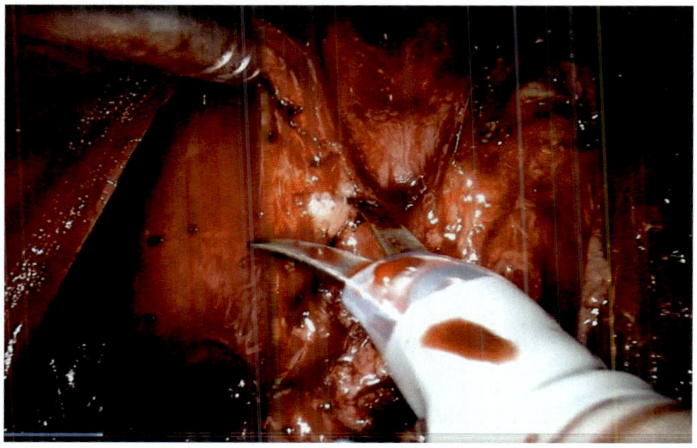

Fig. 32.5 Dissection of the apex

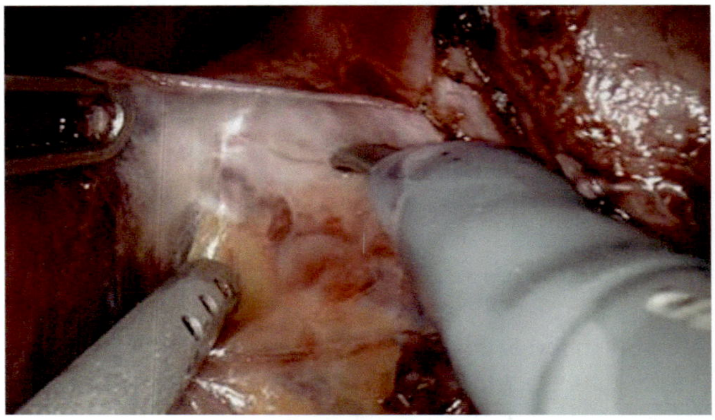

Fig. 32.6 Dissection of the lateral lobes

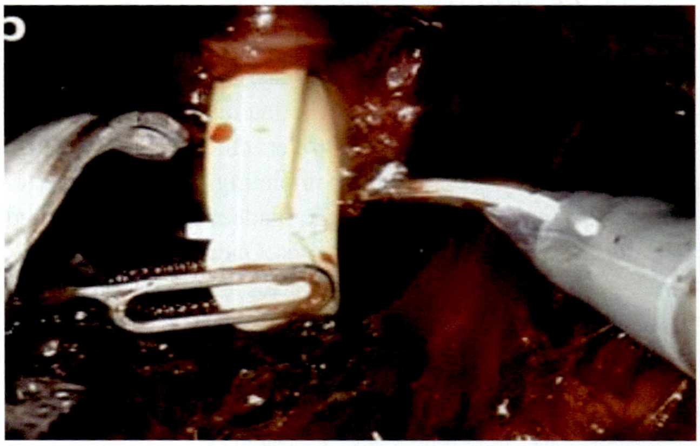

Fig. 32.7 Placing the clip in and cutting the urethral catheter

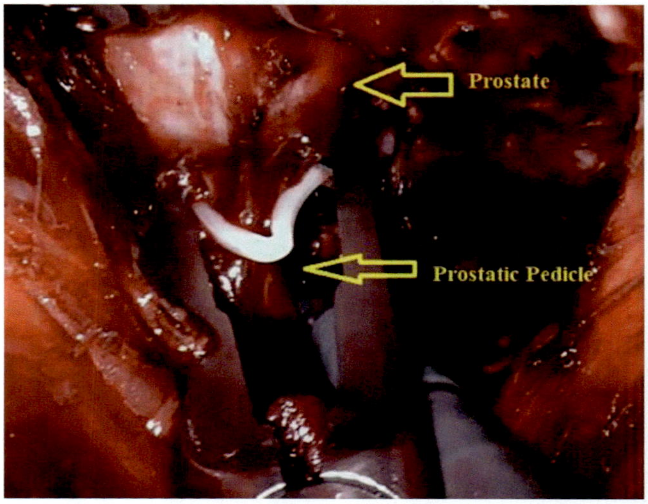

Fig. 32.8 Ligation of the prostatic pedicles

Step III: Bilateral Robotic Pelvic Lymph Node Dissection

After r-RPP is completed and the prostate removed, pelvic lymph node dissection is performed before vesicourethral anastomosis. Initially, when the bladder is medialized, the levator ani muscles are lateralized to the contralateral side and the dissection is extended towards the cranial side of the perivesical area. After passing this stage, endopelvic fascia is revealed (Fig. 32.9). After the endopelvic fascia is gently dissected and medialized, the obturator fossa is exposed and dissection is expanded to this region. When the dissection is continued in this area, the obturator nerve is first visualized at the bottom and most lateral side. When we dissect towards more upwardly and medially, the obturator venous ring may be visible. The obturator artery can be seen if dissection is extended to the lateral side of the obturator venous ring and into fatty planes (Fig. 32.10). When the dissection is performed superiorly, the external iliac vein and the external iliac artery are dissected. The dissection is terminated when the ureteral crossing over the external iliac artery is reached. Thus, obturator lymph nodes and iliac lymph node groups are included in the dissection area (Fig. 32.11). After completion of dissection of pelvic anatomical landmarks, pelvic

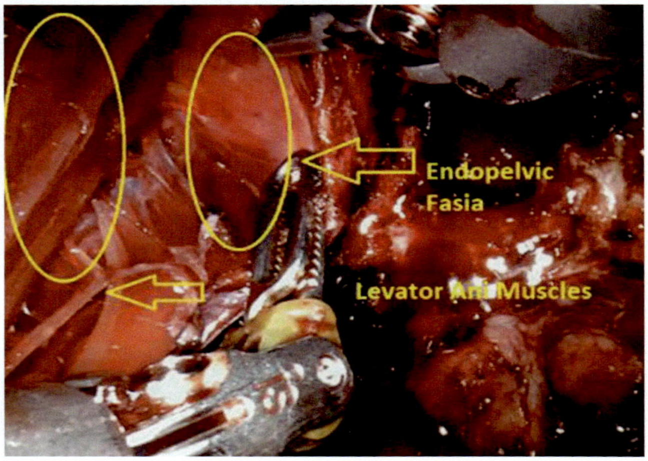

Fig. 32.9 Dissection of the endopelvic fascia

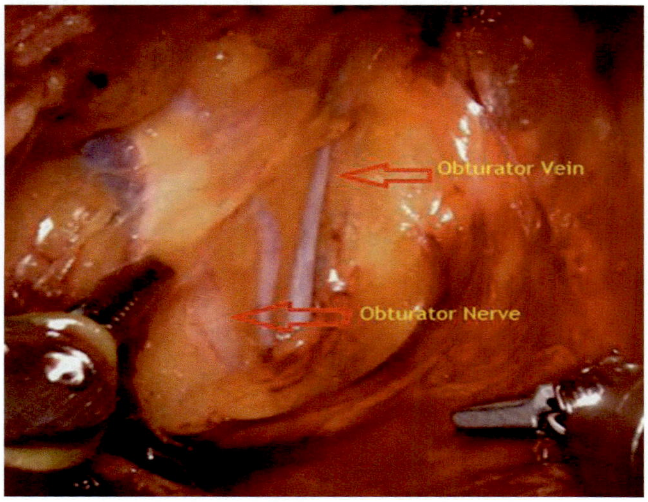

Fig. 32.10 Dissection of the obturator nerve and vein

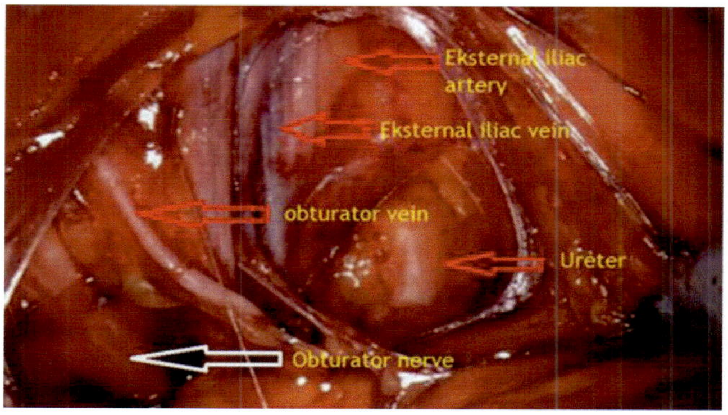

Fig. 32.11 Dissection of the iliac vessels up to crossing ureter

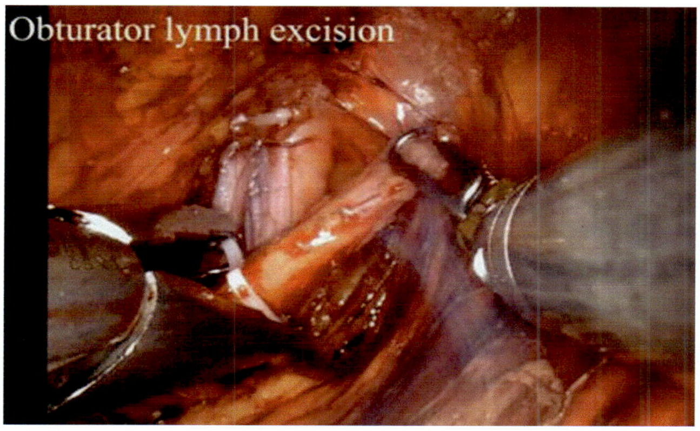

Fig. 32.12 Obturator lymph node excision

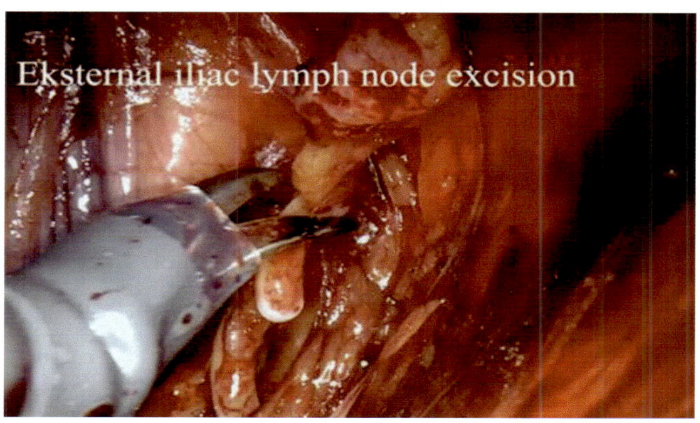

Fig. 32.13 Iliac lymph node excision

lymph node excision is continued. Obturator and Iliac lymph nodes are released and traced, and excision is performed by placement of the Hem-o-loc® clip for safety purposes (Figs. 32.12 and 32.13).

Step IV: Vesico-Urethral Anastomosis

After completing pelvic lymph node dissection, the intraoperative pressure was reduced to 5 mm Hg to perform the vesicourethral anastomosis. The two 4/0 V-Loc™ (Covidien,

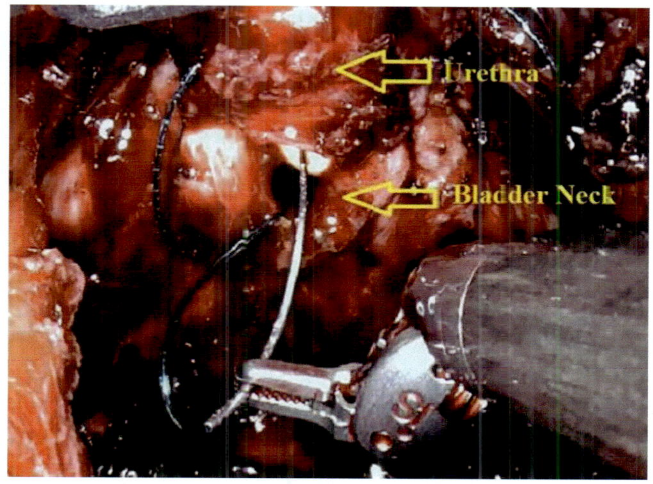

Fig. 32.14 Vesicouretera anostomosis

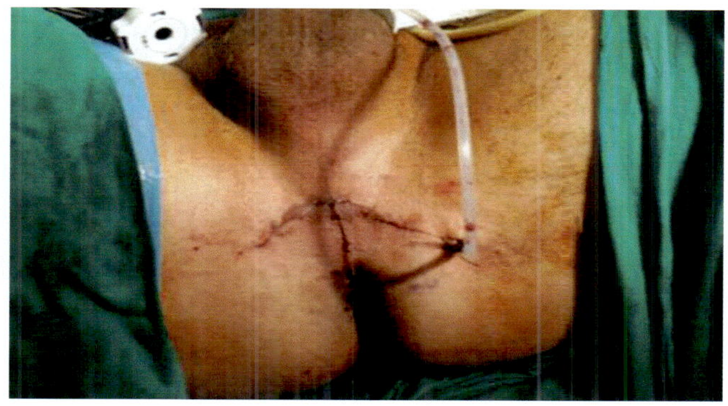

Fig. 32.15 The Jackson Pratt drain is placed

Mansfield, MA, USA) sutures are used in a running fashion starting from the Retzius side to the rectal side of the bladder neck (Fig. 32.14). The first suture is started at 12 o'clock on the bladder neck from outside to inside and then continued to the urethra from inside to outside in a clockwise fashion down to 6 o'clock. A second barbed suture is used in the same setting but reverses a clockwise fashion. Once the anastomosis is completed a 22 Ch urethral catheter is replaced. The bladder is filled with 200 cc saline to test the anastomosis for leakage. After observing the anastomosis is watertight, the robotic system is undocked and, the skin and subcutaneous tissues are approximated over a Jackson Pratt drain are placed before completion of The Tugcu Bakirkoy Robotic Perineal Radical Prostatectomy Technique (Fig. 32.15).

Postoperative Care

The postoperative care path is similar to that following standard robotic prostatectomy, including immediate diet resumption, minimization of narcotic pain medications, and early ambulation. Patients are observed postoperatively and discharged home within 24–48 h in routine cases. The perineal drain is removed before discharge, and the urethral catheter is removed after 1 week.

Conclusion

The Tugcu Bakırkoy technique is new and we have demonstrated in this procedure that pelvic lymph node dissection can be performed safely in vivo. The Tugcu Bakirkoy technique allows for dissection of the pelvic lymph node with less morbidity than other techniques and with superior cosmetic, and equivalent oncological results. This technique doesn't affect the intestines and there is no need to intervene intraabdominal adhesions developed due to previous surgery. Therefore the patient can return to the daily life earlies. Thanks to the development of technology and performing a greater number of operations with this technique, this technique will be gradually used in daily practice.

References

1. Young HH. The early diagnosis and radical cure of carcinoma of the prostate. Being a study of 40 cases and the presentation of a radical operation which was carried out in four cases. 1905. J Urol. 2002;168:914–21.
2. Belt E, Turner RD. A study of 229 consecutive cases of total perineal prostatectomy for cancer of the prostate. J Urol. 1957;77:62–77.
3. Millin T. Retropubic prostatectomy. J Urol. 1948;59:267–80.
4. Walsh PC, Lepor H, Eggleston JC. Radical prostatectomy with preservation of sexual function: anatomical and pathological considerations. Prostate. 1983;4:473–85.
5. Lowrance WT, Eastham JA, Savage C, et al. Contemporary open and robotic radical prostatectomy practice patterns among urologists in the United States. J Urol. 2012;187:2087–92.
6. Ficarra V, Cavalleri S, Novara G, Aragona M, Artibani W. Evidence from robot-assisted laparoscopic radical prostatectomy: a systematic review. Eur Urol. 2007;51:45–55. discussion 56.
7. Heidenreich A, Bastian PJ, Bellmunt J, et al. EAU guidelines on prostate cancer. Part 1: Screening, diagnosis, and local treatment with curative intent—update 2013. Eur Urol. 2014;65:124–37.
8. Ficarra V, Novara G, Artibani W, et al. Retropubic, laparoscopic, and robot-assisted radical prostatectomy: a systematic review and cumulative analysis of comparative studies. Eur Urol. 2009;55:1037–63.
9. Wirth MP, Hakenberg OW. Surgery and marketing: comparing different methods of radical prostatectomy. Eur Urol. 2009;55:1031–3.
10. Nargund VH, Zaman F. Radical prostatectomy—too soon to abandon the perineal approach? Nat Rev Urol. 2011;8:179–80.
11. Wronski S. Radical perineal prostatectomy—the contemporary resurgence of a genuinely minimally invasive procedure: procedure outline. Comparison of the advantages, disadvantages, and outcomes of different surgical techniques of treating organ-confined prostate cancer (PCa). A literature review with a special focus on perineal prostatectomy Central European. J Urol. 2012;65:188–94.
12. Li-Ming S, Scott MG, Joseph AS Jr. Laparoscopic and robotic-assisted laparoscopic radical prostatectomy and pelvic lymphadenectomy. In: Campbell-Walsh Urology, vol. 2. 11th ed. Philadelphia: Elsevier; 2016. p. 663–8.
13. Tasci AI, Simsek A, Tugcu V, Bitkin A, Sonmezay E, Torer BD. Abdominal wall hemorrhage after robotic-assisted radical prostatectomy: is it a complication of robotic surgery? Actas Urol Esp. 2013;37(10):634–9.
14. Matsubara A, Yoneda T, Nakamoto T, Maruyama S, Koda S, Goto K, et al. Inguinal hernia after radical perineal prostatectomy: comparison with the retropubic approach. Urology. 2007;70(6):1152–6.
15. Di Pierro GB, Grande P, Mordasini L, Danuser H, Mattei A. Robot-assisted radical prostatectomy in the setting of previous abdominal surgery: perioperative results, oncological and functional outcomes, and complications in a single surgeon's series. Int J Surg. 2016;36(Pt A):170–6.
16. Horuz R, Goktas C, Cetinel CA, et al. Simple preoperative parameters to assess technical difficulty during a radical perineal prostatectomy. Int Urol Nephrol. 2013;45:129–33.
17. Kaouk JH, Akca O, Zargar H, Caputo P, Ramirez D, Andrade H, et al. Descriptive technique and initial results for robotic radical perineal prostatectomy. Urology. 2016;94:129–38.
18. Tugcu V, Akca O, Simsek A, Yigitbasi I, Sahin S, Tasci AI. Robot-assisted radical perineal prostatectomy: first experience of 15 cases. Turk J Urol. 2017;43(4):476–83.
19. Tugcu V, Eksi M, Sahin S, Colakoğlu Y, Simsek A, Evren I, Ihsan Tasci A. Robot-assisted radical perineal prostatectomy: a review of 95 cases. BJU Int. 2020;125(4):573–8.
20. Tugcu V, Simsek A, Yigitbasi I, Yenice MG, Sahin S, Tasci AI. Robotic perineal radical prostatectomy with high prostate volume. Arch Ital Urol Androl. 2018;90(1):65–7.
21. Tugcu V, Simsek A, Yigitbasi I, Yenice MG, Sahin S, Tasci AI. Robot-assisted perineal radical prostatectomy in a post-kidney transplant recipient. J Endourol Case Rep. 2018;4(1):21–4.
22. Yenice MG, Yigitbasi I, Sam E, Simsek A, Tugcu V. Robotic perineal radical prostatectomy in a patient with a pre-existing three piece inflatable penile prosthesis. Aktuelle Urol. 2020. Online ahead of print 2020 Jan 28. https://doi.org/10.1055/a-0945-2489.
23. Tugcu V, Akca O, Şimşek A, Yigitbasi I, Sahin S, Yenice MG, Tasci AI. Robotic-assisted perineal versus transperitoneal radical prostatectomy: a matched-pair analysis. Turk J Urol. 2019;45(4):265–72.
24. Saito S, Murakami G. Radical perineal prostatectomy: a novel approach for lymphadenectomy from perineal incision. J Urol. 2003;170:1298–300.
25. Keller H, Lehmann J, Beier J. Radical perineal prostatectomy and simultaneous extended pelvic lymph node dissection via the same incision. Eur Urol. 2007;52:384–8.
26. Ramirez D, Maurice MJ, Kaouk JH. Robotic perineal radical prostatectomy and pelvic lymph node dissection using a purpose-built single-port robotic platform. BJU Int. 2016;118(5):829–33.
27. Tugcu V, Akca O, Simsek A, Yigitbasi İ, Yenice MG, Sahin S, Tasci AI. Robotic perineal radical prostatectomy and robotic pelvic lymph node dissection via a perineal approach: the Tugcu Bakirkoy Technique. Turk J Urol. 2018;44(2):114–8.

Bari Technique for Robotic Radical Perineal Prostatectomy

33

Pasquale Ditonno, Umberto Carbonara, Paolo Minafra, Giuseppe Papapicco, Michele Battaglia, and Antonio Vitarelli

Introduction

The ideal procedure for surgical treatment of localized prostate cancer would provide complete oncological eradication maintaining continence and recovery of the erectile function. In the past years, several efforts have been made to find a surgical technique that could achieve all these goals.

Historically, the use of radical prostatectomy to treat prostate cancer began in 1905 when Hugh Hampton Young first published the description of the **perineal radical prostatectomy** (RPP) in Annals of Surgery [1, 2]. Young's radical perineal prostatectomy persisted as the preferred approach for many decades, until 1948, when Millin redefined the procedure using retropubic access through an abdominal incision from the umbilicus to the pubis [3]. Millin's retropubic approach was further improved by Walsh in 1987, which made the procedure safer improving oncological and functional results [4].

In the past years, the robotic has become an integral tool in urologic surgery as well as other specialties [5]. Advantages of the robotic system include improved ergonomics, wristed instrumentation, and magnified, three-dimensional visualization facilitating suturing and dissection during minimally invasive prostatectomy [6]. Moreover, robot assistance reduced many of the challenges associated with open and laparoscopic prostatectomy with the result that "standard" robot-assisted radical prostatectomy following Walsh's method was rapidly adopted for the treatment of localized prostate cancer [7].

Currently, the use of the robotic platform leads to resume several surgical approaches that were poorly used by open surgery such as perineal radical prostatectomy allowing to reduce some technical challenges as ergonomic issues affecting the surgeon, deep and narrow operative field characteristic [6].

P. Ditonno (✉) · U. Carbonara · P. Minafra · G. Papapicco
M. Battaglia · A. Vitarelli
Urology Unit, Department of Emergency and Organ Transplantation, University of Bari, Bari, Italy
e-mail: pasquale.ditonno@uniba.it; michele.battaglia@uniba.it

Surgical and Functional Anatomy

The anatomical features during **robotic radical perineal prostatectomy** (r-RPP) represent peculiar aspects that require in-depth understanding, even for expert surgeons. An extensive discussion of the pelvic and prostatic surgical anatomy is beyond the aim of the present chapter. Key a few anatomical points are illustrated in Figs. 33.1, 33.2, and 33.3 for a better comprehension of the reader.

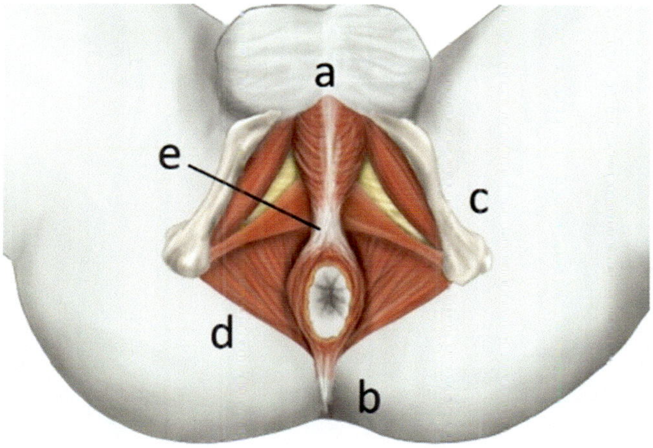

Fig. 33.1 Perineal region. The perineal region presents a diamond shape delimited by (**a**) the inferior margin of the pubic symphysis anteriorly, (**b**) the tip of the coccyx posteriorly, (**c**) the inferior margin of ischiopubic rami and ischial tuberosities anterolaterally, (**d**) the sacrotuberous ligaments posterolaterally. The **perineal body** (**e**) occupies the middle point of the interischial line. It is a fundamental landmark during the perineal prostatectomy since giving attachment to the superficial and deep portions of the external anal sphincter posteriorly, as well as bulbospongiosus, and superficial transverse perineal muscles anteriorly

S. Ren et al. (eds.), *Robot-Assisted Radical Prostatectomy*, https://doi.org/10.1007/978-3-031-05855-4_33

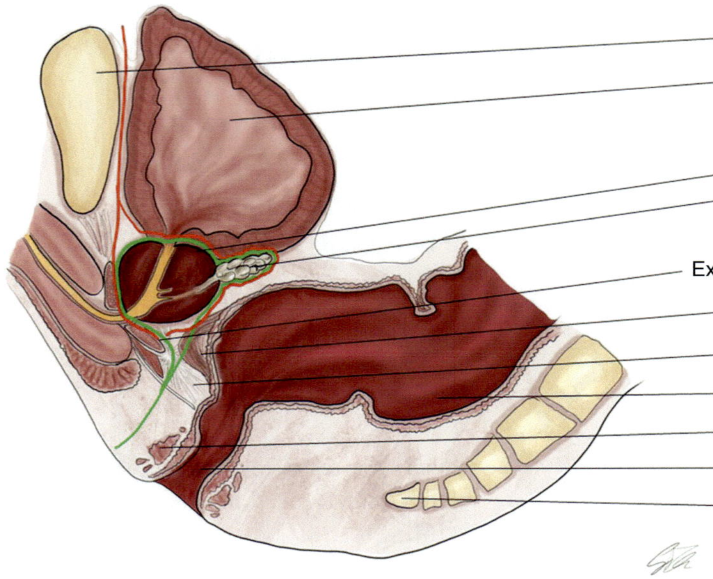

Fig. 33.2 Sagittal section of the male pelvis. The **external anal sphincter** surrounds the anal canal in the lower part. In Young's approach, the incision is made to fall outside the external urinary sphincter directly towards the perineal body, whereas the approach described by Belt is subsphincteric and can cause sphincter-stretching with consequent greater risk of fecal incontinence. The **rectourethralis muscle** is a fundamental landmark for perineal procedures. It is a thin Y-shaped smooth muscle with two branches arising from the anterolateral surface of the rectal wall that merge medially and extend inferiorly towards the perineal body and the bulb of the urethra. The rectal-anal junction is located at the level of the rectourethralis muscle and here the rectum is at the closest point to the prostate apex, since caudally the anal canal folds backward. Therefore, the division of the rectourethralis muscle is the most common cause of rectal injuries during perineal prostatectomy. **The green line identifies the radical perineal prostatectomy route. The red line identifies the "standard" transperitoneal route**

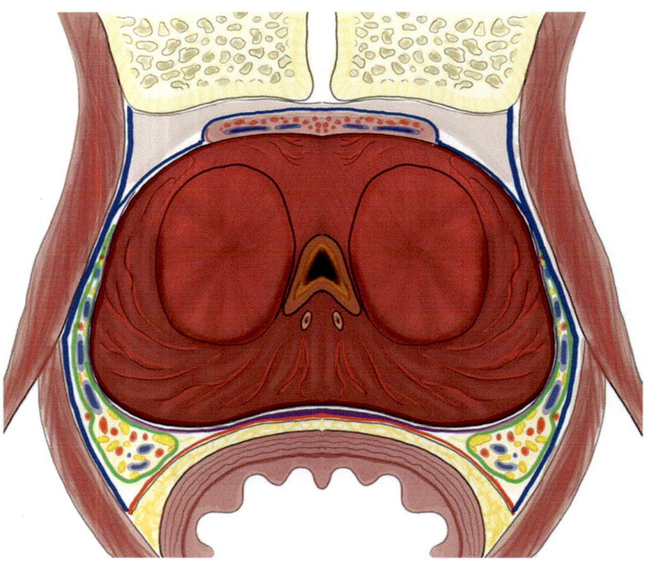

Fig. 33.3 Prostatic fasciae. The **endopelvic fascia (blue line),** the **Denonvilliers' fascia (red line)**, and the **lateral prostatic fascia (purple line)** are the three main fascial structures surrounding the prostate gland. The **neurovascular bundle (green line)** and the prostatic pedicles are present in a virtual space that is delimitated by the prostate gland, the lateral prostatic fascia, and Denonvilliers' fascia

Table 33.1 Suitable candidates per robotic radical perineal prostatectomy

Suitable characteristics	Unsuitable characteristics
• Small or medium prostate weight (<80 ml)	• High-risk prostate cancer[a]
• Low or intermediate risk prostate cancer	• >5% of Briganti's nomogram[a]
• Obese men (BMI > 39)	
• Cardiac comorbidities	
• Post renal transplant recipients	
• Prior mesh repair of inguinal hernia	
• Prior abdominal surgery	

[a]The present contraindications can be overcome if robotic lymphadenectomy with perineal access is performed [9]

Surgical Indications

In the preoperative assessment, some criteria should be considered before selecting the patient for robotic radical perineal prostatectomy (Table 33.1).

Overall, men with **small and medium-volume prostate** (less than 80 ml) represent the suitable candidate for the robotic perineal radical prostatectomy. Nevertheless, performing this surgical procedure in "*very*" small prostate (<20 g), as well as, large prostate (>80 g) is challenging but not contraindicated.

Another preoperative selection criterion is the risk of positive nodes less than 5% according to Briganti's nomogram (low-risk) in men with low or intermediate-risk prostate cancer non-suitable for active surveillance [8]. Nevertheless, the development of the robotic pelvic lymphadenectomy allows overcoming this limitation and including almost all patients choosing surgical treatment for localized prostate cancer [9].

The patient's characteristics to be considered are prior abdominal surgery, and inflammatory bowel disease (representing relative contraindications to transperitoneal surgery), as well as cardiovascular or respiratory comorbidity, and obesity (representing relative contraindication to the pneumoperitoneum).

Robotic System and Instruments

Herein we provide in detail the **Bari technique** of robotic radical perineal prostatectomy performed with *da Vinci Xi® system* (Intuitive Surgical, Sunnyvale, CA, USA) that represents the fourth generation of the robotic system. The Xi® characteristics facilitate the perineal approach by maximizing freedom of movement, minimizing instrument clashing, and providing good ergonomics during the critical steps of the procedure, even comparing to the Si® platform [10].

The following robotic and laparoscopic instruments can be used to perform Bari technique r-RPP:

- 30° Endoscope with camera
- Monopolar curved scissor
- Fenestrated/Maryland Bipolar Forceps
- Medium/large Needle Driver
- AirSeal Access Port
- GelPOINT®

To note, the Bari technique provides the use of the AirSeal® system as an assistant port. This type of insufflation system responds immediately to the slightest changes in pressure maintaining a continuous smoke evacuation, and CO_2 recirculation, and ensuring visibility during the procedure. The AirSeal® access can be used also as a laparoscopic port for the assistant surgeon at the surgical table.

GelPOINT® is the single-port device allowing instruments introduction through a single perineal incision. Three robotic trocars are placed through its jelly top in a triangular disposition, being the optic trocar upwards (Fig. 33.4).

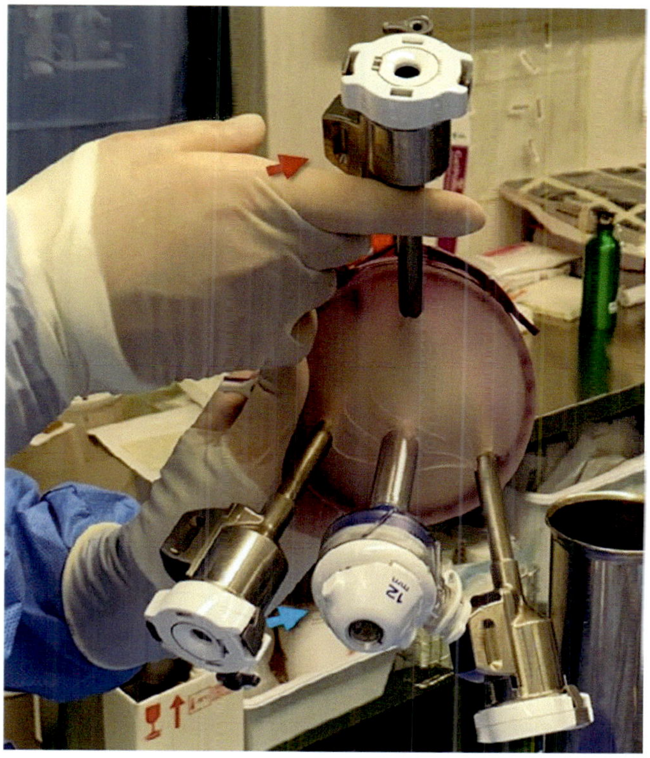

Fig. 33.4 GelPOINT® for the robotic perineal prostatectomy access. Three robotic trocars are placed through its jelly top in a triangular disposition, being the optic trocar upwards (red arrow) and the AirSeal at the base (blue arrow)

Bari Technique

Overall, the Bari technique is robotic radical perineal prostatectomy performed with nerve-sparing attempt.

Patient's Positioning and Operative Room Disposition

The patient is positioned in an **exaggerated lithotomy position** with buttocks protruding from the table, and stirrups for leg support. 15° Trendelenburg tilt is applied, and a cushion stabilizes the pelvis into a 45° plane (Fig 33.5). Pressure points are covered with soft tissues to avoid compartment syndrome. A rectal shield is placed to allow constant rectal examinations during the phase of open surgical access to the prostate, to avoid injuries to the rectal wall.

Perineal Dissection and GelPOINT Port Placement

A semicircular incision of about 7 cm is performed 2 cm above the anus, medial from one ischial tuberosity to the

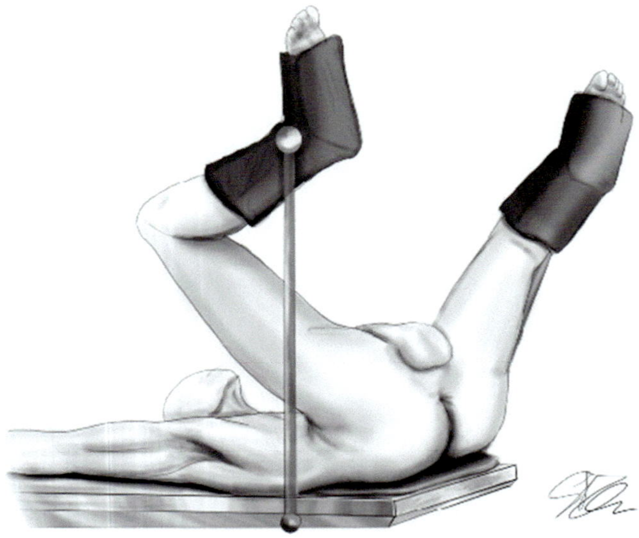

Fig. 33.5 Patient positioning. The patient is placed in an exaggerated lithotomy position, with a 15° Trendelenburg tilt. A cushion under the sacrum further lifted the pelvis

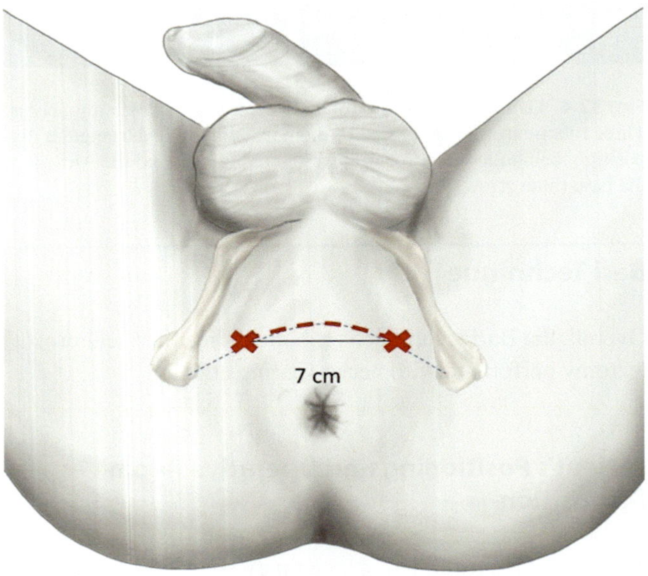

Fig. 33.6 Skin incision. A semicircular landmark is drawn between the ischial tuberosities and 2 cm above the anus (black dashed line). A line of about 7 cm is measured as a subtender chord of the previous line (black line). The red dashed line shows the skin incision

other (Fig. 33.6). The dissection plane is conducted anteriorly to the fibers of the external anal sphincter, and towards the perineal body.

The surgical field is exposed applying traction to the lower skin flap by stay suture or with an Allis forceps, as well as placing Langenbeck retractors at the level of the superior flap.

In the midline, the subcutaneous prolongations of the muscular fibers of the external anal sphincter may be encountered and should be transacted with electrocautery.

On both sides, the surgeon bluntly opens the fibrous septum separating the superficial and deep portion of the ischiorectal fossae. After the opening of these spaces, downward traction of the anal canal is performed. The perineal body becomes apparent and can be gradually divided with a combination of sharp and blunt dissection (Fig. 33.7). The rectourethralis muscle is the last attachment of the rectum to the prostatourethral junction. The recto-anal junction is placed at this level of dissection and here the rectum is located at the point closest to the apex of the prostate. To note, the division of the rectourethralis muscle is the most common cause of rectal injuries during perineal prostatectomy and the plane of dissection should be conducted slightly upwards rather than parallel to the pelvic floor for avoiding rectal lesion. The superior landmark is represented by the spongy urethra. The combination of sharp and blunt dissection and digital guidance through the rectal shield allow the correct plane of dissection to be defined, and the rectourethralis muscle is incised in little increments as dissection progresses.

Once the rectourethralis muscle has been divided, the median edge of the levator ani muscles are lateralized by placing stay sutures (usually with Vicryl® 0) and the rectum can be swept off the prostate. The prostatic dorsal surface covered by the whitish layer of the Denonvilliers' fascia is visualized (Fig. 33.8).

A subcutaneous pouch in the thickness of the adipose tissue facilitates the GelPOINT® placement (Fig. 33.9).

The robot platform is docked to the left side of the patient's legs and a bedside assistant takes part in the surgical procedure.

Bari Nerve-Sparing Technique

The decision of performing the nerve-sparing approach is based on clinical staging, *Gleason* score, localization of the disease, and preoperative erectile function [8].

After the development of the plane between Denonvilliers' fascia and the rectum, the isolation of the lateral aspects of the prostate is performed. Denonvilliers' fascia is coldly incised in the midline with monopolar scissors (Fig. 33.10). The dissection of the prostate along the intrafascial plane is then carried on in a mediolateral direction taking care not to cause any damage to the neurovascular bundles and preserving periprostatic nervous fibers. Small vessels tethering the neurovascular bundles to the prostatic gland can be controlled with the use of small Hem-o-Lock® clips avoiding electrocautery and any form of traction.

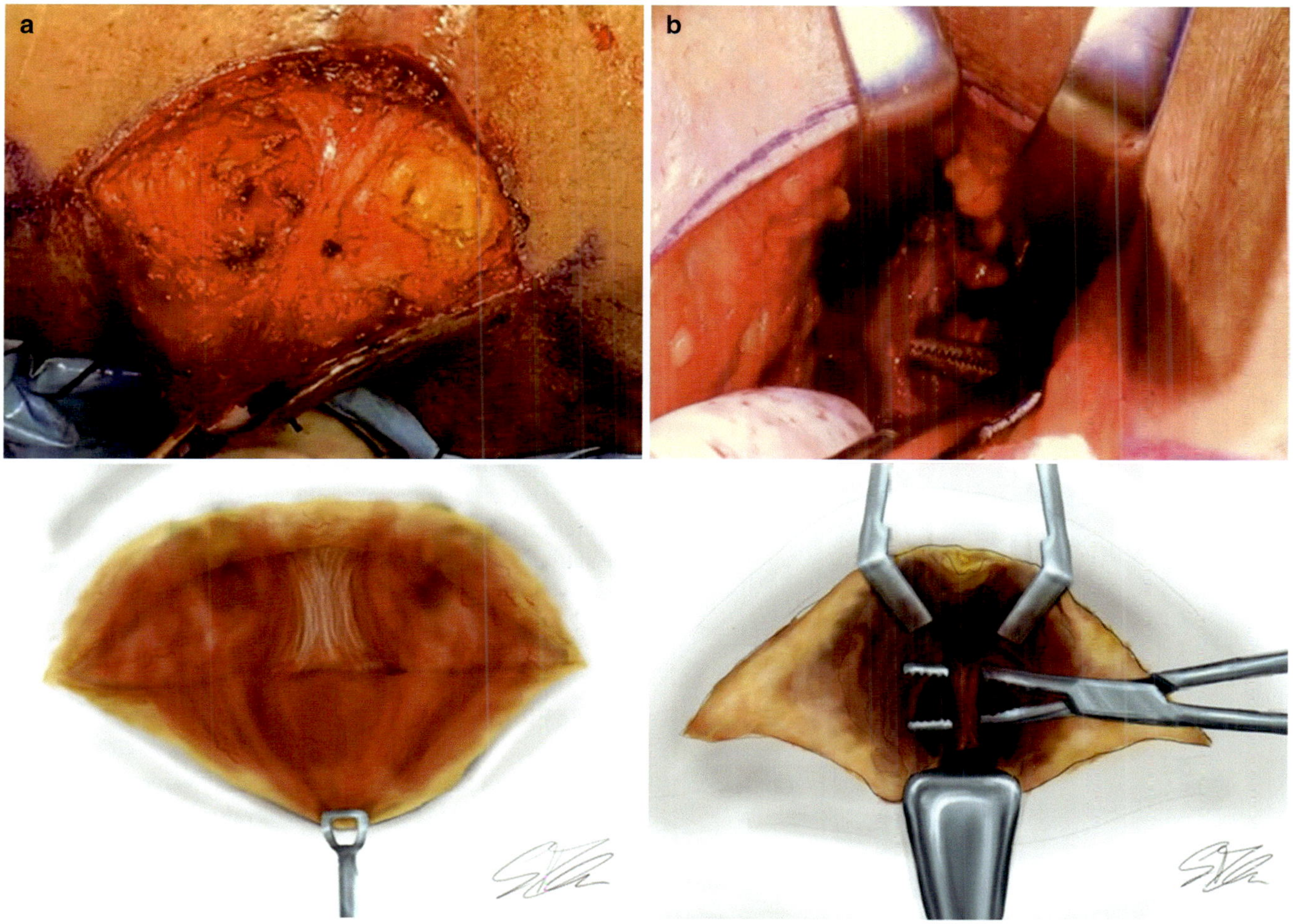

Fig. 33.7 Section of (**a**) perineal body and (**b**) rectourethralis muscle

The dissection of the neurovascular bundles is continued cranially towards the apex and caudally to the seminal vesicles. The vascular vases are clamped and cutted bilateraly.

Vas Deferens and Seminal Vesicles Dissection

The *vas deferens* and the *seminal vesicles* are identified and dissected free with blunt and sharp dissection on either side. First, the vas deferens are ligated and divided. The seminal vesicle is carefully freed by applying controlateral traction on the vas deferens. The isolation of the dorsal aspect of the prostate is completed by tractioning both seminal vesicles and vas deference cranially. To note, caution should be taken during nerve-sparing prostatectomy to avoid damaging the nerve plexus by dissecting laterally to the tips of the seminal vesicles.

Prostate Apex and Membranous Urethra Isolation

The membranous urethra is gently separated from the external urinary sphincter. The isolation of the prostate apex is carefully conducted for keeping the membranous urethra as long as possible. The urethra is incised with cold scissors and the catheter is clipped before being cut for anchoring the inflated catheter balloon to the bladder (Fig. 33.11).

Anterior Dissection and Preservation of the Support of the Bladder Neck

Once the urethra has been transected, the anterior aspect of the prostate is isolated by sweeping off the structures of the puboprostatic complex ventrally. In this way, the retropubic space of Retzius and the anterior suspensory mechanism of the bladder are preserved.

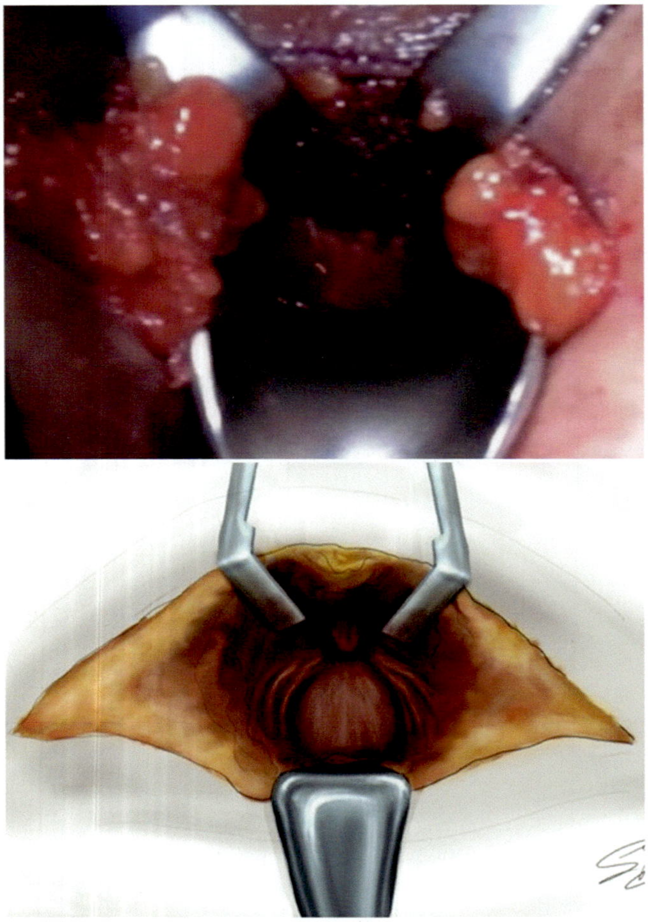

Fig. 33.8 The posterior surface of the prostate. The open phase ends with the exposure of the dorsal face of the prostate covered by the whitish layer of the Denonvilliers' fascia

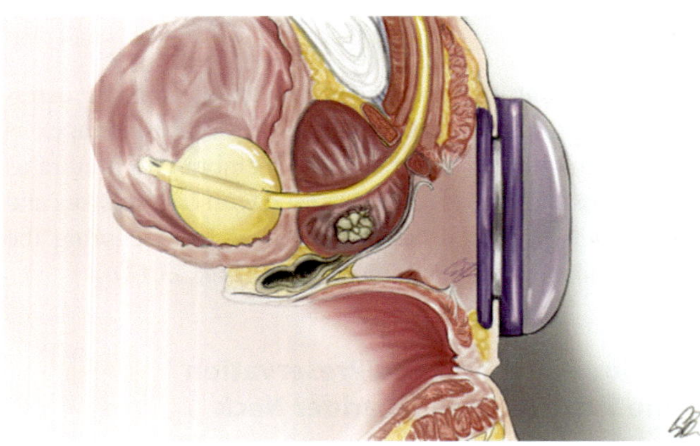

Fig. 33.9 GelPOINT® placement. GelPOINT® is the single-port device allowing instruments introduction through a single perineal incision. A subcutaneous pouch is created in the thickness of the adipose for its placement

The base of the prostate gland is separated from the circular fibers of the anterior margin of the bladder neck. The catheter is then removed and the incision of the bladder neck is completed on lateral and dorsal margins (Fig. 33.12a).

When the gland is completely separated, the robot platform is temporarily undocked. The GelPOINT® is pulled out allowing to remove the prostate specimen.

Vesicourethral Anastomosis

After re-docking of the robotic platform, the anastomosis is carried out in a running fashion with a double V-lock® 3-0 suture anchored to the tail. The perineal approach ensures an excellent visualization of the bladder neck during anastomosis with the urethra. The suture step starts passing both the needles through the ventral side of the urethra with all the passages directed "outside-in" at the bladder and "inside-out" at the urethra (Fig. 33.12b). A 20 French catheter is placed when the suture is almost completed. When the vesicourethral anastomosis is completed, the water test is performed filling with 150–200 ml of saline solution to check water tightness.

Pelvic Floor and Skin Closure

After the drain placement, the pelvic floor is reconstructed in multiple layers by readapting the levator ani muscles in the midline. The skin is closed with intradermic suture and metal clips.

Postoperative Management and Follow-Up

Prolonged antibiotics therapy is not required postoperatively, whereas intravenous fluids and pain drugs are used as needed. Daily blood tests are run to evaluate hemoglobin levels and kidney function. The drain is removed on the first postoperative day, whereas the catheter can be removed 7–10 days after surgery allowing the bladder defect closure. If concerns regarding anastomosis healing are present, a cystography is recommended before catheter removal.

Results

After Jihad H. Kaouk published the first paper describing the robotic radical perineal prostatectomy, other groups published their first experience [11–13]. A recent review of literature summarized the available evidence underlying the feasibility and safety of robotic perineal prostatectomy, as well as reported all issues relevant to the outcomes of r-RPP, including intraoperative and postoperative complications, as well as functional and oncological results.

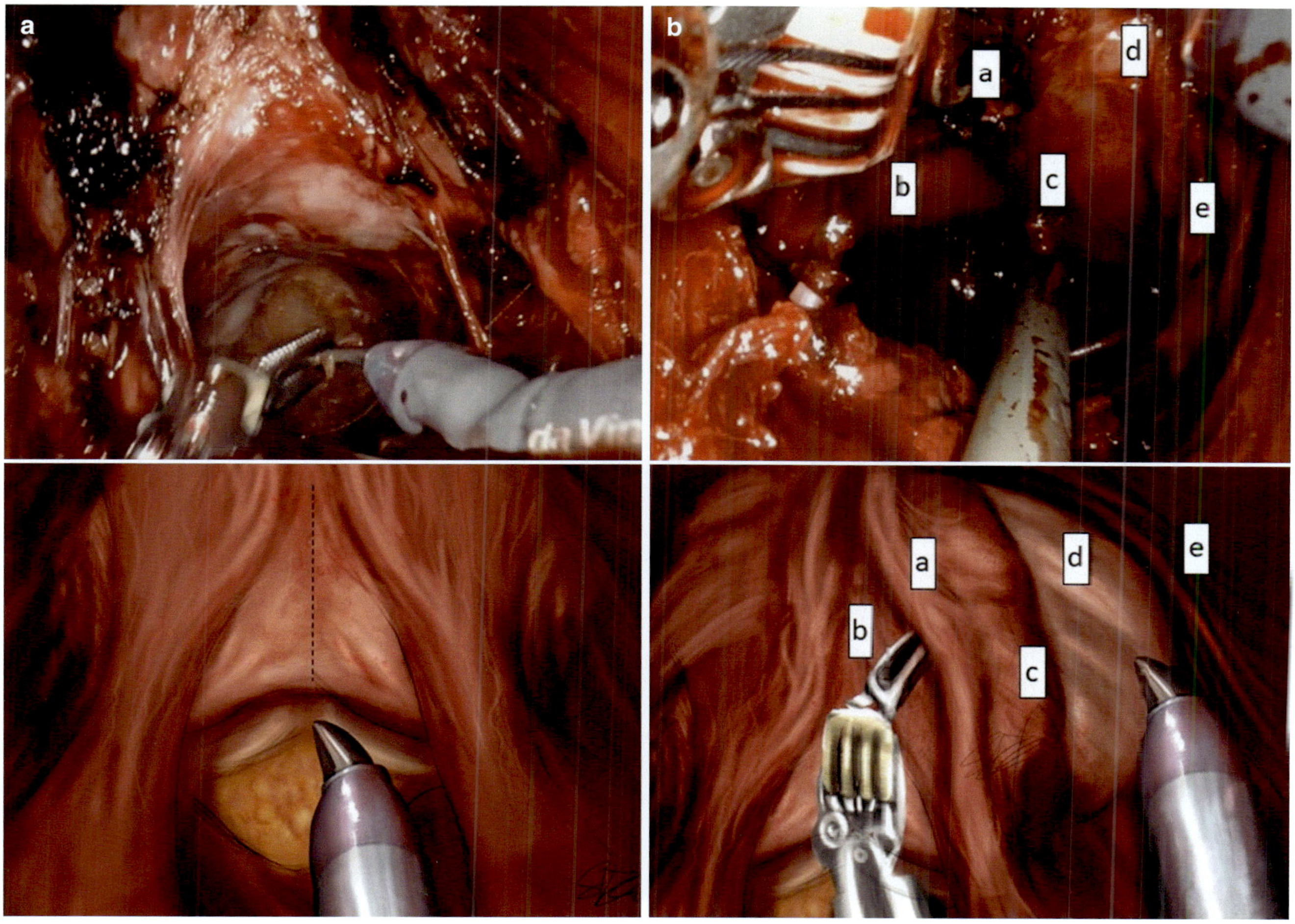

Fig. 33.10 Intrafascial dissection of the neurovascular bundle. In Bari technique nerve-sparing robotic radical perineal prostatectomy. (**A**) The Denonvilliers' fascia is incised in the midline (dotted line) with cold scissors. (**B**) The intrafascial dissection of the neurovascular bundle is performed in medial-laterally direction. The following structures are identified: (**a**) neurovascular bundle; (**b**) posterior prostatic surface; (**c**) lateral aspect of the prostate covered by the neurovascular bundle; (**d**) endopelvic fascia; (**e**) levator ani muscle

Oncological Results

The absence of positive surgical margins is one of the main goals of performing radical prostatectomy with any surgical approach. In a study looking at the association of prostate weight with several pathological and oncological outcomes after radical prostatectomy, Freedland et al. have reported that prostate weight was significantly inversely associated with positive margin rate [14]. As the specific characteristic of the technique allows the selection of patients with small or medium prostate weight, it is no surprise to find a high rate of positive margins among patients undergoing r-RPP.

In the largest series published, Volkan Tuğcu retrospectively analyzed the outcomes of 95 patients undergoing r-RPP at *the University of Health Sciences Bakırkoy Dr. Sadi Konuk Training and Research Hospital* between November 2016 and September 2018 [9]. In this study, the median prostate volume was 52 mL with 26 (27.3%) and 54 (56.8%) patients reported cT2b and cT2c, respectively. Overall, 8 (8.4%) of the men undergoing r-RPP reported positive surgical margins at the pathological analysis, and only three patients (3.1%) developed biochemical recurrence (defined as PSA level >0.2 ng/mL at two consecutive measurements). The authors did not provide any specific details on positive margin location.

In the open approach, the location of surgical margins is more commonly toward the apex in all retropubic approaches and the anterior surface and bladder neck in the perineal approach [15]. This difference could be explained as the apex is the most difficult region to access in retropubic approaches as well as the bladder neck is the farthest and poorly visualized region during the RPP approach. Nevertheless, the robotic radical perineal approach seems to increase the risk of positive margin only at the lateral aspects of the prostate as the and magnified, three-dimensional visualization facilities the dissection of the anterior surface [6].

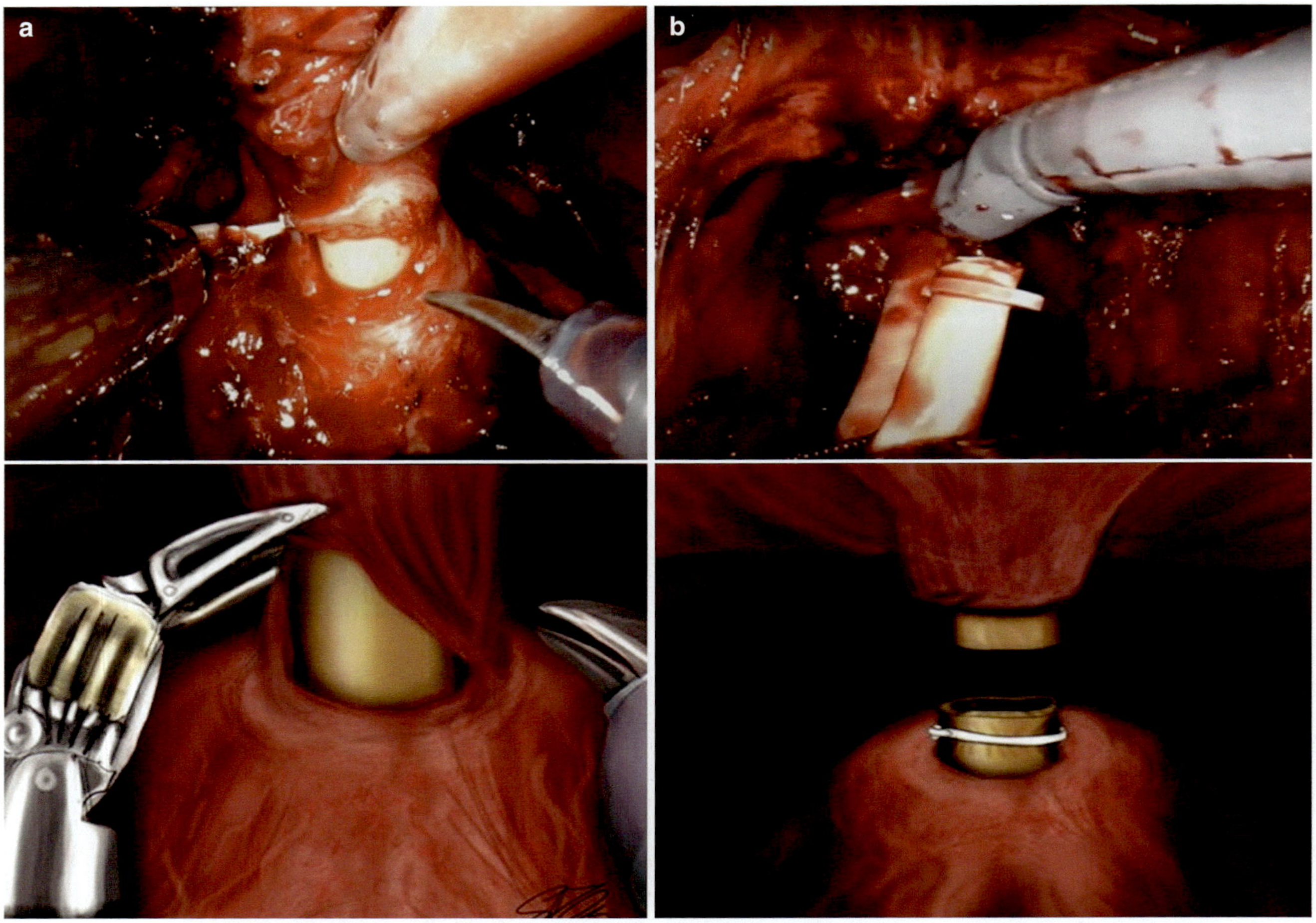

Fig. 33.11 Dissection of the prostatic apex and membranous urethra. The membranous urethra is gently separated from the external urinary sphincter. (**a**) The urethra is incised with cold scissors and (**b**) the catheter is clipped before being cut, to keep the balloon inflated inside the bladder

Functional Results

Overall, the robotic radical perineal prostatectomy reported good early recovery of continence even if few studies on functional outcomes are available to date as this represents an innovative robotic approach [6].

In an initial experience, Kaouk and colleagues reported a high rate of immediate urinary continence after catheter removal [11]. In the largest series available in the literature, recovery of urinary continence was descriptive for 41%, and 91% of the patients immediately and at 12 months, respectively [9].

These results showed a promising early recovery function but further studies need to better address these findings.

The puboprostatic complex (puboprostatic ligaments, dorsal venous complex, anterior detrusor apron, and pubourethral ligament), the arcus tendinous, and the accessory pudendal arteries are maintained untouched during robotic RPP. The integrity of these anatomical structures composing the anterior suspensory mechanism of the pelvic prevents the prolapse of the vescico-urethral anastomosis [16]. These anatomic characteristics are correlated with the functional outcomes and have been first observed after performing open radical perineal prostatectomy [17]. Moreover, the perineal prostatectomy allows optimal preservation of the bladder neck location less distant to the superior edge of the pubic symphysis, as well as, meticulous dissection of the prostate apex from the membranous urethra to keep it as long as possible that could contribute to better continence rates [18–20].

Nerve-Sparing Approach and Erectile Function Recovery

The practice of open nerve-sparing RPP is relatively new, if compared to the first RPP technique description by Young [21]. In Weldon's experience, the potency rate after nerve-sparing open radical perineal prostatectomy in selected men was about 70%. During perineal prostatectomy, the neuro-

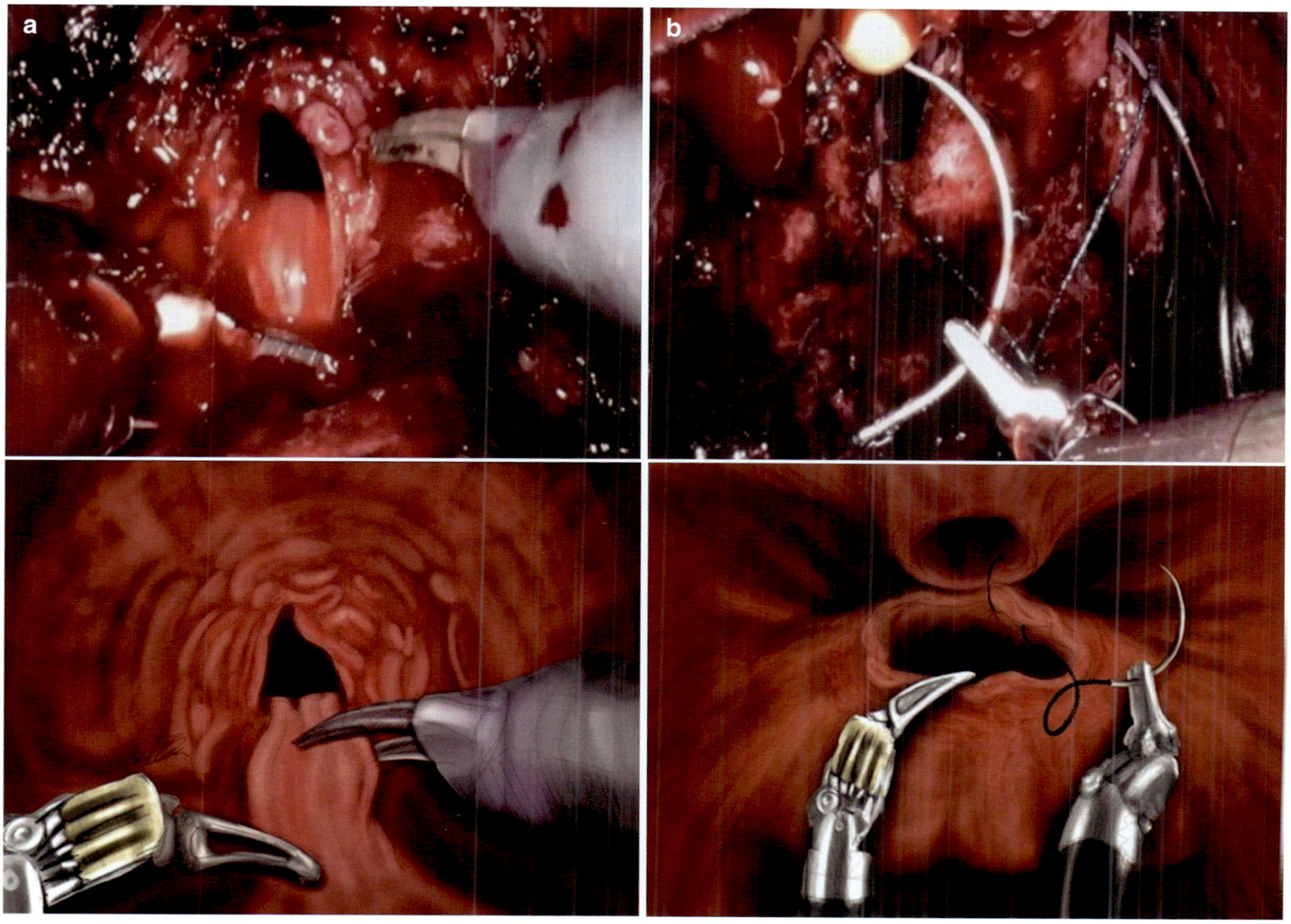

Fig. 33.12 Isolation of the bladder neck and vesicourethral anastomosis. (**a**) The incision of the bladder neck is completed on lateral and dorsal margins. (**b**) The anastomosis is carried out in a running fashion with a double V-lock 3-0 suture. The suture starts from the ventral side of the urethra; all the passages are directed "inside-out" at the urethra and "outside-in" at the bladder

vascular tissue is subjected to few manipulations and stretching (even after dissection from the fascia) while trying to deliver the gland thereby reducing the risk of laceration of the neurovascular tissue.

Regarding the robotic approach, Laydner and colleagues evaluated the feasibility of the nerve-sparing approach in cadaveric models [22]. It was successfully completed in three cadavers with a median total operative time of 89 min. The authors reported that the prostate capsule was grossly intact and histopathology examination was negative for prostatic tissue in all distal urethral sections and two of three bladder neck sections.

The first clinical experience showed that a bilateral nerve-sparing r-RPP in 64 men allowed the preservation of erectile function in 49%, 69%, and 77% after 3, 6, and 12 months, respectively [9]. However, not many studies have reported on nerve-sparing, and literature on results is yet to evolve.

Complications

Excluding major and minor complications that could occur during robotic prostatectomy, specific complications of robotic radical perineal prostatectomy are represented to rectal injury and fecal incontinence.

Although the incidence of rectal injury could be higher compared to the standard approach, when it is intraoperatively identified and sutured, it does not result in further consequences. In the experience of the University of Bari, 2 of 26 patients presented rectal injury but no further complications occurred after intraoperative management [6].

No univocal data on the risk of fecal incontinence after robotic perineal prostatectomy are reported in the literature, but there are some evidences of a higher rate of fecal incontinence after open RPP compared to the standard approach [23]. Notably, several confounding factors can affect the incidence of anorectal dysfunction, such as pre-existing causes or subsequent elements (post-surgical radiotherapy or tumor recurrence). In conclusion, fecal incontinence seems to be rarely directly associated with this type of surgery but more often with the personal history of the patient [23].

Conclusion

Robotic radical perineal prostatectomy is a "*novel*" surgical technique for the treatment of localized prostatic cancer representing a valid alternative approach in selected patients with a history of previous abdominal surgery, cardiology or pulmonary comorbidity, or high body mass index. Moreover, Bari technique robotic radical perineal prostatectomy ensures a *nerve-sparing* approach to these subsets of patients with the aim of preserve erectile function. Nevertheless, expertise in perineal surgery is a limiting factor to the spread of robotic radical perineal prostatectomy. Further studies with a large cohort are needed for evaluating the real advantages in terms of functional outcomes.

References

1. Young HH. Conservative perineal prostatectomy: the results of two years' experience and report of seventy-five cases. Ann Surg. 1905;41:549–57.
2. Young HH. The cure of cancer of the prostate by radical perineal prostatectomy (prostato-seminal vesiculectomy): history, literature and statistics of Young's peration. J Urol. 1945;53:188–252.
3. Millin T. Retropubic prostatectomy a new extravesical technique. Report on 20 cases. Lancet. 1945;246:693–6.
4. Walsh PC. Radical prostatectomy for the treatment of localized prostatic carcinoma. Urol Clin North Am. 1980;7(3):583–91.
5. Koukourikis P, Rha KH. Robotic surgical systems in urology: what is currently available? Investig Clin Urol. 2021;62:14–22.
6. Minafra P, Carbonara U, Vitarelli A, Lucarelli G, Battaglia M, Ditonno P. Robotic radical perineal prostatectomy: tradition and evolution in the robotic era. Curr Opin Urol. 2021;31:11–7.
7. Ficarra V, Novara G, Artibani W, et al. Retropubic, laparoscopic, and robot-assisted radical prostatectomy: a systematic review and cumulative analysis of comparative studies. Eur Urol. 2009;55:1037–63.
8. EAU Guidelines. Edn. presented at the EAU Annual Congress Amsterdam 2022. ISBN 978-94-92671-16-5. EAU Guidelines Office, Arnhem, The Netherlands. http://uroweb.org/guidelines/compilations-of-all-guidelines/
9. Tuğcu V, Ekşi M, Sahin S, Çolakoğlu Y, Simsek A, Evren İ, İhsan Taşçı A. Robot-assisted radical perineal prostatectomy: a review of 95 cases. BJU Int. 2020;125:573–8.
10. Francavilla S, Veccia A, Dobbs RW, Zattoni F, Vigneswaran HT, Antonelli A, Dal Moro F, Autorino R, Simeone C, Crivellaro S. Radical prostatectomy technique in the robotic evolution: from da Vinci standard to single port—a single surgeon pathway. J Robot Surg. 2022;16(1):21–7. https://doi.org/10.1007/s11701-021-01194-8.
11. Kaouk JH, Akca O, Zargar H, Caputo P, Ramirez D, Andrade H, Albayrak S, Laydner H, Angermeier K. Descriptive technique and initial results for robotic radical perineal prostatectomy. Urology. 2016;94:129–38.
12. Tuğcu V, Akça O, Şimşek A, Yiğitbaşı İ, Şahin S, Taşçı Aİ. Robot yardımlı perineal radikal prostatektomi: Ilk 15 vaka. Turk J Urol. 2017;43:476–83.
13. Chang Y, Xu W, Lu X, Zhou Y, Ji M, Xiao YT, Sun Y, Ren S. Robotic perineal radical prostatectomy: initial experience with the da Vinci Si robotic system. Urol Int. 2020;104:710–5.
14. Freedland SJ, Isaacs WB, Platz EA, Terris MK, Aronson WJ, Amling CL, Presti JC, Kane CJ. Prostate size and risk of high-grade, advanced prostate cancer and biochemical progression after radical prostatectomy: a search database study. J Clin Oncol. 2005;23:7546–54.
15. Inoue S, Shiina H, Sumura M, Urakami S, Matsubara A, Igawa M. Impact of a novel, extended approach of perineal radical prostatectomy on surgical margins in localized prostate cancer. BJU Int. 2010;106:44–8.
16. Cui J, Guo H, Li Y, et al. Pelvic floor reconstruction after radical prostatectomy: a systematic review and meta-analysis of different surgical techniques. Sci Rep. 2017;7:2737. https://doi.org/10.1038/s41598-017-02991-8.
17. Abou-Elela A, Reyad I, Morsy A, Elgammal M, Bedair AS, Abdelkader M. Continence after radical prostatectomy with bladder neck preservation. Eur J Surg Oncol. 2007;33:96–101.
18. Olgin G, Alsyouf M, Han D, Li R, Lightfoot M, Smith D, Nicolay L, Ruckle H, Duane Baldwin D. Postoperative cystogram findings predict incontinence following robot-assisted radical prostatectomy. J Endourol. 2014;28:1460–3.
19. Nyarangi-Dix JN, Radtke JP, Hadaschik B, Pahernik S, Hohenfellner M. Impact of complete bladder neck preservation on urinary continence, quality of life and surgical margins after radical prostatectomy: a randomized, controlled, single blind trial. J Urol. 2013;189:891–8.
20. Cameron AP, Suskind AM, Neer C, Hussain H, Montgomery J, Latini JM, Delancey JO. Functional and anatomical differences between continent and incontinent men post radical prostatectomy on urodynamics and 3T MRI: a pilot study. Neurourol Urodyn. 2015;34:527–32.
21. Weldon VE, Tavel FR. Potency-sparing radical perineal prostatectomy: anatomy, surgical technique and initial results. J Urol. 1988;140:559–62.
22. Laydner H, Akça O, Autorino R, et al. Third prize: Perineal robot-assisted laparoscopic radical prostatectomy: feasibility study in the cadaver model. J Endourol. 2014;28:1479–86.
23. Kirschner-Hermanns R, Borchers H, Reineke T, Willis S, Jakse G. Fecal incontinence after radical perineal prostatectomy: a prospective study. Urology. 2005;65:337–42.

Single Port Robotic Perineal Radical Prostatectomy

34

Zeyad R. Schwen and Jihad Kaouk

Introduction

From the beginning, starting with Hugh Hampton Young in 1904, the perineal radical prostatectomy was the preferred surgical approach for prostate cancer [1]. The operation was originally designed for curing obstructive urinary symptoms due to benign prostate disease. The perineal prostatectomy was later adapted as a radical operation for treating prostate cancer. In 1945, the retropubic approach was described by Millin, and later transitioned to become the dominate approach after being popularized by Patrick Walsh after demonstrating the ability to preserve the neurovascular bundle as well as more efficiently control the dorsal venous complex [2, 3]. Moreover, the retropubic approach provided easier access for the pelvic lymphadenectomy. Still, the open perineal approach offered advantages over the retropubic approach including a reduced perioperative morbidity and faster recovery in the form of a shorter hospital stay and reduced pain [4]. Additionally, it was the preferred approach in the morbidly obese as well as for those with prior abdominal surgeries. With the introduction of the robotic assisted radical prostatectomy (RARP), the open radical perineal prostatectomy became less-commonly performed and, practically speaking, a "lost art" [5].

The perineal radical approach was again revitalized with the introduction of the muti-arm robotic platforms [6, 7]. However, there were significant limitations with adapting the multi-arm robots for single-site surgery with instrument clashing as the primary drawback. The development of a purpose-built DaVinci SP platform features intracorporeal triangulation of the instruments which effectively eliminates external clashing which encourages its use in tight surgical fields making it an ideal design for the perineal space [8]. While the SP robot expands the versatility of the surgical approaches for curative surgical therapy for prostate cancer, the perineal approach represents a select indication for patients who are not otherwise candidates for traditional retropubic robotic approaches [9].

Indications

While the principal approach for a radical prostatectomy, robotic or open, continues to be through a retropubic access, the perineal approach is effective for those select patients for whom a retropubic access would be either high-risk or impossible due to a hostile abdomen. We offer a robotic perineal approach for those who have significant surgical adhesions primarily due to extensive prior abdominal or pelvic surgeries such as abdominal perineal resection and total proctocolectomy with J-pouch. While the extra-peritoneal approach may avoid certain dense peritoneal adhesions, any infraumbilical surgical scar typically limits the success of developing the extraperitoneal space. Furthermore, those with prior pelvic radiotherapy as well as those with anatomic obstructions in the pelvis such as a history of inguinal mesh, colostomies or ileostomies, or kidney transplants also may benefit from a perineal approach. Avoiding the potential for unintended injury to surrounding organs as well as eliminating the time-consuming lysis of adhesions with the perineal approach is a way to effectively reduce the risk of complications as well as decrease the operative time. Many of these patients may also be declared unfit for radiotherapy in the form of either external beam radiation or brachytherapy including those with inflammatory bowel disease and prior pelvic radiation. Contraindications include those with prior perineal surgeries and large >80 g prostates.

Z. R. Schwen · J. Kaouk (✉)
Glickman Urological and Kidney Institute, Cleveland Clinic Foundation, Cleveland, OH, USA
e-mail: schwenz2@ccf.org; kaoukj@ccf.org

S. Ren et al. (eds.), *Robot-Assisted Radical Prostatectomy*, https://doi.org/10.1007/978-3-031-05855-4_34

Description of Technique

Preoperative

Preoperative workup and management of patients are largely similar to the other robotic prostatectomy approaches. Patients must obtain standard preoperative labs including type and screen, basic metabolic panel, complete blood count, and urinalysis and culture. We do not require patients to perform a mandatory preoperative bowel regimen or enema as we find little benefit to these practices to improve the operative conditions. We use standard perioperative antibiotic prophylaxis according to guidelines and administer subcutaneous heparin preoperatively which is continued until discharge as part of deep venous thromboembolism prophylaxis. Patients have sequential compressive devices placed bilaterally on the lower extremities. Patients are positioned in a high lithotomy position (Fig. 34.1) with the arms tucked and a 15° Trendelenburg. The perineal skin is cleared of hair using a clipper. The patients are prepped and draped in a standard fashion.

Intraoperative

Perineal Access and SP Docking

A 20F Foley catheter is placed into the bladder and placed to gravity drainage. Next, a finger from a modified sterile glove

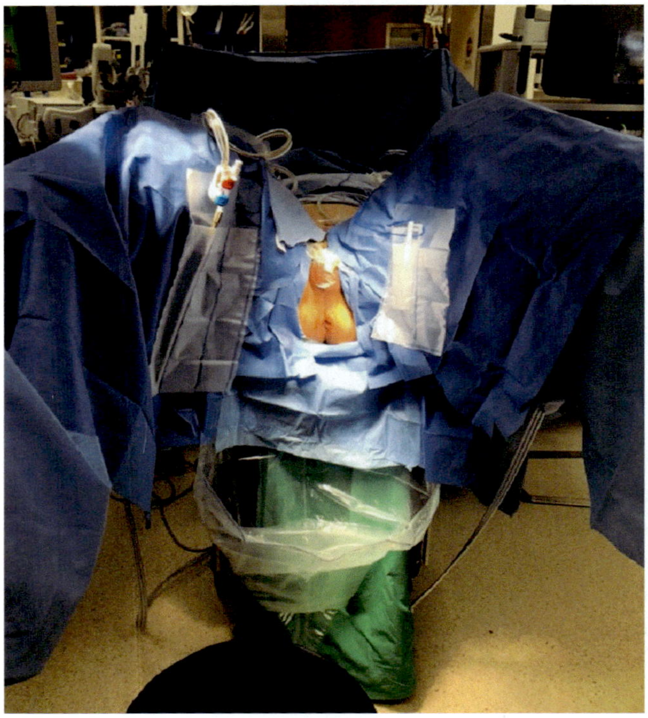

Fig. 34.1 Patient positioning

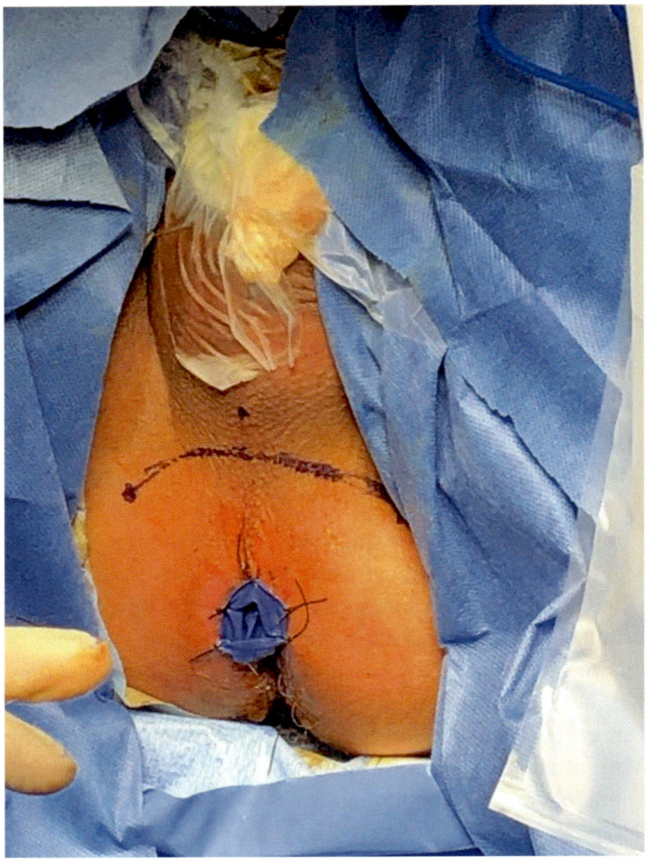

Fig. 34.2 Initial incision with rectal glove

is placed into the rectum and sutured in place to the peri-anal skin to permit easy tactile checking of the rectum without breaking sterility during the procedure (Fig. 34.2). Using the ischial tuberosities as landmarks, a 3 cm inverted semilunar incision is made and the subcutaneous tissue is incised using electrocautery (Fig. 34.3). The central tendon is next identified and incised to expose the rectourethralis and levator ani muscles which are each divided to expose the prostate. Next, to accommodate the inner ring of Alexis wound retractor, subcutaneous space is developed circumferentially and the Gelpoint Mini Advanced Access Platform is deployed to permit the floating dock technique as previously described [10]. Stay sutures are placed anteriorly to lift the subcutaneous flap. Air docking is required for this approach to optimize the working distance for the SP platform robotic arms due to the close proximity of the prostate to the perineal skin (Fig. 34.4a). Through the Gelpoint, a 12 mm Airseal® port (ConMed, Utica, NY, USA), dedicated 25 mm multi-port SP cannula, and ROSI flexible suction tubing are inserted and the perineal space is insufflated to 12 mmHg. The SP robot is side-docked in a camera-up orientation with the robotic scissors (right), Cadiere graspers (left), and Maryland bipolar (down) (Fig. 34.4b).

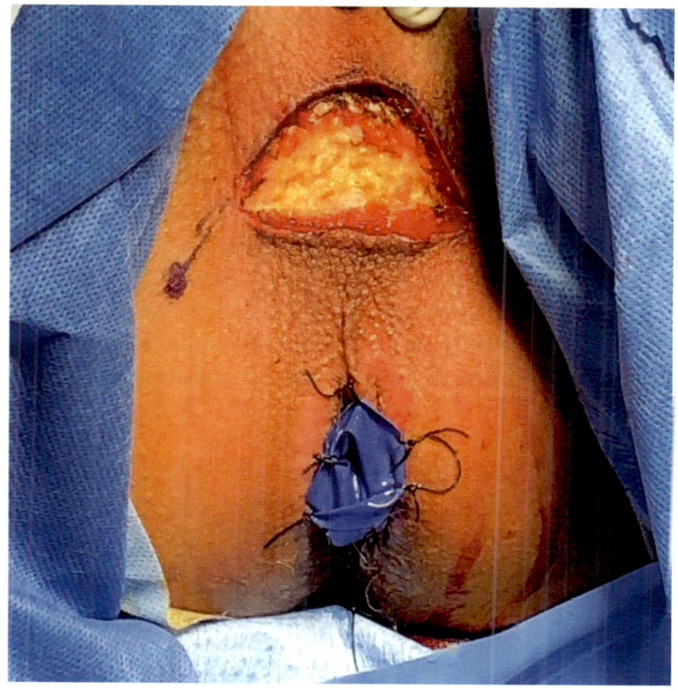

Fig. 34.3 Semilunar perineal incision

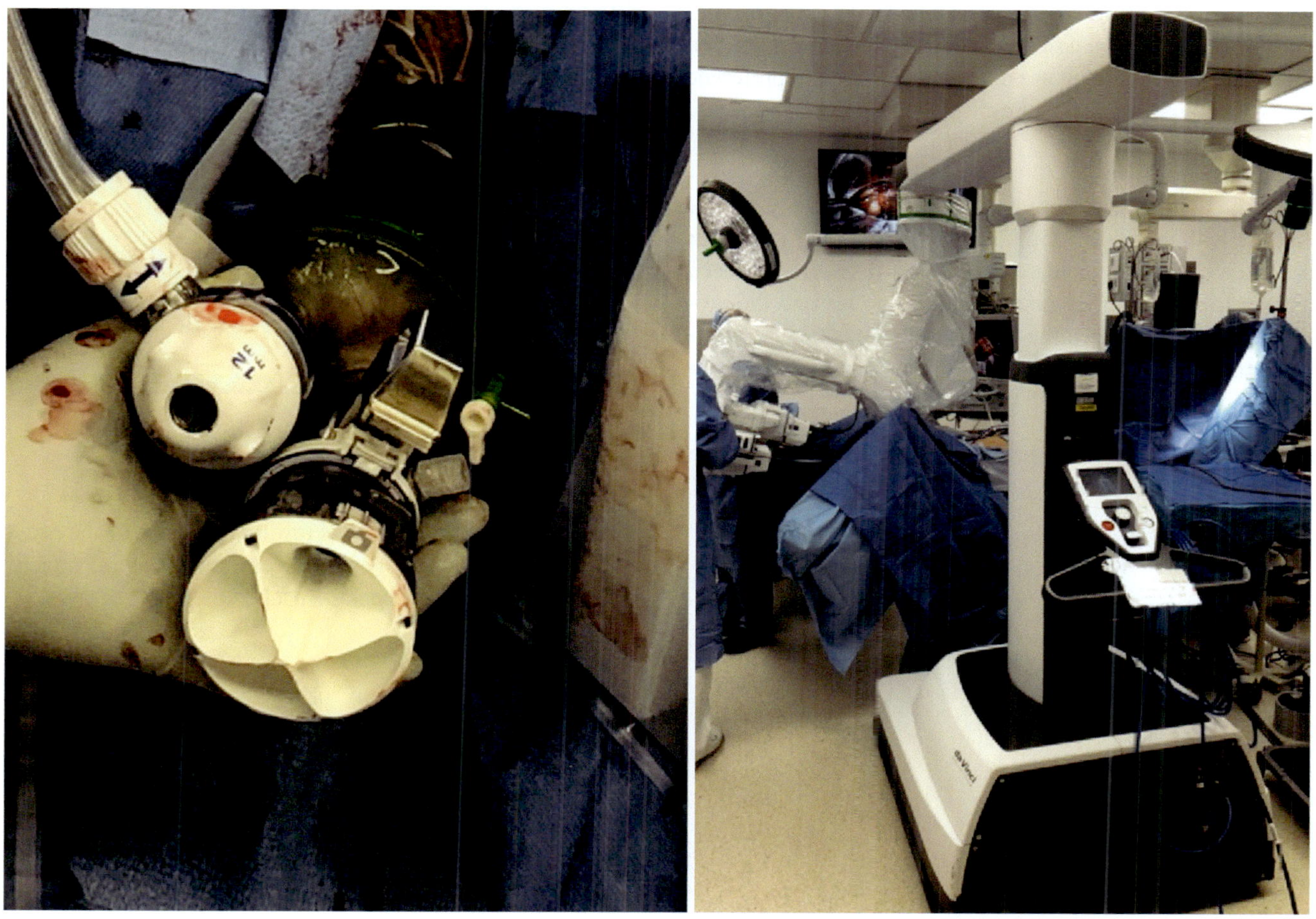

Fig. 34.4 Port placement and SP docking

Posterior Dissection and Seminal Vesical and Vasa Deferentia

Once the robotic instruments are advanced into the developed perineal space, the posterior plane is developed by exposing the levator ani muscle fibers and. Denonvillier's fascia is identified and opened, continuing to bluntly develop the posterior plane towards the base of the prostate and sweeping the neurovascular bundles laterally. As the development of the posterior plane continues cephalad, the seminal vesicles and vasa deferentia are identified, isolated, and controlled with Weck clips using the SP robotic clip applier to minimize the use of cautery near the neurovascular bundles (Fig. 34.5).

Vascular Pedicle and Nerve Sparing

Following the release of the seminal vesicles and prior to the bladder neck transection, the vascular pedicles to the prostate and neurovascular bundles are addressed. Starting from the base of the prostate and working apically, the pedicles are sequentially clipped in packets with the robotic clip applier (Fig. 34.6). Exposure and traction on the vascular pedicles are optimized by anteromedial retraction of each seminal vesicle using the Cadiere grasper. Once the vascular pedicles are controlled, the release of the neurovascular bundles continues apically, avoiding use of electrocautery and preferencing robotic-applied Weck clips.

Apical Dissection

Next, the urethral is exposed at the apex and sharply divided, starting with the posterior urethral plate (Fig. 34.7). Once the urethra is completely released, the apical dissection proceeds anteriorly between the dorsal venous complex and the prostate. In those with apical lesions, extra care is taken to avoid entry into the prostate and avoid a positive surgical margin.

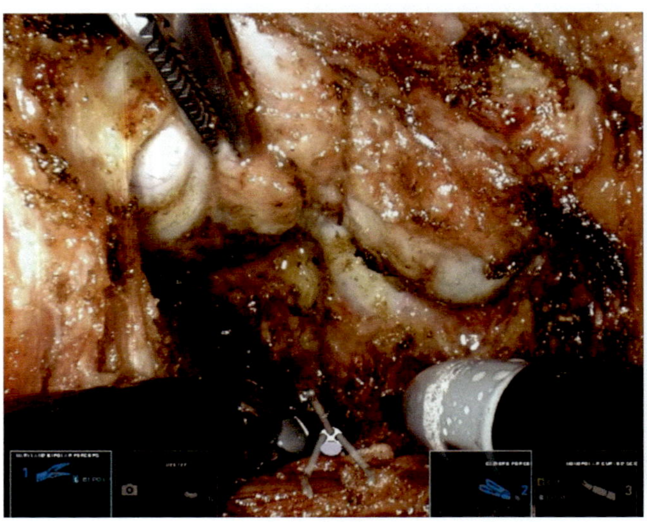

Fig. 34.5 Seminal vesical dissection

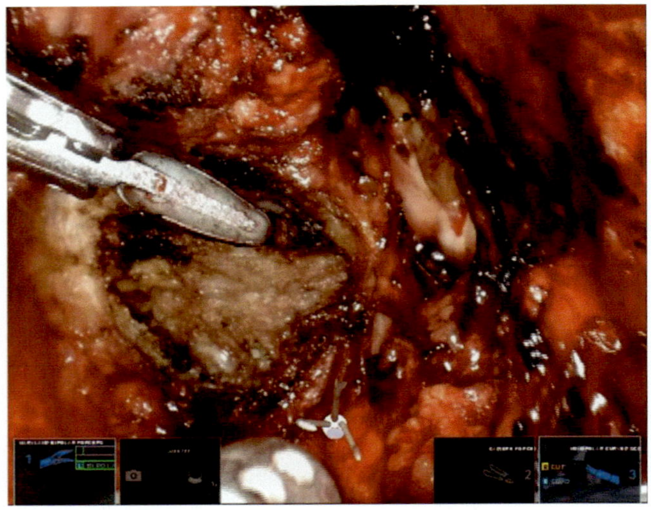

Fig. 34.6 Right vascular pedicle

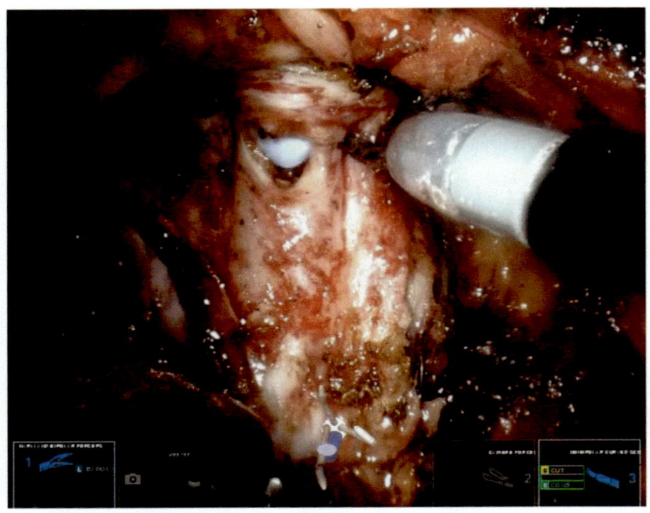

Fig. 34.7 Apical dissection and urethral transection

The apical dissection proceeds towards the base of the prostate while simultaneously freeing the anterolateral attachments until the bladder neck is reached.

Bladder Neck

At the 12-o'clock position, using the Foley balloon as a guide, the anterior bladder neck is opened and the bladder is entered (Fig. 34.8). The bladder neck dissection then proceeds posteriorly in a circumferential fashion. Once the final attachments to the prostate at the posterior bladder neck are free, the SP robot can be undocked for larger specimens that occupy significant space in the limited surgical field and the specimen is extracted through the GelPoint prior to beginning the lymph node dissection and anastomosis. The SP is immediately redocked again using the floating dock.

Pelvic Lymph Node Dissection

For those who require a pelvic lymphadenectomy based on preoperative predictive nomograms, the perineal approach permits access to the pelvic lymph nodes through the same approach. The obturator fossa can be developed by dissecting laterally to the bladder. Typically the obturator nerve, vein and artery are visualized first through this approach and the dissection proceeds anterolaterally towards the inferior aspect of the external iliac vein and pelvic sidewall (Fig. 34.9). The lymph node packed is removed in a caudal-to-cranial fashion, using clips to ligate lymphatics and electrocautery as needed.

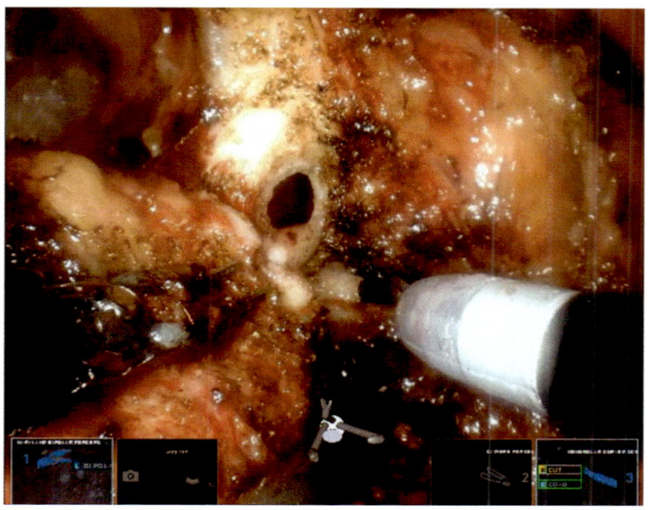

Fig. 34.8 Bladder neck transection

Vesicourethral Anastomosis and Closure

The vesicourethral anastomosis is performed using two 4-0 barbed sutures in a running fashion (Fig. 34.10). Similar to the Retzius sparing approach, the anastomosis is above the camera. As a result, the anastomosis begins anteriorly and proceeds posteriorly. Once the anastomosis is complete, a final 20F Foley is inserted, with 15 cc in the balloon. The anastomosis is then confirmed to be water-tight and the perineum is closed in two layers. In the majority of cases, a drain is not placed.

Postoperative

Postoperative care is similar to our standard robotic prostatectomy pathway including early ambulation, immediate diet resumption, and minimal use of perioperative narcotics. Patients are observed postoperatively and discharged home after the drain is removed with a Foley catheter for 1 week without the need for a cystogram. Similar to open perineal radical prostatectomy compared to open retropubic approaches, patients who undergo SP robotic perineal prostatectomy typically experience significantly less postoperative pain compared to traditional robotic approaches and are candidates for same-day and opioid-free discharge pathways. Routine cases are otherwise discharged within 24 h. Patients with risk factors for postoperative venous thromboembolism including those with NCCN (National Comprehensive Cancer Network) high or very high risk prostate cancer are discharged with 28 days of prophylactic dose enoxaparin. While drain use is infrequent and Foley catheters are typi-

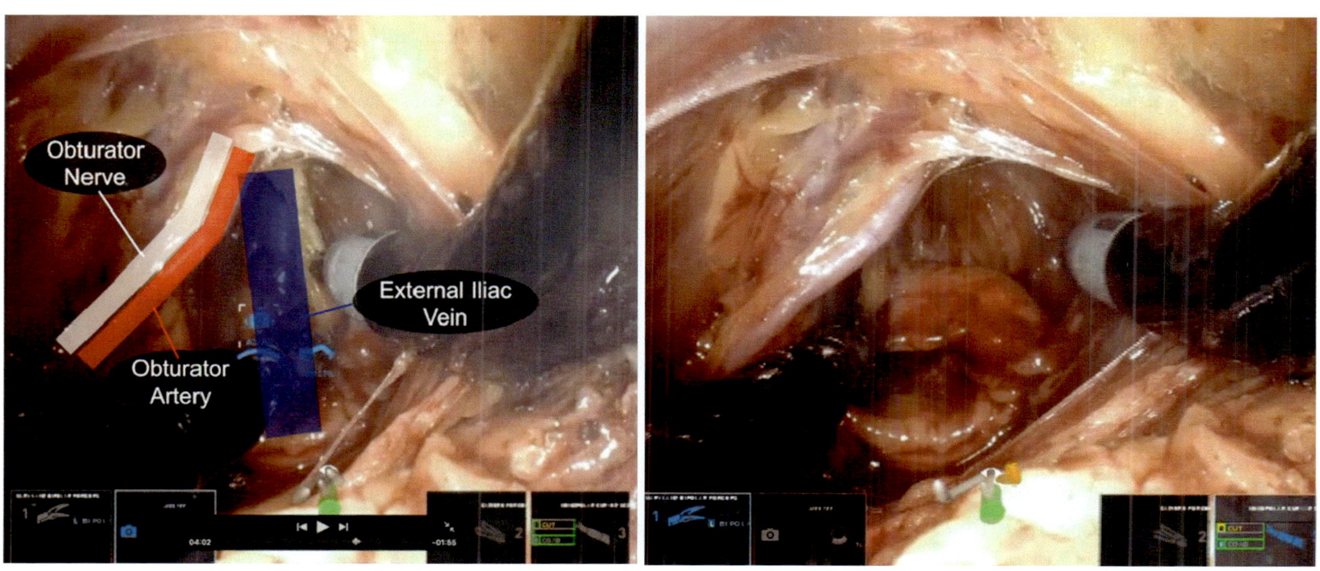

Fig. 34.9 Lymph node dissection

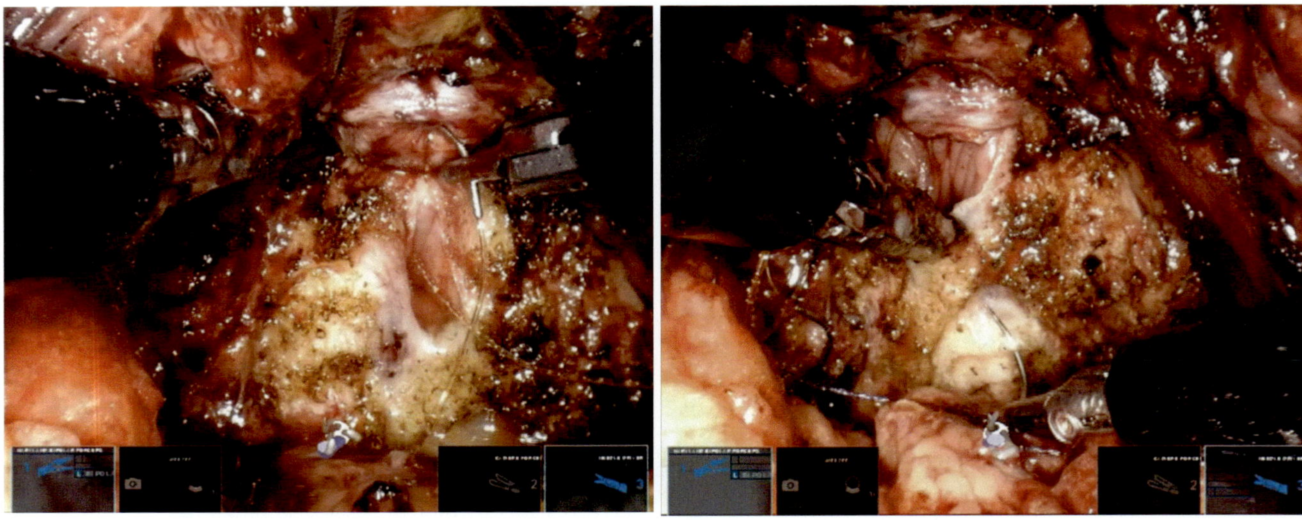

Fig. 34.10 Vesicourethral anastomosis

cally removed, the strategic use of a drain and Foley duration should be individualized due to the complex patient population requiring a perineal prostatectomy.

Outcomes

Intraoperative and Perioperative

As with the open approach, the SP robotic perineal prostatectomy affords a favorable morbidity profile relative to the standard multiport retropubic approach. Much of the reduced morbidity is owing to the minimal pain experienced with a perineal incision in addition to the discomfort related to peritoneal insufflation and bladder and bowel mobilization. Furthermore, the perineal approach avoids steep Trendelenburg, multiple incisions, and in the vast majority of cases, a surgical drain which further minimizes the morbidity of the operation. In a matched comparison to multiport transperitoneal radical prostatectomy, the SP perineal approach offered reduced opioids at discharge (92.3% vs. 50%, $p = 0.016$), shorter hospital length of stay (23 h vs. 27 h, $p = 0.02$), and a reduced estimated blood loss (100 mL vs. 200 mL, $p = 0.007$) [11]. A significantly reduced length of stay and blood loss was similarly seen with open and multiport perineal approaches relative to retropubic counterparts [4, 12]. From our institution, avoidance of a drain was also observed, with only 1 patient (4.8% of 26 patients) requiring a drain [11]. SP perineal radical prostatectomy, however had significantly longer operative times compared to standard multiport approaches (255 vs. 163 min, $p < 0.001$) which may be due to longer time to gain perineal access and learning curve disparities in the initial cases [11]. In a larger multiport matched comparison between perineal and retropubic robotic approaches showed no significant difference between operative time, suggesting the learning curve likely plays a significant factor in the observed operative time differences in our institution's series [12].

Oncologic

Prior series investigating open perineal radical prostatectomy, prior to the introduction and widespread use of active surveillance, demonstrated a lower oncologic risk patient cohort compared to current robotic series. For example, in our series of 26 patients, 46.1% (12/26) of patients were ≥pT3 and 42.3% (11/26) were found to have ≥grade group 3 prostate cancer after pathological analysis of the prostatectomy specimen [11]. Still, relative to traditional retropubic approaches, the positive surgical margin rate (>3 mm) was significantly higher in the perineal approach (38.5% vs. 7.7%, $p = 0.006$). It is unclear whether this higher PSM rate is clinically significant, however, given the greater need for intracorporeal manipulation of the prostate with the perineal approach which may produce artifactual margins and capsular incisions. Reassuring is the finding that at 1 year, the rate of biochemical recurrence (PSA recurrence >0.1 ng/mL) was similar between the approaches (1 vs. 3 patients, $p = 0.3$) [11]. Similarly, there was no significant PSM rate observed in the substantially lower-risk cohort comparing multiport perineal to multiport retropubic (12.5% vs. 10%, $p = 0.65$) [12]. Longer oncologic follow-up and larger multi-institutional series are required to better delineate the oncologic outcomes with this approach. Other explanations for the increased rate of PSMs include the fact that the Retzius space is preserved, maintaining a surgical plane below the dorsal venous complex which is not preserved in the traditional robotic retropubic approaches. The PSM rate in our institution's perineal approach is similar to many early robotic Retzius-sparing cohorts, which reported higher rates of anterior PSMs [13].

An advantage of the robotic perineal approach includes the ability to perform a pelvic lymphadenectomy in those patients who have a high preoperative risk of nodal disease. In our matched comparison, pelvic lymphadenectomy was performed in 62.5% of patients [11]. Not surprisingly, nodal yield was significantly lower in the perineal approach (median 3 nodes vs. 6 nodes, p = 0.015) likely due to the reduced access to the pelvic sidewall and inability to perform an extended template lymphadenectomy. However, the obturator fossa is reliably accessed with the perineal approach for staging purposes in select patients.

Functional

With the preservation of the space of Retzius and anterior support structures which are vital to the continence mechanism, the perineal approach affords high rates of early continence which has been well-demonstrated in the robotic and open experiences [4, 12, 14]. In a low-risk patient population, Tugcu et al., identified a significantly higher continence rate at 6 months with a robotic perineal approach (94.2% vs. 72%, p = 0.001) [12]. In our institution's perineal experience with the SP platform, there was no significant difference in the 6- or 12-month complete continence rate compared to the multiport retropubic approach, which was 75% and 80%, respectively [10]. In context, however, these patients represented highly comorbid patients, often with prior pelvic pathology which could greatly influence continence rates. Longer follow-up is required to demonstrate the true continence rates in this select patient population as well as the need for additional intervention.

The ability to perform a nerve-sparing radical prostatectomy is not hindered with the SP perineal approach. In our series, 2/3rds of patients underwent a nerve-sparing approach, which was lower compared to the traditional robotic approach only due to the extent of disease and presence of erectile dysfunction preoperatively rather than technical feasibility. While the learning curve for nerve-sparing with the perineal approach may be higher due to the unfamiliar view, release of the neurovascular bundle is not any more challenging from a technical standpoint. Given the high degree of preoperative erectile dysfunction and significant comorbidities in the patient population undergoing SP perineal radical prostatectomy, erectile outcomes were not assessed in our matched analysis. Similarly, longer follow-up is required to accurately assess recovery of erections for the approach. In a multiport perineal comparison, using the International Index of Erectile Function-5 (IIEF-5), the perineal approach had significantly higher erectile function rates at 9 months relative to traditional robotic retropubic approaches (75% vs. 66%, p = 0.001) [12].

Complications

The SP perineal robotic approach experiences a significant reduction in perioperative morbidity, which has been well-demonstrated in the open and multi-port experiences. In the current era, SP perineal radical prostatectomy is offered only to those who are otherwise poor surgical candidates who have often significant comorbidities including prior radiation, malignancy, prior pelvic surgeries, as well as a immunodeficiency. As a result, patients are at risk for poor wound healing and significant adhesions in the surgical field. Not surprisingly, our matched series compared to an otherwise healthy patient cohort, we experienced higher rates of perioperative complications (52% vs. 8%), however the majority were Clavien grade 1 and only six patients experienced higher-grade complication (Clavien 3a) [11]. Three patients experienced anastomotic leakages which were managed with urethral catheter reinsertion or suprapubic tube placement, two anastomotic strictures which required endoscopic dilation or incision, and a single lymphocele which required drain placement. While these complications are higher, none were life threatening and the vast majority are manageable with conservative treatment with longer catheterization or small well-tolerated procedures to allow for adequate anastomotic healing. In the largest multiport robotic perineal series in less-comorbid patients, complication rates were low, reporting only a complication rate of 5%, which were all Clavien grade 1 [14]. Notably, as expected, no patient in the perineal group experienced a postoperative ileus or blood transfusion as opposed to 10% and 2.5% of patients, respectively, in the standard transperitoneal retropubic robotic approach [12].

Conclusions

The SP robotic perineal radical prostatectomy is an effective therapeutic option for select patients who are not ideal candidates for standard robotic approaches or radiation therapy. The SP platform optimizes the approach with its ability to avoid external instrument clashing and work in confined spaces. While further investigation and longer follow-up is required to better evaluate the long-term functional and oncologic outcomes, our institution's early experience is very favorable, particularly for those without alternative treatment options. The advantages of the perineal approach are well known due to the long history of open as well as multiport robotic techniques, with a reduced perioperative morbidity, equivalent oncologic outcomes, and improved early continence outcomes due to the preservation of the space of Retzius. Furthermore, the perineal approach allows for replication of the nerve-sparing and pelvic lymphadenectomy of the retropubic approaches. The SP platform simplifies the perineal robotic approach and provides access in those deemed high-risk and poor surgical candidates.

References

1. Scott WW. Origins of radical perineal and nerve-sparing retropubic prostatectomy. Prostate. 1997;32(2):149–51.
2. Millin T. Retropubic prostatectomy; a new extravesical technique; report of 20 cases. Lancet. 1945;2(6380):693–6.
3. Walsh PC, Donker PJ. Impotence following radical prostatectomy: insight into etiology and prevention. J Urol. 1982;128(3):492–7.
4. Janoff DM, Parra RO. Contemporary appraisal of radical perineal prostatectomy. J Urol. 2005;173(6):1863–70.
5. Shay BF, Schmidt JD, Thomas R, Monga M. Urology practice patterns after residency training in radical perineal prostatectomy. Urology. 2002;60(5):766–9.
6. Kaouk JH, Akca O, Zargar H, Caputo P, Ramirez D, Andrade H, et al. Descriptive technique and initial results for robotic radical perineal prostatectomy. Urology. 2016;94:129–38.
7. Garisto J, Bertolo R, Wilson CA, Kaouk J. The evolution and resurgence of perineal prostatectomy in the robotic surgical era. World J Urol. 2020;38(4):821–8.
8. Kaouk J, Garisto J, Bertolo R. Robotic urologic surgical interventions performed with the single port dedicated platform: first clinical investigation. Eur Urol. 2019;75(4):684–91.
9. Kaouk JH, Bertolo R. Single-site robotic platform in clinical practice: first cases in the USA. Minerva Urol Nefrol. 2019;71(3):294–8.
10. Lenfant L, Kim S, Aminsharifi A, Sawczyn G, Kaouk J. Floating docking technique: a simple modification to improve the working space of the instruments during single-port robotic surgery. World J Urol. 2021;39(4):1299–305.
11. Lenfant L, Garisto J, Sawczyn G, Wilson CA, Aminsharifi A, Kim S, et al. Robot-assisted radical prostatectomy using single-port perineal approach: technique and single-surgeon matched-paired comparative outcomes. Eur Urol. 2021;79(3):384–92.
12. Tugcu V, Akca O, Simsek A, Yigitbasi I, Sahin S, Yenice MG, et al. Robotic-assisted perineal versus transperitoneal radical prostatectomy: a matched-pair analysis. Turk J Urol. 2019;45(4):265–72.
13. Rosenberg JE, Jung JH, Edgerton Z, Lee H, Lee S, Bakker CJ, et al. Retzius-sparing versus standard robotic-assisted laparoscopic prostatectomy for the treatment of clinically localized prostate cancer. Cochrane Database Syst Rev. 2020;(8):CD013641.
14. Tugcu V, Eksi M, Sahin S, Colakoglu Y, Simsek A, Evren I, et al. Robot-assisted radical perineal prostatectomy: a review of 95 cases. BJU Int. 2020;125(4):573–8.

Part XI

Single-Port RALP

Different Access of Single-port Robotic Prostatectomy on da Vinci Si: Changzheng Hospital Technique

35

Yifan Chang, Xiaofeng Zou, Qingyi Zhu, and Shancheng Ren

Introduction

The concept of performing laparoscopic surgery via a single abdominal incision can be dated back to several decades ago. At that time, gynecologic surgeons adopted a "1-incision" technique to perform female sterilization or needle biopsy under the observation of laparoscope [1]. Although literature showed that 3600 sterilizations were performed in 4 years [2], such technique was still reserved for limited application. It was not until 2008 when new robotic instruments and single-port devices were designed had single-port surgery gained popularity in urological surgery. Since then, the term laparoendoscopic single-site surgery (LESS) has been used to describe such surgical concept and technique [3]. Apart from the most popular terminologies of "single-port" and "LESS", various other names have been adopted in the literature, including single-incision, single-site, single-access, one-port, and keyhole surgery, as well as acronyms of SILS (single-incision laparoscopic surgery), SPLS (single-port laparoscopic surgery), and TUES (Transumbilical endoscopic surgery) [4] (by descending order of popularity). Although nomenclatures vary, three key components are shared, i.e., access (to the intracorporeal cavity), single (the number of the access), and laparoscopy (platform to perform the surgery). And at the same year, the Laparoendoscopic Single-Site Surgery Consortium for Assessment and Research (LESSCAR) had reached a consensus that LESS be used as the official nomenclature [5]. Also in the similar time period, new ports such as the R-Port (Olympus Surgical, Orangeburg, NY, USA), TriPort (Olympus Winter & Ibe, Hamburg, Germany), SILS Port (Covidien, Hamilton, Bermuda), and GelPoint (Applied Medical, Rancho Santa Margarita, CA, USA), combined with new pre-bent or articulated laparoscopic instruments, had enabled urologists to successfully perform partial nephrectomy [6], donor kidney transplantation [7], adrenalectomy [8], radical prostatectomy [9] and varicoselectomy [10]. Notably, in 2008, Kaouk et al. [11] first reported LESS radical prostatectomy in a pure laparoscopic way, but also showed major drawbacks such as significantly prolonged operative time, clashing of laparoscopic instruments, limited working space, and challenging dissection and ligation procedures. The first study of robotic LESS radical prostatectomy (r-LESS RALP), or single-port robotic-assisted radical laparoscopic prostatectomy (spRALP) was published shortly afterwards by the same team in 2009, but the robotic version of spRALP at its initial phases of development failed to address the aforementioned difficulties, Therefore, only a scarce number of centers have successfully performed spRALP to date.

Nowadays, the advent of da Vinci SP platform (Intuitive Surgical Inc., Sunnyvale, CA, USA) and single-port devices rekindled urologists' interest in re-exploring these urological operations [12–15]. However, because the SP platform is still not available in mainland China, urologists in Changzheng Hospital have made a series of innovations based on the da Vinci Si platform to perform spRALP. Different accesses of transperitoneal, extraperitoneal, transvesical and perineal route have been carried out with their respective optimal indications, which is introduced as follows.

Y. Chang
Department of Urology, Changhai Hospital, Naval Medical University, Shanghai, China

X. Zou
Department of Urology, The First Affiliated Hospital of Gannan Medical University, Ganzhou, Jiangxi, China

Q. Zhu
Jiangsu Province Hospital of Chinese Medicine, Nanjing, Jiangsu, China

S. Ren (✉)
Department of Urology, Changhai Hospital, Naval Medical University, Shanghai, China

Department of Urology, Changzheng Hospital, Naval Medical University, Shanghai, China

S. Ren et al. (eds.), *Robot-Assisted Radical Prostatectomy*, https://doi.org/10.1007/978-3-031-05855-4_35

Transperitoneal

In our center, the transperitoneal approach was first attempted in 2018 as a preliminary investigation to assess the safety and feasibility of spRALP [16]. We successfully carried out the transperitoneal approach on a 60-year-old male with a clinical stage of $cT_{2b}N_0M_0$ and a prostate volume of 33.8 ml. With use of a commercially-available quadri-channel port (Lagiport, Lagis Inc., Taiwan, China), a semicircular incision with a diameter of 6 cm was made above the umbilicus. Access was made transperitoneally, with the robotic camera placed at 6 o'clock (caudal side of the patient), placing 30° upward; robotic arms 1 and 2 were placed laterally (arm 3 was spared), with monopolar Hotshears scissors and Maryland bipolar forceps installed for dissection procedures, respectively, and large needle drivers installed for ligation of deep venous complex (DVC) and anastomosis; assistant's access was placed at 12 o'clock (Fig. 35.1a, b). Intraoperative procedures were the same as a conventional multi-port RALP, as reported previously [17]. The operative time was 152 min, including a console time of 131 min and anastomosis time of 21 min. Estimated blood loss was 100 ml. No additional ports were being placed. The patient was ambulant on post-op day 2 and was discharged on post-op day 4.

Based on the current robotic platform and standard 8-mm da Vinci Si robotic instruments, the transformation from the conventional multi-port RALP to transperitoneal spRALP with an umbilical incision faces tremendous difficulties, among which the biggest challenge was instrument clashing, both inside and outside the peritoneal cavity. First, in order to overcome exterior clashing, a 30-degree lens was adopted, and was set at 30°-up throughout the procedure; also, the camera was kept physically afar from the surgical field, in which case the visual distance was compensated with a 4× digital zooming at the console, in order to give room to the robotic arms 1 and 2. Also, because we didn't use pre-curved cannulae or articulated instruments, nor did we cross the instruments inside (i.e., the "chopsticks" phenomenon proposed by Joseph et al. [18]) which is being practiced by some centers, slight modifications were made by docking the robotic arms 1 and 2 at a wider angle on the proximal joint, and the robotic arms were operated with a lower amplitude and higher movement frequency. All of these modifications contributed to reduced clashing and acceptable operative triangle.

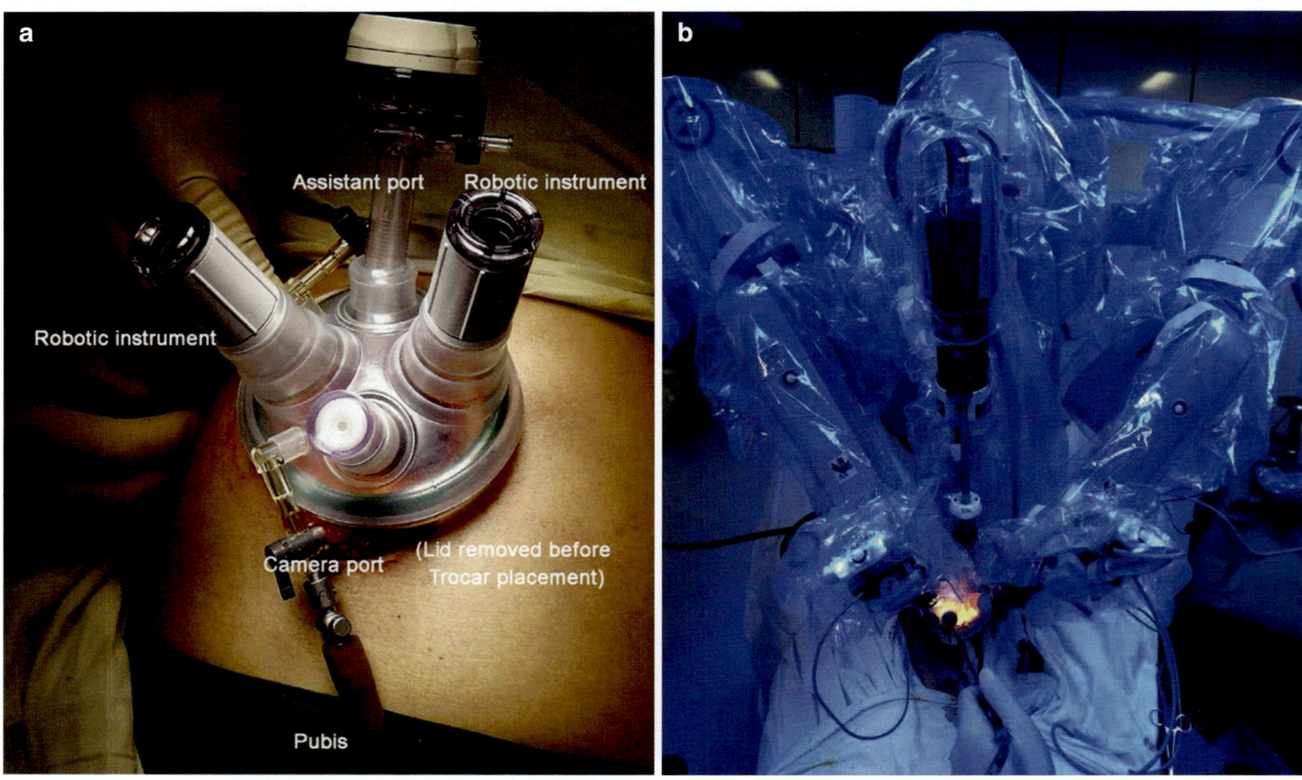

Fig. 35.1 Port installation and trocar placement before and after docking. (**a**) placement of a commercially available quadri-channel port, in which the camera port was placed at 6 o'clock, robotic arm 1 at 9 o'clock, robotic arm 2 at 3 o'clock, and assistant's port at 12 o'clock. (**b**) external view after docking, in which a 30° lens was placed looking upward and farther from the surgical field throughout the procedure, while the robotic arms were installed with more abduction at the proximal joint. (Figures excerpted from Chang et al., Asian J Urol 2019 [16], reprint permission granted by the Asian Journal of Urology editorial office)

However, because we believe that it is the relatively long distance from the umbilicus to the surgical area, i.e., the prostate that results in the frequent clashing, loss of maneuverability and most likely, a steep learning curve, we seek to update the surgical techniques by moving the port lower and closer to the surgical field, in order to make LESS-RALP easier to perform, hence the extraperitoneal spRALP, which is introduced as follows.

Extraperitoneal

To the best of our knowledge, extraperitoneal spRALP is only reported by a limited number of studies, and all with the adoption of the da Vinci SP robotic platform [12, 19, 20]. With the experience from our previous study of transperitoneal spRALP, we have successfully carried out extraperitoneal spRALP (espRALP) with use of the most widely installed da Vinci Si platform worldwide.

Different from the transumbilical incision in the transperitoneal spRALP, the extraperitoneal single-port RALP (espRALP) moves the incision lower, which is approximately 5 cm above the pubis symphysis (Fig. 35.2a, b). With a more customizable port (GelPort, Applied Medical, Rancho Santa Margarita, CA, USA)) installed at this level, the preperitoneal surgical space was first established with a homemade balloon. Other surgical steps were largely similar compared to a transperitoneal spRALP. Still the lens was put at 30°-up and farther from the surgical field (compensated by a 4× digital zoom) throughout the procedure (Fig. 35.2c) [21], but with a port placed at this level, the maneuverability of robotic arms can be markedly improved, with minimal clashing of instruments, and more rookie-friendly. The surgeons may find it much easier to readjust themselves from their habits to perform a conventional RALP to an espRALP. Additionally, more complex techniques, such as bilateral intrafascial nerve-sparing, or super-veil nerve-sparing that was reported in Vattikuti Institute Prostatectomy

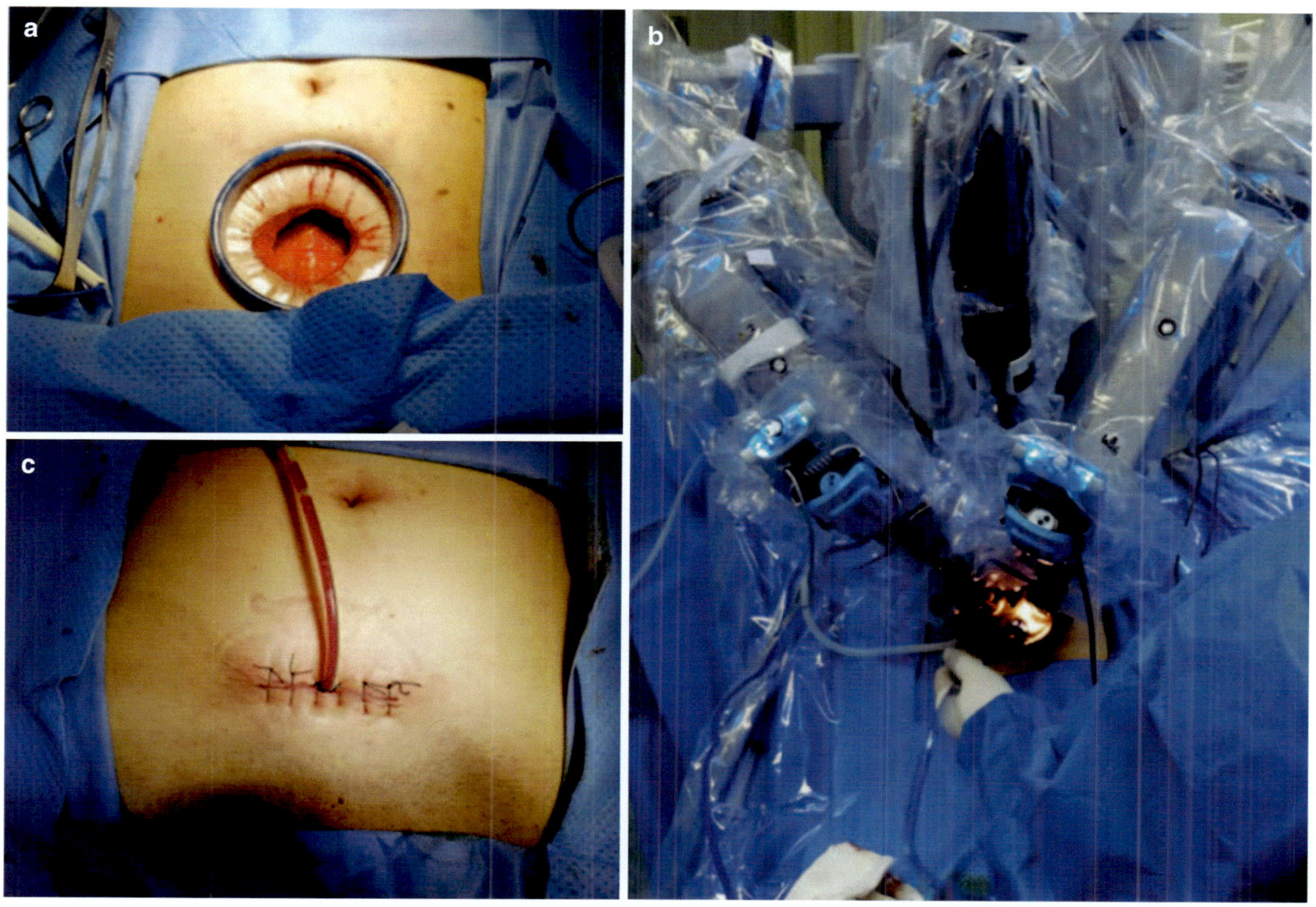

Fig. 35.2 Illustration of Extraperitoneal single-port robotic-assisted radical prostatectomy. (**a**) Abdominal incision and port placement with a 5-cm transverse incision 5 cm above the pubic symphysis; (**b**) External view after docking. Access to the port was identical to the Transperitoneal approach. (**c**) Wound closure with a Jackson-Pratt drainage (optional) placed in the same incision. (Figures excerpted from Chang et al., Chin Med J 2020 [21], reprint permission granted by the Chinese Medical Journal editorial office)

(VIP) [22] that can provide complete periprostatic anatomy preservation, can now be performed safely. Possible potential benefit in continence and potency outcomes requires further perspective controlled studies.

In our opinion, the espRALP may have several advantages compared with conventional RALP for selected patients, for it can provide improved post-op recovery and lower risk to bowel-related and anesthesia-related comorbidities and complications, because the peritoneal disturbance is minimal, and a much less steep Trendelenburg position is required (usually 10–15° vs >30°). Further comparative studies are on the way.

Nevertheless, for a certain patient population, e.g., patients with previous history of lower abdominal or pelvic surgery or radiation, it may be regretful to abandon surgery for early-stage disease, but whether transperitoneal or extraperitoneal access may increase surgical time (such as the need to perform adhesiolysis) or lead to serious intraoperative complications remains inconclusive, according to the literature [23–25]. Therefore, we also investigated alternative routes based on our current single-port robotic platform.

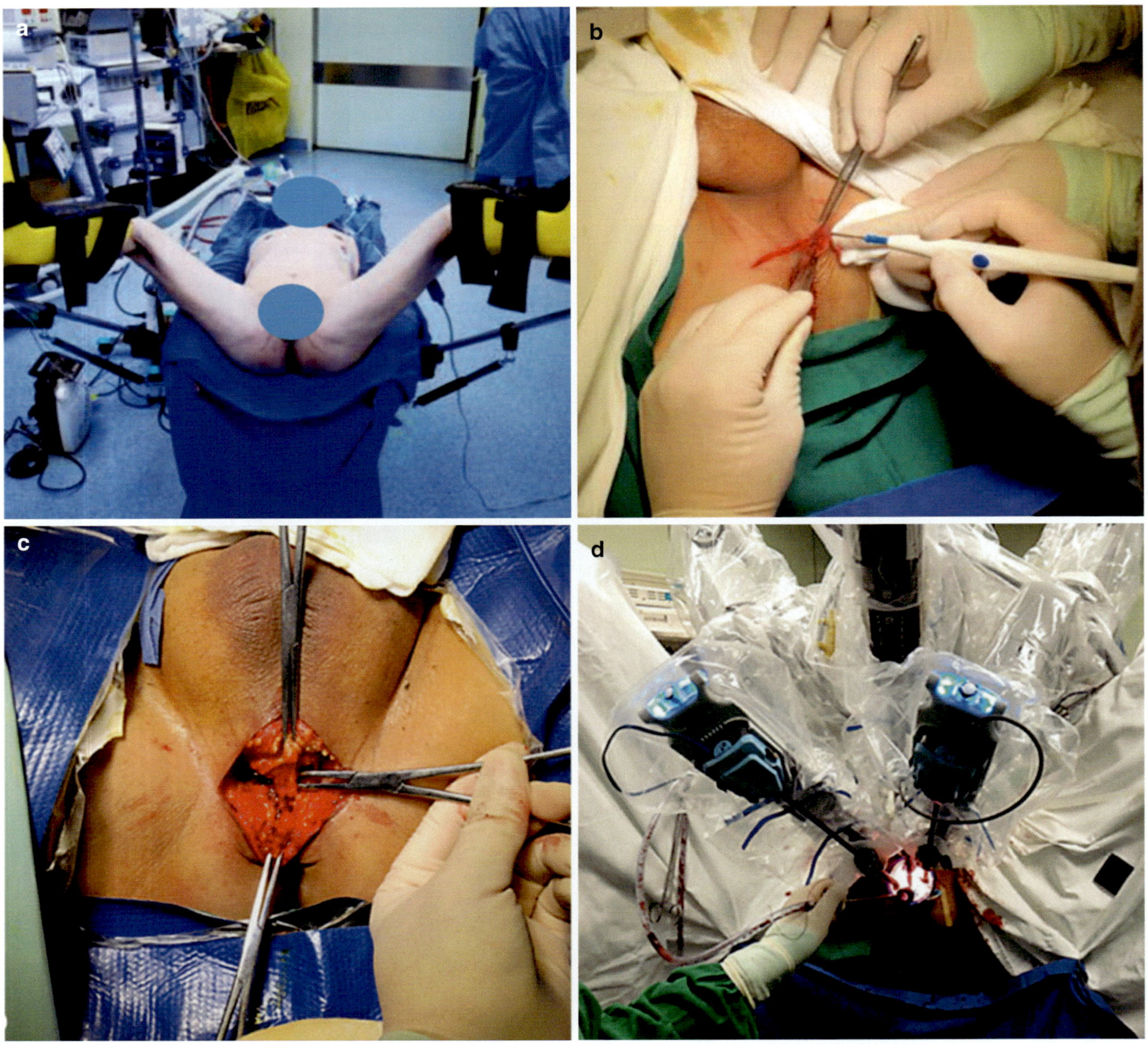

Fig. 35.3 Preoperative preparations to a robotic perineal radical prostatectomy (RPRP). (**a**) patient position, adopting an exaggerated lithotomy with slight Trendelenburg position; (**b**) Incision made at the perineal region approximately 2 cm above the anus to reach the ischial tuberosities at both sides; (**c**) The central tendon was identified, exposed and transected; (**d**) External view after docking. (Figures excerpted from Chang et al. Urol Int 2020 [28], reprint permission granted by the Urologia Internationalis editorial office)

Perineal

Perineal radical prostatectomy was the earliest form of this surgical approach, which can be traced back to over 150 years ago, and outperformed other forms of prostatectomy after Hugh Hampton Young modified this approach in 1905 [26], and continued to serve as the standard approach for the next 40 plus years. However, its popularity was soon lost after the advent of retropubic radical prostatectomy in 1945, which continued to serve as the mainstream worldwide in the laparoscopic and robotic era. In modern times, although the perineal approach comprises only about 5% of the total cases of radical prostatectomies, it is still being adopted as an alternative approach, especially when robotic platform and single port devices are being used for this approach. Introduced by Kaouk et al. [27], robotic perineal prostatectomy (RPP) was believed to be a solution for selected patients with safer surgical profiles, such as those with a history of major open abdominal surgery or obese patients.

In our center, we successfully performed RPP in 2018, and this approach has been offered to obese patients and those with history of open lower-abdominal surgery, with unrestricted hip joint movement [28]. The patient should adopt an exaggerated lithotomy position, with a hip flexion of over 90° and a 0–15° slight Trendelenburg position (Fig. 35.3a). Intrarectal rinsing should be applied two to three times with iodine. An upper-curved incision was made at the perineal region, approximately 2 cm above the anus (Fig. 35.3b), reaching the ischial tuberosities at both sides. Next, the subcutaneous tissue was dissected to expose the central tendon (Fig. 35.3c), which was then transected. Further dissections were made to expose and dissect deeper fascial and muscular structures such as the rectourethralis muscle and the deep transverse perineal muscle. With the assistant's index finger placed inside the rectum, the space between the anterior rectal wall and the posterior apex of the prostate can be identified and divided. A 75-mm single-site quadri-channel surgical port (Freeport, SensCure Biotech Ltd., Ningbo, Jiangsu, China) was placed followed by docking of the da Vinci Si robotic platform, trocar arrangement of which was similar with our extraperitoneal access (Fig. 35.3d). In this case, the 12-o'clock channel was used as camera port, in which the lens was also placed at 30°-up. The 3- and 9- o'clock channel was used as robotic arms 1 and 2, respectively, and the 6 o'clock channel was used as assistant's port. Notably, the Robotic cart was placed at the patient's right hand side with a 45° angle between the axis of the robot and the surgical bed. The assistant was seated at the foot of the bed.

After docking, an Airseal insufflator (Surgiquest Inc., Milford, CT, USA) was connected to maintain a more stable intraperineal pressure at 12 mm mmHg, and is more tolerable to reflux of suction fluid compared to the Olympus UHI-3 insufflator used in transperitoneal and extraperitoneal RALP. Incision of the Denonvilliers' fascia was made first to control the lateral prostatic pedicles with hem-o-lok clips. At this level, the neurovascular bundles were also dissected either extrafascially or intrafascially, according to the patient's eligibility for nerve-sparing procedures (Fig. 35.4a). Further exposure was made at the posterior plane to dissect the vas deferens and seminal vesicles (Fig. 35.4b). After fully mobilizing the posterior plane of the prostate, the apical urethra was then identified and transected, followed by further dissection at the ventral plane of the prostate in a retrograde fashion, until the bladder neck was reached and transected (Fig. 35.4c). At this point, the prostate can be fully mobilized and removed. Vesicourethral anastomosis was then performed after intraperineal pressure was lowered to 5 mmHg to reduce tension. A 3–0 two-way barbed suture was adopted to make continuous sutures starting at the mid-point. The posterior wall was first reapproximated, and the two-way suture was rejoined at the anterior midline (Fig. 35.4d). Finally, Jackson-Pratt drainage was placed before wound closure.

Transvesical

The transvesical approach to perform RALP was first reported by Desai et al. [29] in 2008, adopting both multiport and single-port access. This access was made suprapubically to gain access directly from the Retzius space. Alternatively, the transvesical approach was also reported with trocar placement similar to that of a conventional multiport RALP, and the surgical access was made transperitoneally to open the bladder wall at the dome, followed by dissection of the prostate inside the bladder. In this section we will mainly focus on our technique which was similar to the study of Desai et al., using a single-port device and a direct percutaneous access suprapubically.

First, a 6-cm incision was made transversely, approximately 5 cm above the pubis symphysis. The incision was further extended down to the anterior rectus sheath. The bladder was then filled with 300 ml saline via the Foley catheter for better identification of the incision plane. Then the anterior bladder wall was incised vertically to allow for insertion of the wound protector that was secured in place (Fig. 35.5), followed by fixation of a single-port device (GelPort, Applied Medical, Rancho Santa Margarita CA, USA) above. Port configurations were the same with the extraperitoneal access discussed above. For transvesical RALP, ureteric orifices should be identified and well

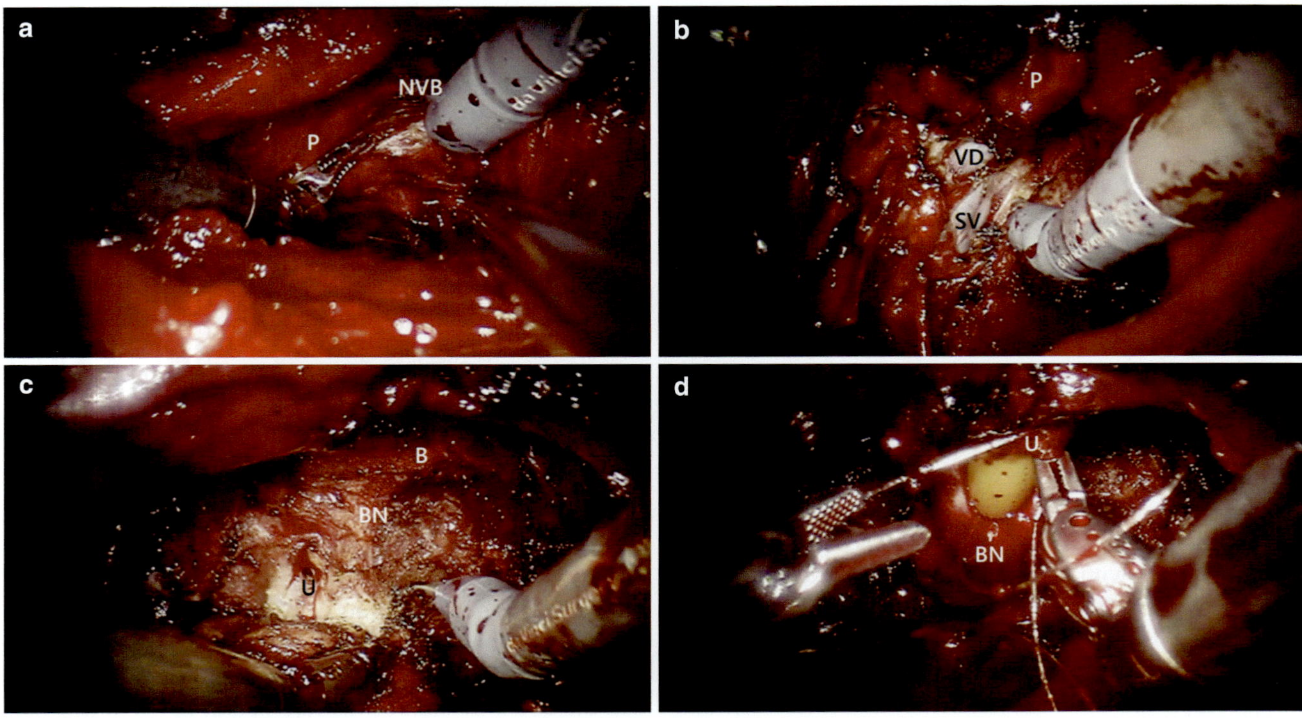

Fig. 35.4 Intraoperative view during different steps of a robotic perineal radical prostatectomy (RPRP). (**a**) Dissection of the neurovascular bundles; (**b**) Dissection of the vas deferens and seminal vesicles; (**c**) Transection of the bladder neck; (**d**) Vesicourethral anastomosis. *P* prostate, *NVB* neurovascular bundles, *VD* vas deferens, *SV* seminal vesicle, *B* bladder, *BN* bladder neck, *U* urethra. (Figures excerpted from Chang et al. Urol Int 2020 [28], reprint permission granted by the Urologia Internationalis editorial office)

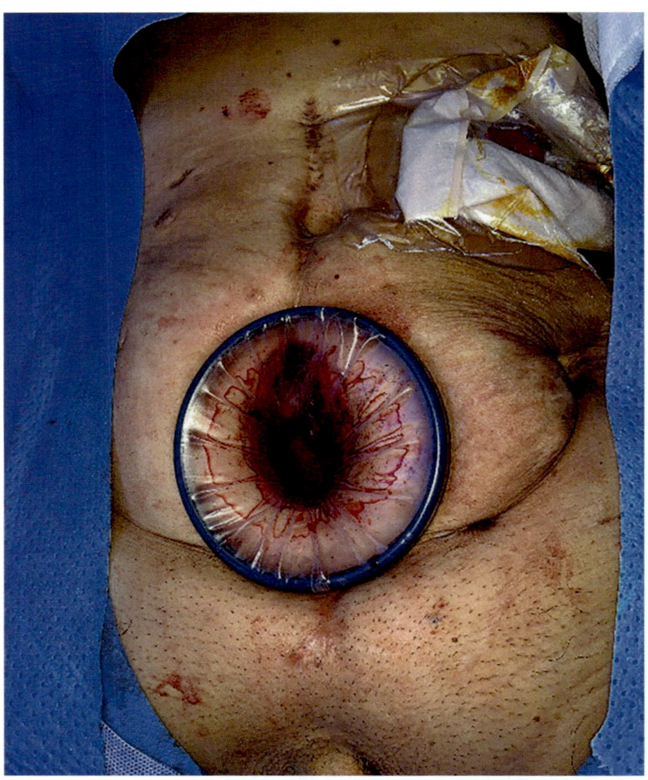

Fig. 35.5 Port placement of transvesical spRALP. The patient had previous open surgery for rectal cancer and a permanent stoma, therefore a regular transperitoneal access may be of high intraoperative risk (data unpublished)

protected. In initial operations, bilateral D-J stents were placed preoperatively for a precautious intent.

The bladder neck junction was cauterized circumferentially to mark the contour of the prostate (Fig. 35.6a). Further dissection was made to divide the ventral plane of the prostate until the apex was reached (Fig. 35.6b). Then, the prostate was suspended upwards to expose and dissect the vas deferens and seminal vesicles (Fig. 35.6c), followed by ligation of the prostatic pedicles with hem-o-lok clips, and dissection of the neurovascular bundles (NVB) (Fig. 35.6d). When both sides of the NVB dissection reached the prostatic apex, the apical urethra was isolated and transected (Fig. 35.6e). Final steps of the surgical procedures were vesicourethral anastomosis, in which case 3–0 two-way barbed suture was used. The posterior wall of the urethra and the posterior lip of the bladder neck were first realigned with 3–4 stitches, and continued at both sides. Then, the bladder neck was cinched at 9 and 3 o'clock with 3–4 stitches before finishing the reapproximation between the anterior urethra and the bladder neck. The two-way stiches were finally joined at 12 o'clock (Fig. 35.6f). After retrieval of the prostate specimen, the bladder wall was closed by the bedside assistant with two layers of 3–0 running sutures, followed by confirmation of water-tight closure by injecting 200 ml saline via the Foley catheter. Finally, the anterior rectus sheath, subcutaneous tissue and skin were closed sequentially.

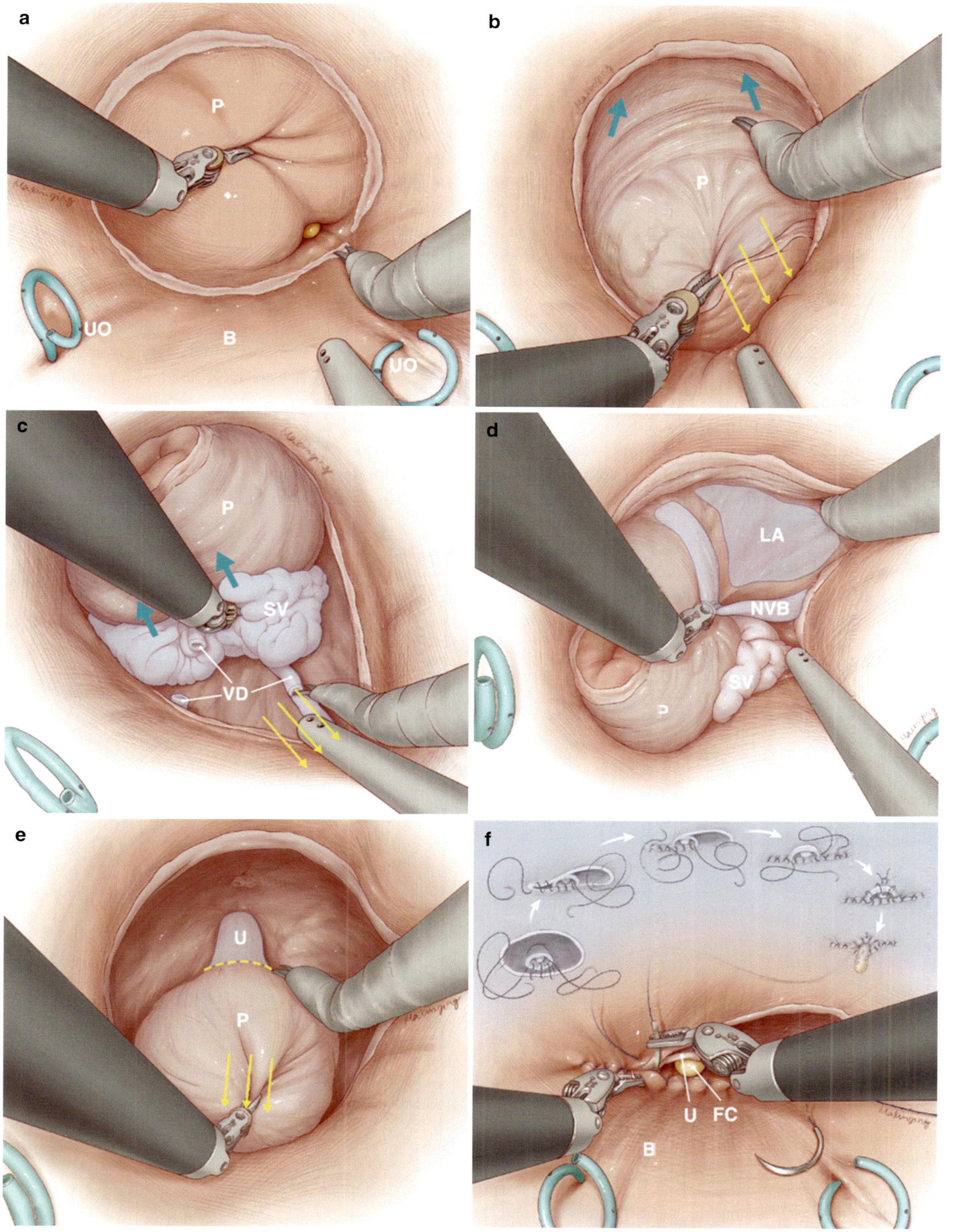

Fig. 35.6 Intraoperative depiction of transvesical single-port robotic radical prostatectomy. (**a**) Circumferential incision of the bladder neck junction; (**b**) Dissection of the ventral plane of the prostate, with the left robotic arm retracting the prostate; (**c**) Dissection of the vasa deferentia and the seminal vesicles; (**d**) Dissection of the neurovascular bundles; (**e**) Transection of the distal urethra; (**f**) Anastomosis of the vesicourethral junction. *B* bladder, *FC* Foley catheter, *LA* levator ani fascia, *NVB* neurovascular bundle, *P* prostate, *SV* seminal vesicles, *U* urethra, *UO* ureteric orifice, *VD* vasa deferentia (data unpublished)

Outcomes

From May 2018 to June 2020, a total of 116 patients underwent spRALP of different routes in our center, in which 1 was transperitoneal, 92 were extraperitoneal, 10 were perineal, and 13 were transvesical (Table 35.1). The transperitoneal case was regarded as a pilot study and was not included in the final analysis. The patients averaged 67 years (range, 52–84) with a body mass index of 24.44 kg/m^2 (range, 19.52–32.33). Among these patients, 111 were < cT3a, 4 were cT3a and none were > cT3a. Preoperative androgen deprivation therapy (ADT) was given to 7 patients with a median time of 4 months (range, 3–12). Preoperative prostate-specific antigen (PSA) was 9.77 ng/ml (IQR, 6.54, 15.32). Thirteen patients had previous undergone lower abdominal or pelvic surgery (6 in extraperitoneal group, 1 in perineal group and 6 in transvesical group). All operations were carried out successfully without open conversion or addition of trocars. Mean operative time was 91.8 min (range, 40–200) with an estimated blood loss of 91.8 ml (range, 45–400). No blood transfusion was documented. Patients were ambulant on postop day 1 except for perineal access, in which one additional day was required before the patients were instructed to be off-bed. Mean postop length of stay was 3 days (range, 1–7). Nineteen patients in the extraperitoneal group had surgery on the day of admission and resumed liquid diet 6 h postoperatively and were encouraged to be off-bed. Drainage was removed on the next day.

For postoperative complications, 1 patient in the extraperitoneal group reported anastomotic leakage on postop day 2, and recovered with conservative treatment. Another patient in the same group reported incision dehiscence after the sutures were removed, and was treated at clinic. One patient in perineal group reported pelvic infection after discharge, and was readmitted followed by systematic antibiotic treatment.

Pathologic staging showed 70 patients to be <pT3a and 45 to be ≥pT3a. Overall positive surgical margin (pSM) was 17.4% (20/115), in which 31.1% (14/45) in ≥pT3a patients, and 8.6% (6/70) in <pT3a patients. Four patients were not applicable for pathological Gleason scoring due to preoperative ADT. Others with pathological Gleason Score of 6, 3 + 4, 4 + 3 and ≥ 8 were 6, 45, 52 and 8 patients, respectively. Final pathology all showed prostatic adenocarcinoma. Mean follow-up time was 10.4 months (range, 3–21). Median PSA on 1-month follow-up was 0.03 ng/ml (IQR, 0.014, 0.05). Continence recovery was recorded in 102 patients (88.7%) 3 months postoperatively (Table 35.2).

Table 35.1 Patient Demographics

	Extraperitoneal	Perineal	Transvesical
n	92	10	13
Age[mean(range), years]	67(52–84)	65(54–73)	68(61–75)
BMI[mean(range), kg/m^2]	24.58(19.53–32.33)	24.85(19.81–27.55)	23.12(20.05–26.45)
PSA[median(IQR), ng/ml]	9.89(6.43. 15.66)	9.52(7.56, 13.75)	9.77(6.54, 15.60)
Clinical stage[n(%)]			
<cT3a	89(96.7)	10(100.0)	12(92.3)
cT3a	3(3.3)	0(0)	1(7.7)
>cT3a	0(0)	0(0)	0(0)
Gleason score[n(%)]			
6	12(13.0)	4(40.0)	0(0)
3 + 4	38(41.3)	4(40.0)	7(53.8)
4 + 3	34(37.0)	2(20.0)	4(30.8)
8	8(8.7)	0(0)	1(7.7)
9/10	0(0)	0(0)	1(7.7)
Previous surgery(n)			
Abdominal	6	1	0
Pelvic	0	0	6

BMI body mass index, *IQR* interquartile range, *PSA* prostate-specific antigen (Data excerpted from Du et al. Chin J Urol, 2020, 41(11): 815–819. DOI: 10.3760/cma.j.cn112330-20200909-00657) (Article in Chinese, reprint permission granted by the Chinese Journal of Urology editorial office) [30]

Table 35.2 Perioperative and follow-up parameters

	Extraperitoneal	Perineal	Transvesical
n	92	10	13
Operative time[mean(range), min]	88.0(40–200)	132.5(90–190)	87.3(60–150)
EBL[mean(range), ml]	77.6(50–200)	178(80–400)	70.4(45–150)
Pathological stage[n(%)]			
<pT3a	58(63.0)	4(40.0)	8(61.5)
≥pT3a	34(37.0)	6(60.0)	5(38.5)
Gleason score[n(%)]			
N/A	3(3.3)	0(0)	1(7.7)
6	5(5.4)	1(10.0)	0(0)
3 + 4	35(38.0)	6(60.0)	4(30.8)
4 + 3	43(46.7)	3(30.0)	6(46.2)
8	6(6.5)	0(0)	1(7.7)
9/10	0(0)	0(0)	1(7.7)
pSM[n(%)]	16(17.4)	2(20.0)	2(15.3)
<pT3a	6(10.3)	0(0)	0(0)
≥pT3a	10(27.8)	2(33.3)	2(40.0)
Post-op length of stay[mean(range), day]	2.9(1–5)	2.1(1–4)	4.8(4–7)
Post-op PSA(1mo) [median(IQR), ng/ml]	0.031(0.017, 0.051)	0.025(0.012, 0.046)	0.017(0.002, 0.045)
Postoperative continence(3 mo) [n(%)]	82(89.1)	9(90.0)	11(84.6)

EBL estimated blood loss, *N/A* not applicable, *pSM* positive surgical margin, *IQR* interquartile range, *PSA* prostate-specific antigen (Data excerpted from Du et al. Chin J Urol, 2020, 41(11): 815–819. DOI: 10.3760/cma.j.cn112330-20200909-00657) (Article in Chinese, reprint permission granted by the Chinese Journal of Urology editorial office) [30]

Discussion

Laparoendoscopic single-site surgery (LESS) in the modern robotic era is explored with the aim of minimizing postoperative pain and perioperative complications, and to achieve better postoperative recovery and cosmesis outcomes. Initially, LESS and robotic-LESS surgery had been successfully attempted in various urological operations including adrenalectomy, pyeloplasty, nephrectomy (including radical, partial, and donor transplantation), radical cystectomy, and radical prostatectomy [6–9, 11, 31]. Interestingly, studies of either LESS or robotic-LESS concerning the upper urinary tract (e.g., nephrectomy and partial nephrectomy), are attempted by a growing number of centers, while single-port radical prostatectomy and radical cystectomy appeared to "fade away" from public attention, and it was not until the birth of da Vinci SP robotic platform has robotic LESS surgery of the lower urinary tract regained urologists' interest. Initially, LESS-RALP was performed via an umbilical incision, therefore the much longer distance between the port and the surgical area, compared to that in an adrenalectomy or a nephrectomy, is one major culprit to instrument criss-crossing, clashing, and loss of triangulation and maneuverability. Earlier experiences included use of articulated or pre-bent instruments, or 5-mm harmonic scalpel which is thinner in diameter, as well as use of 30° lens looking upward to reduce clashing and partially regain triangulation, but the pre-bent or articulating instruments were deemed "nonergonomic and counterintuitive" [32]. Our initial experience of the transperitoneal spRALP also showed extensive clashing and loss of triangulation. By adopting a 30°-up lens throughout the procedure and keeping the lens afar from the surgical field compensated with digital zoom, triangulation was partially regained, and the instruments gave room to each other. Even so, we find it difficult to believe that the transperitoneal spRALP had the value of being widely popularized. It was the change in surgical access that made a genuine difference. Shifting the procedure from an umbilical incision and transperitoneal access to a suprapubic incision and extraperitoneal access allowed the entire procedure to be performed smoothly with minimal clashing and more operator-friendly. Following similar principles, the perineal and transvesical could also be carried out smoothly for routine performance on a da Vinci Si model, without additional trocar placement.

With all these alternative accesses of spRALP, the next step would be to determine the optimal indication for each access. Although the extraperitoneal, perineal and transvesical accesses can all be deemed as extraperitoneal in nature, their applications vary in different patients. We believe that the extraperitoneal is best indicated for patients with localized disease to provide fast recovery, lower perioperative complications and reduced pain, and even allow for outpatient surgery, as reported by Wilson et al. [19]. Patients eligible for perineal and transvesical spRALP somewhat overlap, since they both are feasible alternatives for obese patients and those with previous abdominal or pelvic surgery, in order to minimize incision-related complications, anesthesia-related complications due to steep Trendelenburg position required in a conventional RALP, as well as time and risk spent in potential adhesiolysis procedures. However, our experience showed that patients with larger prostate volume may not be best indicated for perineal robotic spRALP, since tension may be encountered during vesico-urethral anastomosis. Also, the surgeon may find it more challenging coping with pelvic anatomy and more reluctant to perform such procedure. A transvesical spRALP does not require a huge paradigm shift for transition from a conventional RALP mode. However, note that these interpretations are merely based on clinical observation, and perspective controlled studies are mandatory before any definitive conclusions are made. Also, for more challenging cases such as locally advanced prostate cancer that required extended pelvic lymph node and extensive periprostatic invasions may be encountered, we believe that the multiport RALP is still the ultimate choice for most urologists.

References

1. Wheeless CR Jr. Laparoscopy. Clin Obstet Gynecol. 1976;19:277–98.
2. Wheeless CR Jr, Thompson BH. Laparoscopic sterilization. Review of 3600 cases. Obstet Gynecol. 1973;42:751–8.
3. Liatsikos E, Kallidonis P, Kyriazis I, Al-Aown A, Stolzenburg JU. Urologic laparoendoscopic single-site surgery. Nat Rev Urol. 2009;6:654–9.
4. Box G, Averch T, Cadeddu J, et al. Nomenclature of natural orifice translumenal endoscopic surgery (NOTES) and laparoendoscopic single-site surgery (LESS) procedures in urology. J Endourol. 2008;22:2575–81.
5. Gill IS, Advincula AP, Aron M, et al. Consensus statement of the consortium for laparoendoscopic single-site surgery. Surg Endosc. 2010;24:762–8.
6. Aron M, Canes D, Desai MM, Haber GP, Kaouk JH, Gill IS. Transumbilical single-port laparoscopic partial nephrectomy. BJU Int. 2009;103:516–21.
7. Gill IS, Canes D, Aron M, et al. Single port transumbilical (E-NOTES) donor nephrectomy. J Urol. 2008;180:637–41. discussion 41
8. Castellucci SA, Curcillo PG, Ginsberg PC, Saba SC, Jaffe JS, Harmon JD. Single port access adrenalectomy. J Endourol. 2008;22:1573–6.
9. Kaouk JH, Goel RK, Haber GP, Crouzet S, Stein RJ. Robotic single-port transumbilical surgery in humans: initial report. BJU Int. 2009;103:366–9.
10. Kaouk JH, Palmer JS. Single-port laparoscopic surgery: initial experience in children for varicocelectomy. BJU Int. 2008;102:97–9.
11. Kaouk JH, Goel RK, Haber GP, Crouzet S, Desai MM, Gill IS. Single-port laparoscopic radical prostatectomy. Urology. 2008;72:1190–3.

12. Covas Moschovas M, Bhat S, Rogers T, et al. Applications of the da Vinci single port (SP) robotic platform in urology: a systematic literature review. Minerva Urol Nephrol. 2021;73:6–16.
13. Agarwal DK, Hebert KJ, Gettman MT, Viers BR. How to perform a robotic pyeloplasty utilizing the da Vinci SP platform: tips and tricks. Transl Androl Urol. 2020;9:919–24.
14. Kim KH, Song W, Yoon H, Lee DH. Single-port robot-assisted radical prostatectomy with the da Vinci SP system: a single surgeon's experience. Investig Clin Urol. 2020;61:173–9.
15. Khalil M, Cranwell A, Ouyang J, Alam Z, Joseph J. Single-port robot assisted concomitant hemi-nephrectomy, ureterectomy and radical prostatectomy using the da vinci SP platform. Urol Case Rep. 2021;36:101550.
16. Chang Y, Lu X, Zhu Q, Xu C, Sun Y, Ren S. Single-port transperitoneal robotic-assisted laparoscopic radical prostatectomy (spRALP): initial experience. Asian J Urol. 2019;6:294–7.
17. Chang Y, Qu M, Wang L, et al. Robotic-assisted laparoscopic radical prostatectomy from a single Chinese center: a learning curve analysis. Urology. 2016;93:104–11.
18. Joseph RA, Goh AC, Cuevas SP, et al. "Chopstick" surgery: a novel technique improves surgeon performance and eliminates arm collision in robotic single-incision laparoscopic surgery. Surg Endosc. 2010;24:1331–5.
19. Wilson CA, Aminsharifi A, Sawczyn G, et al. Outpatient Extraperitoneal Single-Port Robotic Radical Prostatectomy. Urology. 2020;144:142–6.
20. Kaouk J, Valero R, Sawczyn G, Garisto J. Extraperitoneal single-port robot-assisted radical prostatectomy: initial experience and description of technique. BJU Int. 2020;125:182–9.
21. Chang YF, Gu D, Mei N, et al. Initial experience on extraperitoneal single-port robotic-assisted radical prostatectomy. Chin Med J. 2020;134:231–3.
22. Ghani KR, Trinh QD, Menon M. Vattikuti institute prostatectomy-technique in 2012. J Endourol. 2012;26:1558–65.
23. Bernstein AN, Lavery HJ, Hobbs AR, Chin E, Samadi DB. Robot-assisted laparoscopic prostatectomy and previous surgical history: a multidisciplinary approach. J Robot Surg. 2013;7:143–51.
24. Milone M, de'Angelis N, Beghdadi N, et al. Conversions related to adhesions in abdominal surgery. Robotic versus laparoscopic approach: a multicentre experience. Int J Med Robot. 2021;17:e2186.
25. Di Pierro GB, Grande P, Mordasini L, Danuser H, Mattei A. Robot-assisted radical prostatectomy in the setting of previous abdominal surgery: perioperative results, oncological and functional outcomes, and complications in a single surgeon's series. Int J Surg. 2016;36:170–6.
26. Young HH. The early diagnosis and radical cure of carcinoma of the prostate. Being a study of 40 cases and presentation of a radical operation which was carried out in four cases. 1905. J Urol. 2002;167:939–46. discussion 47
27. Kaouk JH, Akca O, Zargar H, et al. Descriptive technique and initial results for robotic radical perineal prostatectomy. Urology. 2016;94:129–38.
28. Chang Y, Xu W, Lu X, et al. Robotic perineal radical prostatectomy: initial experience with the da Vinci Si robotic system. Urol Int. 2020;104:710–5.
29. Desai MM, Aron M, Berger A, et al. Transvesical robotic radical prostatectomy. BJU Int. 2008;102:1666–9.
30. Du W, Xu W, Yang Y, et al. Single-port robot-assisted laparoscopic radical prostatectomy through different approaches: initial experience and outcomes. Chin J Urol. 2020;41:815–9. (Article in Chinese)
31. Horstmann M, Kugler M, Anastasiadis AG, Walcher U, Herrmann T, Nagele U. Laparoscopic radical cystectomy: initial experience using the single-incision triangulated umbilical surgery (SITUS) technique. World J Urol. 2012;30:619–24.
32. White MA, Haber GP, Autorino R, et al. Robotic laparoendoscopic single-site radical prostatectomy: technique and early outcomes. Eur Urol. 2010;58:544–50.

Single Port Extraperitoneal Radical Prostatectomy

36

Zeyad R. Schwen and Jihad Kaouk

Introduction

As the trend towards further reducing the morbidity of minimally-invasive surgery continues, significant developments have been made in the robotic assisted radical prostatectomy (RARP) to improve the outcomes of patients with clinically localized prostate cancer (PCa). The Da Vinci Single Port platform is the latest iteration of that drive, with the hopes of reducing the operative burden while expanding the access for various urologic surgeries [1]. The single port extraperitoneal robotic radical prostatectomy represents an archetypal demonstration of the additive benefit of the Single Port platform when applied to the extraperitoneal approach in an effort to improve patient outcomes.

The advantages of the extraperitoneal approach are significant and well-described, as demonstrated in the multiport robotic experience [2–5], avoiding the peritoneal cavity to avoid potential bowel adhesions, reduce the rates of postoperative ileus, obviate the need for steep Trendelenburg position, as well as reduce the rate of hernia formation compared to the transperitoneal approach. In short, these many benefits sum to a reduction in operative time, reduction in hospital length of stay, as well as provide a safer access for those with significant prior bowel surgery [5]. In the multiport extraperitoneal experience, however, gaining access can be time-consuming and cumbersome, increasing the potential for clashing as well as unintended peritoneal insufflation with each additional port required. Similarly, the advantages of the single port platform include the ease of operating in smaller spaces, fewer abdominal incisions, and lack of a need for an assistant port [1]. These benefits translate to a further reduction in patient morbidity, a shorter hospital stay length of stay, as well as less postoperative pain and need for opioids [1, 6, 7].

Our experience with the additive value of the SP extraperitoneal radical prostatectomy has been overwhelming positive [8–11]. Now beyond 200 cases, we have shown that outpatient radical prostatectomy has become a more attainable goal, with our same-day discharge rate > 95% and median hospital length of stay of 4.2 hours [8, 11]. Similarly, patients rarely require opioids and early functional and oncologic outcomes are equivalent to multiport and transperitoneal approaches [9, 11].

Indications

The indications for SP extraperitoneal radical prostatectomy are identical for patients undergoing a traditional multiport or transperitoneal robotic radical prostatectomy who have clinically localized prostate cancer according to the National Comprehensive Cancer Network (NCCN) guidelines [12]. Patients who can particularly benefit from a extraperitoneal approach are those patients with extensive prior abdominal surgeries who have not entered the extraperitoneal space. Open midline incisions or exploratory laparotomies that extend well below the umbilicus may make extraperitoneal access more challenging and have a higher risk of unintended entry and insufflation of the peritoneal space. Other patients who are particularly well suited for extraperitoneal approach include those who are unable to tolerate peritoneal insufflation due to restrictive lung disease or those with peritoneal dialysis catheters or ventriculoperitoneal shuts. Additionally, those patients who are unable to tolerate Trendelenburg positioning from significant respiratory disease and glaucoma who are at risk for increased intraocular pressures.

Contraindications to the SP extraperitoneal approach are those who have had prior surgeries that have obliterated the space of Retzius such as laparoscopic inguinal hernia repairs with mesh or major open or laparoscopic pelvic surgeries that requires entry into the extraperitoneal space such as abdominoperitoneal resections or renal transplantations. Relative contraindications include those patients who are morbidly obese or with massive >100 cc prostates which are

Z. R. Schwen · J. Kaouk (✉)
Glickman Urological & Kidney Institute, Cleveland Clinic Foundation, Cleveland, OH, USA
e-mail: schwenz2@ccf.org; kaoukj@ccf.org

S. Ren et al. (eds.), *Robot-Assisted Radical Prostatectomy*, https://doi.org/10.1007/978-3-031-05855-4_36

slightly more technically challenging, primarily due to the increased difficulty with SP access and reduced strength of the robotic arms required for retraction, respectively.

Description of Technique

Preoperative

Preoperative workup is identical to the traditional robotic prostatectomy approaches. Patients are required to provide preoperative laboratory workup including type and screen, basic metabolic panel, complete blood count, and urinalysis and culture. We do not require any bowel prep or enemas prior to surgery as they are of little benefit and may result in dehydration and are often poorly tolerated. We use standard perioperative antibiotic prophylaxis according to guidelines and administer subcutaneous heparin preoperatively which is continued until discharge as part of deep venous thromboembolism prophylaxis. In those patients with NCCN high-risk disease, prophylactic low molecular weight heparin is continued until 28 days postoperatively. Patients have sequential compressive devices placed bilaterally on the lower extremities.

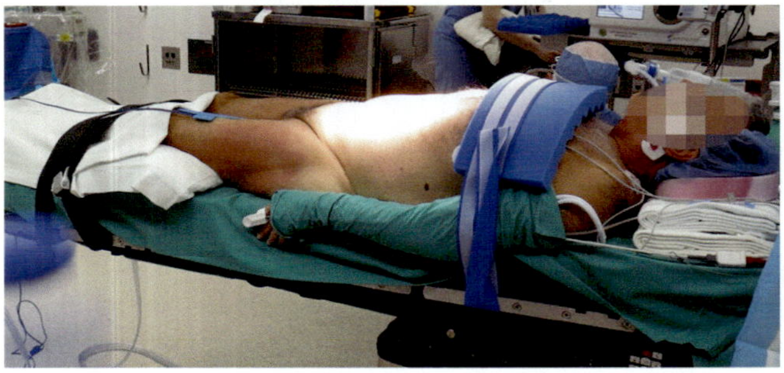

Fig. 36.1 Patient positioning

Patients are positioned in the supine position and Trendelenburg or lithotomy positioning is not required (Fig. 36.1). Because Trendelenburg is not necessary and the SP robot is able to easily side-dock, arm tucking is optional. Patients are prepped and draped in a standard fashion.

Intraoperative

Extraperitoneal Access and SP Docking

A 20F 2-way foley catheter is placed into the bladder and a 3 cm midline, infraumbilical incision is made and continued down to the fascia (Fig. 36.2a and b). A 3 cm anterior rectus fasciotomy is made in the midline, being careful to not go beyond the posterior rectus fascia, particularly at the cranial aspect of the incision to avoid unintended entry into the peritoneum. For those patients with prior midline scars, the incision should be slightly lateralized to avoid prior scar tissue which can distort the anatomy and increase the likelihood of a peritonotomy. Using blunt finger dissection, the space of Retzius is partially developed to accommodate insertion of the kidney-shaped balloon dilator (Spacemaker™ balloon, Covidien, Dublin, Ireland) (Fig. 36.3a and b). The balloon dilator is introduced and positioned below the pubic bone, the rigid plastic introducer is removed, and the balloon is inflated with approximately 400 mL of air (around 30 pumps) to develop the extra-

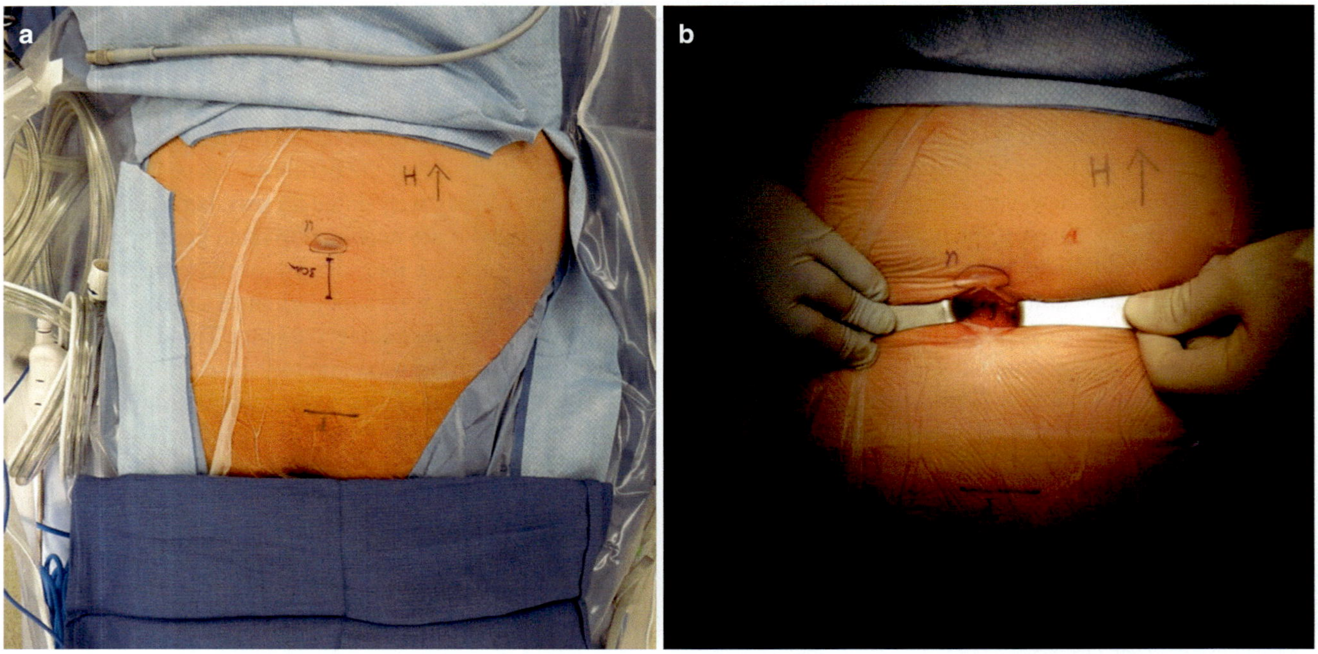

Fig. 36.2 A 3 cm midline infraumbilical incision is marked (**a**) and the incision is extended down to the fascia (**b**). Skin incision and fascial exposure

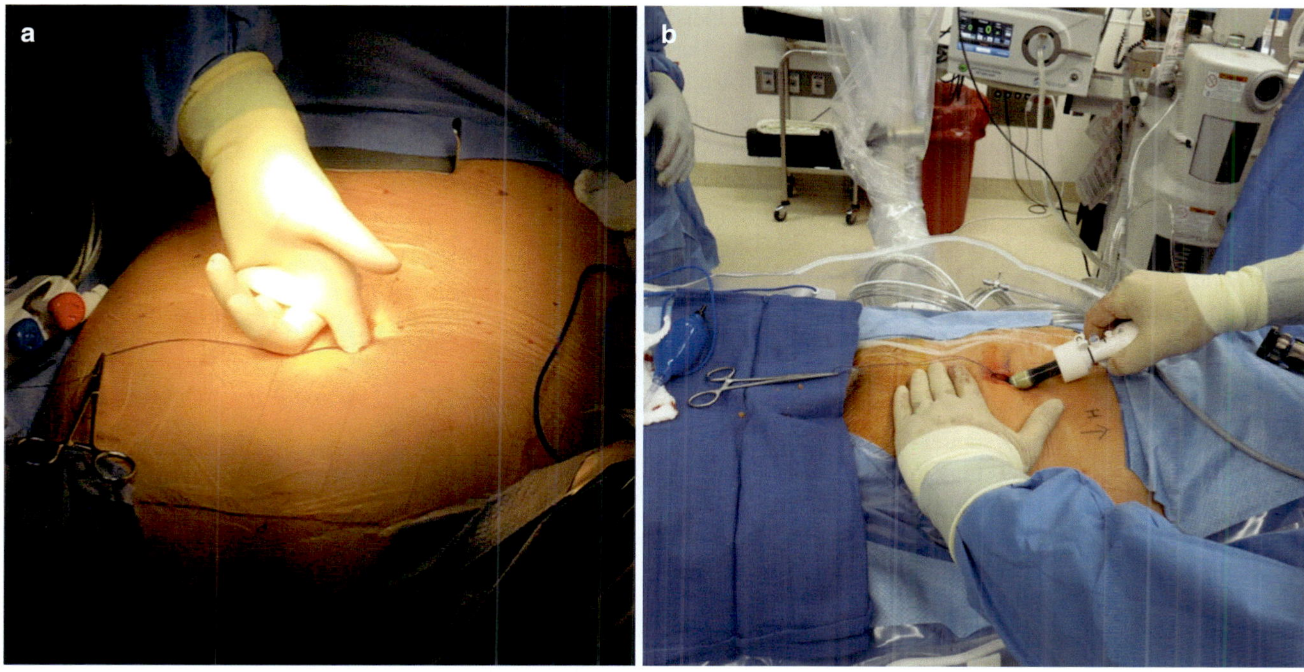

Fig. 36.3 Blunt finger dissection is used to open the initial space down to the pubic bone (**a**). Next, the balloon dilator is inserted and advanced below the pubic bone into the space of Retzius (**b**). Development of extraperitoneal space

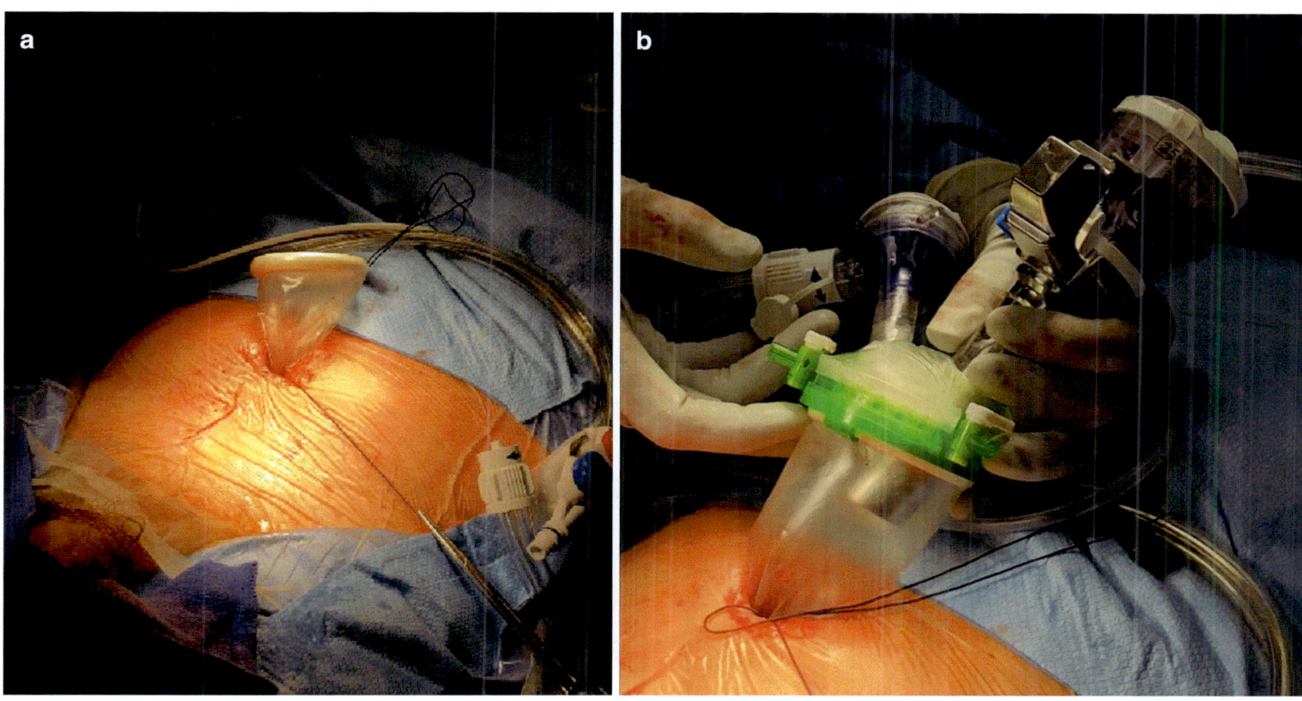

Fig. 36.4 A wound retractor is inserted through the incision so that the inner ring is within the space of Rezius (**a**). Next, (**b**) the ports and ROSI suction are inserted through the Gelpoint and attached to the wound retractor. Floating dock technique

peritoneal space. To provide for an adequate working distance for the SP robotic arms to "fan" out and avoid internal clashing, the "floating dock" technique is applied [13], using a combination of an Alexis wound retractor and a GelPoint Mini (Applied Medical, Similarly, the "floating dock" allows for the omission of a separate lateral assistant port which reduces the incisional burden as well as reduces the likelihood of accidental entry into the peritoneum. The inner ring of the wound retractor is placed below the level of the fascia and into the developed extraperitoneal space (Fig. 36.4a). Next, the 25-mm SP multichannel port, 12-mm Airseal (CONMED, Largo, FL) assistant port, and a ROSI (Remotely Operated Suction Irrigation, Vascular

Technology Inc., Nashua, NH) flexible suction tubing are individually inserted through the GelPOINT cap and insufflate the extraperitoneal space to a pressure of 12 mmHg (Fig. 36.4b).

The SP robot is then side-docked and attached to the multichannel SP port. The SP instruments are brought into the wound retractor by the bedside assistant with the camera (up), monopolar scissor (right), Caidere grasper (left), and the Maryland bipolar (down) positions (Fig. 36.5). The surgeon on the console then brings the robotic arms through the fascia and into the extraperitoneal space. The ROSI flexible suction tubing is activated with a foot pedal by the bedside assistant but controlled entirely by the console surgeon. We typically will hold the ROSI tubing with the Maryland bipolar arm to allow for active suctioning and simultaneous retraction throughout the case (Fig. 36.6).

The extraperitoneal space development continues, exposing and removing the periprostatic fat to reveal the endopelvic fascia and bladder neck. For the remainder of the operation, we attempt to replicate the steps of the standard multiport or SP RARP, next incising the endopelvic fascia and releasing the puboprostatic ligaments.

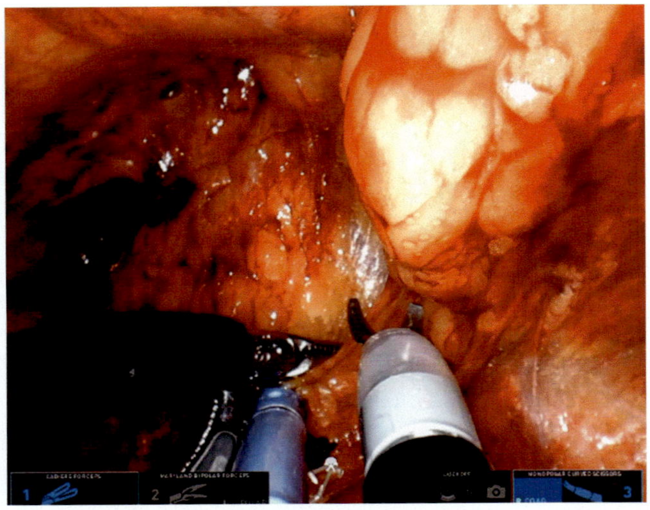

Fig. 36.6 Continuous use of ROSI as suctioning and retractor

Bladder Neck Transection, Seminal Vesicle and Vasa Deferentia Dissection

In the standard fashion, using the Maryland bipolar and ROSI suction to retract the bladder cranially, the anterior bladder neck is opened, revealing the foley catheter (Fig. 36.7a). The urethral catheter is deflated and lifted anteriorly using the Cadiere grasper to provide sufficient anterior traction for the posterior bladder neck dissection (Fig. 36.7b).

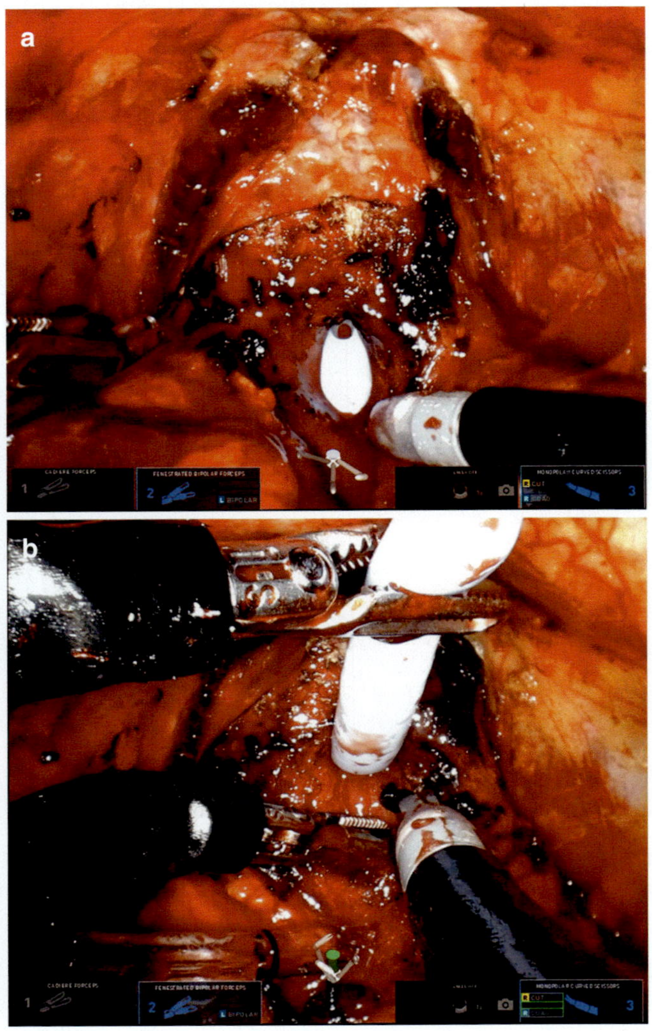

Fig. 36.7 The anterior bladder neck is opened (**a**) so that the foley catheter is visible. Next, (**b**) the catheter is retracted anteriorly using the Cadiere grasper to allow for transection of the posterior bladder neck. Bladder neck transection

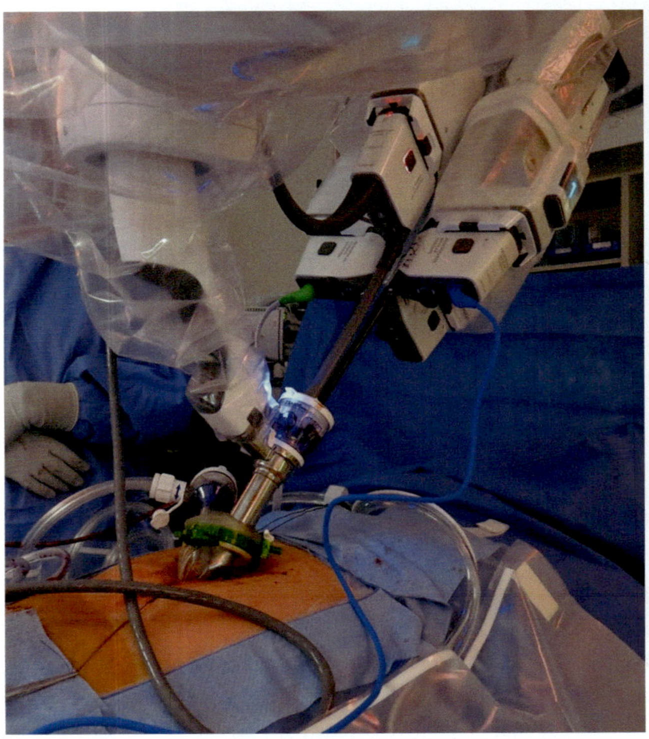

Fig. 36.5 SP robotic docking and instrument insertion

The posterior bladder neck dissection proceeds to reveal the vasa deferentia and seminal vesicles. Lifting anteriorly with the Cadiere, the bilateral vasa and seminal vesicles are dissected free, minimizing the use of electrocautery. The vascular supply to the seminal vesicles are ligated with Weck clips using the SP robotic clip applier (Fig. 36.8). Next, the posterior plane is developed to the prostatic apex, lifting the seminal vesicles anteriorly.

Ligation of the Prostatic Vascular Pedicles and Nerve Sparing

Following the opening of the posterior plane, the ligation of the vascular pedicles to the prostate and nerve sparing is performed. Using the Cadiere to lift the prostate anterolaterally, the vascular pedicles are clipped with the robotic clip applier, continuously switching with the monopolar scissors by the bedside assistant (Fig. 36.9). The limit operative time waste during this step, the bedside assistant will need to be efficient with the SP instrument exchange and anticipate the need for a robotic clip. A primary limitation of the SP platform is the reduction in arm strength relative to the multiport robotic platforms. During the vascular pedicles, it may be difficult to create a packet for clipping for larger packets and those patients with thicker peri-prostatic tissue. To overcome this difficulty, we suggest reducing the thickness and size of packets when necessary, maximizing the anterior retraction with the Cadiere grasper, and judicious use of bipolar electrocautery particularly when far away from the neurovascular pedicles. The nerve sparing proceeds towards the apex following the release of the neurovascular bundles on the lateral aspect of the prostate.

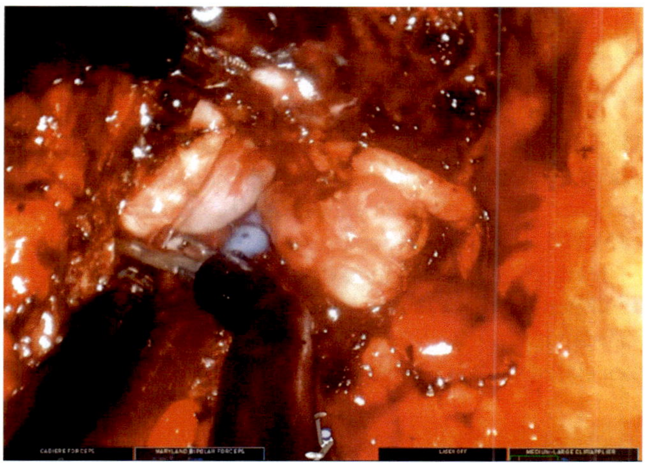

Fig. 36.8 Seminal vesicle dissection

Apical Attachments and Urethral Division

Once the vascular pedicles are released and the nerve sparing has reached the apex, the dorsal venous complex is ligated with a 0-vicryl suture (Fig. 36.10). The prostatic apex and urethra is divided, preserving maximal urethral length. The final apical and posterior attachments are divided, fully releasing the prostate which is temporarily placed cranially. At this time suction tubing is attached to the urethral catheter which is used for the remainder of the case as a dual suctioning device (Fig. 36.11a and b).

Next, the pelvic lymphadenectomy begins, rotating the SP boom laterally towards the pelvic sidewall. The peritoneum is gently released laterally and cranially, avoiding an unintended peritonotomy which can result in transperitoneal insufflation. A standard template pelvic lymphadenectomy is performed, often requiring repositioning of the flexible camera using the "cobra" function to optimize visibility. Lymphatics are clipped again using the SP robotic clip applier as needed.

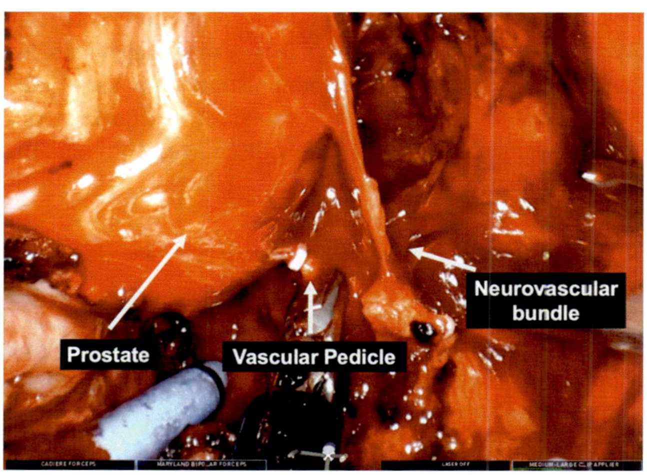

Fig. 36.9 Ligaion of vascular pedicles

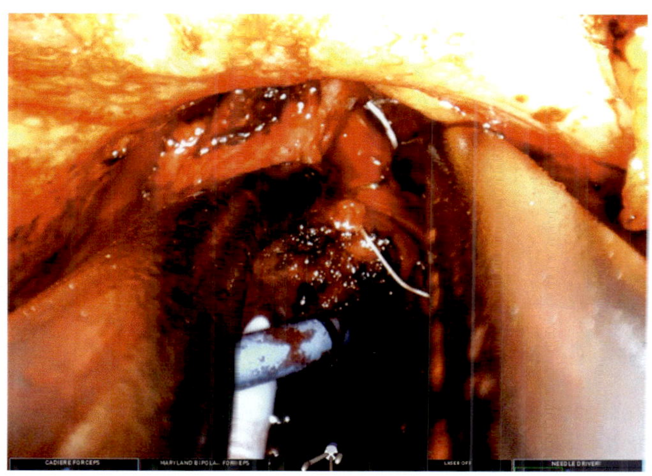

Fig. 36.10 Ligation of the dorsal venous complex

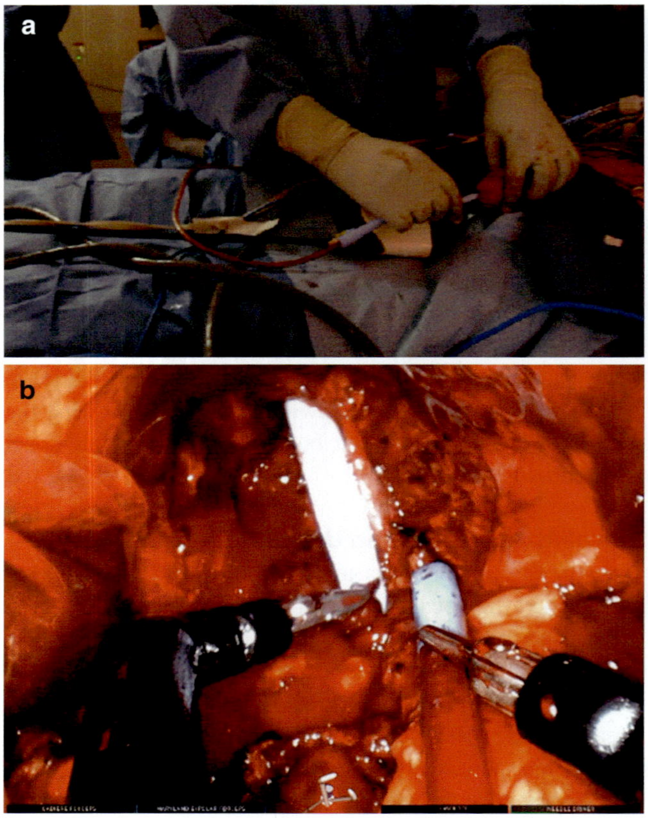

Fig. 36.11 The urethral catheter is attached to continuous suction to allow for a second suctioning device (**a**) which is directed using the SP instuments (**b**), particularly during the anastomosis. Use of urethral catheter as suctioning device

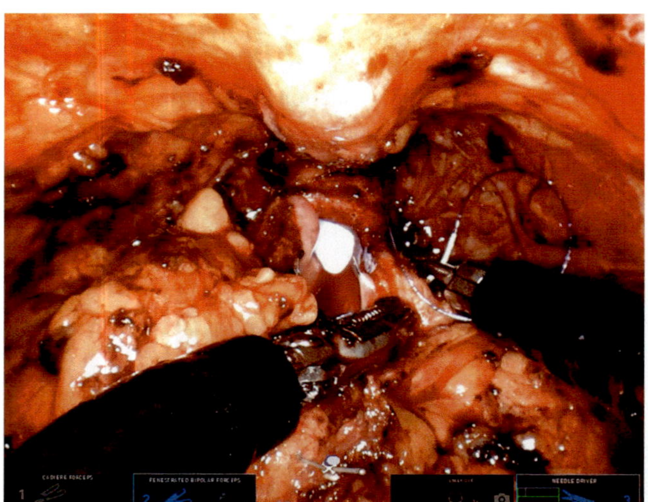

Fig. 36.12 Vesicourethral anastomosis

Vesicourethral Anastomosis, Extraction, and Closure

Next, our attention is turned to the vesicourethral anastomosis which begins with a posterior reconstruction in a "Rocco" fashion using 4–0 V-lok sutures in a running fashion (Fig. 36.12).

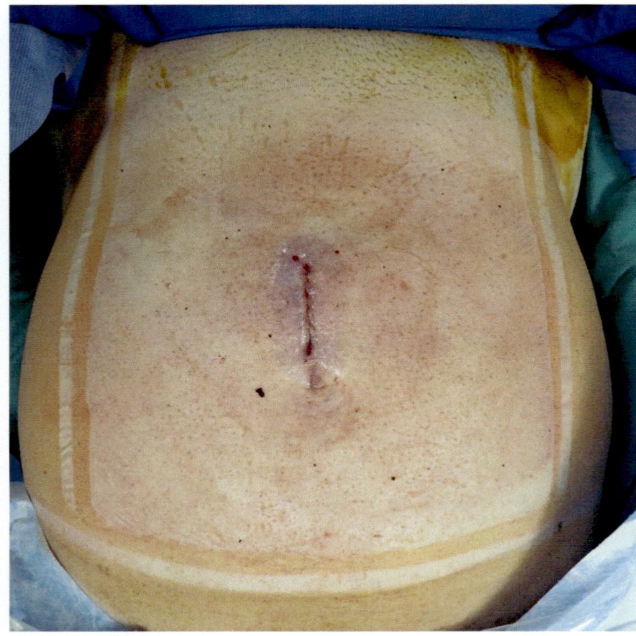

Fig. 36.13 Final incision

The anastomosis is tested to ensure it is water-tight and 15 cc is placed in the catheter balloon. The lymph nodes and the prostate specimen are placed in an endocatch bag and the SP robot is undocked. The wound retractor and specimen bag are removed. At this time, to prevent lymphocele formation postoperatively, a small peritoneal window is made to allow for transperitoneal reabsorption of the accumulating fluid. The fascia and skin are then closed without placement of a drain (Fig. 36.13).

Postoperative

Postoperative care is similar to our standard post-prostatectomy care. Patients are transported to a postoperative recovery area to evaluate if they will be candidates for same-day discharge. Opioid administration is used judiciously and only after NSAIDs are unable to adequately control pain. Patients are not routinely discharged with opioids. Urethral catheters are continued for 5–7 days.

Outcomes

From the vast RARP experience using multiport platforms prior to the introduction of the SP, the outcomes of the extraperitoneal robotic radical prostatectomy has been well-studied and extensively compared to the transperitoneal approach [5]. Additionally, our institution have reported on the early perioperative, oncologic, and functional outcomes with the SP extraperitoneal approach which have been overwhelmingly favorable relative to the transperitoneal approach [9, 11]. Still, our outcomes are maturing and our experience thus far is an improvement in overall outcomes as the learning curve is surpassed. The SP extraperitoneal approach has clear advantages over the transperitoneal approach, chiefly in the intraoperative and perioperative period, which has reduced the morbidity of the operation.

Intraoperative and Perioperative

Prior to the SP experience, multiport extraperitoneal radical prostatectomy was found to have significantly reduced operative times, less blood loss, and shorter hospital stay relative to the transperitoneal approaches [3–5]. In our SP extraperitoneal experience, relative to the SP transperineal approach, we identified similar benefits. Operative times were significantly less in the SP extraperitoneal group by over 45 minutes (201 ± 37.5 vs 248.2 ± 42.3 minutes, $p < 0.00001$), likely due to the lack of a need to lyse bowel adhesions or drop the bladder [9]. Time saved with the SP extraperitoneal approach also likely occurs during extraction and closure, not requiring any time to extend the fascial incision or close additional robotic or assistant ports. Additional measurable differences include a dramatic reduction in postoperative pain as measured by a reduced need for opioids in the extraperitoneal group (30.8% versus 95.6%, $p < 000001$) [9], likely the result of the discomfort related to peritoneal insufflation, bowel irritation, and steep Trendelenburg [6]. Relative to the multiport approaches, the SP reduction in pain likely can be also accounted for by a reduction in the ports and incisional burden as well as our practice of not leaving a postoperative drain. The summation of these benefits translates to a reduced hospital length of stay (4.3 vs 25.7 h $p < 0.0001$), which accounts for an impressive 88% same-day discharge rate, opening the door for a routine outpatient radical prostatectomy [8, 9, 13]. In a similar study, comparing 100 patients who underwent SP extraperitoneal prostatectomy to 110 patients who had a multiport transperitoneal RARP, SP extraperitoneal prostatectomy had dramatically reduced postoperative pain scores as well as half the rate of requiring opioids during their hospitalization (32% vs 63.6%, $p < 0.001$) as well as at discharge (35% vs 87.3%, $p < 0.001$) [13].

Other unmeasurable perioperative benefits include the reduction in the rate of unintended transperitoneal insufflation relative to the multiport extraperitoneal experience. Anecdotally, we believe that placement of the lateral robotic and assistant ports in the multiport approach account for the majority of accidental insufflation into the peritoneum, which greatly increases the difficulty of the operation and requires steep Trendelenburg to mitigate.

Oncologic

The long-term oncologic outcomes of the multiport extraperitoneal experience are well-documented and equivalent to standard transperitoneal multiport RARP in the literature, including the rates of positive surgical margins and biochemical recurrence. In our early SP extraperitoneal series, we similarly have shown favorable early oncologic outcomes. In our series, we reported no difference in rates of positive surgical margins (26.9% vs 41.3%, $p = 0.13$) or 90-day undetectable PSA (94.2% vs 84.2%, $p = 0.12$) relative to the SP transperitoneal approach. Notably, over 80% of patients who had positive surgical margins had high risk features (extraprostatic extension, Gleason score 8–10 or positive nodes) on final surgical pathology [9]. A primary critique of the extraperitoneal approach, however is the reduced ability to perform an extended lymph node dissection, which some have reported a reduced nodal yield. A large meta-analysis of nearly 4000 patients, however demonstrated no significant difference between nodal yield comparing extraperitoneal versus transperitoneal. Similarly, in our large series comparing SP to multiport transperitoneal RARP, there was no difference in the lymph node yield (5 vs 6 nodes, $p = 0.32$) or rate of positivity (4% vs 7%, $p = 0.42$) between the two approaches [11]. At 12 months, there were similar rates of biochemical recurrence, however there was a trend favoring a reduced biochemical recurrence rate for the SP extraperitoneal prostatectomy (3% versus 9%, $p = 0.052$). Because the SP platform offers an ability to replicate the oncologic principles of the traditional extraperitoneal and transperitoneal approach, it is not surprising that the early oncologic outcomes are equivalent to the SP and multiport transperitoneal approaches.

Functional

The early functional outcomes for the SP extraperitoneal approach were favorable and comparable to traditional approaches. It is our opinion that the SP extraperitoneal approach replicates the ability to perform nerve-sparing, create a tight bladder neck, and preserve urethral length for the preservation of erectile function and continence. Our institution has demonstrated similar continence and erectile function outcomes compared to the SP and multiport transperitoneal approach. The continence rate, defined as no pads or 1 safety pad, was 69%, 80%, and 85% at 3, 6, and 12 months, respectively, which was not significantly different from the multiport approach of 73.2%, 84%, and 87.8%, respectively. Importantly, this study represents the early experience of our first 100 cases. Currently, we have completed over 200 cases and our updated outcomes will soon be published. Longer follow-up is needed to assess the rate of post-prostatectomy incontinence as well as intervention rate of these patients to truly assess continence outcomes.

The SP extraperitoneal approach does not limit the ability to perform a nerve sparing procedure, as evidenced by the high rate of nerve sparing reported. Including those patients who had a preoperative SHIM >21, 70% versus 63% of patients reported no erectile dysfunction and 50% versus 38% of patients reported mild to moderate erectile dysfunction at 12 months for patients undergoing SP extraperitoneal prostatectomy and multiport transperitoneal prostatectomy, respectively [9, 11]. Longer follow-up and a more in-depth assessment of erectile function after SP extraperitoneal radical prostatectomy is warranted before conclusions can be drawn.

Complications

Previous literature comparing multiport extraperitoneal approaches to transperitoneal radical prostatectomy have demonstrated a few differences in the patterns of complications between the two approaches. While there is no significant difference in total complications between the approaches (RR 0.6, 95% CI 0.3, 1.2, $p = 0.12$)., there was a significantly decreased risk of ileus (RR 0.2, 95% CI 0.1, 0.7, $p = 0.009$) and inguinal hernia formation (RR 0.2, 95% CI 0.1, 0.5, $p = 0.001$) compared to the transperitoneal approach [5]. Notably, however, it is well-documented that the extraperitoneal approach results in greater rates of symptomatic lymphoceles (RR 1.8, CI 1.0, 3.3, $p = 0.05$), likely related to the confined space and reduction in reabsorption of lymphatic fluid in the extraperitoneal compartment compared to the peritoneum [8]. Our very initial series of SP extraperitoneal prostatectomy similarly experienced a higher rate of lymphoceles requiring interventional radiology drain placement (6 patients versus 1 patient) [9]. To prevent accumulation of lymphatic fluid in the extraperitoneal space, we adjusted our technique to include fenestration of the peritoneum at the completion of the case to allow for transperitoneal reabsorption of the lymphatic fluid to prevent lymphocele accumulation and subsequent infection. Since we have made this modification, we have not experiences any symptomatic lymphoceles.

Conclusions

The SP extraperitoneal prostatectomy represents an important iteration in the quest to minimize the morbidity of the surgical management of prostate cancer. The combined benefits of the SP platform and the extraperitoneal approach has permitted a dramatic improvement of the perioperative recovery, reducing postoperative pain and need for opioids, allowing for routine outpatient radical prostatectomy to be considered. Early outcomes are exceedingly favorable, however longer follow-up will need to be required to evaluate oncologic and functional outcomes.

References

1. Garisto J, Bertolo R, Reese SW, Bove P, Kaouk J. Minimizing minimally invasive surgery: current status of the single-port robotic surgery in urology. Actas Urol Esp. 2021;45(5):345–52.
2. Akand M, Erdogru T, Avci E, Ates M. Transperitoneal versus extraperitoneal robot-assisted laparoscopic radical prostatectomy: a prospective single surgeon randomized comparative study. Int J Urol. 2015;22(10):916–21.
3. Lee JY, Diaz RR, Cho KS, Choi YD. Meta-analysis of transperitoneal versus extraperitoneal robot-assisted radical prostatectomy for prostate cancer. J Laparoendosc Adv Surg Tech A. 2013;23(11):919–25.
4. Madi R, Daignault S, Wood DP. Extraperitoneal v intraperitoneal robotic prostatectomy: analysis of operative outcomes. J Endourol. 2007;21(12):1553–7.
5. Uy M, Cassim R, Kim J, Hoogenes J, Shayegan B, Matsumoto ED. Extraperitoneal versus transperitoneal approach for robot-assisted radical prostatectomy: a contemporary systematic review and meta-analysis. J Robot Surg. 2022;16(2):257–64.
6. Sawczyn G, Lenfant L, Aminsharifi A, Kim S, Kaouk J. Predictive factors for opioid-free management after robotic radical prostatectomy: the value of the SP(R) robotic platform. Minerva Urol Nefrol. 2021;73:591–9.
7. Vigneswaran HT, Schwarzman LS, Francavilla S, Abern MR, Crivellaro S. A comparison of perioperative outcomes between single-port and multiport robot-assisted laparoscopic prostatectomy. Eur Urol. 2020;77(6):671–4.
8. Wilson CA, Aminsharifi A, Sawczyn G, Garisto JD, Yau R, Eltemamy M, et al. Outpatient extraperitoneal single-port robotic radical prostatectomy. Urology. 2020;144:142–6.
9. Kaouk J, Aminsharifi A, Wilson CA, Sawczyn G, Garisto J, Francavilla S, et al. Extraperitoneal versus transperitoneal single port robotic radical prostatectomy: a comparative analysis of perioperative outcomes. J Urol. 2020;203(6):1135–40.
10. Kaouk J, Valero R, Sawczyn G, Garisto J. Extraperitoneal single-port robot-assisted radical prostatectomy: initial experience and description of technique. BJU Int. 2020;125(1):182–9.
11. Lenfant L, Sawczyn G, Aminsharifi A, Kim S, Wilson CA, Beksac AT, et al. Pure single-site robot-assisted radical prostatectomy using single-port versus multiport robotic radical prostatectomy: a single-institution comparative study. Eur Urol Focus. 2021;7(5):964–72.
12. Schaeffer E, Srinivas S, Antonarakis ES, Armstrong AJ, Bekelman JE, Cheng H, et al. NCCN guidelines insights: prostate cancer, version 1.2021. J Natl Compr Cancer Netw. 2021;19(2):134–43.
13. Lenfant L, Kim S, Aminsharifi A, Sawczyn G, Kaouk J. Floating docking technique: a simple modification to improve the working space of the instruments during single-port robotic surgery. World J Urol. 2021;39(4):1299–305.

UIC Technique

37

Marcin Zuberek and Simone Crivellaro

Introduction

Radical prostatectomy has been in the armamentarium of urologists and has been used for over 100 years to treat different conditions affecting the prostate, mostly prostate cancer [1]. The original open approach has evolved over the years into laparoscopic and eventually robotic. Overall, the treatment of prostate cancer has recently been controversial due to long term health effects and questioning of the mortality of the disease. Since the advent of robotic surgery, the mortality of this operation has significantly decreased with a more favorable side effect profile. However, recent technical developments, such as single port surgery seem to have allowed to further decrease the invasiveness of this procedure. In this book chapter we will describe the robotic radical prostatectomy techniques utilized at University of Illinois Hospital and Health Science System. Particular relevance is given to the comparison of our techniques with previously available robotic techniques, how the advent of Single port robotic surgery pertains to patient care, and unique challenges that are faced while using the single port.

History

The first origins of robotic surgery begin around the 1980s with orthopedics and hip replacement. During this timeline there was a concurrent development of a robot for prostate surgery [2]. Neurosurgery and ENT were also working on their specific computer assistant surgery systems [2]. The original goal was to give doctors the ability to provide surgical care in theaters of war. The first touch system was the green telepresence surgery system developed by Stanford research institute or SRI [2]. This was considered the grandfather of the current surgical systems. The system was originally intended for open surgery, but it was quickly adapted towards laparoscopic surgery due to high-definition stereoscopic vision, trauma reduction dexterity, and decreasing human physical limitations. The SRI was the steppingstone for the private industry to develop initial endeavors into robotic applications for commercial use. The first one was by computer motion in 1992 where Dr. Wang created a robot—AESOP—which obtained the FDA clearance for use in human beings [3] (Fig. 37.1). The surgical system used voice

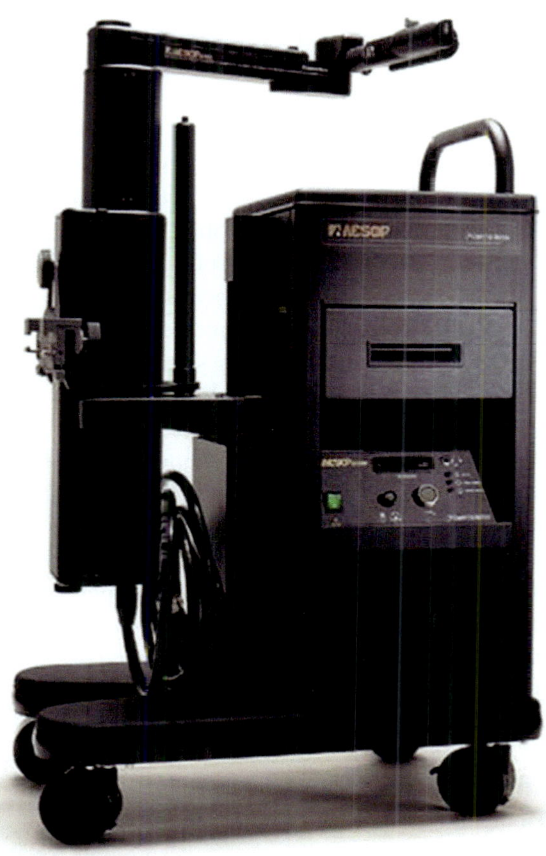

Fig. 37.1 AESOP Robotic System

M. Zuberek (✉) · S. Crivellaro
The University of Illinois Hospital & Health Sciences System, Chicago, IL, USA
e-mail: crivesim@uic.edu

S. Ren et al. (eds.), *Robot-Assisted Radical Prostatectomy*, https://doi.org/10.1007/978-3-031-05855-4_37

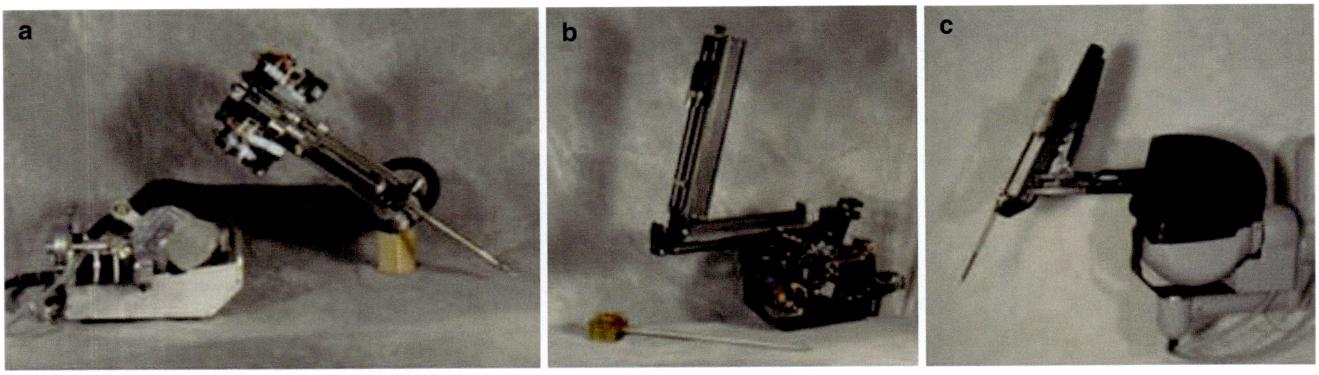

Fig. 37.2 LENNY Robotic System

commands for manipulation. The system went through multiple iterations and the final version was named Zeus which was intended for thoracic surgery. In 1995 Dr. Mo and Dr. Freund created Intuitive surgical and the first prototype named Lenny was built from the SRI's intellectual property and added a 7° of freedom with grasping [2] (Fig. 37.2). Intuitive went through several iterations as well, adding exchange of instruments mechanism, stereoscopic visualization, and improving the patient positioning. This evolution led to the first usable and commercialized prototype of the da Vinci surgical system. Human trials for the system happened in 1998 and were mostly conducted within the scope of thoracic surgery. Only in the year 2000 the da Vinci surgical system was able to be used for general surgeon cases in the United States as it obtained FDA approval. In 2003 the first prospective comparison of robotic assisted and retropubic prostatectomy was published, firmly cementing the technique in the arsenal of a modern urologist [4]. Until then, the only minimally invasive technique was laparoscopic radical prostatectomy, which had a difficult learning curve and less than optimal ergonomics providing significant burden to surgeon fatigue [5, 6]. Development of first da Vinci surgical systems allowed for the surgeon biomechanics to be optimal and patient outcomes to be significantly better than open or laparoscopic techniques. The main limitation of the robotic platform in obtaining complete remote control was the necessity of a trained assistant present for manipulation of the robot and appropriate surgical retraction. One of the goals of the current iteration of the da Vinci surgical system is attempting to bring complete independence to the surgeon through the single port platform.

Available Technology

Currently available robotic surgical systems allow for multiple degrees of freedom in the operating room theater. The market is dominated now by intuitive surgical and their da Vinci platform. Some companies such as CMR are already present with alternative choices and multiple other companies such as Medtronic and J&J are in the process of creating their own platforms. Previous generations of the da Vinci platform included the commercially available da Vinci Is and Si platforms. The inter-generational differences mostly included differences in patient positioning, surgical cart control, and surgeon visualization. The current da Vinci surgical system Xi further improves surgical cart positioning, customization of ergonomics for a given surgery type, and improvements in visualization. Introduction of the single port platform (available in the USA since 2019) allowed for a completely novel way of approaching robotic surgery. Instead of multiple arms as in the previous iterations of the da Vinci surgical system the surgical cart consists of a single boom with an extending single arm connected to a 27 mm trocar (Fig. 37.3). This trocar allowed for insertion of a camera and three articulated instruments. The new camera design allows for multiple degrees of freedom and angulation just like previous endowrist instruments. This differs from the previous generations, where the endoscope was rigid and controlled by the surgical arm. In this case the angulation is controlled by the surgeon at the console allowing for better and closer visualization of the surgical operative areas. Additionally, the novel camera system is in the proximity to the instruments allowing for access to more confined areas and cavities (like the posterior plane of prostatic resection) that were previously almost impossible to effectively reach without the help of the assistant retracting tissue. Bringing these features together advances the modern robotic surgeon closer to the ideal of performing independent and remote surgery, which was the original goal intended for these systems.

Patient Selection

As with all surgical procedures patient selection and exclusion is paramount for the success of the operation. The benefit of the single port platform allows for more versatile port

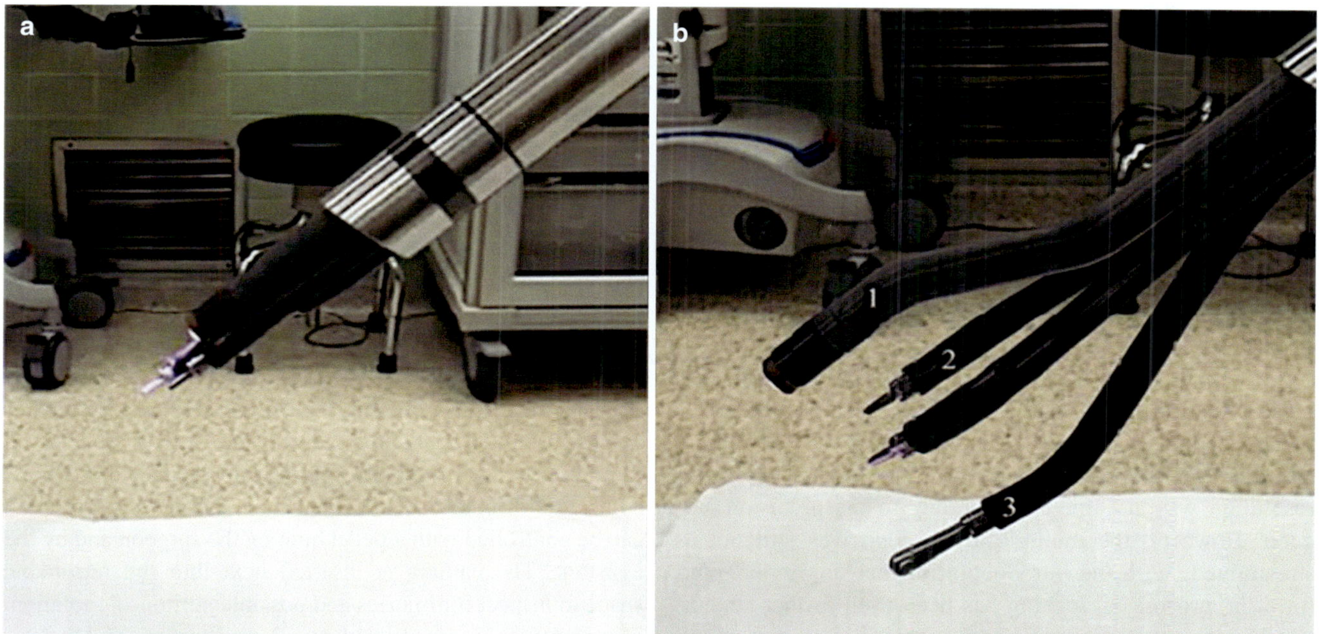

Fig. 37.3 Single Trocar System (**a**) Single Port Trocar with arms (**b**) Surgical instruments in the trocar (1) Camera (2) Needle Driver (3) Forceps

placement due to the instruments approaching the area of operation from a single point instead of multiple entry points. The flexible camera, controlled by the surgeon, and a single trocar allow for unprecedented versatility of the intraperitoneal surgical approach in patients with multiple surgical wounds where adhesions can prove difficult to conduct robotic procedures with multiple ports. Additionally, because of the smaller size and the superior performance in small spaces it allows the routine use of different anatomic approaches such as extraperitoneal or intravesical. Overall, it broadens the application of robotic surgery to multiple clinical situations, reducing absolute contraindications to an historical minimal number.

Financial Considerations

Currently robotic surgery is the standard of practice for radical prostatectomy. Earlier robotic surgical procedures were associated with longer operative time and hospital stays [7]. As the surgeons became more familiar with the robotic platform, operating rooms staff became more familiar with the technology, the hospital facilities became more familiar with instrument processing and consequently the operative times and hospital stays have decreased. However, with the previous generations of robotic platform outpatient setup was not common practice. With the advent of a single port robotic platform and a single incision there is a higher chance for the implementation of robotic surgery in a real outpatient setting [8, 9]. Ability of the surgeon to readily place a trocar externally to the peritoneum decreases the overall invasiveness of the procedure and the necessity for prolonged hospitalization. The initial cost of the disposable material associated with a single port platform is, as to be expected for new technologies, slightly higher than the previous generations. It has been shown though that the single port platform is overall cheaper or at least comparable to multiport when the length of stay and the operating room time is factored in [10]. The main concern in early users was the lack of sturdiness of the instruments. In our preliminary series of single port robotic cases compared to multiport robotic cases there was no significant difference in instrument damage or instrument replacement. With the decreased hospital stay, decreased operative time related to the faster set up, the faster recovery leading to decreased time off the initial and continuous cost of the new single port robotic platform can be offset in comparison to previous laparoscopic or open procedures.

Generational Difference

The generational difference between intuitive surgical systems that are currently used its increasing overtime. The first da Vinci S System presented the surgeon a unique challenge of proper cart positioning. The surgeon had to plan specifically ahead to decide where the surgical cart is going to be placed for what type of surgery. The surgical cart positioning was rather difficult as there was no targeting system, and the arms were difficult to manipulate. Additionally, the latching system of the surgical instruments was hard to engage. The camera resolution of the early systems, and poor visualization, was also contributing to the lack of optimization of the surgical technique [11–13]. The S was a good starting point for development of the Si System. The second generation of the da Vinci platform brought an improvement in visualization offering high-definition cameras and stereoscopic vision. The card maneuverability was improved, and the insertion system of the instruments was streamlined. The cart positioning was also improved by allowing a greater maneuverability by the surgical tech. The generational improvement to the Xi system proved paramount in terms of surgical planning and ease of setting up the system. The novel targeting system allows the surgeon to be worry free about location restraints as the cart was able to be brought to either side of the patient or between the legs. The viewer resolution was also increased adding to the precision surgeon. However, the multiple arm set up was still not as streamlined. With the introduction of the Single port platform the process of docking has been even further streamlined because of the use of a single cannula Port that allows insertion of Instruments from one central arm. There is only one attachment point between the surgical cart in the port itself. This facilitates the ease of targeting the necessary anatomy, allows for surgeon flexibility in port placement based on patient's previous surgical history, and allows for targeting multiple anatomical structures without the necessity of port replacement (i.e., during nephroureterectomy). The single arm construction allows for an even easier cart maneuvering making it even easier for the surgical staff to bring it to the targeted anatomy.

Current Surgical Set up

After standard general anesthesia has been given a 16 Fr Foley is placed in the urethra. Patient position varies depending on the approach and is described in the following sections (extraperitoneal and intraperitoneal retzius sparing). In order to obtain proper trocar placement a 3-cm incision has to be measured and made. Location of the incisions and trocar set up varies again based on the approach and it's described in detail in the following sections.

Radical Prostatectomy

Extraperitoneal (See Video)

The extraperitoneal approach is the preferred approach for SP radical prostatectomy at UIC. It has the benefit of potential same day discharge of the patient due to lack of violation of the peritoneum, faster bowel function return, no need of Trendelenburg and decreased invasiveness. The extraperitoneal approach requires the so-called "floating dock" which is described in detail. A 3 cm horizontal incision Is made approximately 4 fingerbreadth superior to the symphysis, 2 cm inferior to the umbilicus and carried down to the fascia. Fascia is incised. Blunt digital dissection of the retropubic space is carried out. If the patient is obese use of the space making balloon is warranted. The green circle of the Alexis retractor (Mini Gelpoint) is inserted into the retropubic space and the retractor itself is left unrolled. A 5 mm trocar (so-called sidecar) is inserted through the same skin incision, through a different fascial incision and through the plastic of the Alexis retractor (see Figs. 37.4 and 37.5). Eventually the gel cap of the Mini GelPoint is attached to the Alexis retractor and the robotic trocar and a 5 mm Airseal trocar are inserted through the gel. A remotely operated flexible suction (ROSI) is inserted through the side-car trocar, suction and irrigation can be controlled with a pedal both by the surgeon and by the assistant. The camera is inserted next into the retropubic space to inspect for injuries and possible peritoneal violation. The abdomen is insufflated to 12 millimeters of Mercury through the 5 airseal trocar. The robotic trocar is at this point docked to the robot itself completely outside of the abdomen, but still inside the vestibule created by the Mini Gel Point (hence floating dock). This setup allows the surgeon to decrease the length from the target required to articulate the instruments from 10 cm to at least half of it, making it possible to perform complex procedures in shallow spaces.

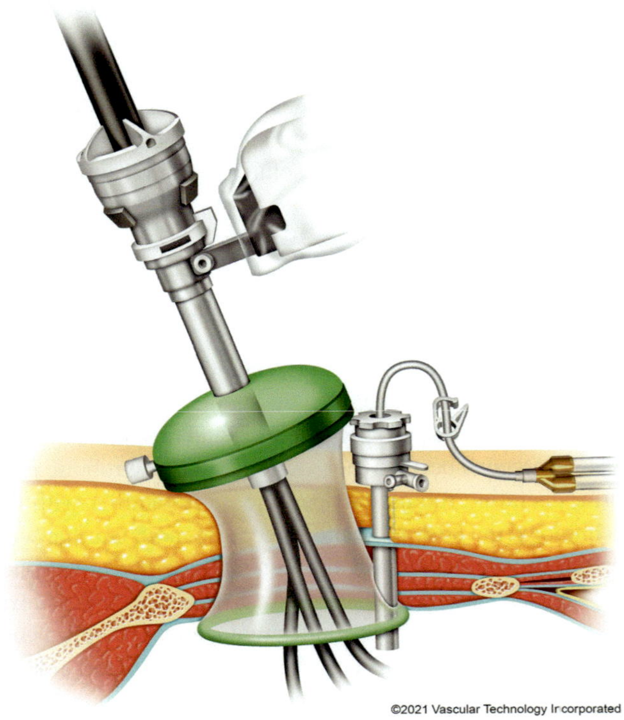

Fig. 37.4 Illustration of the GelPoint set up with side-car assistant port

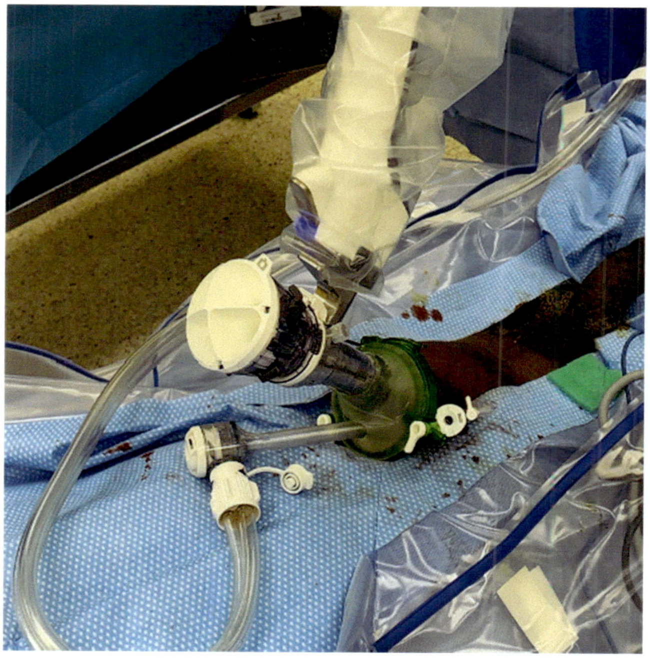

Fig. 37.5 GelPoint side-car in-vivo with 5 mm Airseal inserted through the gel to provide insufflation

The procedure starts with Monopolar scissors at 3 o'clock, Cadiere at 6 o'clock, and Fenestrated bipolar at 9 o'clock. Camera is at 12 o'clock. The relative position of the camera and the instruments can be checked in real time through the navigator. In regard to the camera position at the beginning of each surgical steps the surgeon needs to look for what is called "cobra mode", a particular position which gives the best possible visualization guaranteeing at the same time free movement of the instruments.

The first step of the procedure is to de-fat the prostate with a combination of bipolar retraction and mono polar blunt dissection is utilized to remove the excess fat from the prostate. After defatting the prostate, the endopelvic fascia is divided and separated from the prostate. This allows for the dorsal venous complex to be exposed and tied with a 2–0 vicryl on a SH needle. Note that RB1 and SH needles can easily be passed through the sidecar trocar or the robotic trocar itself after removal of one of the robotic instruments. The flexible camera allows an unprecedented view of the anterior prostate and identification of the correct resection plane. Once reaching the Foley catheter, the fenestrated bipolar and the cadiere are switched to put the foley itself on traction to further expose the posterior bladder neck. The bladder neck dissection is carried down until the Seminal vesicles are encountered. Again, the flexible camera is used to provide excellent visualization of the posterior dissection plane. After dissecting of deferens and seminal vesicles the instruments are flipped and the camera is moved from 12:00 o'clock to 6:00 o'clock position.

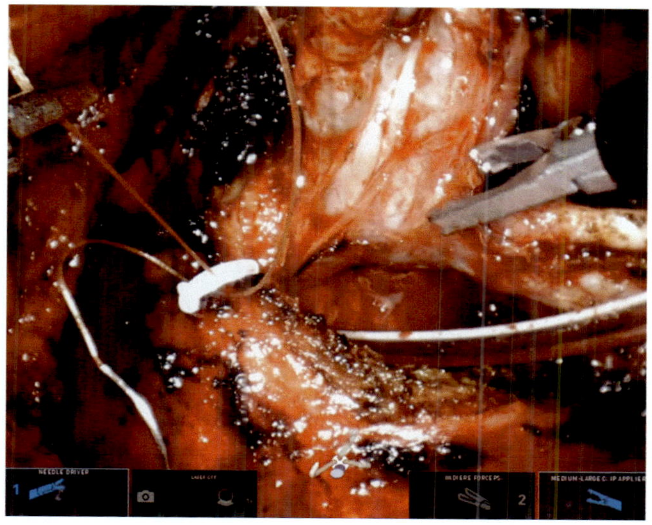

Fig. 37.6 Robotic Hemolock application

This allows the optimal dissection as the cadiere forceps is utilized to elevate the Seminal vesicles and provide traction to the posterior resection. The posterior plane is then developed using a combination of blunt and electrocautery. This is carried out until the apex of the prostate is reached. During this time again the flexible camera allows for the unprecedented view of the posterior of the prostate. At this point one can proceed in either the nerve sparing or not nerve sparing approach. The first one involves the use of a 2–0 vicryl, 15 cm long suture on an SH needle and a little loop at the end. The suture is passed around the base of the pedicle, through the loop and tied with a robotically applied medium-small hemolock (Fig. 37.6).

At that point the nerve sparing dissection is carried out with cold scissors at 3 o'clock and bipolar at 9'oclock.

Alternatively, the non-nerve sparing option will involve the use of the bipolar to coagulate the base of the pedicle and monopolar to section it all the way to the apex. At this point the camera is relocated again at 12 o'clock for the apical dissection (Fig. 37.7).

Cadiere is holding the base of the prostate at 6 o'clock, monopolar at 3 and bipolar at 9 are carrying out the dissection of the apex until the prostate is free. The prostate itself is placed to the side using the cadiere. The lymphadenectomy is carried out in a standard fashion using the relocation feature to reach proximally or medial as much as needed. The posterior reconstruction is performed with a 3–0 V-Loc suture, using 2 needle drivers at 3′ and 9′ while the cadiere at 6′ is holding the specimen proximally and on the side. A double armed 3–0 stratafix suture is used to complete a running anastomosis between urethra and bladder neck. Attention needs to be paid to the fact that the wrists of the SP instruments are not articulated, the elbow and the shoulder are (Fig. 37.8).

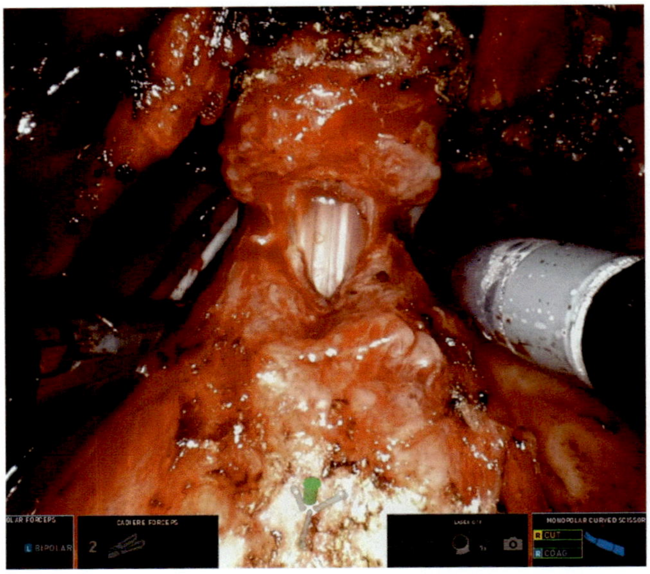

Fig. 37.7 Apical dissection of the prostate with the camera at 12 o'clock

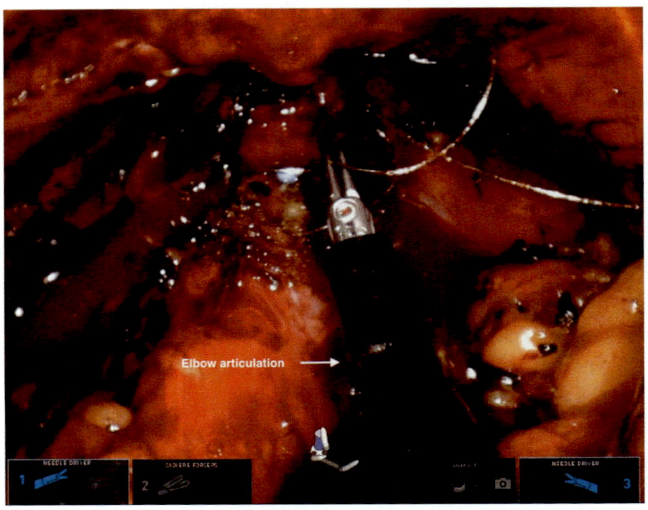

Fig. 37.8 Points of articulation of the robotic elbow on the DaVinci SP system

This produces the necessity of a minimal adjustment from the multiport version. Once the SP platform is undocked, the robotic trocar is removed from the gelpoint. A 5 mm laparoscopic camera is introduced through the 5 mm sidecar trocar. A laparoscopic grasper is used through the gelpoint to retrieve the lymphadenectomy packages. A 10 mm endobag is introduced through the gel as well to retrieve the prostate.

Intraperitoneal Retzius Sparing (Needs Video)

Retzius sparing radical prostatectomy allows for dissection of the pedicles as a first step, minimal manipulation of the bladder neck and total respect for the periprostatic structures. The entire prostatectomy is performed from the Douglas cavity in a very limited space, which is specifically the perfect environment for the Single Port platform. Thanks to the flexible camera, the possibility of relocating camera and instruments around its axis and smaller footprint Single Port make this otherwise technically challenging technique much more approachable.

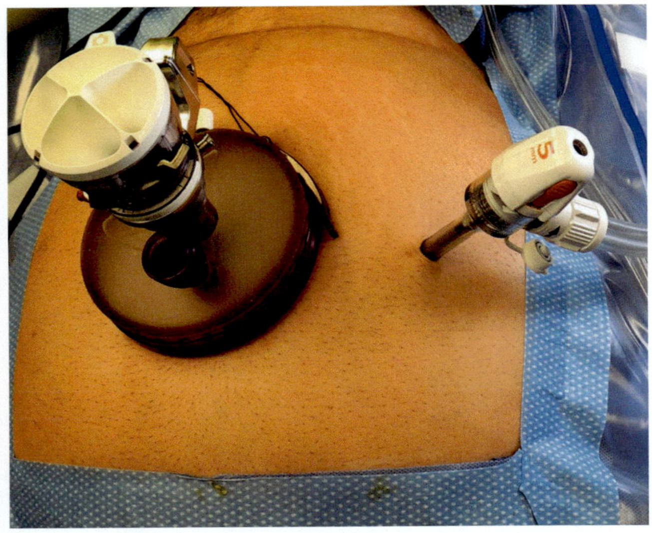

Fig. 37.9 Trocar positioning for the retzius sparing prostatectomy. Please note the difference between the side-car and plus-one trocar placement

The access involves a 3 cm vertical incision above the umbilicus on the midline After access to the peritoneal cavity is gained through a Hasson technique a Mini Gel point Alexis retractor is inserted and rolled completely. The robotic trocar and the 5 mm Airseal trocar are inserted through the gel and the gel cap is connected to the Alexis. A "plus one" 5 mm airseal trocar is required for retzius sparing SP as it is a rigid suction (Fig. 37.9).

At this point the abdomen is insufflated at 12 mmHg, and the robotic trocar is docked. The instruments utilized for the surgery are mono polar scissors at 3 'BI polar fenestrated graspers at 9′, and cadiere grasper for retraction 12′. The camera is positioned from the beginning of the procedure at 6′. A 10 cm long peritoneal incision is performed at the bottom of the douglas cavity. Seminal vesicles and vases are dissected bilaterally and held up by the Cadiere at 12′. The posterior plane between prostate and rectum is developed with the instruments at 3′ and 9′ according to the plan of doing nerve or not nerve sparing. The right seminal vesicle is held by the cadiere at 12′ and the pedicle is clipped mediolaterally with 5 mm titanium clips applied by the assistant through the 5 mm lateral trocar (Fig. 37.10).

The distance from the prostate to where applying the clips marks the difference between nerve or not nerve sparing. In case the latter approach is required a plan lat-

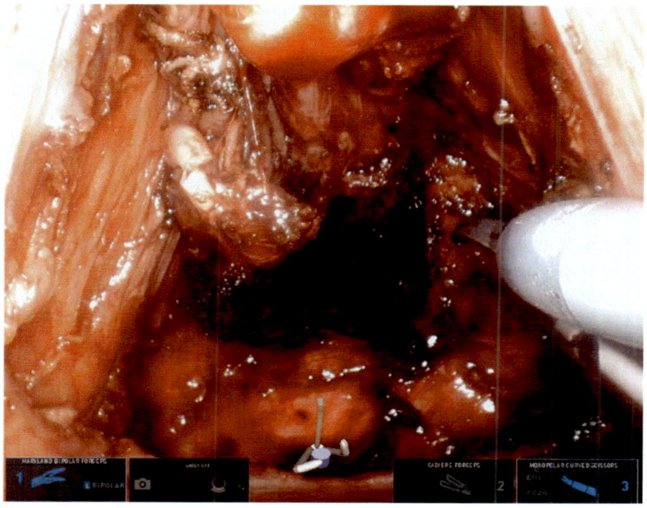

Fig. 37.10 Clip application by the assistant

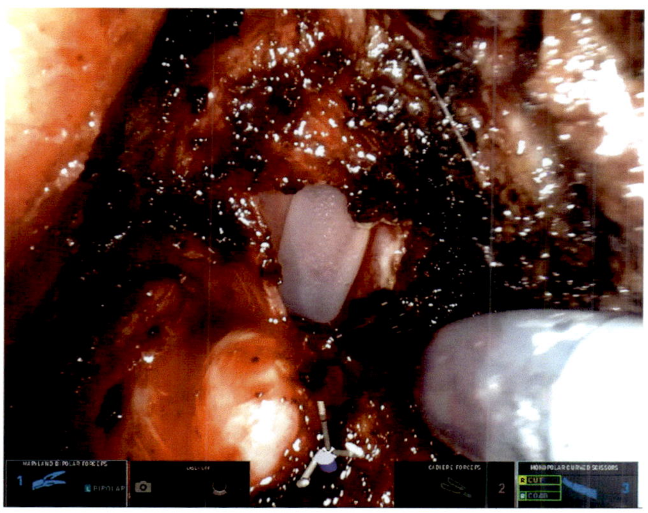

Fig. 37.11 Posterior bladder neck dissection

eral to the pedicle can be developed. It's imperative to have a good traction provided by the cadiere at 12′ in this phase. Similar maneuver is performed contralaterally. At this point attention is turned to the bladder neck with the same disposition of instruments and camera. The cadiere is holding up the bladder neck and the monopolar at bipolar carry on the posterior approach to the bladder neck itself (Fig. 37.11).

It's important in this phase to approach the bladder neck from lateral to medial and the traction provided at 12 o'clock by the cadiere is vital. Eventually the anterior prostate and the apex is dissected, and the prostatectomy is concluded. Pelvic lymphadenectomy is typically performed at this point with the same instrument location leaving the medial umbilical ligament intact. Anastomosis is performed in a running fashion with Stratafix 3/0 double arm starting from the anterior edge of the bladder neck. No posterior reconstruction is required. The flexible camera at 6 o'clock and the 12 o'clock cadiere for retraction are particularly useful to achieve a good visualization throughout the entire anastomosis. Once the robot is undocked, a 5 mm laparoscopic camera is introduced through the 5 mm plus one trocar and the specimen is retrieved via a laparoscopic grasper and a 10 endobag through the Gelpoint.

Post-operative Management

After an SP extraperitoneal or Retzius sparing prostatectomy, the drain is typically not placed and the patient is typically discharged the same day after ensuring in the post anesthesia care unit that he recovered well. Patients are discharged with a Foley catheter and a bag, minimal amount of opioid pain medication, bowel regimen, and instructions for follow up and return. The patient is seen in the clinic within 10–14 days to remove the catheter and then 14 days later to discuss the pathology report and further possible treatment or surveillance. We do not routinely order cystograms or retrograde urethrograms. However, if there is a question about the integrity of the anastomosis, intra-operative difficulty with bladder neck reconstruction, or unforeseen cystotomy, these patients will often obtain additional imaging prior to catheter or drain removal.

Conclusion

The UIC experience has shown that the single port platform makes the extraperitoneal and the retzius spring approach more feasible. The chance to perform different approaches in a safe and effective way gives the urologist the unique opportunity to adapt the technique to the anatomy of the patient, and not the other way around.

References

1. Sriprasad S, Feneley MR, Thompson PM. History of prostate cancer treatment. Surg Oncol. 2009;18(3):185–91. https://doi.org/10.1016/j.suronc.2009.07.001.
2. George EI, Brand TC, LaPorta A, Marescaux J, Satava RM. Origins of robotic surgery: from skepticism to standard of care. JSLS. 2018;22(4):e2018.00039. https://doi.org/10.4293/JSLS.2018.00039.
3. Mendivil A, Holloway RW, Boggess JF. Emergence of robotic assisted surgery in gynecologic oncology: American perspective. Gynecol Oncol. 2009;114(2 Suppl):S24–31. https://doi.org/10.1016/j.ygyno.2009.02.002.
4. Tewari A, Srivasatava A, Menon M, Members of the VIP Team. A prospective comparison of radical retro-

pubic and robot-assisted prostatectomy: experience in one institution. BJU Int. 2003;92(3):205–10. https://doi.org/10.1046/j.1464-410x.2003.04311.x.
5. Finkelstein J, Eckersberger E, Sadri H, Taneja SS, Lepor H, Djavan B. Open versus laparoscopic versus robot-assisted laparoscopic prostatectomy: the European and US experience. Rev Urol. 2010;12(1):35–43.
6. Vickers AJ, Savage CJ, Hruza M, Tuerk I, Koenig P, Martínez-Piñeiro L, Janetschek G, Guillonneau B. The surgical learning curve for laparoscopic radical prostatectomy: a retrospective cohort study. Lancet Oncol. 2009;10(5):475–80. https://doi.org/10.1016/S1470-2045(09)70079-8.
7. Chin JL, Luke PP, Pautler SE. Initial experience with robotic-assisted laparoscopic radical prostatectomy in the Canadian health care system. Can Urol Assoc J. 2007;1(2):97–101.
8. Vigneswaran HT, Schwarzman LS, Francavilla S, Abern MR, Crivellaro S. A comparison of perioperative outcomes between single-port and multiport robot-assisted laparoscopic prostatectomy. Eur Urol. 2020;77(6):671–4. https://doi.org/10.1016/j.eururo.2020.03.031.
9. Abaza R, Murphy C, Bsatee A, Brown DH Jr, Martinez O. Single-port robotic surgery allows same-day discharge in majority of cases. Urology. 2021;148:159–65. https://doi.org/10.1016/j.urology.2020.08.092.
10. Lenfant L, Sawczyn G, Kim S, Aminsharifi A, Kaouk J. Single-institution cost comparison: single-port versus multiport robotic prostatectomy. Eur Urol Focus. 2020;7(3):532–6. https://doi.org/10.1016/j.euf.2020.06.010.
11. Lanfranco AR, Castellanos AE, Desai JP, Meyers WC. Robotic surgery: a current perspective. Ann Surg. 2004;239(1):14–21. https://doi.org/10.1097/01.sla.0000103020.19595.7d.
12. Camarillo DB, Krummel TM, Salisbury J. Robotic technology in surgery: past, present, and future. Am J Surg. 2004;188(4):2–15. https://doi.org/10.1016/j.amjsurg.2004.08.025.
13. Ashrafian H, Clancy O, Grover V, Darzi A. The evolution of robotic surgery: surgical and anaesthetic aspects. Br J Anaesth. 2017;119:i72–84. https://doi.org/10.1093/bja/aex383.

38 Fudan Zhongshan Technique: Single-Port Suprapubic Transvesical Robotic Assisted Radical Prostatectomy

Shuai Jiang, Jiajun Wang, Yu Xia, Hang Wang, and Jianming Guo

Introduction

With the aging of the domestic population and lifestyle change, the incidence of prostate cancer is increasing year by year, and it has become one of the most common malignant tumors among men [1]. Robot-assisted laparoscopic radical prostatectomy showed advantages of less bleeding and faster recovery compared with open or laparoscopic radical prostatectomy, and it has become the first choice for radical prostatectomy [2–5]. The surgical approaches of conventional robot-assisted radical prostatectomy include transabdominal and extraperitoneal retropubic approaches. However, a considerable number of patients still suffer from complications such as urinary incontinence and sexual dysfunction after surgery [6–9].

In 2008, Desai et al. firstly reported single-port transvesical enucleation of the prostate (STEP) to treat benign prostatic hyperplasia (BPH) [10]. Their initial experience appeared encouraging that STEP could be applied for surgical treatment of large-volume BPH (>80 g) [10]. In 2011, Gao et al. firstly reported single-port transvesical laparoscopic radical prostatectomy (STLRP) for prostate cancer, and the initial results showed that STLRP can minimize the nerve injury and obtain better and faster postoperative functional recovery than intrafascial endoscopic extraperitoneal radical prostatectomy (IEERP), and may be an effective treatment for low-risk organ-confined prostate cancer [11]. In 2020, the same team of Gao et al. reported the long-term effect of STLRP on erectile function and urinary continence compared to IEERP [12]. They found STLRP can minimize the nerve injury and obtain better and faster postoperative functional recovery than IEERP, which indicated STLRP may be another effective treatment for low-risk organ-confined prostate cancer [12]. These previous studies suggest that the single port laparoscopic technique combined with transvesical approach to treat benign prostatic hyperplasia or prostate cancer is technically feasible, and may also have the advantages of less trauma, faster recovery, and improved urinary control. However, anastomosis in single port technique needs a long learning curve, which confines the spread of STLRP. Up until now, there is still no report on the application of robotic system combined with single port technique and transvesical approach in radical prostatectomy yet.

Zhongshan hospital Fudan University firstly applied single-port suprapubic transvesical robotic assisted radical prostatectomy (SPSV-RARP) in patients with organ-confined prostate cancer since 2019 [13]. All the SPSV-RARP operations were successfully performed, which showed technical feasibility. Most of the patients also achieved good 6-months urinary continence outcomes. Here we introduce the basic techniques of SPSV-RARP.

Patient Selection

Indications and Contraindications

SPSV-RARP should be performed in organ-confined prostate cancer.

Indications to SPSV-RARP include:

1. Pathologically confirmed prostate cancer
2. Clinically confined within the prostate (stage T1 or T2)
3. Gleason score ≤ 7
4. PSA <20 ng/mL

Contraindications to SPSV-RARP include:

1. Cancer extends beyond the margins of the prostate (T3 or T4)
2. Gleason score ≥ 8

S. Jiang · J. Wang · Y. Xia · H. Wang · J. Guo (✉)
Zhongshan Hospital Fudan University, Shanghai, China
e-mail: jmguo@fudan.edu.cn

S. Ren et al. (eds.), *Robot-Assisted Radical Prostatectomy*, https://doi.org/10.1007/978-3-031-05855-4_38

3. Suspicious lymphoid metastasis
4. Potential metastasis
5. Conventional contraindications to RARP procedures or anesthesia

Preoperative Evaluations

Preoperative evaluations for SPSV-RARP include:

1. Baseline clinical evaluation, including patient age, body mass index and DRE
2. Preoperative PSA level
3. Prostate volume
4. Pelvic MRI or CT
5. Prostate biopsy and Gleason score
6. ECT

Instrumentation

1. da Vinci HD Surgical System
2. Endowrist Maryland or Fenetrited bipolar forceps
3. Endowrist curved monopolar scissors
4. Endowrist large needle drivers
5. In Site Vision System with 30-degree lens
6. Single port multi-channel system: Beijing Hangtian Kadi Technology Development Institute single port kit (a single-use multi-channel laparoscopic surgical approach system), including both ends of the ring fixator and the middle multi-channel system, consisting of two 12 mm channels and two 8 mm channels.
7. 18-Fr three cava balloon urinary catheter
8. Polymer Ligating clips
9. 2–0/3–0 barb stitches anastomosis

Surgical Technique

Patient Positioning and Port Placement

The patient is taken the steep Trendelenburg position after general anesthesia, and underwent routine disinfection. A transverse incision is made 8 cm over the pubic symphysis. The length of the incision is around 3–4 cm. Fill the bladder with saline through the urinary catheter, and the bladder is found in extraperitoneal space. Insert a single port (HK-FDDC-4FGD, Beijing Hang Tian Technology R&D Institute) (Fig. 38.1a) to establish an pneumobladder. The da Vinci camera and arms were established through the ports on the single port. There were separate channels for insufflation and venting on the single port.

Circular Incision of the Bladder Neck

We observed the bladder neck through the bladder. The first step was to identify the border of the prostate. Next, we made a circular incision around the bladder neck. The ureteric orifices were clearly identified and protected. Then we divided the entire thickness of the posterior bladder neck close to the posterior lip of the prostate, and the vas deferens and seminal vesicles were exposed easily.

Dissection of Vas Deferens and Seminal Vesicles and Separation of Denonvillier's Fascia

We used the vas deferens and seminal vesicles as anatomical marks of Denonvillier's fascia. After the Denonvillier's fascia was incised, we separated Denonvillier's fascia along the posterolateral surface of the prostate to the prostatic apex, maintaining a completely intrafascial plane.

Separation of Lateral Ligaments and Nerve-Sparing

For separation of bilateral lateral ligaments, the incision of the bladder neck was deepened around the prostate border. The anterior and lateral space were divided along the prostate surface. The incision also provided additional space for critical dissection of the pedicles. Bilateral neurovascular bundles were clipped and anterograde cut by an intrafascial nerve-sparing approach with a combination of sharp and blunt dissection.

Control of the Dorsal Vein Complex (DVC) and Dissection of the Urethra

Deeper dissection was performed along the anterior surface of the prostate to expose the posterior dorsal vein complex. The puboprostatic ligaments were identified and divided by dissection close to the prostate surface. The DVC was then dissected ventrally in a ligation-free method, and the prostate apex was dissected dorsally to expose the underlying urethra. The anterior aspect of the urethra was incised with cold scissors, the tip of the urethral catheter was withdrawn, and the posterior urethral wall was transected sharply. Complete dissection of the prostate apex was accomplished in a retrograde way. The completely mobilized prostate was extracted into the bladder and examined grossly for adequacy of excision. We can remove the specimen from the single port in 1–2 min and rebuild the single port system very quickly.

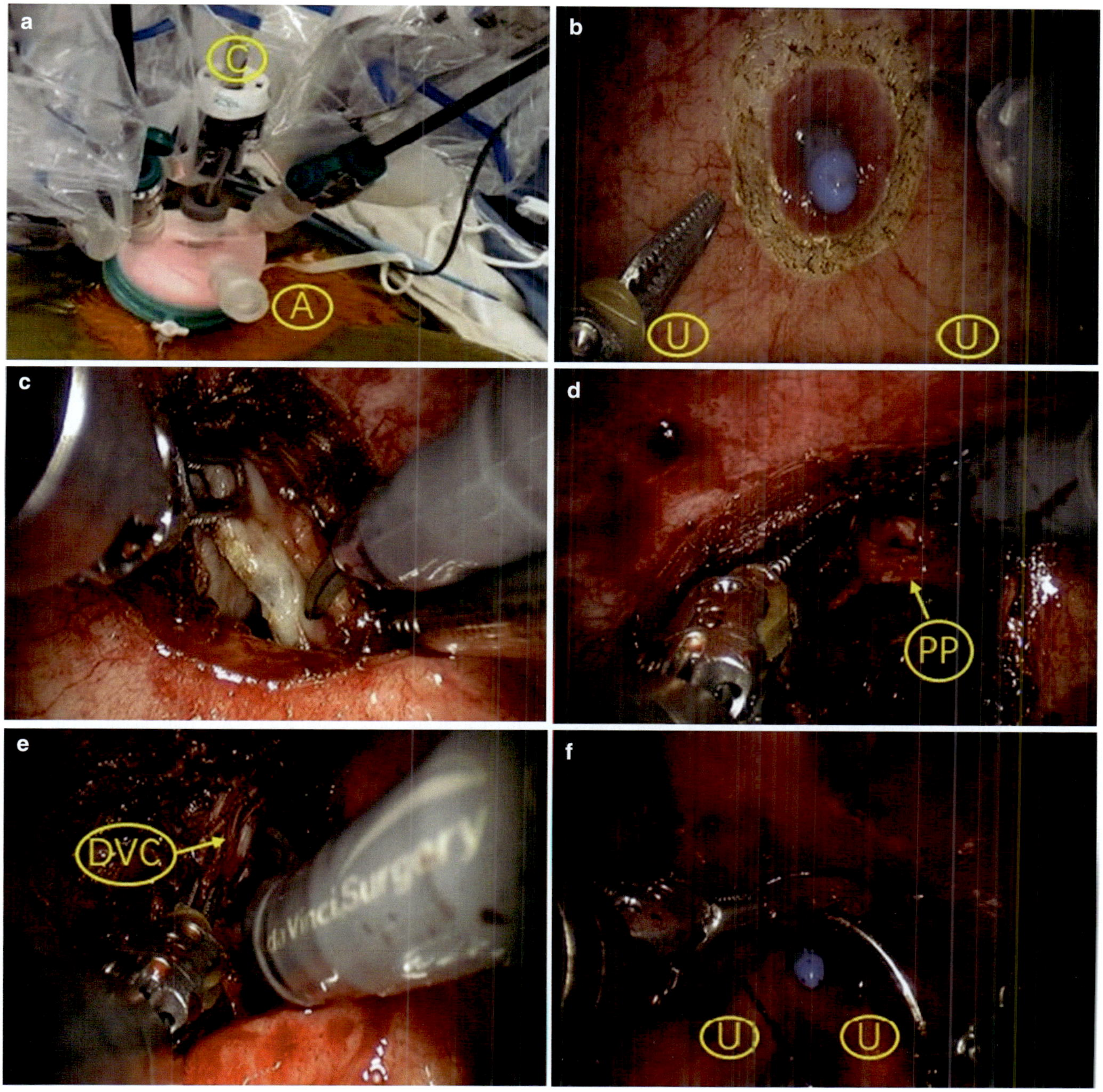

Fig. 38.1 Schematic diagram of surgical procedures. (**a**) Establishment of single port system. (**b**) Circular incision of the bladder neck. (**c**) Dissection of vas deferens and seminal vesicles. (**d**) Separation of lateral ligaments and nerve-sparing technique. (**e**) Dissection of the dorsal venous complex in a ligation-free approach. (**f**) Vesico-urethral anastomosis. *PP* prostate pedicle. *U* ureteric orifice. *DVC* dorsal venous complex

Vesico-Urethral Anastomosis

Bipolar coagulation was used to stop errhysis accurately on the wound surface. Bleeding on the NVB was sutured and ligated avoiding thermal injury. The bladder neck and urethra were anastomosed continuously with a 2–0 bidirectional barbed knotless absorbable suture, which maintains the running suture line tension. The first needle run clockwise from 6 to 12 o'clock. To promote the efficiency of the running sutures, the needles were passed outside-in the bladder and inside-out the urethra in one pass. Another needle at the other end of the barbed suture was run counterclockwise from 6 to 0 o'clock. The anastomosis was completed using the running suture, and the two ends of the suture were pulled out with an appropriate tension. Thus, a complete vesico-urethral mucosa approximation was achieved. An 18-Fr three-lumen Foley urinary catheter was then introduced into the bladder under direct laparoscopic monitoring. All the instruments were withdrawn from the single-port channel. The bladder wall incision was closed with a 2–0 barbed knotless absorbable suture. The wound was closed layer by layer with absorbable thread, and no drainage tube or bladder fistula was used.

Discussion

With the gradually popularity of Da Vinci robotic surgery, more and more centers have performed robotic surgery. The Da Vinci robotic surgical techniques were also improved in China in the recent years. Our institute firstly performed RARP in 2009, and we are still carrying out improvements of the surgical techniques.

The conventional approach for radical prostatectomy is the retropubic approach [14]. This approach is familiar to most urologists, and has become the classic approach for radical prostatectomy. However, this procedure destroys pelvic structures around the prostate, and may affect postoperative urinary control and sexual function [14]. Conventional laparoscopic or robotic-assisted radical prostatectomy requires 4 to 6 incisions, and the range of intraoperative separation is relatively large. In order to reduce trauma, single-port laparoscopic technology is gradually introduced for the field of radical prostatectomy. In 2008, Desai et al. reported transvesical single-port surgery for the treatment of benign prostatic hyperplasia, which obtained preliminary experience [10]. Afterwards, they completed 2 cases of transvesical robot-assisted radical prostatectomy for prostate cancer on the cadaver [15]. In China, Gao et al. began to explore transvesical single-port laparoscopic radical prostate cancer surgery in 2011 and accumulated preliminary experience [11, 12]. However, single-port laparoscopic technology has a long learning curve and requires special equipment assistance. Moreover, the vesico-urethral anastomosis procedure is relatively difficult to operate during single-port laparoscopic radical prostatectomy, which affects the further promotion of single port technology.

Based on the relatively large number of robotic surgery experience at the early stage, our group firstly conducted a preliminary exploration of SPSV-RARP, which combined the advantages of single-port, trans-bladder approach and suprapubic robotic laparoscopic surgery [13]. In our preliminary experience, selected patients with prostate cancer (T1-2cN0M0) received SPSV-RARP. Since all cases of SPSV-RARP were performed successfully, we believe SPSV-RARP was technically feasible in all cases. The Perioperative and postoperative outcome indicated that SPSV-RARP was technically feasible and could achieved good 6-months urinary continence outcomes for patients with organ-confined prostate cancer. Compared with the traditional retropubic approach, SPSV-RARP showed several advantages: it maximally minimized the destruction of the structure around the prostate, its procedures were closer to the prostatic fibrous capsule, and it protects the surrounding structures such as blood vessels and nerves to the greatest extent. These advantages of SPSV-RARP may lead to lower rate of urinary incontinence or erectile dysfunction after surgery.

However, this new approach is relatively unfamiliar to urologists and requires higher level of evidence base data to prove its efficacy. Compared with the transperitoneal approach, the SPSV approach showed advantages such as less intestinal complications and faster recovery after surgery, especially in patients with extreme obesity or abdominal surgery history [16]. Traditional robotic laparoscopic surgery requires 5–6 incisions on the abdominal wall. The single-port technique only needs one incision, which further reduces trauma. However, due to the relatively smaller operating space, the flexibility and freedom of instruments and operation are greatly influenced.

The combination of the Da Vinci device and the single-port transvesical approach could lead to less trauma and more flexible operation. There is no need for drainage tube or bladder fistula after surgery, leading to less surgical trauma and less bleeding. After surgery, the patient's lower abdomen has only one small transverse incision of about 4 cm length, surpassing traditional open surgery or RARP. The patients started eating 4–6 h after surgery, and got out of bed at the same day of the surgery. The length of stay after surgery ranged from 1 to 4 days. The time for removal of the urinary catheter was 5–7 days after surgery. Nearly all patients could get rid of pad after 12 weeks of surgery, indicating that the operation had quicker recovery and better protection of urinary control. All tumor specimens had negative margins, and no patients had complications such as urinary fistula. The post-operative results were encouraging for further studies [13].

Conclusions

In conclusion, SPSV-RARP is technically feasible for patients with organ-confined prostate cancer, and achieved promising perioperative and postoperative outcomes. Longer survival and functional data and randomized prospective studies in larger cohorts are still needed for validations.

References

1. Siegel RL, Miller KD, Jemal A. Cancer statistics, 2020. CA Cancer J Clin. 2020;70(1):7–30. https://doi.org/10.3322/caac.21590.
2. Merseburger A, Herrmann T, Shariat S, Kyriazis I, Nagele U, Traxer O, et al. EAU guidelines on robotic and single-site surgery in urology. Eur Urol. 2013;64(2):277–91. https://doi.org/10.1016/j.eururo.2013.05.034.
3. Koizumi A, Narita S, Nara T, Takayama K, Kanda S, Numakura K, et al. Incidence and location of positive surgical margin among open, laparoscopic and robot-assisted radical prostatectomy in prostate cancer patients: a single institutional analysis. Jpn J Clin Oncol. 2018;48(8):765–70. https://doi.org/10.1093/jjco/hyy092.
4. Pompe RS, Beyer B, Haese A, Preisser F, Michl U, Steuber T, et al. Postoperative complications of contemporary open and robot-assisted laparoscopic radical prostatectomy using standardised reporting systems. BJU Int. 2018;122(5):801–7. https://doi.org/10.1111/bju.14369.
5. Miller J, Smith A, Kouba E, Wallen E, Pruthi RS. Prospective evaluation of short-term impact and recovery of health related quality of life in men undergoing robotic assisted laparoscopic radical prostatectomy versus open radical prostatectomy. J Urol. 2007;178(3 Pt 1):854–8.
6. Novara G, Ficarra V, Rosen R, Artibani W, Costello A, Eastham J, et al. Systematic review and meta-analysis of perioperative outcomes and complications after robot-assisted radical prostatectomy. Eur Urol. 2012;62(3):431–52. https://doi.org/10.1016/j.eururo.2012.05.044.
7. Ficarra V, Novara G, Ahlering T, Costello A, Eastham J, Graefen M, et al. Systematic review and meta-analysis of studies reporting potency rates after robot-assisted radical prostatectomy. Eur Urol. 2012;62(3):418–30. https://doi.org/10.1016/j.eururo.2012.05.046.
8. Novara G, Ficarra V, Mocellin S, Ahlering T, Carroll P, Graefen M, et al. Systematic review and meta-analysis of studies reporting oncologic outcome after robot-assisted radical prostatectomy. Eur Urol. 2012;62(3):382–404. https://doi.org/10.1016/j.eururo.2012.05.047.
9. Ficarra V, Novara G, Rosen R, Artibani W, Carroll P, Costello A, et al. Systematic review and meta-analysis of studies reporting urinary continence recovery after robot-assisted radical prostatectomy. Eur Urol. 2012;62(3):405–17. https://doi.org/10.1016/j.eururo.2012.05.045.
10. Desai MM, Aron M, Canes D, Fareed K, Carmona O, Haber G-P, et al. Single-port transvesical simple prostatectomy: initial clinical report. Urology. 2008;72(5):960–5. https://doi.org/10.1016/j.urology.2008.06.007.
11. Gao X, Pang J, Si-tu J, Luo Y, Zhang H, Li L-y, et al. Single-port transvesical laparoscopic radical prostatectomy for organ-confined prostate cancer: technique and outcomes. BJU Int. 2013;112(7):944–52. https://doi.org/10.1111/bju.12225.
12. Yang Y, Hou G, Mei H, Zhang X, Han X, Pang J, et al. The effect of single-port transvesical laparoscopic radical prostatectomy on erectile function and urinary continence compared to Intrafascial endoscopic extraperitoneal radical prostatectomy. Urol J. 2020;17(6):592–6. https://doi.org/10.22037/uj.v16i7.6355.
13. Jiang S, Xu P, Yao J, Zhao Q, Xia Y, Guo J. Preliminary report of suprapubic transvesical single-port robot assisted radical prostatectomy for prostate cancer. J Chin Clin Med. 2019;26(02):215–7. https://doi.org/10.12025/j.issn.1008-6358.2019.20190289.
14. Ficarra V, Novara G, Artibani W, Cestari A, Galfano A, Graefen M, et al. Retropubic, laparoscopic, and robot-assisted radical prostatectomy: a systematic review and cumulative analysis of comparative studies. Eur Urol. 2009;55(5):1037–63. https://doi.org/10.1016/j.eururo.2009.01.036.
15. Desai MM, Aron M, Berger A, Canes D, Stein R, Haber G-P, et al. Transvesical robotic radical prostatectomy. BJU Int. 2008;102(11):1666–9. https://doi.org/10.1111/j.1464-410X.2008.08004.x.
16. Ragavan N, Dholakia K, Ramesh M, Stolzenburg JU. Extraperitoneal vs. transperitoneal robot-assisted laparoscopic radical prostatectomy-analysis of perioperative outcomes, a single surgeon's experience. J Robot Surg. 2019;13(2):275–81. https://doi.org/10.1007/s11701-018-0850-1.

Part XII

Special Situations in RALP

Large Median Lobe: Robot-Assisted Radical Prostatectomy (RARP)

39

Xu Zhang and Xin Ma

Introduction

With prostate-specific antigen (PSA) screening worldwidely, the incidence of prostate cancer has risen significantly [1]. Robot-assisted radical prostatectomy (RARP) is popular for localized prostate cancer with benefits of a minimally invasive approach as well as good oncologic outcomes [2]. The operative technique of RARP is currently standardized, and multiple medical centers have approved the feasibility and safety of the procedure. In addition, excellent functional and oncologic outcomes have been reported in large RARP cohort [3]. Nevertheless, challenges arises when the anatomy varies such as obese patients, large prostates, previous prostatic surgeries, and large median lobe in their clinical practice. An enlarged median lobe is about 8–18% of the total cases during RARP [4]. The presence of a ML may disturb the clear visualization between the prostate and the bladder neck, making this dissection technically challenging. Therefore, positive surgical margin (PSM) rates at the bladder neck and perioperative outcomes, such as estimated blood loss (EBL) and operative time, and the incidence of ureteral orifices injury could be hypothetically affected by the presence of a large median lobe. In addition, the generated larger bladder neck defect reconstruction in patients with a ML could also potentially affect the recovery of urinary continence after RARP. We describe the approach to the large median lobe and highlight the specific skills that may be beneficial in prevention the related injury and managing this anatomic variant.

Perioperative Results

The effect of a median lobe on perioperative outcomes has been reported by different groups and the results were controversial, including PSM rates, operation time, EBL and early continence outcomes. Several centers reported an increase in operative times, EBL, and hospital stay in men with large median prostate lobes, however, the oncological outcomes, urinary continence, and complications were similar, no difference were found in oncological outcomes in men with and without median prostate lobes [5, 6]. The overall surgical margin rate (10–11%) is comparable with rates previously reported for RARP (9.4–15%) with a 40% positive margin rate for T3 stage [7, 8]. Joshua J et.al reported that of the 154 patients, patients with large median lobes (18%) were older, but had similar PSA, body mass index, clinical and pathologic stage, biopsy and prostatectomy Gleason grade, tumor volumes, and surgical margin rate compared with men without median lobes [9] Yet, prostate weight, estimated blood loss, and hospital stay was significantly greater in men with large median lobes. The overall operative time for the RALP was longer in patients with a large median lobe due to an increased time required for bladder neck and seminal vesicle dissection. No difference were demonstrated in complications such as urine leaks, bladder neck contractures, and migration of Hem-o-lok clips into the bladder. Continence at 3 and 6 months after RARP were statistically similar between the groups. Rafael F et al. reported that the patients with and without large median lobe had similar EBL, length of hospital stay, pathologic stage, complication rates, anastomotic leakage rates, overall PSM rates, and PSM rate at the bladder neck. The median overall operative time was greater in patients with ML (80 vs 75 min, $P < 0.001$); however, no difference was found in the surgical time when calibrating this result by prostate weight. Continence rates were also similar between patients with and without ML at 1 week (27.8% vs 27%, $P = 0.870$), 4 weeks (42.3% vs 48%, $P = 0.136$), 12 weeks (82.5% vs 86.8%, $P = 0.107$), and 24 weeks (91.5% vs 94.1%, $P = 0.183$) after catheter removal [10]. Finally, the median time to recovery of continence had no difference between the groups. Several adverse outcomes, such as higher PSM rates at the bladder neck, longer operative time, higher EBL and ureteral injury rates, could be potentially maximized by the presence of a

X. Zhang (✉) · X. Ma
Chinese PLA Genenal Hospital, Beijing, China

S. Ren et al. (eds.), *Robot-Assisted Radical Prostatectomy*, https://doi.org/10.1007/978-3-031-05855-4_39

median lobe. In an process attempting to remove the median lobe completely, a wide excision of the bladder neck usually results in a larger bladder defect which is potentially associated with lower continence rates after RARP. Because bladder neck preservation has been associated with better recovery of continence after RARP in some previous studies.

Management and Prevention

Presurgical Assessment

The protruding of prostatic median lobe into the bladder is one anatomic challenge during RARP.

Preoperative magnetic resonance imaging (MRI) evaluation is necessary including tumor status (tumor location, staging, tumor extracapsular extension, bladder neck or Denovilliers fascia, seminal vesicle invasion, and lymph node metastasis), describing pelvic and prostate morphology (for example, narrow pelvis, deep or large prostate, intravesical protrusion, and apical configuration), and the assessment for abnormalities (for example, prostate abscess, large seminal vesicle cyst, and urinary bladder lesion). This information helped the surgeon who to make the proper decision (such as preserving the neurovascular bundle) and also helped refine operative details. Large median lobe and intravesical protrusion is prominent in MRI image and crucial for presurgical evaluation. In this way, intravesical prostatic protrusion (IPP) was introduced and was used for guiding the operative strategy and prediction the urinary continence after RARP. A retrospective analysis was performed when the following parameters were assessed in all patients: age, body mass index (BMI), PSA, MRI and pressure-flow studies findings. The impact of preoperative and intraoperative factors on postoperative urinary incontinence (UI) was assessed using multivariate logistic regression analysis. The patients were divided into groups to evaluate the effects of IPP according to the IPP length.

Multivariate analyses showed that IPP and nerve-sparing (NS) were significant factors related to UI in the first month after RARP [11]. Twelve months after RARP, multivariate analyses revealed that only NS is a factor related to postoperative UI. In summary, IPP affects early postoperative UI. IPP does not related to UI incidence in the long run.

Intraoperative Management

RARP approach in optional and we take antegrade manner for example. Standard robotic four-ports placement and an anterior approach were applied. Endopelvic fascia was routinely dissected bilaterally and the dorsal vein complex was stitched. Intraoperatively, large prostatic lobes can be assessed by using the indwelling Foley catheter that was placed at the beginning of the operation. Repeated traction on the catheter can show displacement of the balloon to either side, or deep within the bladder, suggesting an intravesical protruding of prostatic lobe. Therefore the bladder and prostate outline can be precautionary evaluated.

Dissection starts along the ventral portion of the vesicoprostatic junction energetically. The bladder is opened anteriorly, The mucosa overlying the midportion of the median lobe is incised transversely, and the plane between the bladder and the median lobe is developed using the sharp and blunt mobilization. Once this plane has established, the median lobe is identified. The median lobe is grasped and elevated using the fourth arm with the prograsper (Fig. 39.1). The inside of the bladder is then checked, and the UOs were identified. Regarding the accurate position of the UOs, intravenous indigo carmine or diuretics can be given (Figs. 39.2 and 39.3).

UOs injuries during RARP are rare, with a incidence between 0.1% and 0.3% [12]. This complication may result in additional postoperative morbidity, prolonged hospital stay, even re-admitting treatment requirements. It is reported

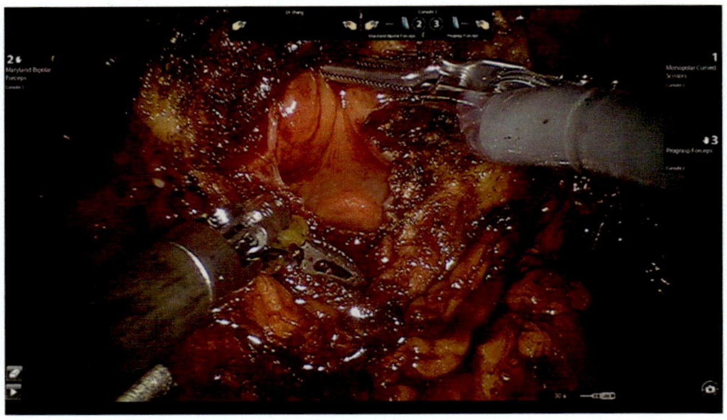

Fig. 39.1 The dissection of the bladder neck and exposure of the large median lobe

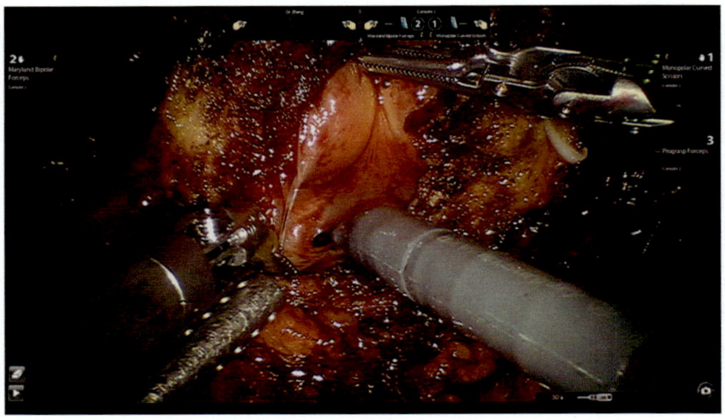

Fig. 39.2 The inspection of the ureteral orifice

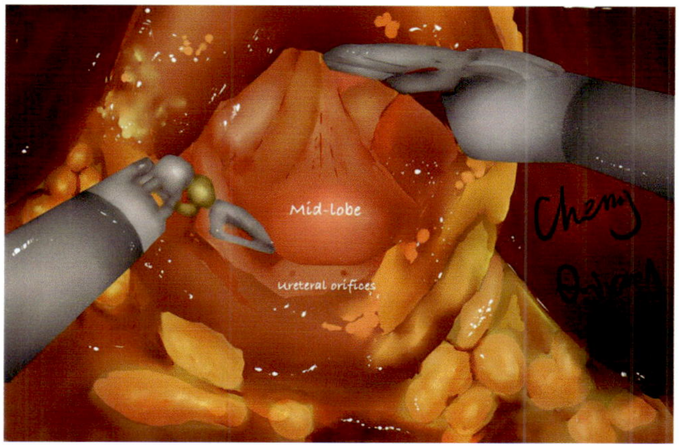

Fig. 39.3 The relationship of ureteral orifices and large median lobe

that for those surgeons who are early in their learning curve for RARP, a cystoscopy before the surgery may allow them to avoid cases with large median lobes until they gain more experience or may allow them to better visualize the UOs before the procedure. However, this measure is not adcpted and recommendated for all patients because of the pain derived from the cystoscopy and unnecessary cost. The lobe is then gradually circumscribed along its surface until it is freed.

Frequent adjustment of the fourth arm maintains traction during the dissection and ensures that the size of the bladder neck is minimized. As the orifice were placed closely to the bladder neck, extreme care was focused to continue the posterior dissection toward Denonvillier's fascia and separate the fascia from the seminal vesicles, without damaging the bladder or orifices. The plane between the posterior part of the seminal vesicles and the posterior layer of the Denonvillier fascia is entered, and the plane between the rectum and the prostate is then developed. The bladder is once again thoroughly inspected to ensure that there has been no injury to the UOs from backwards of the bladder. The bladder neck may requires reconstruction when a large defect is present. Close the bladder neck by placing stitches inferiorly in the bladder neck (ie, tennis racquet closure). This method can move the UOs away from the vesicourethral anastomosis, so as to avoid urine leak or inadvertent injury. In another manner, interrupted sutures may be adopted at 3 and 6 o'clock on each side of the bladder neck, closing it in a "fish mouth" shape, this approach often involves placing sutures very close to the UOs [13].

Of note, the large size needle is not commended to finish the above stitch, because contralateral UO may be injured by the long scale of the needle. Once the bladder neck is complete, a standard running vesicourethral anastomosis is performed using one or two 3-0 5/8 curved suture.

If the UOs were unexpected injured during RARP particularly in patients with an enlarged median lobe [14]. After accurate diagnosis during the operation, this can be effectively treated with intraoperative Double-J stent implantation into the ureter.

Considering the extent of the UOs injury, vesicoureteral reimplantation is required in certain situations.

Conclusion

RARP has become the chosen treatment option for patients with localized prostate cancer. Preoperative MRI evaluation is necessary for precaution and surgical strategy making. Using the technique we have described for the dissection of the median lobe permits a clear visualization of the important dissection planes and Ureteral orifices identification. If UOs injury occurs, intraoperative Double-J stent implantation into the ureter is safe and effective. Reconstruction of the bladder neck is also very crucial for functional outcome.

References

1. Siegel RL, Miller KD, Jemal A. Cancer statistics, 2020. CA Cancer J Clin. 2020;70(1):7–30.
2. Mottet N, et al. EAU-EANM-ESTRO-ESUR-SIOG guidelines on prostate cancer-2020 update. Part 1: screening, diagnosis, and local treatment with curative intent. Eur Urol. 2021;79(2):243–62.
3. Ilic D, et al. Laparoscopic and robotic-assisted versus open radical prostatectomy for the treatment of localised prostate cancer. Cochrane Database Syst Rev. 2017;9(9):Cd009625
4. Patel SR, Kaplon DM, Jarrard D. A technique for the management of a large median lobe in robot-assisted laparoscopic radical prostatectomy. J Endourol. 2010;24(12):1899–901.
5. Ou YC, et al. Prevention and management of complications during robotic-assisted laparoscopic radical prostatectomy following comprehensive planning: a large series involving a single surgeon. Anticancer Res. 2016;36(4):1991–8.
6. Veeratterapillay R, et al. Radical prostatectomy for locally advanced and metastatic prostate cancer. Ann R Coll Surg Engl. 2017;99(4):259–64.
7. Smith JA Jr, et al. A comparison of the incidence and location of positive surgical margins in robotic assisted laparoscopic radical prostatectomy and open retropubic radical prostatectomy. J Urol. 2007;178(6):2385–9; discussion 2389-90
8. Patel VR, Thaly R, Shah K. Robotic radical prostatectomy: outcomes of 500 cases. BJU Int. 2007;99(5):1109–12.
9. Meeks JJ, et al. Impact of prostate median lobe anatomy on robotic-assisted laparoscopic prostatectomy. Urology. 2009;73(2):323–7.
10. Coelho RF, et al. Does the presence of median lobe affect outcomes of robot-assisted laparoscopic radical prostatectomy? J Endourol. 2012;26(3):264–70.
11. Hikita K, et al. Intravesical prostatic protrusion may affect early postoperative continence undergoing robot-assisted radical prostatectomy. BMC Urol. 2020;20(1):164.
12. Bedir F, et al. Diagnosis and conservative Management of Ureteral Orifice Injury during Robotic Prostatectomy for a large prostate with a prominent median lobe. J Endourol Case Rep. 2019;5(2):39–41.
13. Rehman J, et al. Management of an enlarged median lobe with ureteral orifices at the margin of bladder neck during robotic-assisted laparoscopic prostatectomy. Can J Urol. 2009;16(1):4490–4.
14. Sarle R, et al. Robotic-assisted anatomic radical prostatectomy: technical difficulties due to a large median lobe. Urol Int. 2005;74(1):92–4.

Large Volume Gland with Small Pelvis

40

Chin-Heng Lu and Yen-Chuan Ou

Introduction

A large prostate size and a narrow pelvic cavity pose treatment challenges among men with prostate cancer in many ways. In radiation therapy, a large prostate size affects and limits adequate dose delivery for brachytherapy. Furthermore, the radiation may affect adjacent organs and cause radiation-related complications, including radiation proctitis or cystitis. Pre-treatment with androgen deprivation to decrease prostate size may be needed in some patients [1, 2].

In surgical treatment, a larger prostate volume occupies more pelvic space, which can reduce surgical mobility in the pelvis, decrease the surgical field, and impair visualization. These technical challenges cause adverse effects, including increased blood loss and operative times, worse surgical and oncological outcomes, and lower quality of life [3–5]. For example, prostate cancer patients with prostate volumes over 60 g have reported worse sexual function recovery after conventional radical retropubic prostatectomy [4]. The adverse effects of a large prostate size on treatment options and outcomes should be considered. In this era, radical prostatectomy via robotic-assisted surgery may mitigate these adverse effects. Stereoscopic visualization, magnification, robot dexterity, and the pressure of CO_2 exertion are associated with better surgical margins, nerve sparing, outstanding functional outcomes, and less blood loss [6–9]. Given these advantages, robotic-assisted laparoscopic prostatectomy may surmount the obstacles presented by a large prostate size and provide better treatment options for patients.

The most difficult and challenging step in dealing with a large prostate size and narrow pelvic cavity is vesico-urethral anastomosis (VUA) in RALP. Samavedi et al. proposed many technical modifications to facilitate VUA in patients with a narrow pelvis. In addition to the techniques described here, we present our own experiences and skills in managing the challenges presented by a large prostate size and narrow pelvis.

C.-H. Lu · Y.-C. Ou (✉)
Tungs' Taichung Metroharbor Hospital, Taichung City, Taiwan

Tips and Tricks in RALP for Vesico-Urethral Anastomosis and Posterior Reconstruction in Cases Involving A Large Prostate Size and/or Narrow Pelvis

Tips and tricks in RALP for patients with large prostate size and/or narrow pelvis are as follows and details are described in Table 40.1.

1. Patient preparation
2. Surgical field creation
3. Reconstruction skills
4. Confirm security

RALP, Robotic-Assisted Laparoscopic Prostatectomy

Some habitus may be challenging for RALP even for the most experienced surgeons. These conditions include a deeper or narrowed pelvic cavity, sometimes combined with exostosis of the pubic symphysis. These anatomies complicate apical dissection, intra-pelvic urethra preservation, and VUA. More effort in peri-prostatic fat dissection is needed for visual field and surgical working space. Large prostate sizes not only limit the working space in the pelvis but also increase blood loss, widen and weaken the bladder neck, and widen the gap between the urethra and bladder neck after prostate resection.

Some maneuvers that can help maximize the surgical field are described subsequently. First, a steep Trendelenburg position can prevent the bowels and fat from moving into the operative field. The protection of the patient is important for this position. Gel pads, bean bags, tapes, and other stabilizing or restraining facilities are used to prevent positioning-related adverse events, pressure sore formation, nerve injury, compartment syndrome, and other related complications. The usual angle of the position is head down about 25°. The angle can be extended to 30° if difficulty is encountered dur-

S. Ren et al. (eds.), *Robot-Assisted Radical Prostatectomy*, https://doi.org/10.1007/978-3-031-05855-4_40

Table 40.1 Tips and tricks in RALP for patients with large prostate size and/or narrow pelvis. Solutions for problems that may encountered in different stages are described in this table

Steps	Problems	Solutions
1. Patient preparation		
	Steep Trendelenburg position: pressure sores, increased intra-abdominal pressure, heart and lung compression [9]	1. Cushion pad and facilities for patient protection 2. Air seal trocar technology [10] 3. Decreased intra-operative Trendelenburg positioning angle
	Narrow abdominal or pelvic cavity	Alterations in trocar placement [11]
	Acute port angle [11]	1. Alterations in trocar placement 2. More proximal port placement 3. Shifting port laterally
	Obese patients [11]	Bariatric camera and robotic port
	Instrument clashing [11]	1. A minimum distance of 8 cm; 2. Depressing the fourth arm, elevating the third arm, and medially rotating the third arm
2. Surgical field creation [3, 11]		
	Huge omentum and mesenteric fat, bowel distension	1. Steep Trendelenburg positioning 2. Air seal technology [10] 3. Adjustment intra-abdominal pressure
	Urinary bladder distension	1. Foley insertion and urine drainage 2. Anchoring the bladder to pelvic wall by sutuing
	Fat on the bladder or peritoneum	1. Fat excision 2. Retraction by assistant or robotic arm
	Large prostate or predominant middle lobe	Suturing the elarged part of prostate and traction
	Peritoneum restricture	Dissect bilateral peritoneum widely
	Inability to approach for robotic or assistive device	Advancing the trocars more intra-peritoneally
3. Reconstruction skills: Barbed suture, modified posterior reconstruction [11]		
	Wide bladder neck [12, 13]	Bladder neck plication
	Overriding pubic bone	1. Adjusting the camera port 2. Shifting lens from 30° to 0°
	Difficult anastomosis due to large urethra and bladder neck gap [14–17]	1. Release of lateral bladder attachments 2. Posterior reconstruction to decrease tension 3. Decreased angle of Trendelenburg positioning 4. Pushing the proximal part of the bladder 5. Barbed suture
	Fragile bladder neck or urethra cutting end [18, 19]	6. Posterior reconstruction 7. Awareness of force applied and ensuring enough tissue for traction
	Retracting urethra [20]	1. Apical stitch 2. Perineal pressure 3. Posterior reconstruction
4. Confirm security		
	Bladder injection testing	Injection of 150–200 mL normal saline from foley after anastomosis for testing

ing operation. A camera is positioned at 30° when dissecting the prostate. The camera angle is then changed from 30° to 0° for the dissection of the apex and anastomosis in challenging cases, or in visualizing the bladder neck and sphincter complex, which can be difficult to visualize.

In some situations, the pathway of the assistive instrument may be obstructed by the peritoneum, a protruding pubic symphysis, or a pelvic brim in narrow pelvis cases. Port placement should be adjusted in surgeries involving a deep or small pelvis. Trocars should be shifted above the umbilicus and farther away from the surgical target for a better angle and deeper reach. Ports should be inserted further from the pubic symphysis after insufflation. Depressing the robotic arms can also avoid the instruments from hitting pelvic cavity structures. In addition, robotic trocars should be inserted deeper to avoid flattening the working angle. Air seal trocar® technology [10] has been used in laparoscopic procedures. The equipment can maintain intra-abdominal pressure at less than 8 mmHg and help preserve working space especially in surgeries involving narrow pelvises or large prostate sizes.

The goals for an ideal VUA are absence of urine leakage intra- and post- operation with an earlier return of continence. Persistent efforts have been made to reduce the urinary extravasation and achieve urinary continence both in open surgery and in minimally invasive prostatectomy [21]. The dexterity and stereoscopic visualization of the robotic assistant can facilitate complex reconstruction in the deep pelvis. Furthermore, watertight anastomosis is most important for VUA. Failure to achieve this during VUA causes complications including perioperative urinary leakage, paralytic ileus, peritonitis, prolonged catheterization, possibly re-intervention, bladder neck contracture, and delayed continence [21, 22]. Several methods of VUA have been proposed in the past to reduce the risk of peri-operative urine leak and its consequences. An experienced surgeon should choose the most appropriate method in which he or she is competent. These methods include interrupted sutures, two independent running sutures [14], bidirectional pre-tied running sutures, and the bidirectional van Velthoven method [15]. With the use of barbed sutures, either unidirectional [16, 17] or bidirectional [18, 19], the quality and water tightness are improved. In addition, the use of barbed sutures also reduces the anastomotic time and decrease the difficulty of keeping tension and knocking tight for operator and assistant especially in challenging cases [19].

Numerous techniques have been used to improve the early return of and overall continence after RALP. Most of these skills can decrease tension in VUA and increase bladder and urethral stability. These skills are important especially in cases involving a large prostate size and a narrow pelvis. A wide bladder neck is a common problem after prostate resection of a large prostate. Surgical skills in bladder neck intussusception and preservation [12, 13] can manage this issue. However, an increased gap between the urethral cutting ends to the bladder neck can also ensue after resections of a large prostate size. Surgical reconstruction techniques using RALP may help. One useful method is posterior reconstruction, also named Rocco's stitch, which was presented by Rocco et al. in 2001 [20]. Posterior reconstruction is the suturing of the posterior rhabdo-sphincter to the posterior Denonvilliers' fascia. These two layers are then fixed to about 1–2 cm cranial to the new bladder neck of the bladder wall. The method can avoid caudal retraction and decrease the tension of the urethra cutting end to the new bladder neck. The posterior reconstruction technique is important in surgeries involving large prostate, narrow and steep pelvic, and obese individuals.

These methods can facilitate VUA in robotic-assisted radical prostatectomy (RARP). The dexterity of the robotic assistant and technical modifications help surgeons accomplish VUA in challenging anatomical features. Most importantly, every surgeon should make sure every procedure and condition of surgery is carefully controlled. The robotics operator's experience is the critical factor for outcomes especially in technically challenging cases. A surgeon in the initial phase of the learning curve should avoid such cases at best.

Studies and Outcomes in Narrow Pelvis Cases

Surgical cases involving a large prostate size and a narrow or deep pelvis were predicted to be more difficult. Many articles report various degrees of difficulties in patients with a narrow pelvis undergoing RARP. Mason et al. used preoperative magnetic resonance imaging (MRI) to predict surgical difficulty [23]. They calculated the pelvic cavity index (PCI, the pelvic inlet multiplied by the interspinous distance [ISD] and divided by the pelvic depth) and prostate volume (PV). PCI was used to evaluate the robotic working space in RARP. They found that a higher PV/PCI ratio statistically predicted a longer operation time and more blood loss. A higher body mass index (BMI) was also associated with increased blood loss. However, the PV/PCI ratio could not predict positive surgical margins or transfusion risk. Hong et al. investigated the use of preoperative MRI to predict surgical difficulty [24]. They measured the ISD at the pelvic midplane and the inter-tuberous diameter at the pelvic outlet. These two parameters could evaluate the cross-sectional width of the pelvic cavity. The anteroposterior diameters at the pelvic outlet and mid plane were also measured. Furthermore, the apical depth indicates the cranio-caudal length from the most proximal symphysis pubis margin to the prostatic apex on the mid-sagittal MRI. These parameters can classify a wide and shallow pelvis from a narrow and deep one. Hong et al. revealed pelvic cavity might influence surgical outcome, although not significantly. On the other hand, BMI and PV were significantly correlated with pelvic anatomy parameters. Some studies [24–26] showed pelvic dimensions had no significant impact on positive surgical margins or medical or surgical complications. Although no significant differences were found in medical or surgical outcomes, two technically challenging issues were noted in RARP involving narrow pelvises: A smaller intra-pelvic working space and robotic instruments clashing internally or externally especially the third and fourth arms. The incidence is more common in procedures involving a smaller body size or a narrower pelvis. A distance of at least 8 cm can decrease the rate of instrument clashing. Other steps included depressing the fourth robotic arm elevating the third robotic arm, or medially rotating the third robotic arm. If clashing still occurred after robotic arm adjustment, shifting to a three-arm robot with elective assistant ports can resolve the problem.

Studies and Outcomes in Large Prostate Size Cases

Operation Time, Blood Loss, Transfusion Rates, and Surgical Margin

PV is an important consideration in developing the treatment strategy. Studies have shown the effect of a large prostate size on radical prostatectomy outcomes, including greater blood loss, longer operation time, and higher transfusion rates. Studies vary in statements about biochemical recurrence rate and functional outcomes [27]. Pettus et al. reported smaller prostates have a higher risk of positive surgical margin (SM). After tumor grade, stage, and preoperative prostate-specific antigen (PSA) are adjusted, the results are the same that smaller prostates have a higher risk of positive SM [27]. Hsu et al. reported similar findings that PV was significantly inversely related to a positive SM rate ($p = 0.03$). A larger PV is also associated with greater blood loss ($p = 0.021$) and a higher blood transfusion rate ($p = 0.011$). No significant findings were obtained on operative time ($p = 0.121$), continence ($p = 0.227$), or potency rate ($p = 0.900$) in large PV compared to small ones [3]. Levinson et al. reported that a large prostate size was associated with greater blood loss, longer surgical duration, longer hospital stay, and more perioperative complications. However, the blood transfusion rate was not significantly increased. They also found that a smaller prostate increased the positive SM rate ($p = 0.07$) [28]. Link et al. defined a prostate gland >70 g as a large prostate, which was associated with a longer operation time, longer hospital stay, and greater blood loss. The blood transfusion rate, however, was not related to prostate size. Furthermore, a large prostate size was associated with a lower 1-year continence rate ($p = 0.001$) [29].

Biochemical Recurrence (BCR)

Some studies reported that prostate size was not significantly associated with biochemical recurrence (BCR) especially adjusted PSA, pathologic stage, and grade [11, 29]. However, Freedland et al. reported BCR was associated with a large prostate size even after adjusting for adverse factors [30].

Potency and Continence

Several studies report potency and continence are not significantly associated with prostate size [3, 11, 31, 32]. Foley et al. categorized 450 prostate specimens as over or less than 75 g [33]. The result revealed no significant difference in potency or continence between the two groups. However, the BCR was less in the <75 g group. Furthermore, no significant difference was observed between prostate size and positive surgical margins.

Postoperative urinary health-related quality of life (HRQOL).

Levinson et al. reported no significant difference between prostate size and postoperative urinary health-related QOL (HRQOL). The study performed the assessment using the Expanded Prostate Cancer Index Composite questionnaire [34]. In addition, they found that if PV > 70 g, operative times were longer and blood loss was greater. Levinson et al. reported similar findings that no association between prostate size and postoperative urinary HRQOL [35]. However, Samavedi et al. reported that a small prostate size (<40 g) was associated with worse urinary continence at 1 year [11]. No consensus has been reached with regards the relationship between prostate size and HRQOL.

While we have discussed many outcomes after radical prostatectomy, reports still vary on the effects of PV and pelvic size on surgical outcomes. The differences may be due to methodology. Surgeon experience, cohort size, design, follow-up periods, and other factors vary across studies. In our experience, a larger prostate size was associated with greater blood loss and longer console time. Furthermore, although the pelvic size increased the surgical difficulty, it did not significantly affect surgical outcomes.

Conclusions

PV affects surgical difficulty in the aspect of blood loss and operation time. There were many skills to decrease surgical difficulty. Challenging conditions do increase difficulty but not significantly induce worse oncological and functional results. Some studies reported that a smaller prostate size was associated with positive SM. Still, no consensus has been reached on whether oncological and functional outcomes are associated with challenging conditions. Further larger-scale and well-designed investigations should be performed to elucidate answers.

References

1. Locke J, Ellis W, Wallner K, Cavanagh W, Blasko J. Risk factors for acute urinary retention requiring temporary intermittent catheterization after prostate brachytherapy: a prospective study. Int J Radiat Oncol Biol Phys. 2002;52:712–9.
2. Stone NN, Stock RG. Prostate brachytherapy in patients with prostate volumes >/= 50 cm(3): dosimetic analysis of implant quality. Int J Radiat Oncol Biol Phys. 2000;46:1199–204.
3. Hsu EI, Hong EK, Lepor H. Influence of body weight and prostate volume on intraoperative, perioperative, and postoperative outcomes after radical retropubic prostatectomy. Urology. 2003;61:601–6.
4. Hollenbeck BK, Dunn RL, Wei JT, Montie JE, Sanda MG. Determinants of long-term sexual health outcome after radical prostatectomy measured by a validated instrument. J Urol. 2003;169:1453–7.
5. Konety BR, Sadetsky N, Carroll PR. Recovery of urinary continence following radical prostatectomy: the impact of prostate volume--analysis of data from the CaPSURE Database. J Urol. 2007;177:1423–5; discussion 1425–6
6. Menon M, Tewari A, Baize B, Guillonneau B, Vallancien G. Prospective comparison of radical retropubic prostatectomy and robot-assisted anatomic prostatectomy: the Vattikuti Urology Institute experience. Urology. 2002;60:864–8.
7. Menon M, Shrivastava A, Kaul S, Badani KK, Fumo M. Bhandari M, Peabody JO. Vattikuti Institute prostatectomy: contemporary technique and analysis of results. Eur Urol. 2007;51:648–57; discussion 657-8
8. Ficarra V, Novara G, Artibani W, Cestari A, Galfano A, Graefen M, Guazzoni G, Guillonneau B, Menon M, Montorsi F, Patel V, Rassweiler J, Van Poppel H. Retropubic, laparoscopic, and robot-assisted radical prostatectomy: a systematic review and cumulative analysis of comparative studies. Eur Urol. 2009;55:1037–63.
9. Patel VR, Thaly R, Shah K. Robotic radical prostatectomy: outcomes of 500 cases. BJU Int. 2007;99:1109–12.
10. Horstmann M, Horton K, Kurz M, Padevit C, John H. Prospective comparison between the AirSeal® System valve-less Trocar and a standard Versaport™ Plus V2 Trocar in robotic-assisted radical prostatectomy. J Endourol. 2013;27:579–82.
11. Samavedi S, Abdul-Muhsin H, Pigilam S, Sivaraman A, Patel VR. Handling difficult anastomosis. Tips and tricks in obese patients and narrow pelvis. Indian J Urol. 2014;30:418–22.
12. Deliveliotis C, Protogerou V, Alargof E, Varkarakis J. Radical prostatectomy: bladder neck preservation and puboprostatic ligament sparing--effects on continence and positive margins. Urology. 2002;60:855–8.
13. Walsh PC, Marschke PL. Intussusception of the reconstructed bladder neck leads to earlier continence after radical prostatectomy. Urology. 2002;59:934–8.
14. Hoznek A, Salomon L, Rabii R, Ben Slama MR, Cicco A, Antiphon P, Abbou CC. Vesicourethral anastomosis during laparoscopic radical prostatectomy: the running suture method. J Endourol. 2000;14:749–53.
15. Van Velthoven RF, Ahlering TE, Peltier A, Skarecky DW, Clayman RV. Technique for laparoscopic running urethrovesical anastomosis:the single knot method. Urology. 2003;61:699–702.
16. Tewari AK, Srivastava A, Sooriakumaran P, Slevin A, Grover S, Waldman O, Rajan S, Herman M, Berryhill R Jr, Leung R. Use of a novel absorbable barbed plastic surgical suture enables a "self-cinching" technique of vesicourethral anastomosis during robot-assisted prostatectomy and improves anastomotic times. J Endourol. 2010;24:1645–50.
17. Chapman S, Turo R, Cross W. Vesicourethral anastomosis using V-Loc™ barbed suture during robot-assisted radical prostatectomy. Cent European J Urol. 2011;64:236.
18. Valero R, Schatloff O, Chauhan S, HwiiKo Y, Sivaraman A, Coelho RF, Palmer KJ, Davila H, Patel VR. Bidirectional barbed suture for bladder neck reconstruction, posterior reconstruction and vesicourethral anastomosis during robot assisted radical prostatectomy. Actas Urol Esp. 2012;36:69–74.
19. Zorn KC, Widmer H, Lattouf JB, Liberman D, Bhojani N, Trinh QD, Sun M, Karakiewicz PI, Denis R, El-Hakim A. Novel method of knotless vesicourethral anastomosis during robot-assisted radical prostatectomy: feasibility study and early outcomes in 30 patients using the interlocked barbed unidirectional V-LOC180 suture. Can Urol Assoc J. 2011;5:188–94.
20. Rocco F, Gadda F, Acquati P, Carmignani L, Favini P, Dell'Orto P, Ferruti M, Avogadro A, Casellato S, Grisotto M. Personal research: reconstruction of the urethral striated sphincter. Arch Ital Urol Androl. 2001;73:127–37.
21. Tyritzis SI, Katafigiotis I, Constantinides CA. All you need to know about urethrovesical anastomotic urinary leakage following radical prostatectomy. J Urol. 2012;188:369–76.
22. Froehner M, Litz R, Manseck A, Hakenberg OW, Leike S, Albrecht DM, Wirth MP. Relationship of comorbidity, age and perioperative complications in patients undergoing radical prostatectomy. Urol Int. 2001;67:283–8.
23. Mason BM, Hakimi AA, Faleck D, Chernyak V, Rozenblitt A, Ghavamian R. The role of preoperative endo-rectal coil magnetic resonance imaging in predicting surgical difficulty for robotic prostatectomy. Urology. 2010;76:1130–5.
24. Hong SK, Chang IH, Han BK, Yu JH, Han JH, Jeong SJ, Jeong H, Byun SS, Lee HJ, Lee SE. Impact of variations in bony pelvic dimensions on performing radical retropubic prostatectomy. Urology. 2007;69:907–11.
25. Hong SK, Lee ST, Kim SS, Min KE, Hwang IS, Kim M, Jeong SJ, Byun SS, Hwang SI, Lee SE. Effect of bony pelvic dimensions measured by preoperative magnetic resonance imaging on performing robot-assisted laparoscopic prostatectomy. BJU Int. 2009;104:664–8.
26. von Bodman C, Matsushita K, Matikainen MP, Eastham JA, Scardino PT, Akin O, Rabbani F. Do pelvic dimensions and prostate location contribute to the risk of experiencing complications after radical prostatectomy? BJU Int. 2011;108:1566–71.
27. Pettus JA, Masterson T, Sokol A, Cronin AM, Savage C, Sandhu JS, Mulhall JP, Scardino PT, Rabbani F. Prostate size is associated with surgical difficulty but not functional outcome at 1 year after radical prostatectomy. J Urol. 2009;182:949–55.
28. Levinson AW, Ward NT, Sulman A, Mettee LZ, Link RE, Su LM, Pavlovich CP. The impact of prostate size on perioperative outcomes in a large laparoscopic radical prostatectomy series. J Endourol. 2009;23:147–52.
29. Link BA, Nelson R, Josephson DY, Yoshida JS, Crocitto LE, Kawachi MH, Wilson TG. The impact of prostate gland weight in robot assisted laparoscopic radical prostatectomy. J Urol. 2008;180:928–32.
30. Freedland SJ, Aronson W, Presti JC Jr, Kane CJ, Terris MK, Elashoff D, Amling CL. Should a positive surgical margin following radical prostatectomy be pathological stage T2 or T3? Results from the SEARCH database. J Urol. 2003;169:2142–6.
31. Frota R, Turna B, Santos BM, Lin YC, Gill IS, Aron M. The effect of prostate weight on the outcomes of laparoscopic radical prostatectomy. BJU Int. 2008;101:589–93.
32. Zorn KC, Orvieto MA, Mikhail AA, Gofrit ON, Lin S, Schaeffer AJ, Shalhav AL, Zagaja GP. Effect of prostate weight on operative and postoperative outcomes of robotic-assisted laparoscopic prostatectomy. Urology. 2007;69:300–5.

33. Foley CL, Bott SRJ, Thomas K, Parkinson MC, Kirby RS. A large prostate at radical retropubic prostatectomy does not adversely affect cancer control, continence or potency rates. BJU Int. 2003;92:370–4.
34. Freedland SJ, Terris MK, Platz EA, Presti JC Jr. Body mass index as a predictor of prostate cancer: development versus detection on biopsy. Urology. 2005;66:108–13.
35. Levinson AW, Bagga HS, Pavlovich CP, Mettee LZ, Ward NT, Link RE, Su LM. The impact of prostate size on urinary quality of life indexes following laparoscopic radical prostatectomy. J Urol. 2008;179:1818–22.

41 Robot Assisted Laparoscopic Radical Prostatectomy in Kidney Transplant Recipients

Brendan Dias and Homayoun Zargar

Introduction

Renal transplantation is the gold-standard treatment for patients with end-stage renal failure. Compared to dialysis, it provides better results in terms of quality of life and survival [1]. Advancements in immunosuppressive therapy over the past few decades have resulted in a longer and better quality of life for kidney transplant recipients (KTRs). The development of malignancies is one of the leading causes of morbidity and mortality in KTRs [2]. The increased risk of cancer in KTRs has been attributed to the activation of oncogenic viruses, chronic inflammation, and nonspecific immunosuppression [2]. Newer and more potent immunosuppressive agents have improved long-term survival but have also raised concern regarding increased rates of cancer. Genitourinary malignancies have been reported as the second most common malignancies after skin cancer in the KTR population. Prostate cancer (PCa) is the most common genitourinary malignancy seen in post-transplant males [3]. However, with the increased KTR lifespan and recipient age at the time of transplantation, and better screening practices, PCa is seen at a higher frequency in KTRs compared to that in the general population [2, 4–6]. The incidence of prostate cancer in KTRs has not been extensively studied, but the available data report an incidence rate of 0.72% to 3.1% [7–11]. Although usually found early, prostate cancer in KTRs may have more malignant potential and progress because of chronic immunosuppression if left untreated [12]. Aggressive therapeutic interventions in the appropriate clinical setting should not be withheld in renal transplant patients with prostate cancer. Age, general state of health, and clinical risk group remain critically important in determining the proper treatment for localized prostate cancer [13]. Treatment options include the same interventions as in the general population [14]. However, only few patients with a kidney transplant receive radiation therapy due to the potential harm of the graft by a radiation-induced stenosis of the transplanted ureter [15]. Therefore, most transplant patients undergo radical prostatectomy (RP) [13, 14, 16, 17]. RP can be challenging in these patients. Problems may occur due to scarring in the operative field and immunosuppressive therapy. This includes cytostatic agents, as well as biological modifiers and glucocorticoids, to suppress immune response. It is known that immunosuppression may interfere with wound healing and postoperative infections [18].

In this chapter we outline the surgical approaches to radical prostatectomy in a renal allograft recipient with a focus on the robotic approach to radical prostatectomy in this subgroup of patients.

Surgical Approaches to Radical Prostatectomy in KTRs

In 1991 Kinahan et al. described radical prostatectomy in renal allograft recepients. They described their technique of open retropubic radical prostatectomy with bilateral pelvic node dissection in 3 cases of localized prostate cancer post deceased donor renal transplant. In 2 out of the three cases lymph node dissection on the side of the graft was avoided. The authors concluded that the increasing survival of rate of transplanted patients, the potential risk for rapid cancer growth with immunosuppression and the lack of suitable treatment alternatives in these patients argue for early aggressive surgery for localized prostate cancer [19].

In 1999 Yiou et al. described a perineal approach to radical prostatectomy in renal allograft recipients. They did not perform a pelvic node dissection and demonstrated the feasibility of the perineal approach in this subgroup of patients [20].

These initial reports [19, 20] demonstrated that open radical prostatectomy in KTRs is feasible however, challenges in

B. Dias · H. Zargar (✉)
Western Health, Melbourne, Australia

University of Melbourne, Melbourne, Australia

S. Ren et al. (eds.), *Robot-Assisted Radical Prostatectomy*, https://doi.org/10.1007/978-3-031-05855-4_41

managing prostate cancer in this patient cohort do exist. The main challenges include:

1. Watchful waiting in this cohort has the potential for a poorer outcome due to immunosuppression.
2. Radiation therapy has the potential risk for radiation nephritis in the allograft and the risk of radiation injury to the bladder and the site of ureteric reimplantation.
3. Pelvic lymph node dissection on the side of the allograft is technically challenging.
4. Radical prostatectomy in KTRs could potentially increase the complication rates for future transplants due to violation of the contralateral iliac fossa.
5. There is potential for injury to the transplant ureter.
6. There is potential for injury to the renal allograft.
7. The impaired bladder descent could potentially make vesicourethral anastomosis challenging thereby affecting continence and bladder neck contracture rates following radical prostatectomy.

Hafron et al. demonstrated the feasibility of perineal radical prostatectomy in localized prostate cancer in seven consecutive KTRs. The authors advocated that the perineal approach should be preferred in KTRs as it offers several advantages over the retropubic approach in these patients [21].

Antonopoulos et al. demonstrated the feasibility of radical retropubic prostatectomy in eight patients diagnosed with prostate cancer following kidney transplantation. They concluded that radical retropubic prostatectomy in renal transplant patients is safe, effective, and can be easily performed in the same manner as described by Walsh, regardless of the presence of the allograft. The only necessary technical modification is the avoidance of ipsilateral lymphadenectomy to prevent damage to the transplanted organ [16].

In 2000, Laparoscopic Radical Prostatectomy (LRP) emerged as a minimally invasive alternative to open surgery. In 2006 the first case of LRP in a KTR was described by Shah et al. [22]. The authors performed a four-port transperitoneal nerve-sparing laparoscopic radical prostatectomy, with the assistance of the AESOP robotic camera arm. The transperitoneal approach avoided the adhesions present in the retroperitoneal space surrounding the graft.

Thomas et al. [23] from the Cleveland clinic subsequently demonstrated the safety of LRP in three cases. The authors found that the surgical challenges of the present cases were similar to those of standard laparoscopic radical prostatectomies. Furthermore, it was not necessary to catheterize the transplanted ureter to identify the ureteroneocystostomy as previously described in open radical prostatectomy [19]. The bladder descent for the vesicourethral anastomosis was not affected by the presence of a transplanted kidney and perioperative outcomes were comparable to outcomes of open and laparoscopic radical prostatectomy in patients without renal allografts.

Robot-assisted Laparoscopic Radical Prosatectomy (RALP) in KTRs was first described by Jhaveri et al. in 2008 [24]. The patient was a 54 year old male who had prior bilateral nephrectomies for fulminant bilateral ascending pyelonephritis through a midline abdominal approach at the age of 27 followed by a living donor kidney transplant 6 months later. The patient also had a left inguinal herniorraphy performed at age 42. The patient was diagnosed to have gleasons 6 (3 + 3) prostate cancer after a transrectal ultrasound guided biopsy of his prostate was performed for an elevated PSA of 8.5 ng/mL. The following technical modifications to the standard robotic retropubic approach were performed in this patient:

- Since the patient had a midline scar, the camera port was placed at the superior aspect of the scar.
- A surgical da Vinci 3-arm robotic platform was used for the procedure with two bedside assistants and a 6-port transperitoneal approach.
- Port placement modifications:
  1. The right robotic port was inserted superiolaterally to the standard port site under direct visual guidance to avoid allograft injury. Once the port track was established, this was switched to an extended length (5–12 mm caliber) bariatric port (VersaPortTM plus V2, Tyco Healthcare Group LP, Norwalk, CT) to deliver the robotic instrument past the allograft into the pelvis.
  2. The left robotic port was placed inferiorly and slightly laterally as well, to prevent instrument collisions and provide full access to pelvic lymph nodes.
- A deliberate effort was made during development of the retropubic space to avoid the right anterior surface of the bladder where the transplanted ureter and ureteroneocystostomy was expected to lie. Instead, the retropubic space was developed contralaterally with transection of the median umbilical ligament.
- Pelvic node dissection was carried out on the left side. While on the right side on a limited dissection of the obturator nodes was performed due to intense adhesions.

The authors did not catheterize the transplanted ureter in this case and advocated (1) the use of an extended length bariatric port to bypass the allograft site and deliver the ipsilateral robotic instrument directly into the pelvis; (2) development of the retropubic space from the contralateral side; and (3) meticulous posterior dissection of the seminal vesicles via the medial avascular plane to avoid injury to the proximal neurovascular plate.

Robert et al. [25] described their outcomes in 9 cases of LRP in KTRs using the extraperitoneal approach. While surgical time, blood loss, transfusion rate, and bladder injury were similar in comparison to their experience in non-KTR patients, the incidence of rectal injury was 22.2%. Also in one patient there was thrombosis of the iliac vein with extension into and loss of the renal allograft. The authors concluded that posterior dissection of the prostate was more difficult in KTRs when compared to other patients.

Ghazi et al. [12] demonstrated the feasibility of an extraperitoneal robot-assisted radical prostatectomy post kidney transplant in 2012. The authors demonstrated the following modifications to the extraperitoneal approach to RALP in KTRs:

1. The approach was modified to a 3-arm, 5-trocar arrangement rather than the routine 4-arm, 6-port technique. A single robotic trocar was placed medial to the right epigastric vessels, which avoided passage of instruments across the path of the nonvisualized graft ureter. All other trocars were placed on the contralateral side. This modified arrangement avoided dissection over the transplanted kidney.
2. The pressure was maintained at 10 mm Hg, to avoid impairing venous drainage from the renal allograft.
3. The bladder was dissected off the prostate, leaving the bladder neck attached, while the seminal vesicles were dissected from the left lateral aspect of the bladder. Preserving the vesico-prostatic junction enabled suspension of the prostate cephalad and to the right. This facilitated dissection of the left seminal vesicle, prostatic pedicle, neurovascular plane, and the posterior rectal plane, without the need of an assistant port on the right side, which could lead to injury to the graft ureter, during passage of laparoscopic or robotic instruments.
4. The da Vinci Hem-o-lock applier was used for control of vascular pedicles, allowing a precise application of clips within a confined pelvic space, without the need of a 10-mm, laparoscopic applier.
5. The V-Lock Wound Closure Device (Covidien, Mansfield, MA) was used to complete the posterior reconstruction prior to the anastomosis. This self-anchoring suture does not allow the suture to be retracted, thereby maintaining tension without the need of further assistance to hold the bladder in place until the knot tying is complete.

Jenjitranant et al. [26] described the utilization of the retzius sparing RALP technique in a 73 year old patient diagnosed to have prostate cancer post kidney transplant. While the retzius sparing technique does offer theoretical advantages in the form of avoiding bladder dropping and hence the potential for injury to the transplant kidney and ureter, the drawbacks include a higher rate of positive surgical margins which has curtailed the widespread adoption of the technique. In fact the patient in this case report had a positive surgical margin and pT2c disease [26].

More recently, Tugcu et al. [27] demonstrated the utility of robotic perineal radical prostatectomy in KTRs. Potential advantages of the perineal approach include:

- Avoidance of pneumoperitoneum thereby preserving renal blood flow and eGFR.
- Avoidance of bladder drop and dissection in the region of the renal allograft minimizes the risk of damage to the transplanted kidney and/or transplant ureterneocystostomy.
- Earlier mobilization with earlier return to daily life thereby optimizing postoperative transplant kidney function.

Table 41.1 summarizes the various technical modifications to the standard technique of robot assisted radical prostatectomy in KTRs.

Outcomes Following RALP in KTRs

Perioperative Outcomes

The feasibility of RALP in KTRs was first reported in 2008 [24] and since then the evidence in literature is limited to a few case series. Zeng et al. [28] recently published a systematic review on the safety and clinical outcomes of RALP in KTRs. They analyzed a total of 35 patients who underwent RALP following kidney transplantation. They found the overall complication rate to be 17.1% which was higher than what is described for RALP in literature. The authors also demonstrated longer operating times and higher blood loss in this group of patients. They hypothesized that the increased patient comorbidities, difficulty of operation and learning curve of variations to standard technique contributed to the differences in perioperative outcomes in their review when compared to previous studies for standard RALP. Felber et al. [29] recently published the largest case series to date of RALP in KTRs. They included 39 patients who underwent RALP following a kidney transplant and compared them to a control group consisting of patients undergoing RALP without a prior history of kidney transplant. They demonstrated that median operating time and blood loss did not differ significantly between the two groups. However, surgical difficulties were encountered more frequently in the kidney transplant patients undergoing RALP (30.8% vs. 8.2%; $P < 0.0001$) and so were overall complications (51.2% vs. 8.2%; $P < 0.0001$). The occurrence of Clavien grade ≥ 3 was also significantly higher in the kidney transplant patient group (10.2% vs. 0.8%; $P < 0.0001$).

Similarly Leonard et al. [30] compared perioperative and oncological outcomes following RALP in KTRs. They com-

Table 41.1 Summary of perioperative/functional outcomes of RALP in renal transplant patients

Study	No. of Cases	Age (years)	BMI (kg/m^2)	Approach			Perioperative Outcomes						Functional Outcomes			
				Standard	Retzius-Sparing	Extra-peritoneal	Operative time (mins)	Blood Loss (mL)	Length of Stay (days)	Overall Complications (n)	Clavien grade ≥3 (n)	Conversion to open	Continent at 3 months	Continent at 1 year	Errections at 6 months	Graft dysfunction (n)
Jhaveri et al.	1	54	27.3	1	0	0	200	400	2	1	0	0	1	1	1	0
Smith et al.	3	48	NR	1	0	0	244	50	2	0	0	0	NR	1	NR	0
		54	NR	1	0	0	400	100	2	0	0	0	NR	1	NR	0
		61	NR	1	0	0	322	75	3	0	0	0	NR	1	NR	0
Ghazi et al.	1	68	26	0	0	1	130	125	1	0	0	0	NR	NR	NR	0
Wagener et al.	1	71	NR	1	0	0	220	300	NR	0	0	0	1	1	1	0
Polcari et al.	7	63.3	25.7	7	0	0	186	NR	1.8	3	0	0	NR	NR	NR	0
Le Clerc et al.	12	61.9	26.8	12	0	0	241.3	587.9	NR	5	2	1	NR	NR	NR	2
Plagakis et al.	1	60	NR	1	0	0	139	190	2	0	0	0	0	1	0	0
Moreno et al.	4	61.3	NR	4	0	0	196	NR	3.2	1	1	0	NR	3	NR	0
Izuka et al.	3	59	NR	1	0	0	163	75	8	1	0	0	NR	NR	NR	0
		60	NR	1	0	0	195	30	9	0	0	0	NR	NR	NR	0
		67	NR	1	0	0	127	50	7	0	0	0	NR	NR	NR	0
Jenjitrant et al.	1	73	NR	0	1	0	210	250	6	0	0	0	1	1	NR	0
Zeng et al.	1	65	NR	1	0	0	207	500	3	1	0	0	NR	NR	NR	0
Iwamoto et al.	9	61	22.6	9	0	0	111	50	6	0	0	0	NR	NR	NR	0
Mistretta et al.	9	60	25.7	4	5	0	160	100	4	1	0	0	0	7	5	0
Leonard et al.	27	63.3	25.6	27	0	0	244	571.3	5.7	8	2	0	7	23	NR	0
Felber et al.	39	62	25	39	0	0	180	150	4	20	4	0	NR	24 (Continent at 6 months)	4	0

pared outcomes in 27 patients who underwent RALP following a kidney transplant to a matched 1:1 control group of patients undergoing RALP. They found no significant difference between the groups concerning the operative time and intraoperative blood loss. Hospital stay was incidentally shorter in the transplanted group of patients (4.4 days vs. 5.7 days; P = 0.041). No significant differences in early complications were noticed between the groups according to Clavien-Dindo (29.6 vs. 22.2%; P = 0.279).

Table 41.1 summaries the perioperative outcomes following RALP in KTRs in published case series.

Functional Outcomes

Felber et al. [29] compared outcomes following 39 RALPs in KTRs with a matched control group of 282 non transplanted patients who underwent RALP for localized Prostate Cancer. Recovery of continence at 6 months occurred in 68.6% of patients in the KTR group vs. 65% in the control group. Normal erectile function was reported in 12.9% of patients in the KTR group vs. 31.4% in the control group at 6 months post RALP. However this difference in post-operative potency could be attributed to the fact that only 37.5% of patients in the KTR group reported normal erectile function pre-operatively vs. 86% of patients in the control group. Additionally, only 41% of patients in the KTR group underwent either a unilateral or bilateral nerve sparing procedure vs. 73% in the control group.

Leonard et al. [30] compared 27 patients who underwent RALP following a kidney transplant to a matched control group of 27 non transplanted patients who underwent RALP. Continence rates were 25.9%, 59.2%, and 83.3% at 3, 6, and 12 months following RALP in the kidney transplant group. No difference in continence rates was found between the two groups.

Very few studies have reported potency outcomes following RALP in KTRs. Table 41.1 summaries the functional outcomes following RALP in KTRs.

Oncological Outcomes

Table 41.2 summaries the oncological outcomes reported in various studies on RALP in KTRs.

Zeng et al. [28] reported a positive surgical margin (PSM) rate of 32.5% in their systematic review of 35 cases reported in literature on RALP in KTRs. They hence concluded that RALP in KTRs is inferior in regard to PSM rates which could be attributed to the limited number of cases published in literature. This is significant especially given that the role of adjuvant or salvage radiation for biochemical recurrence in this population is controversial given the risk of radiation induced damage to kidney function.

Leonard et al. [30] compared 27 RALPs in KTRs to a match control of 27 non transplanted RALPs and found no difference in the PSM rates (44% vs. 37%; P = 0.58). While the rate of biochemical recurrence (BCR) was similar in both groups (7.4% vs. 11.1%; P = 0.639), the BCR-free survival was significantly shorter in the KTR group (26.9 months vs. 49.3 months; P = 0.018). Mutltivariate analysis revealed that history of a renal allograft was an independent risk factor for a shorter BCR-free survival (hazard ratio = 4.291; 95% confidence interval, 2.102–8.761 and P < 0.001).

More recently Felber et al. [29] compared outcomes following 39 RALPs in KTRs from a multi instituitional database. The rate of positive surgical margins was comparable in both groups: 13.2% for transplant patients vs. 18.1%

Table 41.2 Pathological outcomes of RALP in renal transplant patients

Study	ISUP Grade					PSA	Stage					PSM	BCR	F/U
	I	II	III	IV	V		≤ pT2a	pT2b	pT2c	pT3a	pT3b			
Jhaveri et al.	0	1	0	0	0	8.5	0	0	1	0	0	0	0	6 weeks
Smith et al.	3	0	0	0	0	NR	0	0	3	0	0	1	0	13 months
Ghazi et al.	0	1	0	0	0	6.93	0	1	0	0	0	0	0	NR
Wagener et al.	0	1	0	0	0	12.4	0	0	1	0	0	0	0	9 months
Polcari et al.	2	4	0	0	1	6.17	0	0	4	3	0	2	1	16 months
Le Clerc et al.	8	4	0	0	0	7.34	0	1	8	2	0	4	2	31.2 months
Plagakis et al.	0	1	0	0	0	13	0	0	1	0	0	0	0	10 years
Moreno et al.	3	1	0	0	0	7.1	4	0	0	0	0	2	1	33 months
Izuka et al.	0	1	2	0	0	12.06	3	0	0	0	0	0	1	23 months
Jenjitrant et al.	0	0	1	0	0	11.53	0	0	1	0	0	1	0	1 month
Zeng et al.	0	0	0	0	1	6.65	0	0	0	0	1	1	1	3 months
Iwamoto et al.	0	7	0	2	0	8.58	9	0	0	0	0	2	1	27 months
Mistretta et al.	4	3	2	0	0	5.6	1	0	6	1	1	2	2	42 months
Leonard et al.	12	8	5	0	2		15	9	2	1	0	12	2	34.9 months
Felber et al.	14	18	4	0	3	6.8	5	2	21	9	2	5	3	47.9 months
TOTAL	46	50	14	2	7	8.68 (mean)	37	13	48	16	4	32	14	28.75 (Mean F/U)

(P = 0.65). The BCR rate was also similar in both groups (7% vs. 8.5%; P = 0.84). Progression-free survival (PFS) at 4 years was 96.4% in the KTR group vs. 90.6% in the control group.

Graft Outcomes

Iwamoto et al. [31] reported good postoperative graft function in all 12 patients undergoing RALP following a kidney transplant. Similarly reports by Felber et al. [29] and Leonard et al. [30] demonstrated no significant change in renal function following RALP in KTRs. This was despite changes to immunosuppressive regimens in up to 68% of patients in one study [30].

Authors Take

This chapter summarizes the current evidence for RALP in KTRs. While the initial experience was restricted to case series and isolated case reports, data from Felber et al. [29] and Leonard et al. [30] suggest that RALP can be safely performed in KTRs with comparable outcomes to non-transplanted patients using little to no modifications to the standard approach of trans peritoneal RALP. With the increasing life expectancy of KTRs [32], it is expected that RALP will increasingly feature as a treatment option in this cohort of patients. Moreover, the higher incidence of prostate cancer in this cohort of patients [4, 6] combined with the concerns around watchful waiting and active surveillance and the significant side effects of radiotherapy in this population would make RALP as the treatment of choice for localized prostate cancer in KTRs.

While various prostatectomy techniques and modifications have been described we feel that RALP in KTRs can be performed safely with the following caveats:

1. Surgeon experience: RALP in KTRs has higher rates of overall complications and initial case series have revealed inferior PSM rates. While the reasons for these are multifactorial and surgeon factors such as case volume and learning curve are controversial, we do believe that surgeon experience in RALP is paramount to achieving good outcomes following RALP in the transplant population.
2. Da Vinci Xi (Intuitive Surgical Inc. Sunnyvale, CA): The earlier robotic systems had working distances of 25 cm which made it challenging to perform RALP in KTRs since many of these patients have intraabdominal adhesions due to previous surgery and/or peritonitis (especially in those patients undergoing peritoneal dialysis).

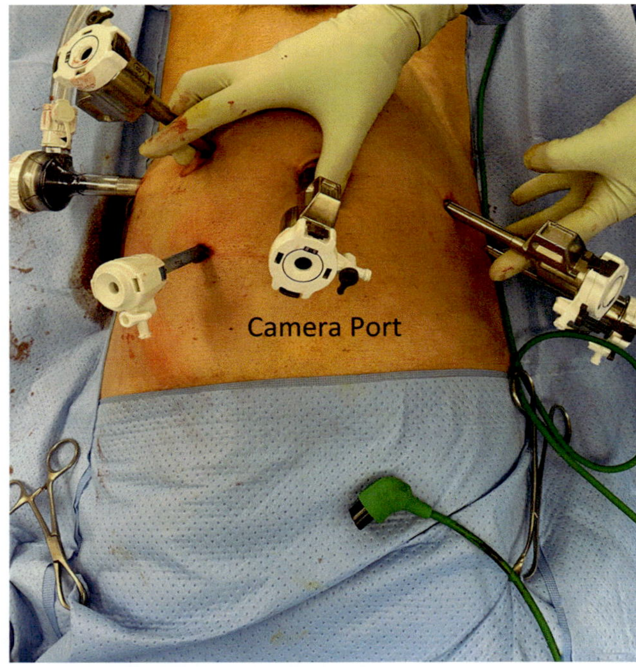

Fig. 41.1 Looking from the head of the table demonstrating our port placements

   The Da Vinci Xi system is more flexible and allows for more cranial placement of ports (Fig. 41.1) since working length is not an issue thereby counteracting some of the challenges in port placements in this cohort of patients.
3. Involvement of renal physicians/surgeons: Best outcomes following surgical interventions in complex patients involves a collaborative approach and hence early involvement of renal physicians and surgeons in the oncological care of transplanted patients enables optimal perioperative and graft outcomes in this patient cohort.
4. Port placement modifications: Although contemporary studies have demonstrated that modifications in port placement are seldom necessary, we believe that more cranial placement of ports, medialization of working port on the side of the transplant and avoidance of assistant ports on the side of the renal allograft does help in ensuring allograft safety and optimal intraoperative outcomes.
5. Posterior approach: In our experience the transplanted ureter and neocystostomy is seldom an issue during RALP using the standard technique. The retzius—sparing approach does offer theoretical advantages in patients who have had multiple renal transplants and patients who have had combined kidney—pancreas transplants (especially those in whom the pancreas drain into the bladder) as it avoids the bladder drop that has the potential for transplant ureteric injury. The perineal approach to radical prostatectomy also offers similar advantages in our opinion. While using the standard approach we recom-

mend development of the retzius space from the contralateral side to avoid transplant ureteric injuries. We do not recommend pre-stenting the transplant kidney ureter as we do not believe that it reduces the incidence of ureteric injury.

References

1. Wolfe RA, Ashby VB, Milford EL, Ojo AO, Ettenger RE, Agodoa LY, et al. Comparison of mortality in all patients on dialysis, patients on dialysis awaiting transplantation, and recipients of a first cadaveric transplant. N Engl J Med. 1999;341(23):1725–30.
2. Vasudev B, Hariharan S. Cancer after renal transplantation. Curr Opin Nephrol Hypertens. 2007;16(6):523–8.
3. Saran R, Robinson B, Abbott KC, Bragg-Gresham J, Chen X, Gipson D, et al. US Renal Data System 2019 Annual Data Report: Epidemiology of Kidney Disease in the United States. Am J Kidney Dis. 2020;75(1 Suppl 1):A6–7.
4. Kessler M, Jay N, Molle R, Guillemin F. Excess risk of cancer in renal transplant patients. Transpl Int. 2006;19(11):908–14.
5. Cormier L, Lechevallier E, Barrou B, Benoit G, Bensadoun H, Boudjema K, et al. Diagnosis and treatment of prostate cancers in renal-transplant recipients. Transplantation. 2003;75(2):237–9.
6. Kasiske BL, Snyder JJ, Gilbertson DT, Wang C. Cancer after kidney transplantation in the United States. Am J Transplant. 2004;4(6):905–13.
7. Carvalho JA, Nunes P, Dinis PJ, Antunes H, Parada B, Marconi L, et al. Prostate cancer in renal transplant recipients: diagnosis and treatment. Transplant Proc. 2017;49(4):809–12.
8. Yanik EL, Gustafson SK, Kasiske BL, Israni AK, Snyder JJ, Hess GP, et al. Sirolimus use and cancer incidence among US kidney transplant recipients. Am J Transplant. 2015;15(1):129–36.
9. Piselli P, Serraino D, Segoloni GP, Sandrini S, Piredda GB, Scolari MP, et al. Risk of de novo cancers after transplantation: results from a cohort of 7217 kidney transplant recipients, Italy 1997–2009. Eur J Cancer. 2013;49(2):336–44.
10. Hall EC, Pfeiffer RM, Segev DL, Engels EA. Cumulative incidence of cancer after solid organ transplantation. Cancer. 2013;119(12):2300–8.
11. Sampaio MS, Cho YW, Qazi Y, Bunnapradist S, Hutchinson IV, Shah T. Posttransplant malignancies in solid organ adult recipients: an analysis of the U.S. National Transplant Database. Transplantation. 2012;94(10):990–8.
12. Ghazi A, Erturk E, Joseph JV. Modifications to facilitate extraperitoneal robot-assisted radical prostatectomy post kidney transplant. JSLS. 2012;16(2):314–9.
13. Kleinclauss FM, Neuzillet Y, Tillou X, Terrier N, Guichard G, Petit J, et al. Morbidity of retropubic radical prostatectomy for prostate cancer in renal transplant recipients: multicenter study from Renal Transplantation Committee of French Urological Association. Urology. 2008;72(6):1366–70.
14. Heidenreich A, Pfister D, Thissen A, Piper C, Porres D. Radical retropubic and perineal prostatectomy for clinically localised prostate cancer in renal transplant recipients. Arab J Urol. 2014;12(2):142–8.
15. Mouzin M, Bachaud JM, Kamar N, Game X, Vaessen C, Rischmann P, et al. Three-dimensional conformal radiotherapy for localized prostate cancer in kidney transplant recipients. Transplantation. 2004;78(10):1496–500.
16. Antonopoulos IM, Nahas WC, Piovesan AC, Falci R Jr, Kanashiro H, Alvarez GA, et al. Radical retropubic prostatectomy for localized prostate cancer in renal transplant patients. Urology. 2008;72(6):1362–5.
17. Hoda MR, Hamza A, Greco F, Wagner S, Reichelt O, Heynemann H, et al. Management of localized prostate cancer by retropubic radical prostatectomy in patients after renal transplantation. Nephrol Dial Transplant. 2010;25(10):3416–20.
18. Bootun R. Effects of immunosuppressive therapy on wound healing. Int Wound J. 2013;10(1):98–104.
19. Kinahan TJ, McLoughlin MG, Manson AD. Radical prostatectomy for localized prostatic carcinoma in the renal transplant patient. J Urol. 1991;146(1):104–7.
20. Yiou R, Salomon L, Colombel M, Patard JJ, Chopin D, Abbou CC. Perineal approach to radical prostatectomy in kidney transplant recipients with localized prostate cancer. Urology. 1999;53(4):822–4.
21. Hafron J, Fogarty JD, Wiesen A, Melman A. Surgery for localized prostate cancer after renal transplantation. BJU Int. 2005;95(3):319–22.
22. Shah KK, Ko DS, Mercer J, Dahl DM. Laparoscopic radical prostatectomy in a renal allograft recipient. Urology. 2006;68(3):672 e5.
23. Thomas AA, Nguyen MM, Gill IS. Laparoscopic transperitoneal radical prostatectomy in renal transplant recipients: a review of three cases. Urology. 2008;71(2):205–8.
24. Jhaveri JK, Tan GY, Scherr DS, Tewari AK. Robot-assisted laparoscopic radical prostatectomy in the renal allograft transplant recipient. J Endourol. 2008;22(11):2475–9.
25. Robert G, Elkentaoui H, Pasticier G, Couzi L, Merville P, Ravaud A, et al. Laparoscopic radical prostatectomy in renal transplant recipients. Urology. 2009;74(3):683–7.
26. Jenjitranant P, Sangkum P, Sirisreetreerux P, Viseshsindh W, Patcharatrakul S, Kongcharoensombat W. Retzius Space Preservation Technique for Robotic-Assisted Laparoscopic Radical Prostatectomy in a Kidney Transplant Patient: First Case in Thailand and Our First Experience. Transplant Proc. 2016;48(9):3130–3.
27. Tugcu V, Simsek A, Yigitbasi I, Yenice MG, Sahin S, Tasci AI. Robot-Assisted Perineal Radical Prostatectomy in a Post-Kidney Transplant Recipient. Journal of endourology case reports. 2018;4(1):21–4.
28. Zeng J, Christiansen A, Pooli A, Qiu F, LaGrange CA. Safety and clinical outcomes of robot-assisted radical prostatectomy in kidney transplant patients: a systematic review. J Endourol. 2018;32(10):935–43.
29. Felber M, Drouin SJ, Grande P, Vaessen C, Parra J, Barrou B, et al. Morbidity, perioperative outcomes and complications of robot-assisted radical prostatectomy in kidney transplant patients: A French multicentre study. Urol Oncol. 2020;38(6):599. e15-e21
30. Leonard G, Pradere B, Monleon L, Boutin JM, Branchereau J, Karam G, et al. Oncological and postoperative outcomes of robot-assisted laparoscopic radical prostatectomy in renal transplant recipients: a multicenter and comparative study. Transplant Proc. 2020;52(3):850–6.
31. Iwamoto K, Iizuka J, Hashimoto Y, Kondo T, Takagi T, Hata K, et al. Radical prostatectomy for localized prostate cancer in renal transplant recipients: 13 cases studied at a single center. Transplant Proc. 2018;50(8):2539–44.
32. Poggio ED, Augustine JJ, Arrigain S, Brennan DC, Schold JD. Long-term kidney transplant graft survival-making progress when most needed. Am J Transplant; 2020.

Patients with Previous BPH Surgery

42

Ng Chi Fai Anthony and Chiu Ka-Fung Peter

Introduction

Prostate cancer (PCa) and benign prostatic hyperplasia (BPH) are both common in middle age to elderly men and so it is not uncommon to have patients with both conditions. With the increase in aging population, there is more and more opportunities to encounter patients diagnosed to have localized PCa with previous BPH surgery performed. Therefore, there are increasing chance to perform robotic assisted radical prostatectomy (RARP) in patients with previous surgery for BPH. There are two common scenarios resulted in these challenging situations, either incidental finding of PCa in pathological specimen of TURP or patients with history of BPH surgery were diagnosed to have PCa due to raised PSA in subsequent follow-up. As BPH surgery will results in many changes in prostate and lower urinary tract, there is a need to understand these potential effects and how to manage this more complicated surgical situation.

Effects of BPH Surgery on Prostate

The effect of BPH surgery is not just limited to the prostate but the whole lower tract could be affected.

For prostate itself, because of surgery (no matter what energy platforms were used), there will be increase in peri-prostatic scarring, in particular if there is perforation of capsule during surgery or bladder neck incision done This scarring will not only affect the precision of surgical dissection, for nerve sparing dissection. These will inevitably increase in blood lost, post-surgery erectile dysfunction, or even margin involvement.

The resection of bladder neck during TURP or even bladder neck incision will result in wide bladder neck junction, which may increase in need for bladder neck reconstruction, increase difficult in anastomosis. All these will lead to increase in catheter time, increase in post-operative urine leak and poorer continence function.

The distortion of bladder neck/trigone anatomy may increase difficulty in identifying the ureteric orifices, or the ureteric orifice may close to the bladder neck cut edge. This may increase the risk of ureteric injury during prostatectomy.

Finally, the instrumentation related to endoscopic procedure or urethral catheterization may also increase the risk of urethral stricture which may also affect subsequent surgery or voiding outcomes.

Surgical Outcomes of Prostatectomy in Patients with Previous BPH Surgery

Transurethral resection of prostate (TURP) is probably the most performed procedure and so most studies' results were based on the surgical outcomes of robotic assisted radical prostatectomy (RARP) after TURP [1, 2]. In an earlier report of the result 26 cases having RARP after TURP, there was significant increase in blood loss, bladder neck reconstruction and operative time, when compared with those patients with no previous TURP [1]. Treatment outcomes for those patients with previous TURP were also poorer, including higher margin positive rate and biochemical recurrence, as well as higher incontinence rates.

In another matched study between patients with previous history of BPH surgery and those without, similar observations were found, i.e., longer operative time, anastomotic time, need of bladder neck reconstruction, and more blood loss in the former group [2]. The were also more perioperative and postoperative complications reported in the group of patients with prior BPH surgery (40%), compared to no prior surgery group (25%). In particular, more perioperative urine leakage and later urethral stricture were reported. This probably reflect the more requirement of bladder neck reconstruc-

N. C. F. Anthony (✉) · C. K.-F. Peter
SH Ho Urology Centre, Department of Surgery, The Chinese University of Hong Kong, Shatin, Hong Kong
e-mail: ngcf@surgery.cuhk.edu.hk; peterchiu@surgery.cuhk.edu.hk

S. Ren et al. (eds.), *Robot-Assisted Radical Prostatectomy*, https://doi.org/10.1007/978-3-031-05855-4_42

tion and more challenges in anastomosis. However, functional outcomes of the two groups were similar in this report.

Holmium Laser enucleation of prostate (HoLEP) is another option of endoscopic treatment for large prostate (>80 g). In a recent report about the outcomes of RARP in patients with HoLEP performed, operating time and need of bladder neck reconstruction was significantly increased compared to HoLEP-naïve group [3]. The time to continence was also significantly longer in HoLEP group. They also compare the experience of post-HoLEP RARP (before 2015) and those from later series, later group has improved operating time, blood loss, time to continence than earlier series. Therefore, experience of surgeons did translate to improvement in surgical outcomes.

Open retropubic prostatectomy for BPH is less commonly performed in current minimally invasive surgery era. In a small series (5 cases) on the surgical outcomes of RARP after prostatic surgery, more adhesion was encountered during surgery [2]. As expected these patients required longer operation time and had more blood loss than those patients having TURP prior to RARP. Fortunately, the overall perioperative, oncological, and functional outcomes seem to be comparable between the two groups.

However, despite these potential pitfalls of RARP in patients after previous BPH surgery, RARP was shown to have better outcomes than open radical prostatectomy in patients with previous TURP [4]. RARP had significantly less blood loss and transfusion, shorter hospital stays and catheterization time, and less postoperative complications. Therefore, it was still the recommended surgical procedure for patients with PCa.

Management

Prevention

Ideally, we should diagnose patients with clinical BPH for any possible co-existing PCa. For patients with reasonable life expectancy, a proper informed discussion on prostate cancer screening should be discussed. If patient agreed, additional serum prostate specific antigen (PSA) measurement should be done, besides digital rectal examination, for prostate cancer detection. Certainly, there may be falsely elevated serum PSA due to BPH or its related complications, such as retention of urine, urinary tract infection, or other manipulation, such as urethral catheter insertion etc. However, this would help to detect potential patients with coexisting PCa and allow proper preoperative investigation done. This would be important for patients planned to undergo ablative type BPH surgery, like green light laser, bipolar vapourization etc., as no tissue for histological assessment would be available after surgery. If patient was finally diagnosed to have prostate cancer, he maybe benefited from more definitive treatment for PCa and avoid the potential poorer functional outcomes later.

Preoperative Assessment

For patients with history of BPH surgery and diagnosed to have PCa, a proper counselling is needed for possible treatment options, the potential poorer surgical, functional, and oncological outcomes [1, 2]. A more appropriate expectation of the outcomes would help to avoid unnecessary patient's frustration and complaints.

If the patient has decided to undergo RARP, proper preoperative assessment would be needed. Any pre-existing lower tract urinary symptoms need to document and investigated. Poor uroflow might be related to regenerated prostate (which might result in difficulty in urethral catheter insertion, irregular bladder neck anatomy etc.), urethral stricture etc. Preoperative storage symptom might be related to pre-existing overactive bladder secondary to bladder outlet obstruction and might increase risk of urge incontinence after RARP. Presence of stress incontinence might be related to possible damage to external sphincter during BPH surgery and could be deteriorate further after RARP. Also baseline sexual function need to be documented before surgery.

Uroflowmetry might help to detect possible urethral stricture. Preoperative MRI imaging would help to provide more information about the prostate lumen and bladder neck anatomy. A flexible cystoscopy would be recommended to assess the anatomy. The "J-maneuver" of flexible cystoscopy would provide a view of the bladder neck from cranio-caudal direction, which would be similar to the robotic view after opening up the bladder neck (Fig. 42.1). This view would help to allow the surgeon to have a better preoperative image of the bladder neck anatomy and the relationship of the ureteric ori-

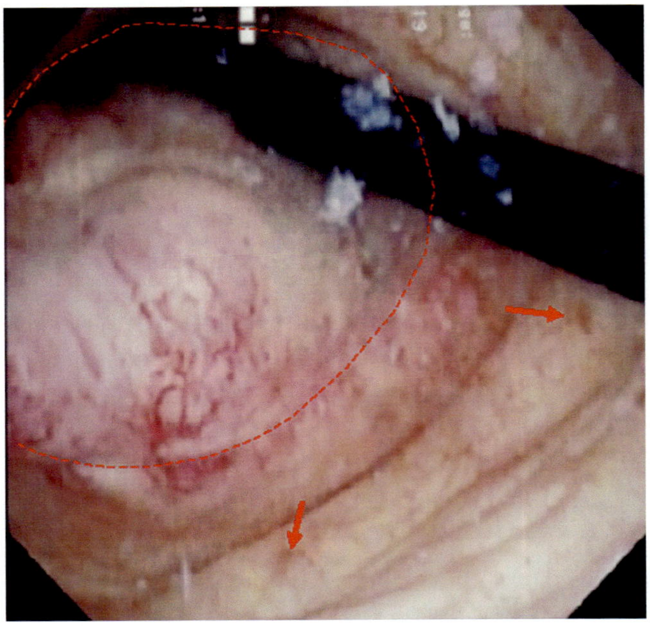

Fig. 42.1 The "J-maneuver" of flexible cystoscopy of the bladder neck. Red dotted line—bladder neck; Red arrows—Ureteric orifices

fices to bladder neck. This will help a better planning of subsequent surgery.

Earlier introduction of pelvic floor exercise might help to have earlier recovery of continence after RARP and should be introduce to patients once they have decided for surgery.

As the difficulty of dissection and potential blood loss were expected to be increased, it would be better to stop all antiplatelet and anticoagulants prior to surgery. Blood might also need to be reserved for possible transfusion if needed.

Intraoperative

If ureteric orifices were found to be close to bladder neck, ureteric stenting might help to allow easier recognition of ureteric orifices during surgery.

While the port placements and surgical steps were similar to usual RARP, more careful dissection of the bladder neck would be important to avoid creating a large bladder neck opening and also damaging the ureteric orifices. The dissection of posterior plane of prostate, as well as nerve dissection might be challenging due to periprostatic scarring after BPH surgery.

After complete dissection of prostate, there would be likely size discrepancy between bladder neck and urethra, (Fig. 42.2) and bladder neck reconstruction will usually be needed. There are many ways to reconstruct the bladder neck. For cases with ureteric orifices close to cut-edge, a posterior tennis-racket reconstruction might help to protect the orifices from caught up during subsequent anastomosis. Other approaches including anterior tennis racket reconstruction or bilateral fish-mouth reconstruction. While studies did not find any different in the outcomes between different approaches, [5] posterior reconstruction might result in bulkiness at the posterior part of bladder neck and result in more difficulty in urethral anastomosis. Due to the requirement of bladder neck reconstruction, water-tightness testing and postoperative drainage to pelvic/anastomotic area were recommended.

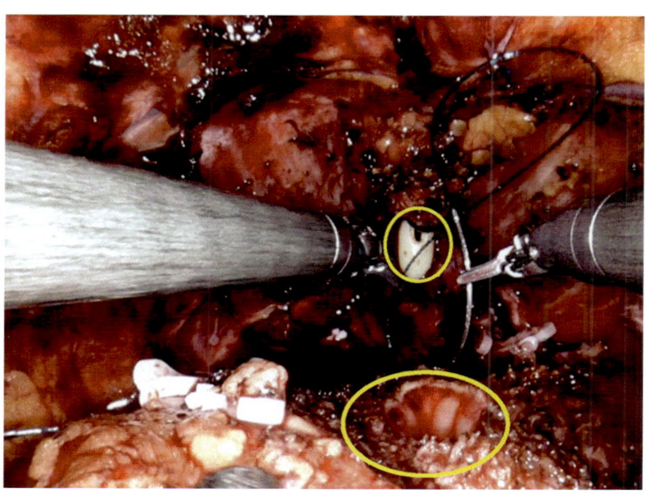

Fig. 42.2 Size discrepancy between bladder neck and urethra. Smaller circle—urethra; Larger circle—bladder neck

Postoperative Care

Depend on the confidence of the surgeon on the anastomosis, longer postoperative catheter time might be needed. If there was concern about the healing of the anastomosis and reconstruction, cystogram might be needed to confirm no contrast leaking before catheter removal.

Conclusion

While there are increasing chance of having patients with previous BPH surgery undergoing radical prostatectomy, careful preoperative assessment and counseling will help to have better surgical planning and proper patient's expectation, which will result in better clinical outcomes.

References

1. Gupta NP, Singh P, Nayyar R. Outcomes of robot-assisted radical prostatectomy in men with previous transurethral resection of prostate. BJU Int. 2011;108(9):1501–5. https://doi.org/10.1111/j.1464-410X.2011.10113.x. Epub 2011 Mar 10
2. Tugcu V, Atar A, Sahin S, et al. Robot-assisted radical prostatectomy after previous prostate surgery. JSLS. 2015;19(4):e2015.00080. https://doi.org/10.4293/JSLS.2015.00080.
3. Abedali ZA, Calaway AC, Large T, Koch MO, Lingeman JE, Boris RS. Robot-assisted radical prostatectomy in patients with a history of holmium laser enucleation of the prostate: the Indiana University Experience. J Endourol. 2020;34(2):163–8. https://doi.org/10.1089/end.2019.0436.
4. Martinschek A, Heinzelmann K, Ritter M, Heinrich E, Trojan L. Radical prostatectomy after previous transurethral resection of the prostate: robot-assisted laparoscopic versus open radical prostatectomy in a matched-pair analysis. J Endourol. 2012;26(9):1136–41. https://doi.org/10.1089/end.2012.0074. Epub 2012 May 31
5. Zhang S, Liang C, Qian J, Liu Y, Lv Q, Li J, Li P, Shao P, Wang Z. The impact of three different bladder neck reconstruction techniques on urinary continence after laparoscopic radical prostatectomy. J Endourol. 2020;34(6):663–70. https://doi.org/10.1089/end.2020.0064. Epub 2020 May 5

Salvage Robot-Assisted Radical Prostatectomy

43

Camille Berquin, Arjun Nathan, Ruben De Groote, and Senthil Nathan

Introduction

This chapter describes the perioperative, oncological and functional outcomes of salvage robot assisted radical prostatectomy (sRARP). Further, we compare the procedure to primary robot assisted radical prostatectomy (RARP) to ascertain the feasibility of the operation.

Non-surgical primary treatment for prostate cancer includes whole gland therapies such as brachytherapy or radiotherapy and focal gland therapies such as High Intensity Focused Ultrasound (HIFU), cryotherapy or electroporation. Cancer recurrence rates of these non-surgical primary treatments may vary from 20–60%. The recurrence is often limited to the prostate and is therefore potentially curable by sRARP or salvage radiotherapy [1, 2].

As focal therapy options are gaining in popularity due to the attractive post treatment toxicity profile, the total number of patients experiencing failure and requiring salvage therapy are also expected to rise. Therefore, it is important for urologists and the multidisciplinary team to understand about salvage curative treatments best suited for these patients. At the outset we will discuss the feasibility of sRARP) and discuss the safety profile of this complex surgery. Further, we shall differentiate the outcomes of sRARP after focal therapy compared to whole-gland primary therapy. Furthermore, we will discuss the key technical considerations to be aware of when performing sRARP after different modalities of primary treatment.

Historically, open salvage radical prostatectomy had less favorable oncological and functional outcomes compared to primary radical prostatectomy, including higher rates of urinary incontinence, erectile dysfunction and peri-operative morbidity. The unfavorable outcomes were due to technical hazards such as fibrosis, adhesions, poor tissue quality, very small prostate, and abnormal surgical planes during salvage surgery. The procedure was considered controversial with minimal uptake by urological surgeons. Even with the advent of strict guidelines the procedure did not gain popularity leaving some patients resigned to non-curative hormonal manipulation. Salvage prostatectomy with the introduction of the robotic platform is gaining popularity and we shall discuss the current evidence of vastly improved outcomes probably due to improved vision and enhanced dexterity [1–4].

Is the procedure safe and comparable? Salvage robot-assisted radical prostatectomy vs. primary robot-assisted radical prostatectomy.

The largest series of propensity matched study were described by Nathan et al. where they compared 135 patients who underwent sRARP to an equal number of patients who underwent primary RARP. The preoperative demographics were controlled with the use of propensity score matching, there were no statistical differences between age, BMI, ASA, Charlson Co-Morbidity Index (CCI), pre-operative PSA, T-stage and Gleason score between both groups. [3].

Some of the peri-operative outcomes were significantly different in both groups, such as the median operation time of 165 vs. 140 min in sRARP vs. primary RARP ($p = 0.004$). It was also noted that nerve sparing was significantly less feasible in the sRARP group. The feasibility of unilateral and bilateral nerve sparing: 23% and 3.7% in the salvage group vs. 28.1% and 20.7% in the primary group ($p < 0.001$) was statistically different and is likely the reason for the inferior erectile function outcomes related to salvage surgery. The reduced nerve-sparing rate may be due to prioritization of oncological control by a wide excision of the prostate or due to challenging difficult and congealed tissue planes. No statistical differences were described in estimated blood loss, blood transfusion or length of hospital stay. Neither was there a statistically significant difference in the 30-day

C. Berquin (✉)
Urology department, UZ Ghent, ORSI Academy, Melle, Belgium

R. De Groote
OLV Hospital, Aalst Belgium, ORSI Academy, Melle, Belgium

A. Nathan · S. Nathan
University College London, London, UK
e-mail: arjun.nathan1@nhs.net; s.nathan@nhs.net

S. Ren et al. (eds.), *Robot-Assisted Radical Prostatectomy*, https://doi.org/10.1007/978-3-031-05855-4_43

Clavien-Dindo grade III and IV complication rates (respectively 1.5 vs. 0%). The high-grade complications described were rectal injury and a hematoma requiring re-operation. Although these complication rates might not be statistically different between both groups, they are clinically relevant as it reflects the poor dissection planes which one could encounter during sRARP [3].

Oncological outcomes such as positive surgical margins (PSM), recurrence rates and recurrence-free survival were all worse in the salvage group compared to the primary group. When comparing patients with recurrence to recurrence-free patients they found preoperative PSA and T-stage to be higher in the recurrence group. EAU guidelines currently suggest referral for salvage therapy at a PSA level < 10 ng/mL, however the results of Nathan et al. suggest referral for salvage therapy should occur earlier after biochemical failure [3, 5].

Functionally, early continence is better in primary RARP however at the one- and two-year time intervals SRARP after focal therapy provides similar continence outcomes to primary RARP. However, SRARP after whole-gland therapy results in inferior continence outcomes compared to primary RARP. Erectile dysfunction was significantly higher in the salvage group (94.8% vs. 76.3%) at last follow-up [3].

Comparing Salvage Options After Focal Therapy Failure

Nathan et al. published the first paper comparing different salvage treatments after focal therapy failure. They investigated the effectiveness of sRARP to salvage radiotherapy after focal therapy failure in a large cohort of 200 patients. They showed that in men with high-risk recurrent disease, salvage radiotherapy may result in better biochemical recurrence (BCR) free survival compared to sRARP at medium term follow up. They highlight this may be due to the ongoing effect of concomitant Androgen Deprivation Therapy used for salvage radiotherapy in the medium-term follow up setting. There was no difference in BCR free survival for men with intermediate risk disease. Unlike sRARP, salvage radiotherapy results in worse toxicity compared to primary radiotherapy and requires the use of concomitant Androgen Deprivation Therapy with its own adverse side effects. Interestingly of note, continence after the early phase was similar between both treatment options. This may be due to improved surgical techniques such as retzius-sparing or anterior reconstruction techniques whilst salvage radiotherapy was associated with increased urinary and bowel toxicity. As expected, erectile function was significantly inferior after sRARP compared to salvage radiotherapy. These novel results are important when considering and counselling patients for the optimum salvage modality to be used for patients after focal therapy failure. Currently there is equipoise on the ideal treatment option and further follow up and studies are needed [6].

Salvage Robot-Assisted Radical Prostatectomy After Whole Gland Therapy vs. Focal Therapy

The study of Nathan et al. also focused on the difference in outcomes between sRARP after focal therapy versus whole gland therapy. The patient characteristics did not differ significantly in age, BMI, ASA or CCI. However, their series contained more high-risk patients in the whole gland salvage group versus the focal gland salvage group, which may account, in part, for the differences observed [3].

Unilateral and bilateral nerve sparing were feasible in 8.2% and 2% of the whole group to 31.4% and 4.7% of the focal group ($p = 0.001$). Complication rates were significantly higher in the whole gland group (22%) compared to the focal group (8%) ($p = 0.025$). Other peri-operative outcomes, such as estimated blood loss, blood transfusion or length of stay did not show statistically significant differences between both groups [3].

Overall survival at last follow-up showed a statistically significant difference with 89.8% in the whole gland group versus 98.8% in the focal group ($p = 0.014$). Other oncological outcomes, such as PSM rates and recurrence rates did not differ statistically between both groups. Concerning, recurrence rates of the salvage group after whole gland therapy compared with the matched primary cohort, a significantly higher recurrence rate was observed in the whole gland salvage group. However, this was not the case for salvage surgery after focal gland therapy [2, 3].

With regards to functional outcomes, continence rates were better in the focal group compared to the whole gland group at 3, 6, 12 and 24 months. At one-year, full continence was achieved by 78% after focal compared to 49% after whole-gland. At two-years, full continence was achieved by 89% after focal compared to 53% after whole-gland. Erectile dysfunction however was high in both groups and did not show a statistically significant difference between groups. [3] These results reflect other literature which suggest that sRARP after focal therapy has better outcomes than compared to sRARP after whole-gland therapy.

Technical Considerations & Recommendations

Due to the consequences of technical hazards such as fibrosis, adhesions, poor tissue quality and abnormal anatomy and surgical planes during sRARP, one could anticipate that the surgical technique of salvage surgery would need to be adapted to the presenting circumstances. De Groote et al. suggested various adaptive strategies based on the primary treatment modality [1].

Post Radiotherapy

Due to neo-vascularization near the anterior bladder neck after radiotherapy, one needs to be careful when performing the bladder drop as it can bleed significantly. The incision of the endopelvic fascia should occur close to the prostate to avoid damage to the sphincter. Due to prior hormonal treatment the seminal vesicles may be more adherent and excessive traction should be avoided. Posterior adhesion of the prostate to the rectum should be released with careful sharp dissection. Lateral dissection of the neurovascular bundles might be more difficult as adhesions can lead to entry into the wrong plane causing injury to the vascular structures. Due to irradiation damage, healing of tissues might take more time and therefore they advise to use a 3-0 PDS for the vesico-urethral anastomosis, taking care not to put too many throws to avoid ischemic damage [1].

Post Brachytherapy

sRARP in this patient population has the worse oncological and functional outcomes. Bladder neck dissection tends to be rather easy, whereas the apex tends to be more adherent which leads to sphincter damage. It is therefore recommended to dissect from base to apex in the midline first and then the stuck pedicles. Excessive traction might lead to fracture of the prostate along the brachytherapy seed lines [1].

Post HIFU

Here the shockwaves are focused from the rectum towards the prostate from midline in a circular arc. This leads to fibrotic adhesions in the midline. The dissection should be performed from lateral to medial in the extra-fascial plane on the treated side. The midline rectum should be dissected last. The treated area will present as a cavity without fibrosis, so gentle dissection is crucial not to enter these cavities with viable tumor [1].

Post Cryotherapy

Again, similar to brachytherapy, the apex might be stuck and thus dissection should be done from the midline to lateral [1].

Post Electroporation

The prostate tends to be irregular and asymmetrical, due to the treatment effect which is quite similar to a Transurethral Resection of the Prostate (TURP).

Conclusion

Salvage robot-assisted radical prostatectomy is proving to be a feasible treatment option for local recurrence after primary non-surgical treatment for prostate cancer. However, the outcomes tend to be marginally worse in salvage surgery due to technical hazards such as fibrosis, adhesions, poor tissue quality and abnormal surgical planes.

Recent studies show similar perioperative comorbidity compared to primary RARP. However, patients should be counselled that functional and oncological outcomes after sRARP are inferior to primary RARP. Salvage RARP after whole gland therapy has worse outcomes than after focal therapy. Knowledge of the different primary treatment options is key for an adaptive strategy for salvage surgery. As sRARP is a technically more challenging procedure, it would be advisable to centralize these surgeries to high-volume centers with highly experienced surgeons.

References

1. De Groote R, Nathan A, De Bleser E, et al. Techniques and outcomes of salvage robot-assisted radical prostatectomy (sRARP). Eur Urol. 2020;78(6):885–92.
2. Kaffenberger S, Smith J. Salvage robotic radical prostatectomy. Indian J Urol. 2014;30(4):429–33.
3. Nathan A, Fricker M, De Groote R, et al. Salvage versus primary robot-assisted radical prostatectomy: a propensity-matched comparative effectiveness study from a high-volume tertiary centre. Eur Urol Open Sci. 2021;27:43–52.
4. Stephenson AJ, Scardino PT, Bianco FJ Jr. Morbidity and functional outcomes of salvage radical prostatec- tomy for locally recurrent prostate cancer after radiation therapy. J Urol. 2004;172(6):2239–43.
5. Mottet N, Comford P, van den Bergh RCN, EAU Guidelines," edn. Presented at the EAU Annual Congress Milan, 2021.
6. Nathan A, Ng A, Mitra A, Sooriakumaran P, Davda R, Patel S, Fricker M, Kelly J, Shaw G, Rajan P, Sridhar A, Nathan S, Payne H. Comparative effectiveness analyses of salvage prostatectomy and salvage radiotherapy outcomes following focal or whole-gland ablative therapy (High Intensity Focused Ultrasound (HIFU), cryotherapy or electroporation) for localised prostate cancer. Clin Oncol (R Coll Radiol). 2022;34(1):e69–78.

Super-Extended Robot Assisted Radical Prostatectomy in Locally Advanced Prostate Cancer

44

Elio Mazzone, Alberto Briganti, and Francesco Montorsi

Introduction

The adoption of prostate-specific antigen (PSA)-based prostate cancer (PCa) screening led to a stage migration towards more favorable disease at the time of PCa diagnosis [1, 2]. However, a reverse stage migration towards more advanced disease was observed in more contemporary PCa patients [3–5] probably due to the decreased use of PSA-based screening [6, 7] following the US Preventive Services Task Force recommendations [8] and the discordant findings provided by the Prostate, Lung, Colorectal and Ovarian (PLCO) [9, 10], the European Randomized study of Screening for Prostate Cancer (ERSPC) and the Cluster Randomized Trial of PSA Testing for Prostate Cancer (CAP) screening trials [11–13]. Indeed, among men diagnosed with PCa during the period 2010–2016, 12 and 4% harbored locally-advanced and metastatic disease, respectively [14]. The management of these groups of PCa patients is one of the most compelling contemporary challenges. Historically, radical prostatectomy (RP) was reserved for PCa patients with organ-confined disease due to the concerns about inadequate disease control in more advanced cases, as well as the related side effects [15]. In the last decade, despite the lack of randomized controlled trials testing the role of RP in high-risk setting, RP has been increasingly employed in the management of high-risk PCa patients [16–18] and good oncologic outcomes were reported [19–25]. As such, in the setting of locally advanced PCa, the European Association of Urology (EAU) [26] and the National Comprehensive Cancer Network (NCCN) [27] guidelines recommend to perform radical prostatectomy as part of multi-modal therapy in highly selected patients who may benefit of this surgical procedure [28].

In this context, it is noteworthy that robot-assisted radical prostatectomy (RARP) has become the most common surgical approach performed in patients with localized PCa [29, 30]. Moreover, multiparametric magnetic resonance imaging (MRI) has significantly changed the diagnostic pathway of PCa patients [31–33] and, in the context of surgical planning, it has become a key tool to assess the clinical relevance and the local extent of disease in PCa patients [34, 35] to guide the decision-making process towards the treatment choice [36, 37]. During the last years several variations of the original description of RARP have been described [38] and remarkably technological refinements of the robotic platform and of its tools have been observed [28]. However, evidence supporting the oncological efficacy of RARP in locally advanced PCa are still sparse. In this regard, several retrospective studies explored the role of extended surgery in the context of locally advanced PCa. Among these, Gandaglia et al. [39], relying on a multi-institutional database, demonstrated that RARP is a safe and oncological effective procedure in PCa patients with locally advanced disease. However, the authors [39] included in the study cohort patients with T3 disease as defined by MRI or rectal examination. To date, the outcomes of RARP in a pure cohort of patients with ECE at MRI were explored only in a recent single centre study [40]. As such, the feasibility and efficacy of RARP exclusively on locally advanced PCa patients with extracapsular extension (ECE) at MRI, who often are considered as inoperable patients, was partially explored so far. Based on this premise, we aim to describe current technique and outcomes of super-extended RARP (SE-RARP) for locally advanced PCa patients.

E. Mazzone · A. Briganti · F. Montorsi (✉)
Division of Oncology/Unit of Urology, URI, IRCCS Ospedale San Raffaele, Milan, Italy

Vita-Salute San Raffaele University, Milan, Italy
e-mail: mazzone.elio@hsr.it; Briganti.alberto@hsr.it; montorsi.francesco@hsr.it

S. Ren et al. (eds.), *Robot-Assisted Radical Prostatectomy*, https://doi.org/10.1007/978-3-031-05855-4_44

Main Body of the Chapter

Surgical Technique for Super-Extended Robot-Assisted Radical Prostatectomy

RARP procedures described in the literature are performed with a DaVinci system (Intuitive Surgical, Sunnyvale, CA, USA) through a six-port transperitoneal approach. This robotic approach begins with the incision of the parietal peritoneum lateral to the lateral umbilical ligaments. The bladder is released and the space of Retzius developed. Subsequently, after complete bladder detachment with the median umbilical ligament preservation [41], bilateral endopelvic fascia incision is performed in order to identify the borders of the prostate. Alternatively, the endopelvic fascia can be preserved, but this might result in lower prostatic mobility and might render the prostatic dissection more difficult in case of larger prostates [42].

Fourth arm maintaining bladder retraction or suspension suture can be placed on the prostate to facilitate the bladder neck dissection. An initial postero-lateral incision of the bladder neck between bladder and prostate is performed and continues towards the mid-line following the peri-prostatic fat. After identification of the vas deferens, the peritoneum is incised at the level of the rectovesical pouch. The vas deferens is dissected, the peritoneum is pushed downwards, the Denonvillier's fascia (DVF) with some perirectal fat is dissected free and pushed upwards with the specimen so that they remain on the posterior surface of the seminal vesicles (Fig. 44.1a). As results of the dissection, the seminal vesicle is not visible, as completely covered by the DVF and the perirectal fat. The dissection is carried forwards to the anterior face of the rectum, pushing the perirectal fat and DVF upwards with the specimen. Notably, preoperative multiparametric MRI use can optimize local staging and surgical planning. Indeed, SE-RARP can be performed with unilateral or bilateral DVF resection according to the extension of the disease at MRI. If the tumour is unilateral, the seminal vesicle on the side without tumour burden is released in a standard fashion leaving DVF attached to the rectum (Fig. 44.1b).

Regarding the degree of preservation of the neurovascular bundle (NVB), this can be preserved in toto (intrafascial dissection) or partly (interfascial dissection), or dissected completely (extra-fascial dissection). In the context of locally advanced PCa, an extrafascial dissection with Hem-o-lock clips is typically carried out laterally to the levator ani fascia. In case of extracapsular extension of PCa is localized at one side, a mono-lateral preservation of NVB can be performed [40]. In this case, recent introduction of preoperative MRI can help in defining the correct location of ECE for surgical planning.

The dissection of the prostatic apex can be carried out with a sharp and direct division of the membranous urethra at the level of the urethroprostatic junction. Alternatively, apical dissection of the prostate can be performed according to the "Collar technique" [43]. Such technique has been demonstrated to reduce the rate of positive margin at the level of the apex and, therefore, may be particularly useful in the context of locally advanced PCa. Finally, posterior reconstruction and urethrovescical anastomosis are performed [44]. In case of unilateral DVF resection, partial monolateral posterior reconstruction is generally performed before urethrovescical anastomosis.

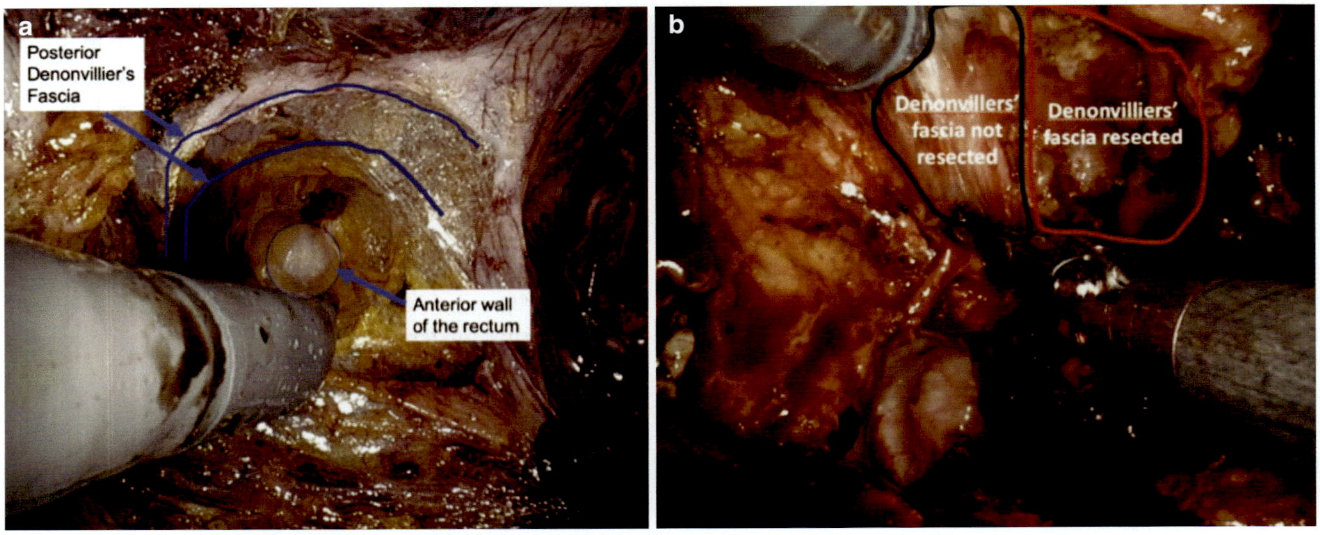

Fig. 44.1 (**a**) Posterior Denonvillier's fascia is dissected and pushed upwards with the specimen. (**b**) Monolateral resection of Denonvillier's fascia left on the posterior surface of the seminal vesicles and of the prostate [40]

Technique for Extended and Super-Extended Pelvic Lymph Node Dissection

Template definitions for extended or super-extended pelvic lymph node dissection (PLND) rely on those previously defined by consensus panels [45]. Generally accepted indications to perform super-extended template are: (1) preoperative Briganti risk score for lymph node invasion ≥30% [46]; (2) positive node at external iliac level at frozen pathology [47]. Regarding the technique, after incision of the peritoneum, release of the bladder laterally to the endopelvic fascia, and localization of the ureter, the dissection of the lymphatic tissue is performed adopting the split and roll technique. The external iliac artery is localized behind the peritoneum. The peritoneal incision is prolonged following the external iliac artery up to the vas deferens, which is exposed and then cut. The fibrofatty tissue along the external iliac vein is dissected, the lateral limit being the genitofemoralis nerve and the distal limit being the deep circumflex vein. Proximally, extended PLND is performed up to and included the crossing between the ureter and common iliac vessels. Once the external iliac vessels are freed, the obturator nerve is approached. The dissection is performed from lateral to medial up to the umbilical artery and the bladder wall that represents the medial limit of the extended PLND. Lymph nodes along as well as medially and laterally to the internal iliac vessels are also removed. The obturator fossa is also accessed lateral to the external iliac artery and the lymphatic tissue freed from the pelvic wall. Smaller vessels are coagulated and cut, and dissection is continued until the deep obturator fossa is reached. All fibrofatty tissue within the obturator fossa is removed. The Marcille's triangular lumbosacral fossa is dissected free. This area is delimited laterally by the medial border of the psoas, medially by the body of the fifth lumbar vertebra, and inferiorly by the border of the sacral wing (Fig. 44.2) [48].

Recently, Mattei et al. [49] described a revised technique for "en-bloc" excision of the lymph nodes. The starting point is a 10-step monoblock template which was first described in 2013 [50]. After this extended template, the authors proposed an additional super-extended template delineated by the following boundaries: cranially, the aortic and caval bifurcation; caudally, the ureter crossing over the common iliac artery laterally and the promontorium medially; laterally, the common iliac vessels; dorsally, the sacral bone; and ventrally, the peritoneum covering the sigma. Considering the anatomical limits, this "en-bloc" approach for super extended PLND was divided into 5 steps: first, mobilization of the sigma and development of right lateral boundary; second, dissection of the cranial boundary; third, dissection of the left lateral boundary; fourth, development of the ventral boundary; fifth, development of the dorsal boundary (Fig. 44.3).

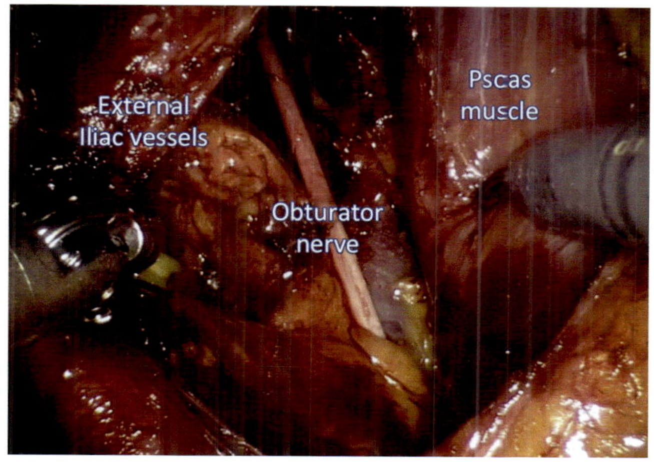

Fig. 44.2 Access to the Marcille's triangle during robot-assisted extended pelvic lymph node dissection. The psoas muscle, external iliac vessels, and obturator nerve are clearly identifiable [39]

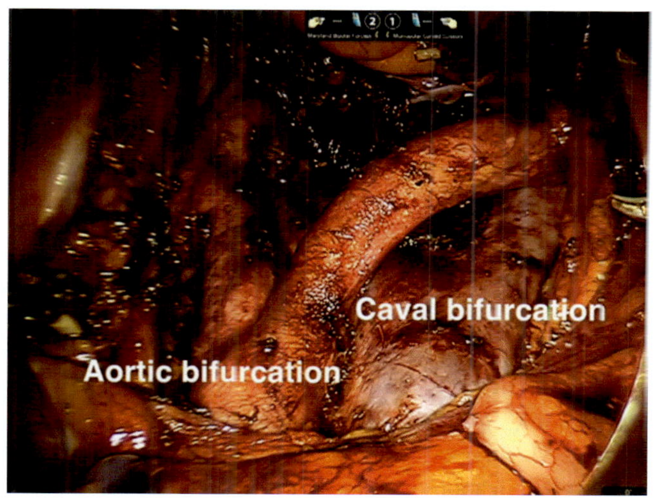

Fig. 44.3 Intraoperative sight from a Da-Vinci 0-degree camera, placed supraumbilically, after having performed a superextended pelvic lymph node dissection including all common lymphatic landing sites of the prostate around the common iliac vessels up to the aortic and caval bifurcation as well as the presacral region [49]

Postoperative Outcomes

Surgical Outcomes

Several authors have demonstrated optimal perioperative outcomes for RARP in advanced PCa cases. Operative time and estimated blood loss in high-risk PCa patients treated with RARP ranged from 111 to 199 min and from 84 to 284 mL, respectively [28, 39, 40, 48, 51, 52]. Transfusion rate ranged between 0 and 5.9%. Length of stay and catheterization time ranged from 1 to 4 days and from 4.7 to 8 days, respectively [39, 40, 48, 51, 52]. Only one study reported a mean catheterization time of 15 days [40]. Overall complication rate ranged from 4 to 28%, while major complication rate ranged from 0.6 to 9.1% [39, 40, 48, 51, 52]. In studies comparing RARP to the open approach, high-risk PCa patients treated with RARP have shorter length of stay, lower estimated blood loss, lower transfusion rates and comparable postoperative complication rates relative to those treated with open radical prostatectomy (ORP) [51, 53, 54]. For example, Gandaglia et al. [54] provided evidence that patients treated with RARP had lower risk of prolonged length of stay compared with those who underwent ORP (≥3 days: odds ratio [OR] 0.18, $p < 0.001$; ≥5 days: OR 0.42, $p = 0.02$) and failed to observe statistically significant difference in terms of 30-day overall postoperative complications between RARP and ORP, after accounting for different confounders (OR: 0.94; $p = 0.6$). However, patients treated with RARP were less likely to receive blood transfusion compared to those treated with ORP (OR: 0.25; $p = 0.002$). These findings suggested that RARP is a relatively safe procedure when performed in high-risk PCa, and not worse with respect to perioperative outcomes when compared with ORP. However, also in contemporary high-risk patients treated with RARP the overall rate of complications is not negligible and in the worst-case scenario may reach 28% [54]. In consequence, there is still a need to improve and surgical expertise is the major determinants of decreased risk of postoperative complications.

Recently, Mazzone et al. [40] described the feasibility of RARP in locally advanced PCa with ECE at preoperative MRI. Here, RARP technique was not associated with increased rate of postoperative complications after surgery compared to previous RARP series on locally advanced cases [39]. This evidence further supports the feasibility and safety profile of this approach in patients with posterior ECE at MRI. Notably, the robustness of these results on postoperative complications is supported by the use of standardized methodology provided by the EAU [55]. Indeed, by fulfilling all the suggested criteria, the high reliability of data report on postoperative complications was ensured.

Functional Outcomes

To date, few studies evaluated functional outcomes in high-risk PCa patients treated with RARP and are limited by the relatively short follow-up and by the lack of standardization on urinary incontinence and erectile dysfunction assessment which make difficult to accurately assess these outcomes in patients who underwent robotic approach. In these studies, urinary continence (UC) recovery at 12 months using 0–1 pad definition ranged from 78 to 85.2% [39, 40, 52, 56–60]. Overall, it is noteworthy that no major functional impairment after wide excision of the posterior plane was reported, when UC was considered. Notably, average early continence rate was 34%. In general, high-risk patients are less likely to undergo neurovascular bundle preservation due to their advanced disease. Indeed, nerve sparing can be challenging in these patients and may expose to higher irsk of positive surgical margins, however in selected individuals it is certainly feasible without compromising cancer control [40, 56, 57]. The rate of nerve sparing reported in this subset of patients treated with RARP is highly variable, ranging from 19.7 to 98.3%. However, in studies relying on preoperative MRI for PCa staging and local extension assessment [40, 59], UC rate at 1 year of follow-up was higher (84%) than those reported for locally-advanced PCa in previous mixed [61] or purely RARP [39] series. This result might be explained by the fact that, differently from previous series, the definition of disease extension at MRI allowed to perform a certain degree of inter-fascial nerve-sparing approach, which has been demonstrated to have a protective effect on early continence recovery [61–63]. Indeed, in the recent study by Mazzone et al. [40], the overall rate of any inter-fascial nerve-sparing was high (75%) and this further supports the recorded differences in UC rate compared to previous analyses [64, 65]. Lastly, no significant difference in UC recovery rates was recorded in the literature between patients with apical or non-apical lesions with suspected ECE at MRI (82 vs 86%, $p = 0.5$) [40]. This data confirms the efficacy of SE-RARP approach combined with the "collar" technique for apical dissection which allows to preserve sphincteric structures of the urethral complex even in case with suspected ECE at apical level [43].

Regarding erectile function (EF), the 12-month recovery rate ranged between 33.8 and 60% [52, 56, 57]. Kumar et al. [57] reported a 12-month EF recovery of 91.4% in high-risk patients who underwent complete nerve sparing. However, the definition of potency recovery used is questionable. Rogers et al. [52] were the first to assess EF recovery at approximately 24 months in contemporary high-risk PCa patients treated with RARP, reporting a rate of 33.3%. However, the authors [52] exclusively focused on men aged ≥70. To date, only few studies assessed functional outcomes of RARP in high-risk PCa setting beyond 1 year after surgery without age restriction. Of note, Abdollah et al. [56] reported Kaplan-Meier estimates of UC and EF recovery at 12, 24 and 36 months were 85.2, 89.1, 91.2% and 33.8, 52.3 and 69%, respectively. In consequence, the authors provided evidence that UC and EF outcomes continue to improve beyond 1-year after surgery and are promising at 3 years of follow-up.

Oncological Outcomes

Current RARP studies in high-risk PCa patients reported positive surgical margins (PSMs) rate ranging from 12 to 53.3% [23, 39, 40, 51, 54, 57–59, 66]. The majority of the studies that assessed the rate of PSMs according to the type of surgical approach, failed to observe a benefit in terms of PSMs of RARP relative to ORP [51, 54, 67–70]. However, all these studies were population-based [54] or assessed a small sample size [51, 67–70]. The two largest studies assessing the rate of PSMs according to surgical approach provided evidence that RARP is associated with lower risk of PSMs relative to ORP in high-risk PCa patients [71, 72]. Mazzone et al. [40] observed that positive surgical margins [73] and the high grade of the disease were independent predictors of biochemical recurrence (BCR) (hazard ratio [HR] 5.86 and 3.17, respectively) and of additional treatment use (HR 5.23 and 5.63, respectively) in multivariable Cox regression models adjusted for pathological covariates. These findings suggest that patients with negative surgical margins and low-grade disease might be the optimal candidates for this surgical treatment without the need for additional therapy at mid-term follow-up.

With respect to BCR, it occurred in 5–50% of patients at last follow-up. These heterogeneous BCR rates reported are mainly related with large differences in the length of follow-up of the studies available (Range: 4–68 months), that is generally short. Long-term oncologic outcomes data available on high-risk PCa treated with RARP is limited since many surgeons are still reluctant to perform RARP in this subset of patients. The first study that reported long-term cancer control in PCa patients treated with RARP was published by Diaz et al. [74] who assessed 483 patients with a median follow-up of 10 years. The Authors reported 10-year BCR-free survival rate of 43.2% in high-risk PCa patients (n = 36, 7.5%). Thereafter, Abdollah et al. [66] published the largest RARP series for high-risk PCa (n = 1100) and observed that at a median follow-up of 48.5 months the 10-year BCR-free and clinical-recurrence (CR)-free survival rates were 50 and 87%, respectively. However, a significant percentage of patients (37%) required salvage therapy. These findings are in line with those reported by previous studies originating from ORP [20, 75]. Moreover, Abdollah et al. [66] identified 5 novel risk-groups within the high-risk patients based on BCR risk and preoperative characteristics. The 10-year BCR-free, CR-free survival and salvage therapy rates ranged from 86 to 26%, from 99 to 55% and from 9.8 to 64%. In consequence, RARP provides sustained long-term oncologic benefit in most high-risk PCa patients. However, some patients should be candidate to a multimodal approach given the high-rate of salvage treatment. In the most recent paper by Mazzone et al. [40], the rate of BCR at 1 and 2-year follow-up were 33 and 45%, respectively. These relatively high rates are in line with previous studies on locally advanced PCa [23, 28], however, might be explained by the low number of adjuvant treatments received by our patients in favour of a strategy based on observation and subsequent salvage treatment.

The Role of Pelvic Lymph Node Dissection

The role of PLND has been largely discussed in the literature [45, 76]. To date, it is known that PLND still represents the most accurate approach for nodal staging of PCa patients. However, it is limited by the weight of potential perioperative morbidity. A recent systematic review and meta-analysis confirmed the aforementioned evidence on complications [76]. Of note, Cacciamani et al. [76] explored the role of PLND and its extent of perioperative morbidity. Remarkably, the authors concluded that the extent of PLND was the strongest predictor of postoperative complications. Therefore, in patients with high-risk disease, the extent of PLND should be balanced in the light of optimizing staging accuracy without excessively increase the risk for complications. In this regard, Gandaglia et al. have identified a cut-off of 30% risk of lymph node invasion based on Briganti nomogram to offer a super extended PLND template [46]. Decision making process should, therefore, be based on predictive tool to balance the risk of complications and the accuracy for staging.

Moreover, there is lack of prospective evidence corroborating the efficacy of PLND on oncological outcomes. Previous retrospective analyses have reported a potential effect of PLND on oncological outcomes, particularly in patients with extensive or low volume metastatic disease [77, 78]. However, prospective evidence has failed to confirm this benefit, as reported in a previous systematic review [45]. Lastly, recently published randomized trial, despite its limitation on study design, failed to demonstrate a benefit for extended PLND template compared to standard template in high risk patients, corroborating the lack of survival benefit associated with PLND [79]. In summary, PLND is to date a key phase of RARP in patients with high-risk disease considering their risk of lymph node invasion. However, PLND extent should be balanced in the light of potential risk of complications without compromising staging accuracy.

Conclusion

Taken together, we outlined specific technical features and outcomes of super extended RARP for locally advanced PCa. Specifically, recent studies described a step-by-step RARP procedure focusing on technical refinements in the DVF dissection for advanced cases, which might play a crucial role in the reduction of PSM risk and in the consequent optimization of cancer-related outcomes. A RARP technique combining the high visual definition of the DaVinci system features with the preoperative possibility of accurately staging advanced cases with MRI allows to perform a safe procedure with limited impact on perioperative complications risk and optimal functional recovery. However, future prospective comparative studies with long follow-up are needed to confirm whether super extended RARP allows maximum oncological control without compromising functional outcomes.

Acknowledgements

Disclosure The authors declare no conflict of interest.

Formatting of Funding Sources This research did not receive any specific grant from funding agencies in the public, commercial, or not-for-profit sectors.

Financial Disclosures Elio Mazzone certifies that all conflicts of interest, including specific financial interests and relationships and affiliations relevant to the subject matter or materials discussed in the manuscript (e.g., employment/affiliation, grants or funding, consultancies, honoraria, stock ownership or options, expert testimony, royalties, or patents filed, received, or pending), are the following: None.

References

1. Galper SL, Chen M-H, Catalona WJ, et al. Evidence to support a continued stage migration and decrease in prostate cancer specific mortality. J Urol. 2006;175:907–12.
2. Shao Y-H, Demissie K, Shih W, et al. Contemporary risk profile of prostate cancer in the United States. J Natl Cancer Inst. 2009;101:1280–3.
3. Reese AC, Wessel SR, Fisher SG, Mydlo JH. Evidence of prostate cancer "reverse stage migration" toward more advanced disease at diagnosis: Data from the Pennsylvania Cancer Registry. Urol Oncol. 2016;34(335):e21–8.
4. Budäus L, Spethmann J, Isbarn H, et al. Inverse stage migration in patients undergoing radical prostatectomy: results of 8916 European patients treated within the last decade. BJU Int. 2011;108:1256–61.
5. Bandini M, Mazzone E, Preisser F, et al. Increase in the annual rate of newly diagnosed metastatic prostate cancer: a contemporary analysis of the surveillance, epidemiology and end results database. Eur Urol Oncol. 2018;1:314–20.
6. Sammon JD, Abdollah F, Choueiri TK, et al. Prostate-specific antigen screening after 2012 US preventive services task force recommendations. JAMA. 2015;314:2077–9.
7. Zeliadt SB, Hoffman RM, Etzioni R, et al. Influence of publication of US and European prostate cancer screening trials on PSA testing practices. J Natl Cancer Inst. 2011;103:520–3.
8. Grossman DC, Curry SJ, Owens DK, et al. Screening for prostate cancer: us preventive services task force recommendation statement. JAMA. 2018;319:1901–13.
9. Andriole GL, Crawford ED, Grubb RL 3rd, et al. Mortality results from a randomized prostate-cancer screening trial. N Engl J Med. 2009;360:1310–9.
10. Pinsky PF, Prorok PC, Yu K, et al. Extended mortality results for prostate cancer screening in the PLCO trial with median follow-up of 15 years. Cancer. 2017;123:592–9.
11. Schröder FH, Hugosson J, Roobol MJ, et al. Screening and prostate-cancer mortality in a randomized European study. N Engl J Med. 2009;360:1320–8.
12. Schröder FH, Hugosson J, Roobol MJ, et al. Screening and prostate cancer mortality: results of the European Randomised Study of Screening for Prostate Cancer (ERSPC) at 13 years of follow-up. Lancet (London, England). 2014;384:2027–35.
13. Martin RM, Donovan JL, Turner EL, et al. Effect of a low-intensity psa-based screening intervention on prostate cancer mortality: the CAP randomized clinical trial. JAMA. 2018;319:883–95.
14. Siegel RL, Miller KD, Fuchs HE, Jemal A. Cancer statistics, 2021. CA Cancer J Clin. 2021;71:7–33.
15. Tewari A, Sooriakumaran P, Bloch DA, et al. Positive surgical margin and perioperative complication rates of primary surgical treatments for prostate cancer: a systematic review and meta-analysis comparing retropubic, laparoscopic, and robotic prostatectomy. Eur Urol. 2012;62:1–15.
16. Cooperberg MR, Carroll PR. Trends in management for patients with localized prostate cancer, 1990–2013. JAMA. 2015;314:80–2.
17. Surcel CI, Sooriakumaran P, Briganti A, et al. Preferences in the management of high-risk prostate cancer among urologists in Europe: results of a web-based survey. BJU Int. 2015;115:571–9.
18. Gray PJ, Lin CC, Cooperberg MR, Jemal A, Efstathiou JA. Temporal trends and the impact of race, insurance, and socioeconomic status in the management of localized prostate cancer. Eur Urol. 2017;71:729–37.
19. Ward JF, Slezak JM, Blute ML, Bergstralh EJ, Zincke H. Radical prostatectomy for clinically advanced (cT3) prostate cancer since the advent of prostate-specific antigen testing: 15-year outcome. BJU Int. 2005;95:751–6.
20. Yossepowitch O, Eggener SE, Serio AM, et al. Secondary therapy, metastatic progression, and cancer-specific mortality in men with clinically high-risk prostate cancer treated with radical prostatectomy. Eur Urol. 2008;53:950–9.
21. Mitchell CR, Boorjian SA, Umbreit EC, et al. 20-Year survival after radical prostatectomy as initial treatment for cT3 prostate cancer. BJU Int. 2012;110:1709–13.
22. Dell'Oglio P, Karnes RJ, Joniau S, et al. Very long-term survival patterns of young patients treated with radical prostatectomy for high-risk prostate cancer. Urol Oncol. 2016;34(234):e13–9.
23. Poelaert F, Joniau S, Roumeguère T, et al. Current management of pT3b prostate cancer after robot-assisted laparoscopic prostatectomy. Eur Urol Oncol. 2019;2:110–7.
24. McKay RR, Xie W, Ye H, et al. Results of a randomized phase II trial of intense androgen deprivation therapy prior to radical prostatectomy in men with high-risk localized prostate cancer. J Urol. 2021;206(1):80–7.
25. Hajili T, Ohlmann CH, Linxweiler J, et al. Radical prostatectomy in T4 prostate cancer after inductive androgen deprivation: results of a single-institution series with long-term follow-up. BJU Int. 2019;123:58–64.
26. EAU Prostate Guidelines. Edn. presented at the EAU Annual Congress Amsterdam 2020. ISBN 978-94-92671-07-3. 2020.
27. Aslam N, Nadeem K, Noreen R. JAC Prostate cancer prostate cancer. Abeloff's Clin Oncol. 2015;5/E:938–44.
28. Dell'Oglio P, Stabile A, Gandaglia G, et al. New surgical approaches for clinically high-risk or metastatic prostate cancer. Expert Rev Anticancer Ther. 2017;17:1013–31.
29. Gandaglia G, Karakiewicz PI, Sun M, et al. Comparative effectiveness of robot-assisted and open radical prostatectomy in the post-dissemination era. J Clin Oncol. 2014;32:1419–26.
30. Mazzone E, Mistretta FA, Knipper S, et al. Contemporary national assessment of robot-assisted surgery rates and total hospital charges for major surgical uro-oncological procedures in the United States. J Endourol. 2019;33:438–47.
31. Dell'Oglio P, Stabile A, Dias BH, et al. Impact of multiparametric MRI and MRI-targeted biopsy on pre-therapeutic risk assessment in prostate cancer patients candidate for radical prostatectomy. World J Urol. 2019;37:221–34.
32. Valerio M, Donaldson I, Emberton M, et al. Detection of clinically significant prostate cancer using magnetic resonance imaging-ultrasound fusion targeted biopsy: A systematic review. Eur Urol. 2015;68:8–19.

33. Fütterer JJ, Briganti A, De Visschere P, et al. Can Clinically significant prostate cancer be detected with multiparametric magnetic resonance imaging? a systematic review of the literature. Eur Urol. 2015;68:1045–53.
34. Stabile A, Dell'Oglio P, Soligo M, et al. Assessing the clinical value of positive multiparametric magnetic resonance imaging in young men with a suspicion of prostate cancer. Eur Urol Oncol. 2019:1–7.
35. Costa DN, Goldberg K, de Leon AD, et al. Magnetic resonance imaging–guided in-bore and magnetic resonance imaging-transrectal ultrasound fusion targeted prostate biopsies: an adjusted comparison of clinically significant prostate cancer detection rate. Eur Urol Oncol. 2019;2:397–404.
36. Spahn M, Fehr JL. Multiparametric magnetic resonance imaging for prostate-specific antigen recurrence after radical prostatectomy: are we leaving the "one treatment fits all approach" and moving towards personalized imaging-guided treatment? Eur Urol. 2018;73:888–9.
37. Preisser F, Marchioni M, Nazzani S, et al. Trend of adverse stage migration in patients treated with radical prostatectomy for localized prostate cancer. Eur Urol Oncol. 2018;1:160–8.
38. Costello AJ. Considering the role of radical prostatectomy in 21st century prostate cancer care. Nat Rev Urol. 2020;17:177–88.
39. Gandaglia G, De Lorenzis E, Novara G, et al. Robot-assisted radical prostatectomy and extended pelvic lymph node dissection in patients with locally-advanced prostate cancer. Eur Urol. 2017;71:249–56.
40. Mazzone E, Dell'Oglio P, Rosiello G, et al. Technical refinements in superextended robot-assisted radical prostatectomy for locally advanced prostate cancer patients at multiparametric magnetic resonance imaging. Eur Urol. 2020:1–9.
41. Mottrie A, Van Migem P, De Naeyer G, et al. Robot-assisted laparoscopic radical prostatectomy: oncologic and functional results of 184 cases. Eur Urol. 2007;52:746–51.
42. Martini A, Tewari AK. Anatomic robotic prostatectomy: current best practice. Ther Adv Urol. 2019;11:1–7.
43. Bianchi L, Turri FM, Larcher A, et al. A novel approach for apical dissection during robot-assisted radical prostatectomy: the "collar" technique. Eur Urol Focus. 2018;4:677–85.
44. Gratzke C, Dovey Z, Novara G, et al. Early catheter removal after robot-assisted radical prostatectomy: surgical technique and outcomes for the aalst technique (ECaRemA Study). Eur Urol. 2016;69:917–23.
45. Fossati N, Willemse PPM, Van den Broeck T, et al. The benefits and harms of different extents of lymph node dissection during radical prostatectomy for prostate cancer: a systematic review. Eur Urol. 2017;72:84–109.
46. Gandaglia G, Zaffuto E, Fossati N, et al. Identifying candidates for super-extended staging pelvic lymph node dissection among patients with high-risk prostate cancer. BJU Int. 2018;121:421–7.
47. Briganti A, Suardi N, Capogrosso P, et al. Lymphatic spread of nodal metastases in high-risk prostate cancer: The ascending pathway from the pelvis to the retroperitoneum. Prostate. 2012;72:186–92.
48. Sagalovich D, Calaway A, Srivastava A, Sooriakumaran P, Tewari AK. Assessment of required nodal yield in a high risk cohort undergoing extended pelvic lymphadenectomy in robotic-assisted radical prostatectomy and its impact on functional outcomes. BJU Int. 2013;111:85–94.
49. Mattei A, Würnschimmel C, Baumeister P, et al. Standardized and simplified robot-assisted superextended pelvic lymph node dissection for prostate cancer: the monoblock technique. Eur Urol. 2020;78:424–31.
50. Mattei A, Di Pierro GB, Grande P, Beutler J, Danuser H. Standardized and simplified extended pelvic lymph node dissection during robot-assisted radical prostatectomy: The monoblock technique. Urology. 2013;81:446–50.
51. Punnen S, Meng MV, Cooperberg MR, et al. How does robot-assisted radical prostatectomy (RARP) compare with open surgery in men with high-risk prostate cancer? BJU Int. 2013;112:E314–20.
52. Rogers CG, Sammon JD, Sukumar S, et al. Robot assisted radical prostatectomy for elderly patients with high risk prostate cancer. Urol Oncol. 2013;31:193–7.
53. Dell'Oglio P, Mottrie A, Mazzone E. Robot-assisted radical prostatectomy vs. open radical prostatectomy: Latest evidences on perioperative, functional and oncological outcomes. Curr Opin Urol. 2020;30:73–8.
54. Gandaglia G, Abdollah F, Hu J, et al. Is robot-assisted radical prostatectomy safe in men with high-risk prostate cancer? Assessment of perioperative outcomes, positive surgical margins, and use of additional cancer treatments. J Endourol. 2014;28:784–91.
55. Mitropoulos D, Artibani W, Graefen M, et al. Reporting and grading of complications after urologic surgical procedures: An ad hoc EAU guidelines panel assessment and recommendations. Eur Urol. 2012;61:341–9.
56. Abdollah F, Dalela D, Sood A, et al. Functional outcomes of clinically high-risk prostate cancer patients treated with robot-assisted radical prostatectomy: a multi-institutional analysis. Prostate Cancer Prostatic Dis. 2017;20:395–400.
57. Kumar A, Samavedi S, Bates AS, et al. Safety of selective nerve sparing in high risk prostate cancer during robot-assisted radical prostatectomy. J Robot Surg. 2017;11:129–38.
58. Ou YC, Yang CK, Wang J, et al. The trifecta outcome in 300 consecutive cases of robotic-assisted laparoscopic radical prostatectomy according to D'Amico risk criteria. Eur J Surg Oncol. 2013;39:107–13.
59. Wang J-G, Huang J, Chin AI. RARP in high-risk prostate cancer: use of multi-parametric MRI and nerve sparing techniques. Asian J Androl. 2014;16:715–9.
60. Koo KC, Jung DC, Lee SH, et al. Feasibility of robot-assisted radical prostatectomy for very-high risk prostate cancer: surgical and oncological outcomes in men aged ≥70 years. Prostate Int. 2014;2:127–32.
61. Suardi N, Moschini M, Gallina A, et al. Nerve-sparing approach during radical prostatectomy is strongly associated with the rate of postoperative urinary continence recovery. BJU Int. 2012;11:717–22.
62. Srivastava A, Chopra S, Pham A, et al. Effect of a risk-stratified grade of nerve-sparing technique on early return of continence after robot-assisted laparoscopic radical prostatectomy. Eur Urol. 2013;63:438–44.
63. Michl U, Tennstedt P, Feldmeier L, et al. Nerve-sparing surgery technique, not the preservation of the neurovascular bundles, leads to improved long-term continence rates after radical prostatectomy. Eur Urol. 2016;69:584–9.
64. Dell'Oglio P, Mazzone E, Lambert E, et al. The effect of surgical experience on perioperative and oncological outcomes after robot-assisted radical cystectomy with intracorporeal urinary diversion: Evidence from a high-volume center. Eur Urol Suppl. 2019;18:e2637–9.
65. Bravi CA, Tin A, Vertosick E, et al. The impact of experience on the risk of surgical margins and biochemical recurrence after robot-assisted radical prostatectomy: a learning curve study. J Urol. 2019;202:108–13.
66. Abdollah F, Sood A, Sammon JD, et al. Long-term cancer control outcomes in patients with clinically high-risk prostate cancer treated with robot-assisted radical prostatectomy: results from a multi-institutional study of 1100 patients. Eur Urol. 2015;68:497–505.
67. Busch J, Magheli A, Leva N, et al. Matched comparison of outcomes following open and minimally invasive radical prostatectomy for high-risk patients. World J Urol. 2014;32:1411–6.
68. Pierorazio PM, Mullins JK, Eifler JB, et al. Contemporaneous comparison of open vs minimally-invasive radical prostatectomy for high-risk prostate cancer. BJU Int. 2013;112:751–7.
69. Harty NJ, Kozinn SI, Canes D, Sorcini A, Moinzadeh A. Comparison of positive surgical margin rates in high risk prostate cancer: open versus minimally invasive radical prostatectomy. Int Braz J Urol. 2013;39:638–9.

70. Lee D, Choi S-K, Park J, et al. Comparative analysis of oncologic outcomes for open vs. robot-assisted radical prostatectomy in high-risk prostate cancer. Korean. J Urol. 2015;56:572–9.
71. Hu JC, Gandaglia G, Karakiewicz PI, et al. Comparative effectiveness of robot-assisted versus open radical prostatectomy cancer control. Eur Urol. 2014;66:666–72.
72. Suardi N, Dell'Oglio P, Gallina A, et al. Evaluation of positive surgical margins in patients undergoing robot-assisted and open radical prostatectomy according to preoperative risk groups. Urol Oncol. 2016;34(57):e1–7.
73. Martini A, Gandaglia G, Fossati N, et al. Defining clinically meaningful positive surgical margins in patients undergoing radical prostatectomy for localised prostate cancer. Eur Urol Oncol. 2019:1–7.
74. Diaz M, Peabody JO, Kapoor V, et al. Oncologic outcomes at 10 years following robotic radical prostatectomy. Eur Urol. 2015;67:1168–76.
75. Joniau S, Briganti A, Gontero P, et al. Stratification of high-risk prostate cancer into prognostic categories: a European multi-institutional study. Eur Urol. 2015;67:157–64.
76. Cacciamani GE, Maas M, Nassiri N, et al. Impact of pelvic lymph node dissection and its extent on perioperative morbidity in patients undergoing radical prostatectomy for prostate cancer: a comprehensive systematic review and meta-analysis. Eur Urol Oncol. 2021;4:134–49.
77. Mazzone E, Preisser F, Nazzani S, et al. The effect of lymph node dissection in metastatic prostate cancer patients treated with radical prostatectomy: a contemporary analysis of survival and early post-operative outcomes. Eur Urol Oncol. 2019;2:541–8.
78. Preisser F, Bandini M, Marchioni M, et al. Extent of lymph node dissection improves survival in prostate cancer patients treated with radical prostatectomy without lymph node invasion. Prostate. 2018;50:1–7.
79. Lestingi JFP, Guglielmetti GB, Trinh Q-D, et al. Extended versus limited pelvic lymph node dissection during radical prostatectomy for intermediate- and high-risk prostate cancer: early oncological outcomes from a randomized phase 3 trial. Eur Urol. 2021;79:595–604.

Prostatectomy in Oligometastatic Prostate Cancer

45

Tushar Aditya Narain, Mohammad Alkhamees, and Prasanna Sooriakumaran

Introduction

Surgery and radiotherapy are both the standard of care for patients with localized prostate cancer, while patients with metastatic prostate cancer at the time of diagnosis are treated with systemic therapy, typically Androgen Deprivation Therapy (ADT) or chemotherapy [1, 2]. Owing to advances and accuracy of new imaging modalities, an intermediate state of metastasis was proposed by Hellman and Weichselbaum in 1995 [3]. This was the stage of oligometastasis, and was initially considered an intermediary stage in the chain of progression from being a localized disease to being a widely metastatic one. This stage of the disease garnered much attention from clinicians as it reopened a window of opportunity to provide complete cure by directing therapy to the prostate and the limited sites of metastases [4].

The genomics and molecular biology of various primary cancers have much been deciphered over the past two decades, and it is now clear that the biology of oligo metastatic and widely metastatic cancer is much different [5–7]. These revelations support the possibility of a true oligometastatic biology, very different from one in which a few clinically apparent lesions are the initial manifestation of a more aggressive and widespread disease entity. Although it is difficult to distinguish easily the biology of this new entity from that of a widely metastatic one due to limitations in the molecular diagnostic techniques, it would be prudent to separate the oligometastatic entity from their more aggressive counterparts, as radical curative therapies could offer cure from disease for these patients as against a palliative treatment for the metastatic disease [8].

Paralleling the advancements in understanding of the biology of prostate cancer, was a paradigm shift in the treatment of locally advanced and advanced prostate cancer [9]. Historically, radical surgery or radiotherapy with a curative intent was offered only to patients having localized disease and the slightest evidence of metastatic disease-even a single pelvic lymph node-precluded curative therapeutic approach, and these patients were offered systemic therapy in the form of Androgen Deprivation Therapy (ADT) [10]. Over the past one decade, sufficient data has emerged supporting survival benefit in men receiving curative therapy for their prostate cancer in the presence of metastatic disease or disease in their lymph nodes [11–15]. Similar benefits were seen when patients were offered metastatic directed therapy with a curative intent rather than a palliative intent [16].

Defining Oligometastatic Prostate Cancer

One of the major hindrances in evaluating the outcomes of treatment of oligometastatic prostate cancer is the definition used to christen this entity. Various authors have used different parameters such as the number of metastatic lesions, the temporal association with the primary tumor of the metastatic sites, the imaging modality used for detection of these lesions, and whether the metastatic lesions were osseous or visceral. Till this date, there is no consensus on the number or sites or oligometastatic prostate cancer. A panel of experts in The Advanced Prostate Cancer Consensus Conference (APCCC) 2017 could not draw final conclusions on what should constitutes an oligometastatic disease. The majority of panelists (66%) believed that three metastases define this entity [17]. Many studies proposed different definitions regarding the site and number of metastatic deposits (Table 45.1).

T. A. Narain
Robotic Pelvic Uro-Oncology, University College London Hospital NHS Foundation Trust, London, UK

M. Alkhamees
Robotic Pelvic Uro-Oncology, University College London Hospital NHS Foundation Trust, London, UK

Majmaah University, Majmaah, Saudi Arabia
e-mail: m.alkhamees@mu.edu.sa

P. Sooriakumaran (✉)
Robotic Pelvic Uro-Oncology, University College London Hospital NHS Foundation Trust, London, UK

Cleveland Clinic, London, UK
e-mail: psoori@santishealth.org

S. Ren et al. (eds.), *Robot-Assisted Radical Prostatectomy*, https://doi.org/10.1007/978-3-031-05855-4_45

Table 45.1 Studies defining oligometastatic prostate cancer

Author	N	Number of metastases	Site of metastasis	Radiological modality
Jereczek-Fossa, et al. (2014) [18]	69	≤1	LN	18F-FDG PET/CT, 11C-choline PET/CT, CT
Ponti, et al. (2015) [19]	16	≤2	LN	11C-choline PET/CT, CT, bone scan
Berkovic, et al. (2013) [20]	24	≤3	Bone or LN	Bone scan, 18F-FDG PET/CT, 11C-choline PET/CT
Decaestecker, et al. (2014) [21]	50	≤3	Bone or LN	18F-FDG PET/CT, 18F-choline PET/CT
Ost, et al. (2016) [22]	119	≤3	Any	18F-FDG PET/CT, 18F-choline PET/CT
Schick, et al. (2013) [23]	50	≤4	Not specified	Bone scan, 18F-choline PET/CT, 11C-acetate PET/CT
Ahmed, et al. (2013) [24]	17	≤5	Not specified	11C-choline PET/CT, CT, MRI
Tabata, et al. (2012) [25]	35	≤5	Bone <50% size of vertebral body	Bone scan

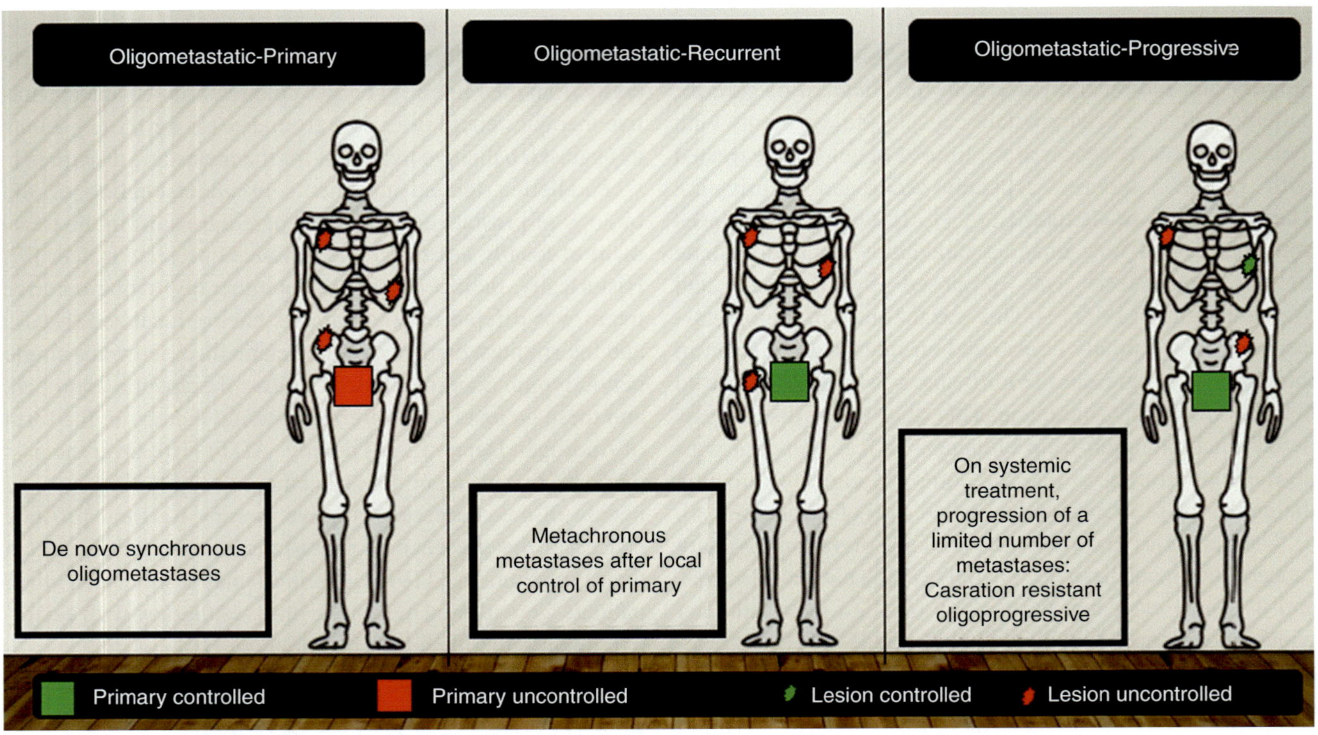

Fig. 45.1 Definitions of oligo-metastatic disease

Based on temporal association, the following three groups have been described (Fig. 45.1):

1. Oligometastatic-Primary: The prostate (primary) and the metastatic lesions are newly discovered and neither of them treated
2. Oligometastatic-Recurrent: The prostate (primary) has been treated and new metastatic lesions have developed later
3. Oligometastatic-Progressive: The prostate (primary)and the metastatic sites have been previously treated and there are new metastatic lesions

It is imperative to distinguish these three different entities of oligometastatic prostate cancer as they have a different tumor biology and express different phenotypes and aggressiveness. The oligometastatic primary is the one which would benefit from a curative surgery and would be considered for the rest of the discussion to follow.

Curative Therapy for Oligometastatic Prostate Cancer

The treatment of oligometastatic prostate cancer is tri-pronged which involves treatment of the primary tumor and metastatic directed therapy, besides long term systemic therapy. The rationale behind this aggressive approach is that it would prolong the overall survival. Treatment of the primary tumor has shown to decrease the need for palliative treatment for locally advanced disease [26, 27]. Besides this, one of the biggest obvious benefits of local therapy is that it delays the initiation of ADT, which is, in most cases life long, and has its own set of detrimental side effect, besides ensuring a delay in the setting in of the castration resistant stage.

Rationale for Local Curative Therapy

The idea of treating the prostate in an oligometastatic setting stems from the belief that the primary tumor serves as a niche for generating circulating tumor cells which result in development of new metastatic sites. This hypothesis is supported by the theory of "seed and soil' proposed by Paget et al. in 1889. The primary tumor produces the seeds, the circulating tumor cells and the distant metastatic sites provide the fertile soil [28]. Control of the primary tumor would reduce the production of the circulating tumor cells and would prevent the progression from an oligometastatic state to a widely metastatic state. Supporting this hypothesis was the hypothesis put forward by Kaplan et al., which described the presence of a "pre-metastatic niche" in which the non-malignant bone marrow cells have the potential to sensitize the target tissues towards the circulating tumor cells and recruiting them, resulting in development of metastatic lesion [29]. Some researchers believe that the primary tumor, besides producing the circulating tumor cells, also produce some endocrine factors which have some control over the extent of metastases. This theory was supported by the works of Weckermann et al., who evaluated the bone marrow aspirates from PCa patients, those who had their primary tumors treated and also those who had not received any therapy for their primary tumor, and found that despite the presence of circulating tumor cells in both groups of patients, development of metastases was seen only in patients who had their primary tumor intact. The authors concluded that there were certain circulating cytokines secreted by the primary tumor which facilitated the development of new metastatic sites [30].

Besides the genesis of new metastatic sites theory, local treatment of prostate in a metastatic setting has shown to reduce the need for palliative treatment requirements arising from the locally advanced nature of the disease. A group of oncologists from Sydney evaluated 263 men with Castrate Resistant Prostate Cancer and evaluated them for their complications arising from the locally advanced disease depending on whether they had previously received any local therapy to the prostate or not, before progressing to the castration resistant stage. The primary treatment to the prostate included both surgery and external beam radiotherapy, and the risk of developing serious local complications later were significantly low as compared to patients who had not received any local therapy (32.6% vs. 54.6%, $p = 0.001$). In a sub set analysis, they found that patients receiving surgery as the local treatment had even lower risk of complications as compared to those receiving radiotherapy(20% vs. 47.6%, $p = 0.007$) [15].

Rationale for Metastatic Directed Therapy

It was believed before that metastasis is a one-way process from the primary tumor to distant sites. However, Kim et al. [31], suggested a "tumor self-seeding" hypothesis, where circulating tumor cells serve as an origin of new metastatic focus. The authors believed that the local therapy of primary tumor and metastatic sites might alter the tumor microenvironment and prevent further metastatic deposition. This approach is proposed in oligometastatic prostate cancer based on the belief that the biology of such a disease is different from that of high volume metastatic prostate cancer.

Tumor debulking and treatment of metastatic sites has been proven to improve OS in various malignancies, including liver metastases from colorectal cancer, and lung metastases from various primary tumors [32, 33]. Applying these findings to oligometastatic PCa, tumor debulking might theoretically prolong the duration to development of aggressive tumor burden, as patients with low volume metastasis tend to have local progression, while those with high volume metastasis have distant progression [34]. Stereotactic body radiation therapy (SBRT) for oligometastatic bony lesions in the setting of castration-resistant PCa was found to provide optimal metastatic control [35]. Moreover, metastatic directed therapy is a good strategy to delay the treatment of metastatic disease with ADT and preventing the side effects of castration.

Surgical Management of Oligometastatic Prostate Cancer

Surgery for Locally Advanced Disease

Historically, patients with locally advanced disease in the form of positive pelvic lymph nodes were deemed unfit for surgery and were offered systemic ADT. This was first challenged in 1993 when Cheng at al evaluated the overall survival in patients receiving surgery or radiotherapy for the primary tumor besides systemic ADT and compared it with those receiving only ADT. They reported a cause-specific survival rate of 91% and 78% for surgery and 84% and 54% for radiotherapy at 5 and 10 years respectively, which was 66% and 39% ($p = 0.037$) [36]. The authors concluded that local therapy for the prostate besides ADT had better survival rates than just systemic ADT as a stand-alone therapy in patients with positive lymph nodes. Frohmuller et all, two years later had similar observations when they evaluated 139 patients with histologically proven lymph node positive disease. Fifty-two patients underwent radical prostatectomy followed by ADT while 87 patients received ADT alone. The DFS and OS were 70.7% and 50.8% for the first group while it was 32.1% and 29.7% respectively. The group also reported lower rates of intervention required for palliation of symptoms resulting from locally advanced disease in patients who had a prostatectomy [37]. Subsequently, several retrospective series have demonstrated a survival benefit in patients who went on to have a prostatectomy despite testing positive for tumor cells in lymph nodes on frozen section analysis [38–40]. These studies brought about a paradigm shift in the practices of surgical management of locally advanced prostate cancer and the practice of aborting surgery in the presence of a positive lymph node was abolished. These practices were supported by the systematic analysis on the role of surgery in locally advanced prostate cancer by Gakis et al. who showed a 10 year cancer-specific survival ranging between 70% and 85% in these patients [41]. Reyes et al. analyzed the Munich Cancer Registry database and compared the survival of patients with positive lymph node disease who had a prostatectomy with those in whom a prostatectomy was abandoned in view of positive lymph nodes. A multivariate analysis negating the cofounders revealed prostatectomy to be independently associated with improved survival in these patients [42].

There are two major randomized control trials that have evaluated the response with immediate versus delayed ADT in patients with lymph node positive disease. Because the major difference between these two trials is that patients in one of these had radical prostatectomy while those in the other had ADT alone, these two trials can be compared to bring out the survival difference attributable to radical prostatectomy. While the Eastern Cooperative Oncology Group (ECOG) 3886 trial which included patients who had a prostatectomy reported a 10 year OS of 45% for prostatectomy alone and 64% for addition of adjuvant ADT to RP, the ECOG 30846 trial which included patients receiving only ADT reported a 10 year OS of only 30% [43, 44]. These studies provide strong evidence in support of surgery for locally advanced prostate cancer, and patients with positive lymph nodes are no longer subjected to ADT monotherapy any more.

Having said that, it has to be understood that all patients with locally advanced disease cannot be blindly offered a therapy with the aim of cure, as the disease biology varies even in patients with just lymph node positive disease. Moschini et al. evaluated 1011 lymph node positive patients who had a radical prostatectomy and used multivariate Cox regression model to predict factors portending a poor survival. They found that three or more lymph nodes (HR 1.75, $p = 0.003$), pathological Gleason score 7 vs. 6 (HR 1.74, $p = 0.04$) and 8–10 vs. 6 (HR 2.63, $p = 0.001$) and positive surgical margins (HR 1.96, $p = 0.001$) were independently associated with increased cancer specific mortality, while adjuvant radiotherapy (early) (HR 0.40, $p = 0.008$) was associated with decreased cancer specific mortality. The authors used these four variables to stratify patients according to their prognoses, and found a 20-year cancer specific mortality to be 19%, 34% and 46% ($p < 0.001$) for low, intermediate and high risk categories respectively [45]. Montorsi, in a very interesting letter to the editor, in response to the systemic analysis of Gakis et al., published in the European Urology journal, highlights the importance of a digital rectal examination to determine the feasibility of extirpation of the prostate, before subjecting every patient with a locally advanced disease to surgery [46].

Surgery for Oligometastatic-Primary Prostate Cancer

Moving a step beyond the positive lymph nodes, several researchers have evaluated the role of surgery in de novo metastatic prostate cancer. Culp et al. identified 8185 patients diagnosed with metastatic prostate cancer at the time of initial diagnosis using the Surveillance Epidemiology and End results (SEER)(2004–2010) and divided them on the basis of the primary therapy received (Radical prostatectomy (RP) = 245, Brachytherapy (BT) = 129 and no surgery or radiation therapy (NSR) = 7811) The 5 year overall survival and disease free survival were each statistically better in patients undergoing RP (67.4% and 75.8%, respectively) or BT (52.6 and 61.3%, respectively) compared with NSR patients (22.5% and 48.7%, respectively) ($p < 0.001$). RP and BT were each independently associated with decreased cancer specific mortality ($p < 0.01$). The authors concluded that definitive treatment of the prostate in men diagnosed with metastatic disease had survival advantages and that prospective studies should be done to strengthen this conclusion [47]. In the same year, Gatzke et al. published their analysis of data from the Munich Cancer Registry wherein they compared the treatment outcomes of patients with metastatic prostate cancer treated with surgery versus those treated with primary RT or ADT. Patients undergoing radical prostatectomy had a significantly higher 5 year overall survival compared to their non-surgical counterparts (55% vs. 21%) [48]. In a multicentric retrospective analysis of 106 newly diagnosed metastatic prostate cancer patients who underwent radical prostatectomy, Sooriakumaran et al. evaluated the perioperative outcomes and short-term complications. In their series, 79.2% of patients did not suffer any complications; the rates of positive-margin were 53.8%, lymphocele 8.5%, and wound infection were 4.7%, all of which were not higher than in a meta-analysis of open radical prostatectomy performed for standard indications. At a median follow-up of 22.8 months, 94/106 (88.7%) men were still alive. The authors concluded that radical prostatectomy for men with locally resectable, distant metastatic prostate cancer was safe in expert hands and the overall and specific complication rates related to the surgical extirpation were not more frequent than when radical prostatectomy was performed for standard indications [49]. Although being retrospective in nature, this paper established the safety of radical prostatectomy in a metastatic setting, and its strength being that it had data from the biggest centers with experienced surgeons performing radical prostatectomies. Jang et al. specifically chose a cohort of 79 patients with oligometastatic prostate cancer (defined as the presence of five or fewer hot spots detected by preoperative bone scan) and evaluated the peri-operative and oncological outcomes of robot assisted radical prostatectomy in these patients. They also did not find a higher incidence of peri-operative complications than in those in whom surgery was performed for traditional indications. The progression free survival and cancer specific survival were longer in surgery cohort as compared with patients receiving systemic hormonal therapy (median PFS: 75 vs. 28 months, $P = 0.008$; median CSS: not reached vs. 40 months, $P = 0.002$). Multivariate analysis further identified RARP as a significant predictor of PFS and CSS (PFS: hazard ratio [HR] 0.388, $P = 0.003$; CSS: HR 0.264, $P = 0.004$) [50]. Heidenreich et al. performed a feasibility and the first case controlled study evaluating the role of cytoreductive radical prostatectomy in prostate cancer with low volume skeletal metastases. Twenty-three patients with biopsy proven prostate cancer, minimal osseous metastases (3 or fewer hot spots on bone scan), absence of visceral or extensive lymph node metastases and prostate specific antigen decrease to less than 1.0 ng/mL after neoadjuvant androgen deprivation therapy were included in the intervention group, while 38 men with metastatic prostate cancer who were treated with androgen deprivation therapy without local therapy served as the control group. The surgery group demonstrated longer progression free survival as compared to the control group (39 vs. 28 months), increased time to castration resistant stage (40 vs. 29 months) and improved cancer specific survival (96% vs. 84%), but similar overall survival rates. The authors concluded that cytoreductive radical prostatectomy was feasible in well selected men with metastatic prostate cancer who respond well to neoadjuvant androgen deprivation therapy [16].

Conclusion

Oligometastatic prostate cancer is an independent entity with a tumor biology different from its widely metastatic counterpart. Surgery in an oligometastatic setting is feasible with no higher rates of complications than when done for the traditional indications. Moreover, curative surgery for the prostate accompanied by stereotactic radiotherapy to the oligometastatic sites improves overall and cancer specific survival with reduced interventions for palliation of symptoms arising from the locally advanced disease.

References

1. Alcaraz A. Management of prostate cancer: global strategies. Eur Urol Suppl. 2006;5(18):890–9.
2. Van den Bergh RC, et al. Timing of curative treatment for prostate cancer: a systematic review. Eur Urol. 2013;64(2):204–15.
3. Hellman S, Weichselbaum RR. Oligometastases. J Clin Oncol. 1995;13:8–10.
4. Weichselbaum RR, Hellman S. Oligometastases revisited. Nat Rev Clin Oncol. 2011;8(6):378–82.
5. Lussier YA, Xing HR, Salama JK, Khodarev NN, Huang Y, Zhang Q, Khan SA, Yang X, Hasselle MD, Darga TE, Malik R. MicroRNA expression characterizes oligometastasis (es). PLoS One. 2011;6(12):e28650.
6. Tamoto E, Tada M, Murakawa K, Takada M, Shindo G, Teramoto KI, Matsunaga A, Komuro K, Kanai M, Kawakami A, Fujiwara Y. Gene-expression profile changes correlated with tumor progression and lymph node metastasis in esophageal cancer. Clin Cancer Res. 2004;10(11):3629–38.
7. Wuttig D, Baier B, Fuessel S, Meinhardt M, Herr A, Hoefling C, Toma M, Grimm MO, Meye A, Rolle A, Wirth MP. Gene signatures of pulmonary metastases of renal cell carcinoma reflect the disease-free interval and the number of metastases per patient. Int J Cancer. 2009;125(2):474–82.
8. Rubin P, Brasacchio R, Katz A. Solitary metastases: illusion versus reality. Semin Radiat Oncol. 2006;16(2):120–30.
9. Bayne CE, Williams SB, Cooperberg MR, Gleave ME, Graefen M, Montorsi F, Novara G, Smaldone MC, Sooriakumaran P, Wiklund PN, Chapin BF. Treatment of the primary tumor in metastatic prostate cancer: current concepts and future perspectives. Eur Urol. 2016;69(5):775–87.
10. Perlmutter MA, Lepor H. Androgen deprivation therapy in the treatment of advanced prostate cancer. Rev Urol. 2007;9(Suppl 1):S3.
11. James ND, Spears MR, Clarke NW, Dearnaley DP, Mason MD, Parker CC, Ritchie AW, Russell JM, Schiavone F, Attard G, De Bono JS. Failure-free survival and radiotherapy in patients with newly diagnosed nonmetastatic prostate cancer: data from patients in the control arm of the STAMPEDE trial. JAMA Oncol. 2016;2(3):348–57.
12. Scott E. Androgen deprivation with or without radiation therapy for clinically node-positive prostate cancer. Lin CC, Gray PJ, Jemal A, Efstathiou JA, Surveillance and Health Services Research Program, Intramural Research, American Cancer Society, Atlanta, GA (CCL, AJ); Department of Radiation Oncology, Massachusetts General Hospital, Harvard Medical School, Boston, MA (PJG, JAE); e-mail: jefstathiou@ partners. org. J Natl Cancer Inst. 2015 May 9; 107 (7). pii: djv119.[Print 2015 Jul. InUrologic Oncology: Seminars and Original Investigations 2017 Mar 1 (Vol. 35, No. 3, pp. 122-123). Elsevier.
13. Tward JD, Kokeny KE, Shrieve DC. Radiation therapy for clinically node-positive prostate adenocarcinoma is correlated with improved overall and prostate cancer-specific survival. Pract Radiat Oncol. 2013;3(3):234–40.
14. Rusthoven CG, Carlson JA, Waxweiler TV, Raben D, Dewitt PE, Crawford ED, Maroni PD, Kavanagh BD. The impact of definitive local therapy for lymph node-positive prostate cancer: a population-based study. International Journal of Radiation Oncology* Biology* Physics. 2014;88(5):1064–73.
15. Aoun F, Peltier A, Van Velthoven R. A comprehensive review of contemporary role of local treatment of the primary tumor and/

or the metastases in metastatic prostate cancer. Biomed Res Int. 2014;2014:501213.

16. Ost P, Bossi A, Decaestecker K, De Meerleer G, Giannarini G, Karnes RJ, Roach M III, Briganti A. Metastasis-directed therapy of regional and distant recurrences after curative treatment of prostate cancer: a systematic review of the literature. Eur Urol. 2015;67(5):852–63.
17. Gillessen S, Attard G, Beer TM, Beltran H, Bossi A, Bristow R, Carver B, Castellano D, Chung BH, Clarke N, Daugaard G, Davis ID, de Bono J, Borges Dos Reis R, Drake CG, Eeles R, Efstathiou E, Evans CP, Fanti S, Feng F, Fizazi K, Frydenberg M, Gleave M, Halabi S, Heidenreich A, Higano CS, James N, Kantoff P, Kellokumpu-Lehtinen PL, Khauli RB, Kramer G, Logothetis C, Maluf F, Morgans AK, Morris MJ, Mottet N, Murthy V, Oh W, Ost P, Padhani AR, Parker C, Pritchard CC, Roach M, Rubin MA, Ryan C, Saad F, Sartor O, Scher H, Sella A, Shore N, Smith M, Soule H, Sternberg CN, Suzuki H, Sweeney C, Sydes MR, Tannock I, Tombal B, Valdagni R, Wiegel T, Omlin A. Management of Patients with Advanced Prostate Cancer: The Report of the Advanced Prostate Cancer Consensus Conference APCCC 2017. Eur Urol. 2018;73(2):178–211. https://doi.org/10.1016/j.eururo.2017.06.002. Epub 2017 Jun 24
18. Jereczek-Fossa BA, Piperno G, Ronchi S, Catalano G, Fodor C, Cambria R, Fossati Ing P, Gherardi F, Alterio D, Zerini D, Garibaldi C, Baroni G, De Cobelli O, Orecchia R. Linac-based stereotactic body radiotherapy for oligometastatic patients with single abdominal lymph node recurrent cancer. Am J Clin Oncol. 2014;37(3):227–33. https://doi.org/10.1097/COC.0b013e3182610878.
19. Ponti E, Ingrosso G, Carosi A, Di Murro L, Lancia A, Pietrasanta F, Santoni R. Salvage Stereotactic Body Radiotherapy for Patients With Prostate Cancer With Isolated Lymph Node Metastasis: A Single-Center Experience. Clin Genitourin Cancer. 2015;13(4):e279–84. https://doi.org/10.1016/j.clgc.2014.12.014. Epub 2014 Dec 30
20. Berkovic P, De Meerleer G, Delrue L, Lambert B, Fonteyne V, Lumen N, Decaestecker K, Villeirs G, Vuye P, Ost P. Salvage stereotactic body radiotherapy for patients with limited prostate cancer metastases: deferring androgen deprivation therapy. Clin Genitourin Cancer. 2013;11(1):27–32. https://doi.org/10.1016/j.clgc.2012.08.003. Epub 2012 Sep 24
21. Decaestecker K, De Meerleer G, Lambert B, Delrue L, Fonteyne V, Claeys T, De Vos F, Huysse W, Hautekiet A, Maes G, Ost P. Repeated stereotactic body radiotherapy for oligometastatic prostate cancer recurrence. Radiat Oncol. 2014;12(9):135. https://doi.org/10.1186/1748-717X-9-135.
22. Ost P, Jereczek-Fossa BA, As NV, Zilli T, Muacevic A, Olivier K, Henderson D, Casamassima F, Orecchia R, Surgo A, Brown L, Tree A, Miralbell R, De Meerleer G. Progression-free Survival Following Stereotactic Body Radiotherapy for Oligometastatic Prostate Cancer Treatment-naive Recurrence: A Multi-institutional Analysis. Eur Urol. 2016;69(1):9–12. https://doi.org/10.1016/j.eururo.2015.07.004. Epub 2015 Jul 16
23. Schick U, Jorcano S, Nouet P, Rouzaud M, Vees H, Zilli T, Ratib O, Weber DC, Miralbell R. Androgen deprivation and high-dose radiotherapy for oligometastatic prostate cancer patients with less than five regional and/or distant metastases. Acta Oncol. 2013;52(8):1622–8. https://doi.org/10.3109/0284186X.2013.764010. Epub 2013 Apr 2
24. Ahmed KA, Barney BM, Davis BJ, Park SS, Kwon ED, Olivier KR. Stereotactic body radiation therapy in the treatment of oligometastatic prostate cancer. Front Oncol. 2013;22(2):215. https://doi.org/10.3389/fonc.2012.00215.
25. Tabata K, Niibe Y, Satoh T, Tsumura H, Ikeda M, Minamida S, Fujita T, Ishii D, Iwamura M, Hayakawa K, Baba S. Radiotherapy for oligometastases and oligo-recurrence of bone in prostate cancer. Pulm Med. 2012;2012:541656. https://doi.org/10.1155/2012/541656. Epub 2012 Sep 9
26. Won AC, Gurney H, Marx G, De Souza P, Patel MI. Primary treatment of the prostate improves local palliation in men who ultimately develop castrate-resistant prostate cancer. BJU Int. 2013;112:E250–5.
27. Heidenreich A, Pfister D, Porres D. Cytoreductive radical prostatectomy in patients with prostate cancer and low volume skeletal metastases: results of a feasibility and case-control study. J Urol. 2015;193(3):832–8.
28. Paget S. The distribution of secondary growths in cancer of the breast. Lancet. 1889;133(3421):571–3.
29. Kaplan RN, Rafii S, Lyden D. Preparing the "soil": the premetastatic niche. Cancer Res. 2006;66(23):11089–93.
30. Weckermann D, Polzer B, Ragg T, Blana A, Schlimok G, Arnholdt H, Bertz S, Harzmann R, Klein CA. Perioperative activation of disseminated tumor cells in bone marrow of patients with prostate cancer. J Clin Oncol. 2009;27(10):1549–56.
31. Kim MY, Oskarsson T, Acharyya S, Nguyen DX, Zhang XH, Norton L, Massagué J. Tumor self-seeding by circulating cancer cells. Cell. 2009;139(7):1315–26. https://doi.org/10.1016/j.cell.2009.11.025.
32. Fong Y, Fortner J, Sun RL, Brennan MF, Blumgart LH. Clinical score for predicting recurrence after hepatic resection for metastatic colorectal cancer: analysis of 1001 consecutive cases. Ann Surg. 1999;230(3):309–18; discussion 318–21. https://doi.org/10.1097/00000658-199909000-00004.
33. Pastorino U, Buyse M, Friedel G, Ginsberg RJ, Girard P, Goldstraw P, Johnston M, McCormack P, Pass H, Putnam JB Jr. International Registry of Lung Metastases. Long-term results of lung metastasectomy: prognostic analyses based on 5206 cases. J Thorac Cardiovasc Surg. 1997;113(1):37–49. https://doi.org/10.1016/s0022-5223(97)70397-0.
34. Furuya Y, Akakura K, Akimoto S, Inomiya H, Ito H. Pattern of progression and survival in hormonally treated metastatic prostate cancer. Int J Urol. 1999;6(5):240–4. https://doi.org/10.1046/j.1442-2042.1999.00060.x.
35. Muldermans JL, Romak LB, Kwon ED, Park SS, Olivier KR. Stereotactic body radiation therapy for oligometastatic prostate cancer. Int J Radiat Oncol Biol Phys. 2016;95(2):696–702. https://doi.org/10.1016/j.ijrobp.2016.01.032. Epub 2016 Jan 29
36. Cheng CW, Bergstralh EJ, Zincke H. Stage D1 prostate cancer. A nonrandomized comparison of conservative treatment options versus radical prostatectomy. Cancer. 1993;71(S3):996–1004.
37. Frohmüller HG, Theiss M, Manseck A, Wirth MP. Survival and quality of life of patients with stage D1 (T1-3 pN1-2 MO) prostate cancer. Eur Urol. 1995;27:202–6.
38. Engel J, Bastian PJ, Baur H, Beer V, Chaussy C, Gschwend JE, Oberneder R, Rothenberger KH, Stief CG, Hölzel D. Survival benefit of radical prostatectomy in lymph node–positive patients with prostate cancer. Eur Urol. 2010;57(5):754–61.
39. Steuber T, Budäus L, Walz J, Zorn KC, Schlomm T, Chun F, et al. Radical prostatectomy improves progression-free and cancer-specific survival in men with lymph node positive prostate cancer in the prostate-specific antigen era: a confirmatory study. BJU Int. 2011;107:1755–61.
40. Ghavamian R, Bergstralh EJ, Blute ML, Slezak J, Zincke H. Radical retropubic prostatectomy plus orchiectomy versus orchiectomy alone for pTxN+ prostate cancer: a matched comparison. J Urol. 1999;161(4):1223–8.
41. Gakis G, Boorjian SA, Briganti A, Joniau S, Karazanashvili G, Karnes RJ, Mattei A, Shariat SF, Stenzl A, Wirth M, Stief CG. The role of radical prostatectomy and lymph node dissection in lymph node–positive prostate cancer: a systematic review of the literature. Eur Urol. 2014;66(2):191–9.
42. Reyes DK, Pienta KJ. The biology and treatment of oligometastatic cancer. Oncotarget. 2015;6(11):8491.

43. Messing EM, Manola J, Yao J, Kiernan M, Crawford D, Wilding G, di'SantAgnese PA, Trump D, Eastern Cooperative Oncology Group study EST 3886. Immediate versus deferred androgen deprivation treatment in patients with node-positive prostate cancer after radical prostatectomy and pelvic lymphadenectomy. Lancet Oncol. 2006;7(6):472–9.
44. Schröder FH, Kurth KH, Fossa SD, Hoekstra W, Karthaus PP, De Prijck L, Collette L. Early versus delayed endocrine treatment of T2-T3 pN1–3 M0 prostate cancer without local treatment of the primary tumour: final results of European Organisation for the Research and Treatment of Cancer protocol 30846 after 13 years of follow-up (a randomised controlled trial). Eur Urol. 2009;55(1):14–22.
45. Moschini M, Sharma V, Zattoni F, Boorjian SA, Frank I, Gettman MT, Thompson RH, Tollefson MK, Kwon ED, Karnes RJ. Risk stratification of pN+ prostate cancer after radical prostatectomy from a large single institutional series with long-term followup. J Urol. 2016;195(6):1773–8.
46. Montorsi F, Gandaglia G. Re: Georgios Gakis, Stephen A. Boorjian, Alberto Briganti, et al. The role of radical prostatectomy and lymph node dissection in lymph node-positive prostate cancer: a systematic review of the literature. Eur urol 2014 66: [illegible]91-9. Eur Urol. 2014;66(6):e107–8.
47. Culp SH, Schellhammer PF, Williams MB. Might men diagnosed with metastatic prostate cancer benefit from definitive treatment of the primary tumor? A SEER-based study. Eur Urol. 2014;65(6):1058–66.
48. Gratzke C, Engel J, Stief CG. Role of radical prostatectomy in metastatic prostate cancer: data from the Munich Cancer Registry. Eur Urol. 2014;66(3):602–3.
49. Sooriakumaran P, Karnes J, Stief C, Copsey B, Montorsi F, Hammerer P, Beyer B, Moschini M, Gratzke C, Steuber T, Suardi N. A multi-institutional analysis of perioperative outcomes in 106 men who underwent radical prostatectomy for distant metastatic prostate cancer at presentation. Eur Urol. 2016;69(5):783–94.
50. Jang WS, Kim MS, Jeong WS, Chang KD, Cho KS, Ham WS, Rha KH, Hong SJ, Choi YD. Does robot-assisted radical prostatectomy benefit patients with prostate cancer and bone oligometastases? BJU Int. 2018;121(2):225–31.

Inguinal Hernia Repair During Robot-Assisted Radical Prostatectomy

46

Abdullah Erdem Canda, Arif Özkan, and Emre Balık

Introduction

Nelsen and Walsh [1] showed 33% incidental inguinal hernia (IH) rate in their retropubic radical prostatectomy (RRP) series (n = 430). Lepor et al. [2] reported 11% rate of IH repair in the same procedure with RRP. Nilsson et al. [3] reported that patients treated with radical prostatectomy (RP) exhibited a four fold increased risk of requiring a subsequent IH repair compared with the control group. Various reasons may led to development of IH after prostatectomy such as prolonged stretching of the rectus abdominis and transversalis fascia during the procedure that weakens the inguinal floor and inguinal ring, and subclinic hernias may manifest themselves after surgery [4].

Previous IH history, lower body mass index, older age and bladder neck stenosis were reported as the risk factors related with the diagnosis of an IH during robot-assisted radical prostatectomy (RARP) [5]. The presence of lower urinary tract dysfunction significantly correlates with the risk of IH development [6]. It was reported that patients with moderate to severe urinary symptoms had a 22.4% chance of requiring IH repair compared to 5% in patients with minimally urinary system symptoms [6]. Apart from these reports, in some concurrent hernia repair and prostatectomy series interestingly in 50% of patients the physical examination could be normal before the surgery [7]. Therefore, in patients with moderate to severe urinary symptoms, patients should be informed regarding the possibility to have an IH and requirement of concurrent repair during the RARP procedure [6].

Supplementary Information The online version contains supplementary material available at [https://doi.org/10.1007/978-3-031-05855-4_46].

A. E. Canda (✉) · A. Özkan
School of Medicine, Department of Urology, Koç University, Istanbul, Turkey
e-mail: arozkan@kuh.ku.edu.tr

E. Balık
School of Medicine, Department of General Surgery, Koç University, Istanbul, Turkey
e-mail: ebalik@ku.edu.tr

Inguinal Hernia Repairing During Radical Prostatectomy

IH repair in patients with previous RP history is often complicated by preperitoneal space scaring with longer operative time and increased morbidity [5]. The effectiveness and the safety of IH repair during RP has been published before [8]. If the IH is not repaired in the same session during the RARP procedure, it might be more difficult to repair it via laparoscopic or robotic surgery after the RARP procedure as there might be severe intra-abdominal adhesions. In addition, this would be a second surgical impact on the patient with additional anesthesia exposure.

The procedure could be performed via extraperitoneal approach (TEP) or transperitoneal approach (TAPP) according to the surgeon's preference. The use of mesh for IH repair during RP was firstly described by Choi et al. in 1999 [9]. Teber et al. [10] reported that patients who underwent IH repair in laparoscopic radical prostatectomy (LRP) required greater analgesic during postoperative period due to additional dissection around the spermatic cord and foreign body reaction around the mesh. Finley et al. [7] published the first series of concurrent transperitoneal RARP and TAPP with 40 patient and 49 concurrent hernia repairs and there were not any significant differences between combined surgery and prostatectomy only regarding blood loss, analgesic usage, duration of hospital stay and, mesh-related complications. The IH repair procedure was reported to add an average of 12–15 min on total surgery time [8, 11].

Mourmouris et al. [12] described "Darning technique"which is a non-prosthetic and tissue based technique regarding IH repair during RARP. They describes the technique for direct hernias, excluded all patients with indirect hernias, in which a prolene suture was used to approximate lateral edge of the rectus muscle sheath to the Coopers'

S. Ren et al. (eds.), *Robot-Assisted Radical Prostatectomy*, https://doi.org/10.1007/978-3-031-05855-4_46

ligament. Although in this study the risk of mesh infection would be eliminated, it was reported that the potential risk of mesh infection is extremely low during the RARP procedure with concomitant IH repair [4, 13]. Although some authors favored [14] extraperitoneal approach others showed that intraperitoneal approach was equally safe with an almost negligible rate of bowel injury and low risk of recurrence [7, 15, 16]. Particularly in extraperitoneal approach, no sutures or tacks are required to fix the mesh, rather the cord and the peritoneum itself stabilized the mesh as the preperitoneal space is collapsed [17].

Major complications rate related with IH repair was reported to be around 1% that includes hernia recurrence, chronic pelvic or scrotal pain, bleeding requiring transfusions, mesh infection requiring removal, bowel or bladder injuries, fistulas or erosions, vascular or nerve injuries, gonadal vessels damages leading to testicular atrophy or loss. Although theoretical concerns regarding mesh infection with concurrent repair requirement exist, the available literature suggests that mesh infections or erosions are extremely rare occasions [6].

The risk of infection arises from the possibility that the mesh may contact with urine in the presence of a vesicourethral anastomotic leakage. Contrary, recent previous studies have showed that concomitant IH repair with mesh during RP is safe and there were no instances of mesh infection or groin pain reported [7, 14]. Mesh is a foreign body and there is a risk for adhesions to intraperitoneal structures. Reducing this risk can be achieved with two methods. First, reperitonealization may be safely achieved after the completion of prostatectomy to avoid contact of mesh with intraperitoneal structures. Second, using adhesion-resistant, coated mesh is another solution that reduces risk of adhesion formation while avoiding related postoperative complications [16]. Another concern regarding RARP with IH repair is lymphatic drainage and seroma formation. The symptomatic lymphocele (requiring drainage) development rate during minimal invasive RP and concurrent IH repair is up to 5%, and seroma formation rate is very low in current literature [14, 16]. The main concern in lymphocele development and seroma formation is a risk of mesh infection that can leads to a mesh removal. Preventing seroma formation can be achieved with good hemostasis, sufficient drainage and fixing the mesh material with running absorbable sutures to prevent the formation of dead space [18].

Preoperative Management

Urinalysis and urine culture should be performed in all cases before the surgical procedure, in case of any urinary tract infection the procedure should be postponed till the sterile urine culture is obtained. Prior to the procedure a single dose of second generation cephalosporine antibiotic is administered intravenously during anesthesia induction.

Surgical Technique

In our technique, RARP is performed by using five abdominal ports (four 8-mm sized robotic ports and one 10-mm sized assistant port) via transperitoneal approach. Da Vinci Xi surgical robot (Intuitive Surgical, Sunnyvale, CA) is used. Maryland bipolar forceps ($n = 1$), large needle driver ($n = 1$), monopolar curved scissors ($n = 1$), and Prograsp forceps ($n = 1$) are used for the whole procedure. We perform the RARP procedure via anterior approach as we described previously and extended pelvic lymph node dissection (ePLND) if indicated. An edited video of an IH repair with mesh application following a RARP procedure can be accessed at: https://drive.google.com/file/d/1CBYk1gg3jl-TtSJQ1yaBqkJcIlkdLgYz/view?usp=sharing

Patient is taken to 30° Trendelenburg position. We use fourth-arm of the robot on the very right side. When we perform a Martini-Klinik NeuroSAFE RARP procedure, we place a small sized Alexis port (Applied Medical©) above the umbilicus in order to take out the prostate to be sent for intraoperative frozen pathological evaluation. In that case, camera port is introduced through the Alexis port into the abdomen (Fig. 46.1).

The procedure starts with making an incision on the anterior peritoneal covering of the Douglas' pouch about 1 cm above the deepest part. Seminal vesicles and vas deferentia are identified and dissected. Thereafter, Denonvillier's fascia is opened. By using monopolar scissors, incisions are made lateral to the medial umbilical folds in order to detach the urinary bladder from the abdominal wall. If ePLND is performed, initially peritoneum covering the ureter where it

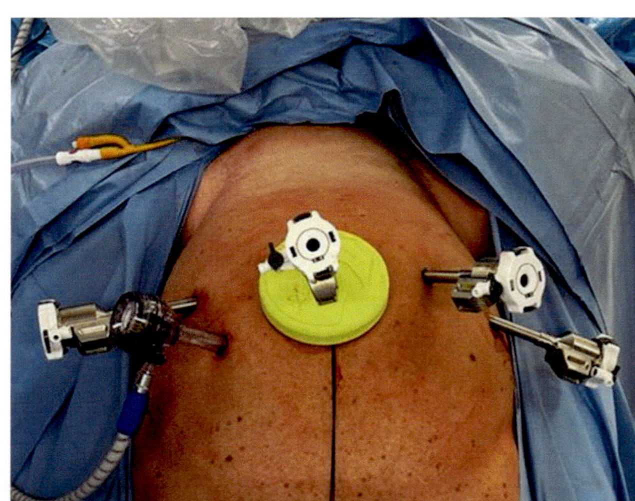

Fig. 46.1 Abdominal port placement

crosses the iliac artery is incised and this incision is extended up to the lateral side of the medial umbilical fold on both sides. The ePLND exposes the area including the genitofemoral nerve running lateral to the iliac artery on the lateral side, preserved neurovascular bundle (NVB) on the medial side, ureter crossing iliac artery superiorly and Cloquet lymph node inferiorly.

Following completion the prostatectomy, anastomosis between urinary bladder and urethra is completed using a running double-armed 3/0 barbed monofilament suture. Following the anastomosis, a 20F Foley catheter is inserted. It is important to have a watertight anastomosis therefore we check the anastomosis by filling the bladder with sterile saline given through the urethral catheter. After a watertight anastomosis is confirmed, we check the surgical field in terms of obtaining a sufficient hemostasis by decreasing the intra-abdominal pressure to 5 mmHg. Particularly in patients with preserved NVBs, we do not apply monopolar and/or bipolar cautery in order not to cause possible thermal injury for the small bleeders. However, we prefer applying hemostatic agents around the NVBs that lead to sufficient hemostasis for most of the cases. We can also apply selective suturing for further bleeders using 4/0 or 5/0 vicryl sutures that will cause minimal or no damage to the preserved NVBs.

The same five trocars used for the RARP procedure are also used for the hernia repair procedure. The epigastric vessels, ductus deferens and spermatic vessels that are the anatomic landmarks of the inguinal region, the hernia defect and the hernia sac should be identified at the beginning of the procedure (Fig. 46.2). After the indentification of the sac and the defect, mobilization, dissection, isolation and reduction of the sac are completed with sufficient mobilization of the peritoneum (Figs. 46.3, and 46.4). Mesh is kept in its sterile box until it is the time to use it for the hernia repair. Surgeon decides about the size and the type of mesh material to be used for the hernia repair. Before opening sterile mesh, the bedside assistant and nurse change their gloves to decrease contamination risk and an appropriate size of the mesh is chosen according to the defect size and inserted to the abdomen via assistant port.

The sterile mesh is introduced into the abdomen through the assistant port and is laid over the defect covering completely. A laparoscopic tacker is applied on the lateral borders of the mesh to fix the mesh material over the hernia defect, to the Cooper's ligament and the rectus/transversalis muscles avoiding the spermatic cord, epigastric and iliac vessels (Fig. 46.5). An absorbable suture can also be used to fix the mesh instead of using a laparoscopic tacker. It is also important to check the triangle of pain that includes femoral nerve, genitofemoral nerve and alteral cutaneous nerve of thigh.

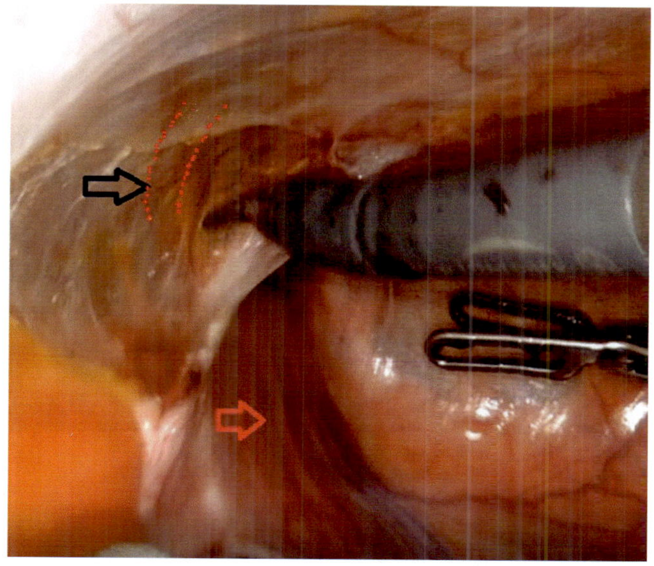

Fig. 46.2 Identification of the landmarks of the inguinal region and the hernia defect. Black arrow: epigastric vessels; Red arrow: spermatic vessels and ductus deferens

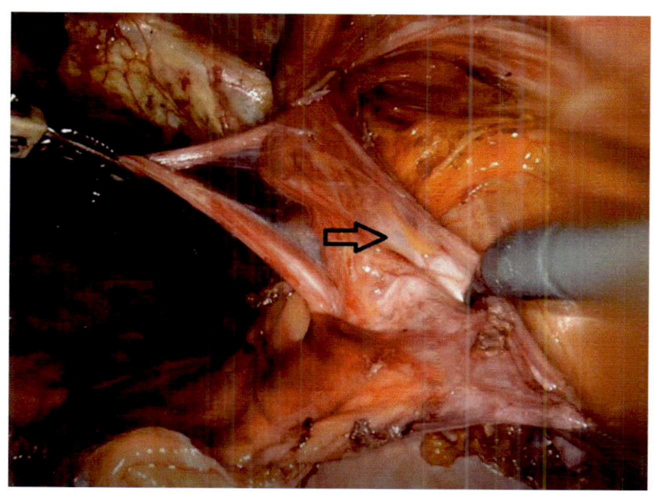

Fig. 46.3 Mobilization, dissection and isolation of the hernia sac (arrow: hernia sac)

The decision to cover the peritoneum over the surgical field including the mesh material is made according to mesh type used. If polypropylene mesh is used, a 3/0 barbed suture is used in order to cover and secure the peritoneum over the mesh material and Retzius space (Figs. 46.6 and 46.7). A soft silicon 24F drain can be inserted into the Retzius space that can be removed on postoperative day-1. Lastly, the specimen is removed through the supraumbilical port incision, and all trocars are removed under direct visualization. Although urologists can perform inguinal hernia repair with mesh

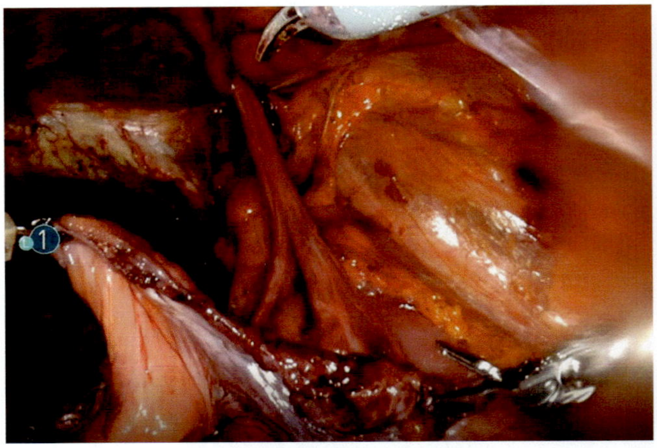

Fig. 46.4 Complete reduction of the hernia sac

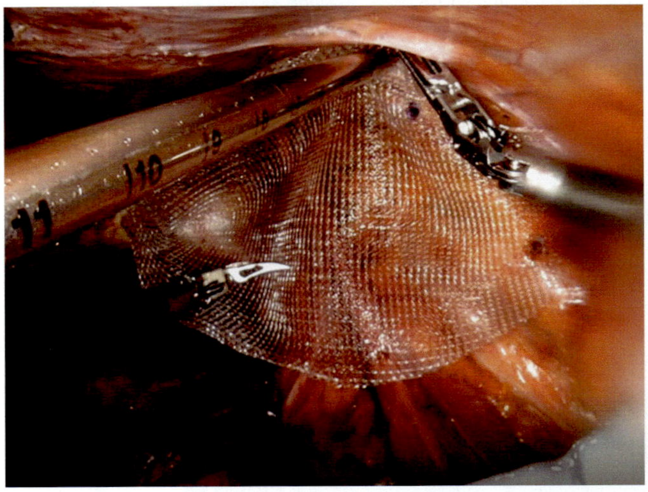

Fig. 46.5 Covering the area of hernia with the mesh material and fixing it at its corners by applying laparoscopic absorbable tackers

application in addition to a RARP procedure in the same session, taking the opinion and suggestions of the laparoscopic and/or robotic general surgeons particularly in large and complex inguinal hernias is very useful and increases collaboration.

Postoperative Management

Oral diet with mobilization is initiated after 6 hours postoperatively. Most patients are discharged on postoperative day-2 or 3 and drains are removed prior to discharge. Postoperative cystography is performed on postoperative day-7 and if no leakage is observed urethral Foley catheter is removed.

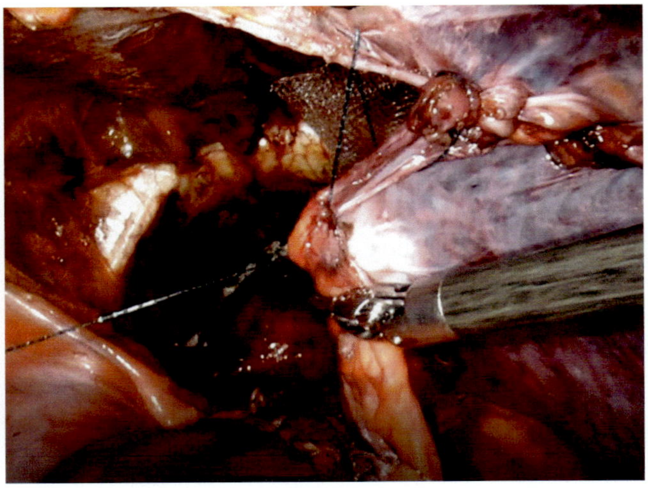

Fig. 46.6 Retroperitonealization of the Retsiuz space in order to secure the mesh. Peritoneum is covered over the mesh material by using an absorbable barbed suture

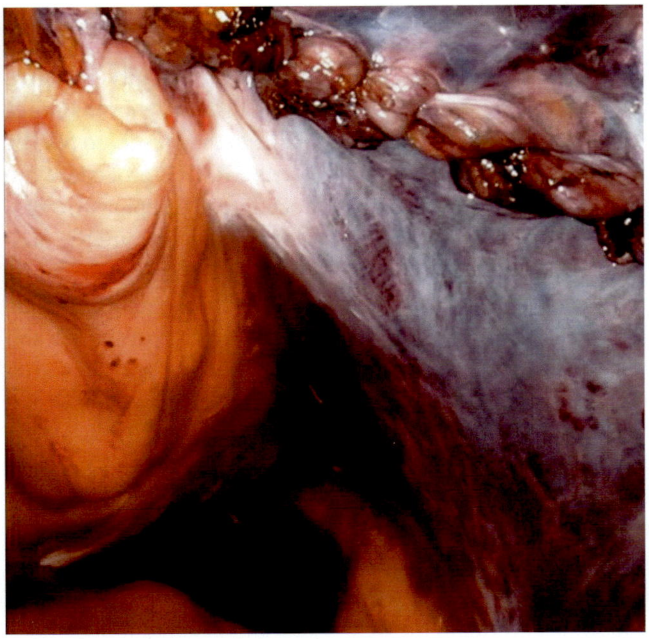

Fig. 46.7 Appearance of the completed RARP procedure with right sided inguinal hernia repair with mesh application

Conclusion

According to literature approximately 10% of patients who undergo RP will need a simultaneous IH repair. The overall risk of identification of a hernia at the time of prostatectomy is 5% in patients without lower urinary tract dysfunction and is 20% in patients with moderate-severe lower urinary tract symptoms regardless of prostate size. Concomitant IH repair with mesh application during RARP is a safe and effective procedure that can be performed following specific precautions are taken.

References

1. Nielsen ME, Walsh PC. Systematic detection and repair of subclinical inguinal hernias at radical retropubic prostatectomy. Urology. 2005;66(5):1034–7.
2. Lepor H, Nieder AM, Ferrandino MN. Intraoperative and postoperative complications of radical retropubic prostatectomy in a consecutive series of 1,000 cases. J Urol. 2001;166(5):1729–33.
3. Nilsson H, Stranne J, Stattin P, Nordin P. Incidence of groin hernia repair after radical prostatectomy: a population-based nationwide study. Ann Surg. 2014;259(6):1223–7.
4. Regan TC, Mordkin RM, Constantinople NL, Spence IJ, Dejter SW Jr. Incidence of inguinal hernias following radical retropubic prostatectomy. Urology. 1996;47(4):536–7.
5. Wauschkuhn CA, Schwarz J, Bittner R. Laparoscopic transperitoneal inguinal hernia repair (TAPP) after radical prostatectomy: is it safe? Results of prospectively collected data of more than 200 cases. Surg Endosc. 2009;23(5):973–7.
6. Soto-Palou FG, Sánchez-Ortiz RF. Outcomes of Minimally Invasive Inguinal Hernia Repair at the Time of Robotic Radical Prostatectomy. Curr Urol Rep. 2017;18(6):43.
7. Finley DS, Rodriguez E Jr, Ahlering TE. Combined inguinal hernia repair with prosthetic mesh during transperitoneal robot assisted laparoscopic radical prostatectomy: a 4-year experience. J Urol. 2007;178(4 Pt 1):1296–9.
8. Rogers T, Parra-Davila E, Malcher F, Hartmann C, Mastella B, de Araújo G, Ogaya-Pinies G, Ortiz-Ortiz C, Hernandez-Cardona E, Patel V, Cavazzola LT. Robotic radical prostatectomy with concomitant repair of inguinal hernia: is it safe? J Robot Surg. 2018;12(2):325–30.
9. Choi BB, Steckel J, Denoto G, Vaughan ED, Schlegel PN. Preperitoneal prosthetic mesh hernioplasty during radical retropubic prostatectomy. J Urol. 1999;161(3):840–3.
10. Teber D, Erdogru T, Zukosky D, Frede T, Rassweiler J. Prosthetic mesh hernioplasty during laparoscopic radical prostatectomy. Urology. 2005;65(6):1173–8.
11. Joshi A, Spivak J, Rubach E. Concurrent robotic transabdominal pre-peritoneal (TAP) herniorrhaphy during robotic-assisted radical prostatectomy. Int J Med Robot. 2010;6(3):311–4.
12. Mourmouris P, Argun OB, Tufek I, et al. Nonprosthetic direct inguinal hernia repair during robotic radical prostatectomy. J Endourol. 2016;30(2):218–22.
13. Lee DK, Montgomery DP, Porter JR. Concurrent transperitoneal repair for incidentally detected inguinal hernias during robotically assisted radical prostatectomy. Urology. 2013;82(6):1320–2.
14. Ludwig WW, Sopko NA, Azoury SC, et al. Inguinal hernia repair during Extraperitoneal robot-assisted laparoscopic radical prostatectomy. J Endourol. 2016;30(2):208–11.
15. Sanchez-Ortiz RF, Andrade-Geigel C, Lopez-Huertas H, Cadillo-Chavez R, Soto-Aviles O. Preoperative International Prostate Symptom Score Predictive of Inguinal Hernia in Patients Undergoing Robotic Prostatectomy. J Urol. 2015;195(6):1744–7.
16. Atmaca AF, Hamidi N, Canda AE, Keske M, Ardicoglu A. Concurrent Repair of Inguinal Hernias with Mesh Application During Transperitoneal Robotic-assisted Radical Prostatectomy: Is it Safe. Urol J. 2018;15(6):381–6.
17. Qazi HA, Rai BP, Do M, et al. Robot-assisted laparoscopic total extraperitoneal hernia repair during prostatectomy: technique and initial experience. Cent European J Urol. 2015;68(2):240–4.
18. Birolini C, de Miranda JS, Utiyama EM, Rasslan S. A retrospective review and observations over a 16-year clinical experience on the surgical treatment of chronic mesh infection. What about replacing a synthetic mesh on the infected surgical field? Hernia. 2015;19(2):239–46.

Robot Assisted Partial Prostatectomy for Anterior Cancer

47

Arnauld Villers and Jonathan Olivier

Introduction

Complications of radical prostatectomy have been well documented in current literature such as erectile dysfunction, chronic urinary incontinence, and the occasional bladder neck contracture. These complications arise because of the close proximity of the neurovascular bundle and the rhabdosphincter to the surgical dissection plane which increase the risk of injury to these structures. Potentially these structures could be preserved if surrounding prostatic tissue was indeed benign. Another approach to preserve these structures is to leave part of the prostate itself free from cancer to obtain a margin of benign tissue which protects even more neurovascular bundle and rhabdosphincter. This partial gland ablation (PGA) can be performed with thermo-ablative energies or radiation or surgery [1]. The goal of PGA is to completely ablate target tissue, which in men with prostate cancer is malignant, and to delay or altogether avoid radical therapy, perhaps indefinitely, through treatment, possible re treatment and surveillance [2]. Surgical techniques for PGA are technically challenging. They need to preserve the vesicourethral continuity; So far two different techniques were described. Partial anterior prostatectomy and a novel surgical technique, the precision prostatectomy.

Robotic partial prostatectomy for isolated anterior cancer was reported in 2016 with a 2 years (range 0.5–8) median follow up [3]. The technique consisted in a en-block template surgical excision of this part of the gland preserving intact the posterior-lateral parts of the distal urethra, peripheral zone (PZ), and periprostatic tissues Technique was feasible, with excellent functional results and 76% biochemical-recurrence free survival at upto 8 years maximal follow-up. Partial prostatectomy maybe a potential option for highly-selected men with anterior cancers who are not candidates for focal ablative therapy.

A. Villers (✉) · J. Olivier
Department of Urology, CHU Lille, Université de Lille, Lille, France
e-mail: arnauld-villers@univ-lille.fr

The precision prostatectomy technique reported in 2019 would allow for maximal prostatic tissue extirpation without affecting the functional reserve [4]. In this approach, all prostatic tissue is removed except for a 5–10-mm rim of glandular (pseudo-capsule) prostate PZ on the side contralateral to the dominant lesion (>90% of prostatic tissue is removed). Furthermore, as an additional fail-safe step, the remnant prostatic capsule is biopsied intraoperatively to ensure the absence of cancer. If cancer is present on frozen intraoperative sections, the operation is converted to radical prostatectomy.

APP Patients Selection

Inclusion criteria comprised an MRI-targeted biopsy-proven predominant APC based on MRI findings, i.e. at a distance of at least 17 mm (biopsy core length) from rectal surface, with negative posterior 12 systematic biopsy series (Fig. 47.1) Since 2008 on a 12 years period, 28 patients fulfilled entry criteria and signed the consent form. This represents roughly 2 patients/year. in a center performing 150 robotic prostatectomies/year. The first part of the series of 17 patients (2008–2015) was published in 2016 [3]. Thirteen patients (76%) had no progression at 1 year MRI and/or repeat biopsy and during follow-up. Four patients (24%) with positive posterior margin had PSA-recurrence at upto 30mo and underwent an uncomplicated completion robotic prostatectomy, with undetectable PSA. At that time of first analyses, we looked for clinical and morphometric criteria which could improve the rate of success. The cancer volume density (cancer volume at MRI/prostate volume) was the most discriminant criteria to separate success from failures. The higher the prostate gland volume, and the smaller the cancer volume, the longest the thickness of safety margin of benign tissue posterior to the APC Out of the 17 cases, 4 cases recurred, and 3 of them had cancer volume density < 0.15 and. None of the remaining 13 cases who did not recurred/progressed had cancer volume density < 0.15. Therefore, for the next

S. Ren et al. (eds.), *Robot-Assisted Radical Prostatectomy*, https://doi.org/10.1007/978-3-031-05855-4_47

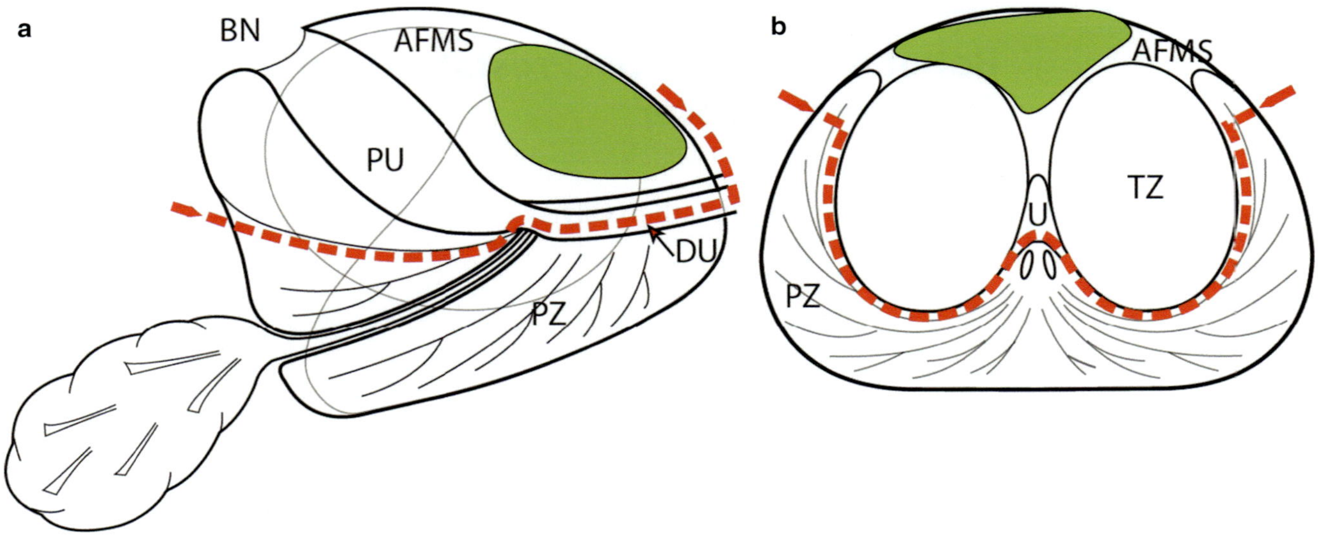

Fig. 47.1 Schematic view of the prostate. (**a**) Sagittal and (**b**) Transverse at the mid-gland. The red dotted line shows the dissection plane of the APP. The average APC anterior to urethra and in the anterior fibro-muscular stroma (AFMS) is depicted in green. The protocol comprises en-bloc template excision of the anterior part of the prostate including the AFMS, prostate adenoma (TZ and median lobe) with the proximal urethra (PU), the anterior part of the distal (sub-montanal) urethra (DU), the most anterior apical parts of the PZ, and the anterior bladder neck (BN)

patients we excluded cases with cancer volume density < 0.15. The rest of the exclusion criteria comprised MR-documented APC located within 5 mm of the posterior TZ boundary, GS ≥8, clinically significant cancer outside the APC or in the PZ lateral horns and previous local or systemic therapy. PSA, was not used as a criteria provided the cancer was localized at imaging. All patients underwent PSA monitoring at 3 and 6 months and then 6-monthly and MRI at 6–12 months. At 6 months, protocol-based 12-core and/or targeted biopsies were performed in the first 7 patients; since biopsies were negative when MRI was not suspicious, only for-cause biopsies were performed in the remaining 21 patients. Self-administered questionnaires assessed urinary function (IPSS), continence (ICS1-2) and potency (IIEF-5) at months 6 and 12. In case of cancer progression, from index tumor or de novo cancer in the PZ, robotic completion of prostatectomy was performed.

Step-by-Step description with video was described in 2016 [5]. APP was performed in all cases in 5 steps in the following order.

Patient positioning and robotic approach. All procedures were performed using a Da Vinci surgical system (Intuitive Surgical, Sunnyvale, CA, USA) in the four arm configuration via a transperitoneal approach. Patient positioning and port placement were identical to transperitoneal RARP procedure. Prevesical space was developed. Surgical protocol comprised en-bloc template excision of the anterior part of the prostate comprising of the anterior fibromuscular stroma AFMS, prostate adenoma Transition zone (TZ) and median lobe with the proximal urethra, anterior part of the distal (sub-montanal) urethra and the anterior bladder neck. Postero-lateral PZ and peri-prostatic tissues were preserved intact. (Fig. 47.1).

Retrograde dissection of PZ and TZ at the apex. The prostate was exposed leaving the fatty tissue anterior to the gland to avoid anterior positive margins at this level (Fig. 47.2). A 1 cm opening of the endopelvic fascia was performed on each side at the prostato-urethral junction. Neurovascular bundles were not exposed, since the plane of dissection remains anterior to the 3 and 9 o'clock location and lateral to the urethra. Dorsal venous complex was secured and divided (Fig. 47.2). The anterior half of urethra was transected at apex. Lateral walls of distal urethra length as well as PZ lobes were divided, at 3 and 9 o'clock with cold scissors using a retrograde approach without significant bleeding requiring hemostasis. Apical TZ lobes were also enucleated up to the verumontanum. The verumontanum and posterior half of urethra and PZ were maintained intact.

Antegrade dissection of TZ lobe at bladder neck. Anterior and posterior bladder neck was divided. The specimen was retracted anteriorly. Ureteral orifices were exposed. Posterior bladder neck incision was made up to the glandular surface of adenoma. Adenoma enucleation plane was developed bluntly and sharply, posteriorly up to the verumontanum. The anterior and anterolateral aspects of adenoma lobes were not enucleated. The anterior and anterolateral

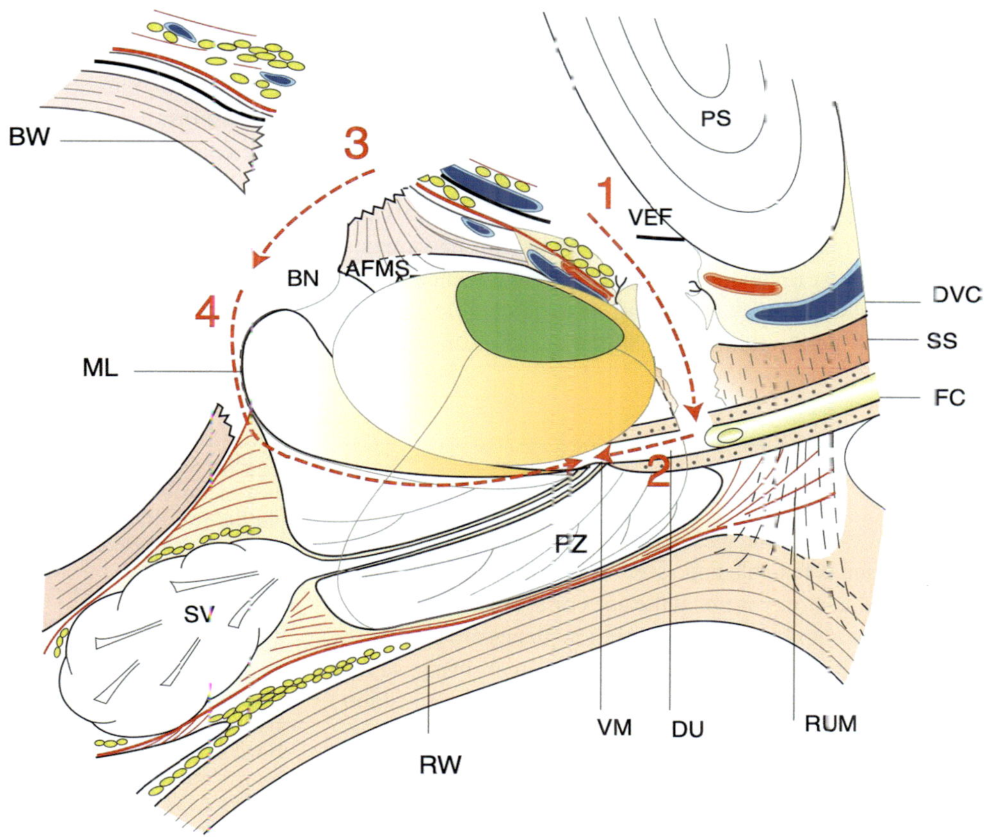

Fig. 47.2 Sagittal section of prostate, bladder, seminal vesicles, urethra and periprostatic fascia. The average APC is depicted in green. The red dotted line shows the dissection plane of the APP. Step 1 [1], retrograde (R): division of dorsal venous complex (DVC) (1—arrow) and anterior half of the urethra at the apex (Step 2—arrow). Step 3, antegrade (A): division of the anterior BN (3—arrow), division of the posterior neck and median lobe enucleation (4—arrow). *BW* bladder wall, *DA* detrusor apron, *DU* distal urethra, *VPF* ventral endopelvic fascia, *FC* Foley catheter, *ML* TZ median lobe, *PS* pubic symphysis, *PU* proximal urethra, *RUM* rectourethralis muscle, *RW* rectum wall, *SS* striated sphincter, *SV* seminal vesicles, *VM* verumontanum

aspects of adenoma were not dissected which allowed us to keep the anterior attachments to the AFMS intact (Fig. 47.2).

Lateral sectioning of PZ. The lateral parts of the PZ were divided at mid-gland, and specifically excised along a coronal plane crossing the verumontanum. This was joined to the previous retrograde adenoma enucleation plane and PZ sectioning at mid-gland along the incision line (Fig. 47.1). The specimen was placed in a bag and extracted for pathologic evaluation. Inspection of the remaining part of PZ was made to assess hemostasis in the prostatic bed, and to evaluate any residual adenoma lobules were remaining. Edges of the PZ were located.

Bladder suturing to urethra and PZ. Reconstruction was performed by suturing the edges of the bladder opening, and advancing an anterior bladder flap to the anterior remaining half of the urethra using two 3/0 V-lock running sutures. The bladder neck was then sutured to the edges of PZ to obtain a watertight urethro prostatovesical anastomosis. An 18 French Foley catheter was left for 7 days without irrigation. A suction drain was placed in the retropubic space.

Robotic completion of prostatectomy was performed in 7 cases due to cancer recurrence. In these cases complete nerve-sparing prostatectomy was performed as during RARP procedure. Anterior aspect of bladder wall was divided at the level of the PZ upper limit at a distance of 3 cm from the urethral rhabdosphincter. The endopelvic fascia was incised laterally, and a margin of the bladder wall covering PZ (previously sutured to PZ lateral edges) was excised to ensure removal of APC recurrence site. Posterior bladder neck was then divided and posterior and lateral dissection of PZ performed. Urethral wall was incised as the prostate-urethral junction at the level of previous bladder suturing.

Results

The current series comprises 25 patients, including the 14 cases with cancer volume density < 0.15 from the first analyses; Median PSA was 11 ng/ml (IQR: 7–12). Median prostate volume was 63 cc (IQR: 46–71). Median cancer volume at MRI was 2.11 cc (IQR: 0.97–3.67). No intra-operative complications were identified during APP or salvage RARP. Perioperative complications included Clavien-Dindo grade II only. These complications were as follows: anastomotic leak (12%), urinary tract infection (6%), and transient intestinal ileus in one case (6%). At

3 months, continence and potency rates were 92% and 83%, respectively. At 12 months, continence rate was 96%. Median nadir PSA was 0.4 ng/ml (IQR: 0.24–0.68). For the whole series of 25 patients full filling the modified exclusion criteria, at a median follow-up of 6 years, 4 patients recurred/progressed at 2, 3, 6 and 4 years respectively. All but one had undetectable PSA after salvage completion radical prostatectomy. One patient had a positive margin at the level of the APC site recurrence at the posterior bladder neck, resulting in a detectable PSA at 0.33 ng/ml post-operatively. Salvage radiation therapy was performed.

Discussion

Our initial experience with robotic APP demonstrated that the technique is feasible and safe. The technical challenge of partial prostatectomy is not at the apex or at the antero-lateral aspect of the gland where the dissection planes are similar to RP; the challenge is to ensure negative margins postero-laterally at PZ site. This is why we modified the selection criteria in 2016, taking into account cancer density at MRI. The specific role of prostate volume in the technique was not prospectively evaluated. However, as for open simple prostatectomy, the enucleation plane is easier to find and develop in high volume glands (>40–50 cc).

Conclusion

Our results of anterior partial prostatectomy show good functional results and 21 out of 25 patients are under remission at a median follow-up of 6 years. Technique is reversible to whole gland prostatectomy. One patient had biological recurrence after completion radical prostatectomy. These results validate the concept of surgical partial gland ablation for these APC.

References

1. Gross MD, Sedrakyan A, Bianco FJ, Carroll PR, Daskivich TJ, Eggener SE, Ehdaie B, Fisher B, Gorin MA, Hunt B, Jiang H, Klein EA, Marinac-Dabic D, Montgomery JS, Polascik TJ, Priester AM, Rastinehad AR, Viviano CJ, Wysock JS, Hu JC. SPARED collaboration: patient selection for partial gland ablation in men with localized prostate cancer. J Urol. 2019;202(5):952–8.
2. Sivaraman A, Barret E. Focal therapy for prostate cancer: an “À la Carte” approach. Eur Urol. 2016;69(6):973–5.
3. Villers A, Puech P, Flamand V, Haber GP, Desai MM, Crouzet S, Leroy X, Chopra S, Lemaitre L, Ouzzane A, Gill IS. Partial prostatectomy for anterior cancer: short-term oncologic and functional outcomes. Eur Urol. 2017;72(3):333–42.
4. Sood A, Abdollah F, Jeong W, Menon M. The precision prostatectomy: “waiting for Godot”. Eur Urol Focus. 2020;6(2):227–30.
5. Villers A, Flamand V, Arquímedes RC, Puech P, Haber GP, Desai MM, Crouzet S, Ouzzane A, Gill IS. Robot-assisted partial prostatectomy for anterior prostate cancer: a step-by-step guide. BJU Int. 2017;119(6):968–74.

Complications in Robotic-Assisted Laparoscopic Radical Prostatectomy: Prevention and Management

48

Laura C. Perez, Aref S. Sayegh, Anibal La Riva, Charles F. Polotti, and Rene Sotelo

Abbreviations

CK	Creatine kinase
CO_2	Carbon dioxide
CT	Computerized tomography
DVT	Deep venous thrombosis
ICP	Intracranial pressure
PE	Pulmonary embolism
RALP	Robot-Assisted Laparoscopic Radical Prostatectomy

Complications of Patient Positioning

Patient positioning has been widely studied due to its critical role in preventing complications even before the surgical procedure has started [1]. The surgical team must have a deep understanding of the potential complications from various positions. To increase effectiveness, having the same team position the patient for every surgery is recommended [2].

Postoperative complications due to positioning can go as high as 13% of patients undergoing robotic-assisted laparoscopic radical prostatectomy (RALP) [1]. Most of them being postoperative pain and neuromuscular injuries [3]. In an extensive multi-center review, the most common injuries identified were abdominal wall neuralgia, sensory and motor nerve deficit, rhabdomyolysis, shoulder pain, and back pain [4].

During RALP, lithotomy and 30° Trendelenburg position are required to allow adequate pelvic exposure. This steep head-down position for several hours can cause significant changes in cerebral hemodynamic physiology and increase intracranial pressure (ICP). Postoperative corneal abrasions have been observed in 0.1–0.6%, together with postoperative ischemic optic neuropathy (Fig. 48.1). Careful monitoring should be done to prevent delirium as well as short-term cognitive changes postoperatively [5, 6].

Safe fixation of the patient by increasing support and well-distributed friction using a soft mattress is mandatory to avoid sliding. Vacuum mattresses may also be used. However, unnoticed gas leakage may lead to compression injuries [7]. Sliding-associated complications include incisional wound tear, postoperative incisional hernia, and increase postoperative pain due to overstretching of the abdominal wall. Other maneuvers used in the past to prevent sliding, such as shoulder and body straps, restraints, or headrests, should be avoided.

During the preoperative assessment, protective padding is intended to protect the patient from peripheral neuropathies and muscle compression injuries (Fig. 48.1). In severe cases, muscle compression may lead to rhabdomyolysis and compartment syndrome, with incidence being particularly higher in patients with cardiovascular risk factors such as obesity, diabetes, hypertension, or peripheral vascular disease and those placed in Trendelenburg position for extended periods of time. These patients should be meticulously evaluated clinically and have an immediate assessment of serum creatinine and creatine kinase (CK) levels in order to prevent renal damage [8].

It is crucial to use well-padded armrests designed explicitly for Trendelenburg positioning to distribute the patient's weight evenly. Generally, these cushions have a notch stabilizing the patient's head without compression and limiting rotation or lateral flexion of the neck, preventing brachial plexus neuropathies [9].

The arms should be in an anatomically neutral position limiting abduction of the arm to 90° and flexion/extension of the elbows and hands, preventing any excessive nerve stretching [10, 11] (Fig. 48.1).

Sciatic nerve injury has been reported in up to 1% of cases due to lower extremity overextension and separation of 30° during extreme lithotomy [12]. Considering the sciatic

L. C. Perez · A. S. Sayegh · A. L. Riva · C. F. Polotti · R. Sotelo (✉)
The Catherine and Joseph Aresty Department of Urology, USC Institute of Urology, Keck School of Medicine, University of Southern California, Los Angeles, CA, USA
e-mail: rene.sotelo@med.usc.edu

S. Ren et al. (eds.), *Robot-Assisted Radical Prostatectomy*, https://doi.org/10.1007/978-3-031-05855-4_48

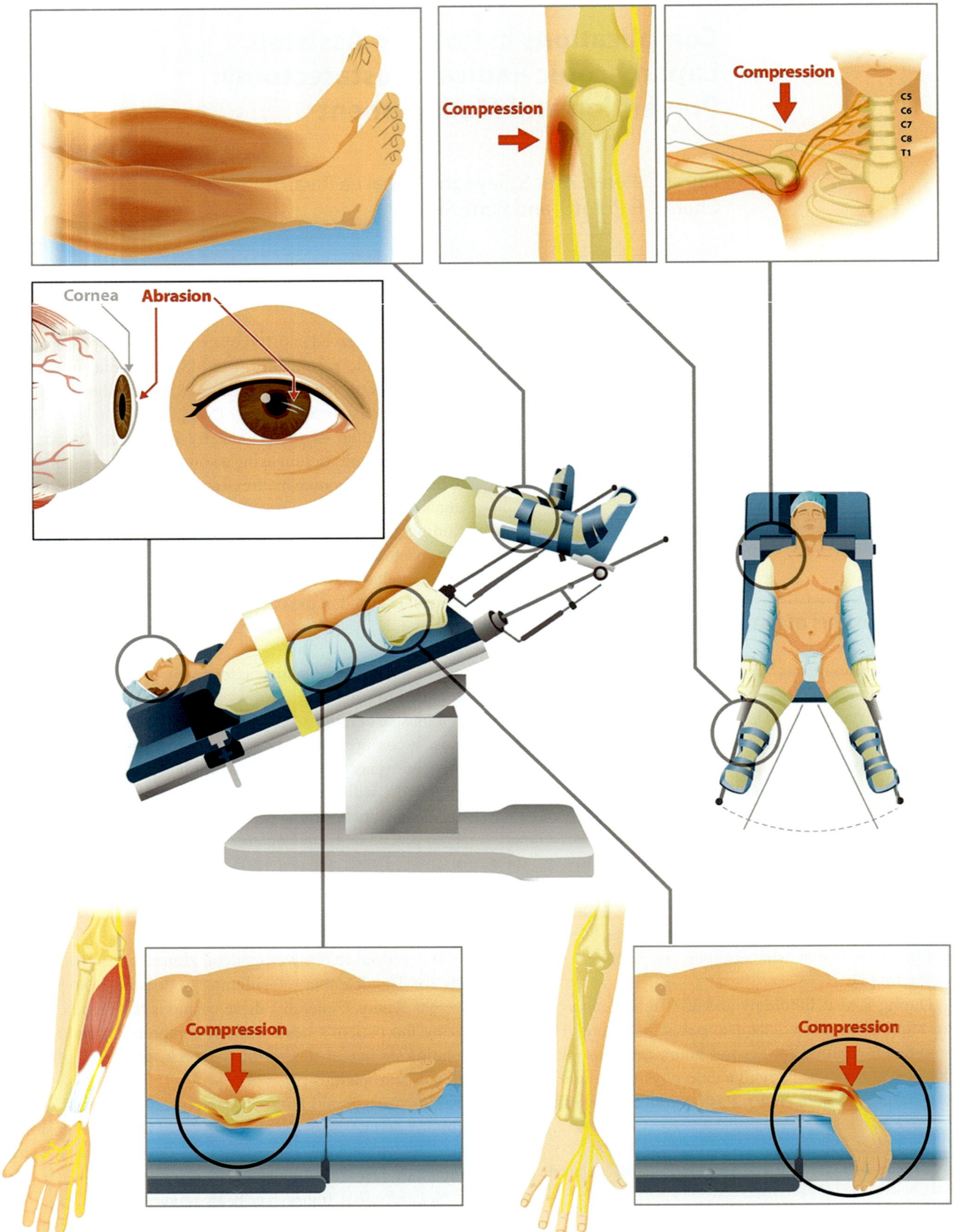

Fig. 48.1 Complications of Patient Positioning. Schematic drawing represents patient positioning-related complications, including corneal abrasions, muscle compression injuries, and brachial plexus, ulnar, radial, and common peroneal neuropathies

nerve or its branches cross both the hip and the knee joints, it is important to assess these joints' extension and flexion when determining the degree of hip flexion. When possible, excessive stretch of the hamstring muscle group should be avoided. Most nerve injuries are caused by stretching rather than direct nerve transections during the surgery itself [4]. In addition, specific padding to limit the pressure of a hard surface against the fibular head may be used to decrease the risk of peroneal neuropathy (Fig. 48.1).

Periodic perioperative assessments may be performed to ensure maintenance of the desired position. Of note, postoperative pain in the areas described should serve as a warning sign.

Care must be taken with the position and movement of the robotic arms during surgery, especially when one of the arms is placed outside the field of view. The drape must be kept free of surgical instruments as unrecognized compression injuries can occur, leading to intramural hematomas or thrombosis due to blood stasis.

Face masks, metallic bars, foam pads, and glasses can be used to protect the patients from any injury on the face and eyes due to the robotic ports' proximity.

Complications During Port Positioning

An essential component for performing a safe and effective robotic surgery is optimal port placement. Although complications associated with port-site placement are rare, devastating consequences can be seen, with most injuries involving either visceral or vascular organs. Ideally, the best method to manage those complications is prevention [13].

A pre-incisional checklist should be done to rule out any equipment malfunctions and the availability of all necessary resources, including preparation for open conversion [14].

Access Complications

Blind Veress needle insertion and insufflation followed by the blind camera trocar placement is the technique most widely used. Abdominal wall scars should be avoided as excessive force may be required, and adhesions can be present beneath these scars. The Veress needle should be inserted by bracing the hand on the patient to avoid pushing too deep, commonly at 2 cm above the umbilicus. The angle of insertion can vary from 45° in non-obese patients to 90° in those who are obese. The double-click test indicates the two resistance points (anterior and posterior rectus fascia). After passing through the second point, an aspiration and hanging drop test are used to identify any vascular or visceral lesions and verify the intraperitoneal position [14].

Next, the needle is attached to an insufflator, and the CO_2 opening pressure should be <10 mmHg if it is appropriately placed. Flow rate must be low until a symmetrical distention is well-documented. Then a 12–15 mmHg pneumoperitoneum is established. The camera trocar is then carefully introduced, and immediate camera inspection is done for early injury identification.

In patients with history of previous abdominal surgeries with presumed adhesions, an open laparoscopic trocar placement is recommended.

Vascular Injuries

The incidence of vascular injuries during access is low, with an estimated incidence of 0.03–0.3% [15]. Major or unrecognized vascular injury may cause a significant increase in morbidity and mortality. Most vascular injuries are caused by the Veress needle or the initial trocar placement, as these are often performed without visual confirmation. The most common vessel injuries are those located in the abdominal wall, particularly epigastric vessels. Otherwise, intra-abdominal vascular injury sites include the iliac vein, greater omental vessels, inferior vena cava, aorta, pelvic vessels, superior mesenteric veins, and lumbar veins [16].

Trendelenburg position should be avoided until port placement is completed because it causes promontory rotation and places the aortic bifurcation closer to the umbilicus, increasing the likelihood of vascular injury.

Direct compression of the bleeding site is the quickest and safest way to gain initial control of blood loss, especially with a venous injury. Small, non-expanding lesions can be managed with clips or pinpoint electrocautery. Increasing pneumoperitoneum pressure by up to 5–10 mmHg higher can be helpful, but frequent monitoring during the entire procedure is recommended as lesions partially controlled can rebleed. In those cases where cautery or clips are not sufficient, a figure-of-eight suture should be placed for adequate control.

If the hematoma expands, additional trocars should be placed, and the system docked. Robotic-assisted immediate repair with exploration and bleeding site exposure should be the preferable approach. Alternative strategies include compression, gauze insertion, and U stitches using a suture passer. Also, a Foley catheter can be inserted and inflated, doing gentle traction to tamponade the bleeding site [13] (Fig. 48.2). If the robotic attempt is not successful, the bleeding site is challenging to detect, or the patient is unstable, a prompt laparotomy should be performed.

Of note, at the end of the procedure, all ports should be visualized after trocars removal to ensure that there is no bleeding that was tamponade by the trocar itself.

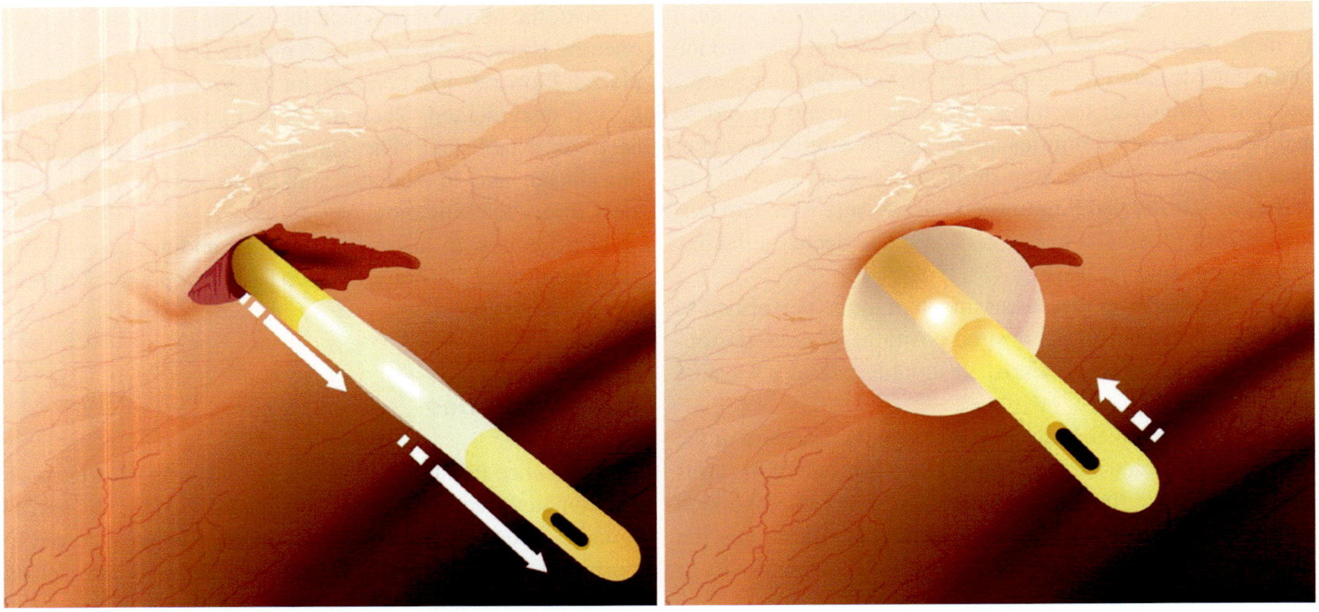

Fig. 48.2 Foley Catheter Balloon Tamponade. Schematic drawing shows balloon tamponade for temporary bleeding control after an abdominal wall vessel injury

Visceral Injuries

Bowel injuries during port placement are uncommon, ranging from 0.04% to 0.09%. However, 30–50% of them are not recognized intraoperatively, leading to a mortality rate of up to 30% [17, 18]. Once identified, it must be repaired. The trocar should be left in place, and another trocar should be inserted to explore and determine the extent of injury (Fig. 48.3). Depending on surgeon expertise and defect size, a primary intracorporeal closure can be done with a purse-string or double-layer suture. Alternatively, the bowel can be externalized and repaired through a small incision. Major injuries requiring bowel resection can be managed by stapling or may require laparotomy.

Colon injuries should be immediately treated by primary repair, in which case drainage is always recommended. The decision to perform primary anastomosis or colostomy should be individualized considering the patient's condition and the primary procedure to be performed.

Liver or spleen injury management includes compression primarily using an instrument or by introducing gauze into the abdominal cavity. Increasing the pressure of the pneumoperitoneum may help control hemostasis in venous injuries. The use of dry hemostatic agents or thrombin sealants should be considered if bleeding control is not achieved. Suture use should be carefully assessed as it could cause larger tears.

Bladder injuries may also occur. The use of a Foley catheter may reduce the risk of injury and allow early diagnosis by air or blood in the collection bag. The diagnosis is made by instilling dye into the bladder. If the damage was caused by a Veress needle and is less than 5 mm, it can be managed by leaving a Foley catheter up to 10 days. More extensive injuries will require primary two-layer closure.

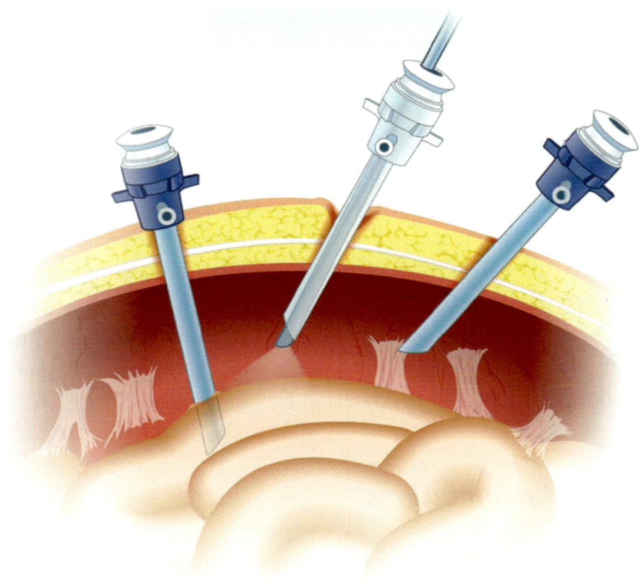

Fig. 48.3 Visceral Injury. Schematic drawing depicts trocar visceral injury, and secondary trocar placement to explore, and determine the extent of injury

Secondary Trocar Placement Complications

Subsequent trocars must always be placed under direct vision. The optimal sites of trocar placement should be marked after a full pneumoperitoneum has been established.

Transillumination may help visualize subcutaneous vessels; however, the epigastric vessels at the rectus muscle's lateral border are often undetectable.

After placement of the camera, adhesions are identified and avoided. The degree of adhesions is unpredictable, ranging from extensive after previous minor surgeries to nonexistent despite major abdominal interventions. If adhesions are present, subsequent trocars are placed in a position that allows manual laparoscopic adhesiolysis.

Despite direct port placement visualization, vascular injury can still occur. Lower abdominal wall vessels, notably inferior epigastric vessels, and intra-abdominal (aorta or iliac vessels) can be involved in 35% and 30% of cases, respectively [19].

Intraoperative Complications

Bowel Injury During Instrument Exchange

Robotic-assisted surgery occurs with the primary surgeon working on the console, apart from the operating table. Therefore, many steps must be synchronously performed with the bedside team, generally, another surgeon, scrub nurse, or surgical physician assistant. Most surgical procedures require a variety of instruments to accomplish each step. Hence, a constant exchange between the instruments has to occur [20].

During instrument insertion, a bowel injury can occur as previously mentioned; this is preventable by following the simple rule of inserting any instrument always under direct visualization. Some robotic platforms have instrument exchange memory where the instrument returns to just short of its previous location, but this may not always be reliable. Manual repositioning of the robotic arm resets this memory when the new instrument is inserted, causing it to go further than expected and cause an organ lesion, most commonly a bowel injury. If a bowel injury is suspected, careful inspection of the bowel surface must follow. If it is recognized, it must be properly managed depending on the extent of the damage.

Vascular Lesions

Arterial injuries are prevented by understanding the dissection boundaries and the specific risky steps that involve the iliac vessels. If an arterial injury occurs, immediate clamping with a grasper should follow. Gauze can be passed through one of the assistant ports for compression. Clip placement may be helpful, but this cannot be blindly placed, as it could represent a risk for a future complication. Suturing may be necessary if entry into a larger arterial vessel occurs. If hemostasis is not achieved by the described methods, the bedside team can apply external compression to momentarily control the bleeding while the surgical team prepares for conversion to open surgery.

Generally, a venous lesion can be controlled by increasing pneumoperitoneum up to 25 mmHg; this should be the first maneuver to attempt after recognition. If pneumoperitoneum alone does not resolve the bleeding, the following most crucial step is the visual identification of the vein's particular injury site to achieve hemostasis by clip or suture ligation. It is recommended to limit suction as this could significantly decrease pneumoperitoneum. In an iliac vein injury, ipsilateral sequential compression devices should be stopped to avoid worsening the bleeding and allow appropriate control. If it is difficult to determine the exact location of the injury, temporary clamping of distal branches may allow a window of no bleeding to determine the lesion location. Venous injury complications rarely go beyond this point. However, it is always recommended to be prepared to escalate the decision-making process in real time.

Rectal Injury

Rectal injury is an infrequent complication of RALP, generally reported in <1% of the procedures [21]. The vast majority occurred during the early phase of the surgeon's robotic learning curve. It can be avoided by limiting aggressive electrocautery and blunt dissection during the posterior plane dissection that occurs just above the rectum. If a rectal injury is recognized, closure of the defect with a 3-0 V-Loc suture in two layers is recommended as depicted in the picture (Fig. 48.4). It is crucial to make sure the edges of the injury are well vascularized, and this could be ensured using indocyanine green. It is also essential to be aware of the rectal lumen diameter during the repair as rectal stenosis and stricture are possible complications. A chest tube inserted in a retrograde fashion while placing the sutures can ensure proper diameter, or a rectoscopy can be performed by another team simultaneously. Some authors recommend the interposition of tissue between the rectum and the bladder to avoid the possibility of rectovesical fistula development, seen in 1% of the cases [22].

Obturator Nerve Injury

Obturator nerve injury is an uncommon complication of RALP reported in 0.2–5.7% of the cases [23]. The injury occurs due to the proximity of the nerve to the nodal packet. It can be preventable by clearly separating the bladder pedicle from the lateral pelvic wall and ensuring that the obturator nerve is always visualized. Generally, an obturator lesion

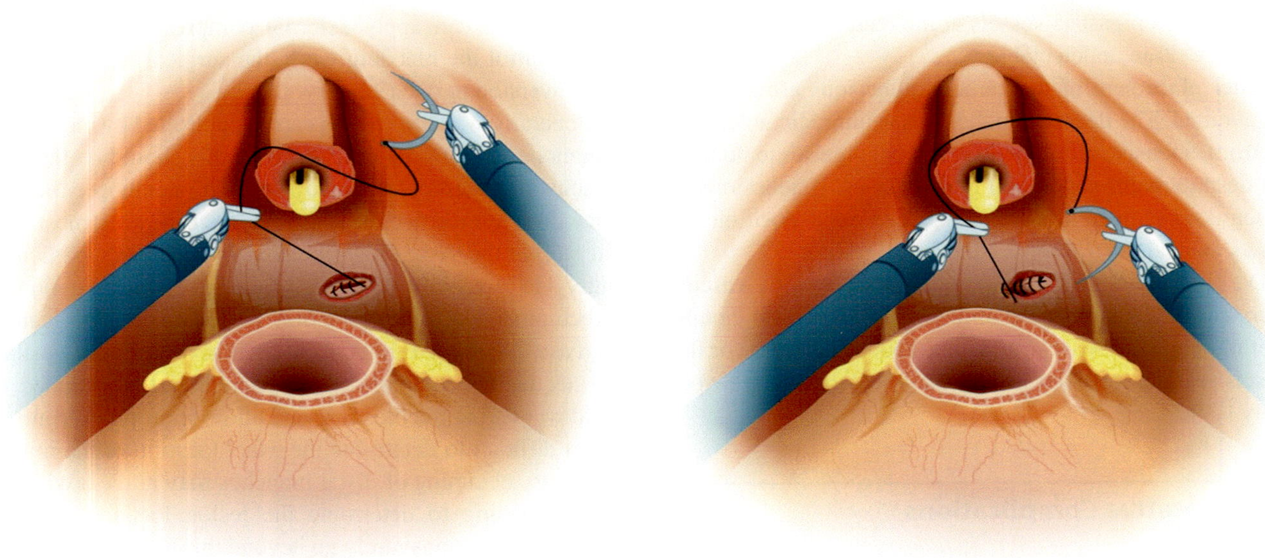

Fig. 48.4 Rectal Injury Repair. Schematic drawing exhibits a rectal repair in a two-layer running fashion with 3-0 V-Loc suture after iatrogenic injury during posterior plane dissection

could be caused by direct thermal injury, stretching, or transection.

In pelvic lymph node dissection, visual identification at every step is critical to avoid blind use of electrocautery and direct thermal damage. Stretching nerve injury generally occurs due to forceful traction of the tissues. Therefore, gentle management of them is encouraged. A total or partial transection could happen as the lymph node dissection occurs.

All these lesions may result in neuropraxia, characterized by gait disturbance, weakness, and atrophy of the adductor muscles. If identified intraoperatively, the best way to manage is by approximating and suturing both ends of the nerve together. In some circumstances, they will not reach each other if the patient is supine and extended; for these cases, thigh flexion may help reduce tension. Otherwise, a neural graft has to be used.

Urinary Tract Injuries

The incidence of ureteral injury during RALP is reported in <1% of cases [24–26]. Some steps pose a risk for unintentional ureteric injuries to occur. During the downward dissection between the prostate and the bladder in the anterior approach, the bladder neck can be injured if the detrusor muscle thickness is reduced. Therefore, it is crucial to constantly check detrusor muscle thickness while performing this dissection. If a bladder neck lesion happens, it is recommended to close the defect with a 3-0 V-Loc suture and do not remove the urethral catheter before a cystogram is performed to rule out any urinary leak. Less frequently, a large defect could compromise the ureteric orifices. In this case, both ureters should be stented with double J stents to remain in place for at least 21 days. Again, a cystogram is mandatory before catheter removal.

The posterior approach for radical prostatectomy described by Guillonneau et al. poses a significant risk to the distal ureter during the seminal vesicles' dissection. If there is no proper identification of the structures, the distal ureter can be confused for the seminal vesicles as they lie posterior to the vas deferens. Distal ureteral injuries can be partial or complete. If a partial ureteral injury is intraoperatively identified, a ureteral stent placement followed by suture with 5-0 Monocryl is recommended. If there is a complete transection of the ureter, ureteral reimplantation will be the next step.

Lastly, during extended lymph node dissection of the pelvic lymph nodes, the middle third of the ureter can be injured. This type of injury occurs as the ureter runs with the psoas muscle and crosses anterior to the common iliac vessels at the bifurcation level. To prevent this, it is vital to visualize the ureter at all times during pelvic lymph node dissection.

Complications from Technical Errors and Robotic Malfunction

Electrocautery or Thermal Energy Injuries

A robot is still a machine with mechanical parts and accessories, and their errors or malfunction can cause significant injuries. Monopolar instruments failure such as tip cover

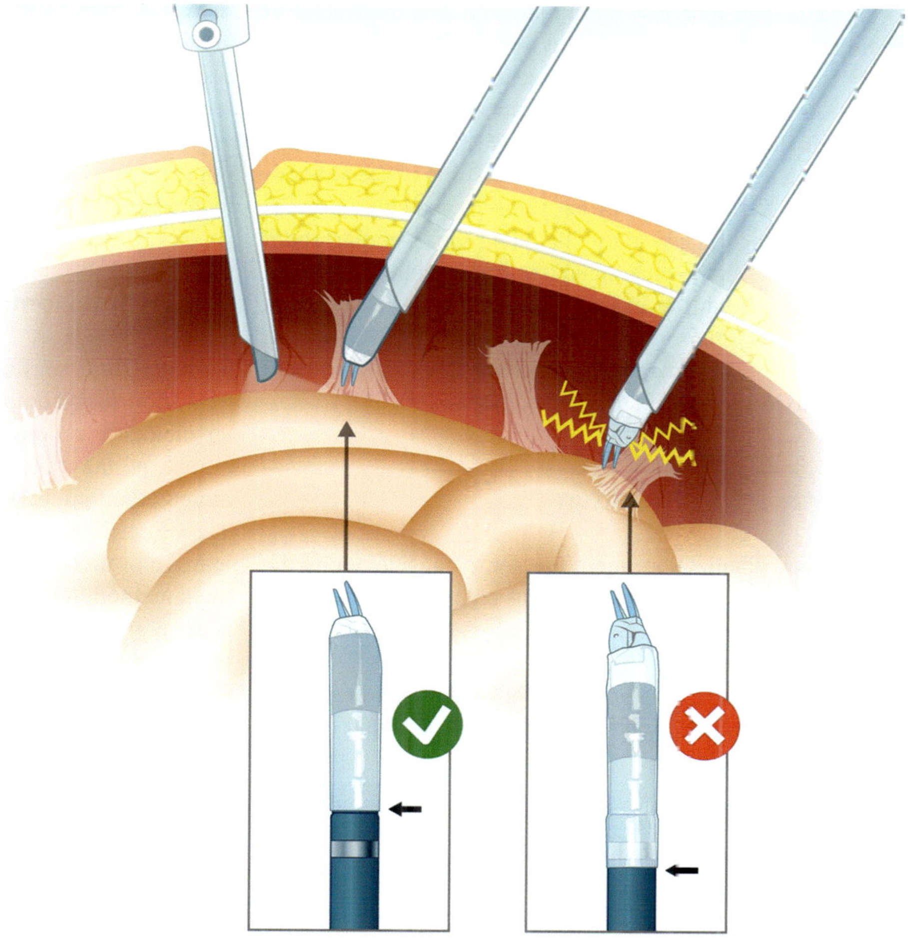

Fig. 48.5 Electrocautery or Thermal Energy Injuries. Schematic drawing represents a thermo-electrical injury due to cover tip failure

failure can result in dissipation of monopolar electrical current leading to significant damage [27]. Blood vessels and intestinal injury can be caused directly by electrosurgical arcs and thermal energy (Fig. 48.5). These electrical arcs may go over from the tip of the scissor to the non-isolated parts of the instrument or to a suction cannula, leading to visceral or bowel injury. Therefore, surgeons must take greater care and ensure the insulation's integrity, preventing broad dissipation of monopolar electric current, allowing a safe dissection in proximity to blood vessels, nerves, and bowel.

Instrument Malfunction

Different events of instrument malfunction can occur before or during surgery. Breaking of the endo-wrist wire and instrument jaws is the most common scenario of instrument malfunction. In cases where this happened, the instrumentation can be removed without difficulty [28]. Other common events that can be encountered are broken or disintegrated instruments, which can get lost intra-abdominally during surgery. In many cases, the broken instrument is easily retrieved with graspers. If the instrument cannot be simply visualized, imaging techniques as fluoroscopy can facilitate the location. Lastly, if fluoroscopy fails or is unavailable, open conversion is necessary to retrieve the part [29].

Needle Loss

Intraoperative retained instruments have been reported in up to 0.11% of the surgical cases. One in five surgeons will encounter needle loss during surgery over their entire professional career [30]. For this reason, needle loss is an important matter. Needle loss during robotics procedures can occur, and the retrieval can pose a challenge due to laparoscope visual field limitation.

In order to avoid this situation, preventive measures can be followed. Ideally, only one needle at a time inside the cavity, except in cases when double-armed sutures are used. Besides, a needle holder must be used instead of a grasper for needle insertion or retrieval. Needle retrieval and counts should be confirmed verbally; therefore, clear communication between the surgical team is essential in these scenarios.

In cases of needle loss during surgery, it is imperative to avoid any instrumental movement that may lead further hiddenness of the needle. During the searching process, examination of the surgical field by quadrants must be performed, starting in the last area manipulated. If there is no presence of the needle, a systematic inspection of the rest of the abdominal quadrants is done. If still not found, a searching process outside the abdominal cavity, including the operating room floor, is done. On the other hand, the trocar's lumen and suction devices should be inspected and, in some cases, even X-rayed. Lastly, fluoroscopy imaging or abdominal X-ray can be used. Moreover, magnetic searching devices have been reported to locate and aid in needle retrieval [30, 31].

Final Steps Consideration

During case finalization, there are some considerations the surgeons should make. Subcutaneous emphysema should be assessed, as it can easily be misled with generalized edema. Pneumoperitoneum must be reduced by 5 mm Hg to inspect for bleeders masked by high levels of insufflation pressures. Finally, the scrotum should be free of gas to avoid epidermolysis and skin lesions.

Postoperative Complications

The first three hours postoperative are the most crucial to assess the patient exhaustively, owing to the fact that early postoperative complications are the most common complications encountered. The overall incidence of postoperative complications is 1.9–9% [24, 32].

Assessment includes:

- Vital signs
- Inspection of skin coloration
- Level of consciousness
- Character and volume of catheter and drain outputs
- Abdominal tenderness

Hemorrhage

The incidence reported for blood transfusions is less than 1.5% [24, 32]. Blood transfusions represent the most critical immediate complication seen in the open approach. Indications for transfusions and reintervention are based on clinical findings. This is particularly important in patients presenting with hypotension, tachycardia, and abdominal distension, where immediate reintervention is the standard of care.

A CT scan with contrast will aid in determining the urgency of reintervention for patients experiencing postoperative hemorrhage, evidenced by a decrease in hemoglobin levels. In cases when active bleeding is encountered, reintervention is imperative. In contrast to cases where active bleeding is not present, the necessity of re-intervention is decided by the hematoma's size and location.

Urinary Anastomotic Leakage

Vesicourethral anastomotic leaks are one of the most common short-term complications of radical prostatectomy, with an incidence reported of 0.3–15.4% [33]. Increased drain output is the initial sign of urinary leakage. However, increased output can be indicative of ureteral injury as well. Therefore, to differentiate the origin between anastomotic leakage or ureteral injury, cystography is the easiest assessment method. A cystography shows either partial or total disruption of the anastomosis. Furthermore, to differentiate urine leak from an anastomosis or a ureteral lesion, the gold standard is a CT urogram. In order to confirm the presence of urine drainage, drain fluid creatinine must be higher than serum creatinine.

Retrograde pyelogram is an alternative method that adds the benefit of identifying and treating ureteral lesions. In cases where the defect is minor, and guidewire passage is possible, ureteral stent placement for 4–6 weeks is the treatment to follow. But, if retrograde pyelogram shows a larger defect, or in cases when the passage of a guidewire is not achievable, reintervention, combined with percutaneous renal drainage, is imperative.

Port Site Hernia

Port site hernia is a rare but existing complication with an incidence reported ranging from 0.04% to 0.47% due to multiple incision sites and large trocars [34]. For this reason, fascia should be closed on ports larger than 10 mm as a preventative measure. However, 5–8 mm port-site hernias have been described in the literature due to a cone effect in the abdominal incision caused by the trocar's movement [14].

Stricture and Bladder Neck Contracture

Stricture and bladder neck contracture represent an uncommon, late complication following radical prostatectomy, with an incidence of 0.7–1.4%, presenting with symptoms of urinary retention [34–37]. To avoid the incidence of these complications, an ideal mucosa-to-mucosa, watertight, and tension-free anastomosis should be made.

Lymphoceles

Lymphoceles are considered the most common long-term complication, with an incidence of up to 50% in patients who underwent RALP with pelvic lymphadenectomy [38]. Pelvic pain, pressure, leg edema, thrombosis formation, and even abdominal distension are typical signs. Lymphatic collections are diagnosed with ultrasound. Doppler sonography of the lower extremities should exclude deep venous thrombosis (DVT) [39, 40]. The modality of choice to treat lymphocele is CT-guided percutaneous drainage. Those who do not resolve or continue to recollect after drainage, may require a laparoscopic fenestration [41].

Thromboembolic Events

Thromboembolic events refer to those complications caused by a triad of predisposing factors, such as Virchow's triad (hypercoagulability, venous stasis, endothelial injury), specifically DVT, which can lead to pulmonary embolism (PE). They have been reported in <1% of the cases [24]. Nonetheless, prophylaxis is recommended with low molecular weight heparin and compressive devices.

Conclusions

Robotic-assisted laparoscopic prostatectomy represents a safe and feasible procedure in experienced surgeons. Complications are inherent to surgery, yet immediate recognition and reporting contribute significantly to the prevention of complications during the surgeon's learning curve in addition to improving patient outcomes.

References

1. Haese A, Sotelo R. Simple prostatectomy. In: Sotelo R, Arriaga J, Aron M, editors. Complications in robotic urologic surgery. Cham: Springer; 2018. https://doi.org/10.1007/978-3-319-62277-4_25.
2. Chitlik A. Safe positioning for robotic-assisted laparoscopic prostatectomy. AORN J. 2011;94(1):37–48. https://doi.org/10.1016/j.aorn.2011.02.012.
3. Azhar R, Elkoushy M. Complications of patient positioning. In: Complications in robotic urologic surgery. Cham: Springer; 2018. https://doi.org/10.1007/978-3-319-62277-4_9.
4. Permpongkosol S, Link RE, Su LM, et al. Complications of 2,775 urological laparoscopic procedures: 1993 to 2005. J Urol. 2007;177(2):580–5. https://doi.org/10.1016/j.juro.2006.09.031.
5. Chen K, Wang L, Wang Q, et al. Effects of pneumoperitoneum and steep Trendelenburg position on cerebral hemodynamics during robotic-assisted laparoscopic radical prostatectomy: a randomized controlled study. Medicine (Baltimore). 2019;98(21):e15794. https://doi.org/10.1097/MD.0000000000015794.
6. Weber ED, Colyer MH, Lesser RL, Subramanian PS. Posterior ischemic optic neuropathy after minimally invasive prostatectomy. J Neuroophthalmol. 2007;27(4):285–7. https://doi.org/10.1097/WNO.0b013e31815b9f67.
7. Klauschie J, Wechter ME, Jacob K, et al. Use of anti-skid material and patient-positioning to prevent patient shifting during robotic-assisted gynecologic procedures. J Minim Invasive Gynecol. 2010;17(4):504–7. https://doi.org/10.1016/j.jmig.2010.03.013.
8. Reisiger KE, Landman J, Kibel A, Clayman RV. Laparoscopic renal surgery and the risk of rhabdomyolysis: diagnosis and treatment. Urology. 2005;66(5 Suppl):29–35. https://doi.org/10.1016/j.urology.2005.06.009
9. Sawyer RJ, Richmond MN, Hickey JD, Jarrratt JA. Peripheral nerve injuries associated with anaesthesia. Anaesthesia. 2000;55(10):980–91. https://doi.org/10.1046/j.1365-2044.2000.01614.x.
10. Zhang J, Moore AE, Stringer MD. Iatrogenic upper limb nerve injuries: a systematic review. ANZ J Surg. 2011;81(4):227–36. https://doi.org/10.1111/j.1445-2197.2010.05597.x.
11. American Society of Anesthesiologists Task Force on Prevention of Perioperative Peripheral Neuropathies. Practice advisory for the prevention of perioperative peripheral neuropathies: an updated report by the American Society of Anesthesiologists Task Force on prevention of perioperative peripheral neuropathies. Anesthesiology. 2011;114(4):741–54. https://doi.org/10.1097/ALN.0b013e3181fcbff3.
12. Di Pierro GB, Wirth JG, Ferrari M, Danuser H, Mattei A. Impact of a single-surgeon learning curve on complications, positioning injuries, and renal function in patients undergoing robot-assisted radical prostatectomy and extended pelvic lymph node dissection. Urology. 2014;84(5):1106–11. https://doi.org/10.1016/j.urology.2014.06.047.
13. Sanchez A, Medina L, Husain F, Sotelo R. Complications of robotic surgical access. In: Robotic urology. Springer; 2018. https://doi.org/10.1007/978-3-319-65864-3_46.
14. Sotelo RJ, Haese A, Machuca V, et al. Safer surgery by learning from complications: a focus on robotic prostate surgery. Eur Urol. 2016;69(2):334–44. https://doi.org/10.1016/j.eururo.2015.08.060.
15. Simforoosh N, Basiri A, Ziaee SA, et al. Major vascular injury in laparoscopic urology. JSLS. 2014;18(3):e2014.00283. https://doi.org/10.4293/JSLS.2014.00283.
16. Pemberton RJ, Tolley DA, van Velthoven RF. Prevention and management of complications in urological laparoscopic port site placement. Eur Urol. 2006;50(5):958–68. https://doi.org/10.1016/j.eururo.2006.06.042.
17. Vilos GA, Ternamian A, Dempster J, Laberge PY, CLINICAL PRACTICE GYNAECOLOGY COMMITTEE. Laparoscopic entry: a review of techniques, technologies, and complications. J Obstet Gynaecol Can. 2007;29(5):433–47. https://doi.org/10.1016/S1701-2163(16)35496-2.
18. Wind J, Cremers JE, van Berge Henegouwen MI, Gouma DJ, Jansen FW, Bemelman WA. Medical liability insurance claims on entry-related complications in laparoscopy. Surg Endosc. 2007;21(11):2094–9. https://doi.org/10.1007/s00464-007-9315-8
19. Chandler JG, Corson SL, Way LW. Three spectra of laparoscopic entry access injuries. J Am Coll Surg. 2001;192(4):478–91. https://doi.org/10.1016/s1072-7515(01)00820-1.
20. Menon M, Tewari A, Peabody JO, et al. Vattikuti Institute prostatectomy, a technique of robotic radical prostatectomy for management of localized carcinoma of the prostate: experience of over 1100 cases. Urol Clin North Am. 2004;31(4):701–17. https://doi.org/10.1016/j.ucl.2004.06.011.
21. Wedmid A, Mendoza P, Sharma S, et al. Rectal injury during robot-assisted radical prostatectomy: incidence and management. J Urol. 2011;186(5):1928–33. https://doi.org/10.1016/j.juro.2011.07.004.

22. Mundy AR, Andrich DE. Posterior urethral complications of the treatment of prostate cancer. BJU Int. 2012;110(3):304–25. https://doi.org/10.1111/j.1464-410X.2011.10864.x.
23. Gözen AS, Aktoz T, Akin Y, Klein J, Rieker P, Rassweiler J. Is it possible to draw a risk map for obturator nerve injury during pelvic lymph node dissection? The Heilbronn experience and a review of the literature. J Laparoendosc Adv Surg Tech A. 2015;25(10):826–32. https://doi.org/10.1089/lap.2015.0190.
24. Tewari A, Sooriakumaran P, Bloch DA, Seshadri-Kreaden U, Hebert AE, Wiklund P. Positive surgical margin and perioperative complication rates of primary surgical treatments for prostate cancer: a systematic review and meta-analysis comparing retropubic, laparoscopic, and robotic prostatectomy. Eur Urol. 2012;62(1):1–15. https://doi.org/10.1016/j.eururo.2012.02.029.
25. Teber D, Gözen AS, Cresswell J, Canda AE, Yencilek F, Rassweiler J. Prevention and management of ureteral injuries occurring during laparoscopic radical prostatectomy: the Heilbronn experience and a review of the literature. World J Urol. 2009;27(5):613–8. https://doi.org/10.1007/s00345-009-0428-7.
26. Jhaveri JK, Penna FJ, Diaz-Insua M, Jeong W, Menon M, Peabody JO. Ureteral injuries sustained during robot-assisted radical prostatectomy. J Endourol. 2014;28(3):318–24. https://doi.org/10.1089/end.2013.0564.
27. Lorenzo EI, Jeong W, Park S, Kim WT, Hong SJ, Rha KH. Iliac vein injury due to a damaged Hot Shears™ tip cover during robot assisted radical prostatectomy. Yonsei Med J. 2011;52(2):365–8. https://doi.org/10.3349/ymj.2011.52.2.365.
28. Park SY, Ahn JJ, Jeong W, Ham WS, Rha KH. A unique instrumental malfunction during robotic prostatectomy. Yonsei Med J. 2010;51(1):148–50. https://doi.org/10.3349/ymj.2010.51.1.148.
29. Park SY, Cho KS, Lee SW, Soh BH, Rha KH. Intraoperative breakage of needle driver jaw during robotic-assisted laparoscopic radical prostatectomy. Urology. 2008;71(1):168.e5-6. https://doi.org/10.1016/j.urology.2007.09.052.
30. Medina LG, Martin O, Cacciamani GE, Ahmadi N, Castro JC, Sotelo R. Needle lost in minimally invasive surgery: management proposal and literature review. J Robot Surg. 2018;12(3):391–5. https://doi.org/10.1007/s11701-018-0802-9.
31. Small AC, Gainsburg DM, Mercado MA, Link RE, Hedican SP, Palese MA. Laparoscopic needle-retrieval device for improving quality of care in minimally invasive surgery. J Am Coll Surg. 2013;217(3):400–5. https://doi.org/10.1016/j.jamcollsurg.2013.02.035.
32. Novara G, Ficarra V, Rosen RC, et al. Systematic review and meta-analysis of perioperative outcomes and complications after robot-assisted radical prostatectomy. Eur Urol. 2012;62(3):431–52. https://doi.org/10.1016/j.eururo.2012.05.044.
33. Tyritzis SI, Katafigiotis I, Constantinides CA. All you need to know about urethrovesical anastomotic urinary leakage following radical prostatectomy. J Urol. 2012;188(2):369–76. https://doi.org/10.1016/j.juro.2012.03.126.
34. Filip V, Pleşa C, Târcoveanu E, Bradea C, Moldovanu R. Eventraţiile după chirurgia laparoscopică [Incisional hernias after operative laparoscopy]. Rev Med Chir Soc Med Nat Iasi. 2000;104(4):83–6.
35. Parihar JS, Ha YS, Kim IY. Bladder neck contracture-incidence and management following contemporary robot assisted radical prostatectomy technique. Prostate Int. 2014;2(1):12–8. https://doi.org/10.12954/PI.13034.
36. Breyer BN, Davis CB, Cowan JE, Kane CJ, Carroll PR. Incidence of bladder neck contracture after robot-assisted laparoscopic and open radical prostatectomy. BJU Int. 2010;106(11):1734–8. https://doi.org/10.1111/j.1464-410X.2010.09333.x.
37. Msezane LP, Reynolds WS, Gofrit ON, Shalhav AL, Zagaja GP, Zorn KC. Bladder neck contracture after robot-assisted laparoscopic radical prostatectomy: evaluation of incidence and risk factors and impact on urinary function. J Endourol. 2008;22(1):97–104.
38. Orvieto MA, Coelho RF, Chauhan S, Palmer KJ, Rocco B, Patel VR. Incidence of lymphoceles after robot-assisted pelvic lymph node dissection. BJU Int. 2011;108(7):1185–90. https://doi.org/10.1111/j.1464-410X.2011.10094.x.
39. Khoder WY, Trottmann M, Buchner A, et al. Risk factors for pelvic lymphoceles post-radical prostatectomy. Int J Urol. 2011;18(9):638–43. https://doi.org/10.1111/j.1442-2042.2011.02797.x.
40. Keegan KA, Cookson MS. Complications of pelvic lymph node dissection for prostate cancer. Curr Urol Rep. 2011;12(3):203–8. https://doi.org/10.1007/s11934-011-0179-z.
41. Raheem OA, Bazzi WM, Parsons JK, Kane CJ. Management of pelvic lymphoceles following robot-assisted laparoscopic radical prostatectomy. Urol Ann. 2012;4(2):111–4. https://doi.org/10.4103/0974-7796.95564.

Part XIII

Functional Recovery After RALP

Functional Recovery After RALP: Erectile Function

49

Giacomo Rebez, Ottavia Runti, Michele Rizzo, Giovanni Liguori, Andrea Lissiani, and Carlo Trombetta

Introduction

The radical prostatectomy is associated with different grades of erectile function loss due to the damage of the autonomic cavernous nerves injured during the surgery because of their anatomical position [1]. The reported incidence of long-term erectile dysfunction (ED) after radical prostatectomy ranges from approximately 14–90% [2]. In recent years, the new laparoscopic and robotic-assisted techniques have established their role in prostate cancer surgery, with a comparable or even slightly lower reported erectile dysfunction incidence of 7–33% [3]. The concept of erectile function and potency has eventually changed during the past two decades, after the introduction of Sildenafil on the market in 1998. The 'Viagra' has played an important role in the awareness of the erectile function for both men and society itself. Nowadays, patients are aware of different therapeutic choices over erectile dysfunction and are more demanding and conscious of them [4]. As awareness of potency was growing in the last two decades so was mini-invasive surgery that has changed the surgical approach to radical prostatectomy [5].

Robot-assisted radical prostatectomy (RALP), is a well-established method for treating localized prostate cancer, and potency outcome has become an important outcome both for patients and researchers. Over the last 10 years, the diagnostic pathway of prostate cancer has changed significantly by the advent of multiparametric magnetic resonance imaging (mpMRI) which is the best technique to detect and localize suspicious areas for clinically significant prostate cancer, and it allows performing MRI targeted biopsy [6]. Therefore, many patients have a diagnosis of prostate cancer at an early stage and mini-invasive procedures can be easily performed. The ability to have a satisfactory erection and sexual function play a significant role in the overall quality of life of patients and their partners.

Pathophysiology of ED After Radical Prostatectomy

The surgical removal of the prostate gland provokes damage to the neurovascular mechanism that initiates the erection causing the ED. The nerve-sparing technique is the result of an evolution of radical prostatectomy started 30 years ago. During this procedure, a postoperative defect in sexual function is usually common. However, patients are usually impaired in the early postoperative period recovering the erectile function in the next months. This happens because of a neuropraxia provoked on the neurovascular bundles during the surgical dissection. The mechanism of cavernous nerve-fibre injury in part involves, Wallerian degeneration with a loss of normal nerve tissue connections to the corpora cavernosal and associated neuroregulatory functions. Both of these processes cause cavernosal tissue degeneration and atrophy [7, 8]. Besides, some authors implicate arterial insufficiency as a possible contributory cause of ED. Polascik and Walsh reported that the preservation of the accessory pudendal artery was associated with a significant increase in potency rates. They showed that the time for recovery of a spontaneous erection was significantly less in the vascular preservation group [9]. ED in patients with arterial insufficiency is most likely provoked by collagen accumulation and the resulting fibrosis which provoke venous leakage. The contribution of prolonged tissue hypoxia to permanent ED to date remains open to further investigation [10].

In summary, ED after radical prostatectomy is likely to have a multifactorial aetiology and also a psychological component. Altered vascular factors and neuropraxia lead to absence of erection and therefore absence of oxygenation of cavernosal tissue. Penile hypoxia is the most important precipitating factor in cavernosal fibrosis [10] which with the collagen accumulation may result in a veno-occlusive dysfunction [11].

G. Rebez (✉) · O. Runti · M. Rizzo · G. Liguori · A. Lissiani
C. Trombetta
Urology Clinic, Department of Medical, Surgical and Health Science, University of Trieste, Trieste, Italy

S. Ren et al. (eds.), *Robot-Assisted Radical Prostatectomy*, https://doi.org/10.1007/978-3-031-05855-4_49

Robotic Surgery

It seems that adequate surgical technique during neurovascular bundles preservation leads to a successful recovery of erections in patients with good preoperative sexual function [12]. A focal point of both techniques is the nerve-sparing surgery. Nerve-sparing can be unilateral or bilateral but clearly, bilateral nerve-sparing has been proven better than unilateral (see Table 49.1). There are numerous different nerve-sparing surgical techniques. Different approaches in RALP and different techniques are mainly related to the surgical anatomy of periprostatic fascia and their role in ED after RALP.

Robotic Nerve-Sparing Surgery: Anatomy

Walsh and Donker initially described the dorsolateral location of the neurovascular bundle (NVB) and proposed its contribution to potency in 1982 [13] and subsequently developed the technique of anatomic nerve-sparing radical prostatectomy to preserve postoperative potency in patients [14]. Recently, many studies have updated the anatomical knowledge of cavernous nerves and the classically described NVB, given that periprostatic nerves disperse on the ventrolateral and dorsal surfaces of the prostate, instead of in a confined single dorsolateral "bundle." [15]. Such dispersion of periprostatic nerve fibres can range up to the 2 o'clock and 10 o'clock positions over the lateral prostate [16]. Inoue et al. evaluated the distance between cancer and the NVB at the classical 5 o'clock and 7 o'clock position in prostates without nerve-sparing. In patients without extra prostatic extension, they found a mean distance of 3.3 mm (standard deviation [SD]: 2.6), 3.4 mm (SD: 2.7), and 3.7 mm (SD: 2.4) at the apex, mid gland, and base, respectively. In patients with extra prostatic extension, the distance between cancer and the NVB was 2.0 mm (SD: 1.9), 1.9 mm (SD: 1.9), and 1.8 mm (SD: 2.1) at the apex, mid gland, and base, respectively. A note in this study was that in an individual case, the nerves could be in direct contact with the NVB. Preservation of these fibres may have a positive effect not only on the preservation of the patient's erectile function but also on the recovery of continence following prostatectomy [17, 18]. In the current understanding of the neurovascular anatomy, conventional nerve-sparing radical prostatectomy has undergone some modifications and refinements, developed to maximize preservation of periprostatic nerves, and consequently, enhance the potential for recovery of potency [19]. Anyway, the main goal is to avoid positive margins of resection balanced with a satisfactory nerve-sparing [20].

Robotic Surgical Techniques to Preserve Sexual Function

The surgeon can't reproduce the same surgical dissection in every patient because of different interindividual anatomic variations. Anyway, the multi-layered character of the periprostatic fascia allows choice in the dissection between nerves and prostate pseudo capsule. The aim of leaving a more or less thick tissue layer on the prostate as a safety margin can be the objective of the urologist during the prostatectomy. The chosen plane can vary: in cases with a low risk of extra prostatic extension (EPE), a closer dissection can be performed while in cases with a higher risk of EPE a wider dissection plane should be preferred [21, 22]. Surgeons

Table 49.1 Potency rate after RALP

Study	No. of patients	Inclusion criteria	Surgical technique	Definition of Potency	Potency pre %	Potency post %	Treatment
Ahlering et al. (2008) [25]	90	41–65 years and IIEF-5 ≥22	RALP nerve sparing	Adequate erection for penetration	100	TOT 92 BNS 83 UNS 68	5-PDE inhibitors beginning immediately postoperatively and continuing for 1 year
Chien et al. (2005) [45]	56	At least 3 months follow-up	RALP nerve sparing and non-nerve sparing	Adequate erection for penetration	–	TOT 40 BNS 50 UNS 44	5-PDE inhibitors
Van der Poel and de Blok (2009) [46]	107	Little or no ED and/or IIEF >19	RALP nerve-sparing and non-nerve sparing	Little or no ED and/or IIEF >19	–	TOT 53 BNS 59 UNS 36	5-PDE inhibitors
Mendiola et al. (2008) [47]	227	SHIM >20	RALP nerve-sparing and non-nerve sparing	Adequate erection for penetration	100	TOT 57 BNS 76 UNS 63	–
Haglind et al. (2015) [48]	1847	IIEF score 21 = some erectile function	RALP nerve-sparing and non-nerve sparing	IIEF>21	72	70	–
Nyberg et al. (2018) [49]	1847	IIEF score 21 = some erectile function	RALP nerve-sparing and non-nerve sparing	IIEF>21	–	85	–

are aware that EPE is in most cases only a matter of millimetres, which could allow a nerve-sparing procedure in selected cases with focal EPE [22]. Depending on the dissection plane chosen during the procedure three different surgical dissection planes are described (Fig. 49.1).

The intrafascial dissection is considered a dissection that follows a plane on the pseudo capsule, remaining internal to the prostatic fascia at the anterolateral and posterolateral aspect of the prostate and anterior to the PPF/SVF. The intrafascial approach allows whole-thickness preservation of the NVB [16].

The interfascial dissection of the NVB is considered a dissection within the thickness or between the leaves of the periprostatic fascia and includes incremental nerve-sparing. Depending on anatomic variations, the NVB might be prone to partial resection. This approach allows a greater safety margin around the prostate relative to the intrafascial dissection, presumably resulting in an oncologically safer approach [23, 24].

The extrafascial dissection is a dissection carried out lateral to the elevator ani fascia and posterior to the PPF/SVF. In this case, the NVB will be completely resected. This approach results in the largest amount of tissue surrounding the prostate and thus is the most oncological safe dissection, but it carries with its probable complete erectile dysfunction if done bilaterally [23].

According to Wang meta-analysis, intrafascial prostatectomy led to a statistically higher postoperative potency rate at 3, 6 and 12 months with a potency rate of 42.2%, 54.2%, 72.2% respectively, compared with the interfascial technique with 32.2% at 3 months, 40.1% at 6 months and 58.7% at 12 months [19] (Table 49.2).

The choice of surgical instruments can play a key role in the intraoperative technique. For example, by avoiding the thermal energy damage on neurovascular bundles during NS procedure. Indeed, Ahlering in his study [25] shows that by avoiding thermal energy patients gained a nearly a fivefold improvement of potency recovery at 3 and 9 months (see Table 49.1). Moreover, their data suggest that the volume of

Table 49.2 Nerve-sparing to preserve erectile function

Study	No. of patients	Nerve-sparing technique (n)	Potency rate %	Follow up time
Ahlering et al. (2008) [25]	500	BNS 165 UNS 33	83% 68%	24 months
Chien et al. (2005) [45]	56	BNS 28 UNS 20	50% 44%	12 months
Van der Poel and de Blok (2009) [46]	107	BNS 58 UNS 49	59% 36%	6 months
Mendiola et al. (2008) [47]	227	BNS 80 UNS 40	76% 53	12 months

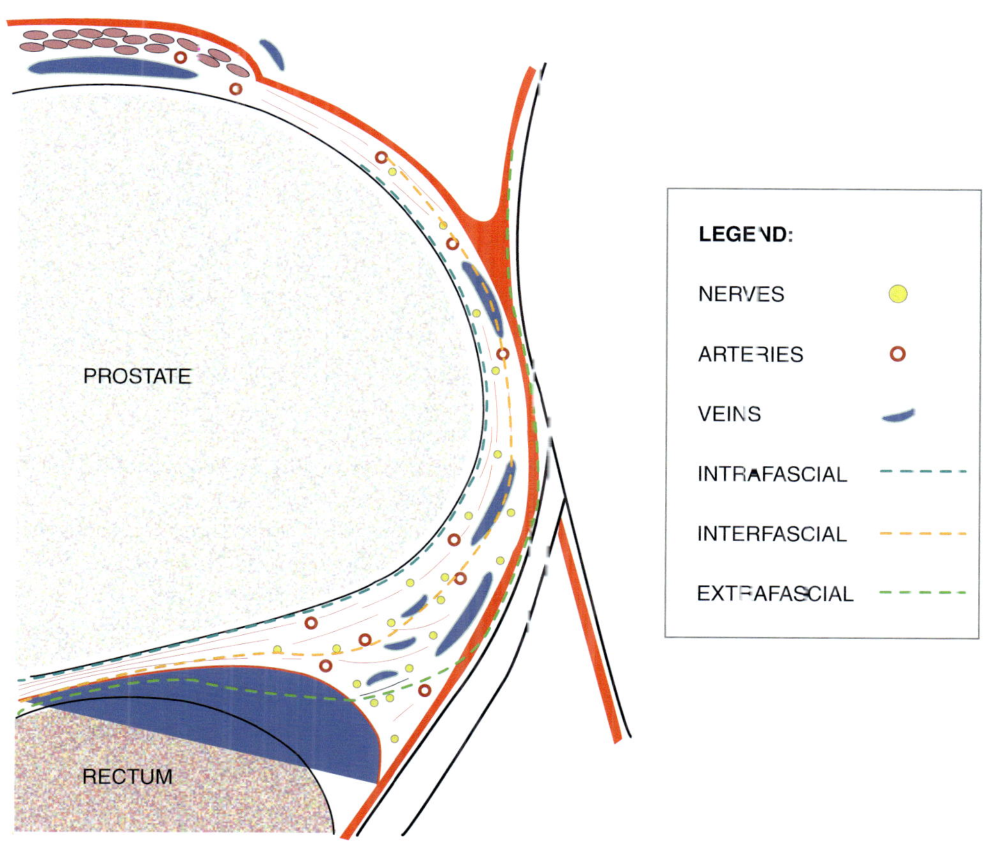

Fig 49.1 The three prostate dissection planes

nerve preservation is not as critical as initially believed. As noted, increasing volume of nervous tissue by 100% from one to two nerves only improved potency recovery rates by approximately 1.2-fold. This finding seems to suggest the benefit of an intrafascial dissection with the potential total preservation of the nerves while other techniques that attempt to preserve 2–5% more nerve tissue would likely have little chance of increasing potency recovery and would certainly be outweighed by the risk of a positive surgical margin [25].

Bearing in mind that the anatomy of the nerves may vary substantially, the concept of different dissection planes aims to an incremental security margin on the prostate. This is made to avoid positive surgical margins (PSMs) more than for true incremental nerves sparing. Moreover, the selection of patients for such an incremental safety margin approach depends on patient and cancer characteristics and is the fundamental concern with this technique. The main problem for surgeons offering an aggressive nerve-sparing approach is the lack of strategy that can ensure oncological safety, intraoperative frozen-section analysis of the excised prostate specimen during a radical prostatectomy has the potential to help to solve the issue. Mirmilstein et al. showed how NeuroSAFE techniques allow the possibility to do an NS in higher-risk patients, reducing positive surgical margins rates and at improving potency rates at 12 months [26].

The new potential role of dehydrated human amniotic membrane (dHAM) positioned around nerve bundles (NVB) during robotic-assisted laparoscopic radical prostatectomy (RALP) was explored by Radzam in a recent publication [27]. Radzam et al. studied potency outcomes in 1400 patients who underwent full bilateral nerve-sparing RALP performed by a single surgeon, wherein 700 patients had dHAM allograft wrapped around the NVB and 700 did not. It is hypothesized that dHAM use would lead to better potency outcomes and results seem promising since the first noticeable erection sufficient enough for satisfactory penetrative intercourse was significantly earlier ($p < 0.01$; 34.6 ± 3.6 days) in the group treated with dHAM.

Another new scientific field is the stem cell-based therapy which has recently received a lot of attention for erectile function recovery. Multiple types of stem cells have been employed in animal models in the study of organic erectile dysfunction. Most studies involved mesenchymal stem cells, neural crest cells, embryonic ones, endothelial progenitor cells and muscle-derived stem cells [28]. Transplantation of these types of cells provides cells capable of restoring normal function after injury or deterioration and restoring nervous capacity. Depending on the cell type, these transplanted cells display a paracrine effect on surrounding penile tissues and may differentiate into smooth muscle, endothelium, and neuronal tissues. The therapeutic efficacies of stem cells in research models will need more human trials to deeply understand their role in the treatment of erectile dysfunction in particular in surgical-induced neuropraxia.

Penile Rehabilitation

The vast majority of men will experience an initial complete loss of erectile function following radical prostatectomy, regardless of whether or not the nerves were spared during surgery. Nonetheless, many of these men will ultimately regain erectile function. To improve the regain of erectile function after prostatectomy the first step is rehabilitation [10]. The concept of penile rehabilitation has been first introduced in 1997 by Montorsi et al. which demonstrated that the use of the vacuum device or any drug after radical prostatectomy could increase the recovery of erectile function in terms of quality and time needed [11]. Therapeutically, maintaining regular oxygen-rich blood flow to corpora seems to promote smooth muscle integrity and prevent fibrotic changes [29]. The recent literature suggests to start the rehabilitation immediately after surgery, without going past 1 year postoperatively [10]. Furthermore pre-surgery rehabilitation is emerging: Santa Mina et al. [30] reported promising outcomes of preoperative pelvic floor training and moderate with physical and psychological benefits. However, the rehabilitation after robotic prostate cancer surgery is mainly based on restoring erectile function along with continence. The most common pharmacological therapies are phosphodiesterase type 5 (PDE-5) inhibitors, intraurethral prostaglandin E1 (PGE-1) gel or intracavernous PGE1 injection (Table 49.3). Some surgeons promote the use of mechanical devices like vacuum pumps with or without constriction rings. Combinations of these modalities can be also effective as a rehabilitation program. Anyway, early postoperative penile rehabilitation/stimulation of erectile function appears to optimize the outcome [31]. The different non-invasive penile rehabilitation strategies are described in the following paragraphs.

Vacuum Erection Devices

Vacuum erection devices (VED) work by creating a vacuum around the penis, drawing blood into the corpora cavernosa. It can be used both for rehabilitation and therapy. During rehabilitation patient without spontaneous erection or with partial tumescence can use this device to improve blood flow inside the penis. If reducing tissue hypoxia-induced fibrosis and loss of smooth muscle cells are the main target of penile rehabilitation therapy, VED may be beneficial as they would permit erections earlier than PDE- 5 inhibitors alone [10]. Moreover, as highlighted in a review by Wang, the majority

Table 49.3 Different methods of rehabilitation

Study	Study typology	Method of rehabilitation	Dosage	No. of patients	Outcomes	% Patients achieving the outcome	Abandon rate
Jo (2018) [33]	Prospective randomized trial	Sildenafil right after catheter removal	100 mg twice a week	58	IIEF >17 after 12 months	41%	–
Jo (2018) [33]	Prospective randomized trial	Sildenafil after 3 months	100 mg twice a week	62	IIEF>17 after 12 months	17%	–
Montorsi (2008)[50]	Randomised, double-blind double-dummy, multicentre, parallel-group study	Nightly vardenafil 14 days after surgery	10 mg	210	IIEF >22 after 9 months	32%	35%
Montorsi et al. (2014) [51]	Randomized placebo-controlled study	Tadalafil once daily	5 mg	139	IIEF>22 after 13.5 months	32.4%	29%
Kohler (2007) [52]	Pilot study	VED used daily 1 month after surgery		28	IIEF>12 after 6 months	38%	0%
Polito 2012 [53]		ICI of PGE1 after 1 month		273	IIEF>20 after 6 months	77%	19%
Nandipati (2006) [54]	Prospective study	Combination of Sildenafil and ICI of Alprostadil	Sildenafil 50 mg daily Alprostadil 4 mcg 2–3 times weekly	22	Sexually active patients after 6 months	96%	–
Engel (2011) [55]	Randomized clinical trial	Combination PDE5 + VED		13	Hard enough for vaginal penetration after 12 months	92%	

of blood entering the penis while using a VED is arterial in source [32]. VED can also be used for short periods, multiple times per day, which may be more physiologically relevant than intracavernosal injection as men usually have several erections per 24-h period [10]. Moreover, VED is a drug-free programme with limited side effects and good compliance [27]. VED can also be used as a therapy to get enough erection to be able to have sexual intercourse. In this context constriction rings can be placed at the base of the penis, causing a trapping of blood and a prolonged tumescence.

Intracavernosal Injections

Intracavernous injections (ICI) work by local stimulation of the erectogenic mechanism, by causing vasodilation and therefore an increased inflow. Prostaglandins (PGE1) analogues, such as alprostadil, are available for use both intracavernous injection as well as intraurethral administration. ICI can give a rigid erection by increasing arterial inflow into the penis, similar to a natural erection, resulting in increased delivery of oxygenated blood and stretching of the penis. Therefore, if reducing tissue hypoxia-induced fibrosis and loss of smooth muscle cells are the main target of penile rehabilitation therapy, ICI can be very effective at the beginning when PDE5 are still ineffective. A specific postoperative programme of ICI administration does not exist at the moment but the majority of authors recommend at least 1 injection per week for the first postoperative period [19].

Phosphodiesterase-5 Inhibitors

These drugs work by improving cavernous oxygenation, thereby limiting the development of hypoxia-induced tissue damage. There are different molecules on the market nowadays and it seems that there are no great differences between them in the outcome of penile rehabilitation. Various administration methods and side effects can make the patient choice between one molecule and another.

Sildenafil

Early treatment is thus aimed at minimizing cavernous hypoxia by the active use of PDE5 inhibitors [33]. Clinical data to suggest that earlier rehabilitation with phosphodiesterase type 5 inhibitors can contribute to the recovery of erectile function after radical prostatectomy in the clinical setting. Patients who underwent bilateral or unilateral nerve-sparing had a better response than patients who underwent a non-nerve-sparing. A work showed that most patients who initially respond to sildenafil continue to use the drug long term [34]. All patients who undergo RP are routinely started on a dose of 50–100 mg of sildenafil daily or an on-demand dose of 100 mg of sildenafil and 200 mg of avanafil. After

6 months of treatment, patients in the two groups showed no significantly different sexual function scores.

Combination Therapy

Various combinations of treatment can be used. By reviewing the current literature, it seems that usually association is between PDE5 with either VCD or ICI.

The benefit of combination VED/PDE5 inhibitor therapy was demonstrated in a study of men undergoing penile rehabilitation following total mesorectal excision for rectal cancer (which tends to be a younger age group than prostate cancer) [35]. This study was done in rectal cancer patients undergoing radical prostatectomy and demonstrated that VED promoted early erectile recovery. This suggests that attaining an erection as soon as possible may yield the best results and supports combination therapy for penile rehabilitation. As seen in previous studies without a washout period, nightly low-dose sildenafil was associated with significant improvement in IIEF-5 scores at 3, 6, and 12 months post-surgery compared to no intervention. Combination sildenafil with daily VED use had even greater improvements, particularly at the earlier time points. These data suggest that increasing blood delivery and stretching the penis with VED is superior to waiting for spontaneous PDE5 inhibitor-assisted erections to take place. Also, in RP alone, Chen et al. found that combination of sildenafil and a VED resulted in greater satisfaction, as documented by a significant improvement in IIEF scores, compared with either agent alone [36].

Moncada et al. evaluate the data on the combination of a PDE5I with alprostadil in patients who have previously failed therapy with either drug [37]. The results indicate that the combination therapy resulted in an improved outcome compared with either of the drugs as monotherapy. This was demonstrated by the increased total International Index of Erectile Function (IIEF) scores as well as IIEF erectile function domain scores. Soodong et al. [38] performed penile duplex ultrasound in most of the patients after prostatectomy and found that over 50% of the men who had either arterial insufficiency or a normal exam would respond to PDE5 inhibitors. By contrast, only 1 individual with venous leak responded. Penile ultrasound performed soon after RALP may help delineate who is likely to respond to PDE5 alone and who may benefit from combination therapy.

Other Experimental Therapies for ED

Preclinical studies are divided by the outcome: some of them have largely focused on regaining erectile function after nerve damage has occurred while other, however, has been focusing on preventing the nerve loss and regeneration in the immediate period following nerve damage [10].

The regenerative properties of platelet-rich plasma (PRP) and stem cells have been investigated in animal models of bilateral nerve crush injury, a model of nerve injury that closely approximates radical prostatectomy. Currently, no studies have reported outcomes of PRP injection in men with post-surgical ED. Injection of bone marrow-derived stem cells into the corpora of men with severe post-prostatectomy ED has previously been shown to improve erectile function and blood flow [39]. Preclinical and forthcoming clinical trials in regenerative medicine therapies may expand rehabilitation and allow for the damage incurred by surgery to be reversed. As the regenerative studies reported to date have largely been preclinical, most surgeons stick to the classic rehabilitation methods.

ED Therapy: Prosthesis

Dr. Brantley Scott revolutionized the treatment of ED in 1973 with the three-piece silicone IPP consisting of a reservoir, pump, and Dacron-reinforced corporal cylinders. Whenever other conservative strategies do not work, penile prosthesis surgery is a last-line treatment to regain erectile function after radical prostatectomy (RP) for localized prostate cancer [40]. Men in this series who underwent penile prosthesis surgery after RP generally reported good sexual function and 94% of men reported optimal satisfaction with a penile prosthesis and so did their partners. Penile prosthesis placement can be performed simultaneously with the radical prostatectomy in the 'one solution technique'. The ideal candidates for simultaneous penile prosthesis implantation are those who report pre-existent refractory ED and patients in whom there is a high risk of extracapsular diseases, such as any cT2c or cT3, and undergo non-nerve sparing RP. To the best of our knowledge, to date, there is no series of such procedures performed during RALP. Anyway, synchronous implantation seems a safe and effective treatment option but future studies are needed to explore this field in robotic surgery [41].

Conclusions/Discussion

Restoring erectile function does not always solve all the sexual problems associated with erectile dysfunction; up to 60% of the patient will discontinue their erectile dysfunction treatment within 2 years, even if it is pharmacologically successful [42]. This means that the rehabilitation programme after radical prostatectomy should not only be focused on the penile function but should involve a clinical psychosexologist to manage the sexual rehabilitation more effectively. This can lead to address other side effects of the surgery such as loss of ejaculate, penile shortening, change in orgasmic feeling, alteration of body image and various type of anxiety [43]. All these problems should be counted during the preoperative discussion with the patient. A specific programme for rehabilitation after surgery in which every patient should fit doesn't exist. Every person is different and so should be the rehabilitation programme; it should be created specifically for every patient. Anyway, most important prognostic factors include the age of the patient, the quality of the spared neurovascular bundles and the baseline sexual function status [44]. More rigorous prospective trials are needed to deeply understand the role of rehabilitation post RALP in different patients and different surgical techniques. Preoperative counselling should be emphasized to understand patient wills and objectives before planning a therapeutic path, bearing in mind that as physicians we should seek cancer survivorship but we can't forget the importance of quality of life. Every patient has different needs which should be satisfied whenever possible. The introduction of a quality assurance programme should improve the quality of prostate cancer care in terms of consistency of patient selection and outcomes of surgery during a period of a major reorganisation of cancer services.

References

1. Basal S, Wambi C, Acikel C, Gupta M, Badani K. Optimal strategy for penile rehabilitation after robot-assisted radical prostatectomy based on preoperative erectile function. BJU Int. 2013;111:658–65.
2. Burnett AL, Aus G, Canby-Hagino ED, et al. Erectile function outcome reporting after clinically localized prostate cancer treatment. J Urol. 2007;178(2):597–601. https://doi.org/10.1016/j.juro.2007.03.140.
3. Tewari A, Rao S, Martinez-Salamanca JI, et al. Cancer control and the preservation of neurovascular tissue: how to meet competing goals during robotic radical prostatectomy. BJU Int. 2008;101:1013–8.
4. Akhvlediani ND, Matyukhov IP. Current role of sildenafil in the management of erectile dysfunction. Urologiia. 2018;(2):142–6. https://doi.org/10.18565/urology.2018.2.142-146.
5. Humphreys MR, Gettman MT, Chow GK, Zincke H, Blute ML. Minimally invasive radical prostatectomy. Mayo Clin Proc. 2004;79(9):1169–80. https://doi.org/10.4065/79.9.1169.
6. Stabile A, Giganti F, Kasivisvanathan V, Giannarini G, Salomon G, Turkbey B, Villeirs G, Barentsz JO. Factors influencing variability in the performance of multiparametric magnetic resonance imaging in detecting clinically significant prostate cancer : a systematic literature review. Eur Urol Oncol. 2020;3(2):145–67. https://doi.org/10.1016/j.euo.2020.02.005.
7. Moreland RB. Is there a role of hypoxemia in penile fibrosis: a viewpoint presented to the society for the study of impotence. Int J Impot Res. 1998;10(2):113–20. https://doi.org/10.1038/sj.ijir.3900328.
8. User HM, Hairston JH, Zelner DJ, McKenna KE, McVary KT. Penile weight and cell subtype specific changes in a postradical prostatectomy model of erectile dysfunction. J Urol. 2003;169(3):1175–9. https://doi.org/10.1097/01.ju.0000048974.47461.50.
9. Rogers CG, Trock BP, Walsh PC. Preservation of accessory pudendal arteries during radical retropubic prostatectomy: surgical technique and results. Urology. 2004;64(1):148–51. https://doi.org/10.1016/j.urology.2004.02.035.
10. Gabrielsen JS. Penile rehabilitation: the "up"-date. Curr Sex Health Rep. 2018;10(4):287–92. https://doi.org/10.1007/s11930-018-0174-1.
11. Montorsi F, Guazzoni G, Strambi LF, da Pozzo LF, Nava L, Barbieri L, Rigatti P, Pizzini G, Miani A. Recovery of spontaneous erectile function after nerve-sparing radical retropubic prostatectomy with and without early intracavernous injections of alprostadil: results of a prospective, randomized trial. J Urol. 1997 158(4):1408–10. https://doi.org/10.1016/S0022-5347(01)64227-7.
12. Orvieto MA, Coelho RF, Chauhan S, Mathe M, Palmer K, Patel VR. Erectile dysfunction after robot-assisted radical prostatectomy. Expert Rev Anticancer Ther. 2010;10:747–54.
13. Walsh PC, Donker PJ. Impotence following radical prostatectomy: insight into etiology and prevention. J Urol. 1982,128:492–7
14. Walsh PC. Anatomic radical prostatectomy: evolution of the surgical technique. J Urol. 1998;160(6 Pt 2):2418–24. https://doi.org/10.1016/S0022-5347(01)62202-X.
15. Ganzer R, Blana A, Gaumann A, Stolzenburg J, Rabenalt R, Bach T, Wieland WF, Denzinger S. Topographical anatomy of periprostatic and capsular nerves: quantification and computerised planimetry. Eur Urol. 2008 54:353–61.
16. Walz J, Burnett AL Costello AJ, et al. A critical analysis of the current knowledge of surgical anatomy related to optimization of cancer control and preservation of continence and erection in candidates for radical prostatectomy. Eur Urol. 2010;57:179–92.
17. Costello AJ, Brooks M, Cole OJ. Anatomical studies of the neurovascular bundle and cavernosal nerves. BJU Int. 2004;94(7):1071–6.
18. Kaul S, Savera A, Badani K, Fumo M, Bhandari A, Menon M. Functional outcomes and oncological efficacy of Vattikuti Institute prostatectomy with Veil of Aphrodite nerve-sparing: an analysis of 154 consecutive patients. BJU Int. 2006;97(3):467–72. https://doi.org/10.1111/j.1464-410X.2006.05990.x.
19. Wang X, Wu Y, Guo J, Chen H, Weng X, Liu X. Intrafascial nerve-sparing radical prostatectomy improves patients ' postoperative continence recovery and erectile function: a pooled analysis based on available literatures. Medicine (Baltimore). 2018;97(29):e11297.
20. Tavukçu HH, Aytac O, Atug F. Nerve-sparing techniques and results in robot-assisted radical prostatectomy. Investig Clin Urol. 2016;57:S172–84.
21. Tewari AK, Srivastava A, Huang MW, et al (2011) BJUI anatomical grades of nerve sparing : a risk-stratifi ed approach to neural-hammock. 984–992.
22. Montorsi F, Wilson TG, Rosen RC, et al. Best practices in robot-assisted radical prostatectomy: recommendations of the Pasadena Consensus Panel. Eur Urol. 2012;62:368–81.
23. Dasgupta P. Anatomic considerations during radical prostatectomy. Eur Urol. 2010;57(2):193–5. https://doi.org/10.1016/j.eururo.2009.11.037.
24. Deho' F, Salonia A, Briganti A, Zanni G, Gallina A, Rokkas K, Guazzoni G, Rigatti P, Montorsi F. Anatomical radical retropubic prostatectomy in patients with a preexisting three-piece inflatable prosthesis: a series of case reports. J Sex Med. 2009;6:578–83.
25. Ahlering TE, Rodriguez E, Skarecky DW. Overcoming obstacles: nerve-sparing issues in radical prostatectomy. J Endourol. 2008;22(4):745–50. https://doi.org/10.1089/end.2007 9834
26. Mirmilstein G, Rai BP, Gbolahan O, Srirangam V, Narula A, Agarwal S, Lane TM, Vasdev N, Adshead J. The neurovascular structure-adjacent frozen-section examination (NeuroSAFE) approach to nerve sparing in robot-assisted laparoscopic radical prostatectomy in a British setting – a prospective observational comparative study. BJU Int. 2018;121(6):854–62. https://doi.org/10.1111/bju.14078.

27. Qin F, Wang S, Li J, Wu C, Yuan J. The early use of vacuum therapy for penile rehabilitation after radical prostatectomy: systematic review and meta-analysis. Am J Mens Health. 2018;12:2136–43.
28. Razdan S, Bajpai RR, Razdan S, Sanchez MA. A matched and controlled longitudinal cohort study of dehydrated human amniotic membrane allograft sheet used as a wraparound nerve bundles in robotic-assisted laparoscopic radical prostatectomy: a puissant adjunct for enhanced potency outcomes. J Robot Surg. 2019;13:475–81.
29. Woo SH, Kang DI, Ha YS, Salmasi AH, Kim JH, Lee DH, Kim WJ, Kim IY. Comprehensive analysis of sexual function outcome in prostate cancer patients after robot-assisted radical prostatectomy. J Endourol. 2014;28:172–7.
30. Santa Mina D, Hilton WJ, Matthew AG, et al. Prehabilitation for radical prostatectomy: a multicentre randomized controlled trial. Surg Oncol. 2018;27:289–98.
31. Ljunggren C, Ströberg P. Improvement in sexual function after robot-assisted radical prostatectomy: a rehabilitation program with involvement of a clinical sexologist. Cent Eur J Urol. 2015;68:214–20.
32. Wang R. Vacuum erectile device for rehabilitation after radical prostatectomy. J Sex Med. 2017;14(2):184–6. https://doi.org/10.1016/j.jsxm.2016.12.010.
33. Jo JK, Jeong SJ, Oh JJ, Lee SW, Lee S, Hong SK, Byun SS, Lee SE. Effect of starting penile rehabilitation with sildenafil immediately after robot-assisted laparoscopic radical prostatectomy on erectile function recovery: a prospective randomized trial. J Urol. 2018;199(6):1600–6. https://doi.org/10.1016/j.juro.2017.12.060.
34. Raina R, Lakin MM, Agarwal A, Sharma R, Goyal KK, Montague DK, Klein E, Zippe CD. Long-term effect of sildenafil citrate on erectile dysfunction after radical prostatectomy: 3-year follow-up. Urology. 2003;62(1):110–5. https://doi.org/10.1016/S0090-4295(03)00157-2.
35. Deng H, Liu H, Lan X, Mo J, Mao X, Li G. Phosphodiesterase-5 inhibitors and vacuum erection device for penile rehabilitation after laparoscopic nerve-preserving radical proctectomy for rectal cancer: a prospective, nonrandomized, controlled trial in a single Chinese center. In: Surgical endoscopy and other interventional techniques. Berlin: Springer; 2015.
36. Cathcart P, Sridhara A, Ramachandran N, Briggs T, Nathan S, Kelly J. Achieving quality assurance of prostate cancer surgery during reorganisation of cancer services. Eur Urol. 2015;68(1):22–9. https://doi.org/10.1016/j.eururo.2015.02.028.
37. Moncada I, Martinez-Salamanca J, Ruiz-Castañe E, Romero J. Combination therapy for erectile dysfunction involving a PDE5 inhibitor and alprostadil. Int J Impot Res. 2018;30(5):203–8. https://doi.org/10.1038/s41443-018-0046-2.
38. Kim S, Sung GT. Efficacy and safety of Tadalafil 5 mg once daily for the treatment of erectile dysfunction after robot-assisted laparoscopic radical prostatectomy: a 2-year follow-up. Sex Med. 2018;6(2):108–14. https://doi.org/10.1016/j.esxm.2017.12.005.
39. Yiou R, Hamidou L, Birebent B, et al. Safety of Intracavernous bone marrow-mononuclear cells for postradical prostatectomy erectile dysfunction: an open dose-escalation pilot study. Eur Urol. 2016;69(6):988–91. https://doi.org/10.1016/j.eururo.2015.09.026.
40. Pillay B, Moon D, Love C, Meyer D, Ferguson E, Crowe H, Howard N, Mann S, Wootten A. Quality of life, psychological functioning, and treatment satisfaction of men who have undergone penile prosthesis surgery following robot-assisted radical prostatectomy. J Sex Med. 2017;14(12):1612–20. https://doi.org/10.1016/j.jsxm.2017.10.001.
41. Synchronous penoscrotal implantation of penile prosthesis and artificial urinary sphincter after radical prostatectomy - PubMed. https://pubmed.ncbi.nlm.nih.gov/28422042/. Accessed 10 Apr 2021.
42. Hackett GI. What do patients expect from erectile dysfunction therapy? Eur Urol. 2002;1(8):4–11. https://doi.org/10.1016/S1569-9056(02)00112-4.
43. Benson CR, Serefoglu EC, Hellstrom WJG. Sexual dysfunction following radical prostatectomy. J Androl. 2012;33(6):1143–54. https://doi.org/10.2164/jandrol.112.016790.
44. Catalona WJ, Carvalhal GF, Mager DE, Smith DS. Potency, continence and complication rates in 1,870 consecutive radical retropubic prostatectomies. J Urol. 1999;162(2):433–8. https://doi.org/10.1016/S0022-5347(05)68578-3.
45. Chien GW, Mikhail AA, Orvieto MA, Zagaja GP, Sokoloff MH, Brendler CB, Shalhav AL. Modified clipless antegrade nerve preservation in robotic-assisted laparoscopic radical prostatectomy with validated sexual function evaluation. Urology. 2005;66:419–23.
46. van der Poel HG, de Blok W. Role of extent of fascia preservation and erectile function after robot-assisted laparoscopic prostatectomy. Urology. 2009;73(4):816–21. https://doi.org/10.1016/j.urology.2008.09.082.
47. Mendiola FP, Zorn KC, Mikhail AA, Lin S, Orvieto MA, Zagaja GP, Shalhav AL. Urinary and sexual function outcomes among different age groups after robot-assisted laparoscopic prostatectomy. J Endourol. 2008;22:519–24.
48. Haglind E, Carlsson S, Stranne J, et al. Urinary incontinence and erectile dysfunction after robotic versus open radical prostatectomy: a prospective, controlled, nonrandomised trial. Eur Urol. 2015;68:216–25.
49. Nyberg M, Hugosson J, Wiklund P, et al. Functional and oncologic outcomes between open and robotic radical prostatectomy at 24-month follow-up in the Swedish LAPPRO trial. Eur Urol Oncol. 2018;1:353–60.
50. Montorsi F, Brock G, Lee J, Shapiro JA, van Poppel H, Graefen M, Stief C. Effect of nightly versus on-demand Vardenafil on recovery of erectile function in men following bilateral nerve-sparing radical prostatectomy. Eur Urol. 2008; https://doi.org/10.1016/j.eururo.2008.06.083.
51. Montorsi F, Brock G, Stolzenburg JU, et al. Effects of tadalafil treatment on erectile function recovery following bilateral nerve-sparing radical prostatectomy: a randomised placebo-controlled study (REACTT). Eur Urol. 2014;65(3):587–96. https://doi.org/10.1016/j.eururo.2013.09.051.
52. Köhler TS, Pedro R, Hendlin K, et al. A pilot study on the early use of the vacuum erection device after radical retropubic prostatectomy. BJU Int. 2007;100(4):858–62. https://doi.org/10.1111/j.1464-410X.2007.07161.x.
53. Polito M, D'anzeo G, Conti A, Muzzonigro G. Erectile rehabilitation with intracavernous alprostadil after radical prostatectomy: refusal and dropout rates. BJU Int. 2012;110(11 Pt C):E954–7. https://doi.org/10.1111/j.1464-410X.2012.11484.x.
54. Nandipati K, Raina R, Agarwal A, Zippe CD. Early combination therapy: Intracavernosal injections and sildenafil following radical prostatectomy increases sexual activity and the return of natural erections. Int J Impot Res. 2006;18(5):446–51. https://doi.org/10.1038/sj.ijir.3901448.
55. Engel JD. Effect on sexual function of a vacuum erection device post-prostatectomy. Can J Urol. 2011;18(3):5721–5.

Functional Recovery POST-RALP: Continence

50

Dahong Zhang, Yuchen Bai, and Qi Zhang

Introduction

Prostate cancer (Pca) is the most common cancer in males and one of the significant cause of death [1]. Recently years, Pca prognosis has been improved a lot. Hence, earlier diagnosis and the availability of more effective treatments was the point [2]. Nowadays, radical prostatectomy (RP) and radiotherapy are performed as first-line treatment in patients with localized Pca, alongside with active surveillance in selected patients [3, 4]. However, population-based analyses reveals that there was high rates of interventional treatments has been performed, especially in radical prostatectomy (RP) in patients eligible to active surveillance [5]. Most-recent studies have reveals similar oncological and functional outcomes in open RP (ORP) and robot-assisted RP (RARP) [6, 7]. The most advantage of RARP was that could be more precise and decrease the blood loss during the procedures [8]. However, to date intra-operative advantages cannot be extended to functional outcomes [6, 7].

In order to improve functional outcomes, several surgical techniques have been developed [9]. Unfortunately, incontinence still was one of the major concerns for surgeons and patients Post-RARP and remains one of the most annoying post-operative complication in RARP [10]. RP leading to anatomical variation of the pelvic anatomy, the pelvic floor supported and the dynamics of the urinary flow which might cause inability to hold urine due to a multifactorial failure system. The incontinence considering as really importance in the impact of UIon patients'quality of life (QOL) [11]. UI is one of the most frequent causes of dissatisfaction in patients who treated with RARP [12].

Nowadays, many surgical and conservative UI treatments are available. Surgical treatments and bulking agents are various and commonly been performed, artificial urinary sphincter implants, retro-urethral trans-obturator slings and adjustable male sling systems [13, 14]. On the other hand, conservative management strategies are available as well, which including lifestyle education, pelvic floor training and pharmacological treatments. Considering that RARP causes better preserve anatomical structures which responsible for urinary continence [15]; we might could expect that after RARP UI treatments, especially for conservative treatment. The proportion of continent patients was from 69% to 96% at 12 months after surgery [10]. Although, the time to achieve stable UC after prostatectomy might be changed. Which could lead to different results in the literature, However, those changes could consider associated with inconsistent definitions of urinary continence (UC) and measurement methods (questionnaires, number of pads, pad test). The advantages of RARP stands in as several potentials to develop further surgical technique in order to optimize UC recovery. Proof by facts, robotic-assist surgery has greater precision of exposure and suturing, magnification of the surgery bed and simplicity of movements if compared with conventional surgery. Three steps was important to achieve improvements of the early return of UC post-RAR: preservation, reconstruction and reinforcement. More frequency performed these steps in mini-invasive robotic surgeries, the patients could gain maximal benefit from curative prostatectomy while experiencing early return of UC. We will critically summarize current knowledge of the factors influencing UC and technical innovations to optimize UC recovery post-RARP.

Pathophysiology of Incontinence After Radical Prostatectomy

Postoperative UI presented with a multifactorial etiology, which including both anatomical and functional factors. UC in male more concerns about anatomical (basic structures and organs) and functional. It is the result of the cooperation of single components and dynamic movements of muscles and cavities anchored to the pelvic floor, except the prostate,

D. Zhang (✉) · Y. Bai · Q. Zhang
Department of Urology, Zhejiang Provincial People's Hospital, Hangzhou Medical College, Hangzhou, China

S. Ren et al. (eds.), *Robot-Assisted Radical Prostatectomy*, https://doi.org/10.1007/978-3-031-05855-4_50

which might create physiopathology obstruction. The main urinary structures influencing continence are: puboperinealis muscle [15]: parts of the centrum perinea, the ventral suspension apparatus and the musculofascial plate. Smooth muscle: bladder neck and proximal internal urethral sphincter (vesical sphincter); distal external urethral sphincter (urethral sphincter); neurovascular structures in the pelvis.

Actually, the primary reason for post-RP UI is the incompetence of the external sphincter because which leading to stress urinary incontinence (SUI) [16]. However, some patients can also develop overactive bladder (OAB) in post-surgery, which might require pharmacotherapy [16, 17]. Porena et al. [18] found some degree of detrusor overactivity (DO) up to 77% of cases after RP. Surgical-related damage to anatomic structures or nerves, leading to levels of impairment of the urinary sphincters, that is crucial etiological factor in post-RP UI. The external sphincter is a striatal muscle that is found above the membranous urethra which insert on the anterior prostate and under voluntary control. Moreover, the internal sphincter is located at the level of the bladder neck (BN) and is consist of smooth muscle fibers. The function of internal sphincter consists of maintaining UC under exertion which analogue to an hammock, Because it provides a complementary occlusive effect on the ureter, it is triggered by elevated intra-abdominal pressure [16]. Anatomically, the male anterior support system includes the pubic prostatic ligament and the pubic bladder ligament as well as the so-called intrapelvic fascia and tendon arch (EPF), which represents the thickened band of EPF [19]. The posterior support includes the perineal body, Denonvillier's posterior prostate fascia, rectus urethral muscles, and pelvic diaphragmatic complex [16]. The pudendal nerve provides innervation for the external sphincter. Although it primarily follows an extrapelvic pathway, anatomical evaluation also shows limited intrapelvic trajectories through the neurovascular bundle (NVB), which may help innervate the striated muscle [20]. In fact, NVB injury may be the cause of postoperative UI, and the preservation of NVB during RP can lead to early recovery of UC [21].

Preoperative Setting

1. Identification of the risk factors

   Several risk factors for urinary incontinence has been reported. Their purpose was to comparison of surgical techniques for UC. These factors can be classified as demographic/patient comorbidities, surgeon-related, and due to the patient's anatomy. Patients who receive RARP treatment are often selected based on more favorable tumor and patient characteristics. Therefore, selection bias that may have misleading results cannot be ruled out. As robot experience increases, the options for such patients may decrease. In fact, over time, there has been a clear trend of more unfavorable characteristics.

   A large number of studies recognized age as a fundamental factor for estimating the risk of UI. Mandel et al. [22] analysed data from 8295 RP patients, reveals that the one-year UC rates worsened in older patients. These findings were confirmed in RARP series. The higher probability of UI may be due to some specific characteristics of the elderly subgroup of the RP population, so it takes into account the pre-existing benign prostatic hypertrophy (BPE) and some functional or structural damage of the bladder, urethra, and support system [23, 24].

2. Bodyweight and obesity

   In two large series of open retropubic RP, overweight patients were not found to have worse urinary outcomes compared with their nonoverweight counterParts. Although the reason for the relation between post-RP UI and obesity is not available [25], increased visceral adiposity has been associated with lower urinary tract symptoms (LUTS) in BPE- patients, therefore obese RP-candidates have a higher likelihood of being affected by pre-existing LUTS, which are related to post-RP UI outcomes [16]. Visceral fat cells secrete adipocytokines, which have an adverse effect on the lower urinary tract, because they may directly cause increased sympathetic tone and have a proliferation effect on prostate cells [26]. Among of 2849 RP patients, high BMI levels were predictors of poorer UC outcomes at 6- and 12-month follow-up [27]. Worst UC-outcomes were identified for obese (BMI > 30 kg/m^2) men undergoing RARP at both 12 and 24 months after surgery [28]. Conversely, Xu et al. [29] reveals comparable UC outcomes between obese (BMI > 30 kg/m^2) and non-obese RARP patients, arguing that RARP seemed to promote better functional outcomes even in obese men.

3. Comorbidities

   General health impairment has demonstrated a negative influence on UC recovery. However, only few studies focused on this issue. Teber et al. showed a significant association between diabetes and lower rates of both early (*e.g.*, 0–3 months) and late (*e.g.*, 12–24 months) postoperative UC recovery [30]. Similarly, in a cohort of 308 RARP patients, the Charlson comorbidity index was an independent predictor of the incidence of UC at 12 months [23]. Overall health was described as an independent predictor of UC recovery immediately after RP [31].

4. Prostate surgery before radical prostatectomy

   ExtiRPative surgery in those patients with previous prostate surgeries was technically more challenging and there was significant increase in the operative time; patients should be counseled according to adjust their expectations on functional outcomes following surgery. RP-candidates with a history of previous prostatic surgery has higher likelihood of developing post-RP UI, due to both pre-existing LUTS and the challenging RP procedure in this category of patients [16, 32]. Although several studies showed that previous transurethral resection of the prostate (TURP) did not effect post-RP UC outcomes, Tienza et al. [33] reveals a sixfold higher risk of postoperative UI in those who had already received TURP. In a RARP cohort, Gupta et al. [34] found a 14%-UI rate vs. 11.8% after 6 months, and 25% vs. 8% after 1 year for patients with or without previous TURP, respectively. The results of UC after RARP after holmium laser enucleation of the prostate (HoLEP) were evaluated. Abedali et al. identified 27 RARP patients who had previously received HoLEP. These patients were matched 1:1 with RARP patients who did not have any history of transurethral surgery; in the HoLEP cohort, 27% of patients achieved strict UC, and matched 64% of the control group; however, this comparison is meaningless [35]. Suardi et al. studied the functional results of open radical prostatectomy (ORP) with nerve preservation after HoLEP. In their 1:1 matched study, they failed to describe any significant differences in UC recovery among patients who received RP after HoLEP, TURP, or open simple prostatectomy [32].

5. Prostate volume

   The role of prostate volume (PV) on UC outcomes is controversial. Worst UC outcomes are expected with larger prostates because RP requires substantial urethral damage or because postoperative UI can be associated with antecedent LUTS. In a cohort of 5447 RP patients, Mandel et al. showed that postoperative short-term (1 week–3 months) and long-term (6–12 months) UC was adversely affected by higher PVs [22]. Conversely, in 3067 men PV was identified as an irrelevant factor on 12 months post-RP UC recovery. High prostate volume (≥50 mL) significantly reveals slow recovery of urinary UC [36]. These results can be explained by a wide range of resection and more complicated surgery [37, 38].

6. Membranous urethral length

   The membranous urethral length (MUL), typically measured with magnetic resonance imaging (MRI), may be correlated with post-RP UC recovery. A recent systematic review concluded that larger levels of preoperative MUL were related with a prompt return to UC [39]. In analyzing a large cohort of patients, pre-operative MUL levels were found to be predictors of faster UC recovery post-RARP [38]. A greater preoperative membranous urethral length has a major positive effect on immediate and an overall time to UC recovery [39, 40]. Since a variable portion of the urinary sphincter complex is removed during RP a longer membranous urethral length may increase that continence zone which extends from bladder neck to corpus spongiosum (including internal and external sphincters) [15]. The combination and coordination function of intact smooth muscle fibers and striated sphincter play an important role in UC, support to maintain and increase urethral closure pressure.

7. Variations in the shape of the prostatic apex

   There are some evidence proved that anterior or posterior overlapping of the prostate to the membranous urethra may significantly affect early recovery of UC after RP [41]. Such result suggestion that a longer residual urethral length after RP is associated with a more rapid return of urinary UC after surgery.

8. Angle of the membranous urethra

   Compared with patients who has incontinence during urination or Valsalva maneuvers, the angle of the membranous urethra measured by MRI was found to be significantly wider in non-incontinent patients [42].

9. 3D printing Intraoperative image guided surgical system during RARP

   Although preliminary, 3D printing seems to be the cutting-edge topic with potential implemen- tation in the robotic surgery and possible benefit even for the continence recovery [43]. Virtual reality may become a new field of robotic surgery [44].The benefits of virtual reality to clinicians today include several aspects Such as better surgical planning and patient staging during surgery. Preliminary results showed a potential role of image-guided surgical systems to navigate, accuracy and the real time during the more challenging parts of RP including the apical dissection, the nerve sparing procedure and the bladder neck dissection [45, 46].

Preoperative Preventative Strategies

The typical strategy to prevent UI in RP-candidates is pelvic floor muscle exercise (PFME), this strengthen the pelvic floor muscles, hence possibly improving the urinary sphincters and/or the supportive system. It can be associated with biofeedback, which assists patients' muscles contraction whilst being provided with either a sound or a visual feedback of the correct exercise.

PFME was performed prior and after RARP. Preoperative muscle strength was defined as strong in 77 patients (79%), moderate in 12 (12%) and weak in 9 (9%) patients [47]. Chang et al. [48] performed a meta-analysis which including 739 patients: They found that patients who received preoperative PFME had a significantly lower UI rate 3 months after RP. However, no benefit was observed during the 6-month evaluation. In addition, Yoshida et al. [49] prospectively evaluated 116 men receiving RARP. 21 out of 36 people received ultrasound-guided PFME before and after

RARP. The difference is that 80 patients only received oral guidance from PFME.

Continence recovery was considered achieved when the amount of leakage could be managed with a small pad (20 g) per day. The mean time to continence recovery was shorter in the ultrasound-PfM vs. verbal PFME group (75.6 vs. 121.8 days; $P = 0.037$). Continence recovery rates within 4 weeks were 52.8% (19/36) and 35.4% (28/80) respectively ($P = 0.081$) [49]. Authors reported that the use of ultrasound-PFME was significantly associated with better postoperative continence status. A recent meta-analysis reveals significantly better outcomes for those trials where a preoperative PFME was performed [50]. A finer comprehension of its usefulness will however only be available when studies including standardized protocols will be carried out.

Intraoperative Setting

The basic concept of the intraoperative technique to improve the early recovery of UC after RARP was to maintain the normal anatomy and functional structure of the pelvis as much as possible. Preservation, reconstruction and reinforcement of the bladder-urethral sphincter and suspension components can recreate a new supporting and closing system to ensure ureterovesical pressure dynamics, and thus improve recovery of UC after surgery. On the basis of this concept, three steps can be carried out in order to preserve post-prostatectomy UC with different techniques: (1) preservation; (2) reconstruction; and (3) reinforcement of anatomical structures in the pelvis [51]. Table ii summarizes the surgical technique and the hypothesis of its potential benefit.

Bladder Neck Preservation

BN includes internal sphincter muscles as described earlier, which helps ensure UC. Different methods have been described to obtain the best BN preservation (BNP), including anterior, lateral or anterolateral methods, all of which aim to carefully dissect the bladder from the base of the prostate to preserve the round BN fibers [51, 52].

There are several approaches for the dissection between prostate and bladder, including anterior, lateral and anterolateral approaches. In order to achieve bladder neck preservation (BNP), no matter what method is used, the bladder neck should be sharply dissected from the bottom of the prostate to preserve the round fibers of the bladder neck.

RP-outcomes with and without BNP were compared in an randomized controlled trial (RCT): post-RP UC rates (*e.g.*, wearing 1 safety pad or no-pad at all) at 12 months were 74.8% *vs.* 94.7% for those in the control *vs.* the BNP group, respectively [53]. Long- term follow-up from the same cohort confirmed Such trend [54]. Similarly, in a series of 791 and 276 RARP patients who received and did not receive BNP treatment, the authors found a significant association between BNP and UC recovery time [55]. Finally, Ma et al. [56] analyzed 13 trials, which including 1130 cases and 1154 controls, and confirmed that BNP promoted the occurrence of early recovery levels and better 1-year UC results. However, other studies have not confirmed these data, thus hindering to make final conclusione of this method [10]. A lower bladder neck position visualized by routine postoperative cystography predicts prolonged incontinence. There are several reports assessing that a higher vesical-urethral anastomosis (VUA) location was correlated with recovery of postoperative UC in the short and long term [57, 58]. It is assumed that stabilization and suspension of the urethral sphincteric complex by total reconstruction is an important procedure to achieve a higher bladder neck position.

Bladder Neck Reconstruction

BNP may not be suitable for all patients. In these circumstances, some have shown improved urinary continence with bladder neck reconstruction. Lin et al. [59] published a series of 74 men undergoing RARP who did not undergo BNP for various reasons. Among these men, who underwent bladder neck folding, 12.7% of the men who underwent folding had urinary incontinence after the catheter was removed, and 97.3% had urinary incontinence at 12 months, but the results were not compared with the control group. Similarly, Lee [60] describes a single bladder neck fold suture to improve urinary incontinence. After changing the technique of performing bladder folding, they noticed that in the multivariate analysis, the urination time was shorter and the chance of urination increased significantly at 1 and 12 months.

Nerve-Sparing Approach

The innervation of the penis comes from the pelvic plexus and passes through the NVB near the prostate. During RP, some branches of NVB that supply the striated fascicles may be damaged [61]. The multi-layered feature of the periprostatic fascia allows the anatomy between the nerve and the prostate pseudocapsule to be selected according to the risk of prostate cancer and the T stage. This method is called incremental neural preservation. A systematic review including 13,749 patients concluded that significantly higher rates of UC recovery up to 6 months after surgery were observed in men submitted to NS approach as compared with those treated with non-nerve sparing (NNS) approach. However, at the 12-month follow-up this difference was not significant [62]. Another meta-analysis addressed the issue of functional outcomes after intra-fascial or inter-fascial NS technique [63]. If compared with the inter-fascial technique, the intra-fascial approach was found to be associated with faster UC recovery at the 1-, 3-, and 6-month assessments, but not at the 12-month follow-up. Michl et al. [64] compared long-term UC outcomes in 18,427 patients who had received a primary bilateral NS (BNS) procedure; a primary NNS procedure; or BNS intervention with subsequent resection of NVBs for positive surgical margins. Compared with the NNS group, the latter group is associated with a better 12-month UC rate, which may indicate a careful surgical approach, not just the intention to retain NVB, and is associated with UC recovery.

Maximal Urethral Length Preservation (MULP)

An increased urethral length, associated with higher levels of muscle tissue sparing, can possibly aid in rhabdosphincter's functional rehabilitation. Preservation of the urethral length seems essential to improve postoperative UC. RARP techniques indeed may support in the urethral length preservation as well as avoiding disturbance of the levator muscles. Schlomm et al. [65] described preservation of the entire length of the urethral sphincter by identifying and dissecting the distinct striated and smooth muscle part of the sphincter inside the prostate apex until the colliculus seminalis is encountered. As a result, 50% of cases achieved UC within 1 week after extubation, and 97% at 12 months. Although it seems reasonable to preserve the entire urethral sphincter as much as possible, it is still unclear whether the seminal mound needs to be dissected. Hamada et al. [66] mentioned that the length of the functional sphincter mechanism is preserved by increasing the length of the urethra in the prostate. Their results are very promising, with incontinence rates of 96.6% and 100% at 3 months and 13 months, respectively.

The group of Hakimi et al. [67] intraoperatively measured the urethral stump length in 75 MULP technique-treated patients; a urethral stump length of >2 cm significantly predicted time to pad-free state. With the support of pre- and postoperative MRI, Kadono et al. [68] recorded the location of the distal membranous urethra in 185 patients. These records, in terms of urethral positioning and length, were then analyzed taking into account the chronological changes in UC recovery. It was found that the distal membranous urethra shifted proximally shortly after RP, and returned to its usual pre-RP position 1 year after RP [68].In parallel, the sphincter's function worsened 10 days after RP, but recovered 12 months later. Maximal preservation of the urethral stump's length was associated with the entity of displacement of the membranous urethra and impacted positively on UI after RP.

Endopelvic Fascia Preservation

During the operation, the medial or lateral incision of the pelvic fascial fusion will produce different access to the lateral prostate, and have different results in terms of nerve preservation and fascia preservation. The incision of this fascia just outside the arch of the fascia makes an incision of the levator ani fascia and exposes the muscle fibers of the levator ani muscle and attaches the levator ani fascia to the prostate. An incision of the visceral endopelvic fasciax medial to the fascial tendinous arch results in a dissection plane that leaves the levator ani muscle covered with its fascia without exposure of its fibers. The result is a prostate covered only by prostatic fascia, when present, and not by a layer of levator ani fascia. Avoiding incision of the endopelvic fascia with a medial access during RP may often, combined with an intrafascial nerve-sparing procedure, improve early recovery of urinary continence as well as postoperative erectile function. Endopelvic fascia preservation technique during RARP has been proposed by van der Poel et al. [21] In a prospective study of 151 men, they found that the extent of lateral fascial preservation was the strongest predictor of UC at 5 and 12 months postoperatively [21].

Retzius-Sparing Approach

"Retzius-sparing prostatectomy" is a surgical technique with a direct access to the posterior plane going directly through the Douglas space, aiming at minimizing surgical trauma whilst preserving regional anatomy. The goal of this surgery is to avoid the dissection of the anterior compartment where all the structures involved in the maintenance of UC and potency are present, as well as aphrodite's veil, endopelvic fascia, dorsal vascular complex (DVC) and pubo-urethral ligaments. The results of this technique are very promising in terms of immediate and late UC and effectiveness recovery, with a one-year abstinence rate exceeding 96% [69]. In addition, even the satisfactory rate of immediate continence observed in larger prostates encourages the use of this method in any prostate volume.

The Retzius-sparing method allows the entire RP to be completed through the Douglas capsule. Therefore, the bladder does not descend, and the EPF and pubic prostatic ligament are preserved, thereby improving urethral support. Several papers have compared the so-called "posterior approach" with traditional methods to prove the practicality of this kind of preservation surgery. As a prospective study, Sayyid et al. [70] compared 100 patients undergoing a retzius-sparing and 100 a conventional anterior RARP. The study arm reveals superior rates of post-operative UC achieved, with 20% of patients continent within the first month, compared with 8% of patients in the conventional anterior group. A RCT with 60 patients to each arm, treated either with standard RARP or with retzius-sparing-RARP, found a rapid early return to UC in those patients with low and intermediate-risk localized Pca; 71% of patients with retzius-sparing-RARP were continent (0/1 pad/day) at 1 week after surgery vs. 48% in the standard RARP group [71]. A systematic review concluded that early UC recovery when using this technique as opposed to conventional RARP, is significantly enhanced [72].

Selective Ligature of Dorsal Venous Complex

Optimal dorsal vascular complex (DVC) management, hence avoiding any damage to the rhabdophane's fibres, could influence UC recovery [73]. The standard "ligate and cut" technique can result in an accidental sphincter's damage, whilst the "cut and ligate" technique is instead thought to provide better anatomical control [74]. Therefore, to obtain prompt UC recovery, the venotomies' suture can be performed after DVC section, and in a selective way. Pneumoperitoneum provided by laparoscopy makes selective ligature technique more feasible because it reduces the bleeding and increases the overview vision. Porpiglia et al. [74] identified a selective suture ligature during laparoscopic RP was associated with improved UC at 3 months in a prospective randomized study of 30 patients undergoing selective suture ligature *vs.* 30 patients undergoing complete ligature. Although there was initial benefit in the early post-operative time, no differences were observed at 6 and 12 months. A significant difference in terms of UC outcomes was recorded between the 2 groups, *e.g.*, 53% in group A vs. 80% in group B, after 3 months. In another trial, UC outcomes of 303 patients receiving DVC ligation and eventual section were compared with those of 240 patients who received a selective DVC division with sequent ligature [75]. With respect to the whole ligation, the selective ligature technique was associated with earlier UC-recovery (61.4% vs. 39.6%, $p < 0.001$).

Pubo-Prostatic Ligament Preservation

The pubo-prostatic ligament is the most important supportive element between the pubis and the prostate; in supporting the urethra the ligament concurs in maintaining UC [76]. Hence, the ligament section is expected to worsen the lack of urethral stability, thus negatively influencing UC outcomes. Pubo- prostatic ligament preservation was therefore proposed to hasten UC recovery, with some authors reporting an associated improvement of postoperative UC [77, 78]. Indeed, data of 30 RARP patients treated with pubo-prostatic ligament preservation showed an impressive 80% UC recovery rate after catheter removal, and 100% 1 month after surgery [78].

Anterior Reconstruction

Walsh et al. [79] proposed a technique based on arranging an anterior suspension stitch running through the urethra and then secured to the pubic periosteum [80]. In their cohort of 331 RARP patients, Patel et al. [81] reported that the suspension of the tissues ventral to the urethra on the pubic bone providing anatomical support and stabilization of the urethra, resulted in significantly greater UC rates at 3 months after RARP than a non-suspension technique. Moreover, in the case of suspension, the median interval of UC recovery is shorter, which indicates that the sling during RARP leads to a statistically significant reduction in the interval of UC recovery, and the incidence of UC is higher at 3 months after surgery [51].

Posterior Reconstruction

Rocco et al. [82] described a technique based on the reconstruction of the posterior area of the rhabdophane, thus allowing the positioning of the sphincter in a more natural fashion. The tissue included in this area extends from the retrovesical peritoneum to the central tendon of the perineum. Several RCTs investigated the role of posterior reconstruction (PR) regarding UC recovery [83–89]. In 2011, Patel's group [90] described a modified suturing of the rhabdosphincter applied to RARP. Several studies have been published so far to compare pos- terior reconstruction versus traditional approaches [91]; furthermore, several modified approach to the concept of posterior reconstruction have been proposed. In a meta- analysis, typical data showed a significant advantage associated with the PR in terms of postoperative UC at different time intervals, but not at later follow-ups [92]. A recent RCT examined the usefulness of a 3-layer/2-step RARP technique being carried out using peritoneum, in comparison with the standard RARP technique; 48 patients were subdivided into 2 groups, being treated with either the standard or the 3-layer technique [84]. Four weeks after surgery, UC rates were higher in the experimental (57%) vs. the standard RARP group (26%). Even if its efficacy on early recovery of continence is a common matter of debate, the posterior reconstruction of the rhabdosphincter as described, or with a modified approach, is performed by more than 50% of the robotic surgeons all over Europe. Several papers with various levels of evidence, including randomized control trials, challenged the efficacy of this technique with controversial results. as a matter of facts, three meta-analysis have been published so far, the last out of

2600 patients, reporting a significant advantage in terms of early continence recovery, and a reduction of peri-anastomotic urinary leakages in the first 90 days [10, 92, 93].

In an extensive prospective trial, Tan et al. [94] reported significant advantage for a complete reconstruction (CR) approach as compared with both AR and standard approaches. These results were confirmed in 2 RCTs showing better outcomes for the CR compared to a standard technique at 1-month follow-up [80, 87]. A novel CR approach was proposed by Porpiglia et al. [95]: they reinforced the anastomosis using three posterior and two anterior tissue's layers, in order to re-establish the peri-urethral tissue's anatomy. The last step of the technique involves suture the muscle fibers of the bladder neck with the previously dissected tissue around the urethra, located between the urethra and the DVC, with a barbed needle. Using the same suture, the reconstruction is completed by the connection of the visceral layer of endopelvic fascia that covers the bladder with the endopelvic fascia that covers the DVC, involving the pubo-prostatic ligaments. Results were encouraging, with UC rates of 94.4%, and 98.0% at 12, and 24 weeks post-RARP, respectively. Based on the results of the RCTs [80, 87–89], it seems that CR is associated with better UC outcomes 1 and 3 months after RARP, whereas long-term outcomes are scarcely supported by solid evidence.

Postoperative Setting

Role of Postoperative Length of Catheterization

Many studies [96–99] have associated longer postoperative catheterization time with the worst results of UC. This conclusion comes from non-random, potentially biased studies. Therefore, it is impossible to draw a clear conclusion on this issue.

Diagnostic Work-Up

History should identify possible features of urgency- or mixed-type UI and should include a bladder diary consisting in frequency of micturition; number of UI episodes; voided volumes; and 24-hour urinary output collection of related data. Validated tools, Such as the OAB questionnaire, are considered reliable and useful to evaluate postoperative UC [100]. Due to its replicability, the 24-hour pad test is the most accurate to quantify UI [101]. A urinalysis test should also be performed in order to rule out any infection. Although its routinal adoption is considered controversial [102], urodynamic investigation had been habitually used in the past to assess DO in candidates for corrective treatment.

Conservative Strategies

Conservative care should be appraised before moving to invasive options; in this context patients should be examined on a regular basis to evaluate the improvements. Indeed, UI status can last for more than 1 year after RP [103]. Fluid intake reduction, timed voiding and reduction of bladder irritants (e.g., coffee, hot spices) have been associated with improvement of post-RP urinary symptoms and UC [104].

Pelvic Floor Muscle Exercise

The most established conservative option for dealing with post-RP UI is PFME. However, drawing a definitive conclusion about the advantage of PFME for surgery-related UI may be difficult due to the conflicting results provided by current evidences. There is large heterogeneity between trials regarding both PFME content/delivery (*e.g.*, biofeedback, muscles targeted, and time of commencement of the training) and UC definition (*e.g.*, 1 hour pad test, 24 hour pad test, International Consultation on Incontinence Questionnaire (ICIQ), bladder diary, and number of pads/d) [105]. Over the past decade, several RCTs have been conducted to evaluate the effectiveness of PFME. Although some RCTs support the benefits of PFME, a recent meta-analysis [106] of 45 RCTs does not support PFME as a first-line rehabilitation method for UC recovery after RP. The method proposed here to deconstruct the details of the PFME protocol, as described in a recent review by Hall et al. [105], can help to better understand the usefulness of this strategy. In their analysis, preoperative PFME, use of biofeedback, and UC defined as non-leaky were characteristics associated with successful patient outcomes. Four studies included a total of 655 patients undergoing RARP treatment and investigated the use of PFME to improve recovery from incontinence after RARP [47, 49, 107, 108]. Manley et al. [47] evaluated the improvement of pelvic muscle strength after PfME. They also studied the effect of improving pelvic floor muscle strength on the recovery of urinary incontinence. PfME is performed before and after RARP. Patients were trained by an expert physiotherapist. Preoperative muscle strength was defined as strong in 77 patients (79%), moderate in 12 (12%) and weak in 9 (9%) patients. Authors reported an improvement in all categories of PfM strength from day 4 to day 28 after catheter removal [47]. However, it should be noted that authors reported that most of the patients classified as strong preoperatively were still strong after RARP.

Pharmacological Treatment

DO may be a contributing factor to post-RP UI [109], hence the attempt to improve UC with anti-muscarinics. in the pasted few years, several studies investigated their efficacy on post-RP OAB symptoms. An RCT found that the emergency UI of tolterodine 2 mg was significantly lower than the untreated UI early after catheter removal [110]. Two RCTs reveals a significant effect of the anti-depressant duloxetine on SUI after RP [111, 112]. Although off-label in many European countries, duloxetine is currently recommended by the European Association GUI delines panel as an effective drug for postoperative SUI, but the side effects should be adequately explained to the patient. Also two studies tested the possible use of solifenacin for the treatment of postoperative incontinence [113, 114]. Overall, 662 patients treated with RARP were included. Solifenacin 5 mg daily was dispensed for 3 months. Similarly, Bianco et al. [114] evaluated the efficacy of solifenacin in patients incontinent after 1 to 3 weeks after catheter removal. Authors conducted a randomized, double-blind, phase 4, multicentric trial. Urinary continence was considered achieved if patients did not require the use of pads for at least 3 consecutive days. Gandaglia et al. [115] prospectively assessed a large cohort of RP patients, finding that those who were taking phosphodiesterase type 5 inhibitors (PDE5Is) presented with better UC recovery rates as compared with those left untreated. Conversely, other studies failed to show any benefits after PDE5Is in RP patients [116].

Surgical Treatments

Surgical therapy for post-RP SUI is an option for patients with unsatisfactory improvements after conservative management.

Male Slings

Male slings (MS) are considered a feasible alternative to artificial urinary sphincter (AUS) in a number of cases of mild to moderate post-RP UI. Different types of slings are available, and all of them are meant to appropriately reposition the urethra. Compared with AUS, a obviously advantage of slings was that they do not require the dexterity of the patient, and they are also cheaper [117]. Over- all, slings are divide into adjustable and non-adjustable types. Furthermore, depending on the method of insertion, slings can be divided into retropubic and transobturator categories. Currently, there is a range of adjustable MS commercially available; therefore, it is difficult to express an opinion regarding the superiority of one MS against another, due to significant heterogeneity of the available data and lack of long-term follow-up RCTs. There are many types of sling has already been used to treat post-RP UI. Among of them, the InVance sling is a polyester mesh positioned under the bulbar urethra and anchored to the ischiopubic bone bilaterally, thus restoring continence by urethral compression. The success rate of this system is between 13% and 66% [118], although it is mainly studied for patients with mild to moderate UI. Patients who have previously received radiation therapy result with high failure rate [119].

Re-adjustable sling systems are sub-urethral slings allowing for the regulation of the desired tension, by traction on the threads located in the subcutaneous tissue 2 cm above the pubic bone). Two different types of re-adjustable slings (e.g. *Argus* and *Remeex* system) are currently available, with few reported data showing comparable results in terms of efficacy, but with an overall high explantation rate ranging from 10% to 21% of cases [118].

Rehder and Gozzi [120] was first described the *AdVance* trans-obturator sling, acting via a repositioning of the supporting structures of the sphincter to their former presurgical place. Treatment success rates ranging was between 9% and 73%.According to previously reported, this technique has 20% failure rate, and a higher risk of failure for patients having a 24 h pad-test >200 g/day [121].

Artificial Urinary Sphincter

The artificial urinary sphincter (AUS) is based on a pressure-regulating balloon placed in the prevesical space over the pubis and connected to an inflatable cuff placed around the urethra, with a control pump in the scrotum which allowing the patient to decrease the pressure for voiding the bladder. The AUS reveals the highest success rate ranging from 20% to 89% in several studies and it is currently considered as gold-standard for patients with moderate-to-severe post-RP SUI [122]. However, the high reported complication rate (19.4%) including erosions, infections, and Mechanical failure, coupled with the need for dexterity in operating equipment, makes this option less popular than other options in male UI therapy [116].

Alternative Options

Urethral Bulking Agents

The injection treatment of fillers (e.g. collagen, Teflon, silicone, autologous tissue, hyaluronic acid) is based on the development of tissue masses at the BN level, leading to the latter and/or urethral occlusion. There are only few available data reported the effectiveness of the procedure. Overall, the reported success rate is very low, with only less evidence that the patient's QOL has improved.

Adjustable Balloons

The Pro-Act system depends upon the compression force which is provided by two balloons that are located bilaterally to the BN. Adjustable balloons appear to be a valid alternative for patients with mild to moderate post-RP UI. A recent retrospective single-institution study [123] focusing on 143 patients who received a post-RP Pro-Act implantation showed that, after a median follow-up of 56 months, 64% of patients showed levels of improvement, with daily pad use reduced by ≥50%, and 45% of patients either did not wear any pad or used only one "security" pad per day. The treatment was considered safe, as 90.2% patients showed no complications.

Intravesical Onabotulinum Toxin A Injections

This treatment had been approved for OAB in 2014, following the results of several RCTs. However, there are limited data relating to their use in the post-RP population. In a retrospective series of 11 patients with post-RP OAB, Habashy et al. [124] observed a resolution of urgency-UI in 45% after onabotulinum toxin A intradetrusorial injection.

Conclusions

RP was a major cause of UI in male; Therefore, during the preoperative evaluation, the patient must be informed of the risk of UI after RP. In a long period of time, a large part of patients can regain self-control, but a shorter recovery time is very important to prevent the deterioration of QOL. Patient's individual features should be well kept in mind, with the aim of better assessing the individual risk of UI. in the pasted decade, the advances of surgical technique opened the way to the progress of multiple intraoperative techniques to improve UC outcomes after RP. Robotic approach to RP allows to have a greater precision, when compared to RRP. Therefore, we can expect conservative and surgical treatment after RARP to be more effective than PRP. Since the outcome of UI surgery is affected by many factors, such as the state of the urethra, the type of treatment used, and other patient characteristics, we can expect that conservative treatment will also be affected by the same predictive factors. Future observational and randomized clinical trials should test the hypothesis that the same UI treatment may have different results depending on the RP technology used. Ideally, these studies should be designed to include pelvic and abdominal magnetic resonance imaging to study the anatomical changes that occur after RARP. In addition, it is important to include pelvic floor muscles and bladder system function studies in the research design. This kind of approach could provide important anatomical and functional information and it will allow to tailor the UI management, according to patients' needs. PFME and pharmacotherapy are reasonable conservative approaches for post-RP UI, even if success rates using these techniques have been inconsistent. Several surgical procedures are currently available to treat post-RP UI. Out of these, AUS showed the longest record of safety and efficacy for patients with moderate to severe UI. MS are an alternative approach, with intermediate data supporting their efficacy. Other options, Such as injectable agents or adjustable balloons, should only be considered when more established options are contra-indicated. Further randomized trials should be carried out to compare the different options, and innovation in the field should continue to refine current techniques and produce novel, and possibly more effective treatment methods.

References

1. Siegel RL, Miller KD, Jemal A. Cancer statistics, 2019. CA Cancer J Clin. 2019;69:7–34. https://doi.org/10.3322/caac.21551.
2. Bandini M, et al. Radical prostatectomy or radiotherapy reduce prostate cancer mortality in elderly patients: a population-based propensity score adjusted analysis. World J Urol. 2018;36:7–13. https://doi.org/10.1007/s00345-017-2102-9.
3. Bill-Axelson A, et al. Radical prostatectomy or watchful waiting in early prostate cancer. N Engl J Med. 2014;370:932–42. https://doi.org/10.1056/NEJMoa1311593.
4. Hamdy FC, et al. 10-year outcomes after monitoring, surgery, or radiotherapy for localized prostate cancer. N Engl J Med. 2016;375:1415–24. https://doi.org/10.1056/NEJMoa1606220.
5. Bandini M, et al. Increasing rate of noninterventional treatment Management in localized prostate cancer candidates for active surveillance: a North American population-based study. Clin Genitourin Cancer. 2019;17:72–78.e74. https://doi.org/10.1016/j.clgc.2018.09.011.
6. Coughlin GD, et al. Robot-assisted laparoscopic prostatectomy versus open radical retropubic prostatectomy: 24-month outcomes from a randomised controlled study. Lancet Oncol. 2018;19:1051–60. https://doi.org/10.1016/s1470-2045(18)30357-7.
7. Yaxley JW, et al. Robot-assisted laparoscopic prostatectomy versus open radical retropubic prostatectomy: early outcomes from a randomised controlled phase 3 study. Lancet. 2016;388:1057–66. https://doi.org/10.1016/s0140-6736(16)30592-x.
8. Pompe RS, et al. Postoperative complications of contemporary open and robot-assisted laparoscopic radical prostatectomy using standardised reporting systems. BJU Int. 2018;122:801–7. https://doi.org/10.1111/bju.14369.
9. Manfredi M, Fiori C, Amparore D, Checcucci E, Porpiglia F. Technical details to achieve perfect early continence after radical prostatectomy. Minerva Chir. 2019;74:63–77. https://doi.org/10.23736/s0026-4733.18.07761-1.
10. Ficarra V, et al. Systematic review and meta-analysis of studies reporting urinary continence recovery after robot-assisted radical prostatectomy. Eur Urol. 2012;62:405–17. https://doi.org/10.1016/j.eururo.2012.05.045.
11. Geraerts I, et al. Prospective evaluation of urinary incontinence, voiding symptoms and quality of life after open and robot-assisted radical prostatectomy. BJU Int. 2013;112:936–43. https://doi.org/10.1111/bju.12258.
12. Schroeck FR, et al. Satisfaction and regret after open retropubic or robot-assisted laparoscopic radical prostatectomy. Eur Urol. 2008;54:785–93. https://doi.org/10.1016/j.eururo.2008.06.063
13. Kretschmer A, Nitti V. Surgical treatment of male postprostatectomy incontinence: current concepts. Eur Urol Focus. 2017;3:364–76. https://doi.org/10.1016/j.euf.2017.11.007.
14. Løvvik A, Müller S, Patel HR. Pharmacological treatment of post-prostatectomy incontinence: what is the evidence? Drugs Aging. 2016;33:535–44. https://doi.org/10.1007/s40266-016-0388-8.
15. Zattoni F, et al. Technical innovations to optimize continence recovery after robotic assisted radical prostatectomy. Minerva Urol Nefrol. 2019;71:324–38. https://doi.org/10.23736/s0393-2249.19.03395-2.
16. Heesakkers J, et al. Pathophysiology and contributing factors in postprostatectomy incontinence: a review. Eur Urol. 2017;71:936–44. https://doi.org/10.1016/j.eururo.2016.09.031.

17. Pastore AL, et al. The role of detrusor overactivity in urinary incontinence after radical prostatectomy: a systematic review. Minerva Urol Nefrol. 2017;69:234–41. https://doi.org/10.23736/s0393-2249.16.02790-9.
18. Porena M, Mearini E, Mearini L, Vianello A, Giannantoni A. Voiding dysfunction after radical retropubic prostatectomy: more than external urethral sphincter deficiency. Eur Urol. 2007;52:38–45. https://doi.org/10.1016/j.eururo.2007.03.051.
19. Kojima Y, et al. Urinary incontinence after robot-assisted radical prostatectomy: pathophysiology and intraoperative techniques to improve surgical outcome. Int J Urol. 2013;20:1052–63. https://doi.org/10.1111/iju.12214.
20. Narayan P, et al. Neuroanatomy of the external urethral sphincter: implications for urinary continence preservation during radical prostate surgery. J Urol. 1995;153:337–41. https://doi.org/10.1097/00005392-199502000-00012.
21. van der Poel HG, de Blok W, Joshi N, van Muilekom E. Preservation of lateral prostatic fascia is associated with urine continence after robotic-assisted prostatectomy. Eur Urol. 2009;55:892–900. https://doi.org/10.1016/j.eururo.2009.01.021.
22. Mandel P, Graefen M, Michl U, Huland H, Tilki D. The effect of age on functional outcomes after radical prostatectomy. Urol Oncol. 2015;33(203):e211–08. https://doi.org/10.1016/j.urolonc.2015.01.015.
23. Novara G, et al. Evaluating urinary continence and preoperative predictors of urinary continence after robot assisted laparoscopic radical prostatectomy. J Urol. 2010;184:1028–33. https://doi.org/10.1016/j.juro.2010.04.069.
24. Mendiola FP, et al. Urinary and sexual function outcomes among different age groups after robot-assisted laparoscopic prostatectomy. J Endourol. 2008;22:519–24. https://doi.org/10.1089/end.2006.9845.
25. Wei Y, et al. Impact of obesity on long-term urinary incontinence after radical prostatectomy: a meta-analysis. Biomed Res Int. 2018;2018:8279523. https://doi.org/10.1155/2018/8279523.
26. De Nunzio C, Roehrborn CG, Andersson KE, McVary KT. Erectile dysfunction and lower urinary tract symptoms. Eur Urol Focus. 2017;3:352–63. https://doi.org/10.1016/j.euf.2017.11.004.
27. Matsushita K, et al. Preoperative predictive model of recovery of urinary continence after radical prostatectomy. BJU Int. 2015;116:577–83. https://doi.org/10.1111/bju.13087.
28. Wiltz AL, et al. Robotic radical prostatectomy in overweight and obese patients: oncological and validated-functional outcomes. Urology. 2009;73:316–22. https://doi.org/10.1016/j.urology.2008.08.493.
29. Xu T, et al. Robot-assisted prostatectomy in obese patients: how influential is obesity on operative outcomes? J Endourol. 2015;29:198–208. https://doi.org/10.1089/end.2014.0354.
30. Teber D, et al. Is type 2 diabetes mellitus a predictive factor for incontinence after laparoscopic radical prostatectomy? A matched pair and multivariate analysis. J Urol. 2010;183:1087–91. https://doi.org/10.1016/j.juro.2009.11.033.
31. Hatiboglu G, et al. Predictive factors for immediate continence after radical prostatectomy. World J Urol. 2016;34:113–20. https://doi.org/10.1007/s00345-015-1594-4.
32. Suardi N, et al. Nerve-sparing radical retropubic prostatectomy in patients previously submitted to holmium laser enucleation of the prostate for bladder outlet obstruction due to benign prostatic enlargement. Eur Urol. 2008;53:1180–5. https://doi.org/10.1016/j.eururo.2007.07.027.
33. Tienza A, et al. Prevalence analysis of urinary incontinence after radical prostatectomy and influential preoperative factors in a single institution. Aging Male. 2018;21:24–30. https://doi.org/10.1080/13685538.2017.1369944.
34. Gupta NP, Singh P, Nayyar R. Outcomes of robot-assisted radical prostatectomy in men with previous transurethral resection of prostate. BJU Int. 2011;108:1501–5. https://doi.org/10.1111/j.1464-410X.2011.10113.x.
35. Abedali ZA, et al. Robot-assisted radical prostatectomy in patients with a history of holmium laser enucleation of the prostate: the Indiana University experience. J Endourol. 2020;34:163–8. https://doi.org/10.1089/end.2019.0436.
36. Pettus JA, et al. Prostate size is associated with surgical difficulty but not functional outcome at 1 year after radical prostatectomy. J Urol. 2009;182:949–55. https://doi.org/10.1016/j.juro.2009.05.029.
37. Dommer L, et al. Lower urinary tract symptoms (LUTS) before and after robotic-assisted laparoscopic prostatectomy: does improvement of LUTS mitigate worsened incontinence after robotic prostatectomy? Transl Androl Urol. 2019;8:320–8. https://doi.org/10.21037/tau.2019.06.24.
38. Kitamura K, et al. Significant association between urethral length measured by magnetic resonance imaging and urinary continence recovery after robot-assisted radical prostatectomy. Prostate Int. 2019;7:54–9. https://doi.org/10.1016/j.prnil.2018.06.003.
39. Mungovan SF, et al. Preoperative membranous urethral length measurement and continence recovery following radical prostatectomy: a systematic review and meta-analysis. Eur Urol. 2017;71:368–78. https://doi.org/10.1016/j.eururo.2016.06.023.
40. Coakley FV, et al. Urinary continence after radical retropubic prostatectomy: relationship with membranous urethral length on preoperative endorectal magnetic resonance imaging. J Urol. 2002;168:1032–5. https://doi.org/10.1097/01.ju.0000025881.75827.a5.
41. Lee SE, et al. Impact of variations in prostatic apex shape on early recovery of urinary continence after radical retropubic prostatectomy. Urology. 2006;68:137–41. https://doi.org/10.1016/j.urology.2006.01.021.
42. Soljanik I, et al. Is a wider angle of the membranous urethra associated with incontinence after radical prostatectomy? World J Urol. 2014;32:1375–83. https://doi.org/10.1007/s00345-014-1241-5.
43. Chandak P, et al. Three-dimensional printing in robot-assisted radical prostatectomy - an idea, development, exploration, assessment, long-term follow-up (IDEAL) phase 2a study. BJU Int. 2018;122:360–1. https://doi.org/10.1111/bju.14189.
44. Porpiglia F, et al. Augmented reality during robot-assisted radical prostatectomy: expert robotic surgeons' on-the-spot insights after live surgery. Minerva Urol Nefrol. 2018;70:226–9. https://doi.org/10.23736/s0393-2249.18.03143-0.
45. Kratiras Z, et al. Phase I study of a new tablet-based image guided surgical system in robot-assisted radical prostatectomy. Minerva Urol Nefrol. 2019;71:92–5. https://doi.org/10.23736/s0393-2249.18.03250-2.
46. Porpiglia F, et al. Augmented-reality robot-assisted radical prostatectomy using hyper-accuracy three-dimensional reconstruction (HA3D™) technology: a radiological and pathological study. BJU Int. 2019;123:834–45. https://doi.org/10.1111/bju.14549.
47. Manley L, et al. Evaluation of pelvic floor muscle strength before and after robotic-assisted radical prostatectomy and early outcomes on urinary continence. J Robot Surg. 2016;10:331–5. https://doi.org/10.1007/s11701-016-0602-z.
48. Chang JI, Lam V, Patel MI. Preoperative pelvic floor muscle exercise and postprostatectomy incontinence: a systematic review and meta-analysis. Eur Urol. 2016;69:460–7. https://doi.org/10.1016/j.eururo.2015.11.004.
49. Yoshida M, et al. May perioperative ultrasound-guided pelvic floor muscle training promote early recovery of urinary continence after robot-assisted radical prostatectomy? Neurourol Urodyn. 2019;38:158–64. https://doi.org/10.1002/nau.23811.
50. Marchioni M, et al. Conservative management of urinary incontinence following robot-assisted radical prostatectomy.

Minerva Urol Nefrol. 2020;72:555–62. https://doi.org/10.23736/s0393-2249.20.03782-0.
51. Capogrosso P, et al. Recovery of urinary continence after radical prostatectomy. Expert Rev Anticancer Ther. 2016;16:1039–52. https://doi.org/10.1080/14737140.2016.1233818.
52. Asimakopoulos AD, Mugnier C, Hoepffner JL, Piechaud T, Gaston R. Bladder neck preservation during minimally invasive radical prostatectomy: a standardised technique using a lateral approach. BJU Int. 2012;110:1566–71. https://doi.org/10.1111/j.1464-410X.2012.11604.x.
53. Nyarangi-Dix JN, Radtke JP, Hadaschik B, Pahernik S, Hohenfellner M. Impact of complete bladder neck preservation on urinary continence, quality of life and surgical margins after radical prostatectomy: a randomized, controlled, single blind trial. J Urol. 2013;189:891–8. https://doi.org/10.1016/j.juro.2012.09.082.
54. Nyarangi-Dix JN, et al. Complete bladder neck preservation promotes long-term post-prostatectomy continence without compromising midterm oncological outcome: analysis of a randomised controlled cohort. World J Urol. 2018;36:349–55. https://doi.org/10.1007/s00345-017-2134-1.
55. Friedlander DF, Alemozaffar M, Hevelone ND, Lipsitz SR, Hu JC. Stepwise description and outcomes of bladder neck sparing during robot-assisted laparoscopic radical prostatectomy. J Urol. 2012;188:1754–60. https://doi.org/10.1016/j.juro.2012.07.045.
56. Ma X, et al. Bladder neck preservation improves time to continence after radical prostatectomy: a systematic review and meta-analysis. Oncotarget. 2016;7:67463–75. https://doi.org/10.18632/oncotarget.11997.
57. Jeong SJ, et al. Early recovery of urinary continence after radical prostatectomy: correlation with vesico-urethral anastomosis location in the pelvic cavity measured by postoperative cystography. Int J Urol. 2011;18:444–51. https://doi.org/10.1111/j.1442-2042.2011.02760.x.
58. Olgin G, et al. Postoperative cystogram findings predict incontinence following robot-assisted radical prostatectomy. J Endourol. 2014;28:1460–3. https://doi.org/10.1089/end.2014.0236.
59. Lin VC, et al. Modified transverse plication for bladder neck reconstruction during robotic-assisted laparoscopic prostatectomy. BJU Int. 2009;104:878–81. https://doi.org/10.1111/j.1464-410X.2009.08784.x.
60. Lee DI, et al. Bladder neck plication stitch: a novel technique during robot-assisted radical prostatectomy to improve recovery of urinary continence. J Endourol. 2011;25:1873–7. https://doi.org/10.1089/end.2011.0279.
61. Walz J, et al. A critical analysis of the current knowledge of surgical anatomy of the prostate related to optimisation of cancer control and preservation of continence and erection in candidates for radical prostatectomy: an update. Eur Urol. 2016;70:301–11. https://doi.org/10.1016/j.eururo.2016.01.026.
62. Reeves F, et al. Preservation of the neurovascular bundles is associated with improved time to continence after radical prostatectomy but not long-term continence rates: results of a systematic review and meta-analysis. Eur Urol. 2015;68:692–704. https://doi.org/10.1016/j.eururo.2014.10.020.
63. Wang X, et al. Intrafascial nerve-sparing radical prostatectomy improves patients' postoperative continence recovery and erectile function: a pooled analysis based on available literatures. Medicine (Baltimore). 2018;97:e11297. https://doi.org/10.1097/md.0000000000011297.
64. Michl U, et al. Nerve-sparing surgery technique, not the preservation of the neurovascular bundles, leads to improved long-term continence rates after radical prostatectomy. Eur Urol. 2016;69:584–9. https://doi.org/10.1016/j.eururo.2015.07.037.
65. Schlomm T, et al. Full functional-length urethral sphincter preservation during radical prostatectomy. Eur Urol. 2011;60:320–9. https://doi.org/10.1016/j.eururo.2011.02.040.
66. Hamada A, Razdan S, Etafy MH, Fagin R, Razdan S. Early return of continence in patients undergoing robot-assisted laparoscopic prostatectomy using modified maximal urethral length preservation technique. J Endourol. 2014;28:930–8. https://doi.org/10.1089/end.2013.0794.
67. Hakimi AA, et al. Preoperative and intraoperative measurements of urethral length as predictors of continence after robot-assisted radical prostatectomy. J Endourol. 2011;25:1025–30. https://doi.org/10.1089/end.2010.0692.
68. Kadono Y, et al. Investigating the mechanism underlying urinary continence recovery after radical prostatectomy: effectiveness of a longer urethral stump to prevent urinary incontinence. BJU Int. 2018;122:456–62. https://doi.org/10.1111/bju.14181.
69. Takenaka A, Hara R, Soga H, Murakami G, Fujisawa M. A novel technique for approaching the endopelvic fascia in retropubic radical prostatectomy, based on an anatomical study of fixed and fresh cadavers. BJU Int. 2005;95:766–71. https://doi.org/10.1111/j.1464-410X.2005.05397.x.
70. Sayyid RK, et al. Retzius-sparing robotic-assisted laparoscopic radical prostatectomy: a safe surgical technique with superior continence outcomes. J Endourol. 2017;31:1244–50. https://doi.org/10.1089/end.2017.0490.
71. Dalela D, et al. A pragmatic randomized controlled trial examining the impact of the Retzius-sparing approach on early urinary continence recovery after robot-assisted radical prostatectomy. Eur Urol. 2017;72:677–85. https://doi.org/10.1016/j.eururo.2017.04.029.
72. Phukan C, et al. Retzius sparing robotic assisted radical prostatectomy vs. conventional robotic assisted radical prostatectomy: a systematic review and meta-analysis. World J Urol. 2020;38:1123–34. https://doi.org/10.1007/s00345-019-02798-4.
73. Power NE, Silberstein JL, Kulkarni GS, Laudone VP. The dorsal venous complex (DVC): dorsal venous or dorsal vasculature complex? Santorini's plexus revisited. BJU Int. 2011;108:930–2. https://doi.org/10.1111/j.1464-410X.2011.10536.x.
74. Porpiglia F, Fiori C, Grande S, Morra I, Scarpa RM. Selective versus standard ligature of the deep venous complex during laparoscopic radical prostatectomy: effects on continence, blood loss, and margin status. Eur Urol. 2009;55:1377–83. https://doi.org/10.1016/j.eururo.2009.02.009.
75. Lei Y, et al. Athermal division and selective suture ligation of the dorsal vein complex during robot-assisted laparoscopic radical prostatectomy: description of technique and outcomes. Eur Urol. 2011;59:235–43. https://doi.org/10.1016/j.eururo.2010.08.043.
76. Wimpissinger TF, Tschabitscher M, Feichtinger H, Stackl W. Surgical anatomy of the puboprostatic complex with special reference to radical perineal prostatectomy. BJU Int. 2003;92:681–4. https://doi.org/10.1046/j.1464-410x.2003.04489.x.
77. Stolzenburg JU, et al. Nerve sparing endoscopic extraperitoneal radical prostatectomy--effect of puboprostatic ligament preservation on early continence and positive margins. Eur Urol. 2006;49:103–11; discussion 111–102. https://doi.org/10.1016/j.eururo.2005.10.002.
78. Asimakopoulos AD, et al. Complete periprostatic anatomy preservation during robot-assisted laparoscopic radical prostatectomy (RALP): the new pubovesical complex-sparing technique. Eur Urol. 2010;58:407–17. https://doi.org/10.1016/j.eururo.2010.04.032.
79. Walsh PC. Anatomic radical prostatectomy: evolution of the surgical technique. J Urol. 1998;160:2418–24. https://doi.org/10.1097/00005392-199812020-00010.

80. Hurtes X, et al. Anterior suspension combined with posterior reconstruction during robot-assisted laparoscopic prostatectomy improves early return of urinary continence: a prospective randomized multicentre trial. BJU Int. 2012;110:875–83. https://doi.org/10.1111/j.1464-410X.2011.10849.x.
81. Patel VR, Coelho RF, Palmer KJ, Rocco B. Periurethral suspension stitch during robot-assisted laparoscopic radical prostatectomy: description of the technique and continence outcomes. Eur Urol. 2009;56:472–8. https://doi.org/10.1016/j.eururo.2009.06.007.
82. Rocco F, et al. Personal research: reconstruction of the urethral striated sphincter. Arch Ital Urol Androl. 2001;73:127–37.
83. Cui J, et al. Pelvic floor reconstruction after radical prostatectomy: a systematic review and meta-analysis of different surgical techniques. Sci Rep. 2017;7:2737. https://doi.org/10.1038/s41598-017-02991-8.
84. Ogawa S, et al. Three-layer two-step posterior reconstruction using peritoneum during robot-assisted radical prostatectomy to improve recovery of urinary continence: a prospective comparative study. J Endourol. 2017;31:1251–7. https://doi.org/10.1089/end.2017.0410.
85. Jeong CW, et al. Effects of new 1-step posterior reconstruction method on recovery of continence after robot-assisted laparoscopic prostatectomy: results of a prospective, single-blind, parallel group, randomized, controlled trial. J Urol. 2015;193:935–42. https://doi.org/10.1016/j.juro.2014.10.023.
86. Sutherland DE, et al. Posterior rhabdosphincter reconstruction during robotic assisted radical prostatectomy: results from a phase II randomized clinical trial. J Urol. 2011;185:1262–7. https://doi.org/10.1016/j.juro.2010.11.085.
87. Koliakos N, et al. Posterior and anterior fixation of the urethra during robotic prostatectomy improves early continence rates. Scand J Urol Nephrol. 2010;44:5–10. https://doi.org/10.3109/00365590903413627.
88. Menon M, Muhletaler F, Campos M, Peabody JO. Assessment of early continence after reconstruction of the periprostatic tissues in patients undergoing computer assisted (robotic) prostatectomy: results of a 2 group parallel randomized controlled trial. J Urol. 2008;180:1018–23. https://doi.org/10.1016/j.juro.2008.05.046.
89. Sammon JD, et al. Long-term functional urinary outcomes comparing single- vs double-layer urethrovesical anastomosis: two-year follow-up of a two-group parallel randomized controlled trial. Urology. 2010;76:1102–7. https://doi.org/10.1016/j.urology.2010.05.052.
90. Coelho RF, et al. Influence of modified posterior reconstruction of the rhabdosphincter on early recovery of continence and anastomotic leakage rates after robot-assisted radical prostatectomy. Eur Urol. 2011;59:72–80. https://doi.org/10.1016/j.eururo.2010.08.025.
91. Galfano A, et al. A new anatomic approach for robot-assisted laparoscopic prostatectomy: a feasibility study for completely intrafascial surgery. Eur Urol. 2010;58:457–61. https://doi.org/10.1016/j.eururo.2010.06.008.
92. Grasso AA, et al. Posterior musculofascial reconstruction after radical prostatectomy: an updated systematic review and a meta-analysis. BJU Int. 2016;118:20–34. https://doi.org/10.1111/bju.13480.
93. Rocco B, et al. Posterior musculofascial reconstruction after radical prostatectomy: a systematic review of the literature. Eur Urol. 2012;62:779–90. https://doi.org/10.1016/j.eururo.2012.05.041.
94. Tan G, et al. Optimizing vesicourethral anastomosis healing after robot-assisted laparoscopic radical prostatectomy: lessons learned from three techniques in 1900 patients. J Endourol. 2010;24:1975–83. https://doi.org/10.1089/end.2009.0630.
95. Porpiglia F, et al. Total anatomical reconstruction during robot-assisted radical prostatectomy: implications on early recovery of urinary continence. Eur Urol. 2016;69:485–95. https://doi.org/10.1016/j.eururo.2015.08.005.
96. Tilki D, et al. The impact of time to catheter removal on short-, intermediate- and long-term urinary continence after radical prostatectomy. World J Urol. 2018;36:1247–53. https://doi.org/10.1007/s00345-018-2274-y.
97. Palisaar JR, et al. Predictors of short-term recovery of urinary continence after radical prostatectomy. World J Urol. 2015;33:771–9. https://doi.org/10.1007/s00345-014-1340-3.
98. Cormio L, et al. Prognostic factors for anastomotic urinary leakage following retropubic radical prostatectomy and correlation with voiding outcomes. Medicine (Baltimore). 2016;95:e3475. https://doi.org/10.1097/md.0000000000003475.
99. Tiguert R, Rigaud J, Fradet Y. Safety and outcome of early catheter removal after radical retropubic prostatectomy. Urology. 2004;63:513–7. https://doi.org/10.1016/j.urology.2003.10 042.
100. Moore K, Allen M, Voaklander DC. Pad tests and self-reports of continence in men awaiting radical prostatectomy: establishing baseline norms for males. Neurourol Urodyn. 2004;23:623–6. https://doi.org/10.1002/nau.20067.
101. Karantanis E, Fynes M, Moore KH, Stanton SL. Comparison of the ICIQ-SF and 24-hour pad test with other measures for evaluating the severity of urodynamic stress incontinence. Int Urogynecol J Pelvic Floor Dysfunct. 2004;15:111–6; discussion 116. https://doi.org/10.1007/s00192-004-1123-2.
102. Arcila-Ruiz M, Brucker BM. The role of urodynamics in post-prostatectomy incontinence. Curr Urol Rep. 2018;19:21. https://doi.org/10.1007/s11934-018-0770-7.
103. Xu AJ, Taksler GB, Llukani E, Lepor H. Long-term continence outcomes in men undergoing radical prostatectomy: a prospective 15-year longitudinal study. J Urol. 2018;200:626–32. https://doi.org/10.1016/j.juro.2018.05.005.
104. Goode PS, et al. Behavioral therapy with or without biofeedback and pelvic floor electrical stimulation for persistent postprostatectomy incontinence: a randomized controlled trial. JAMA. 2011;305:151–9. https://doi.org/10.1001/jama.2010.1972.
105. Hall LM, Neumann P, Hodges PW. Do features of randomized controlled trials of pelvic floor muscle training for postprostatectomy urinary incontinence differentiate successful from unsuccessful patient outcomes? A systematic review with a series of meta-analyses. Neurourol Urodyn. 2020;39:533–46. https://doi.org/10.1002/nau.24291.
106. Anderson CA, et al. Conservative management for postprostatectomy urinary incontinence. Cochrane Database Syst Rev. 2015;1:Cd001843. https://doi.org/10.1002/14651858.CD001843.pub5.
107. Neumann PB, O'Callaghan M. The role of preoperative puborectal muscle function assessed by transperineal ultrasound in urinary continence outcomes at 3, 6, and 12 months after robotic-assisted radical prostatectomy. Int Neurourol J. 2018;22:114–22. https://doi.org/10.5213/inj.1836026.013.
108. Oh JJ, et al. Effect of personalized extracorporeal biofeedback device for pelvic floor muscle training on urinary incontinence after robot-assisted radical prostatectomy: a randomized controlled trial. Neurourol Urodyn. 2020;39:674–81. https://doi.org/10.1002/nau.24247.
109. Juszczak K, Ostrowski A, Bryczkowski M, Adamczyk P, Drewa T. A hypothesis for the mechanism of urine incontinence in patients after radical prostatectomy due to urinary bladder hypertrophy. Adv Clin Exp Med. 2019;28:391–5. https://doi.org/10.17219/acem/79935.
110. Mitropoulos D, Papadoukakis S, Zervas A, Alamanis C, Giannopoulos A. Efficacy of tolterodine in preventing urge incontinence immediately after prostatectomy. Int Urol Nephrol. 2006;38:263–8. https://doi.org/10.1007/s11255-005-4031-6.

111. Cornu JN, et al. Duloxetine for mild to moderate postprostatectomy incontinence: preliminary results of a randomised, placebo-controlled trial. Eur Urol. 2011;59:148–54. https://doi.org/10.1016/j.eururo.2010.10.031.
112. Filocamo MT, et al. Pharmacologic treatment in postprostatectomy stress urinary incontinence. Eur Urol. 2007;51:1559–64. https://doi.org/10.1016/j.eururo.2006.08.005.
113. Liss MA, Morales B, Skarecky D, Ahlering TE. Phase 1 clinical trial of Vesicare™ (solifenacin) in the treatment of urinary incontinence after radical prostatectomy. J Endourol. 2014;28:1241–5. https://doi.org/10.1089/end.2014.0342.
114. Bianco FJ, et al. A randomized, double-blind, solifenacin succinate versus placebo control, phase 4, multicenter study evaluating urinary continence after robotic assisted radical prostatectomy. J Urol. 2015;193:1305–10. https://doi.org/10.1016/j.juro.2014.09.106.
115. Gandaglia G, et al. Postoperative phosphodiesterase type 5 inhibitor administration increases the rate of urinary continence recovery after bilateral nerve-sparing radical prostatectomy. Int J Urol. 2013;20:413–9. https://doi.org/10.1111/j.1442-2042.2012.03149.x.
116. Honda M, et al. Impact of postoperative phosphodiesterase type 5 inhibitor treatment on lower urinary tract symptoms after robot-assisted radical prostatectomy: a longitudinal study. Scand J Urol. 2017;51:33–7. https://doi.org/10.1080/21681805.2016.1250810.
117. Radadia KD, et al. Management of postradical prostatectomy urinary incontinence: a review. Urology. 2018;113:13–9. https://doi.org/10.1016/j.urology.2017.09.025.
118. Crivellaro S, et al. Systematic review of surgical treatment of post radical prostatectomy stress urinary incontinence. Neurourol Urodyn. 2016;35:875–81. https://doi.org/10.1002/nau.22873.
119. Giberti C, Gallo F, Schenone M, Cortese P, Ninotta G. The bone anchor suburethral synthetic sling for iatrogenic male incontinence: critical evaluation at a mean 3-year followup. J Urol. 2009;181:2204–8. https://doi.org/10.1016/j.juro.2009.01.022.
120. Rehder P, Gozzi C. Transobturator sling suspension for male urinary incontinence including post-radical prostatectomy. Eur Urol. 2007;52:860–6. https://doi.org/10.1016/j.eururo.2007.01.110.
121. Cornu JN, et al. The AdVance transobturator male sling for post-prostatectomy incontinence: clinical results of a prospective evaluation after a minimum follow-up of 6 months. Eur Urol. 2009;56:923–7. https://doi.org/10.1016/j.eururo.2009.09.015.
122. Tutolo M, et al. Efficacy and safety of artificial urinary sphincter (AUS): results of a large multi-institutional cohort of patients with mid-term follow-up. Neurourol Urodyn. 2019;38:710–8. https://doi.org/10.1002/nau.23901.
123. Noordhoff TC, Scheepe JR, Blok BFM. Outcome and complications of adjustable continence therapy (ProACT™) after radical prostatectomy: 10 years' experience in 143 patients. Neurourol Urodyn. 2018;37:1419–25. https://doi.org/10.1002/nau.23463.
124. Habashy D, Losco G, Tse V, Collins R, Chan L. Botulinum toxin (OnabotulinumtoxinA) in the male non-neurogenic overactive bladder: clinical and quality of life outcomes. BJU Int. 2015;116(Suppl 3):61–5. https://doi.org/10.1111/bju.13110.

Index

S. Ren et al. (eds.), *Robot-Assisted Radical Prostatectomy*, https://doi.org/10.1007/978-3-031-05855-4

R

W

Y

MIX
Papier aus verantwortungsvollen Quellen
Paper from responsible sources
FSC® C105338

If you have any concerns about our products,
you can contact us on
ProductSafety@springernature.com

In case Publisher is established outside the EU,
the EU authorized representative is:
Springer Nature Customer Service Center GmbH
Europaplatz 3, 69115 Heidelberg, Germany

Printed by Libri Plureos GmbH
in Hamburg, Germany

Flies

The term "flies" applies to the insects belonging to the order Diptera, more commonly known as flies, gnats, midges, and leaf miners. They typically possess a pair of antennae, a set of sponging-type mouthparts, two developed forewings for flight, and two hindwings which are used for aerial balance.

Flies occupy unique and diverse roles within our ecosystem: some are pests which affect our agricultural and horticultural crops; other varieties act as vectors that spread diseases within the human and animal population. However, not all flies are harmful to humans: some species of fly play a role in facilitating crop pollination, whilst others are involved in environmental engineering, waste decomposition, and/or nutrient recycling, forming an important component of integrated pest management as effective biocontrol agents. Others even play a role in crime solving within the field of forensic entomology.

Flies: Agricultural and Public-Health Perspectives has been planned with a holistic approach to highlight both the positive and negative aspects of flies. This book starts with a chapter on the introduction to flies, followed by insects of agricultural and horticultural importance, flies as vectors, and beneficial flies. Designed with ease of reader use in mind, each chapter includes "pointwise learning objectives" at the beginning, as well as "conclusions" and "points to remember" at the end.

This book will be useful not only to students of entomology, public health, agriculture, and applied life sciences but also to those involved in policy planning and vector management. In addition, this book will benefit students preparing for competitive examinations as well as the public.

Flies

Agricultural and Public-Health Perspectives

Edited by
Omkar

CRC Press
Taylor & Francis Group
Boca Raton London New York

CRC Press is an imprint of the
Taylor & Francis Group, an **informa** business

Designed cover image: Author's own

First edition published 2025
by CRC Press
2385 NW Executive Center Drive, Suite 320, Boca Raton FL 33431

and by CRC Press
4 Park Square, Milton Park, Abingdon, Oxon, OX14 4RN

CRC Press is an imprint of Taylor & Francis Group, LLC

ISBN: 9781032773445 (hbk)
ISBN: 9781032773476 (pbk)
ISBN: 9781003482581 (ebk)

DOI: 10.1201/9781003482581

Typeset in Times
by codeMantra

Contents

SECTION II Flies of Medical, Veterinary, and Forensic Importance

Preface

The majority of insects are quite useful, and only a small fraction of them are harmful to us. Insects often carry negative connotations due to the presence of cockroaches, flies, fleas, and mosquitoes that we encounter frequently. They can be quite obnoxious and affect human life in various ways. The term "flies" applies to the insects belonging to the order Diptera, which contains approximately 125,000 species. They are commonly known by the terms such as gnats, midges, and leaf miners. They often possess a pair of aristate antennae, a set of sponging-type mouthparts, and two functional and developed forewings, which help in flight, while the two hindwings are reduced to halteres, which serve as balancing organs during flight. Additionally, several other wing-bearing insects, such as whiteflies, dragonflies, caddisflies, mayflies, and mustard sawflies, are commonly termed flies, but their wing structure distinguishes them from true flies. Several flies are pests that affect our agricultural and horticultural crops, significantly reducing the crop yield. Others act as vectors, transmitting various diseases; for example, sand flies, black flies, and tsetse flies cause leishmaniasis, river blindness (onchocerciasis), and sleeping sickness, respectively, in humans. Additionally, flies such as flesh flies have medico-veterinary significance. However, not all flies are harmful. Several species play beneficial roles, such as serving as natural enemies of pests, crop pollinators, decomposers of organic waste, and agents of nutrient recycling, as well as in forensic investigations for solving criminal mysteries.

Due to the great economic value of flies, I have decided to produce a book exclusively devoted to them. Existing books on flies either emphasize their taxonomy and distribution records or their role as vectors for humans and livestock. This book has been planned with a holistic approach to highlight both the positive and negative aspects of flies. Furthermore, each chapter has been designed to contain Pointwise Learning Objectives at the beginning, and Conclusions and Points to Remember at the end. This approach makes this book user-friendly for both students and readers.

This book begins with a chapter on the introduction to flies, followed by insects of agricultural and horticultural importance, flies as vectors of human and veterinary diseases, and beneficial flies. This book will be quite useful not only to students in entomology, public health, agriculture, and applied life sciences but also to those involved in policy planning and vector management. In addition, this book will benefit students preparing for competitive examinations and the general public.

I am highly thankful to various specialists and academicians for kindly taking time from their routines to contribute to the chapters assigned to them. Most of the contributors, being senior specialists, are likely to provide their respective chapters with special emphasis on the topics they cover. I express my thanks to my team members Prof. Geetanjali Mishra, Dr. Tripti Yadav, Dr. Lata Verma, M/S Shriza Rai, Dipali Gupta, Md. Sariq, Sanjeev Kumar, Deeksha, Hera Alam, and Priya Yadav for their support in various ways. I am also thankful to my wife, Mrs. Kusum Upadhyay, for her silent sacrifice.

Omkar
Editor

About the Editor

Omkar, FNASc, is a professor with about 36 years of teaching experience and 44 years of research experience. He is a Former Head of the Department of Zoology at the University of Lucknow and Former Coordinator of UGC-SAP (DRS-II), DST-FIST, DST-PURSE, and Centre of Excellence programmes for the Government of UP. He has worked on ten additional projects funded by the state and central agencies. He specializes in environmental toxicology and entomology, particularly in insect pest management. He is the chief editor of the *Journal of Applied Bioscience*; associate editor of the *International Journal of Tropical Insect Science*, Springer; and president of the International Society of Applied Biology.

He has received several awards, including the Saraswati Samman from the Department of Higher Education, Government of UP; the Prof. T N Ananthakrishanan Foundation Award; the Rescholar Award of Excellence in Agricultural Entomology from the Association of Entomologists; the Prof. G. S. Shukla Gold Medal from The Academy of Environmental Biology; and the Dr. S. Pradhan Memorial Lecture Award from The Division of Entomology, Indian Agricultural Research Institute & The Entomological Society of India, New Delhi. He has also received the ACCLAIM and Uddeepan awards from the University of Lucknow. He is a Fellow of The Entomological Society of India, the Zoological Society of India, the Society for Biocontrol Advancement, and a Fellow of The National Academy of Sciences India (FNASc). He has authored 23 books and published 270 research papers, 12 reviews, 50 book chapters, and 17 popular science articles. He has guided 28 Ph.D. students. He visited the School of Biological Sciences at the University of East Anglia (2006) for 3 months and the Department of Zoology at the University of South Bohemia and the Czech Academy of Sciences, Ceske Budejovice, Czech Republic (May 2016) under INSA bilateral exchange programmes.

List of Contributors

Venkateshaiah Abhishek
Keladi Shivappa Nayaka University of Agricultural and Horticultural Sciences
Shivamogga, India

Meena Agnihotri
Department of Entomology
G.B. Pant University of Agriculture & Technology
Pantnagar, India

U. Amala
Division of Germplasm Conservation and Utilization
ICAR-National Bureau of Agricultural Insect Resources Bengaluru, India

Sanjay M. Bandi
Division of Crop Protection
ICAR-National Institute of Pulses Research
Kanpur, India

Hassan Beg
Department of Entomology
G.B. Pant University of Agriculture & Technology
Pantnagar, India

Anup Chandra
Division of Crop Protection
ICAR-National Institute of Pulses Research
Kanpur, India

Kailash Chandra
Zoological Survey of India
Kolkata, India
and
Mahagun Mezzaria
Noida, India

Keerthi Manikyanahalli Chandrashekara
Division of Crop Protection
ICAR-Indian Institute of Horticultural Research
Bengaluru, India

L. Rajesh Chowdary
Regional Agricultural Research Station, RARS
ANGRAU
Guntur, India

Mani Chellappan
Department of Entomology
College of Agriculture
Kerala Agricultural University
Thrissur, Kerala

Karamankodu Jacob David
Division of Genomic Resources
ICAR-National Bureau of Agriculturally Important Insect Resources
Bengaluru, India

Rajnni Dogra
Department of Entomology
GB Pant University of Agriculture, and Technology
Pantnagar, India

Giri Naga Harish
Agricultural Research Station, Darsi
Prakasan, India

Nandan Jana
Department of Zoology, Sreegopal Banerjee College, Calyptrate Research Centre
Hooghly, India

Jagdish Jaba
Entomology Unit
International Crops Research Institute for the Semi-Arid Tropics
Patancheru, India

Deepika Jeengar
Department of Entomology
GB Pant University of Agriculture, and Technology
Pantnagar, India

Radha Joshi
Department of Entomology
G.B. Pant University of Agriculture & Technology
Pantnagar, India

Ashok Kumar Karedla
Agricultural Research Station
Palnadu, India

Mareppa Hussani Kodandaram
Division of Crop Protection
ICAR-National Institute of Pulses Research
Kanpur, India

Jasti Sri Vishnu Murthy
Department of Entomology
College of Agriculture
Kerala Agricultural University
Thrissur, India

N. R. Noor Mahammed
ICAR-National Bureau of Agriculturally Important Insect Resources
Bengaluru, India

Ranjith Mohanrao
Central Integrated Pest Management Centre
Directorate of Plant Protection Quarantine and Storage
Bengaluru, India

Nishismita Parida
Department of Entomology
Shiksha 'O' Anusandhan (Deemed to be University)
Bhubaneshwar, India

Melur Ashwathappa Rashmi
Rashvee-International Phytosanitary Research and Services Pvt. Ltd.
Bengaluru, India

Ramya Ramesan Syamala
Division of Genomic Resources
ICAR-National Bureau of Agriculturally Important Insect Resources
Bengaluru, India

Revanasidda
Division of Crop Protection
ICAR-National Institute of Pulses Research
Kanpur, India

Shanthamma Salini
ICAR-National Bureau of Agriculturally Important Insect Resources
Bengaluru, India

Rajander S. Sharma
National Expert on Bio Pesticide
Absolute Human Care Foundation
Centre for Medical Entomology
UNIDO, NCDC
Delhi, India

T. M. Shivalingaswamy
Division of Germplasm Conservation and Utilization
ICAR-National Bureau of Agricultural Insect Resources Bengaluru, India

Shuvra Kanti Sinha
Department of Zoology
Calyptrate Research Centre
Sreegopal Banerjee College
Hooghly, India

Devinder Singh
Chandigarh University
Gharuan, India

Swoyam Singh
Department of Entomology
Shiksha 'O' Anusandhan (Deemed to be University)
Bhubaneshwar, India

S. K. Sinha
Department of Zoology
Sreegopal Banerjee College
Mogra, India

Gopalakrishnan Kesharivarmen Sujayanand
Division of Crop Protection
ICAR-National Institute of Pulses Research
Kanpur, India

Shivakumara Kadanakuppe Thammayya
Division of Genomic Resources
ICAR-National Bureau of Agriculturally Important Insect Resources
Bengaluru, India

Ranjith Matta Thodikayiland
Department of Entomology
College of Agriculture
Kerala Agricultural University
Thrissur, India

Naveena Unnikrishnan
Department of Entomology
College of Agriculture
Kerala Agricultural University
Thrissur, India

Vijay Veer
Golden Manor
Dehradun, India

H. S. Venu
Division of Germplasm Conservation and Utilization
ICAR-National Bureau of Agricultural Insect Resources Bengaluru, India

Abraham Verghese
Former Director
ICAR-National Bureau of Agriculturally Important Insect Resources
Bengaluru, India

Bhanvi Wadhawan
Department of Zoology
M. M. Modi College
Patiala, India

Flies: An Introduction

Omkar

LEARNING OBJECTIVES

1. To learn the basic morphology and life cycle of flies.
2. To understand the species diversity of flies.
3. To grasp the ecology and behaviour of flies.
4. To study the economic importance of flies.
5. To understand the measures of fly management.

INTRODUCTION

Flies belong to the order Diptera, which means "two wings" in Greek. They are one of the most diverse and abundant groups of insects on Earth, with over 150,000 described species. The hindwings of flies are reduced to small, knob-like structures called halteres, which function as gyroscopes for balance during flight.

Diptera is one of the largest orders of insects, encompassing a vast array of families, genera, and species. Some of the most common families include Muscidae (houseflies), Culicidae (mosquitoes), Calliphoridae (blowflies), and Drosophilidae (fruit flies). Each family exhibits unique morphological and behavioural characteristics. Flies vary greatly in size, ranging from minute species, like the fruit fly (*Drosophila melanogaster*) to larger ones, such as the robber fly (Asilidae) or the horse fly (Tabanidae). They come in various colours and patterns, often reflecting their habitats and behaviours.

The presence of only "two wings" on the mesothorax distinguishes them from other winged insects that possess four wings, with one pair of forewings on the mesothorax and one pair of hindwings on the metathorax. Flies are characterized by their two wings and remarkable agility in flight. From the common housefly to the delicate fruit fly, these insects are ubiquitous, found in nearly every corner of the globe. Despite their small size, flies have left a significant mark on both the natural world and human culture. Whether admired for their ecological contributions or detested for their pesky presence, these resilient insects continue to fascinate and intrigue scientists, writers, and curious minds alike.

In many cultures, flies have also found their way into folklore, symbolism, and even literature. They are often associated with themes of decay, transience, and impurity, reflecting their tendency to congregate around decaying matter. In the literature, flies have been used as metaphors for corruption, representing the fleeting nature of life or the presence of evil.

One of the most notable features of flies is their adaptability. They thrive in a wide range of environments, from urban settings to rural landscapes, and even inside our houses. Their ability to reproduce quickly ensures their continuous presence, often becoming a nuisance to humans during the warmer months.

Flies have diverse feeding habits. Many species are scavengers, feeding on decaying organic matter; others are predators (like robber flies), parasites (such as tsetse flies), or herbivores (like some fruit flies). Some species are also important pollinators. They are equipped with specialized mouthparts designed for different feeding habits. Some, like the housefly, have sponging mouthparts ideal for lapping up liquids, while others, such as horseflies, possess piercing-sucking mouthparts to feed on blood. This diversity in feeding strategies contributes to their ecological importance.

DOI: 10.1201/9781003482581-1

MORPHOLOGY

The morphology of flies, like that of all insects, is characterized by distinctive features that contribute to their remarkable diversity and ecological success. Some key aspects of fly morphology are given below:

Body segmentation: Flies, like other insects, have three main body segments: the head, thorax, and abdomen. These segments are often fused or specialized for specific functions. For example, the head houses sensory organs, such as compound eyes, antennae, and mouthparts, while the thorax contains the muscles responsible for flight and locomotion.

Head: The head of a fly is typically small and compact, bearing several important sensory structures. These include large compound eyes, which provide a wide field of vision and are composed of numerous individual units called ommatidia. Flies also possess simple eyes called ocelli, which detect changes in light intensity and aid in navigation. Antennae, located between the eyes, are used for detecting chemical cues, including those related to food, mates, and environmental conditions. The mouthparts of flies are adapted to their feeding habits and may be modified for piercing, sucking, sponging, or lapping.

Thorax: The thorax is divided into three segments: the prothorax, mesothorax, and metathorax. Each segment bears a pair of legs, one on either side of the body, resulting in a total of six legs, each typically ending in a clawed footpad that aids in gripping surfaces. The mesothorax bears a pair of wings, while the metathorax bears a pair of reduced wings, called halteres, giving flies their characteristic ability to fly. In addition to wings and legs, the thorax also contains muscles that power flight and locomotion. The wings of flies are membranous structures supported by a network of veins. They are typically transparent or translucent and may be modified in shape and size depending on the species. In some flies, such as mosquitoes and black flies, the wings are adapted for flight over long distances, while in others, such as hoverflies, the wings may be modified for hovering or rapid manoeuvring.

Abdomen: The abdomen of a fly is usually elongated and composed of multiple segments. It contains internal organs, such as the digestive, reproductive, and respiratory systems. In females, the abdomen may also contain specialized structures for egg production and oviposition.

Flies exhibit a wide range of external features that vary depending on the species and ecological niche. These may include bristles, hairs, spines, or other structures used for sensory perception, defence, or communication. For example, some flies have conspicuous bristles on their legs or body, which may aid in detecting vibrations or airborne stimuli.

From a scientific perspective, flies have been subjects of extensive research, particularly the fruit fly, *Drosophila melanogaster*. Its other species and mutants have become model organisms in genetics and developmental biology. Its short lifespan, rapid reproduction, and well-understood genetics make it an invaluable tool for studying various biological processes.

LIFE CYCLE

Flies undergo complete metamorphosis, consisting of four stages: egg, larva, pupa, and adult. The duration of each stage varies depending on factors such as species, environmental conditions, and food availability. The egg stage lasts a few days, after which larvae hatch and begin feeding. Larvae undergo several moults as they grow, eventually entering the pupal stage, during which they undergo metamorphosis into adults. The entire life cycle can range from a few days to several weeks, depending on species and environmental factors.

1. **Egg stage**: Female flies lay eggs in suitable habitats, which vary depending on the species. For example, houseflies may lay eggs in decaying organic matter, while fruit flies lay eggs on ripe fruits. The number of eggs laid by a female fly can vary widely, ranging from just a few to hundreds or even thousands, depending on factors such as species, environmental conditions, and availability of resources. The eggs are typically small and oval shaped, and they may be deposited singly or in clusters, depending on the species and habitat.
2. **Larval stage (maggot)**: Upon hatching from the eggs, larvae emerge and begin feeding on organic matter in their environment. The larvae of flies are commonly referred to as maggots. Fly larvae exhibit a diverse range of feeding habits depending on the species. Some are scavengers, feeding on decaying organic matter, while others are predators or parasites. As larvae grow, they undergo several moults, shedding their exoskeleton to accommodate their increasing size. The duration of the larval stage varies depending on factors such as species, temperature, and food availability. Larvae are often highly mobile and may actively move within their environment in search of food or suitable pupation sites.
3. **Pupal stage**: When larvae complete their growth and development, they typically enter the pupal stage, during which they undergo metamorphosis into adult flies. This stage is characterized by the formation of a protective outer covering called a puparium, which encases the developing fly. The puparium may be soft and membranous or hard and sclerotized, depending on the species. Inside the puparium, the larval tissues undergo a process of reorganization and differentiation, leading to the formation of adult structures. The duration of the pupal stage varies widely among different fly species, ranging from a few days to several weeks, depending on factors such as species, temperature, and environmental conditions.
4. **Adult stage**: After completing metamorphosis, the adult fly emerges from the puparium and begins its brief adult life. Adult flies are typically sexually mature and capable of reproduction shortly after emergence. The primary function of adult flies is to mate and reproduce, although they may also feed on various food sources, depending on the species. The lifespan of adult flies varies greatly among different species, ranging from a few days to several weeks or even months, depending on factors such as species, environmental conditions, and availability of resources.

SPECIES DIVERSITY

There are thousands of species of flies, each with its own unique characteristics, behaviours, and ecological roles. Some common types of flies are outlined below:

1. **Houseflies (*Musca domestica*)**: Houseflies are one of the most common and widespread fly species found worldwide. While they play a role in nutrient recycling by feeding on decaying organic matter, they are significant vectors in human environments due to their potential to spread diseases. Houseflies can transmit pathogens such as bacteria, viruses, and parasites that cause diseases such as cholera, dysentery, and food poisoning.
2. **Fruit flies (*Drosophila* spp.)**: Fruit flies are small flies that are often found near ripe or fermenting fruits and vegetables. While they are not generally harmful to humans, they can be nuisance pests in houses and commercial settings. In scientific research, particularly in genetics and developmental biology, the fruit fly *Drosophila melanogaster* is a widely used model organism due to its short lifespan, rapid reproduction, and well-understood genetics.
3. **Blowflies (Calliphoridae)**: Blowflies are known for their metallic blue or green colouration and are often associated with decomposing organic matter, including carrion and dung. While their larvae play an essential role in decomposition and nutrient recycling, blowflies are also significant in forensic entomology. The presence and development of

blowfly larvae on a corpse can provide valuable information to forensic investigators about the time and location of death.

4. **Mosquitoes (Culicidae)**: Mosquitoes are well-known vectors of diseases such as malaria, dengue fever, Zika virus, and West Nile virus. Female mosquitoes require blood meals for egg production, and in the process, they can transmit pathogens to humans and animals. Mosquito control efforts are essential for preventing the spread of mosquito-borne diseases and for protecting public health.
5. **Hoverflies (Syrphidae)**: Hoverflies are important crop pollinators, often resembling bees due to their yellow and black striped markings. They visit flowers to feed on nectar and pollen, inadvertently transferring pollen between flowers and facilitating pollination. Hoverflies play a valuable role in agricultural ecosystems through their pollination services, contributing to the reproduction of many flowering plants and agricultural crops.
6. **Stable flies (*Stomoxys calcitrans*)**: Stable flies are biting flies that feed on the blood of livestock, including cattle, horses, and poultry. Their bites can cause irritation, blood loss, and reduced productivity in livestock. Stable flies are significant pests in agricultural settings, particularly in livestock production facilities, where they cause economic losses and impair animal welfare.
7. **Black flies (Simuliidae)**: Black flies are small, blood-feeding insects that are notorious pests in many regions of the world. While the bites themselves are painful and irritating, black flies are of particular significance due to their potential role as vectors of diseases such as river blindness (onchocerciasis) and various types of filariasis. In areas where these diseases are endemic, black flies can pose significant public health challenges.
8. **Horseflies and Deerflies (Tabanidae)**: Horseflies and deerflies are large, robust flies known for their painful bites, which they inflict on mammals, including humans, as well as birds. While their bites are primarily a nuisance and can cause discomfort, these flies are also vectors of pathogens such as viruses and protozoa. Additionally, their feeding behaviour can negatively impact livestock and wildlife, leading to reduced productivity and potential health issues.
9. **Gnats (Psychodidae and Ceratopogonidae)**: Gnats are small, non-biting flies that are commonly found near bodies of water, damp soil, and decaying organic matter. While many species of gnats are harmless, some biting midges (Ceratopogonidae) can be significant pests, causing painful bites and skin irritation. Certain species of gnats are known to transmit diseases such as leishmaniasis and Oropouche fever, posing public health concerns in some regions.
10. **Tsetse flies (Glossinidae)**: Tsetse flies are blood-feeding insects found in sub-Saharan Africa, where they are notorious as vectors of African trypanosomiasis, also known as sleeping sickness. The parasites transmitted by tsetse flies infect humans and animals, causing a range of symptoms from fever and fatigue to neurological complications and death. African trypanosomiasis is a significant public health issue in affected regions, impacting human health, agriculture, and economic development.
11. **Sand flies (Psychodidae)**: Sand flies are small, blood-feeding insects found in sandy habitats and are known for their role as vectors of diseases such as leishmaniasis. Leishmaniasis is caused by parasites of the genus *Leishmania*, which are transmitted to humans and animals through the bites of infected sand flies. The disease can manifest in various forms, including cutaneous, mucocutaneous, and visceral leishmaniasis, posing significant public health challenges in many parts of the world.
12. **Flesh flies (Sarcophagidae)**: Flesh flies are commonly found around decaying organic matter, including carrion, faeces, and compost. While they primarily feed on decaying material as adults, their larvae are significant scavengers, aiding in the decomposition process. In forensic entomology, flesh flies play a role in the decomposition of cadavers and

can provide valuable information to forensic investigators about the time and location of death.

13. **Dance flies (Empididae)**: Dance flies are a diverse group of flies known for their distinctive mating behaviour, which involves males presenting females with gifts such as prey items or saliva droplets during courtship. While dance flies are not typically considered pests or disease vectors, their mating behaviour and reproductive biology make them of interest to researchers studying sexual selection and mate choice in insects.
14. **Robber flies (Asilidae)**: Robber flies are predatory insects known for their aggressive hunting behaviour. They are formidable predators of other insects, including flies, bees, and beetles, which they capture in flight or ambush on vegetation. Robber flies are beneficial in agricultural ecosystems as natural enemies of pest insects, helping to regulate populations of potentially damaging species.
15. **Moth flies (Psychodidae)**: Moth flies, also known as drain flies or sewer flies, are small, hairy flies commonly found in damp, humid environments, such as drains, sewage systems, and compost piles. While they are primarily nuisance pests, their presence in indoor environments indicates plumbing or sanitation issues. Moth flies are not known to transmit diseases to humans but can cause annoyance due to their swarming behaviour.
16. **Soldier flies (Stratiomyidae)**: Soldier flies are medium to large-sized flies known for their distinctive appearance, with metallic colours and prominent bristles on their bodies. While adult soldier flies feed on nectar and pollen, their larvae play important roles as decomposers and recyclers of organic matter. Soldier fly larvae are efficient composters and are being explored as a sustainable solution for organic waste management and nutrient recycling.
17. **March flies (Bibionidae)**: March flies are medium-sized flies, commonly found in grassy and wooded habitats. While they are not typically considered pests, certain species of March flies can be significant agricultural pests, particularly in their larval stage. March fly larvae feed on plant roots, causing damage to crops, such as grasses, cereals, and ornamental plants.
18. **Midge flies (Chironomidae)**: Midge flies, also known as non-biting midges, are small flies commonly found near bodies of water, including lakes, ponds, and streams. While most midge species are harmless, their larvae play essential roles in aquatic ecosystems as detritivores, feeding on decaying organic matter and contributing to nutrient cycling. In large numbers, midge flies emerge in swarms, which can be a nuisance to humans, particularly in coastal areas.
19. **Fungus gnats (Sciaridae and Mycetophilidae)**: Fungus gnats are small flies commonly found in damp environments such as soil, compost, and decaying plant material. While adult fungus gnats are primarily nuisance pests and do not bite, their larvae feed on fungi, organic matter, and plant roots. In some cases, fungus gnat larvae can cause damage to the roots of plants, particularly in greenhouse settings or indoor plantings.

ECOLOGY AND BEHAVIOUR

Understanding the biology, behaviour, and ecological roles of flies is essential for effective pest management, disease control, and conservation efforts. By studying these fascinating insects, researchers gain insight into fundamental biological processes, ecological interactions, and the dynamics of natural ecosystems. Some key aspects of the ecology and behaviour of flies are as follows:

1. **Feeding behaviour**: Flies exhibit a diverse range of feeding habits, reflecting their adaptation to various ecological niches. Many species are scavengers, feeding on decaying organic matter, faeces, or carrion. Others are herbivores, feeding on plant material such as sap, nectar, or fruit. Some flies are predators, preying on smaller insects, while others are parasitic, feeding on the blood or bodily fluids of vertebrates or other invertebrates.

The diversity of feeding habits within the order Diptera contributes to their ecological importance and impact on ecosystems. House flies (*Musca domestica*), for example, feed on decaying organic matter and are important decomposers, while fruit flies (*Drosophila* spp.) are often found on fermenting fruits.

2. **Communication and aggregation**: Flies communicate and perceive their environment using a combination of visual, olfactory, and tactile cues. Their compound eyes provide a wide field of view, allowing them to detect movement and navigate their surroundings. Flies also have specialized sensory structures, such as antennae and mouthparts, which enable them to detect chemical signals, locate food sources, and communicate with conspecifics. Flies may use auditory signals, such as wing vibrations or buzzing sounds, for communication or mate attraction.

   Flies often exhibit aggregation behaviour, gathering in large numbers in specific locations where resources such as food, water, or suitable breeding sites are abundant. This aggregation behaviour can vary depending on the species and environmental conditions. For example, houseflies may congregate around decaying organic matter, while fruit flies may gather around ripe fruits. Aggregation sites can serve as focal points for communication among flies, allowing them to exchange information about food sources, mating opportunities, and environmental conditions.
3. **Migration**: Some fly species are known for their impressive migratory behaviour, travelling long distances in search of suitable breeding or feeding sites. For example, the annual migration of the monarch butterfly (*Danaus plexippus*) spans thousands of kilometres. Similarly, certain species of hoverflies (family Syrphidae) undertake extensive migrations to avoid unfavourable conditions or exploit seasonal resources.
4. **Ecological Interactions**: Flies interact with various organisms within their ecosystems. They serve as pollinators for many flowering plants, including some important agricultural crops. Additionally, flies play roles as both predators and prey in food webs, contributing to the regulation of insect populations. Some species also have mutualistic relationships with other organisms, such as certain parasitic wasps that use flies as hosts for their larvae.

   While flies may not exhibit the same complex social structures as some other animals, they do engage in various forms of social behaviour that influence their ecology, reproduction, and interactions with other species, including humans. Flies have significant social and cultural implications for humans, often eliciting strong reactions ranging from fascination to disgust. As vectors of disease and pests of agriculture and livestock, flies can profoundly impact human health, food security, and economic well-being. Additionally, flies have inspired various cultural beliefs, superstitions, and artistic representations throughout history. In literature, art, and popular culture, flies have been used as symbols of decay, transience, and the fragility of life, reflecting their ubiquitous presence and association with death and decomposition.
5. **Role in disease transmission**: While many flies are harmless or even beneficial, some species are vectors of diseases affecting humans, livestock, and wildlife. Mosquitoes (family Culicidae), for example, are infamous for transmitting diseases such as malaria, dengue fever, and the Zika virus. Tsetse flies (genus *Glossina*) are vectors of African trypanosomiasis (sleeping sickness), which affects both humans and animals.
6. **Reproductive behaviour**: Many fly species exhibit elaborate courtship rituals involving visual, auditory, or chemical cues to attract mates.

Like many insects, flies engage in complex mating behaviours that involve communication, courtship rituals, and mate selection. Male flies may use visual, olfactory, and auditory cues to attract females and compete with rival males for mating opportunities. Some fly species engage in elaborate courtship displays, which may include wing movements, pheromone release, or other behaviours designed to impress potential mates. Mating behaviour in flies can be influenced by factors such as population density, resource availability, and environmental conditions. Reproductive behaviour varies among species, with some laying eggs on specific substrates, such as rotting fruit or dung, while others lay eggs directly on or inside host organisms.

Flies communicate through a variety of sensory modalities. Visual cues, such as body movements and colour patterns, play a significant role in courtship and mate recognition. Chemical signals, including pheromones, are also important for attracting mates, marking territories, and identifying suitable oviposition sites.

OVIPOSITION BEHAVIOUR

Oviposition behaviour, or egg-laying behaviour, is a critical aspect of the reproductive ecology of flies. The oviposition process involves the selection of suitable substrates for egg deposition, ensuring the survival and development of the offspring. Some key points on the oviposition behaviour of flies are given below:

1. **Substrate selection**: Different fly species exhibit preferences for specific substrates on which to lay their eggs. These substrates can vary widely and may include decaying organic matter, animal faeces, plant material, carrion, soil, or even living organisms. The choice of substrate is influenced by factors such as nutrient availability, moisture levels, temperature, and the presence of competing or predatory organisms.
2. **Physical characteristics**: The physical characteristics of the substrate play a role in oviposition site selection. Flies may prefer substrates with specific textures, moisture levels, or microbial communities that are conducive to larval development. Some species may also exhibit preferences for ovipositing in shaded or sheltered locations to protect eggs from desiccation or predation.
3. **Chemical cues**: Flies often rely on chemical cues to identify suitable oviposition sites. These cues may include volatile organic compounds released by decomposing organic matter, microbial metabolites, or specific chemicals associated with host organisms. Female flies use their sense of smell to detect these cues and locate appropriate egg-laying sites.
4. **Egg-laying behaviour**: The oviposition behaviour of flies can vary depending on the species and environmental conditions. Some species deposit eggs individually or in small clusters, while others may lay eggs in large masses or egg rafts. Female flies may use specialized structures, such as ovipositors or egg-laying appendages, to insert eggs into the substrate. Oviposition may occur rapidly and repeatedly, with females depositing multiple batches of eggs over their lifespan.
5. **Parental care**: In some fly species, females exhibit varying degrees of parental care following oviposition. This may include guarding the eggs or providing provisions for the developing larvae. In parasitic fly species, females may deposit eggs directly onto or inside host organisms, ensuring that the larvae have access to suitable resources for development.

   While flies are not typically known for extensive parental care, some species exhibit interesting reproductive strategies that involve interactions between parents and offspring. For example, certain species of hoverflies lay their eggs near aphid colonies, where the hatched larvae feed on aphids, providing indirect protection and nutrition for their offspring. In some cases, female flies may choose oviposition sites based on factors such as food availability, substrate suitability, or predator avoidance, demonstrating a form of parental investment in offspring survival.
6. **Competition and predation**: Ovipositing flies may face competition from other individuals of the same or different species vying for access to limited resources. Eggs and newly hatched larvae are vulnerable to predation by predators, such as ants, beetles, or other insects. Some fly species have evolved strategies to minimize predation risk, such as

selecting cryptic oviposition sites or synchronizing egg-laying with periods of low predation pressure.

By studying the factors influencing oviposition site selection and the mechanisms underlying egg-laying behaviour, researchers can develop strategies to manipulate fly populations, mitigate pest damage, and conserve important habitat.

SEASONAL BEHAVIOUR

Flies exhibit seasonal patterns in their activity and abundance. These patterns are often influenced by factors such as temperature, humidity, daylight length, and food availability. Different species of flies may have varying responses to these environmental cues. A general overview of how seasonality affects flies is given below:

1. **Temperature**: Flies are cold-blooded creatures, so their activity levels tend to increase as temperatures rise. In temperate regions, this often means that fly populations peak during warmer months, such as spring and summer, and decline during colder months, like autumn and winter. However, in tropical regions where temperatures are relatively constant throughout the year, fly may not show as pronounced seasonal fluctuations.
2. **Humidity**: Flies, particularly those like fruit flies, are attracted to moist environments. High humidity levels provide suitable conditions for fly breeding and development. Therefore, seasons with higher humidity, such as spring and summer, may see increased fly activity compared to drier seasons.
3. **Daylight length**: Day length also influences the behaviour of flies. Many species are diurnal, meaning they are most active during the day. Longer daylight hours in spring and summer can result in increased activity levels and breeding opportunities for flies.
4. **Food availability**: Flies are attracted to decaying organic matter, faeces, fruits, and other food sources. Seasonal fluctuations in food availability affect the fly populations. For example, ripe fruits and vegetables in the summer can attract more fruit flies, while decaying organic matter in autumn may attract other types of flies.
5. **Breeding cycles**: Some fly species have specific breeding cycles that are tied to seasonal changes. For instance, certain species may lay eggs in spring or summer when temperatures are optimal for larval development, leading to population booms during these seasons.
6. **Migration**: Some fly species exhibit migratory behaviour, moving to different regions in response to changing seasons. This may influence the local abundance of flies in particular areas.

ECONOMIC IMPORTANCE

The economic importance of flies encompasses both positive and negative aspects, depending on their ecological roles and interactions with human activities. The economic significance of flies is given below:

1. **Pollination**: Certain fly species, such as hoverflies and bee flies, play a crucial role as pollinators. They visit flowers to feed on nectar and pollen, inadvertently transferring pollen between flowers, thereby facilitating fertilization and fruit production. This pollination service is vital for the reproduction of many flowering plants, including numerous agricultural crops, such as fruits, vegetables, and oilseed crops. Consequently, flies contribute significantly to agricultural productivity and food security.
2. **Decomposition and nutrient cycling**: Flies, particularly those with larvae that feed on decaying organic matter, are essential contributors to the process of decomposition. They help break down dead animals, plant debris, and other organic materials, accelerating the

recycling of nutrients back into the soil. This decomposition process is critical for maintaining soil fertility and ecosystem health, as it releases essential nutrients that can be utilized by plants for growth. Thus, flies indirectly support agricultural productivity and nutrient cycling in ecosystems.

3. **Biological control**: Some fly species are natural enemies of agricultural pests and can be utilized as biological control agents to manage pest populations. For example, certain parasitic flies lay their eggs on or inside pest insects, such as aphids or caterpillars, leading to the death of the host as the fly larvae develop. Certain hoverflies are predators of aphids and other small, soft-bodied insects. By targeting pest species, these natural enemies help reduce the need for chemical pesticides, thereby lowering production costs and minimizing environmental impacts.
4. **Disease transmission**: Unfortunately, flies also pose significant economic risks as vectors of diseases. Mosquitoes are the primary disease vectors, spreading several dreaded diseases in humans. Houseflies, for instance, are notorious for transmitting pathogens, such as bacteria, viruses, and parasites that cause diseases in humans and livestock. These diseases include foodborne illnesses, such as salmonellosis and dysentery, as well as serious health threats like cholera and typhoid fever. The economic impact of fly-borne diseases includes healthcare costs, lost productivity, and potential damage to livestock industries.
5. **Nuisance and losses in livestock production**: Flies cause economic losses in livestock production by annoying animals, reducing feed intake, and transmitting diseases. For example, stable flies and horn flies are common pests of cattle, causing irritation, blood loss, and decreased milk production. Additionally, certain fly species, such as the screwworm fly, cause severe damage to livestock through their parasitic larvae, which feed on living tissue, leading to economic losses in the meat and dairy industries.
6. **Costs of pest control**: Controlling fly populations in agricultural, residential, and commercial settings can incur significant costs. Integrated pest management (IPM) strategies may involve the use of insecticides, traps, sanitation practices, and biological control agents to manage fly populations effectively. These control measures require financial investments, labour, and ongoing monitoring efforts to mitigate the economic impacts of fly infestations.
7. **Scientific research**: Flies, particularly the fruit fly *Drosophila melanogaster*, have been instrumental in advancing scientific knowledge in fields such as genetics, developmental biology, and neuroscience. *Drosophila*, in particular, has served as a model organism for studying fundamental biological processes, including inheritance, gene expression, and behaviour.

FORENSIC VALUE OF FLIES

Flies, particularly blowflies (Calliphoridae), hold significant forensic importance due to their predictable life cycles and behaviours. The key forensic aspects of flies are provided below:

1. **Post-mortem interval (PMI) estimation**: Flies are among the first insects to colonize a decomposing body, often within minutes to hours after death. By studying the succession of fly species and their developmental stages on a corpse, forensic entomologists can estimate the time since death, known as the PMI. This estimation relies on the predictable patterns of succession and development exhibited by different fly species under varying environmental conditions.
2. **Species identification**: Different fly species have distinct preferences for colonizing decomposing remains, and their presence provides valuable information for forensic investigations. Forensic entomologists can identify the species of flies collected from a crime

scene or a decomposing body to infer details such as the geographical origin of the body, the season of death, and potential environmental conditions at the time of colonization.
3. **Life cycle studies**: Flies undergo predictable developmental stages, from egg to larva (maggot), pupa, and adult. Forensic entomologists study the developmental rates of fly larvae under controlled laboratory conditions to establish temperature-dependent growth models, known as thermal summation or accumulated degree-hour models. These models allow for a more accurate estimation of PMI based on ambient temperature data collected from the crime scene.
4. **Forensic entomotoxicology**: Flies serve as bioindicators of drug or toxin exposure in decomposing remains. By analysing the tissues of fly larvae for the presence of drugs, toxins, or heavy metals, forensic scientists can provide valuable evidence of substance abuse, poisoning, or environmental contamination. This branch can contribute to criminal investigations and provide insights into the circumstances surrounding death.
5. **Case investigations**: Flies and their life stages are commonly encountered in forensic investigations involving human remains, including homicides, suicides, accidents, and mass disasters. By analysing the entomological evidence collected from crime scenes or decomposing bodies, forensic entomologists can reconstruct the sequence of events leading to death, corroborate other evidence, and provide valuable insights into the circumstances surrounding the incident.
6. **Legal significance**: Entomological evidence, including data on fly colonization patterns, developmental stages, and species identification, can have significant legal implications in criminal trials. Forensic entomologists may be called upon to testify as expert witnesses to explain the relevance of entomological evidence, the methodologies used for analysis, and the conclusions drawn regarding PMI estimation and other aspects of the case.

Flies play a crucial role in forensic investigations by providing valuable evidence for estimating PMI, identifying the geographical origin of decomposing remains, detecting drug or toxin exposure, and reconstructing the events surrounding death.

MANAGEMENT OF FLIES

Managing flies, whether in agricultural, residential, or commercial settings, often requires a comprehensive approach that combines multiple strategies to effectively control populations and minimize their impact on human health, livestock, and the environment. The key management techniques for controlling fly populations are provided below:

1. **Education and awareness**: Educating occupants of residential or commercial properties about the importance of sanitation practices, fly biology, and prevention methods can help foster proactive participation in fly management efforts. Providing information on proper waste management, food storage, and exclusion techniques can empower individuals to contribute effectively to fly control efforts.

   By employing a combination of these management strategies tailored to specific environments and circumstances, it is possible to mitigate fly populations and minimize their impact on human health, agriculture, and the environment. Regular monitoring, adaptation of control measures, and collaboration between stakeholders are essential components of successful fly management programmes.
2. **Sanitation practices**: Proper sanitation is fundamental to fly management. Eliminating or reducing breeding sites and food sources can significantly limit fly populations. This includes
   a. Prompt removal and disposal of decaying organic matter, such as garbage, compost, or animal waste.

   b. Regular cleaning of trash receptacles, dumpsters, and other areas where organic waste accumulates.
   c. Proper storage of food and waste in sealed containers to prevent access by flies.
   d. Cleaning up spilled food or liquids promptly to eliminate attractants for flies.
3. **Exclusion measures:** Preventing flies from entering buildings or enclosed spaces is key to reducing indoor infestations. This can be achieved through
   a. Installing and maintaining window screens and door sweeps to prevent entry.
   b. Sealing cracks, gaps, and other entrypoints where flies may gain access to buildings.
   c. Using air curtains or fans at entry ways to create barriers against flying insects.
4. **Physical control:** Physical methods can help reduce fly populations by directly removing or trapping adult flies. Examples include
   a. Using fly swatters or electronic fly zappers to kill adult flies indoors.
   b. Employing sticky traps or fly paper to capture flies in specific areas.
   c. Deploying fly traps baited with attractants, such as food or pheromones, to lure and trap flies.
5. **Chemical control:** Insecticides may be necessary in some situations to control fly populations, especially in cases of severe infestations. It is important to use insecticides judiciously and according to label instructions to minimize risks to humans, animals, and the environment. Some considerations include
   a. Choosing insecticides specifically labelled for fly control and selecting products with minimal environmental impact.
   b. Applying insecticides as directed, targeting areas where flies rest, breed, or congregate.
   c. Rotating between different classes of insecticides to reduce the risk of resistance development in fly populations.
6. **Biological control:** Biological control involves using natural enemies of flies to reduce populations. This can include
   a. Introducing predatory or parasitic insects that feed on fly eggs, larvae, or adults.
   b. Encouraging the presence of natural predators, such as birds, spiders, or predatory insects, in outdoor environments.
   c. Employing microbial agents, such as certain bacteria or fungi, that target fly larvae or pupae.
7. **IPM:** IPM combines multiple control tactics to manage flies effectively while minimizing reliance on chemical insecticides. A holistic IPM approach may include
   a. Regular monitoring of fly populations to assess infestation levels and identify contributing factors.
   b. Implementing cultural, physical, and biological control measures as primary interventions.
   c. Chemicals may be used as a supplementary tactic when other methods are insufficient or when flies pose significant health or economic risks.

CONCLUSION

Their body is typically divided into head, thorax, and abdomen. The head possesses a pair of antennae and siphoning or piercing and sucking mouthparts. They are holometabolous insects, meaning they undergo four stages: egg, larva, pupa, and adult. More than 1,50,000 species of dipterans have been described. Besides transmitting disease-causing organisms from host to host, they also cause damage to our crop plants, and some of them act as biocontrol agents as parasitoids and predators. Their feeding, reproductive, and ovipositional behaviour has been described, in addition to their communication, migration, disease transmission, seasonal behaviour, and role in crop pollination, environmental cleaning, and decomposition. Various measures of their management have also been described.

POINTS TO REMEMBER

1. Flies belong to the insect order Diptera and possess only one pair of forewings.
2. Hindwings are reduced to a spoon-like structure called halteres, which help maintain balance during flight.
3. Over 150,000 species have been described so far.
4. They possess sponging mouthparts ideal for feeding on liquids, for example, houseflies, or piercing and sucking mouthparts, as in horseflies and mosquitoes.
5. They have diverse feeding habits; some feed on decaying organic matter, others are predators like robber flies, some are parasites like tsetse flies, and others are herbivorous like fruit flies.
6. They are holometabolous insects, meaning they undergo four life stages: egg, larva, pupa, and adult.
7. Flies communicate and perceive their environment using a combination of visual, olfactory, and tactile cues.
8. Some fly species are known for their impressive migratory behaviour, travelling long distances for feeding and reproduction.
9. Flies serve as pollinators for some important agricultural crops.
10. Some other herbivorous species act as crop pests.
11. They function as prey and predators in food webs, contributing to the regulation of insect populations. Thus, they can be used in the biocontrol of insects.
12. Some dipterans serve as vectors of diseases.
13. Many flies exhibit elaborate courtship rituals involving visual, auditory and chemical cues.
14. Different fly species have preferences for specific substrates for oviposition.
15. Flies exhibit seasonal patterns in their activity and abundance.
16. Scavenger flies that feed on decaying organic matter contribute to the process of decomposition.
17. Flies cause economic losses in livestock production by annoying animals and transmitting diseases.
18. They play a significant role in scientific advancements and in forensic science.

Section I

Flies as Agricultural and Horticultural Pests

1 Fly Pests of Cereals

Swoyam Singh, Rajnni Dogra, Deepika Jeengar, and Nishismita Parida

LEARNING OBJECTIVES

1. A detailed description of the morphology of each developmental stage, *viz*., egg, larva, pupa, and adult stages of rice gall midge, rice whorl maggot, and sorghum shoot fly
2. Understanding the behaviour of rice gall midge, whorl maggot, and sorghum shoot fly
3. Studying the ecological preferences and habitats of rice gall midge, whorl maggot, and sorghum shoot fly
4. Learning the seasonal occurrence, life cycle, and population dynamics of the above insects
5. The feeding mechanisms of the insect pests on rice plants and the resultant symptoms produced on the host plant
6. Identification of the most successful integrated pest management (IPM) module including cultural, biological, physical, mechanical, host plant resistance and chemical management methods
7. Proper planning and synchronization of different IPM tools for best management.

1.1 INTRODUCTION

Rice and sorghum are two major cereal crops that nourish more than half of the world's population. They are the major source of carbohydrates for more than 90% of the world (Kumar et al., 2012; Desta and Yeshitila, 2024). Both crops are grown on a large scale in South Asian and African countries (Srinivasa et al., 2014; Singh and Tiwari, 2021). The major limiting factor to the production of these cereals is insect pests. Rice and sorghum are reported to be attacked by more than 150 insect pests belonging to various orders, such as Lepidoptera, Coleoptera, Hemiptera, and Thysanoptera (Ul Ane and Hussain, 2015; Okosun et al., 2021), which cause 25% and 30% yield loss in rice and sorghum, respectively (Dhaliwal et al., 2015). However, the literature concerning the damage, symptoms, and management of dipteran pests of sorghum and rice is scarce. Hence, this chapter explores the life cycle, the nature of the damage, the ecological impact, and the strategies for mitigating the major dipteran flies causing economic damage to sorghum and rice.

1.2 PADDY GALL FLY: *ORSEOLIA ORYZAE* (WOOD-MANSON, 1889) (CECIDOMYIIDAE: DIPTERA)

1.2.1 Systematic Position

Phylum – Arthropoda
Class – Insecta
Order – Diptera
Family – Cecidomyiidae
Genus – *Orseolia*
Species – *oryzae*

DOI: 10.1201/9781003482581-3

1.2.2 Distribution

Gall midges primarily affect tropical agriculture as pests of cultivated plants. The rice gall midge (*Orseolia oryzae*) is found mostly in Asian countries that grow rice, especially in Bangladesh, Vietnam, Thailand, India, China, and the Philippines, as the environmental conditions in these areas are ideal for the pest's growth and dissemination (Cramer, 1967). It is also documented in other rice-growing regions of the world, including Europe (Italy), South America (Brazil and Colombia), Malaysia, and Africa (Tanzania, and Uganda). Damage to rice from the gall midge has been reported in different rice-growing areas of Asia, such as China (Lai et al., 1984), India (Kalode and Bentur, 1989), Laos (Inthavong, 2004), Cambodia (Jahn and Bunnarith, 2004), and Thailand (Tayathum et al., 2004).

1.2.3 Identification of Pest

Identifying the rice gall midge (*O. oryzae*) usually entails noticing specific traits:

Egg: The female lays an average of 200 eggs (Wong et al., 1956). The eggs are tiny, elongated, cylindrical, shiny, and whitish or reddish in colour. The eggs laid by the fly are difficult to discern without magnification (Figure 1.1a).

Larvae: With a pointed front/anterior end, the full-grown larvae are pale red (Figure 1.1b), measuring 1 mm in length with 13 distinctly divided segments (Huang, 1957). The larvae are spindle-shaped, bearing two kidney-like spots dorsally on the second body segment (Rajamani et al., 2004).

Pupae: The pupa bears a series of strongly chitinized cephalic horns that bifurcate into a pair of spines pointing backwards (Figure 1.1c). The abdomen of the male pupa is shorter, and the posterior extension of the legs and claspers are visible through the pupal skin at the posterior end of the abdomen, which helps to differentiate it from the female pupa (Perera and Fernando, 1968).

Adult: Adult rice gall midges emerge from the pupa by bursting its skin. The midge crawls out, dries its wings, hangs on to the pupal skin, flies to neighbouring rice plants, mates, and resumes the cycle. The length of an adult rice gall midge is only 1–2 mm (Figure 1.1d). They have transparent wings and a reddish-brown or orange appearance, resembling a mosquito. The male is ash grey. Their bodies are elongated, including long, thin legs and antennae (Joshi et al., 1983).

1.2.4 Life Cycle of Gall Midge

In various grasses, wild rice, regenerated rice plants, and rice stubble, *O. oryzae* larvae overwinter. In the spring, overwintered larvae emerge and mature into pupae and adults. A few midge generations can grow on wild hosts before migrating to cultivated rice. Adult midges typically feed

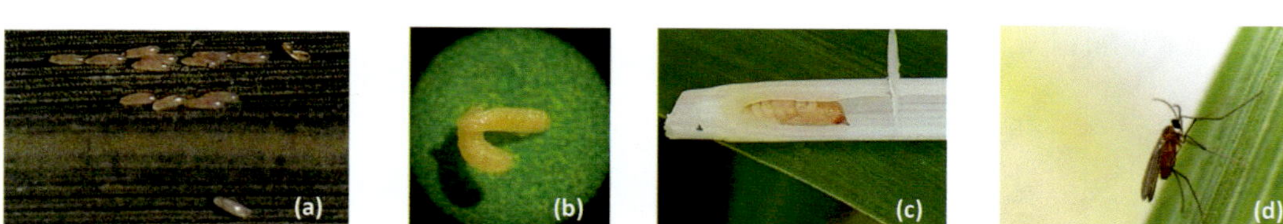

FIGURE 1.1 (a) Eggs, (b) maggots, (c) pupa, and (d) adult of *O. oryzae*.

at night. Males typically emerge between 18:00 and 20:00, while females emerge between 20:00 and 24:00 hours (Rajamani et al., 2004). Mating occurs immediately. While females mate only once, males can mate several times (Wong et al., 1956).

The females lay eggs individually or in clusters of 3–4 on the rice plants, especially on the undersides of the leaf blades, stems, sheaths, base of the plant, leaf ligules, and sometimes even on standing water (Reddy, 1967). The incubation period for the egg stage is 2–4 days at 24°C–35°C (Pathak, 1994).

Upon hatching, the juvenile larvae emerge and move to the shoots, originating from auxiliary buds, consuming the internal tissues of the rice plant. They are believed to secrete a growth hormone while lacerating the plant's apical meristem, which leads to the formation of galls (Sy, 1978). The larva takes 15–20 days to undergo two moults and complete its larval period (Figure 1.2).

After feeding, the larva pupates inside the developed gall (Reddy, 1967). While transforming into a midge, the pupa uses its antennal horn to slither up the gall tube and reach the tip of the silver shoot. It then cuts the tip of the silver shoot to mark its exit. After cutting the tip of the silver shoot, the pupal skin bursts, leading to the emergence of the midge (Fernando, 1962). The pupal stage lasts 3–7 days at 24°C–35°C (Rajamani et al., 2004; Murthy, 1958).

O. oryzae exhibits unisexual progeny, that is, a female gives birth to either all-male or all-female offspring. *Wolbachia* is linked to the species' ability to determine sex (Behura et al., 2000). The ideal temperature and relative humidity for midge development are 26°C–30°C and 82%–88%, respectively (Pathak, 1968). The entire life cycle of *O. oryzae* in India is completed between 14 and 21 days. Males outnumber females in the field and live longer, lasting 1–5 days (Sy, 1978). The insect has five to seven overlapping generations in a year in India (Yen et al., 1941; Li and Chiu, 1951; Wong et al., 1956).

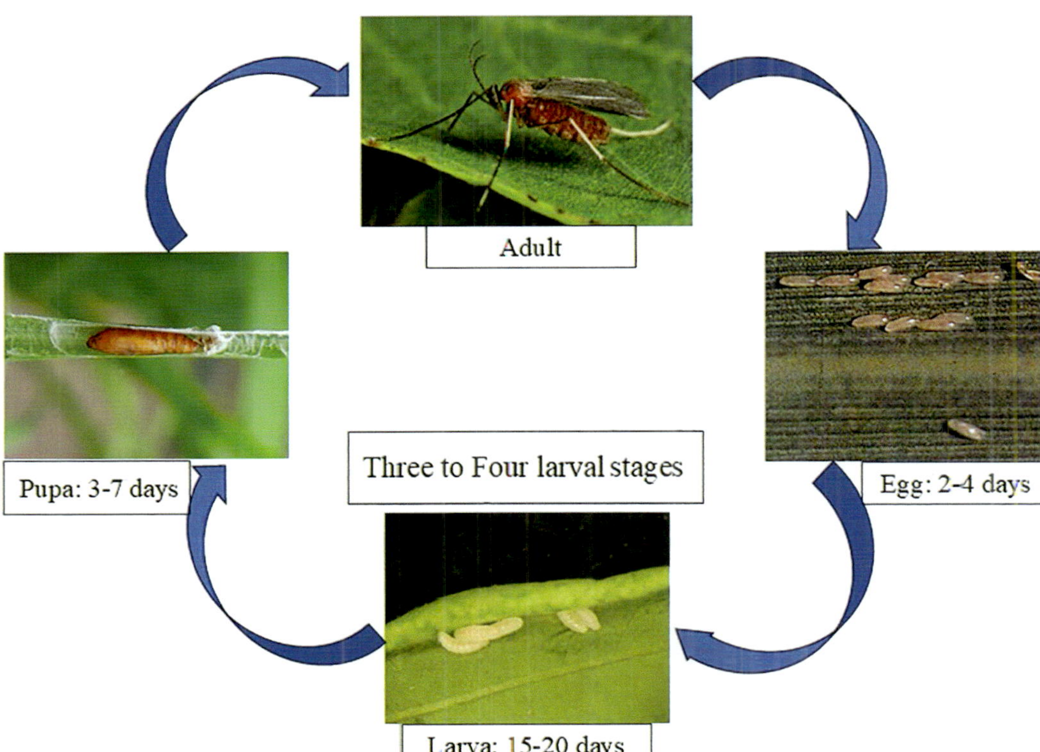

FIGURE 1.2 Life cycle of gall midge in paddy.

1.2.5 Nature of Damage

Galls or swellings on the stalks, leaf sheaths, or panicle bases of rice plants are the most obvious signs of rice gall midge infestation. Typically, elongated and cylindrical, these galls can vary in size from 1 cm wide to 10–30 cm long. When the larvae continue to feed and develop within, they may first appear as small, reddish-brown swellings inside silvery-white hollow tubes, which eventually grow larger. This silvery-white extension of the leaf sheaths is referred to as an "onion leaf" or "silver shoot" (Figure 1.3). The feeding larvae cause stunted growth, a possible symptom of infestation in rice plants. The height and general vigour of the plant may be restricted. Plants infested with midges exhibit rolling, withering, and yellowing of the leaves. This occurs particularly as the larval feeding activity disrupts the intake of nutrients and water.

The gall midge infestation during the flowering stage causes abnormal development of rice panicles, reducing yield. Specifically, when the stem is torn apart, several long, tubular eggs and larvae resembling maggots are found feeding inside growing buds (Figure 1.4). This leads to decreased panicle exertion, inadequate grain filling, and diminished tillering.

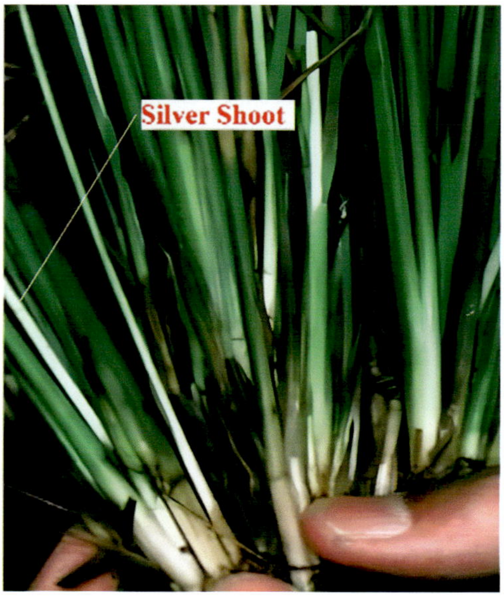

FIGURE 1.3 Onion/silver shoot in rice.

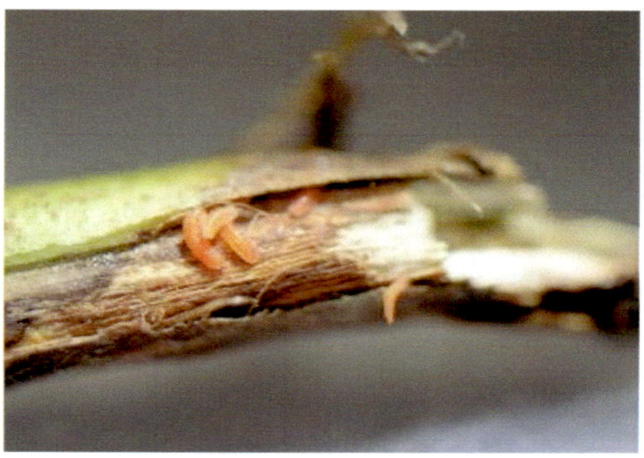

FIGURE 1.4 Maggots found within the stem of rice.

1.2.6 Management of Paddy Gall Fly

Effective and long-lasting management of the paddy gall fly can be achieved by combining chemical, biological, and cultural techniques based on IPM principles. Optimizing control mechanisms to reduce production costs and environmental impacts requires regular monitoring and prompt intervention based on thresholds. By incorporating various tactics into an all-encompassing pest control scheme, farmers may proficiently handle infestations of the paddy gall fly and foster the enduring viability and adaptability of rice-producing systems.

1. **Cultural Practices**
   a. After harvesting the paddy, ploughing should be done as possible.
   b. Planting resistant varieties of rice that naturally resist gall midge infestation can greatly reduce losses.
   c. By alternating rice with non-host crops, rice gall midge populations can be decreased, disrupting their life cycle in following rice crops.
   d. After harvest, removing and discarding crop remnants and alternative hosts can help hinder the life cycle of rice gall midges and lower their overwintering populations.
   e. Applying split applications and limiting the amount of fertilizer applied can slow down population growth rates.
   f. Removing water from rice fields for 5–7 days can significantly reduce the number of gall midges.
   g. Planting rice at the right time of year can reduce infestation levels of rice gall midge by avoiding the period when its activity is highest. Planting early or when insect activity is low can help lower damage from gall fly.
2. **Monitoring and Early Detection**
   a. Consistent field scouting may provide indications of gall formation in rice fields, especially in the initial phases of crop development.
   b. The utilization of either pheromone or infrared light traps can help track and evaluate the dynamics of adult rice gall midge populations.
   c. Adult gall midges are most active from 6 to 10 pm. Therefore, to attract them, light traps should be set up, one per acre, between 6 and 10 pm.
3. **Biological Control**
   a. Encourage the presence of bioagents that parasitize the larvae, such as *Platygaster*, *Eupelmid*, and *Pteromalid* wasps.
   b. Ten days after transplanting, release the *Platygaster oryzae*-parasitized galls at a density of 1 per 10 sq. m.
   c. The application of Phytoseiid mites and spiders will destroy the eggs and adults, respectively.
   d. Introduce natural enemies of the rice gall midge, like as parasitoid wasps, to target and diminish midge populations as an additional method of biological management.
   e. Any plant-based substance, such as 10% extract of neem leaf, 5% neem seed kernel extract, 1% neem oil, 0.3% fish oil resin soap, 3% dasagavya, and 3% herbal plant extract, might be applied to reduce pest numbers in the event of a severe infestation.
4. **Chemical Control**

   Applications of tailored insecticides may be required if infection levels are above economic thresholds and alternative control strategies prove unproductive. To lessen the chance of resistance developing, use insecticides that do not significantly harm non-target organisms and alternate chemical classes.

   a. Maximize the benefits of potash fertilizer recommendations. Provide up to 30 days of protection for germinated seeds by dipping them in a 0.2% chlorpyrifos solution for 3 hours before sowing.

b. Seedlings in transplanted crops may have their roots soaked in a 0.2% chlorpyrifos suspension for a full day before planting.
c. Within 10 days of planting, phorate granules 10G (1.5 kg ai/ha), carbofuran 3G (0.5 kg ai/ha), quinalphos (1.5 kg ai/ha), or chlorpyrifos 10G (0.5 kg ai/ha) may be applied where the pest is frequently observed. Spread the granules in 2–3 cm of water and leave the field pounded for a minimum of 4 days.

1.3 RICE WHORL MAGGOT: *HYDRELLIA PHILIPPINA* FERINO (EPHYDRIDAE: DIPTERA)

1.3.1 Systematic Position

Phylum – Arthropoda
Class – Insecta
Order – Diptera
Family – Ephydridae
Genus – *Hydrellia*
Species – *philippina*, *griseola*, *sasakii*

1.3.2 Distribution

The rice whorl maggot is prevalent in the early phases of crop development and usually stops at the booting stage of the plants. This is most likely because the maggots, which consume the central whorl leaf, lack a suitable environment. After panicle emergence, there is no recorded infestation (Pathak and Khan, 1994). *H. griseola* is found in the USA, Europe, North Africa, Malaysia, and Japan (Emden, 2013). Other species, like *H. prosternalis*, are reported from Africa, *H. wirthi* from Colombia, and *H. tomiokai* from Japan (Litsinger et al., 2013). *H. philippina* is known to be present in the Philippines only (Shepard et al., 1995); however, it is now reported in many other parts, like Assam, India, and is believed to be one of the seven major pests of paddy in both rabi and kharif seasons (Baruah and Dutta, 2023). *Hydrellia* sp. is considered a minor pest of paddy in Varanasi (Kumar et al., 2013), Faizabad (Singh et al., 2013), and Himachal Pradesh (Dumra and Srivastava, 2019), India, and other countries, like Myanmar (Win et al., 2020).

1.3.3 Life Cycle

Three important species of *Hydrellia* are known to infest paddy plants, viz. *Hydrellia philippina* Ferino, *H. griseola* (Fallen), and *H. sasakii* (Emden, 2013).

H. griseola: The adults are greyish in colour. The adults have a black face with a pale bright frontal lunule (the small area between the antennal insertions). The reticulately sculpted, curved eggs are placed singly on leaves close to the water surface, and the larvae that hatch pierce the leaf to start a linear mine. Pupation occurs inside the leaf, and the mine's dark pupae are readily visible. The life cycle lasts 2 and 3 weeks depending on the climate, and there can be between 8 and 11 generations in a year (Emden, 2013).

Hydrellia philippina: The adults are dull grey in colour. Males are slightly shorter than females, which measure about 1.5–3.0 mm in length. Adults prefer locations with plenty of calm water and luxuriant vegetation. They float on the water or perch on floating vegetation in the morning and evening. They lounge around and cling to erect vegetation throughout the daytime hours. Each female lays about 20 eggs. The egg-laying phase lasts 1–8 days (Figure 1.5) (Shepard et al., 1995).

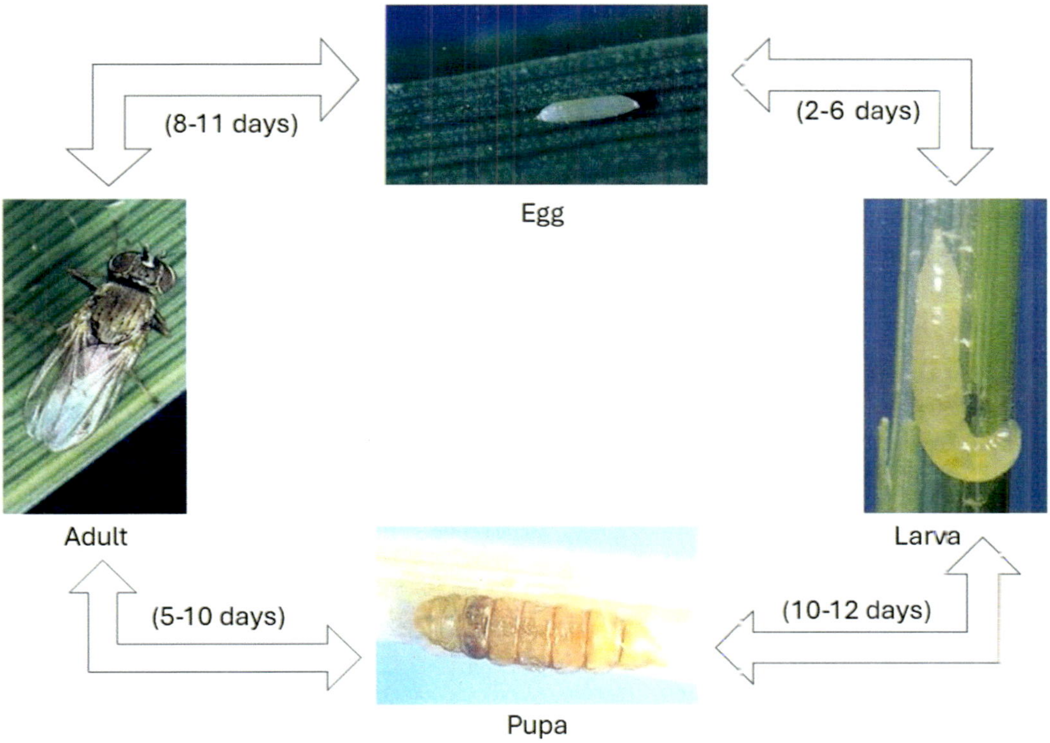

FIGURE 1.5 Life cycle of whorl.

1.3.4 Nature of Damage

Whorl maggots are early vegetative pests of paddy (Shepard et al., 1995). The members are typically stem or leaf miners. The inner margins of unfurled leaves are a source of food for fly maggots. To feed on the mesophyll tissue, the freshly hatched larvae move to the central whorl (Pathak and Khan, 1994).

H. griseola: In order to start a linear mine, the hatchling larvae burrow into the leaf. Later, however, the larvae chew away at the mine's sides, enlarging them into blotch mines. *H. philippina* is rare for a dipteran because the larva does not mine but instead feeds in plain sight on the leaf surface, tearing at the tissues in the paddy plant's unexpanded core whorl of leaves (Emden, 2013).

Symptoms: Small, chewed-up, discoloured spots on the innermost margin of the central whorl are indicators of damage. Damaged leaves typically droop as these places eventually become dry. Significant plant stunting, a lack of tillers, and a delay in panicle initiation and maturity are all effects of severe infestation (Pathak and Khan, 1994).

H. griseola: The harmed leaves typically lie flat on the water and wilt. Plants that are severely harmed may perish. In the case of infestation by *H. philippina*, the plants have a stunted appearance and do not tiller. Their expanded leaves are marred by white spots (Shepard et al., 1995).

1.3.5 Management Measures

The economic threshold level is recognized after the record of 25% damaged leaves.

1. **Monitoring**: Monitoring provides early warning for the infestation of any insect pest. In the case of whorl maggot, checking for eggs is a tedious yet effective way to monitor the fields, but looking for leaf damage is easier and the most sought-out way to monitor the crop by the farmers. Field scouting generally once a week is considered the best way to monitor the fields (Litsinger et al., 2013).
2. **Cultural control**: Since adults are drawn to standing water, it is advised that paddy fields be drained at intervals of 3–4 days during the first 30 days after transplanting to reduce egg laying (Litsinger et al., 2013). However, care should be taken as the drained fields promote the growth of additional weeds. When crops are established in a way that allows the plants to cover the water surface as quickly as possible, whorl maggot damage is minimal. *Azolla* covering the water surface aids in pest control. Several indigenous practices can also be included in IPM; for boro paddy in West Bengal, India, it has been observed that the techniques used in indigenous technology yield good results for rice whorl maggot, and these indigenous practices can be combined with other IPM strategies due to the ease of availability of the materials used and their wide social acceptance (Pokhrel and Laskar, 2020). Since directly seeded fields or seedbeds are not very appealing to adults, direct sowing is advised (Pathak and Khan, 1994). This method shows less incidence than transplantation (Kumar et al., 2017), and in the case of transplanting, using older seedlings reduces exposure to whorl maggots (Yadav et al., 2021). Higher plant densities result in less harm to fields. Close planting reduces oviposition and the potential damage that follows (DPPQS, 2014). Whorl maggot resistance has been found in two wild paddy species (*Oryza brachyantha* and *O. ridleyi*) and one cultivar of paddy (IR40) (Pathak and Khan, 1994). High-yielding paddy varieties, like Jayanti (CR Dhan 502) released in 2012, CR Dhan 505 released in 2014 (Chattopadhyay et al., 2018), CR Dhan 506 released in 2017 and CR Dhan 308, and CR Dhan 309 released by the National Rice Research Institute, show moderate resistance to whorl maggot (NRRI, 2019).
3. **Biological control**: Wasps of the genus *Trichogramma* and flies of the genus *Dolichopus* parasitize and prey upon exposed eggs on plants, respectively. Whorl maggot larvae are parasitized by euphids (such as *Tetrastichus* sp.) and braconids (such as *Opius* sp.). *Chaenusa conjugens* (Nees), a braconid, parasitizes *H. griseola* larvae. *Ochthera brevitibialis* de Meijere, an ephydrid fly, feeds on adult whorl maggots. The oxyopid *Oxyopes javanus* (Thorell) lynx spider, the lycosid *Pardosa pseudoannulata* (Boesenberg and Strand) wolf spider, and the araneid, *Neoscona theisi* (Walckenaer) are among the spiders that feed on adults. A fungus of the genus *Entomophthora* has also been identified as a whorl maggot parasite (Pathak and Khan, 1994). Management through *Bacillus thuringiensis* var. *kurstaki* is also used to control whorl maggot (Singh and Chatterjee, 2021).
4. **Chemical control**: Fipronil 5% SC @50 g a.i./ha and @ 75% a.i./ha are two important doses recommended for whorl maggot (Paul et al., 2018). According to the list of major insecticides used by the Central Insecticide Board and Registration Committee, some insecticides recommended for whorl maggot in paddy include cartap hydrochloride 4% granules a.i./ha, chlorpyrifos 10% G a.i./ha, deltamethrin 11%w/w EC a.i./ha, ethofenprox 10% EC a.i./ha, fipronil 5% SC a.i./ha, fipronil 0.3% GR a.i./ha, and thiamethoxam 25% WG a.i./ha in nursery as soil drenching (CIBRC, 2021).

1.4 SORGHUM SHOOTFLY: *ATHERIGONA SOCCATA* (RONDANI, 1871) (MUSCIDAE: DIPTERA)

1.4.1 Systematics Position

Class: Insecta
Order: Diptera
Family: Muscidae
Genus: *Atherigona*
Species: *soccata*

1.4.2 Distribution

The sorghum shoot fly affects all sorghum cultivation regions. It is widespread in tropical and subtropical regions encompassing Africa, the Mediterranean, the Middle East, and Southeast Asia, with extensions reaching the Philippines (Pont, 1973). In Asia, the sorghum shoot fly emerges as a significant pest of sorghum, particularly in India, notably in Maharashtra, Andhra Pradesh, Tamil Nadu, and Karnataka. The abundance of sorghum shoot flies reaches its maximum levels in the rainy season, typically occurring 20–30 days subsequent to the commencement of monsoon precipitation. Post-rainy season crops sown in September–October witness a notable surge in sorghum shoot fly populations. The pest population remains low during the intensely hot and dry summers in southern India (about 35°C) and the winter season in northern India (about 18°C), gradually diminishing with consistent rainfall (Taneja et al., 1986). During the season when sorghum is not available, the insect sustains itself by utilizing substitute hosts, like *Sorghum* sp., *Echinochloa colonum*, *E. procera*, *Cymbopogon* sp., *Paspalum scrobiculatum*, and *Pennisetum glaucum*, in addition to feeding on tillers of regrown crops and self-sown/fodder sorghum.

1.4.3 Identification of the Pest

Adult: The adult female, characterized by a whitish-grey colour (Figure 1.6d), lays white, cigar-shaped eggs (Figure 1.6a) singly on the lower surface of leaf blades, predominantly during the morning hours. The adult shoot fly bears a striking resemblance to a housefly, with a dark brown body, and males are smaller than females. Typically, adults have a lifespan of 10–20 days, which can vary based on host plant availability and environmental factors.

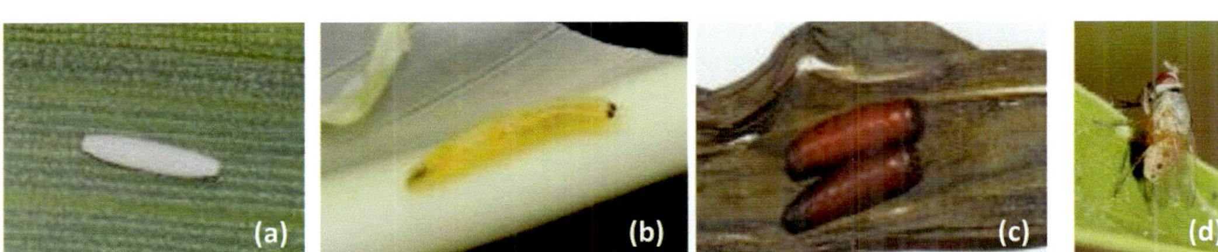

FIGURE 1.6 (a) Eggs, (b) maggots, (c) pupae, and (d) adult of *A. soccata*.

Maggots: The immature stage of the shoot fly, known as maggots, appears dirty white and apodous, with mature larvae reaching about 6 mm in length and displaying a yellow hue (Figure 1.6b). The larval period spans 8–10 days across four larval instars, with pupation occurring at the base of the stem or in the soil for 8–10 days, thereby completing the life cycle in 17–21 days. The female shoot flies are drawn towards host plants by emitted odours to facilitate oviposition. These females are attracted to both volatile and photoactive stimuli emitted by susceptible seedlings, aiding in orientation for oviposition (Nwanze et al., 1998).

1.4.4 Life Cycle

Adults: Female *A. soccata* lays cigar-shaped eggs individually on the lower leaf surface during the 1–7-leaf stage, typically parallel to the midrib. Multiple eggs may be found on the same leaf in the presence of numerous shoot flies, often laid by distinct females. In certain instances, as many as 25 eggs can be found on a single seedling (Singh et al., 2004). The eggs hatch within 2–5 days (Sharma et al., 1996), with an incubation period ranging from 2 to 3 days. Under an average temperature of 27°C, larval instars undergo development within a span of about 7 days. The larva moves towards the upper surface of the leaf, navigating through the leaf whorl towards the growing apex by passing through the leaf sheath. Subsequently, the larva cuts off the growing apex, leading to the withering and drying of the central leaf, a state commonly referred to as the "dead heart". Consumption of decaying plant material occurs by the larva. The dead heart can be readily removed and releases a foul smell. Typically, harm manifests within 1–4 weeks post-seedling emergence. Side tillers emerging from affected plants may also become targets. The larval phase spans 8–10 days, with pupation predominantly occurring at the stem base and sporadically in the soil. Generally, the pupal phase lasts for 7–10 days to reach maturity. Pupal maturation lasts in the southern parts of India and northern regions for about 8 and 14 days, respectively. Optimal conditions for the life cycle duration are 15–18 days at temperatures of 20°C–30°C and relative humidity exceeding 60% (Srivastava, 1985). Populations of sorghum shoot flies persist year-round, yielding 15–16 generations annually (Sharma et al., 1996), though in cooler regions, this may decrease to 5–6 generations (Bene, 1986); however, diapause is absent in this insect during the off-season (Rao and Rao, 1956).

1.4.5 Nature of Damage

Damage caused by *A. soccata* at the seedling stage typically emerges within 5–30 days post-seedling. It is commonly observed that seedlings between the ages of 5–30 days are susceptible to damage caused by maggots of shoot flies. The shoot is targeted by the pest, leading to the characteristic dead heart symptoms. Larvae migrate towards the upper surface of the foliage, advancing through the leaf spiral until they reach the apical meristem, initiating the process of detachment. Consequently, the central leaf desiccates, forming a dead heart that emits a putrid odour and is easily detachable. Usually, damage manifests within 1–4 weeks of seedling emergence. Plants older than 30 days are usually resistant to shoot fly attacks, except under high humidity conditions during the rainy season, which may lead to infestations. Such conditions do not induce dead heart symptoms. Affected leaves become thin and papery, wrapping around other foliage and impeding normal growth. Late-stage shoot fly infestations may trigger rotting or desiccation of affected panicle portions during the formative phase. Injured plants generate side tillers, which are then susceptible to subsequent *A. soccata* infestations. Certain seedlings might not display conventional symptoms;

however, they can produce lateral tillers as a reaction to environmental factors, such as temperature or moisture fluctuations. Specific genetic variations demonstrate an innate capacity to yield extra tillers (Singh et al., 2017).

1.4.6 Management Measures

The economic threshold level is 10% dead hearts or 1 egg/plant.

1. **Cultural Practices**
   a. Integrated farming systems aim to mitigate shoot fly populations by combining agricultural crops or animal husbandry practices. This approach is particularly beneficial for sorghum cultivation in Africa and Asia.
   b. Adjusting the sowing date, such as opting for early sowing, approximately 7–10 days before the monsoon season, can help decrease infestation by avoiding the active phase of shoot fly emergence. Alternatively, a higher seed rate can be employed if early sowing is not feasible, compensating for the later removal of dead hearts from affected fields (Shekharappa and Bhuti, 2007).
   c. The joint application of nitrogen fertilizer and *Azospirillum* biofertilizer is known to impact shoot fly incidence and plant growth significantly.
   d. Utilization of resistant sorghum varieties, such as Co-1, CSH 15R, Maldandi, Hagari, M35-1, Swati, SPV 491, IS-18551, 5566, 5285, 5613, ICSV 700, ICSV 705, Phule Yashoda, CSH 7, and CSH 8, has been shown to be an effective strategy in combating damage caused by shoot fly.
   e. Utilizing a high seeding rate may help mitigate damage caused by maggots, making it less appealing for oviposition, as seedlings cultivated under conditions of high planting density typically exhibit narrow leaves, which are not preferred for oviposition by females.
   f. By practicing inter-cultivation, pest populations can be minimized by exposing pupae to natural enemies and adverse environmental conditions. Infested seedlings and alternate hosts should be removed and destroyed by burning to prevent further infestation.
   g. Utilizing a high seeding rate may assist in mitigating shoot fly damage, since seedlings cultivated under conditions of high planting density typically exhibit narrow leaves that are less appealing for oviposition.
   h. Research has shown a decrease in shoot fly damage when sorghum is grown alongside leguminous crops.
   i. These practices can effectively decrease the carry-over and build-up of shoot fly populations from one season to the next. Field sanitation through fallowing aids in removing insects by enhancing the presence of natural enemies.
2. **Host plant resistance**: Host plant resistance is a crucial aspect of pest management in shoot fly infestation. Trials conducted in southern Africa and Asia have highlighted varying resistance levels among tested varieties, with some showing medium to high resistance to shoot fly attacks.
3. **Biological control**: Limited information and research exist on the activity of natural enemies in managing shoot fly populations. Certain predators, like spiders and parasitoids, such as *Trichogramma simmondsi* and *T. chilonis*, *may* play a significant role in controlling shoot fly eggs and larvae (Singh and Sharma, 2002).
4. **Chemical control**: In India, various chemicals, including imidacloprid, chlorpyrifos, monocrotophos, carbofuran, phorate, and endosulfan, have been utilized for seed treatment, planting, and spraying to combat this pest. However, the recent recommendations are listed below in Table 1.1:

TABLE 1.1
Insecticide Used to Control Shoot Fly (DPPQS, 2023)

Insecticide	a.i (g) doses/ha	Formulation (g/mL) doses/ha
Carbofuran 03% CG	1,000	33,300
Imidacloprid 48% FS	720	1,200
Imidacloprid 70% WS	700	1,000
Thiamethoxam 30% FS	03	10
Oxydemeton-methyl 25% EC	250	1,000

1.5 CONCLUSION

In conclusion, the management of fly pests such as the sorghum shoot fly, paddy gall fly, and rice whorl maggot is critical for ensuring the health and productivity of cereal crops. There have been significant contributions in studying, understanding the behaviour, and managing the fly pests of rice and sorghum. Each of these pests presents unique challenges due to their life cycles, feeding habits, and the specific damage they inflict on their host plants. However, a constant effort is necessary to address emerging problems like pest resurgence and resistance due to unexpected and indiscriminate use of pesticides. Effective management strategies must include a combination of cultural, biological, and chemical controls tailored to the specific needs of each crop and pest. Cultural practices such as crop rotation, timely planting, and proper field sanitation can significantly reduce pest populations. Biological control methods, including natural predators and parasitoids, offer sustainable and environmentally friendly options. When necessary, the judicious use of chemical insecticides can help manage outbreaks, although this should be approached with caution to avoid resistance development and environmental harm. Hence, sustainable and integrated approaches are the sole solution for safeguarding rice and sorghum production against these pests to ensure food security and environmental safety. IPM approaches that combine various strategies will provide the most effective and sustainable solutions for managing these fly pests, ultimately contributing to improved crop yields and food security.

1.6 POINTS TO REMEMBER

1. **Sorghum shoot fly**: Notable for attacking young sorghum plants, causing dead heart symptoms.
2. **Paddy gall fly**: Affects rice, leading to the formation of galls on the leaf sheaths.
3. **Rice whorl maggot**: Targets rice seedlings, damaging central leaves and stunted growth.
4. Understanding the life cycles of each pest is crucial for effectively timing control measures.
5. Sorghum shoot fly lays eggs on the leaves; the larvae burrow into the stem.
6. Paddy gall fly lays eggs on rice plants, and larvae induce gall formation.
7. Rice whorl maggot larvae feed on the whorl of rice seedlings, causing damage to new leaves.
8. Each pest causes significant yield losses if not managed properly.
9. Damage symptoms vary: dead heart in sorghum, galls in rice, and whorl damage in rice seedlings.
10. Early detection and intervention are key to minimizing crop loss.
11. Practices such as crop rotation, timely planting, and field sanitation can reduce pest incidence.
12. Removing and destroying infested plants can help break the life cycle of pests.

13. Utilization of natural predators and parasitoids can effectively reduce pest populations.
14. Encouraging biodiversity and natural habitats for beneficial insects is beneficial.
15. Chemical insecticides should be used judiciously and as a last resort to avoid resistance and environmental damage.
16. Specific insecticides should be selected based on the pest and crop and applied according to guidelines.
17. Combining cultural, biological, and chemical methods provides a holistic approach to pest management.
18. IPM aims for long-term, sustainable pest control while minimizing negative environmental impacts.
19. Regular field monitoring for signs of pest infestation allows for early intervention.
20. The use of traps and scouting techniques can help in tracking pest populations.
21. Rotating insecticides and incorporating non-chemical methods can help prevent the development of resistant pest strains.
22. Educating farmers on resistance management strategies is essential for long-term pest control success.
23. All control methods should be evaluated for their environmental impact and safety on non-target organisms, including humans.
24. The adoption of eco-friendly practices ensures sustainable agriculture.
25. By remembering these points, farmers can effectively manage the fly pests of cereals ensuring healthier crops and better yields.

REFERENCES

Baruah, M., & Dutta, B. C. (2023). Relative abundance of major insect pests and natural enemies in high yielding rice varieties of Assam. *Research Square*, pp. 1–18. https://doi.org/10.21203/rs.3.rs-2756112/v1

Behura, S. K., Sahu, S. C., Nair, S., & Mohan, M. (2000). An AFLP marker that differentiates biotypes of the Indian gall midge (*Orseolia oryzae*, Wood-Mason) is linked to sex and avirulence. *Molecular Genetics and Genomics*, 263, 328–334.

Bene, G. (1986). Notes on the biology of *Atherigona soccata* Rondani (Diptera: Muscidae) in Tuscany and Latium. *Redia*, 69, 47–63.

Central Insecticide Board and Registration Committee (2021). CIBRC0. https://ppqs.gov.in/divisions/cib-rc/major-uses-of-pesticides

Chattopadhyay, K., Reddy, J. N., Pradhan, S. K., Patnaik, S. S. C., Marndi, B. C., Swain, P., Nayak, A. K., Anandan, A., Chakraborty, K., Sarkar, R. K., Bose, L. K., Katara, J. L., Parameswaram, C., Mukherjee, A. K., Mohapatra, S. D., Poonam, A., Mishra, S. K., & Korada, R. R. (2018). Genetic improvement of rice for multiple stress tolerance in unfavourable rainfed ecology. In: H. Pathak, A.K. Nayak, D. Maiti, G.A.K. Kumar, J.N. Reddy, P.C. Rath, P. Swain, & R. Bhagawati (eds.), *Rice Research for Enhancing Productivity, Profitability and Climate Resilience*. ICAR-National Rice Research Institute, Cuttack, Odisha, India, pp. 120–137.

Cramer, H. H. (1967). Plant protection and world crop protection. *Pflanzenschutz Nachr*, 20, 1–524.

Desta, A. G., & Yeshitila, B. H. (2024). The distribution of insect pests and the associated loss of stored sorghum in the Kena district of Konso Zone, South-Western Ethiopia. *PLoS One*, 19(1), e0295833. https://doi.org/10.1371/journal.pone.0295833

Dhaliwal, G. S., Jindal, V., & Mohindru, B. (2015). Crop losses due to insect pests: Global and Indian scenario. *Indian Journal of Entomology*, 77(2), 165–168.

DPPQS (2023). Central Insecticide Board and Registration Committee (CIBRC). https://ppqs.gov.in/divisions/cib-rc/major-uses-of-pesticides

Dumra, N., & Srivastava, A. (2019). Seasonal abundance of rice caseworm and whorl maggot under mid hill conditions of Himachal Pradesh, India. *Journal of Entomology and Zoology Studies*, 7(**4**), 61–66.

Emden, H. F. (2013). *Handbook of Agricultural Entomology*. Wiley-Blackwell, Delhi, India, pp. 117–137.

Fernando, H. E. (1962). *Administrative Report of the Director of Agriculture for 1960*. Entomology Division, Colombo, Ceylon, pp. 204–208.

Huang, C. K. (1957). Study of *Pachydiplosis oryzae* Wood-Mason in Fu-Chien province. *East China Science and Agricultural Journal*, 6, 293–304.

ICAR-National Rice Research Institute (2014). *Contributions of NRRI Varieties to National Food Security*, NRRI Research Bulletin No. 16. ICAR-National Rice Research Institute, Odisha, pp. 7–14.

Inthavong, S. (2004). Status of gall midge in Lao PDR. In: J. Bennett, J. S. Bentur, I. C. Pasalu, & K. Krishnaiah (eds.), *New Approaches to Gall Midge Resistance in Rice.* International Rice Research Institute and Indian Council of Agricultural Research, Hyderabad, India, pp. 77–89.

Jahn, G. C., & Bunnarith, K. (2004). Gall midge in Cambodian lowland rice. In: J. Bennett, J. S. Bentur, I. C. Pasalu, & K. Krishnaiah (eds.), *New Approaches to Gall Midge Resistance in Rice.* International Rice Research Institute and Indian Council of Agricultural Research, Hyderabad, India, pp. 71–77.

Joshi, R. C., Grover, P., & Venugopal, M. S. (1983). The rice gall midge, *Orseolia oryzae*: A brief review. *Cecid Internationale*, 4, 9–21.

Kale, S., Mandawi, N. C., & Sahu, H. (2023). Seasonal incidence and correlation studies between the rice whorl maggot (*Hydrellia philippina* F.) and weather parameters under Bastar Plateau conditions. *International Journal of Advanced Biochemistry Research*, SP-7(**2**), 538–541.

Kalode, M. B., & Bentur, J. S. (1989). Characterization of Indian biotypes of rice gall midge, *Orseolia oryzae* (Wood-mason) (Diptera: Cecidomyiidae). *Insect Science and its Application*, 10, 219–224.

Kumar, A., Ram, L., & Singh, B. (2017). Crop establishment impact on foliage feeders and *Leptocorisa acuta* in rice. *Journal of Entomology and Zoology Studies*, 5(**5**), 2023–2027.

Kumar, D. Raghuraman, M., Singh, J., Waza, S. A., & Kumar, K. (2013). Occurrence of insec-pests and natural enemies in rice (*Oryza sativa* L.) agro-ecosystem. *International Journal of Plant Protection*, 6(**2**), 266–270.

Kumar, G. K. P., Pradeep, S., Sridhara, S., & Manjunatha, M. (2012). Incidence of sucking pests on promising traditional paddy cultivars in organic situation. *Plant Archives*, 12, 23–26.

Lai, K., Tan, Y., & Pan, Y. (1984). Rice gall midge biotypes in Guangdong province. *International Rice Research Notes*, 9, 17–18.

Li, C. S., & Chiu, S. F. (1951). A study of the rice gall midge *Pachydiplosis oryzae* Wood-Mason. *Agricultural Research Taiwan*, 2, 1–13.

Litsinger, J. A., Barrion, A. T., Canapi, B. L., Lumaban, M. D., Pantua, P. C., & Aquino, G. B. (2013). The rice whorl maggot, *Hydrellia philippina* Ferino (Diptera: Ephydridae) in the Philippines: A review. *Philipp Ent Journal*, 27(**1**), 1–57.

Murthy, D. V. (1958). Studies on the bionomics of the paddy gall midge *Pachydiplosis oryzae* (W.M.) Mani. *Mysore Agricultural Journal*, 32, 145– 153.

Nwanze, K. F., Nwilene, F. E., & Reddy, Y. V. R. (1998). Evidence of shoot fly *Atherigona soccata* Rondani (Dipt., Muscidae) oviposition response to sorghum seedling volatiles. *Journal of Applied Entomology*, 122(**15**), 591–594.

Okosun, O. O., Allen, K. C., Glover, J. P., & Reddy, G. V. (2021). Biology, ecology, and management of key sorghum insect pests, *Journal of Integrated Pest Management*, 12(**1**), 4.

Pathak, M. D. (1968). Ecology of common insect pests of rice. *Annual Review of Entomology*, 13(1), 257–294.

Pathak, M. D., & Khan, Z. R. (1994). *Insect Pests of Rice*. IRRI, ICIPE, Philippines, pp. 29–60.

Paul, B., Samanta, S., Sen, K., Manger, A., & Samata, A. (2018). Evaluation of bioefficacy and phytotoxicity of fipronil 5% SC and acetamiprid 20% SP on rice insect pest complex. *Journal of Entomology and Zoology Studies*, 6(**4**), 1410–1416.

Perera, N., & Fernando, H. E. (1968). Infestation of young rice plants by the rice gall midge (*Pachidiplosis oryzae* Wood-Mason) (Dipt., Cecidomyiidae) with special reference to shoot morphogenesis. *Bulletin Entomology Research*, 59, 605–613.

Pokhrel, P., & Laskar, N. (2020). Indigenous technical knowledge (ITK) based pest management practices for Boro paddy in Northern parts of West Bengal. *Journal of Entomology and Zoology Studies*, 8(**2**), 494–498.

Pont, A. C. (1973). A review of the Oriental species of *Atherigona Rondani* (Diptera, Muscidae) of economic importance. In: M. G. Jotwani & W. R. Young (eds.), *Control of Sorghum Shoot Fly*. Oxford and IBH Publishing Company, Delhi, India, pp. 27–102.

Rajamani, S., Pasalu, I. C., Mathur, K. C., Sain, M., Bennett, J., Bentur, J. S., & Krishnaiah, K. (2004). Biology and ecology of rice gall midge. In: J. Bennett, J. S. Bentur, I. C. Pasalu, & K. Krishnaiah (eds.), *New Approaches to Gall Midge Resistance in Rice*. IRRI, Los Baños, Philippines, pp. 7–17.

Rao, P., & Rao, N. D. V. (1956). Studies on the sorghum shoot-borer-fly *Atherigona indica* Malloch (Anthomyiidae - Diptera) at Siruguppa. *Mysore Agriculture Journal*, 31, 158–174.

Reddy, D. B. (1967). *The Rice Gall Midge O. oryzae (W-M): The Major Insect and Pest of Rice Plant*. Johns Hopkins Press, Baltimore, MD, pp. 457–81.

Sharma, M., Kapoor, K. N., & Bharaj, G. S. (1996). Effect of seed treatment of sorghum with some new insecticides for control of shoot fly. *Crop Research (Hisar)*, 11(**1**), 90–92.

Shekharappa, S. & Bhuti, S. G. (2007) Integrated management of sorghum shoot fly, *Atherigona soccata Rondani. Karnataka Journal of Agricultural Sciences*, 20, 535–536.

Shepard, B. M., Barrion, A. T., & Litsinger, J. A. (1995). *Rice Whorl Maggot: Rice-Feeding Insects of Tropical Asia*. IRRI, Philippines, pp. 20–26.

Singh, B., & Chatterjee, S. (2021). Relative efficacy of some biorational and microbial insecticides against yellow stem borer and whorl maggot of *boro* paddy. *Biorational Insecticides against YSB and Whorl Maggot*, 14(**2**), 90–96.

Singh, B., Kumar, N., & Kumar, H. (2017). Seasonal incidence and management of sorghum shoot fly, *Atherigona soccata Rondani-a review. Forage Research*, 42, 218–224.

Singh, B. U., Padmaja, P. G., & Seetharama, N. (2004). Biology and management of sorghum shoot fly, Atherigona soccata (Rondani). *Annual Review of Entomology*, 49, 77–97.

Singh, B. U., & Sharma, H. C. (2002). Natural enemies of Sorghum shoot fly, *Atherigona soccata* Rondani (Diptera: Muscidae). *Biocontrol Science and Technology*, 12(**3**), 307–323.

Singh, S., & Tiwari, S. N. (2020). Sucking Pests of Rice. In Omkar (ed.), *Sucking Pests of Crops*. Springer Nature, Cham, pp. 55–105.

Sontakay, K. R. (1941). The gangai disease of rice caused by *P. oryzae* Mani on the central provinces. Final Report on Schemed Financed by Indian Council Agricultural Research (ICAR), New Delhi, p. 24.

Srinivasa, R. P., Reddy, B. V., Nagaraj, N., & Upadhyaya, H. D. (2014). Sorghum production for diversified uses. In: Y. H. Wang, H. D. Upadhyaya, & C. Kole (eds.), *Genetics, Genomics and Breeding of Sorghum*. CRC Press, Taylor & Francis Group, Boca Raton, FL, pp. 1–27.

Srivastava, K. P. (1985). Sorghum insect pests in India. In: *Proceedings of the International Sorghum Entomology Workshop*, 15–21 July 1984, Texas A&M University and ICRISAT, pp. 65–72.

Sy, A. (1978). *Insect Pests of Economic Importance on Cereal Crops in the Senegal River Basin*, West Africa, Oregon State Uiversity.

Taneja, S. L., Seshu Reddy, K. V., & Leuschner, K., (1986). Monitoring of shoot fly population in sorghum. *Indian Journal of Plant Protection*, 14(**2**), 29–36.

Tayathum, C., Attathom, T., Thongphak, D., & Sripongpankul, K. (2004). Rice gall midge in Thailand: current status and biotype characterization. In: J. Bennett, J. S. Bentur, I. C. Pasalu, & K. Krishnaiah (eds.), *New Approaches to Gall Midge Resistance in Rice*. International Rice Research Institute and Indian Council of Agricultural Research Publications, Los Baños, Philippines, pp. 89–99.

Ul Ane, N., & Hussain, M. (2015). Diversity of insect pests in major rice growing areas of the world. *Journal of Entomology and Zoology Studies*, 4, 36–41.

Win, N. N., Phyu, M. H., Oo, T. T., & Win, K. K. (2020). The abundance of hemiptera and diptera fauna on monsoon rice at Nay Pyi Taw, Myanmar. *International Journal of Environmental and Rural Development*, 11(**2**), 140–145.

Wong, T. C., Lee, J. P., & Huang, C. C. (1956). Research on *Pachydiplosis oryzae* Wood-Mason in Chiang-Hsi Province. *East China Science and Agricultural Journal*, 7, 347–354.

Yadav, P. K., Sharma, S., & Sharma, A. (2021). Management trends of rice insect pests in south Asia: A review. *Food and Agriculture*, 2(**2**), 46–53.

Yen, C. H., Liu, C. Y., & Kuo, K. (1941). A preliminary study on the life history of the rice stem midge *Pachydiplosis oryzae* WoodMason (Dipt.: Cecido) in Kwangsi Province, south China. *Kwangsi Agricultural*, 2, 429–453.

2 Flies Pests of Food Legumes

Sanjay M. Bandi, Jagdish Jaba, Revanasidda, Anup Chandra, Gopalakrishnan Kesharivarmen Sujayanand, and Mareppa Hussani Kodandaram

LEARNING OBJECTIVES

1. What are the major agromyzid pests infesting legume crops?
2. What is the distribution, taxonomy, and biology of agromyzid pests?
3. What are the host plants of agromyzid pests?
4. How do agromyzid pests damage the legume host crops?
5. How to manage agromyzid pests in food legumes?

2.1 INTRODUCTION

Some of the agromyzid flies (Agromyzidae: Diptera) are well-known pests with economic significance worldwide. They are primarily referred to as *leaf miners* or *leaf-mining flies* since 75% of the known agromyzid species (about 2,860) described worldwide infest plant leaves (Spencer, 1973; Thapa, 2011). Larvae also form external stem mines, bore into the stems of herbaceous plants or the cambium of trees, and feed in plant roots or flower heads (Spencer, 1990). The agromyzids are minute to small-sized flies and vary in color from yellow, black, brown, grey, metallic greenish, bluish, to coppery. The larval stages are internal plant feeders and cause damage to leaves, stems, seeds, pods, and even roots of the crops. Agromyzidae are divided into two subfamilies, Agromyzinae and Phytomyzinae (Boucher, 2008), comprising about 28 genera with more than 2,860 described species (Scheffer et al., 2007). Agromyzid flies infest a broad diversity of plant hosts representing 140 plant families (Benavent-Corai et al., 2005). The genera *Melanagromyza* and *Ophiomyia* are potential pests of crops in the tropics, while the leaf-mining genera *Liriomyza* and *Phytomyza* are more dominant in temperate regions. Legume crops suffer heavy losses from agromyzid fly infestations. The pod fly, *Melanagromyza obtusa* (Malloch), is a serious pest of pigeonpea (*Cajanus cajan* (L.) Millsp.) in the oriental regions, including India. Among *Ophiomyia* species, *O. phaseoli* (Tryon) is the most damaging and extensively distributed throughout Asia and Africa. Agromyzids are strictly host-specific, but a few species are oligophagous or polyphagous (Tengecho et al., 1988). The chickpea leaf miner, *Liriomyza cicerina* Rondani, is reported to feed only on plants belonging to the family Fabaceae (Shevtchenko, 1937). Among the polyphagous species, the leaf miner *Phytomyza horticola* (Goureau) [(= *Chromatomyia horticola* (Goureau)] is a pest on field pea.

2.2 PIGEONPEA POD FLY (*MELANAGROMYZA OBTUSA* (MALLOCH))

The pod fly is a major pest of pigeonpea throughout South and Southeast Asia. In India, it is a key pest of late-maturing pigeonpea in the northern parts, particularly Uttar Pradesh, Bihar, and Madhya Pradesh, although it occurs throughout the country. It causes an average of 35% pod damage, which in turn results in 30% grain damage (Srivastava, 1972). Crop losses due to pod fly are estimated to be USD 256 million annually (ICRISAT, 1992).

DOI: 10.1201/9781003482581-4

2.2.1 Distribution

Pod fly is reported to occur mostly in South and Southeast Asia (Lal and Katti, 1997). This pest is widely distributed in India, Sri Lanka, Burma, Bangladesh, Indonesia, Japan, Malaysia, Myanmar, Nepal, Pakistan, the Philippines, Taiwan, Thailand, Papua New Guinea, and Vietnam (Shanower et al., 1999) and has also been reported from the Dominican Republic (Serra et al., 2003) Colombia (Martínez-Alava et al., 2016), Puerto Rico, Florida, Peru, Panama, Haiti, Guadeloupe, etc. (EPPO, 2023). Its presence in eastern and southern Africa is disputed. In India, pod fly is widely distributed throughout the country wherever the pigeonpea crop is grown but is more prevalent in northern than in southern states (Sehgal, 1990). The infestation is higher in central and northern states (Uttar Pradesh, Madhya Pradesh, and Bihar) and moderate in the states of Punjab, Maharashtra, Karnataka, and Andhra Pradesh.

2.2.2 Taxonomy

Pod fly was recorded by Maxwell-Lefroy in 1909 as "Tur pod fly" or "Tur pod *agromyza*". Tur pod fly was subsequently described as *Agromyza obtusa* by Malloch in 1914. De Meijere (1922) described the pest as *Melanagromyza weberi* on pigeonpea and *Flemingia* sp. The species was then redescribed as *Melanagromyza obtusa* by Henning (Lal and Katti, 1997). The genus *Melanagromyza* is one of the largest in the subfamily Agromyzinae, with more than 380 species distributed worldwide (Shi and Gaimari, 2015). Only two species, *M. obtusa* and *M. chalcosoma* Spencer, are reported to infest pigeonpea, and latter is geographically limited to eastern and southern Africa (Spencer, 1973).

2.2.3 Life Stages and Diagnostic Characters

Eggs: Eggs are glistening white, smooth, pear-shaped, tapering posteriorly, and projecting into the pod cavity (Ipe, 1974).

Larva: Freshly emerged larvae are transparent and glistening white, subsequently turning creamy white with a greenish tinge. They are sub-cylindrical and slightly tapering towards either side. The body comprises a head, three thoracic, and eight abdominal segments. Mandibles are stout, hooked, with a single cutting edge (Spencer, 1973). Anterior spiracles are absent in first instars. Anterior and posterior spiracles are present in second and third instars (Ipe, 1974).

Pupa: The puparium is yellowish-white when freshly formed but turns reddish-brown later. There are two pairs of spiracles: the anterior pair on the prothoracic region and the posterior pair on the last abdominal segment.

Adults: Medium-sized flies, green-coppery in colour, with a well-developed green ocellar triangle. The frons is relatively narrow, with numerous fronto-orbital bristles. Antennae have a long arista. Palpi are black, and the proboscis is brown at the apex. The abdomen is glossy black with a metallic or light bronzy surface and a violaceous tinge on a greenish-blue ground. Legs are shiny black. Wings are clear, yellowish at the base. Halteres are black. The basal cone of the ovipositor is conspicuously elongated in females (Lal and Katti, 1997; Spencer, 1973).

2.2.4 Biology

Females copulate 24 hours post-emergence, and oviposition follows quickly. Eggs are laid singly into the lumen of the pod. Females deposit 30–40 eggs, although as many as 79 eggs have been recorded (Ahmad, 1938). The average incubation period is 3.1 days at 23°C–28°C (Spencer, 1973). Partly matured pods are preferred over tender or fully matured pods for oviposition. Maximum eggs are deposited on the ventral pod surface rather than on the lateral and dorsal surfaces (Lal and Katti, 1997). More than one egg (2–10) can be found in a locule or in a single pod, but only one larva develops on each seed. The larval period ranges from 6 to 19 days and includes three instars. A larva completes its life cycle in a single seed. Pupation takes place in or near the mines on the seeds and within the lumen of the pod locule. Pupation lasts for 9–23 days depending on climatic conditions (Singh and Beri, 1971, Rehman et al., 2016). The fly emerges normally in the morning hours, and its average longevity is 12 days (Shanower et al., 1999).

2.2.5 Host Plants

Pod fly has a very restricted host range. It is reported to survive on hosts belonging to five genera (*Cajanus*, *Dunbaria*, *Flemingia*, *Rhynchosia*, and *Tephrosia*) of the Fabaceae (Papilionaceae) family. Shanower et al. (1999) reviewed more than 19 host plant species belonging to the family Fabaceae as pod fly host plants. *F. macrophylla* and *F. semialata* are commercially grown as host crops for the production of lac (Kulkarni, 1966; Jaiswal et al., 2015). The pod fly thrived on *R. minima* and *F. congesta* (=*F. macrophylla*) at Kanpur during May and September (Lal and Katti, 1997).

2.2.6 Nature and Extent of Damage

The maggots are the damaging stage of the pod fly (Figure 2.1a). The larvae, upon hatching, mine into soft seeds to feed on their contents. Later, they mine deeper into the seeds through galleries running just under the seed epidermis. The galleries are filled with larval faecal matter and some uneaten starch, which appears as a dirty white band encircling the galleries (Spencer, 1973) (Figure 2.1b). Second and third instar larvae feed deeper into the seeds, consuming the starchy portion as well as the embryo and depositing their excreta inside. Full-grown larvae come out of the seed and pupate in or near the mines on the seeds and within the pod locule. Before pupation, larvae eat a portion of the pod wall, leaving a thin layer of epidermis intact for the emerging fly to escape.

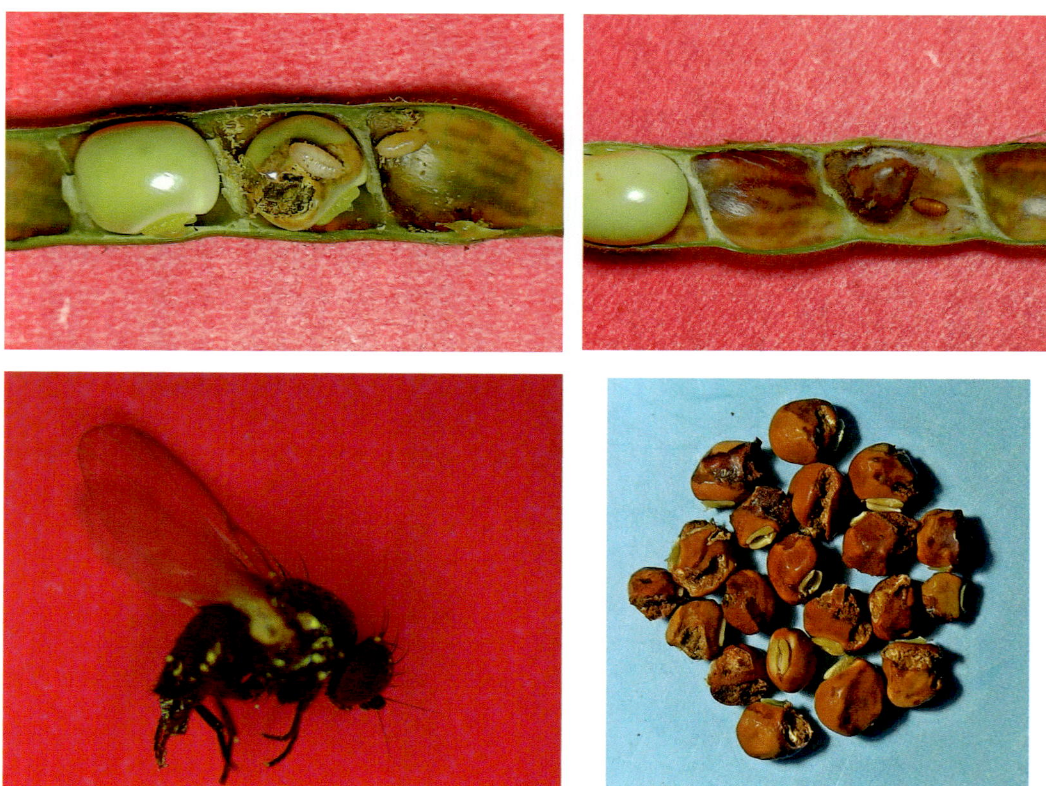

FIGURE 2.1 Pod fly: (a) larvae, (b) pupae, (c) adult, and (d) infested pigeonpea seeds.

Infested pods exhibit pinhead-sized holes indicating the exit holes of flies. When damaged pods are split open, the immature stages can be seen attached to the pod wall or affected seeds. Adult flies feed on the sap that oozes from the oviposition punctures, but this injury does not significantly affect the plant (Talekar and Chen, 1986).

Pod fly causes heavy crop losses, particularly in late pigeonpea. The damaged seeds become unfit for consumption and fail to germinate. The pest was more serious in the northern and central regions of India than in the southern or northwestern areas. Estimates of grain damage by the pod fly ranged from3%–86% in different parts of India, depending on the locations, seasons, and cultivars (Lal and Katti, 1997; Shanower et al., 1999). ICRISAT survey reports pod damage of 22% (north), 21% (central), and 13% (south) in India. Losses are estimated to be USD 256 million annually (ICRISAT, 1992). A survey of farmers' fields reported seed damage of 14%–46% in Uttar Pradesh (Lal et al., 1992), 20% in Madhya Pradesh (Sithanantham and Singh, 1986), and 29%–41% in Maharashtra (Sharma et al., 2011). Pandey et al. (2011) recorded 6%–36% and 3%–18% pod and seed damage in late maturing genotypes at Varanasi. Pod and seed damage by pod fly in different genotypes was estimated to be 5%–28% (Lal and Rathore, 2001) and 23.8% (Gandhi et al., 2017) at Kanpur. In short-duration pigeonpea, pod and seed damage were 37% and 17% under Madhya Pradesh conditions (Jakhmola and Bhaduria, 1998).

2.2.7 Management

1. Pod fly is reported to survive on pigeonpea ratoons and alternate hosts; hence, the destruction of alternate host plants is advised to reduce the carry-over population of the pest.
2. The pod fly multiplication rate is low during winter months (December–February); therefore, early-maturing plant types suffer fewer losses due to pod fly (Bhosale and Nawale, 1985; Lal et al., 1988). Early-sown pigeonpea exhibited low pod fly damage.
3. Indeterminate pigeonpea types (37%–40% grain damage) are more susceptible to pod fly infestation than determinate types (26%–28%) due to the availability of green pods for a longer duration (Lal et al., 1986; Gupta et al., 1991). The adoption of less susceptible plant types can help reduce infestation. However, Moudgal et al. (2008) reported no association between plant growth type and pod fly resistance.
4. More than 25 hymenopterans are known to parasitize the pod fly. Three hymenopteran parasitoids, namely, *Euderus lividus* (Eulophidae), *Ormyrus orientalis* (Ormyridae) and *Eurytoma* sp. (Eurytomidae), were commonly reported in India (Ahmad, 1940; Sithantham et al., 1983; Singh, 1991). Patange et al. (2017) reported 3%–32% larval parasitism of the pod fly by an ecto-parasitoid, *Torymoides* sp. (Torymidae). The larval–pupal ectoparasitoid, *Pseudotorymus* sp. (Torymidae), recorded 2%–4% parasitization in late pigeonpea fields (Singh et al., 1991; Yadav et al., 2012). Parasitization by *Euderus* sp. was reported to be 4%–14% at Kanpur and 26% at Parbhani on the late cultivar BSMR-736 (Badabagni et al., 2019). Conservation and augmentation of these natural enemies can play a role in the natural suppression of the pod fly population.
5. Host resistance is an important component of pest management. *Ecological resistance*: Asynchrony between insect pests and host plants allows the genotype to escape or avoid peak pest infestation. Genotypes that matured early suffered less pod fly infestation than late-maturing genotypes. Early and medium genotypes recorded 4%–11% seed damage (Yadava et al., 1983) compared to 35% seed damage in late-maturing genotypes (Lal et al., 1988). *Genetic resistance*: Several pigeonpea lines have been identified for resistance to pod fly. Pigeonpea lines ICRISAT 16, ICP 7946-1-3-3,ICP 127, SL 12–3-1, ICP3401, ICP 7950, ICP12304 (Lateef and Pimbert, 1990), PDA 88-1E, PDA 88-2E, PDA 88-3E, PDA 89-3E (Lal and Sachan, 1991), ICP 8102, GP 3-3, SI 12-2, ICP 7946, ICP 7151, SL 42-3, ICP 1950, SL 20-2, SL 42-2 (Lal et al., 1986; Lal and Katti, 1997), SL 21-1-3, SL 21-6-2, SL 21-9-2, SL 22-2-3, PDA 93-1E, PDA 92-1E, PDA 89-2E (Lal and Rathore, 2001), and PDA 92-2E

(Durairaj and Ganapathy, 1997) were identified as potential sources of pod fly resistance. Vegetable pigeonpea genotypes ICPL 7035, GAUT 85-K, ICPL 87075, and ICPL 151 were found to be less susceptible (Borad et al., 1991). Sharma et al. (2003) identified pod fly-resistant wild pigeonpea accessions belonging to *C. scarabaeoides*, *C. cajanifolius*, *C. sericeus*, *R. bracteata*, *C. acutifolius*, *C. lineatus*, and *C. albicans*.

6. The immature stages of the pod fly are concealed within the pigeonpea pods; hence, systemic insecticides are reported to provide more effective control than contact insecticides. The pod fly prefers to oviposit on tender green pods, and insecticide spray coinciding with this stage is found to be more effective. Earlier studies found reduced pod fly infestation with 2–3 sprayings. Several studies reported the effectiveness of insecticides registered with CIBRC for use in pigeonpea against pod fly (Sunil Kumar et al., 2016; Chiranjeevi and Patange, 2018; Ravi et al., 2021). Neem-based preparations were also reported to minimize the damage (Sharma et al., 2011). An initial spray with Methomyl 40 SP (0.6 g/L)+jaggery (10 g/L) at the pod formation stage and a second spray with thiamethoxam 25 WG (0.2 g/L) or imidacloprid 17.8 SL (0.2 mL/L)+jaggery (10 g/L) is also suggested to control this pest (UAS, 2021).

2.3 STEM FLY (BEAN FLY) (*OPHIOMYIA PHASEOLI* (TRYON))

Among *Ophiomyia* spp., the most predominant and destructive is *Ophiomyia phaseoli* (Tryon), known as stem fly, bean fly, or bean stem maggot. Bean flies affect the production of common bean (*Phaseolus vulgaris* L.) in tropical and subtropical countries around the world. They infest the stem of young plants, which can die under heavy damage. Immature stages feed in the internal part of the stem, causing external browning and leading to plant death (Ipe, 1987).

2.3.1 Distribution

The bean fly, *O. phaseoli*, has an extensive distribution throughout Asia and Africa. It is also recorded from Australia, America, and Oceania (Spencer, 1973; Boucher, 2008; EPPO, 2023). Bean fly (*Ophiomyia* spp.) has been reported from countries like Australia, Botswana, Burundi, China, Egypt, Ethiopia, India, Indonesia, Japan, Kenya, Malawi, Mozambique, South Korea, Taiwan, Tanzania, Thailand, Uganda, Vietnam, Zambia, and Zimbabwe (Nkhata et al., 2019).

2.3.2 Taxonomy and Diagnostics

The *Ophiomyia* spp. infesting beans in different parts of the world include *Ophiomyia phaseoli* (Tyron), *O. spencerella* (Greathead), and *O. centrosematis* (de Meij). Their distribution varies by location (Abate and Ampofo, 1996), with *O. phaseoli* being the most devastating across Africa, Asia, and Australia (Kayitare, 1993).

Adults: The adults are small, shining black flies. The frons is narrow; orbital setulae are sparse and reclinate; the ocellar triangle is brilliantly shining black and conspicuously elongated; the third antennal segment is small, round, moderately pubescent, and the aristae are long, appearing bare; the abdomen is brilliantly shining black (Spencer, 1973).
Eggs: Pearly-white and oval.
Larva: Slender and long, with paired mouth hooks;
Puparium: Pale yellowish, straw-coloured, or brownish.

2.3.3 Biology

Oviposition occurs on either the upper or lower surface of young bean leaves. Eggs are inserted between the epidermis and spongy parenchyma (Talekar, 1990). A female can lay between 100 and 300 eggs in

2 weeks. The egg period lasts for 2–4 days. The larva initially forms a short leaf mine and then enters the nearest vein to the petiole and down into the stem. The main feeding occurs in the lower cortical layers of the stem, and sometimes larvae penetrate the taproot (Talekar and Chen, 1986). The larva has three instars, and the total larval stage lasts for 8–10 days, with the pupal stage lasting 9–10 days (Kayitare, 1993). The puparium remains beneath the epidermis and near the base of the stem.

2.3.4 Host Plants

Stem fly infests wide range of legumes including the common bean (*Phaseolus vulgaris* L.), soybean (*Glycine max* L.), cowpea (*Vigna unguiculata* (L.) Walp.) (Abul-Nasr and Assem, 1968); mung bean (*Vigna radiata* (L.) Wilczek) (Islam et al., 1984; Gopali et al., 2014), and urad bean (*V. mungo* (L.) Hepper) (Prodhan et al., 2008). The other host crops are sunflower (*Carthamus tinctorius* L.), black-night shade (*Solanum nigrum* L.) (Kayitare, 1993), lima bean (*P. lunatus* L.), and lablab (*Dolichos lablab* L.) (Spencer, 1973).

2.3.5 Nature and Extent of Damage

The nature and extent of damage caused by bean fly depend on seasonal variations, time of planting, growth stage, geographical location, soil fertility, and varietal tolerance. Higher temperatures, relative humidity, and low rainfall conditions are reported to promote bean fly reproduction and infestations. Nkhata et al. (2019) reviewed yield losses to the extent of 8%–100% in legumes. Larval feeding on the seedling stems results in characteristic swelling and cracking just above ground level. The destruction of cortex tissue weakens the stem, resulting in lodging of the plant. Infested plants become yellowish, wilted, and stunted, which may eventually die unless they form adventitious (secondary) roots (Abate, 1993; Abate and Ampofo, 1996). Symptoms of bean fly attack on common bean (*Phaseolus vulgaris* L.) include yellowing of leaves, defoliation, and premature plant death (Figure 2.2).

2.3.6 Management

1. Earth up the plants 3 days after the appearance of cotyledons above the ground, which can suppress bean fly infestation. The production of adventitious roots at the affected basal portion of the stem helps the plant to survive (Talekar, 1990).
2. Cultivation of onion as an intercrop with common bean (*P. vulgaris*) has been found to minimize bean fly infestation (Jemutai, 2008). Intercropping maize and common bean, especially with early planting of maize, is reported to reduce pest incidence (Talekar, 1992; Peter et al., 2009). Adoption of varietal mixtures is also found to be helpful to the farmers (Ssekandi et al., 2016).
3. Crops like moth bean, chickpea, lentil, and cluster bean were suggested as "dead-end trap crops". Bean flies oviposit on these crops, but the eggs fail to hatch (Talekar and Lee, 1988).
4. Conservation of parasitoids (*Opius phaseoli* Fischer; *O. importatus* Fischer; Hymenoptera: Braconidae) and avoiding the use of broad-spectrum insecticides helps in the natural suppression of bean flies (Greathead, 1975; Abate and Ampofo, 1996).
5. Seed treatment using recommended insecticides has been found effective against bean fly (Srinivasan, 2014). A reduction in stem tunnelling and seedling mortality of mung bean was reported when seeds were treated with thiamethoxam 35 FS (3.5 g a.i./kg) and imidacloprid 60 FS (3 g a.i./kg) (Gopali et al., 2014).
6. Genotypes of legume crops identified as sources of resistance to stem fly include Mlama 49, Mlama 127, G22501 (Hillocks et al., 2006); GBK 047810, GBK047866, G3844, BAT 16 (Ojwang et al., 2010); KK 8, Tasha, Chelalang (Kiptoo et al., 2016) in common bean CO-3 (Devasthali and Joshi, 1994), BM 4, Vaibhav (Bhople et al., 2017) in mung bean (Nair et al., 2019); UG 218, PDU 1, PDU 5, AKU 7, CO 305, UP 95-1, and LBG 707 in urad bean (Gupta and Kumar, 2006; Cheema et al., 2017).

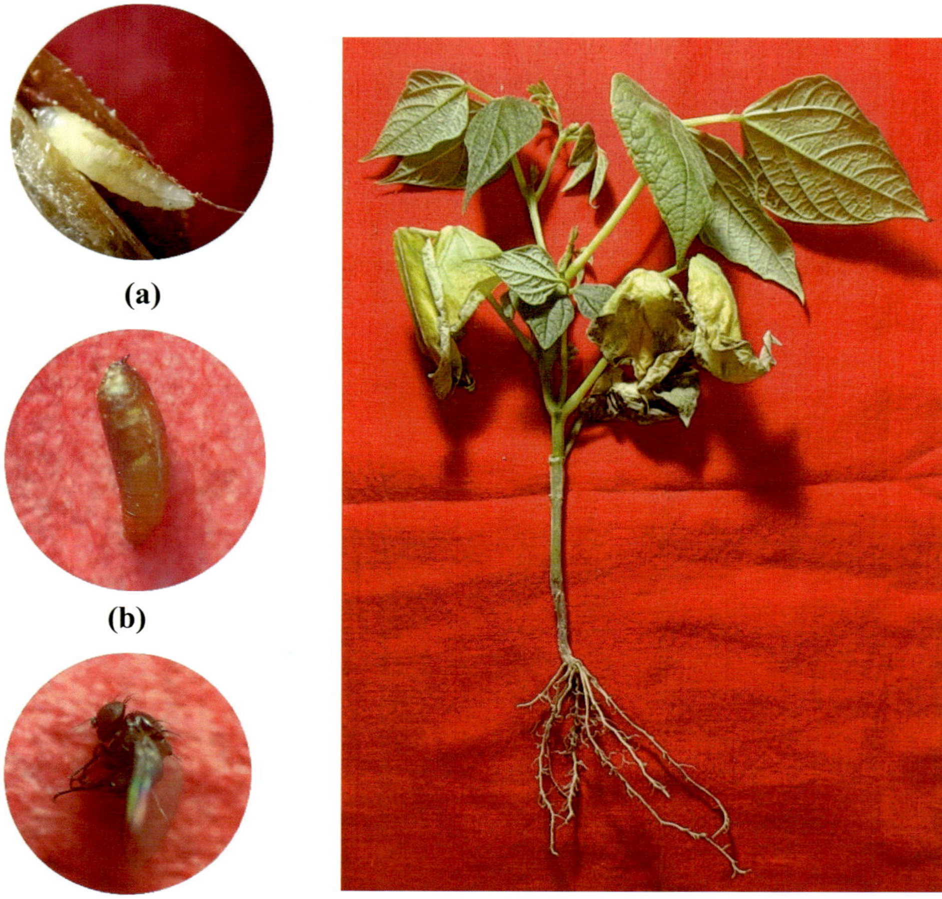

(a) (b) (c) (d)

FIGURE 2.2 Stem fly infestation on urdbean (Source: IIPR, 2020).

2.4 PEA LEAF MINER (*PHYTOMYZA HORTICOLA* GOUREAU)

This is a highly polyphagous and cosmopolitan leaf-mining fly commonly referred to as the pea leaf miner. It was treated as *Chromatomyia horticola*, but the nomenclature was restored to *P. horticola* after the genus *Chromatomyia* was synonymized with *Phytomyza* (Winkler et al., 2009). Hence, most of the description is found under the genus *Chromatomyia* in the world literature. The legume crop, field pea (*Pisum sativum* L.), is severely damaged by this pest in India.

2.4.1 Taxonomy and Diagnostics

Genus *Phytomyza* Fallen: The *Phytomyza* is a species-rich group (>600 species) and is distinguished from other Agromyzids by morphological characters: fronto-orbital setae proclinate; halteres usually white or faintly yellow; costa extending only to vein R_{4+5}, and cross vein *dm-cu* usually absent (Spencer, 1987; Winkler et al., 2009; Kwon et al., 2009).

***Phytomyza horticola* Goureau, 1851**: mesonotum distinctly mat, ash-grey, without acrostichals; frons broad, yellow, slightly darker; third antennal segment small, round, arista appears bare; face greyish black; legs: coxae, femora, tibia, and tarsi black (Spencer, 1973).

2.4.2 Host Range

Pea leaf miner, *P. horticola*, is a polyphagous pest. Cultivated host plants have been found in eight families, viz., Fabaceae, Asteraceae, Brassicaceae, Cucurbitaceae, Lamiaceae, Liliaceae, Linaceae, and Solanaceae (Spencer, 1973, 1990). The most common host plants are reported to be from Brassicaceae, Fabaceae, and Asteraceae (Malipatil and Ridland, 2008). Griffiths (1967) listed an additional 25 plant families that serve as host plants for the pea leaf miner.

2.4.3 Distribution

The pest is distributed in different regions of Africa, Asia, and Europe (Spencer, 1973). In India, it is a serious pest on field pea (*Pisum sativum* L.) (Prasad, 1993) and *Brassica* spp. (Singh and Bakhetia, 1983). Mehta et al. (1994) recorded >20% avoidable yield loss when leaf infestation was >40% in north India.

2.4.4 Biology

Eggs hatch in 2–4 days. The larval period is reported to be 5 days at 23°C–28°C, and the pupal stage lasts for 7–15 days. Aestivation or hibernation of the pupal stage is also on record (Ahmad and Gupta, 1941).

2.4.5 Nature and Extent of Damage

Adult females oviposit into living plant tissue, and the entire larval stage is spent feeding within the mines created as they feed. Larval leaf mines are irregularly linear (Spencer, 1973) (Figure 2.3). Larvae tunnel into the mesophyll and feed on palisade and spongy parenchyma (Sen and Sehgal, 1993), but the upper and lower epidermis remain intact (Srivastava and Singh, 1972). Leaf mining activity destroys chlorophyll content, affecting rates of photosynthesis (Parrella et al., 1985). Leaf mining by larvae results in withering and premature dropping of leaves. Under severe infestations, reduced flowering is observed (Molitas and Gabriel, 1975). The feeding punctures of adult females appear creamy-white, crowded mainly in the central area of the leaf. Oviposition punctures are yellowish-brown along the leaf margins (Singh and Bakhetia, 1983).

Leaf infestation by *P. horticola* ranged between 3.4% and 49.4% on different genotypes of field pea under Kanpur conditions, and genotypes manifested higher leaf infestation (25.7%–61.2%) under late-sown conditions (Yadav et al., 2022). Kooner and Singh (1980) reported up to 32%

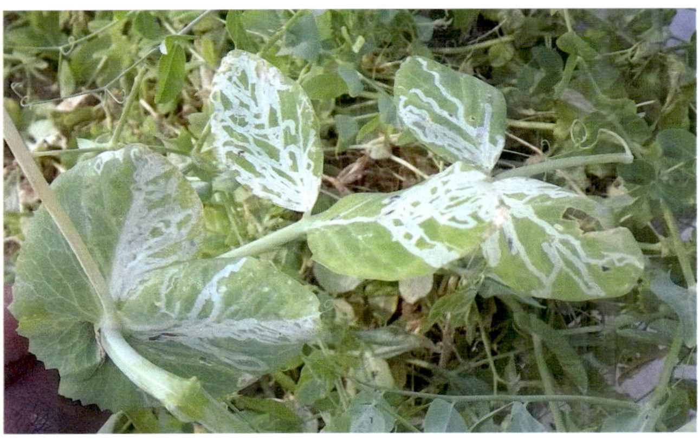

FIGURE 2.3 Leaf miner infestation on field pea.

infestation of leaves on field pea in Punjab. Leaflet infestation of 16%–59% was reported by Thakur and Patial (2019) in the mid-hills of Himachal Pradesh.

2.4.6 Management

1. Leaf infestation in field pea was reported to be higher in late-sown conditions compared to timely sowing (Yadav et al., 2022). Hence, timely sowing of field pea and field sanitation are essential to reduce leaf miner infestations.
2. The use of yellow sticky traps has also been found to reduce the population of adult flies in the field (Salvo and Valladares, 2007).
3. Spraying of neem seed kernel extract (5%) is used to control the leaf miner in brassica crops (TNAU, 2015).
4. Field pea genotypes: IPFD 2021-8, IPFD 2021-9, IPF 5–19, IPF 2021-17, IPF 2021-21 were identified as less susceptible to leaf miner infestation under timely sown conditions (Yadav et al., 2022). IPFD 2021-8 and IPFD 12-2 demonstrated a moderate level of resistance under both timely and late sowing conditions. According to Sen and Sehgal (1993), pea varieties P-200 and P-402 demonstrated resistance to the leaf miner by affecting the growth, longevity, survival, and fecundity of the insect.

2.5 CHICKPEA LEAF MINER (*LIRIOMYZA CICERINA* RONDANI)

Chickpea leaf miner, *L. cicerina*, is one of the major pests infesting chickpea (*Cicer arietinum* L.) from the seedling to podding stage (Toker et al., 2019). This species is reported to be native to the Mediterranean area (Spencer, 1973). It is an oligophagous species, feeding on the plants belonging to the Fabaceae family (Shevtchenko, 1937).

2.5.1 Distribution

Chickpea leaf miner is most widespread in western Asia, northern Africa (Cardona, 1983), and Europe (Toker et al., 2019). It is a serious pest on plants belonging to the Fabaceae family throughout the entire Mediterranean region (Cikman and Civelek, 2006; El-Bouhssini et al., 2008).

2.5.2 Taxonomy and Diagnostics

The genus *Liriomyza* contains more than 300 species and is widely distributed in the New and Old Worlds, but is most dominant in temperate regions (Parrella, 1987). The adults are very small and dark, with a small, round, darkened third antennal segment; in wings, the costa extends to vein M_{1+2}, and the discal cell is small; the frons is orange-yellow; the mesonotum is deep black; the mesopleura is normally black along the lower and front margins, paler above, and more rarely has only a small black patch on the lower margin; the legs are dark, and the femora, while basically yellow, are largely darkened by variable black striations. Larval posterior spiracles each have seven to nine pores, with the two processes widely separated; the puparium is pale brownish-yellow (Spencer, 1973).

2.5.3 Biology

Females insert their eggs just beneath the epidermis of the leaflet. Eggs hatch in about 4 days. Larvae pass through three instars before exiting the leaf to pupate in the soil (Changizi et al., 2012). The pupal stage lasts for 10–12 days. The life cycle is completed in 20–30 days. Generally, two to three overlapping generations occur during one cropping season, depending on the availability of host plants, prevailing temperature, and region (Pastucha, 1996; Cikman and Civelek, 2006).

2.5.4 Host Plants

The host plants of *L. cicerina* primarily belong to the Fabaceae family (CABI, 2009). According to Spencer (1973), the primary host plants of *L. cicerina* are likely to be European plant, including *Ononis* spp. such as *Ononis arvensis* L., *O. hircina* Jacq., *O. repens* L., *O. spinosa* L., and *Hymenocarpus circinnatus* (L.) Savi. This pest switched hosts to chickpea (*Cicer arietinum* L.) when this legume crop was introduced to southern Europe from Asia (Carapelli et al., 2018). The pest was reported on chickpea by Naresh and Malik (1989) from India. It has also been reported on *Melilotus alba* (white sweet clover) and *M. officinalis* (yellow sweet clover) (Robbins, 1983). Recently, *L. cicerina* has been reported as a pest of faba bean (*Vicia faba* L.) in the Damanhur region of Egypt (El-Serwy, 2003).

2.5.5 Nature and Extent of Damage

Female flies of the leaf miner puncture the lower and upper surfaces of leaves for feeding and oviposition (Ceylan et al., 2018), resulting in a stippled appearance of the leaflets (Toker et al., 2019). The major damage results from mining in the leaflets by the larvae. Lower leaves are infested first, and only three to four healthy leaves are found on each stem (CABI, 2009). Larvae create serpentine mines along the parenchyma tissue (Ceylan et al., 2018). These mines are present on both upper and lower leaf surfaces and are linear and shallow (Spencer, 1973). The mines appear whitish and winding irregularly, later forming a secondary blotch. The larvae feed on leaf mesophyll tissue, affecting chlorophyll content and stomatal conductance (Yildirim et al., 2010). This leads to reduced photosynthetic activity, leaf desiccation, and premature leaf fall (El-Bouuhssini et al., 2008). Leaf crop results in a lack of shade and sun scalding of pods (Reed et al., 1987) According to Shevtchenko (1937), infested leaves turn yellow, dry, and fall prematurely.

The chickpea leaf miner can cause up to 40% yield losses, depending on the level of infestation, genotypes, and planting times (Reed et al., 1987; Chen et al., 2011). Sabraoui et al. (2019) reported 25%–43% leaf infestation by the chickpea leaf miner and 20% (winter season) to 42% (spring season) grain yield losses in Morocco.

2.5.6 Management

1. Deep ploughing prior to planting the crop is suggested to destroy the pupal stages of the leaf miner (El-Serwy, 2003).
2. Early-sown chickpeas are found to escape leaf miner damage (Sharma et al., 2006). Chickpeas planted during the spring season had a significantly higher number of infested leaflets than the winter-sown crop (El-Bouhssini et al., 2008).
3. The population density of the pest is found to increase under high humidity and irrigated conditions (Cikman and Civelek, 2006; Carapelli et al., 2018). However, increased infestation under higher irrigation did not result in a loss of yield.
4. Yellow traps have been reported effective in capturing adult leaf miner flies (Cikman and Civelek, 2006).
5. The practice of spreading the harvested plants of faba bean on plastic sheets to facilitate the collection of the accumulated leaf miner pupae was suggested by El-Serwy (2003).
6. Several hymenopteran natural enemies have been reported to reduce the leaf miner population. *Opius monilicornis* F., *O. pygmaeus* F., *O. tersus* Foerster (Braconidae), and *Diglyphus isaea* W., *Diglyphus crassinervis* Erdos, *Diaulinopsis arenaria* E., *Neochrysocharis formosa* (Westwood), *N. ambitiosa* Hansson, *N. sericea* Erdos, and *Pediobius metallicus* (Nees) (Eulophidae) were recorded on *L. cicerina* (Grenouillet et al., 1993; Cikman et al., 2008a; Cikman et al., 2008b; CABI, 2009). Soltani *et al.* (2018) reported 13%–52%

parasitism by *O. monilicornis*, *D. isaea*, and *D. arenaria* in Tunisia. Conservation of these natural enemies would help in naturally suppressing the leaf miner population.

7. Chickpea varieties with larger leaflets are found to be preferred by the leaf miner over those with smaller leaflets. Genotypes ILWC 39, ILC 3800, ILC 5901, and ILC 7738 are reported to be resistant to leaf miner damage in chickpeas (Chen et al., 2011). Among the wild relatives of chickpeas, two accessions of *Cicer cuneatum* (ILWC 40 and ILWC 187) and ten accessions of *C. judaicum* have been reported as highly resistant to leaf miner damage (Singh and Weigand, 1994). The germplasms, including one mutant (3304) and two breeding lines (LMR 140 and LMR 160), were reported as highly resistant to the leaf miner (Ceylan et al., 2018).
8. Spraying of azadirachtin 0.03%, *Bacillus thuringiensis* spores (60×10^6/mg), deltamethrin 50 EC, spinosad 240 SC, and cyromazine 75 WP significantly reduce leaflet damage by leaf miners in chickpea (Cikman et al., 2008b; El-Bouhssini et al., 2008; Cikman et al., 2011).

2.6 CONCLUSIONS

Agromyzids are important crop pests worldwide, and some members of this group are key pests of food legumes. The pigeonpea pod fly, bean (stem) fly, pea leaf miner, and chickpea leaf miner are significant agromyzid pests of food legumes in different parts of the world. The larval stages are internal feeders on leaves, stems, seeds, or pods, causing significant crop losses. Due to their internal mining or feeding habits, the monitoring, sampling, and controlling these pests is difficult until the infestation becomes evident. Future studies should emphasize aspects such as off-season survival and seasonal carry-over of the population, seasonal dynamics, artificial rearing methods, identifying baits/attractants, and sources of resistance for the effective management of agromyzids in legume crops.

2.7 POINTS TO REMEMBER

1. The major agromyzid pests of food legumes belong to the genera *Melanagromyza*, *Phytomyza*, *Liriomyza*, and *Ophiomyia*.
2. The larval stages of agromyzids are internal feeders on leaves, stems, seeds, and pods of various legume crops.
3. Pod flies thrust their eggs into the lumen of the pigeonpea pods.
4. All the immature stages of pod flies are concealed within the pigeonpea pods.
5. Pod flies infest partially matured pods and damage the developing seeds of pigeonpea.
6. Stem flies (bean flies) insert their eggs into the surface of young bean leaves.
7. Stem flies (bean flies) infest and damage the stem portion of young bean plants.
8. Pea leaf miners deposit their eggs into leaf tissues.
9. Pea leaf miners are highly polyphagous pests and infest a wide range of host plants.
10. Chickpea leaf miners insert their eggs just beneath the epidermis of chickpea leaflets.
11. Chickpea leaf miners create serpentine mines on the chickpea leaflets and feed within these mines.

REFERENCES

Abate, T. (1993) Control of other pests and diseases. In: J.R.J. Rowland (ed.), *Dryland Farming in Africa.* Macmillan, London, pp. 9188–9204.

Abate, T. and Ampofo, J.K.O. (1996) Insect pests of beans in Africa: Their ecology and management. *Annu. Rev. Entomol.*, 41(1):45–73.

Abul-Nasr, S. and Assem, M. (1968) Studies on the biological processes of the bean fly, *Melanagromyzaphaseoli* (Tryon) (Diptera: Agromyzidae). *Bull. Soc. Entomol.*, 52:283–295.

Ahmad, T. (1938) The tur-pod fly, *Agromyzaobtusa* Mall., as pest of *Cajanuscajan. Indian J. Agric. Sci.*, 8(1):63–76.

Ahmad, T. (1940) Studies on the biology of *Euderuslividus* (Ashm.), a parasite of *Agromyza obtusa* Mall. *Indian J. Ent.*, 2:59–64.

Ahmad, T. and Gupta, R.L. (1941) The pea leaf-miner, *Phytomyza atricornis* (Meigen) in India. *Indian J. Ent.*, 3(1):37–49.

Badabagni, C., Patange, N.R. and Sagadai, M. (2019) Parasitisation of pigeon pea pod fly *Melanagromyza obtusa* and its population dynamics as influenced by genotypes. *Indian J. Ent.*, 81(3):521–525.

Benavent-Corai, J., Martinez, M. and Jiménez Peydró, R. (2005) Catalogue of the hosts-plants of the world Agromyzidae (Diptera). *Boll. Zool. Agr. Bachic.*, 37(Suppl.):1–97.

Bhople, S.K., Dhandge, S.R., Aravindarajan, G. and Patange, N.R. (2017) Varietal screening of mungbean genotypes for their resistance against pest complex of mungbean. *AGRES*, 6:123–128.

Bhosale, D.J. and Nawale, R.N. (1985) Field screening of pigeonpea germplasm against pod fly *Melanagromyza obtusa* (Malloch). *Indian J. Ent.*, 47:92–97.

Borad, P.K., Patel, J.R. and Patel, M.G. (1991) Evaluation of vegetable pigeonpea (*Cajanus cajan*) genotypes resistant to gram-pod borer (*Helicoverpa armigera*), plume moth (*Marasmarcha liophanes*) and pod fly (*Melanagromyza obtusa*). *Indian J. Agric. Sci.*, 61:682–684.

Boucher, S. (2008) Leaf-miner flies (Diptera: Agromyzidae). In: J.L. Capinera (ed.), *Encyclopaedia of Entomology.* Springer, New York, pp. 2164–2169.

CABI (2009) CABI compendium: *Liriomyza cicerina.* https://www.cabidigitallibrary.org/doi/10.1079/cabicompendium.30953 (accessed 27 June 2023).

Carapelli, A., Soltani, A., Leo, C., Vitale, M., Amri, M. and Mediouni-Ben Jemâa, J. (2018) Cryptic diversity hidden within the leaf miner genus *Liriomyza* (Diptera: Agromyzidae). *Genes*, 9(11):554.

Cardona, C. (1983) Insect pests of faba beans, lentils, and chickpeas in North Africa and West Asia: A review of their economic importance. In: M.C. Saxena and S. Varma (eds.), *Faba Beans, Kabuli Chickpeas, and Lentils in the 1980's.* ICARDA, Aleppo, Syria, pp. 159–167.

Ceylan, F.O., Sari, H., Sari, D., Adak, A., Erler, F. and Toker, C. (2018) Revealing of resistant sources in *Cicer* species to chickpea leaf miner, *Liriomyza cicerina (Rondani). Phytoparasitica*, 46:635–643.

Changizi, S., Goldasteh, S.H., Shoushtari, R.V., Changizi, M. and Najafabadi, S S.M. (2012) Study on biology and population fluctuations of leaf miner *Agromyza* sp. on chickpea in Khomeyn Region (Iran). *Mun. Entomol. Zool.* 7(1):474–480.

Cheema, H.K., Pratap, A. and Sujayanand, G.K. (2017) Breeding for insect resistance in mungbean and urdbean. In: R. Arora and S. Sandhu (eds.), *Breeding Insect Resistant Crops for Sustainable Agriculture.* Springer, Singapore, pp. 353–385.

Chen, W., Sharma, H.C. and Muehlbauer, F.J. (2011) *Compendium of Chickpea and Lentil Diseases and Pests.* American Phytopathological Society, St. Paul, MN, p. 165.

Chiranjeevi, B. and Patange, N.R. (2018) Bio-efficacy of newer insecticides and botanicals against population of pigeonpea pod fly, *Melanagromyza obtusa (Malloch). J. Entomol. Res.*, 42(3):377–382.

Cikman, E. and Civelek, H.S. (2006) Population densities of *Liriomyza cicerina* (Rondani, 1875) (Diptera: Agromyzidae) on *Cicer arietinum* L. (Leguminosae: Papilionoidea) in different irrigated conditions. *Turk. Entomol. Derg.*, 30(1):3–10.

Cikman, E., Civelek, H.S. and Weintraub, P.G. (2008a). The parasitoid complex of *Liriomyza cicerina* on chickpea (Cicer arietinum). *Phytoparasitica*, 36:211–216.

Cikman, E., Civelek, H.S. and Yildirim, E.M. (2011) Effects of spinosad on *Liriomyza cicerina* (Rondani, 1875) (Diptera: Agromyzidae) and its parasitoids in chickpea. *Turk. Entomol. Bult.* 1(2):71–77.

Cikman, E., Kaplan, M. and Cokun, Y. (2008b) The effects of *Bacillus thuringiensis* on larval serpentine leaf miners, *Liriomyza cicerina* (Rondani, 1875) (Dipetera: Agromyzidae) in chickpea. *J. Appl. Sci. Res.*, 4(10):1191–1198.

De Meijere, J.C.H. (1922) Zur Kenntnis Javanischer Agromyzinen. *Bijdr Dierk.* 22:18–23.

Devasthali, S. and Joshi, M. (1994) Infestation and varietal preference of insect pests in green gram. *Ind. Agric.*, 38:263–272.

Durairaj, C. and Ganapathy, N. (1997) Evaluation of pigeonpea (*Cajanus cajan*) entries of late-maturity group for tolerance to pod borers (*Helicoverpa armigera, Maruca testulalis) and pod fly (Melanagromyza obtusa). Indian J. Agric. Sci.*, 67:317–318.

El-Bouhssini, M., Mardini, K., Malhotra, R.S., Joubi, A. and Kagka, N. (2008) Effects of planting date, varieties and insecticides on chickpea leaf miner (*Liriomyza cicerina* R.) infestation and the parasitoid, *Opius monilicornis* F. *Crop Prot.*, 27(6):915–919.

El-Serwy, S.A. (2003) Studies on the leaf miner; *Liriomyza cicerina* (Rondani) and *Liriomyza bryoniae* (Kaltenbach) (Diptera: Agromyzidae) and their parasitoids in faba bean in Egypt. *Egypt. J. Agric. Res.*, 81(4):1581–1593.

EPPO (2023) EPPO (European and Mediterranean Plant Protection Organization) global database: *Melanagromyza obtusa*. https://gd.eppo.int/taxon/MEAGOP (accessed 15 June 2023).

Gandhi, K.B., Bandi, S.M., Naik, S.S.J., Singh, S.K. and Kumar, K. (2017) Character association and assessment of yield loss in pigeonpea cultivars infested by pod fly and bruchid. *Legume Res.*, 42(3):411–415.

Gopali, R.J.B., Hoshmani, A. and Yelshetty, S. (2014) Estimation of avoidable loss due to stem fly, *Ophiomyia phaseoli* (Tryon) and its management by using new molecules as seed dressers in green gram. *Karnataka J. Agric. Sci.*, 27:32–35.

Greathead, D.J. (1975) Biological control of the beanfly, *Ophiomyia phaseoli* [Dipt.: Agromyzidae], by *Opius* spp.[Hym.: Braconidae] in the Hawaiian Islands. *Entomophaga*, 20(3):313–316.

Grenouillet, C., Martinez, M. and Rasplus, J.Y. (1993) Liste des parasitoids et des predateurs des Liriomyza d' importance economique dans le monde (Diptera: Agromyzidae). *"LIRIOMYZA" Colloque sur les mouches mineuses des plantescultive´es* 200:143–156.

Griffiths, G.C.D. (1967) A stem-mining fly (*Ophiomyia*) (Dipt., Agromyzidae) attacking peas (*Pisum sativum* L.). *Entomologist's Mon. Mag.*, 102:135–137.

Gupta, S. and Kumar, S. (2006) Urdbean breeding. In: M. Ali and S. Kumar (eds.), *Advances in Mungbean and Urdbean*. Indian Institute of Pulses Research, Kanpur, pp. 149–168.

Gupta, S.C., Lateef, S.S. and Ariyanayagam, R.P. (1991) Are determinates inferior to in determinates in short duration pigeonpea? *Int. Pigeonpea Newsl.*, 13:11–13.

Hillocks, R., Madata, C.S., Chirwa, R., Minja, E.M. and Msolla, S. (2006) Phaseolus bean improvement in Tanzania. *Euphytica*, 150:215–231.

ICRISAT (1992) *The Medium-Term Plan*, Vol 1. International Crops Research Institute for the Semi-Arid Tropics, Patancheru, India, p. 80.

IIPR (2020) Knowledge platform on pulse crops. https://pest.dalhangyanmanch.res.in/rogKeetPageInfo/5/51/233. (accessed 20 January 2025).

Ipe, I.M. (1974) Morphological, behavioural and biological studies of *Melanagromyza obtusa* (Malloch) (Diptera: Agromyzidae) *on Cajanus indicus Spreng. Zeitschrift für Angewandte Entomologie*, 75(1–4):89–98.

Ipe, I.M. (1987) Biosystematic studies on Agromyzidae from India. *Proc. Indian Acad. Sci. (Animal Sciences)*, 96(5):573–581.

Islam, W., Ahmed, K.N. and Joarder, O.I. (1984) Timing and extent of damage caused by insect pests of green gram (*Vigna radiata* L.) in Bangladesh. *CropProtection* 3(3):343–348.

Jaiswal, A.K., Singh, A.K., Singh, J.P. and Patamajhi, P. (2015) Management of pod fly, *Melanagromyza obtusa* in a bushy lac host, *Flemingia semialata* for quality seed production. *Indian J. Entomol.*, 77(3):278–282.

Jakhmola, S.S. and Bhadauria, N.S. (1998) Response of short-duration pigeonpea (*Cajanus cajan*) genotypes for resistance to pod-fly (*Melanagromyza obtusa*) under protected and unprotected conditions. *Indian J. Agri. Sci.*, 68(1):46–47.

Jemutai, J. (2008) Effect of seed dressing insecticide, intercropping and plant density on bean fly (*Ophiomyia* spp.) infestation in common bean (*Phaseolus vulgaris* L.). M.Sc. Thesis, Egerton University, Kenya, p. 52.

Kayitare, J.S. (1993) Infestation of *Phaseolus vulgaris* (L) by the bean fly, *Ophiomyia* spp. (Diptera: Agromyzidae) and its management by cultural practices. PhD thesis, University of Ghana, Accra.

Kiptoo, M., Kinyua, O., Kiplagat, F., Wanjala, M., Kiptoo, J., and Cheboi, J. (2016) Evaluation of common bean (*Phaseolus vulgaris* L.) varieties for resistance to bean stem maggot (*Ophiomyia* spp.) in Kenya. *Am. J. Exp. Agric.*, 12:1–7.

Kooner, B.S. and Singh, H. (1980) Performance of some cultivars of field-peas against leaf-miner (*Phytomyzahorticola* Gour.). *Indian J. Hortic.*, 37(1):101–102.

Kulkarni, S.M. (1966) Infestation, sex-ratio and damage by *Melanagromyza obtusa* (Diptera: Agromyzidae) to *Moghaniam acrophylla* seeds in the field. *Entomol. Exp. Appl.*, 9(3):323–326.

Kwon, Y.J., Kim, J. and Suh, S.J. (2009) Taxonomy of the genus *Phytomyza* Fallen (Diptera: Agromyzidae) in Korea. *Entomol. Res.*, 39(3):207–213.

Lal, S.S. and Katti, G. (1997) Pod fly, *Melanagromyza obtusa* Malloch: A key pest of pigeonpea. ICAR-IIPR, Kanpur, India, p. 26.

Lal, S.S. and Rathore, Y.S. (2001) Host plant resistance to pod fly (*Melanagromyza obtusa*) in pigeonpea (*Cajanu scajan*). *Indian J. Agric. Sci.*, 71(8):531–534.

Lal, S.S. and Sachan, J.N. (1991) Controlling pod fly, *Melanagromyza obtusa* in late pigeonpea through host-plant resistance. *Int. Pigeonpea Newsl.*, 15:28–30.

Lal, S.S., Yadava, C.P. and Chandra, S. (1986) Suppression of pod fly damage through varietal selection. *Int. Pigeonpea Newsl.*, 5:42–43.

Lal, S.S., Yadava, C.P. and Sachan, J.N. (1988) Studies on some aspects of oviposition and damage of pod fly in relation to the host phenology. *Indian J. Pulses Res.*, 1:83–88.

Lal, S.S., Yadava, C.P. and Sachan, J.N. (1992) Assessment of pod borers damage on pigeonpea in different agroecological zones of Uttar Pradesh. *Indian J. Pulses Res.*, 5:174–178.

Lateef, S.S. and Pimbert, M.P. (1990) The search for host plant resistance to *Helicoverpa armigera* in chickpea and pigeonpea at ICRISAT. In: *Summary Proceedings of the First Consultative Group Meeting on Host Selection Behaviour of Heliothis Armigera*. ICRISAT, Patancheru, India, pp. 25–28.

Malipatil, M. and Ridland, P. (2008) *Polyphagous Agromyzid Leaf Miners. Identifying Polyphagous Agromyzid Leaf Miners (Diptera: Agromyzidae) Threatening Australian Primary Industries*. The Department of Primary Industries, Victoria. https://keys.lucidcentral.org/keys/v3/leafminers/index.htm (accessed 15 June 2023).

Martínez-Alava, J.O., Serna, F. and Pérez, A.L. (2016) *Melanagromyza obtusa* (Diptera: Agromyzidae), a new record for Colombia. *Agronom. Colomb.*, 34(2):292–294.

Maxwell, L.H. (1909) *Indian Insect Life*. Today and Tomorrow Printers and Publishers, New Delhi, India, p. 786.

Mehta, P.K., Sood, P. and Chandel, Y.S. (1994) Extent of losses caused by pea leaf miner, *Chromatomyia horticola* in mid hills of Himachal Pradesh. *Indian J. Plant Protec.*, 22(1):1–4.

Molitas, L.P. and Gabriel, B.P. (1975) Biology of the sweet pea leaf miner *Phytomyza horticola* Goureau (Diptera: Agromyzidae) in the Philippines. *Philip. Entomol.*, 3:89–108.

Moudgal, R.K., Lakra, R.K., Dahiya, B. and Dhillon, M.K. (2008) Physico-chemical traits of *Cajanus cajan* (L.) Millsp. pod wall affecting *Melanagromyza obtusa* (Malloch) damage. *Euphytica*, 161:429–436.

Nair, R.M., Pandey, A.K., War, A.R., Hanumantharao, B., Shwe, T., Alam, A., Pratap, A., Malik, S.R., Karimi, R., Mbeyagala, E.K., Douglas, C.A., Rane, J. and Schafleitner, R. (2019) Biotic and abiotic constraints in mungbean production- Progress in genetic improvement. *Front. Plant Sci.*, 10:1340.

Naresh, J.S. and Malik, V.S. (1989) Observations on the pests of chickpea (*Cicer arientinum* L.) in Haryana. *Bull. Entomol. (New Delhi)*, 27(1):75–77.

Nkhata, W., Shimelis, H., Melis, R., Chirwa, R. and Mzengeza, T.T. (2019) Breeding for bean fly resistance in common bean (*Phaseolus vulgaris* L.): A review. *Acta Agric. Scand. Sec. B Soil Plant Sci.*, 69:275–285.

Ojwang, P.P.O. (2010) Genetic studies on host-plant resistance to bean fly (*Ophiiomyia* spp.) and seed yield in common bean (*Phaseolus vulgaris*) under semi-arid conditions. PhD Thesis. University of KwaZulu-Natal, Pietermaritzburg.

Pandey, V., Srivastava, C.P., Nath, T. and Raha, P. (2011) Chemical traits of pigeonpea (*Cajanuscajan*) pod wall affecting pod fly (*Melanagromyza obtusa*) damage. *Indian J. Agric. Sci.*, 81(11):1059–1062.

Parrella, M.P., Jones, V.P., Youngman, R.R. and Lebeck, L.M. (1985) Effect of leaf mining and leaf stippling of *Liriomyza* spp. on photosynthetic rates of *Chrysanthemum*. *Ann. Entomol. Soc. Am.*, 78:90–93.

Parrella, M.P. (1987) Biology of *Liriomyza*. *Ann. Rev. Entomol.*, 32:201–224.

Pastucha, L. (1996) Bionomy and harmfulness of chickpea leaf miner (*Liriomyza cicerina* Rond.) in Slovakia. *Ved. PrVysk. UstRastl.Vyroby. Piestanoch.*, 26:111–123.

Patange, N.R., Sharma, O.P. and Chiranjeevi, B. (2017) Population dynamics of *Melanagromyza obtusa* (Malloch) (Diptera: Agromyzidae) and its natural parasitization in pigeonpea. *Entomon*, 42(3):201–06

Peter, K.H., Swella, G.B. and Mushobozy, D.M.K. (2009) Effect of plant populations on the incidence of bean stem maggot (*Ophiomyia* spp.) in common bean intercropped with maize. *Plant Protect. Sci.*, 45(4):148–155.

Prasad, C.S. (1993) Assessment of losses by pea Ieaf miner, *Phytomyza horticola* (G.) on pea. *Natl. Acad. Sci. Lett.*, 16(3):119–21.

Prodhan, M.Z.H., Hossain, M.A., Rahman, M.T. and Afroze, M.A. (2008) Incidence of major insect pest of black gram at different dates of sowing. *Int. J Sustain. Crop Prod.*, 3:6–9.

Ravi, S., Singh, R.B., Patel, S., Patel, P.K. and Kumar, S. (2021) Field evaluation of newer insecticides against pod fly (*Melanagromyza obtusa* Malloch) on pigeon pea (*Cajanus cajan*). *J. Entomol. Res.*, 45(4):724–727.

Reed, W., Cardona, C., Sithanantham, S. and Lateef, S.S. (1987) Chickpea insect pest and their control. In: M.C. Saxena and K.B. Singh (eds.), *The Chickpea*. CAB International, Wallingford, UK, pp. 283–318.

Rehman, S.M.A.S., Naik, S., Kumar, K.P., Chakravarthy, A.K. and Gowda, B.H. (2016) Bioecology of pigeonpea pod fly, *Melanagromyza obtusa* Malloch in Karnataka, south India. *Bioscan*, 11(4):2087–2092.

Robbins, J. (1983) Leaf mining insects in Warwickshire. *Proc. Birming. Nat. Hist. Soc.*, 26:46–48.

Sabraoui, A., Lhaloui, S., Bouchelta, A., El Fakhouri, K. and El Bouhssini, M. (2019) Grain yield losses due to leaf miner (*Liriomyza cicerina* R.) in winter-and spring-planted chickpea in Morocco. *Crop Prot.*, 117:115–120.

Salvo, A. and Valladares, G.R. (2007) Leaf miner parasitoids and pest management. *Ciencia E Invest. Agrar.*, 34(3):167–185.

Scheffer, S.J., Winkler, I.S. and Wiegmann, B.M. (2007) Phylogenetic relationships within the leaf-mining flies (Diptera: Agromyzidae) inferred from sequence data from multiple genes. *Mol. Phylogenet. E* 42(3):756–775.

Sehgal, V.K. (1990) Agroecological pest management in chickpea and pigeonpea crops in India. In: *Proceedings of the 3rd International Conference on Plant Protection in the Tropics*, Vol. 5. Malaysian Plant Protection Society, Kuala Lampur, Malaysia, pp. 74–79.

Sen, A. and Sehgal, V.K. (1993) Resistance in peas, *Pisum sativum* L., against pea leaf miner, *Chromatomyia horticola* (goureau) (Diptera: Agromyzidae): Biology, feeding and ovipositional preferences. *Insect Sci. Appl.*, 14(2):185–191.

Serra, C.A., Garcia, S., Segura, Y. and Arias, J. (2003) Dramatic impact of the recently introduced Asian pigeonpea pod fly, *Melanagromyza obtuse* (Malloch) (Diptera: Agromyzidea) in the Dominican Republic. *In: Proceedings of the Caribbean Food Crops Society. No.* 1881-2017-592. 39(2):200–207.

Shanower, T.G., Romeis, J. and Minja, E.M. (1999) Insect pests of pigeon pea (*Cajanus cajan)* and their management. *Ann. Rev. Entomol.*, 44:77–96.

Sharma, H.C., Gaur, P.M., Samineni, S. and Gowda, C.L. (2014) Exploiting host plant resistance for pest management in chickpea. *Legume Perspect.*, 3:25–28.

Sharma, H.C., Gowda, C.L.L., Stevenson, P.C., Ridsdill-Smith, T.J., Clement, S.L., Rao, G.R., Romeis, J., Miles, M. and El-Bouhssini, M. (2006) Host plant resistance and insect pest management in chickpea. In: S. Yadav et al. (eds.), *Chickpea Breeding and Management.* CABI, Wallingford, UK, pp. 527–544.

Sharma, H.C., Pampapathy, G. and Reddy, L.J. (2003) Wild relatives of pigeonpea as a source of resistance to the pod fly (*Melanagromyza obtusa* Malloch) and pod wasp (*Tanaostigmodes cajaninae* La Salle). *Genet. Resour. Crop E* 50:817–824.

Sharma, O.P., Bhosle, B.B., Kamble, K.R., Bhede, B.V. and Seeras, N.R. (2011) Management of pigeonpea pod borers with special reference to pod fly (*Melanagromyza obtusa*). *Indian J. Agric. Sci.*, 81(6):539–543.

Shevtchenko, M. (1937) *Liriomyza cicerina* Rond., and its importance to cultivation of *Cicer arietinum. Plant Prot.*, 12:159–170.

Shi, L. and Gaimari, S.D. (2015) Revision of the genus *Melanagromyza* in California, with descriptions of three new species (Diptera: Agromyzidae). *Zootaxa*, 4005(1):001–102.

Singh, D. (1991) Three hymenopterous parasitoids of *Melanagromyza obtusa* (Malloch), a pest of tur, *Cajanus cajan* (L.) Millsp. *J. Entomol. Res.*, 15(4):282–286.

Singh, K.B. and Weigand, S. (1994) Identification of resistant sources in *Cicer* species to *Liriomyza cicerina. Genetic Resour. Crop Evol.*, 41:75–79.

Singh, P. and Bakhetia, D.R.C. (1983) Comparative development and host selection mechanism of the pea leaf miner, *Phytomyza horticola* Goureau on rapeseed and mustard. In: *Proceedings of VITH International Rapeseed Conference*, Paris, pp. 1135–1141.

Singh, S. and Beri, S.K. (1971) Studies on the immature stages of Agromyzidae (Diptera) from India. *J. Nat. Hist.*, 5(3):241–250.

Singh, S., Singh, S.P., Babu, S.S. and Sebastian, P.C. (1991) Bioecology of Hymenoptera parasites of Agromyzidae (Diptera) pests species in India. *Mem. Sch. Ent.*, 11:1–238.

Sithanantham, S. and Singh, H. (1986) Pod fly damage on late maturity pigeonpea at and around Gwalior. *Intl. Pigeonpea Newsl.*, 5:40–42.

Sithanantham, S., Singh, U., Reed, W. and Jambunathan, R. (1983) Differences of some chemical constituents of pigeonpea pod walls in relation to pod fly susceptibility. *Int. Pigeonpea Newslett.*, 2:68–69.

Soltani, A., Beyareslan, A., Gençer, L., Hamdi, S.H., Bousselmi, A., Amri, M. and Jemâa, J.M.B. (2018) Parasitoids of chickpea leaf miner *Liriomyza cicerina* (Diptera: Agromyzidae) and their parasitism rate on chickpea fields in North Tunisia. *J. Asia-Pac. Entomol.*, 21(4):1215–1221.

Spencer, K.A. (1973) Agromyzidae (Diptera) of economic importance. *Ser. Entomol.*, 9:418.

Spencer, K.A. (1987) Agromyzidae. J.F. McAlpine, B.V. Peterson, G.E. Shewell, H.J. Teskey, J.R. Vockeroth and D. M. Wood (eds.), *Manual of Nearctic Diptera.* Vol. 2. Monograph No. 28, Research Branch, *Agriculture Canada Monograp*, pp. 869–879.

Spencer, K.A. (1990) Host specialization in the world Agromyzidae (Diptera). *Ser. Entomol.* 45:444.

Srinivasan, R. (2014) Insect and mite pests on vegetable legumes: A field guide for identification and management. *AVRDC (Taiwan)*, 14-778:92.

Srivastava, A.S. and Singh, Y.P. (1972) Bionomics and control of pea leaf miner, *Phytomyza atricornis* Meig. (Agromyzidae: Dipt.). *Zeitschrift für Angew. Entomol.*, 70(1-4):437–440.

Srivastava, O.S. (1972) Estimation of loss in T 21 variety of arhar (*Cajanuscajan* L.) due to tur pod fly (*Melanagromyza obtusa* Malloch). *Indian J. Entomol.*, 34(1):82–83.

Ssekandi, W., Mulumba, J., Colangelo, P., Nankya, R., Fadda, C., Karungi, J., Otim, M., De Santis, P., Jarvis, D.I. (2016) The use of common bean (*Phaseolus vulgaris*) traditional varieties and their mixtures with commercial varieties to manage bean fly (*Ophiomyia* spp.) infestations in Uganda. *J Pest Sci.*, 89:45–57.

Sunil Kumar, N.M., Yelshetty, S.D., Rathod, P.S. and Sreenivas, A.G. (2016) Bio-efficacy of insecticides for the management of pod fly, *Melanagromyza obtuse* Malloch (Diptera: Agromyzidae) in pigeonpea. *J. Exp. Zool. India.*, 19(1):591–595.

Talekar, N.S. (1990) *Agronomyzid Flies of Food Legumes in the Tropics*. Wiley Eastern Limited, Delhi, India, p. 297.

Talekar, N.S. (1992) The bean fly pest complex of snap beans in the tropics. In: G. Henry and W. Janssen (eds.), *Cartillas para CIAL Los comités de investigaciónAgrícola local Cartilc*, Vol. 2. CIAT, Cali, pp. 127–130.

Talekar, N.S. and Chen, B.S. (1986) The bean fly pest complex of tropical soybean. In: *International Symposium on Soybean: Soybean in Tropical and Subtropical Cropping Systems*. AVRDC, Tsukuba, Japan, pp. 257–271.

Talekar, N.S. and Lee, Y.H. (1988) Biology of *Ophiomyia centrosematis* (Diptera: Agromyzidae), a pest of soybean. *Ann. Entomol. Soc. Am.*, 6:938–942.

Tengecho, B., Coulson, C.L. and D'Souza, H.A. (1988) Distribution and effect of bean flies, *Ophiomyia phaseoli* and O. spencerella, on beans at Kabete, Kenya. *Insect Sci. Appl.* 9(4):505–508.

Thakur, A. and Patial, M. (2019) Studies on host plant resistance in pea against pea leaf miner, *Chromatomyia horticola* (Goureau). *Intl. J. Tropical Agric.*, 37(2):271–279.

Thapa, R.B. (2011) Description of new species of leaf miners (Diptera Agromyzidae) associated with leguminous host described from northern India. *Nepalese J. Biosci.*, 1:66–82.

TNAU (2015) *Agritech Portal-Crop Protection*. Tamil Nadu Agricultural University, Coimbatore, India. https://agritech.tnau.ac.in/crop_protection/crop_prot.html (accessed on 15 June 2023).

Toker, C., Adak, A., Sari, D., Sari, H., Ceylan, F.O., Canci, H., Ikten, C., Erler, F. and Upadhyaya, H.D. (2019) Registration of AWC 612M chickpea mutant germplasm line resistant to leaf miner (*Liriomyza cicerina*). *J. Plant Regist.*, 13(1):87–90.

UAS (2021) *Improved Agronomic Practices-2021*. University of Agricultural Sciences, Dharwad, India, pp. 102–114.

Winkler, I.S., Scheffer, S.J. and Mitter, C. (2009) Molecular phylogeny and systematics of leaf-mining flies (Diptera: Agromyzidae): Delimitation of *Phytomyza* Fallén sensu lato and included species groups, with new insights on morphological and host-use evolution. *Syst. Entomol.*, 34(2):260–292.

Yadav, A.K, Yadav, S. and Singh, M.K. (2012) Effect of temperature on the population of parasitoids and their impact on the pest, *Melanagromyza obtusa* (Diptera: Agromyzidae). *Ecoscan.* 1:45–50.

Yadav, R.K., Chandra, A., Parihar, A.K., Sujayanand, G.K., Kumar, V., Bandi, S.M., Arya, M. and Usha. (2022) Escape resistance in field pea against *Phytomyza horticola* Goureau, as influenced by sowing time and its correlation with plant metabolites. *Pest Manage. Hortic. Ecosyst.*, 28(2):119–128.

Yadava, C.P., Lal, S.S., Dias, C.A.R. and Nigam, R. (1983) Host evasion- a prospective approach for suppressing *Heliothis* damage. *Int. Pigeonpea Newslett.*, 2:62–64.

Yildirim, E.M., Unay, A. and Civelek, H.S. (2010) The effect of *Liriomyza trifolii* (Burgess) (Diptera: Agromyzidae) on some leaf characteristics of bean (*Phaseolus vulgaris* L.). *J. Food Agric. Environ.*, 8(8):3.

3 Fruit Flies (Diptera: Tephritidae) in India

Karamankodu Jacob David, N. R. Noor Mahammed, Venkateshaiah Abhishek, Shanthamma Salini, Abraham Verghese, and Melur Ashwathappa Rashmi

LEARNING OBJECTIVES

1. To appreciate the diversity and habits of fruit flies.
2. To familiarize oneself with the diagnostic characters of major subfamilies.
3. To know the major pestiferous species in India.

3.1 INTRODUCTION

Tephritidae is one of the most economically important families in Diptera (true flies), with more than 5,000 described species classified into six subfamilies, 500 genera, 40 tribes, and subtribes (Korneyev, 1999; Norrbom et al., 1999; Freidberg, 2006). Of these, nearly 300 species in 84 genera and five subfamilies – namely, Dacinae, Phytalmiinae, Tachiniscinae, Tephritinae, and Trypetinae – have been documented from India (Agarwal and Sueyoshi, 2005; David and Ramani, 2019, 2011; David and Hancock, 2013; David et al., 2013, 2014, 2017, 2019, 2024; Abhishek et al.., 2024a, 2024b). Fruit flies belonging to Tephritidae are characterized by well-developed frontal plates, frontal setae that are significantly longer than the surrounding setulae, the presence of a costal break before the apex of the subcostal veins, two or three spines protecting the break, vein Sc bent and joining the costa at nearly right angles, and a wing cell cup with an acute extension; the wing may be patterned or hyaline (Hardy, 1973; White and Elson-Harris, 1992; Korneyev, 1999b).

3.2 ECONOMIC IMPORTANCE

Fruit flies are among the major pests of quarantine concern across all continents due to their concealed feeding and invasive nature. Most of the pestiferous species in India belong to *Bactrocera*, *Dacus*, and *Zeugodacus* in subfamily Dacinae, and *Carpomya* in Trypetinae. They mainly affect horticultural crops in India, and a few pest species, like *Bactrocera caryae* (Kapoor), are endemic to India. Pest species can cause undesirable economic impacts beyond yield losses and increased management expenses, such as loss of export markets and/or increased costs for the construction and maintenance of fruit treatment and management facilities.

In many countries, strict quarantine regulations significantly restrict the export of most commercially grown fruits to prevent the spread of fruit fly species. About 40 species of Tephritidae have been intentionally or unintentionally introduced by humans outside of their natural ranges. These species include *Bactrocera dorsalis* (Hendel), *B. carambolae* Drew and Hancock, *B. latifrons* (Hendel), *Z. cucurbitae* (Coquillett), and *B. zonata* (Saunders), which have been introduced from the Oriental region to other regions, while *B. oleae* (Rossi) was brought from the Mediterranean region to India (Norrbom et al., 1999).

DOI: 10.1201/9781003482581-5

Apart from pestiferous taxa, fruit flies are also significant as weed biocontrol agents. Over 20 species have been utilized as biological control agents for managing invasive weed species. Most of these introduced fruit fly species belong to the subfamily Tephritinae. To control thistles and knapweeds, several species of *Urophora* were introduced to North America (White and Elson-Harris, 1992). The biological control of certain weeds has been achieved in India through the introduction of *Cecidochares connexa* Macquart on Siam weed, *Chromolaena odorata*, and *Procecidochares utilis* Stone on *Eupatorium adenophorum*, which causes stem galls (Bhumannavar et al., 2004; 2007; Ramani, 2004).

Some tephritids are important models for testing evolutionary or ecological theories (*Rhagoletis* spp. for sympatric speciation, and *C. capitata* for demographic research), and they are important subjects for studying basic biology (Norrbom, 2004). *Ceratitis capitata* is used in molecular biology and genetic research.

3.3 DISTRIBUTION

The family Tephritidae can be found in several environments, from open savannah to rainforests and is widely distributed in tropical, subtropical, and temperate regions, with the exception of the Arctic and Antarctic (Kapoor et al., 1980; Norrbom et al., 1999; Agarwal and Sueyoshi, 2005). In India, fruit flies are distributed across all geographic regions, i.e. northern, southern, central, and eastern regions. Members of the tribe Dacini, namely, *Bactrocera*, *Zeugodacus*, and *Dacus*, are distributed throughout India.

3.4 DIVERSITY

Species diversity across major zoogeographic regions indicates that the tropical regions are the most diverse; the Oriental region seems to have the greatest diversity in both genera and species (975 species, 155 genera), followed by the Afro-tropical region with 929 species and 154 genera. The Palearctic, Australasian, Neotropical, and Nearctic regions exhibit approximately equivalent numbers of genera, with the exception that the Palearctic has fewer than the Australasian.

Out of the six subfamilies, Dacinae is the most common in India, accounting for nearly 42% of the country's fauna with 119 described species. Tephritinae comes second with 69 species, followed by Trypetinae with 65 species. Acanthonevrini is the only tribe that contains 18 species from 10 genera that make up the subfamily Phytalmiinae. Only a single species of the subfamily Tachiniscinae has been reported from India (David and Hancock, 2013).

3.5 BIOLOGY AND NATURE OF DAMAGE

Though fruit flies are generally known as fruit feeders, only species of the subfamily Dacinae (particularly tribe Dacini) and subfamily Trypetinae are frugivorous; the rest of the taxa in Tephritidae exhibit a diverse array of feeding habits, such as bamboo shoot feeders, flower feeders, leaf miners, gall makers, etc. Female flies have an extendible long ovipositor, and usually the eggs are deposited between parts of the host flower/intact fruit/stem/leaves. There are three larval instars and a puparial stage. Larvae of fruit flies develop in seed-bearing plants, and about 35% of species attack soft fruits. Apart from infesting soft fruits, approximately 40% of fruit fly species' larvae develop in Asteraceae flowers, while the rest of the species are typically associated with flowers from diverse plant families, or their larvae mine the leaves, stems, or root tissues (White and Elson-Harris, 1992), and some induce gall formation. Fruit flies are synovigenic, i.e. female flies need a protein-rich diet to mature their eggs and oviposit after emergence. Most of the pestiferous species are multivoltine (10–12 generations per year), except *B. minax*, which is univoltine.

Generally, females lay eggs in the tender soft tissues of fruit, the gynoecia of flowers, stems, leaves, or leaf sheaths by piercing with the ovipositor. After hatching, maggots bore into the pulp tissue and create feeding galleries. Frequently, they introduce different pathogens, which lead to decomposition. The last instar drops into the soil, and pupariation takes place in the soil, except in the case of flower-feeding Tephritinae.

3.6 HOST PLANT ASSOCIATIONS

The majority of fruit flies are highly host-specific, except for saprophytes and polyphagous taxa. Polyphagous species in *Zeugodacus* and *Dacus* are mainly associated with several host plants of the family Cucurbitaceae. Among the pestiferous species, *B. minax* is highly host-specific to Rutaceae. Meanwhile, several monophagous species of *Dacus* are associated with Asclepiadaceae.

In Dacinae, only the tribe Gastrozonini has acquired bamboo as its host. The Gastrozonini are considered to be a monophyletic tribe (Wang and Chen, 2002; Kovac et al., 2006; De Meyer, 2006; Dohm et al., 2014); the larvae of Gastrozonini mainly feed on the shoot meristem or other soft tissues of living or dead bamboo shoots.

Species of Phytalmiinae appear to be saprophagous, although Hardy (1986) and Permkam and Hancock (1995) reported that *Clusiosomina*, *Clusiosoma*, *Cheesmanomyia*, and *Rabaulia* species to infest the fruits of *Ficus* spp. Larvae of *Austronevra*, *Dacopsis*, *Diarrhegma*, *Diarrhegmoides*, *Lumirioxa*, and *Phytalmia* develop in decomposing tree trunks or rotting parts of trees (Hardy, 1986; Permkam and Hancock, 1995). Few species of *Afrocneros* and *Ocnerioxa* have been found under the bark of living trees (Munro, 1967). *Termitorioxa termitoxena* (Bezzi) was found to breed in termite galleries in tree trunks (Hill, 1921).

Regarding larval feeding habits, Trypetinae stands out as the most varied subfamily. Adramini are primarily found in the Old World, except for two *Euphranta* species found in North America (Hardy, 1986; White and Elson-Harris, 1992; Hancock and Drew, 1994). One species, *E. toxoneura* (Loew), is known to feed on sawfly larvae within galls (Kopelke, 1984). According to White and Elson-Harris (1992), the Carpomyini tribe only reproduces in fruits, and the majority of their species are very host-specific.

Toxotrypanini, a tribe in the subfamily Trypetinae restricted to the Neotropical zone, likewise breeds nearly exclusively in fruits or in the seeds they contain; while some species are generalists, many are specialized on particular plant groups, like *Passiflora* or latex-bearing families like Sapotaceae.

3.7 SYSTEMATIC POSITION

Phylum: Arthropoda
Class: Insecta
Order: Diptera
Suborder: Brachycera
Section: Schizophora
Subsection: Acalyptratae
Superfamily: Tephritoidea
Family: Tephritidae

3.7.1 Tephritidae Is Divided into Six Subfamilies

1. Dacinae
2. Phytalmiinae
3. Tephritinae
4. Trypetinae
5. Tachiniscinae
6. Blepharoneurinae

3.7.1.1 Subfamily Dacinae

They are one of the most economically significant groups, with several species as pests of various fruit and vegetable crops. Several of them are of serious concern as quarantine pests. 1,300 species in 51 genera and three tribes – Dacini, Ceratitidini, and Gastrozonini – have been included in this subfamily (Norrbom et al., 1999; Doorenweerd et al., 2018; David et al., 2014, 2016, 2017; David and Hancock, 2017). They are brightly coloured and frequently imitate wasps to avoid predation, as seen in *Dacus*, *Bactrocera*, and *Zeugodacus*. Ceratitidini comprises several genera, of which *Ceratitella sobrina* Zia was recorded from India. Species included in Gastrozonini, commonly known as bamboo-shoot fruit flies, exploit bamboo as their host for development.

3.7.1.2 Subfamily Phytalmiinae

They are predominantly saprophytic, primarily feeding on decaying matter, with a primitive tactile type of aculeus. It is classified into four tribes, with 100 genera and 369 species (Norrbom et al., 1999), of which Acanthonevrini, with 18 species and eight genera, have been reported from India (Agarwal and Sueyoshi, 2005, David and Ramani, 2011). *Rioxoptilona*, *Ptilona*, *Diarrhegma*, *Rioxa*, and *Themara* are the most common genera in India. *Diarrhegma modestum* (Fabricius) has been recorded to breed on the frass of borer-damaged trunks of drumsticks.

3.7.1.3 Subfamily Tephritinae

They are distributed throughout the world, with 219 genera and 1,847 described species (Norrbom et al., 1999). They are characterized by a dense microtrichose grey body, spotted wings, the presence of fine tomentosum on the anepisternum, the absence of scapular setae, which makes the sutures obscure, and the presence of two spermathecae in females (Hardy, 1973, 1974; Hardy and Drew, 1996). They are primarily associated with Asteraceae as flower feeders, gall formers, or stem miners. *Acanthiophilus helianthi* (Rossi) is a pest on safflower; *Cecidochares connexa* Macquart affects siam weed, *Chromolaena odorata* (L.) R. M. King & H. Rob; and *Procedidochares utilis* Stone causes stem galls on *Eupatorium adenophorum* Spreng. *C. odorata and P. utilis* species have been introduced to India for biological control of weeds (White and Elson-Harris, 1992). It is well represented in India, with 34 genera and 70 species (Agarwal and Sueyoshi, 2005).

3.7.1.4 Subfamily Trypetinae

This is a predominantly frugivorous group, although a few species are stem and leaf miners. Many species are economically important pests on commercial fruit crops, such as *Anastrepha* Schiner, *Carpomya* Costa, and *Rhagoletis* Loew (White and Elson-Harris, 1992). Nearly 1,000 species under 229 genera and nine tribes have been described so far from the world, of which 49 species belonging to 19 genera have been reported from India (Agarwal and Sueyoshi, 2005). *Adrama*, *Euphranta*, and *Carpomya* are a few of these commonly found in India.

3.7.1.5 Subfamily Tachiniscinae

It is the smallest subfamily in Tephritidae. The biology of this group not completely known, except for an unidentified *Bibundia* species reared from the larvae of a saturniid moth. In this subfamily, a single species is recorded from India: *Ortalotrypeta isshikii* (Matsumura) from Sikkim (David and Hancock, 2013).

3.7.1.6 Subfamily Blepharoneurinae

This is primarily found in tropical regions and is a relatively small taxon, consisting of 35 species within five identified genera. They are phytophagous which breeds on Cucurbitaceous flowers and stems. They are categorized according to their feeding preferences, such as stems, flowers, or fruits.

Unlike other fruit flies, adult flies of the genera *Hexaptilona*, *Bariglossa*, and *Blepharoneura* have rows of spine-like modified pseudotracheal ring tips on the labella, which are used for rasping flowers or leaves of their host plant (Norrbom and Condon, 1999). This subfamily has not been recorded from India so far, even though *Hexaptilona* has been observed in the Oriental region.

3.8 MAJOR FRUIT FLY PESTS IN INDIA

3.8.1 Oriental Fruit Fly: *Bactrocera (Bactrocera) dorsalis* Hendel (Figure 3.1)

Diagnosis: **Adult**: Face yellowish with two separate black spots. Medium-sized flies with yellow lateral vittae on a black/reddish-brown scutum. Wing with a continuous costal band confluent with vein R_{2+3}. All femora yellow without any fuscous/black markings. Abdomen orange-red with a prominent T-shaped mark (White and Elson-Harris, 1992; Ramani, 1997).

Attractant: Methyl eugenol.

3.8.1.1 Host Plants

Aegle marmelos (L.) Corr. (Bael), *Anacardium occidentale* L. (cashew), *Artocarpus altilis* (Park.) (breadfruit), *A. heterophyllus* Lamk. (jackfruit), *Capsicum frutescens* L. (red pepper), *Carissa carandas* L. (karanda), *Cerbera manghas* L. (honde fruit), *Chrysophyllum cainito* L. (star apple), *Citrus aurantium* L. (sour orange), *C. grandis* Osbeck. (pomelo), *C. medica* L. (citron), *C. nobilis* Lours (orange), *C. reticulata* Blanco (mandarin), *Coffea arabica* L. (Arabian coffee), *C. canephora* Pierre ex Froehner (robusta coffee), *Cydonia oblonga* Mill. (quince), *Diospyros* sp. (persimmon), *Eriobotrya japonica* (Thunb.) (loquat), *Ficus carica* L. (fig), *F. mysorensis* Heyne, *Litchi chinensis* (Gaertn.) Sonn. (litchi), *Malus pumila* Mill. (apple), *Mangifera indica* L. (mango), *Manilkara achras* (Mill.) (sapodilla), *Mimusops elengi* L. (Spanish cherry), *Morus australis* Poir. (common mulberry), *Musa paradisiaca* L. (banana), *Persea americana* Mill. (avocado), *Physalis peruviana* L. (cape gooseberry), *Prunus armeniaca* L. (apricot), *P. avium* L. (sweet cherry), *P. domestica* L. (plum), *P. persica* (L.) (peach), *Psidium guajava* L. (guava), *Punica granatum* L. (pomegranate), *Pyrus communis* L. (pear), *Rubus fruticosus* L. (blackberry), *Santalum album* L. (white sandalwood), *Solanum erianthum* D. Don., *Solanum indicum* L. (Indian nightshade), *S. melongena* L. (eggplant), *S. torvum* Swartz, *Syzygium cumini* (L.) Skeels (jamun), *Terminalia catappa* L. (Indian almond), and *Ziziphus mauritiana* Lamk. (jujube/ber) (White and Elson-Harris,1992; Kapoor, 1993; Ramani, 1997)

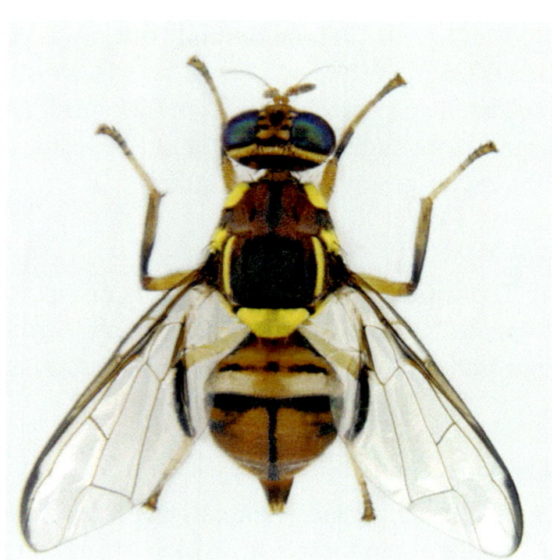

FIGURE 3.1 Habitus (dorsal) of fruit flies: *B. dorsalis.*

Distribution: Assam, Bihar, Delhi, Himachal Pradesh, Jammu & Kashmir, Kerala, Karnataka, Maharashtra, Manipur, Orissa, Punjab, Rajasthan, Sikkim, Tamil Nadu, Uttar Pradesh, and West Bengal (Bhat, 1989; Agarwal and Sueyoshi, 2005).

3.8.1.2 Biology and Ecology

The life cycle of *B. dorsalis* ranges from 21 to 26 days, with an average of 23.5 days. Eggs are laid in clusters of 2–9 in half- to overripe fruits by making punctures using a telescopic ovipositor. The incubation period of the eggs ranges from 24 to 48 hours, with an average of 36 hours. There are three larval instars, which take 2.16, 4.83, and 5.25 days, respectively. Fully matured maggots drop to the soil, and pupation occurs in the soil at a depth of 2–10 cm, with an average of 5.4 cm under field conditions (Belavadi, 1979).

Adults are synovigenic. They were observed to mate after feeding for a few days during the evening hours. Mating usually starts at dusk and lasts from 35 minutes, with an average of 1 hour 10 minutes (Belavadi, 1979).

3.8.2 *Bactrocera (Bactrocera) carambolae* Drew & Hancock (Figure 3.2)

Diagnosis: Face fulvous/yellow with two oval black spots, scutum predominantly black with broad (>0.15 mm) lateral postsutural vittae, fore femur with an elongate black spot, mid and hind femur without spots/markings, wing with costal band overlapping vein R_{2+3} and expanded slightly beyond the apex of R_{2+3}, abdomen orange-brown with a prominent T-shaped pattern and lateral transverse markings on tergites 4 and 5.

Attractant: Methyl eugenol

Host plants: It is known to breed on 75 host plants belonging to 26 families. Ranganath and Veenakumari (1995, 1999) recorded its severe incidence in *Syzygium* spp. in the Andamans. List of host plants: *Alangium griffithii* (Alangiaceae), *Bouea oppositifolia*, *Mangifera indica* (Anacardiaceae), *Annona montana*, *Annona muricata*, *Rollinia pulchrinervis*, *Uvaria grandiflora* (Annonaceae), *Thevetia peruviana* (Apocynaceae), *Argena pinnata* (Arecaceae), *Garcinia atroviridis*, *Garcinia cowa*, *Garcinia griffithii*, *Garcinia mangostana* (Clusiaceae), *Terminalia catappa*, *Terminalia manii*, *Terminalia procera* (Combretaceae), *Baccaurea motleyana*, *Drypetes longifolia* (Euphorbiaceae),

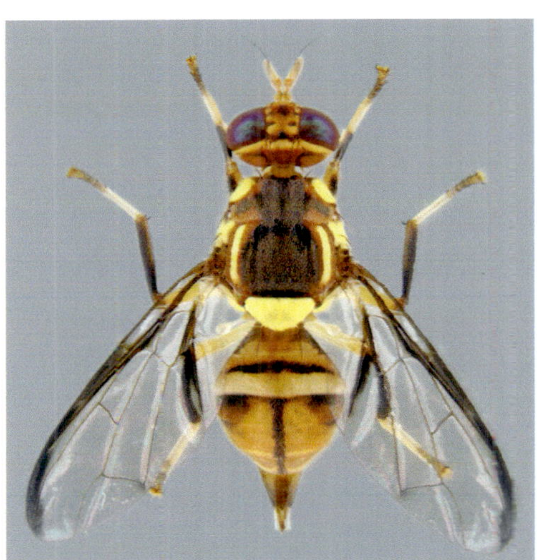

FIGURE 3.2 Habitus (dorsal) of fruit flies: *B. carambolae*.

Persea americana (Lauraceae), *Fagraea ceilanica* (Loganiaceae), *Aglaia dookoo*, *Lansium domesticum*, *Sandoricum koetjape* (Meliaceae), *Artocarpus altilis*, *Artocarpus comeziana*, *Artocarpus elastica*, *Artocarpus heterophyllus*, *Artocarpus integer*, *Artocarpus lakoocha*, *Artocarpus odoratissimus*, *Artocarpus rigidus* var. *asperulus*, *Ficus grossularioides*, *Ficus hispida*, *Pouroma paefolia* (Moraceae), *Knema angustifolia* (Myristaceae), *Eugenia uniflora*, *Psidium cattleianum*, *Psidium guajava*, *Rhodomyrtus tomentosa*, *Syzygium aqueum*, *Syzygium grande*, *Syzygium jambos*, *Syzygium malaccense*, *Syzygium samarangense* (Myrtaceae), *Ochanostachys amentosa* (Olacaceae), *Averrhoa bilimbi*, *Averrhoa carambola* (Oxalidaceae), *Xanthophyllum amoenum* (Polygalaceae), *Punica granatum* (Punicaceae), *Ziziphus jujuba* (Rhamnaceae), *Pellacalyx saccardianus*, *Rhizophora* sp. (Rhizophoraceae), *Citrofortunella mitis*, *Citrus aurantifolia*, *Citrus limon*, *Citrus madurensis*, *Citrus paradisi*, *Citrus reticulata*, *Fortunella margarita*, *Fortunella polyandra*, *Paramignya andamanica*, *Tetractomia majus*, *Triphasia trifolia* (Rutaceae), *Lepisanthes alata* (Sapindaceae), *Chrysophyllum cainito*, *Manilkara littoralis*, *Manilkara zapota*, *Mimusops elengi*, *Planchonella longipetiolatum*, *Pouteria campechiana* (Sapotaceae), *Irvingia malayana* (Simaroubaceae), *Capsicum annuum*, *Lycopersicon esculentum*, *Solanum ferox* (Solanaceae), and *Symplocos cochinchinensis* (Symplocaceae) (Allwood et al., 1999)

Distribution: Peninsular Malaysia, Malaysia, Indonesia, Singapore, Thailand, Borneo, India (Andaman Islands); French Guiana, Suriname, Vietnam (Drew and Hancock, 1994; Drew and Romig, 2016), Bangladesh (Leblanc et al., 2019). It was originally described from Malaysia in 1994 by Drew and Hancock. Ranganath and Veenakumari (1995, 1999) reported the occurrence of *B. carambolae* in the Andaman Islands, India. Hence, this pest cannot be considered an invasive species in India, as it has already been reported from the Andaman Islands. Even though it has been recorded from the Andaman Islands, so far no *B. carambolae* have been encountered in mainland India.

3.8.3 *Bactrocera* (*Bactrocera*) *caryeae* (Kapoor) (Figure 3.3)

Morphology: **Adult**: Narrow, elongate-oval facial dark spots, parallel-sided narrow lateral post-sutural vittae, large dark fuscous black subapical spots on all femora, a narrow anal streak, and a reduced band of microtrichia above the basal cell; apex of aculeus needle-shaped with four pairs

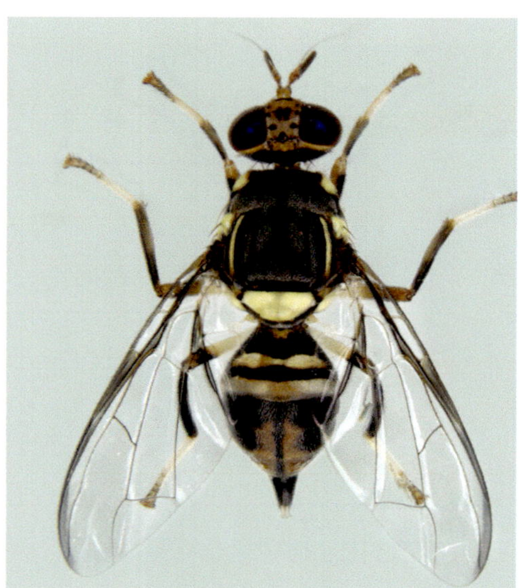

FIGURE 3.3 Habitus (dorsal) of fruit flies: *B. caryeae*.

of subapical setae; spicules at the distal end of the eversible membrane of ovipositor shell-shaped with 9–11 small dentations of uneven size (Ramani, 1997).

Attractant: Methyl eugenol.

Host plants: *Psidium guajava* L., *Mangifera indica* L., *Psidium guajava* L., *Persea americana* Mill., *Malphigia glabra* L., *Syzygium jambos* (L.) Alston, *Aegle marmelos* (L.), *Cassimiroa edulis* La Llave & Lex., *Citrus grandis* Osbeck, *Citrus maxima* Merr., and *Citrus* sp. (Kapoor, 1993; Ramani, 1997).

Distribution: Karnataka, Kerala, and Tamil Nadu (Bhat, 1989; Ramani,1997; Agarwal and Sueyoshi, 2005; David, 2005).

3.8.4 Guava Fruit Fly: *Bactrocera* (*Bactrocera*) *correcta* (Bezzi) (Figure 3.4)

Diagnosis: Adults are medium-sized with the scutum black in colour and broad lateral vittae (>0.15 mm). Wing with a costal band discontinuous beyond vein R_1, sometimes faint, with a narrow apical spot. Abdomen reddish-brown with a prominent T-shaped mark. This species is characterized by the presence of facial spots coalescing to form a transverse line (White and Elson-Harris, 1992, Ramani, 1997).

Attractant: Methyl eugenol.

3.8.4.1 Host Plants

Carrisa carandas L., *Casimiroa edulis* Llave & Lex, *Eugenia uniflora* L., *Mangifera indica* L., *Malphigia glabra* L., *Prunus armeniaca* L., *Santalum album* L., *Vitis vinifera* L., and *Ziziphus mauritiana* Lam. (Kapoor,1993; Ramani, 1997).

Distribution: Bihar, Gujarat, Haryana, Himachal Pradesh, Karnataka, Kerala, Madhya Pradesh, Maharashtra, Punjab, and Tamil Nadu (Bhat, 1989; Agarwal and Sueyoshi, 2005).

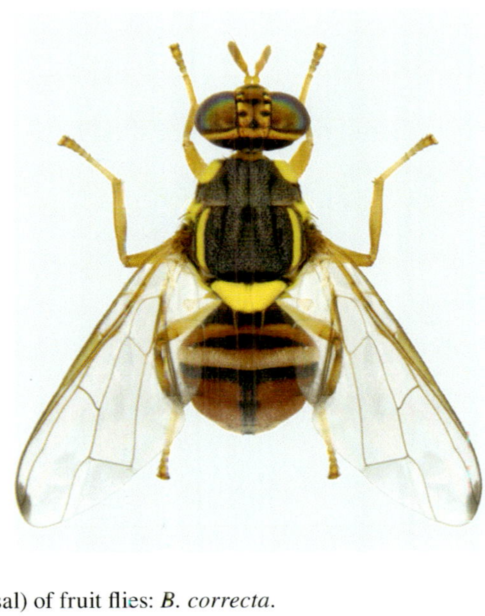

FIGURE 3.4 Habitus (dorsal) of fruit flies: *B. correcta*.

3.8.5 Peach Fruit Fly: *Bactrocera (Bactrocera) zonata* (Saunders) (Figure 3.5)

Diagnosis: Pale orange-brown to red species with lateral post-sutural yellow vittae on the scutum, circular to oval facial spots, anterior supra-alar setae, prescutellar setae, and two scutellar setae present. Wing with a discontinuous costal band forming a spot apically. Abdomen reddish-brown with pecten on the third tergum of males (Ramani, 1997; White and Elson-Harris, 1992)

Attractant: Methyl eugenol.

Host plants: *Aegle marmelos* (L.) Corr. Serr., *Annona squamosa* L., *Careya arborea* Roxb., *Casimiroa edulis* Llave & Lex, *Citrus aurantium* L., *C. grandis* Osbeck., *C. limon* (L.) Burman f., *C. medica* L., *C. nobilis* Lours, *C. reticulata* Blanco, *C. sinensis* (L.), *Cucumis melo* L., *Diospyros blancoi* A. DC, *Ficus carica* L., *Lagenaria siceraria* (Mol.) Standl., *Luffa acutangula* (Roxb.), *Luffa aegyptica* Mill., *Lycopersicum esculentum* (L.) Karst., *Malphigia glabra* L., *Mangifera indica* L., *Prunus persica* (L.) Batsch., *Psidium guajava* L., *Punica granatum* L., *Pyrus communis* L., *Solanum melongena* L., *Syzygium cumini* (L.) Skeels, *S. jambos* (L.) Alston, *Terminalia catappa* L., and *Ziziphus mauritiana* Lamk. (Kapoor, 1993; Ramani, 1997).

Distribution: Andhra Pradesh, Assam, Bihar, Delhi, Gujarat, Haryana, Himachal Pradesh, Punjab, Karnataka, Kerala, Madhya Pradesh, Maharashtra, Tamil Nadu, Uttaranchal, Uttar Pradesh, and West Bengal (Agarwal and Sueyoshi, 2005).

3.8.6 *Zeugodacus (Hemigymnodacus) diversus* Coquillett (Figure 3.6)

Morphology: **Adult**: Small to medium-sized fly with a greenish-black body, featuring both lateral and medial vittae on the thorax. Wings have a costal band confluent with R_{2+3}. Males lack pecten on the third abdominal tergite. Sexual dimorphism is observed in this species. The face of the male is entirely yellow, without facial spots, while the face of the female has a transverse black line above the mouth opening (Ramani, 1997; White and Elson-Harris, 1992).

Attractant: Methyl eugenol.

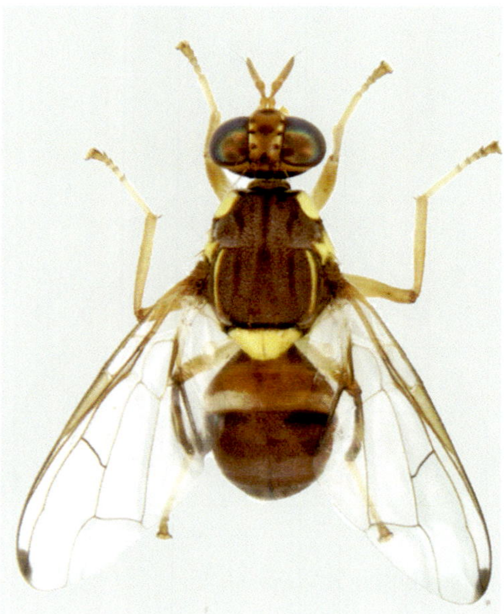

FIGURE 3.5 Habitus (dorsal) of fruit flies: *B. zonata*.

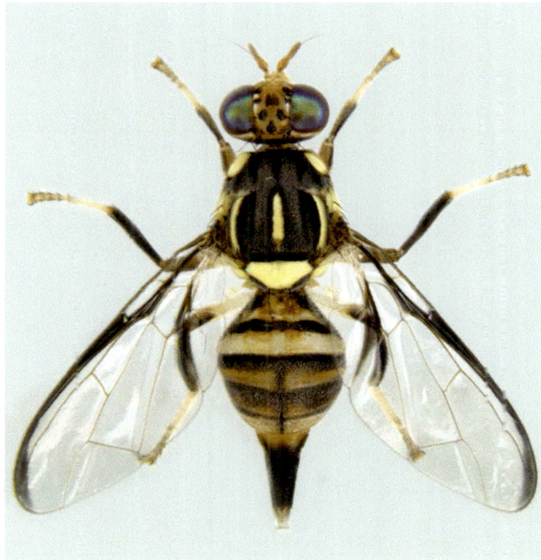

FIGURE 3.6 Habitus (dorsal) of fruit flies: *Z. diversus*.

Host plants: *Benincasa hispida* (Thunb.) Cogn., *Luffa aegyptica* Mill., *Citrus aurantium* L., *C. grandis* Osbeck, *Coccinia grandis* L. Voigt, *Cucurbita maxima* Duch, *Cucurbita pepo* L., *Lagenaria siceraria* (Mol.) Standl, *Musa paradisiaca* L., *Psidium guajava* L., *Syzygium cumini* (L.) Skeels, *S. malaccense* (L.) Merr. & Perr, *Solanum erianthum* D. Don, *Mangifera indica* L., *Myristica beddomei* King, *M. fragrans* Houtt, and *Citrus aurantium* L. (Kapoor,1993).

Distribution: Andhra Pradesh, Bihar, Himachal Pradesh, Karnataka Maharashtra, Meghalaya, Punjab, Tamil Nadu, Uttaranchal, Uttar Pradesh, and West Bengal (Bhat, 1989; Agarwal and Sueyoshi, 2005).

Nature of damage: The female flies lay eggs at the base of the flower and flower buds, near the ovary. In opened flowers, the flies may lay eggs directly into the ovary. The larvae, upon hatching, feed on the reproductive organs of the flower. The affected flowers become unfit for pollination or fruit setting and subsequently drop off and rot (Gavigowda, 1976).

3.8.7 Melon Fly: *Zeugodacus (Zeugodacus) cucurbitae* (Coquillett) (Figure 3.7)

Diagnosis: A predominantly orange-brown species with separate black spots on a fulvous face. The scutum has yellow medial and lateral postsutural vittae, and the wing is characterized by the presence of a broad costal band expanded into an apical spot, along with a radial medial band and subapical band.

Attractant: Cuelure.

3.8.7.1 Host Plants

It is a polyphagous pest with a wide host range. *Benincasa hispida* (Thunb.) Cogn., *Capsicum frutescens* L., *Careya arborea* Roxb., *Coccinia grandis* L. Voigt, *Cucumis melo* L., *C. sativus* L., *Momordica charantia* L., *Momordica dioica* Roxb. ex Wild, *Mukia maderaspatana* (L.) M. Roem., *Trichosanthes cucumerina* L., *T. dioica* (L.), *Luffa* spp., *Citrus* spp., *Psidium guajava* L., and *Carica papaya* L. (Kapoor,1993; Ramani, 1997) are a few of the host plants infested by *Z. cucurbitae*.

Distribution: Widespread in India (Agarwal and Sueyoshi, 2005).

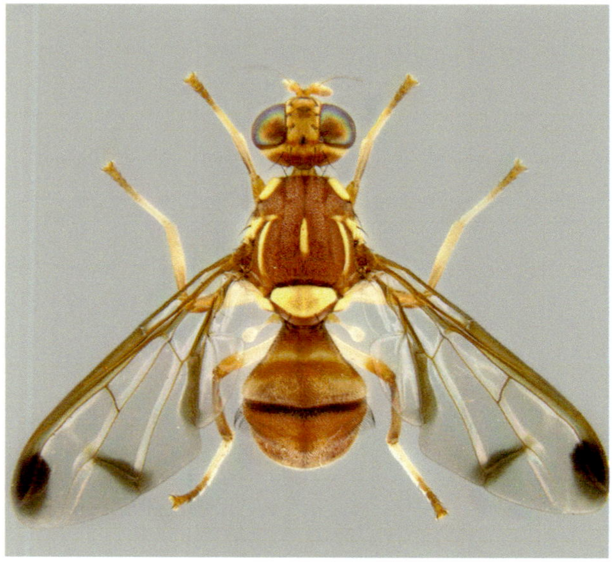

FIGURE 3.7 Habitus (dorsal) of fruit flies: *Z. cucurbitae.*

3.8.7.2 Biology and Ecology

The adult female inserts her eggs singly or in clusters of 4–10 beneath the skin of suitable hosts, especially in tender vegetables. The incubation period ranges from 27 to 28 hours during August and 31–38 hours during May (Back and Pemberton, 1914). Narayanan and Batra (1960) reported durations of 24 hours and 6–9 days for eggs in summer and winter, respectively. There are three larval instars, which last for 1.2, 1.58, and 2.25 days, respectively, and the total larval duration is 5–6 days at a mean temperature of 25.72°C. However, the larval duration varies with the host plant and season. Puparium is formed from the third larval skin; pupation takes place in soil, and the pupal period ranges from 8 to 10 days. Adult life may vary based on nutrition. If given only water, lifespan is prolonged to 3 days; with sucrose, the flies survive for 17 days; with sucrose and water, up to 32 days (Gavigowda, 1976).

3.8.8 *Zeugodacus* (*Zeugodacus*) *tau* (Walker) (Figure 3.8)

Morphology: **Adult**: Scutum dark brown with lateral and medial yellow vittae; oval facial spots, anterior supra-alar setae, prescutellar setae, and four scutellar setae present Wing with a costal band overlapping vein R_{2+3}, expanded apically into a spot. Male with a pecten on the third abdominal tergum (White and Elson-Harris, 1992).

Attractant: Cuelure.

3.8.8.1 Host Plants

Artocarpus heterophyllus Lamk., *Benincasa hispida* (Thunb.) Cogn., *Bryonia lacinosa* L., *Citrullus lanatus* (Thunb.) Mansf., *Citrus grandis* Osbeck, *Cucumis sativus* L., *Cucurbita maxima* Duch., *Lagenaria siceraria* (Molina) Standley, *Luffa acutangula* (L.) Roxb. *Momordica charantia* L., *Passiflora edulis* Sims., *Syzygium samarangensis* (Bl.), *Trichosanthes anguina* L., and *T. palmata* Roxb. (Kapoor, 1993, White and Elson-Harris, 1992; Ramani, 1997).

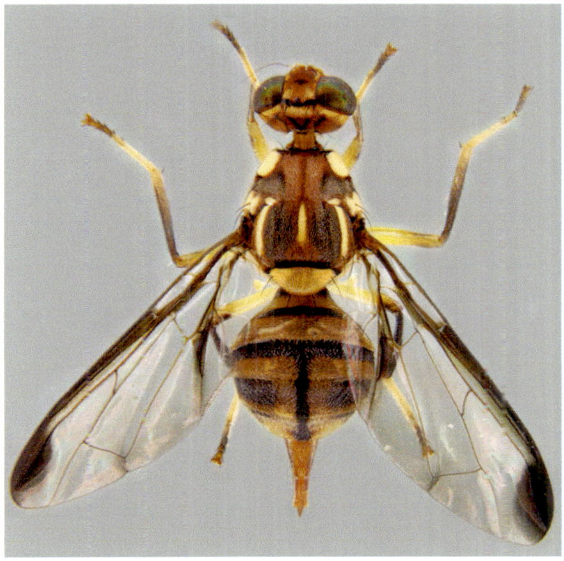

FIGURE 3.8 Habitus (dorsal) of fruit flies: *Z. tau*.

3.8.8.2 Distribution

Andaman and Nicobar Islands, Arunachal Pradesh, Bihar, Haryana, Himachal Pradesh, Jammu and Kashmir, Karnataka, Maharashtra, Meghalaya, Punjab, Sikkim, Tamil Nadu, Uttaranchal, and West Bengal (Bhat, 1989; Agarwal and Sueyoshi, 2005).

3.8.9 Ethiopian Fruit Fly/Lesser Fruit Fly/Cucurbit Fly: *Dacus (Didacus) ciliatus* Loew (Figure 3.9)

Morphology: **Adult**: A predominantly orange species, with facial spots, two scutellar setae, a yellow spot covering most of the katatergite, an anatergite that is orange, mid femur that is yellow or orange-yellow, and a wing with a costal band that is expanded apically to form a spot. Scutum without yellow stripes, anterior supra-alar setae, and prescutellar acrostichal setae (White and Elson-Harris, 1992).

Attractant: Not attracted to any lures.

Host plants: *Momordica charantia* L., *Cucumis sativus* L., *Luffa* spp., *Cucumis melo* L., *Cucurbita maxima* Duch., and *Lagenaria siceraria* (Molina) Standley (Kapoor, 1993).

Distribution: Bihar, Chandigarh, Delhi, Gujarat, Himachal Pradesh, Karnataka, Maharashtra, Meghalaya, Punjab, Tamil Nadu, and Uttar Pradesh (Ramani, 1997; Agarwal and Sueyoshi, 2005).

Biology and ecology: The fly remains active throughout the year, with six generations in equable and subtropical climates, but the number of generations decreases in northern areas due to winter months, as the fly is active only until the end of November. It starts hovering in April in search of cucurbits. During May to June, it attacks cucurbits such as ivy gourd, cucumber, and long melon. Ivy gourd is another preferred host of this fly, as attacks on this continue from May to November (Kapoor, 1993).

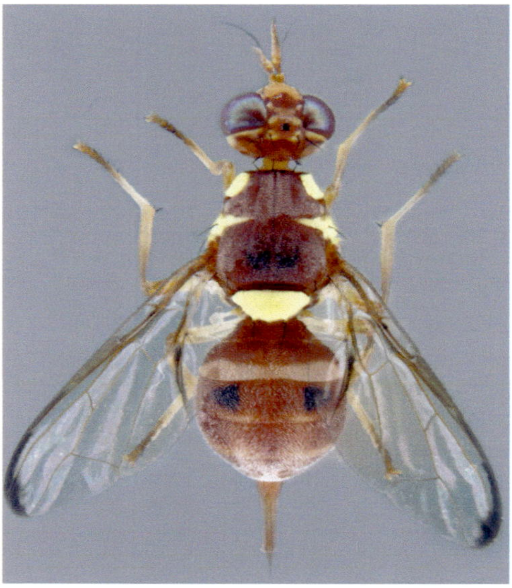

FIGURE 3.9 Habitus (dorsal) of fruit flies: *D. ciliatus*.

3.9 MANAGEMENT STRATEGIES

Fruit flies, *Bactrocera* spp. and *Zeugodacus cucurbitae*, are serious pests of mango, guava, custard apple, dragon fruit, sapota, and other fruit crops; *Z. cucurbitae* is particularly damaging to all cucurbitaceous crops and tomatoes. Previously, the Indian Institute of Horticultural Research (IIHR), Bangalore, developed cost-effective control strategies for integrated pest management (IPM) (Verghese et al., 2002). Now there is an urgent need to phase out traps with insecticide-laced plywood or any other substrate, due to high residual concerns, environmental and air pollution, and impacts on non-target organisms, especially ants. Male annihilation of fruit flies is no longer a control strategy in most fruit ecosystems, and the notion that "more flies in traps means more control" is a myth. However, the same is not true when the fruit fly density is low or in vegetable ecosystems, where the density of the fruit flies is usually low. Parapheromone lures should be used only for fruit fly surveillance and diversity assessment (sticky traps cannot be used for identification in diversity studies). Young males do not respond satisfactorily to Methyl eugenol (ME)+insecticide; hence, male annihilation is not satisfactory. The IPM of fruit flies was vastly improved upon subsequently by Rashvee International Phytosanitary and Research Services (RIPRS), recognized by GoI and DPPQ. Under a BIRAC, DBT program, an insecticide-free liquid lure fruit fly trap, ovipositional deterrence spray, and phagostimulant baits were developed. These fit into the updated export protocols and Good Agricultural Practices in Integrated Fruit Flies Management are as follows:

1. **Sanitation**: Collect fallen fruits into small manure pits (3 ft×3ft×3ft), wet them, and close the pits after harvest (serves as manure); a pit/tree is recommended. Sanitation pits with rotting fruits will attract older females. The collected fallen fruits (which also include infested fruits with maggots) on the ground prevent pupation and subsequent adult emergence.
2. Introduce a non-insecticidal, climate-resilient, anti-evaporant liquid lure (Rashvee fruit fly liquid lure) instead of plywood or other substrate traps. This lure should be used @ 5 mL/100 mL water in used disposable water bottles (any size). The traps have a unique cap resilient to high wind, high rainfall, and high temperature, for which the design is

patented (Figure 3.10a and b). Use a minimum of 8–10 traps/acre in the case of mango and 15 multi-lure traps/acre in the case of cucurbits. In the case of fruit crops, use Rashvee fruit fly liquid ME lure. Traps should be fastened well on lower branches, between 2 metres in height, at least the size of a marble for fruits, or 30 days prior to harvest or earlier.

3. The liquid traps are found to be superior commercial traps in attracting diverse species of fruit flies, as studied by ICAR-NBAIR.
4. RIPRS placement geometry should be followed (Figure 3.11).
5. Based on trap surveillance data, further control can be achieved by female fruit fly deterrence using 2–3 pre-harvest sprays of 1 mL Azadirachtin 10,000 ppm synergized with 1 mL Rashvee Herbal Liquid Soap as an adjuvant 30 days prior to harvest to deter oviposition.
6. If trap catches are high (15/day), a single spray of 0.37 mL/L Spinosad 20 days prior to harvest is recommended.
7. Additionally, Rashvee Phytofer bait splashed on the base of the tree attracts and kills both males and females of the fruit fly.
8. Rashvee Phytofer bait (10% + 2 mL/L decamethrin) should be splashed on the tree trunk. To prepare the bait, take 20 L of water in a bucket and add 1 kg of phagostimulant bait and leave it overnight covered. On the next day, add 40 mL of decamethrin and stir well; using an old brush, splash at the base of the tree. This can be done 10 days before harvest and also repeated 5 days before harvest. In cucurbits Phytofer bait splash on the lower leaves gives good control.
9. Bait sprays on the trunk should be given if the population is high (Verghese et al., 2020).
10. For high-priced varieties, bag with cloth-lined covers 4 weeks prior to harvest to prevent infestation (Rashmi et al., 2025).

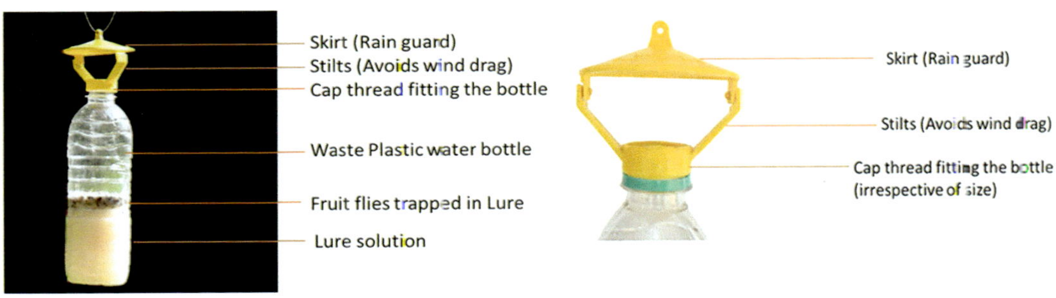

FIGURE 3.10 (a) Rashvee fruit fly liquid lure and (b) climate-resilient caps.

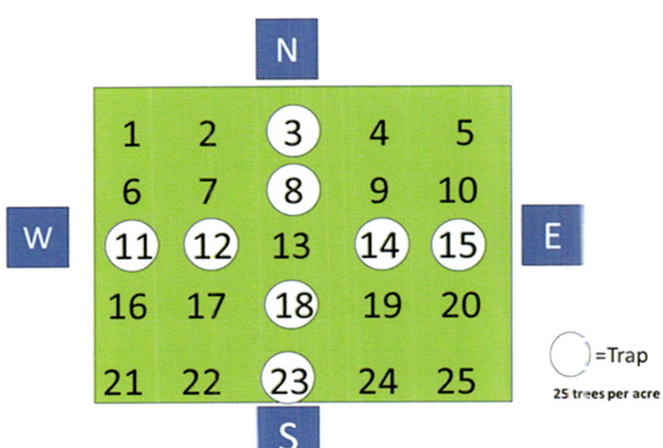

FIGURE 3.11 Rashvee non-insecticidal liquid lure trap placement geometry.

3.9.1 Post Harvest Fruit Fly Management

Establishing a hot water facility (47°C+1°C for 1 hour, ICAR-IIHR) both for export and retail markets in all major markets and mango belts is recommended. Hot water treatment is a successful ICAR-IIHR technology for exports. Hot water plants for fruit fly control have been commercialized in India, with about 52 units in operation. It is pertinent to mention that the above IPM measures are residue-free (Verghese et al., 2024).

3.10 CONCLUSIONS

Fruit flies are one of the major pests of several horticultural crops in India, and many of them are of quarantine concern to other countries as well. They are more diverse in the Oriental region, with the maximum number of species, followed by the Afrotropical region. Apart from frugivory, they exhibit diverse modes of feeding, such as leaf mining, seed feeding, stem feeding, and flower feeding. Most of the current management practices are centred around male annihilation methods, and no female fruit fly attractants have been developed so far in India. Concerted efforts in this direction may help improve the management of fruit flies.

3.11 POINTS TO REMEMBER

1. Only 35% of fruit fly species are frugivorous; the rest are flower feeders, gall makers, bamboo stem feeders, or leaf miners
2. *Bactrocera*, *Zeugodacus*, *Dacus*, and *Carpomya* are the major economically important genera in India
3. In general, fruit flies are multivoltine, but a few species, like *Bactrocera minax*, are univoltine

REFERENCES

Abhishek, V., David, K. J., Hancock, D. L., Pradeep, S., Kalleshwaraswamy, C., Sridhara, S., Satish, K (2024a). New Indian species of *Dacus* Fabricius (Diptera: Tephritidae: Dacinae: Dacini) similar to *Dacus crabroniformis* (Bezzi), endemic to the Western Ghats and Northeastern Himalayas. *Zootaxa*, 5446(3): 366–382.

Abhishek, V., David, K. J., Pradeep, S (2024b). Two new species and a new record of *Bactrocera* Macquart (Diptera: Tephritidae: Dacinae: Dacini) from India with an updated key to species of subgenus *Bactrocera. Zootaxa*, 5486(2): 283–300.

Agarwal, M. L., M. Sueyoshi (2005). Catalogue of Indian fruit flies (Diptera: Tephritidae). *Oriental Insects*, 39: 371–433.

Allwood, A. J., A. Chinajariyawong, R. A. I. Drew, E. L. Hamacek, D. L. Hancock, C. Hengasawad, J. C. Jipanin, M. Jirasurat, C. Kong Krong, S. Kritsaneepaaiboon, C. T. S. Leong, S. Vijaysegaran (1999). Host plant records for fruit flies (Diptera: Tephritidae) in South East Asia. *Raffles Bulletin of Zoology* Supplement, 7: 1–92.

Back, E. A., C. E. Pemberton (1914). Life history of the melon fly. *Journal of Agricultural Research*, 3: 269–274.

Belavadi, V. V. (1979). Bionomics of the Oriental Fruit Fly, *Dacus dorsalis* Hendel (Diptera: Tephritidae) on guava (*Psidium guajava* L.) and its control by male annihilation, M Sc. Agri. Thesis, University of Agricultural Sciences, Bangalore.

Bhat, G. U. (1989). Faunistic and some ecological studies on Fruit flies (Diptera: Tephritidae) of Bangalore and Kodagu districts. M.Sc Thesis, University of Agricultural Sciences, Bangalore, p. 117.

Bhumannavar, B. S., S. Ramani., S. K. Rajeswari et al. (2004). Host specificity and biology of Cecidochares connexa (Macquart) (Diptera: Tephritidae) introduced into India for the biological suppression of *Chromolaena odorata* (Linnaeus) King & Robinson. *Journal of Biological Control*, 18(2): 111–120.

Bhumannavar, B. S., S. Ramani, S. K. Rajeswari et al. (2007). Field release and impact of *Cecidochares connexa* (Macquart) (Diptera: Tephritidae) *on Chromolaena odorata. Journal of Biological Control*, 21(1): 59–64.

David, K. J., Abhishek, V., Kennedy, N., Ajaykumara, K. M., Gracy, R. G., Hissay, C. B (2024). Four new species of *Zeugodacus* Hendel (Diptera, Tephritidae, Dacinae, Dacini) and new records of dacines from India. *ZooKeys*, 1188: 1–26. https://doi.org/10.3897/zookeys.1188.114031

David, K. J. (2005). Diversity and abundance of fruit flies (Diptera: Tephritidae: Dacinae) in Kerala with special reference to Western Ghats. M. Sc. Agri Thesis, University of Agricultural Sciences, Bangalore.

David, K. J., D. L. Hancock (2013). The first record of *Ortalotrypeta isshikii* (Matsumura) and subfamily Tachiniscinae (Diptera: Tephritidae) from India, with re-description of the species. *Australian Entomologist*, 40(3): 131–135.

David, K. J., D. L. Hancock (2017). A new species of *Gastrozona* Bezzi (Diptera: Tephritidae: Dacinae: Gastrozonini) with an updated key to species from India. *Zootaxa*, 4216(1): 55–64.

David, K. J., D. L. Hancock, A. Freidberg, K. Goodger (2013). New species and records of *Euphranta* Loew and other Adramini (Diptera: Tephritidae: Trypetinae) from south and southeast Asia. *Zootaxa*, 3635(4): 439–458.

David, K. J., D. L. Hancock, S. Ramani (2014). Two new species of *Acroceratitis* Hendel (Diptera: Tephritidae) and an updated key for the species from India. *Zootaxa*, 3895(3): 411–418.

David, K. J., D. L. Hancock, S. K. Singh et al. (2017). New species, new records and updated subgeneric key of *Bactrocera* Macquart (Diptera: Tephritidae: Dacinae: Dacini) from India. *Zootaxa*, 4272(3): 386–400.

David, K. J., D. L. Hancock, S. K. Singh, S. Ramani, G. Behere, S. Salini (2017). New species, new records and updated subgeneric key of *Bactrocera* Macquart (Diptera: Tephritidae: Dacinae: Dacini) from India. *Zootaxa*, 4272(3), 386–400.

David, K. J., S. Ramani (2011). An illustrated key to fruit flies (Diptera: Tephritidae) from Peninsular India and the Andaman and Nicobar Islands. *Zootaxa*, 3021: 1–31.

David, K. J., S. Ramani (2019). New species, redescriptions and phylogenetic revision of tribe Dacini (Diptera: Tephritidae: Dacinae) from India based on morphological characters. *Zootaxa*, 4551(2): 101–146.

David K. J., S. Ramani, S. K. Singh (2019). *Taxonomy and Diversity of Indian Fruit Flies* (Diptera: Tephritidae). Indian Insects, 1st edn. CRC Press, London, pp. 305–324.

David, K. J., K. Sachin, D. L. Hancock (2020). A new species of *Acrotaeniostola* Hendel and new records of Gastrozonini and Ceratitidini (Diptera: Tephritidae) from India. *Zootaxa*, 4731(3): 425–432.

David K. J., D. L. Hancock, H. Y. Han, R. G. Gracy, K. Sachin, R. S. Swathi (2021). A new genus in the tribe Acidoxanthini (Diptera: Tephritidae: Trypetinae) from India, with a discussion of its phylogenetic relationships. *Journal of Asia-Pacific Entomology*, https://doi.org/10.1016/j.aspen.2021.06.010

David K. J., D. L. Hancock, R. G. Gracy, K. Sachin (2022). A new genus of fruit fly in subfamily Dacinae (Diptera: Tephritidae) from India. *Zootaxa*, 5195(6): 585–597.

David K. J., V. Abhishek, N. Kennedy, K. M. Ajaykumara, R. G. Gracy, C. B. Hissay (2024). Four new species of *Zeugodacus* Hendel (Diptera, Tephritidae, Dacinae, Dacini) and new records of dacines from India. *ZooKeys,* 1188: 1–26. https://doi.org/10.3897/zookeys.1188.114031

De Meyer, M. (2006). Systematic revision of the fruit fly genus *Carpophthoromyia* Austen (Diptera, Tephritidae). *Zootaxa*, 1235: 1–48.

Dohm, P., D. Kovac, A. Freidberg et al. (2014). Basic biology and host use patterns of Tephritid flies (Phytalmiinae: Acanthonevrini, Dacinae: Gastrozonini) breeding in Bamboo (Poaceae: Bambusoidea). *Annals of Entomological Society of America*, 107(1): 184–203.

Doorenweerd, C., L. Leblanc, A. L. Norrbom et al (2018). A global checklist of the 932 fruit fly species in the tribe Dacini (Diptera: Tephritidae). *Zookeys*, 730: 17–54.

Drew, R. A. I., D. L. Hancock (1994). The *Bactrocera dorsalis* complex of fruit flies (Diptera: Tephritidae: Dacinae) in Asia. *Bulletin of Entomological Research Supplement Series*, 2: 1–68.

Drew, R. A. I., M. C. Romig (2016). *Keys to the tropical fruit flies of Southeast Asia*. CAB International, Wallingford, 485 pp.

Freidberg, A. (2006). Biotaxonomy of Tephritoidea. *Israel Journal of Entomology*, 35–36: 1–597.

Gavigowda (1976). Studies on fruit flies infesting cucurbits with special reference to bionomics of *Dacus cucurbitae* Coquillett (Diptera: Tephritidae) and possibility of utilizing susceptible musk melon in protecting cucurbits from its attack, M Sc. Agri Thesis, University of Agricultural Sciences, Bangalore.

Hancock, D. L., R. A. I., Drew (1994). New species and records of Asian Trypetinae (Diptera: Tephritidae). *Raffles Bulletin of Zoology*, 42: 555–591.

Hardy, D. E. (1973). The fruit flies (Tephritidae: Diptera) of Thailand and bordering countries. *Pacific Insects Monograph*, 31: 1–353.

Hardy, D. E. (1974). The fruit flies of the Philippines (Diptera-Tephritidae). *Pacific Insects Monograph*, 32: 1–266.

Hardy, D. E. (1986). Fruit flies of the subtribe Acanthonevrina of Indonesia, New Guinea and the Bismarck and Solomon Islands (Diptera: Tephritidae: Trypetinae: Acanthronevrini). *Pacific Insects Monograph*, 42: 1–42.

Hardy, D. E., R. A. I. Drew (1996). Revision of the Australian Tephritini (Diptera: Tephritidae). *Invertebrate Taxonomy*, 10: 213–405.

Hill, G. F. (1921). Notes on some Diptera found in association with termites. *Proceedings of Linnaean Society of New South Wales*, 46: 216–220.

Kapoor, V. C. (1993). *Indian Fruit Flies (Insecta: Diptera: Tephritidae)*. International Science Publisher, New York, p. 228.

Kapoor, V. C., D. E. Hardy, M. L. Agarwal et al. (1980). *Fruit Fly (Diptera: Tephritidae) Systematics of the Indian Subcontinent*. Export India Publications, Jalandhar, India.

Kopelke, J. P. (1984). Der erste Nachweis eines Brutparasiten unter den Bohrfliegen. *Naturmuseum Senckenberg*, 114: 1–28.

Korneyev, V. A. (1999). Phylogenetic relationships among higher groups of Tephritidae. In *Fruit Flies (Tephritidae): Phylogeny and Evolution of Behavior*, eds. M. Aluja and A. L. Norrbom, pp. 73–113. CRC Press, Boca Raton, FL.

Kovac, D., P. Dohm, A. Freidberg et al. (2006). Catalog and revised classification of the Gastrozonini (Diptera: Tephritidae: Dacinae). In *Biotaxonomy of Tephritoidea*, ed. A. Freidberg, Entomological Society of Israel, Jerusalem, Israel, pp. 163–196.

Leblanc, L., M. A. Hossain, C. Doorenweerd, S. A. Khan, M. Momen, M. San Jose, D. Rubinoff (2019). Six years of fruit fly surveys in Bangladesh: A new species, 33 new country records and discovery of the highly invasive Bactrocera carambolae (Diptera: Tephroitidae). *Zookeys*, 876: 87–109.

Munro, H. K. (1967). Fruit flies allied to species of Afrocneros and Ocnerioxa that infest Cussonia, the umbrella tree or kiepersol (Araliaceae) (Diptera: Trypetidae). *Annals of the Natal Museum*, 18: 571–594.

Narayanan, E. S., H. N. Batra (1960). *Fruit Flies and their Control*. A monograph by I.C.A.R, New Delhi, p. 66.

Norrbom, A. L. (2004). *Fruit Fly (Diptera: Tephritidae) Classification and Diversity: Fruit Fly Taxonomy Pages*. https://www. sel.barc.usda.gov/diptera/tephriti/TephClas.htm (accessed January 2010.)

Norrbom, A. L., L. E. Carroll, F. C. Thompson et al. (1999). Systematic database of names. In *Fruit Fly Expert Identification System and Systematic Information Database*, ed. F. C. Thompson, Backhuys Publishers, Leiden, the Netherlands, pp. 65–251.

Norrbom, A. L., L. E. Carroll, F. C. Thompson, I. M. White, A. Freidberg (1999). Systematic database of names: Fruit fly expert identification system and systematic information database. *Myia*, 9: 65–251.

Norrbom, A. L., M. A. Condon (1999). Phylogeny of the subfamily blepharoneurinae. In *Fruit Flies (Tephritidae): Phylogeny and Evolution of Behavior*, eds. M. Aluja and A. L. Norrbom, CRC Press, Boca Raton, FL, pp. 135–154,

Permkam, S., D. L. Hancock (1995). Australian Trypetinae (Diptera: Tephritidae). *Invertebrate Taxonomy*, 9: 1047–1209.

Ramani, S. (1997). Biosystematic studies on fruit flies (Diptera: Tephritidae) with special reference to the fauna of Karnataka and Andaman and Nicobar. Ph.D. Thesis, University of Agricultural Sciences, Bangalore.

Ramani, S. (2004). Classical biological control attempts in India. In *Quarantine Procedures and Facilities for Biological Control Agents*, eds. S. Ramani, B. S. Bhumannavar, and R. J. Rabindra, Project Directorate of Biological Control, Bangalore, India, pp. 17–22.

Ranganath, H. R., K. Veenakumari (1999). Notes on the dacine fruit flies (Diptera: Tephritidae) of Andaman and Nicobar islands-II. *Raffles Bulletin of Zoology*, 47(1): 221–224.

Ranganath, H. R., K. Veenakumari (1995). Notes on the dacine fruit flies (Diptera: Tephritidae) of Andaman and Nicobar islands. *Raffles Bulletin of Zoology*, 43(1): 235–238.

Rashmi, M. A., David, K. J., Abraham Verghese (2025). Novel green management strategies for fruit flies (Tephritidae: Diptera) infesting horticultural crops in India: A critical review. *Current Horticulture*, 13(1): 1–13.

Stonehouse, J. M., A. Verghese, J. D. Mumford, J. Thomas, T. Jiji, R. Faleiro, H. R. Sardana (2005). Research conclusions and recommendations for the on–farm IPM of Tephritid fruit flies in India. *Pest Management in Horticultural Ecosystems*, 11(2): 172–180.

Verghese, A., H. S. Madhura, P. D. K. Jayanthi, J. M. Stonehouse (2002). Fruit flies of economic significance in India, with special reference to *Bactrocera dorsalis* (Hendel). In *Proceedings of 6th International Fruit fly Symposium held between*, 6–10 May 2002, Stellenbosch, South Africa, pp. 317–324.

Verghese, A., Nagaraj, D. K., Rashmi, M. A., Singh, J. P. (2024). Ramification of post-harvest thermal disinfestation technology for mango fruit flies [Bactrocera spp. (Diptera: Tephritidae)] across India. *Current Horticulture*, 12(2): 90–93.

Verghese, A., M. Rakshitha, T. N. Shivananda, C. B. Soumya, M. A. Rashmi (2020). A push-pull strategy for the management of the Oriental fruit fly, *Bactrocera dorsalis* (Hendel) in mango. *Pest Management in Horticultural Ecosystems*, 26(2): 269–271.

Wang, X.-J., X.-L. Chen (2002). A revision of the genus *Gastrozona* Bezzi from China (Diptera: Tephritidae). *Acta Entomologica Sinica*, 45(4): 507–515.

White, I. M., M. M. Elson–Harris (1992). Fruit flies of economic significance: Their identification and bionomics. CAB International, Wallingford, UK, p. 601.

4 Flies for Biological Control in Environmental Engineering

Mani Chellappan, Jasti Sri Vishnu Murthy, Ranjith Matta Thodikayil, and Naveena Unnikrishnan

LEARNING OBJECTIVES

1. To efficiently learn about the flies utilized in biological control.
2. To learn and understand the environmental engineering provided by flies and their significance in pollination, decomposition, and nutrient cycling.
3. To effectively understand their services and impact on ecosystem health and agriculture for the benefit of humankind.

4.1 INTRODUCTION

Insects play a pivotal role in environmental engineering and are the main contributors to our planet's services (Schowalter et al., 2018). They provide significant functions such as pest control, pollination, biocontrol, nutrient recycling, cultural services, food and feed, spore dispersal, managing waste products, and enhancing agricultural production (Nichols et al., 2008; Togni et al., 2019). In addition, they play a significant role in maintaining the stability of plant communities by feeding on plants and consuming seeds (Braga et al., 2013; Garibaldi et al., 2016; Schowalter, 2016; Milotić et al., 2018). Insects serve as a nutritional resource for insectivorous birds, mammals, reptiles, and fish. Dipteran flies exhibit remarkable diversity in terms of species richness, habitat exploration, behaviour, and relationships with humans. Researchers such as Hennig (1973), McAlpine et al. (1981, 1987), Papp and Darvas (2000), Brown (2001), Skevington and Dang (2002), Pape (2009), and Marshall (2012) have thoroughly studied this diversity. This is one of the largest orders, after Coleoptera and Hymenoptera, with over 1,50,000 species from 130 families worldwide. Flies are extensively distributed across all continents, including Antarctica, and have adapted to nearly every habitat (aquatic and terrestrial), with the exception of glaciers and the open sea (Teskey, 1976; Ferrar, 1987; Hövemeyer, 2000; Courtney and Merritt, 2008, 2009). Many larval species are aquatic or semi-aquatic because they require a wet environment to survive. They can be found in living plant tissues, decomposing organic debris, as parasites or parasitoids of other animals, or in close proximity to bodies of water. Hence, throughout agricultural history, employing predators, parasites, and pathogens to naturally control pests has been a longstanding practice. This sustainable approach has gained importance due to the limitations of traditional pesticides, such as the emergence of insect resistance, harmful environmental impacts, pest resurgence, and the decline of natural enemies in agricultural ecosystems (Waage, 1989). Biological control, which involves introducing, augmenting, and conserving natural enemies for pest management, is recognized as an effective, environmentally friendly, and economically and socially acceptable method. Among these natural enemies, dipteran predators and parasitoids are particularly important and widely used in agriculture to manage various pest species (Parra, 2002). Therefore, it is critical to prioritize the study and preservation of various dipteran flies and the ecosystem services they offer in order to safeguard their diversity for our own existence. It is essential to recognize the significance of flies in biological control and environmental engineering for the essential ecosystem services

DOI: 10.1201/9781003482581-6

that society and policymakers require. In this chapter, we provide a comprehensive analysis of the diverse ecosystem services offered by flies, exploring their roles in biological control and environmental engineering.

4.2 BIOLOGICAL CONTROL

One sustainable approach to addressing the pest management crisis involves utilizing natural enemies as biological control agents. These natural enemies can co-evolve with pests and effectively adapt to changes in pest populations. For instance, in U.S. agricultural systems, naturally occurring insect predators and parasitoids contribute approximately USD $4.5 billion annually in pest management services. This is achieved through decreased crop losses and cost savings from reduced insecticide use. True flies encompass many predatory or parasitic species that play a vital role as natural enemies of harmful or potentially harmful insects and other invertebrates. This is particularly important for plant pests, where dipterans can act as key biocontrol agents in pest management or control programmes. Some predatory dipterans are generalist feeders, either as adults, larvae, or both, while others are more specialized, such as the aphidophagous midge larvae (family Cecidomyiidae) and hoverfly larvae (family Syrphidae). Parasitic dipterans, especially tachinid flies (family Tachinidae), are specialists, with most being larval parasitoids of lepidopteran caterpillars or pupae (Chandler, 2014).

4.2.1 Predators

4.2.1.1 Asilidae (Robber Flies)

Robber flies, belonging to the family Asilidae, are a large group of predatory dipterans, with the northern robber fly (*Rhadiurgus variabilis*) serving as a typical example. As adults, they bear a resemblance to stiletto flies but are easily distinguished by the grooved vertex (the upper part of the head between the compound eyes) and sturdier legs. Robber flies are opportunistic predators that typically prey on flying insects, chasing them down and ambushing them mid-flight. Upon capturing their prey, they swiftly stab it with their modified piercing mouthparts. The victim is then drained of fluids after being injected with neurotoxins that cause rapid paralysis, along with proteolytic enzymes that dissolve and liquefy its body contents, a process particularly effective in warm, sunny conditions. These adept hunters often take on insects larger than themselves, including formidable adversaries like bees and wasps (Wood, 1981). While they can be found in field crops, grasslands, and open forests, robber flies play a minor and indiscriminate role as predators of crop pests. Their carnivorous larvae, inhabiting soil or dung, feed on various insect larvae and require 1–3 years to complete their development (Dennis et al., 2013) (Figure 4.1).

4.2.1.2 Cecidomyiidae (Gall Midges)

Gall midges, belonging to the family Cecidomyiidae, are diminutive insects characterized by their small size and delicate build. They typically feature broad, often hairy wings with reduced wing venation. Their antennae are commonly bead-like or moniliform, with each segment, technically called a flagellomere, adorned with a basal whorl of hairs. Their legs are elongated and slender, and the male genitalia are easily discernible. Larvae of gall midges possess a small, inconspicuous head and a body that tapers at both the front and the rear. Additionally, they typically have a distinctive sternal spatula, also known as an anchor process or breastbone. Gall midge larvae undergo three developmental stages (instars) and commonly pupate inside small silken cocoons (Chandler, 2014).

In Europe, four species of Aphidoletes are recognized, two of which prey on aphids and two on adelgids. Among these, *A. aphidimyza* is the most prevalent and well-known, with numerous supposedly distinct "species" merged under this name (Gagné, 2010). Adult *A. aphidimyza* are small, gnat-like insects, relatively large for the genus, with females having a wing length of approximately

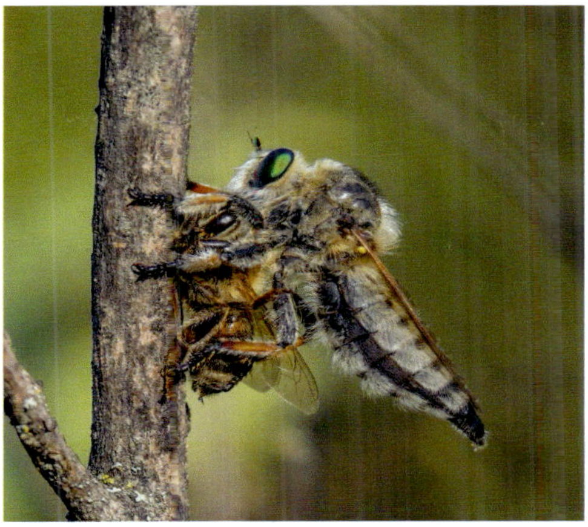

FIGURE 4.1 Robber flies predation.

2.5–3.0 mm (Harris, 1966). *A. aphidimyza* exhibits polyphagy towards aphids, including common pest species associated with greenhouse crops and outdoor plants, both cultivated and uncultivated. Prey species include economically significant aphids like the cabbage aphid (*B. brassicae*) on brassicaceous crops and the mealy plum aphid (*Hyalopterus pruni*) on plum trees. It serves as a predator of aphids on ornamental trees, shrubs, flowers, and in orchards, making it suitable for augmentative and inundative biocontrol programmes due to its favourable biological characteristics (Harris, 1973, 1982).

4.2.1.2.1 *Aphidoletes* spp.

In Europe, four species of *Aphidoletes* are recognized, two of which prey on aphids and two on adelgids. Among these, *A. aphidimyza* is the most prevalent and well-known, with numerous supposedly distinct "species" merged under this name (Gagné, 2010). Adult A. *aphidimyza* are small, gnat-like insects, relatively large for the genus, with females having a wing length of approximately 2.5–3.0 mm (Harris, 1966). *A. aphidimyza* exhibits polyphagy towards aphids, including common pest species associated with greenhouse crops and outdoor plants, both cultivated and uncultivated. Prey species include economically significant aphids like the cabbage aphid (*B. brassicae*) on brassicaceous crops and the mealy plum aphid (*Hyalopterus pruni*) on plum trees. It serves as a predator of aphids on ornamental trees, shrubs, flowers, and in orchards, making it suitable for augmentative and inundative biocontrol programmes due to its favourable biological characteristics (Harris, 1982).

Aphidoletes urticaria is a polyphagous European aphid predator, though it appears to have a more northern distribution than *A. aphidimyza*. Unlike the latter, it is absent from the Mediterranean region. Prey records include various aphid species such as the black bean aphid (*A. fabae*), cherry blackfly (*Myzus cerasi*), and others (Harris, 1973; Harris and Bennett, 2003). *Aphidoletes abietis* is a less commonly encountered species whose larvae prey on adelgids within pineapple-like galls on young spruce trees, notably those cultivated for the Christmas market. Larvae infiltrate closed galls, feeding on adelgids, and later cause premature gall opening, allowing the fully fed predators to escape and pupate (Mitchell and Maksymov, 1977). Adults of this species have been observed to emerge in the spring from larvae collected in autumn (Nijveldt, 1969), with just one generation annually. Another *Aphidoletes* species, *A. thompsoni*, is associated with adelgids, specifically *A. piceae* on silver-fir trees, and has been observed attacking Scots pine adelgid on Scots pine trees in the Isle of Man. Unlike *A. abietis*, A. thompsoni is multivoltine, completing three to five generations annually (Harris, 1973; Harris and Bennett, 2003).

4.2.1.2.2 *Lestodiplosis* sp.

The genus *Lestodiplosis* comprises a group of predatory midges, whose larvae commonly prey on the larvae of other gall midges. *Lestodiplosis* larvae are also known to feed on small beetles and mites (Harris, 1966). For instance, in clover seed crops, various gall midge species, including pests like the clover leaf midge (*Dasineura trifolii*), clover seed midge (*D. leguminicola*), and white clover seed midge (*D. gentneri*), inhabit flower heads. These flower heads may also host larvae of predatory midges, such as *Lestodiplosis trifolii*, which preys on both the clover seed midge and the white clover seed midge (Milne, 1960). Additionally, *Lestodiplosis* larvae have been discovered on oak trees, where they not only coexist with phytophagous gall midge larvae and phytophagous gall mites but are also considered predators of lepidopterous larvae, particularly those of the green oak tortrix moth (*T. viridana*) and winter moth (*O. brumata*) (Cole and Harris, 2002).

4.2.1.3 Chloropidae (Grass Flies)

Grass flies, belonging to the family Chloropidae, are small or very small insects, often shiny and yellow with black markings, primarily associated with grasses of the Poaceae family. As larvae, many species are phytophagous, including economically significant pests of grasslands and cereals, such as the fruit fly, gout fly (*Chlorops pumilionis*), and yellow cereal fly (*Opomyza florum*). However, larvae of a few species are predatory, such as *Thaumatomyia glabra* and *T. notata*, both of which prey on root aphids, including harmful species like the lettuce root aphid (*Pemphigus bursarius*) and sugar beet root aphid (Toth et al., 2006). Thaumatomyia adults overwinter, often invading buildings in large swarms in autumn before hibernating (Kotrba, 2010). This behaviour was formally documented in September 1831, when tens of thousands of flies invaded an upper room of the Provost's Lodge in King's College, Cambridge, entering through an open window (Jenyns, 1832). Adults emerge from hibernation in late March or early April and then seek suitable hosts for breeding. Typically, there are two or more generations annually before young adults search for suitable overwintering sites.

4.2.1.4 Dolichopodidae (Long-Legged Flies)

Long-legged flies, belonging to the family Dolichopodidae, are predominantly small, bluish-metallic or greenish-metallic predatory flies, characterized by their elongated, stilt-like legs and prominently exposed male genitalia. Both adults and larvae of these flies primarily prey on minute insects, including psocids, springtails, thrips, and other Diptera. In northern Germany, several adults per square metre have been documented in emergence traps placed in fields of oilseed rape (Prescher and Buchs, 1998), while in France, adults of numerous long-legged fly species were captured in water traps set in flowering oilseed rape (Brunel et al., 1989). In the context of oilseed rape cultivation, long-legged flies are considered potentially beneficial predators of the brassica pod midge. Examples include Dolichopus acuticornis and the significantly smaller Medetera micacea (adults approximately 2 mm long). Long-legged flies, specifically M. truncorum, also prey on adult fruit flies (Jones, 1969), although Medetera spp. are primarily associated with thrips (Laurence, 1951).

4.2.1.5 Muscidae (Muscid Flies)

As a collective, muscid flies (family Muscidae) encompass several economically significant pests, some of which hold global importance. Examples include house flies (Musca domestica) and false stable flies (*Muscina stabulans*). The larvae of muscid flies exhibit a remarkably diverse range of feeding behaviours, including coprophagous and saprophagous habits, as well as carnivorous, endoparasitic, and phytophagous tendencies (Kutty et al., 2014). Certain species, like the western Palaearctic *Phaonia trimaculata*, have larvae that are predatory on plant pests, rendering them valuable as biocontrol agents (Fritzsche, 1955; Krivesheina, 2013). The larvae of most carnivorous muscid species are monomorphic, emerging from the egg in their final (third) instar. However, in some species with carnivorous larvae (referred to as dimorphic), they hatch and begin feeding during their second instar. Victims targeted by *P. trimaculata* include notable crop pests such as the cabbage root fly (*Delia radicum*), a significant threat to brassicaceous crops, and the cabbage stem weevil (*Ceutorhynchus pallidactylus*), which infests oilseed rape and other brassicaceous crops. Another widely distributed Holarctic species, *Agria affinis*, also preys on lepidopterans, including forestry pests like the black arches moth (*Lymantria monacha*), European gypsy moth (*L. dispar*), and lackey moth (*Malacosoma neustria*) (Schwenke, 1974). In Canada, this species is notably known as a predator of the non-European eastern spruce budworm (*Choristoneura fumiferana*) (Coppel et al., 1959).

4.2.1.6 Phoridae (Scuttle Flies)

Scuttle flies, also known as phorid flies, belong to the family Phoridae and are characterized by their small to very small size, a distinct humped thorax, and reduced wing venation. When disturbed, adults are notable for their tendency to run (scuttle) over surfaces instead of taking flight. The larvae of scuttle flies exhibit various feeding habits (Disney, 1983, 1989), with some species being saprophagous or fungivorous. Additionally, certain species act as parasites, parasitoids, and predators, with a few considered potentially valuable natural enemies of plant pests. For instance, *Borophaga crassata* parasitizes larvae of the St Mark's fly (*Bibio marci*) (Morris, 1922) and preys on the sugar beet root aphid (*Pemphigus fuscicornis*) (Toth et al., 2004).

4.2.1.7 Syrphidae (Hoverflies)

Hoverflies, belonging to the family Syrphidae, are easily distinguished from other dipterans by the presence of a false vein called the vena spuria, which form from remnants of a former longitudinal fold in the wing membrane. Additionally, the wing often features a false margin formed by two submarginal cross-veins running parallel to the true wing margin. Hoverflies frequently mimic bees or wasps and are known to hover in the air, emitting a shrill, bee-like hum. As adults, hoverflies, also referred to as flower flies, avidly feed on nectar, pollen, and honeydew, playing a beneficial role as pollinators of wildflowers and important flowering crops. While the predatory larvae of hoverflies typically feed on aphids, occasionally targeting other soft-bodied invertebrates like coccids and psyllids, some species prey on different types of prey. For instance, larvae of several hoverflies, including *Heringia heringi*, *Meliscaeva auricollis*, and *Scaeva mecogramma*, are associated with psyllids, particularly in southern Europe. Here, hoverfly larvae are known to prey on notable pests such as the bay sucker (*Inoza alacris*) and olive sucker (*Euphyllura olivina*). In the case of *M. auricollis*, which overwinters as an adult, larval development in southern Europe is completed in 2 weeks, with adults emerging from pupae just over a week later (Rojo et al., 1999). *S. mecogramma* exhibits a similarly rapid rate of development. *H. heringi*, which overwinters in the larval stage and displays a broader diet, preys not only on the olive sucker but also on other pests such as the cherry blackfly and peach leaf-roll aphid (*Myzus varians*) on cherry trees, the leaf-curling plum aphid (*Brachycaudus helichrysi*) on plum trees, the pear/bedstraw aphid (*Dysaphis pyri*) on pear trees, and the rosy apple aphid (*D. plantaginea*) on apple trees, at least in Italy (Niccoli and Fagnani, 1994) (Figure 4.2).

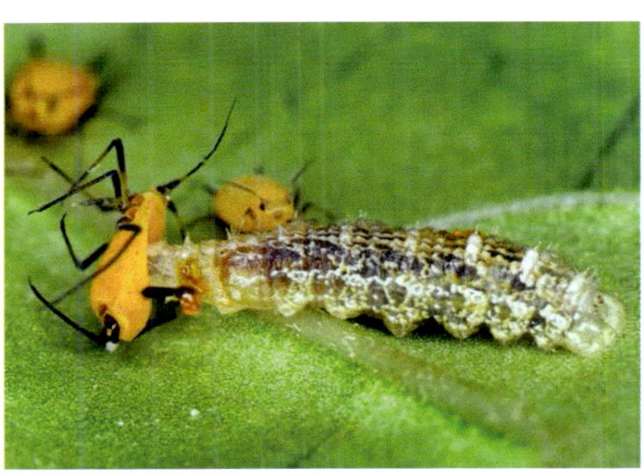

FIGURE 4.2 Syrphid larvae feeding on aphids.

4.2.1.7.1 *Epistrophe* spp.

Epistrophe species are medium-sized hoverflies mainly found in forest or scrubland habitats, with larvae typically being green and dorsoventrally flattened. Several species of Epistrophe are found in Europe, including the widely distributed *E. eligans*. The larvae of *E. eligans* prey on aphids infesting a variety of deciduous plants, including fruit trees, ornamental trees, and shrubs. They have also been observed with black bean aphids (*A. fabae*) on *Vicia* beans (Wojciechowicz-Zytko and Wnuk, 2012), as well as cereal aphids on winter wheat (Chambers et al., 1986). Adults of *E. eligans* are active from April to June, varying according to local conditions, and are often found near blackthorn and hawthorn bushes. Their eggs hatch within 2–3 days, and larvae typically reach full maturity in about 8 days. Subsequently, the larvae enter an extended period of obligatory diapause before overwintering and pupating in spring (Schneider, 1948). Several other Epistrophe species found in European apple orchards, including *E. melanostoma*, *E. nitidicollis*, and possibly E. ochrostoma, are known to prey on aphids. Their prey species include the apple/grass aphid (*Rhopalosiphum insertum*), woolly apple aphid (*Eriosoma lanigerum*), green apple aphid (*A. pomi*), and rosy apple aphid (Lyon and Goldlin de Tiefenau, 1974).

4.2.1.7.2 *Syrphus* spp.

This genus, which currently encompasses nine recognized European species, includes *Syrphus ribesii*, one of the most prevalent, widely distributed, and economically significant aphid-eating hoverflies. Commonly referred to as the currant hoverfly, *S. ribesii* is found in various human-altered environments such as parks, gardens, orchards, and soft-fruit plantations, as well as in broad-leaved woodlands and coniferous forests. Third-instar larvae undergo winter diapause in leaf litter before pupating in spring, resulting in up to four, but typically two to three, annual generations, categorizing *S. ribesii* as an oligovoltine species. At a temperature of 21°C, eggs hatch within 2–3 days, larvae feed for 9 days, and the pupal stage lasts for an additional 10 days (Schneider, 1948). However, in natural settings, a period of facultative summer diapause by larvae may extend this timeframe and reduce the number of annual generations. In northern Europe, adults are active from April to November, with activity peaks in May and August (Speight, 2011), while in southern Europe, adults emerge about a month earlier. *S. ribesii*, like many other species, is a well-known migrant. In addition to *S. ribesii*, two other Syrphus species, *S. torvus* and *S. vitripennis*, are cited as aphid predators in European apple orchards (Lyon and Goldlin de Tiefenau, 1974; Rossi et al., 2006).

4.2.1.8 Sarcophagidae (Flesh Flies)

Flesh flies, members of the family Sarcophagidae, resemble blowflies and were previously considered a subfamily within the Calliphoridae. Several species exhibit parasitic or predatory behaviour, including *Agria mamillata*, a natural enemy of small ermine moths (Yponomeuta spp.). *A. mamillata* targets various hosts, ranging from the apple small ermine moth (*Y. malinellus*), the bird-cherry small ermine moth (*Y. evonymella*), and the common small ermine moth (*Y. padella*) on hawthorn, among others, to the willow small ermine moth (*Y. rorella*). These moths inhabit communal silken webs (tents) formed on their respective arboreal hosts. *A. mamillata* follows a univoltine lifecycle, with adults emerging from overwintered pupae in late spring or early summer. After a prolonged pre-oviposition period, the ovoviviparous females lay eggs on final-instar larvae and pupae. The eggs hatch immediately, and the larvae then prey upon their hosts. Each larva-like predator eliminates around five host larvae or pupae during its development, with the feeding period lasting approximately 9–15 days (Kuhlmann, 1995). Fully fed Agria larvae, measuring about 10 mm in length, typically leave the host's web to pupate in the ground, often triggered by rainfall.

4.2.2 Parasitoids (Table 4.1)

4.2.2.1 Tachinidae

The Tachinidae family is widely utilized as parasitoids and is noted for its relatively low host specificity (Greathead, 1986). Recent studies indicate that around 8,200 species of Tachinidae have been identified, belonging to 1,530 genera (Stireman et al., 2006; Cerretti et al., 2014). Tachinidae are exclusively parasitic and play a crucial role in controlling macrolepidopteran pests. Over 100 species from this family have been incorporated into biological control programmes targeting crop or forest pests, yielding varying degrees of success (Greathead, 1986; Genier, 1988). Many agriculturally significant tachinid species share common host species or utilize alternative hosts in their native habitats, which serve as parasitoid refuges (Marino et al., 2006). One example is *Compsilura concinnata*, initially introduced for gypsy moth control in the northeastern United States. When combined with another tachinid, *Blepharipa scutellata*, they can collectively contribute to a mortality rate of up to 50% in moth populations. *Lydella thompsoni* is a parasitoid of the European corn borer (Figure 4.3).

TABLE 4.1
Tachinid parasitoids

Bio-agent	Insect species	Reported regions
Periscepsia carbonaria	*Agrotis segetum*	Asia
Linnaemya haemorrhoidalis	*Apamea illyria*	Asia
Tratoia monticola	*Cosmorhae ocellata*	Asia
Archytas sp.	*Helicoverpa gelotopoeon*	Europe
Lydella thompsoni	*Ostrinia nubilalis*	Europe
Drino maroccana	*Streblote panda*	Europe
Lixophaga Townsend	*Neoleucinodes elegantalis*	South America
Senometopia illota	*Helicoverpa armigera*	Asia
Archytas marmoratus		
Linnaemya longirostris		
Drino inconspiaoides	*Mythimna separate*	Asia
Compsilura concinnata	*Actias luna*	America
Blepharipa zebina	*Notolophus antiqua*	Asia

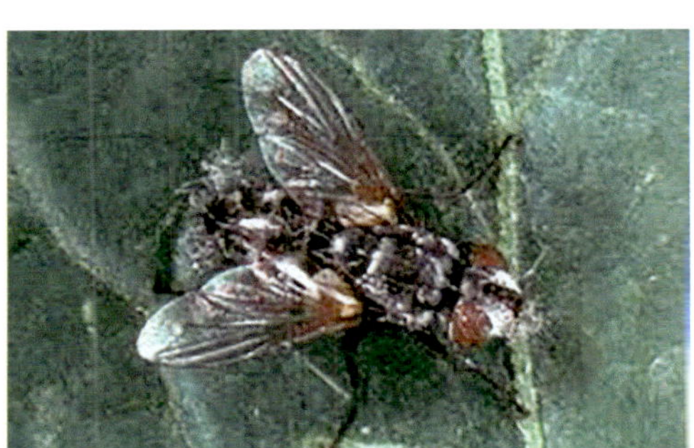

FIGURE 4.3 Parasitoid, *Lydella thompsoni*.

4.3 ENVIRONMENTAL ENGINEERING AND ECOSYSTEM SERVICES

4.3.1 Pollination of Flowers

Worldwide, more than 80% of crops depend on insect pollinators for their productivity. Flies are the world's second-most significant pollinators, next to bees. They exhibit remarkable diversity and are efficient pollinators found in various habitats. They frequently carry large amounts of pollen in both natural and engineered environments. These unmanaged pollinators provide consistent pollination to a wide range of crops. In agriculture, fly species aid in crop pollination and enhance yields. Flies visit flowers to acquire nectar and pollen, which serve as sources of energy and protein, respectively. Flowers also serve as special meeting places for mating and provide a favourable microclimate for flies (Kearns, 2002; Kevan, 2002).Dipteran flies play a significant role in preserving plant diversity by actively participating in pollination (Ssymank et al., 2008). Diptera likely served as one of the earliest pollinators of angiosperms, potentially having a significant impact on the early diversification of these plants (Labandeira, 1998; Endress, 2001). Also known as flower flies, Diptera are highly prevalent insects that frequently visit flowers (Free, 1970). In Belgium, flower flies alone are known to visit around 700 plant species belonging to 94 families (De Buck, 1990). Flies from 86 Diptera families visit over 1,100 plant species. While not all visits result in pollination, the diversity and frequency of these visits suggest that many flies contribute to global plant pollination. Fly families visiting agricultural crops (Table 4.2) include flower flies (Anthomyiidae), march flies (Bibionidae), bee flies (Bombyliidae), blow flies (Calliphoridae), flesh flies (Sarcophagidae), house flies (Muscidae), hover flies (Syrphidae), horse flies (Tabanidae), and bristle flies (Tachinidae). Effective pollinators among flies include blow flies (Calliphoridae), hover flies (Syrphidae), flower flies (Anthomyiidae), and specifically, the house fly, *Musca domestica* Linnaeus 1758 (Muscidae). Flies exhibit a reduced frequency of flower visiting, possess fewer hairs compared to bees, and generally lack unique anatomical adaptations for pollen transportation. However, due to the hairs on their bodies, pollen adheres to flies. Certain fly species have adaptations on their front legs that enable them to collect and consume pollen (Holloway, 1976; Neff et al., 2003). Diptera play a crucial role in the pollination of numerous vital crops, such as apples, cacao, carrots, cashew, cassava, cauliflower, leek, mango, mustard, onions, strawberries, and tea (Heath, 1982, Hansen, 1983, Clement et al., 2007, Mitra and Banerjee, 2007).

The highly specialized flowers of cacao are exclusively pollinated by small midges from the genus Forcipomyia (Young, 1986, 1994). Additionally, more flowering plants are being discovered that rely solely on dipteran pollinators. For example, the seed-for-seed mutualism involving the anthomyiid genus *Chiastocheta*, which pollinates the closed flowers of *Trollius europaeus* (Pellmyr, 1989), and the gall midge pollination of *Artocarpus*, which also involves a parasitic fungus (Sakai et al., 2000). Numerous flowers, including the world's largest flower, *Rafflesia arnoldii*, have specialized in being pollinated by carrion flies (Beaman et al., 1988). Diptera are crucial pollinators for flat to bowl-shaped flowers, especially in habitats and conditions where bees are less active. Many flies have adapted to moist and cool environments, such as cloud forests and arctic and alpine regions, which have a high proportion of dipteran pollinators (Kevan, 1972; Elberling and Olesen, 1999; Kearns, 1992, 2001; Lefebvre et al., 2014). In forest understories, small Diptera might be the primary pollinators, particularly for shrubs with many small, inconspicuous, and dioecious flowers (Larson et al., 2001; Borkent and Harder, 2007) (Table 4.2; Figure 4.4).

4.3.1.1 Calliphoridae (Blow Flies)

Blow flies have a cosmopolitan distribution with over 1,000 species in 150 genera, making them one of the most important pollinators among flies (Saeed et al., 2016; McAlpine, 1987). *Blow flies are major crop pollination insects, along with honey and wild bees.* Blow flies are stout, medium- to large-sized, and exhibit metallic coloration. They visit a wide range of agricultural crops and flowering plants, carrying a significant amount of pollen on their bodies. Blow flies visit plants for

TABLE 4.2
Flies in pollination various agricultural crops

Dipteran flies (Family)	Species	Crop
Anthomyiidae	*Delia* spp.	Pak Choi
(Flower Flies)	*Delia platura*	
	Anthomyia punctipennis	Carrot, Onion, Pak Choi
Bombyliidae	*Comptosia ocellata*	Carrot
(Bee Flies)		
Calliphoridae	*Calliphora* spp.	Avocado,Macadamia, Mango, Onion
(Blow Flies)	*Calliphora vicina*	Avocado Carrot, Lucerne, Leek, Onion, Pak Choi
	Calliphora stygia	Avocado Onion, Pak Choi
	Calliphora augur	Avocado
	Calliphora albifrontalis	Avocado, Blueberry
	Chrysomya spp. *Chrysomya megacephala, Chrysomya saffranea*	Mango
	Chrysomya rufifacies	Avocado, Mango
	Chrysomya varipes	Avocado
	Lucilia sericata	Avocado, Celery, Lychee, Mango, Onion, Pak Choi Strawberry
	Lucilia cuprina	Avocado
Muscidae	*Musca domestica*	Leek, Mango, Onion
(House Flies)	*Hydrotaea rostrate*	Onion, Pak Choi
	Spilogona spp.	Pak Choi
Rhiniidae	*Stomorhina discolour*	Avocado, Macadamia, Mango
(Nose Flies)	*Stomorhina xanthogaster*	Mango
Sarcophagidae		Mango, Onion
(Flesh Flies)	*Oxysarcodexia varia*	Onion, Pak Choi
Stratiomyidae (Soldier Flies)	Odontomyia spp.	Pak Choi
	Odontomyia atrovirens	
Syrphidae	Eristalis spp (Drone Flies)	Mango
(Hover Flies)	*Eristalinus hervebazini*	Mango
	Eristalis tenax	Cranberry, Carrot, Onion, Peppers, Pak Choi
	Melangyna spp	Carrot, Onion, Pak Choi
	Mesembrius bengalensis	Mango
	Simosyrphus grandicornis	Avocado
Tachinidae	Bristle Flies	Avocado
Tabanidae	*Scaptia* spp.	Pak Choi, Onion
(Horse Flies)		

sugars (nectar, honeydew, and sweet liquids) and inadvertently cause pollination during the day. The genera *Chrysomya*, *Lucilia*, and *Calliphora* are significant pollinators for the seed production of vegetables, especially carrots, onions, and leeks (Lisi & Shindler 2011; Woodcock, 2012). Clement et al. (2007) reported that *Calliphora vicina* is an efficient pollinator of leeks. Similarly, *C. vicina* is an effective pollinator of *Medicago citrina* (Lucerne). *Chrysomya megacephala* is the most frequent visitor and significant pollinator of avocados in Mexican orchards (Howlett, 2017; Pérez-Balam et al., 2012). In New Zealand, among native plants, *Metrosideros robusta* is visited by *C. vicina*; *Pittosporum crassifolium* and *Leptospermum scoparium* are visited by *C. sggia*; and

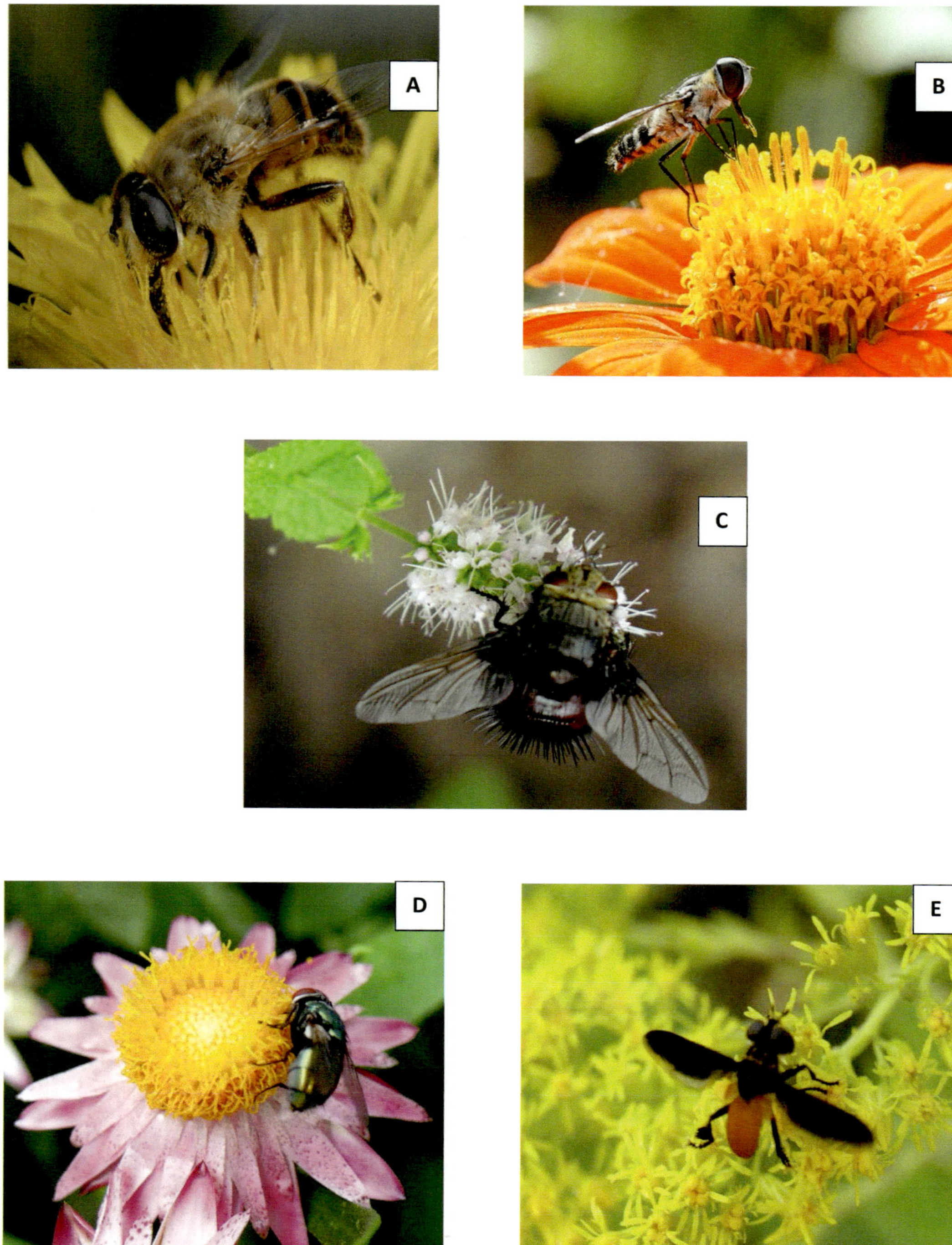

FIGURE 4.4 Flies in pollination (A. Drone fly; B. Hover fly; C. Tachinid fly; D. Blow fly; E. Hairy-legged fly).

Rhopalostylis sapida and *Schefflera disata* are visited by *C. quadrimaculata*. *C. vicina* is also a pollinator of *Hebe* spp. (grass) and at least 18 species of exotic plants. In India, the study of their pollination ability is not comprehensive, although reports indicate that twelve calliphorid flies visit flowers and pollinate them. After wasps and bees, blow flies are the major pollinators of carrot, onion, and cauliflower (Priti, 1998; Priti and Sihag, 1997, 1998). Blow flies regularly visit wild and cultivated plants (Mitra and Parui, 2002). Mitra et al. (2005) identified three calliphorid fly species in West Bengal as pollinators of medicinal plants. Mitra (2010) documented *Lucilia* sp. as a pollinator for the medicinal herb *Ammi majus*. Additionally, Bhatnagar (1986) noted four species of blow flies acting as pollinators for Asclepiadaceae in Central India. As a result, some blow fly species are now commercially available for pollination services, for example, the green blow fly *Lucilia sericata* (Meigen).

4.3.1.2 Syrphidae

The Syrphidae family (hover flies and flower flies) is one of the largest dipteran families, with over 6,000 species described worldwide. Adult syrphids primarily obtain their resources from flowers, visiting for both nectar and pollen. This family exhibits a diverse range of life histories, and the larvae of many species benefit horticultural industries by preying on pest insects such as aphids. Thus, syrphids are considered important pollinators as adults and significant biocontrol agents as larvae. Drone flies, members of the genus *Eristalis* within the Syrphidae, mimic bees and have shown potential for commercial-scale pollination, particularly in orchards, seed crops, and greenhouses.

4.3.2 Scavengers and Decomposers

In most terrestrial and freshwater ecosystems, Diptera outnumber and outweigh other insect decomposers (McLean, 2000). Sarcophagidae, Calliphoridae, and Muscidae are globally recognized as the primary necrophagous dipteran families. However, numerous other families, including Phoridae, Psychodidae, Sepsidae, Stratiomyidae, Fanniidae, Anthomyiidae, Piophilidae, Chloropidae, Ephydridae, Milichiidae, Neriidae, Micropezidae, Drosophilidae, Dixidae, Sphaeroceridae, and Cecidomyiidae, play essential roles in decomposing and recycling decaying organic matter. The significance of Diptera in dung recycling is extensively studied (Laurence, 1953, 1954, 1955; Papp, 1976, 1985; Papp and Garzó, 1985; Skidmore, 1991; O'Hara et al., 1999). The black soldier fly *Hermetia illucens*, a pantropical species breeding in decaying fruit and organic matter (James, 1935), demonstrates the decomposing prowess and ecological importance of flies. The colonization of chicken manure by *Hermetia illucens* often leads to reduced manure volume (Sheppard et al., 1994), fewer house flies (Sheppard, 1983; Axtell and Arends, 1990), and serves as a food source for fish and swine (Newton et al., 1977; Bondari and Sheppard, 1981). Additionally, *H. illucens* and *Ornidia obesa* (Syrphidae) hold potential benefits for the citrus industry by decomposing orange-peel waste, as seen in Costa Rica (Pape, 2009). While effective decomposers, many Diptera pose pest potential by locating and infecting stored human food. Meat products, cheese, and ham are particularly susceptible to infestation by blow fly eggs and cheese skippers such as *Piophila casei*. Flies like *Calliphora*, *Chrysomya*, and *Lucilia* infest dried fish, causing significant losses in tropical and subtropical regions (Haines and Rees, 1989; Esser, 1991; Wall et al., 2001) (Figure 4.5).

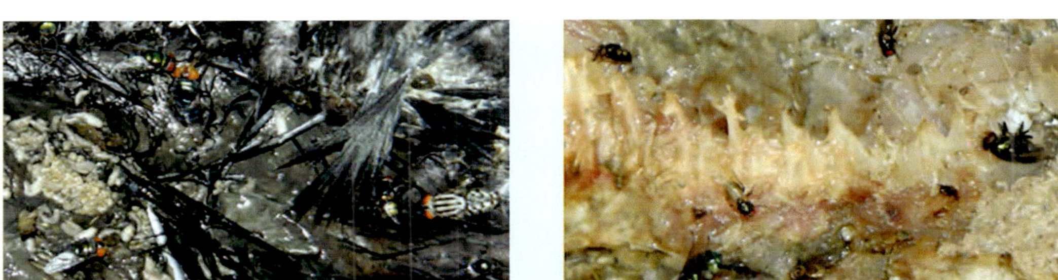

FIGURE 4.5 Necrophagous flies feeding on carcasses.

4.3.2.1 Ecosystem Services Provided by Necrophagous Flies

Decomposers play a vital role in nutrient cycling and maintaining ecological balance within natural and semi-natural habitats. In any ecosystem, including those with producers and consumers, the effective functioning of the nutrient cycle is crucial for sustainability. Decomposers facilitate humus formation in the soil and make nutrients available to plants, contributing significantly to ecosystem health (Galante and Marcos-Garcia, 2004). Necrophagous dipterans, despite their small size and cumulative biomass, exert considerable influence on carbon and nutrient cycling by regulating the quality and quantity of resources entering the detrital food web (Yang and Gratton, 2014). Beyond simply consuming carrion, these flies also facilitate its breakdown, making it accessible to microorganisms. The larvae of flies and other insects liquefy corpse tissues, priming them for microbial decomposition (Galante and Marcos-Garcia, 2004). This process aids in the recycling of carbon and essential nutrients like nitrogen and phosphorus within the ecosystem, enhancing their availability to producers.

4.3.2.2 Necrophagous Flies as Potential Bioindicators for Detecting Environmental Changes

Diptera serve as valuable bioindicators for assessing environmental changes and monitoring forest recovery (Majer, 1987). Their abundance and taxonomic diversity enable the collection of large samples, facilitating the analysis of community-level effects across various species contributions. Dipterans occupy diverse niches and trophic levels, making them widespread in both natural and human-altered habitats, from rural to urban settings (D'Almeida and Lopes, 1983). Due to their ecological diversity, dipteran communities are sensitive indicators of environmental changes, detecting even subtle shifts (Pereira de Sousa et al., 2014; Odat et al., 2015). Species within families like Calliphoridae and Sarcophagidae inhabit various environments but differ in their sensitivity to human impacts. Studies indicate that sites with intermediate disturbance levels harbour greater diversity of these species compared to heavily disturbed or undisturbed areas (Dufek et al., 2016). Similar investigations in India could identify specific necrophagous dipterans as potential bioindicators of environmental changes.

4.3.3 Bioindicators

Biomonitoring involves using living organisms or their responses to assess environmental quality (Rosenberg and Resh, 1993; Resh et al., 1996; Barbour et al., 1999; Moulton et al., 2000; Bonada et al., 2006; Rosenberg et al., 2008). It encompasses surveys conducted before and after impacts, regular sampling for compliance with environmental standards, and large-scale surveys to establish reference conditions or assess biological impairment (Thomson et al., 2005; Yoder and Rankin, 1998; Maret et al., 2003; Klemm et al., 2003; Black and Munn, 2004). Diptera are frequently included in biomonitoring studies, particularly in water quality assessments, due to the presence of their abundance and habitat specificity (Saether, 1979). Chironomidae, commonly known as midges, are widely used dipterans in water quality studies. Their larvae, often called "blood worms" due to haemoglobin in their blood, can survive in poorly oxygenated aquatic habitats (Wiederholm, 1980). Morphological deformities in chironomid larvae, such as changes in sclerite shape, are used to assess environmental stress (Wiederholm, 1984). While many aquatic dipterans are tolerant of environmental impacts, some families, like Blephariceridae and Deuterophlebiidae, are highly sensitive (Lenat, 1993b). Diptera are also employed in laboratory toxicity studies to compare toxicants and predict their environmental effects (Michailova et al., 1998; Karouna-Renier and Zehr, 1999). Their diverse microhabitat requirements make them valuable for habitat-quality assessment and conservation planning (Rotheray et al., 2001). For instance, abundance patterns of stiletto flies (Therevidae) can indicate habitat heterogeneity and successional stage in dry areas (Holston, 2005). Moreover, Diptera, such as flower flies (Syrphidae), are used as bioindicators of environmental stress in various habitats, including ski slopes and landscapes (Haslett, 1988; Sommaggio, 1999). Additionally, saproxylic and fungivorous flies serve as indicators of woodland quality, aiding in forest management strategies (Speight, 1986; Økland, 1994, 1996, 2000; Good and Speight, 1996; Fast and Wheeler, 2004; Økland et al., 2004, 2008). Endemic Dolichopodidae in Hawaii, along with other selected families, can indicate valuable aquatic habitats with high native diversity (Englund et al., 2007).

4.3.4 Diptera as Model Organisms and Research Tools (Figure 4.6)

The functional and physiological similarities between insect flight muscles and human heart musculature provide valuable insights into both insect flight mechanics and human muscular disorders. Research on *Drosophila* wing-muscle myofibrils and the expression of heterologous human cytoplasmic actin in *Drosophila* flight muscles offers promising avenues for understanding human muscular disorders (Chan and Dickinson, 1996; Maughan et al., 1998; Vigoreaux, 2001; Brault et al., 1999). Asynchronous flight muscles, which allow a single nerve impulse to trigger multiple muscle contractions, are essential for the high-frequency wingbeat required for sustained flight in many insects. Studies on Ceratopogonidae have shown wingbeat frequencies exceeding 1,000 Hz, highlighting the efficiency of insect flight mechanics (Sotavalta, 1947, 1953). Understanding the mechanical and physiological aspects of insect flight muscles provides insights into muscle operational design, contractile costs, and energy-saving mechanisms, with implications for both human health and biotechnological advances (Conley and Lindstedt, 2002; Syme and Josephson, 2002). *Drosophila melanogaster*, introduced as a laboratory model organism a century ago, has revolutionized genetic research. Studies using Drosophila have provided profound insights into gene expression, gene regulatory mechanisms, and genomics (Castle, 1906; Ashburner and Bergman, 2005). The sequencing of the Drosophila genome has been highly rewarding, with nearly 75% of candidate human disease genes having homologues in Drosophila. This has opened avenues for improved treatments of human disorders, from diabetes to alcoholism (Reiter et al., 2001; Brogiolo et al., 2001; Leevers, 2001; Campbell et al., 1997; Morozova et al., 2006). Furthermore, discoveries like the Hox genes in *D. melanogaster* have provided insights into how organisms regulate segment identity and body patterning along the embryonic axis (Carroll, 1995; Akam, 1998; Lewis, 1998). The short generation time of Drosophila facilitates studies on age-specific behaviours and age-related memory impairment, contributing to our understanding of aging processes (Carey et al., 2006; Horiuchi and Saitoe, 2005).

4.3.5 Diptera as Part of Our Cultural Legacy

Indeed, flies have woven themselves into the fabric of human culture in multifaceted ways. From ancient folklore to modern literature and cinema, they have left their mark on our imagination. The tale of the brave little tailor, who famously boasted of defeating "seven in one blow", captivates the

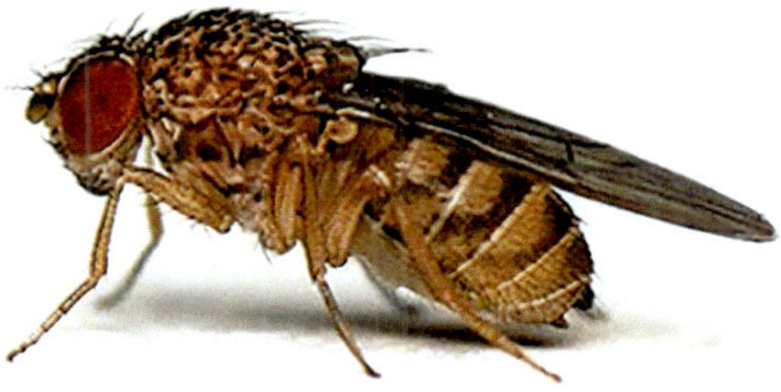

FIGURE 4.6 *Drosophila* sp. as model organism.

minds of countless children, highlighting the enduring fascination with these small creatures (Pape, 2009). Similarly, the comedic trope of finding a fly in one's soup has been a source of amusement for generations, illustrating the common experience of encountering flies in everyday life. Literature and film have also explored the symbolism and intrigue surrounding flies. George Langelaan's "The Fly" and its cinematic adaptations delve into the realm of science fiction, exploring the consequences of human–fly hybridization. This narrative resonates with themes of transformation and the blurring of boundaries between species. Moreover, flies have made their mark in religious and literary contexts. In the biblical story of the plagues, flies are depicted as agents of divine wrath, symbolizing pestilence and disruption. In William Golding's "Lord of the Flies", flies take on a darker symbolism, representing the primal instincts and savagery lurking within humanity. Conversely, William Blake's poem "The Fly" offers a more introspective exploration, using the fly as a metaphor for life's fleeting moments and existential ponderings. Through these diverse portrayals, flies emerge as potent symbols that reflect human fears, desires, and existential inquiries, reminding us of our intertwined existence with the natural world.

Flies, despite their ecological importance, can also be a considerable nuisance, interfering with various human activities and causing discomfort. Mosquitoes, gnats, and other flies can harass individuals, and sometimes their presence reaches nuisance levels. For instance, in Australia, the proliferation of the Australian bush fly in cow dung became a significant issue after European settlement, exacerbated by the absence of native dung beetles. Similar situations have been observed in other regions, with flies like *Thaumatomyia notata* invading homes in large numbers in search of overwintering sites. Indoor proliferation of flies from families like Phoridae and Sphaeroceridae often requires eradication measures due to their nuisance levels. Certain Psychodidae species can also be problematic, with larvae in sewage treatment facilities impeding flow and adults causing respiratory issues when inhaled. Additionally, aquatic fly species, like Chaoboridae and Chironomidae, can form massive swarms, causing inconvenience and even traffic problems in urban areas. While some communities have found ways to utilize swarming midges for food, as seen in East African lakes, the presence of flies like *Sarcophaga aldrichi*, despite their beneficial role as parasitoids, can lead to complaints when their populations become excessive. Moreover, blood-feeding flies such as mosquitoes, black flies, deer flies, and horse flies are notorious for their annoyance and potential disease transmission. Efforts to control these nuisance flies are often significant, particularly in areas where they pose a threat to public health and comfort. Even flies like the common house fly (*Musca domestica*) and eye gnats (*Hippelates* spp.) can disrupt human comfort, with house flies acting as mechanical vectors of pathogens and eye gnats causing irritation by being attracted to bodily secretions. While these nuisance flies may not always pose direct health risks, their presence can significantly impact human well-being and necessitate management strategies to mitigate their effects.

4.4 CONCLUSION

In conclusion, flies play diverse and vital roles in biological control and environmental engineering, exerting significant influence on ecosystems, agriculture, public health, and waste management. As important pollinators, decomposers, and predators, flies contribute to ecosystem functioning and stability. Their role in biological control, particularly in regulating pest populations, highlights their potential as natural allies in agriculture and forestry. Moreover, flies serve as valuable indicators of environmental health, with their abundance, diversity, and behaviour reflecting changes in ecosystems due to natural or anthropogenic factors. Biomonitoring studies utilizing flies provide insights into ecosystem dynamics and aid in assessing the impact of environmental changes. In addition to their ecological significance, flies can also be a nuisance, interfering with human activities and causing discomfort. Efforts to manage nuisance fly populations are crucial for safeguarding public health and well-being. Overall, a comprehensive understanding of flies' ecological roles, coupled with effective management strategies, is essential for harnessing their benefits while mitigating their potential drawbacks. Continued research into fly biology, behaviour, and interactions with the environment will further enhance our ability to utilize flies for biological control and environmental engineering purposes.

4.5 POINTS TO REMEMBER

1. Flies can serve as biological control agents by preying on or parasitizing pest species.
2. Mainly tachinid flies, hoverflies, and robber flies are significant in integrated pest management programmes to reduce reliance on chemical pesticides.
3. Flies play a role in environmental engineering by pollinating crops and wild plants, decomposing organic waste into compost, and scavenging to clean up decaying matter and recycle nutrients.
4. They act as bioindicators to monitor and assess ecosystem health and environmental quality.
5. Flies are used as model organisms in research for studying genetics, developmental biology, and ecological interactions.
6. Flies are an integral part of cultural legacy, symbolizing their historical significance and influence in art, literature, and folklore.

REFERENCES

Akam, M. (1998). Hox genes, homeosis and the evolution of segment identity: No need for hopeless monsters. *International Journal of Developmental Biology*, *42*, 445–451.

Ashburner, M., & Bergman, C. M. (2005). Drosophila melanogaster: A case study of a model genomic sequence and its consequences. *Genome Research*, *15*(12), 1661–1667.

Axtell, R. C., & Arends, J. J. (1990). Ecology and management of arthropod pests of poultry. *Annual Review of Entomology*, *35*, 101–126.

Barbour, M. T., Gerritsen, J., Snyder, B. D., & Stribling, J. B. (1999). *Rapid Bioassessment Protocols for Use in Streams and Wadable Rivers: Periphyton, Benthic Macroinvertebrates and Fish*. United States Environmental Protection Agency, Washington, DC, 202 pp.

Beaman, R. S., Decker, P. J., & Beaman, J. H. (1988). Pollination of *Rafflesia* (Rafflesiaceae). *American Journal of Botany*, *75*(8), 1148–1162.

Black, R. W., Munn, M. D., & Plotnikoff, R. W. (2004). Using macroinvertebrates to identify biota–land cover optima at multiple scales in the Pacific Northwest, USA. *Journal of the North American Benthological Society*, *23*(2), 340–362.

Bonada, N., Prat, N., Resh, V. H., & Statzner, B. (2006). Developments in aquatic insect biomonitoring: A comparative analysis of recent approaches. *Annual Review Entomology*, *51*, 495–523.

Bondari, K., & Sheppard, D. C. (1981). Soldier fly larvae as feed in commercial fish production. *Aquaculture*, *24*, 103–109.

Borkent, C. J., & Harder, L. D. (2007). Flies (Diptera) as pollinators of two dioecious plants: Behaviour and implications for plant mating. *The Canadian Entomologist*, *139*(2), 235–246.

Braga, R. F., Korasaki, V., Andresen, E., & Louzada, J. (2013). Dung beetle community and functions along a habitat-disturbance gradient in the Amazon: A rapid assessment of ecological functions associated to biodiversity. *PLoS One*, *8*(2), e57786.

Brault, V., Reedy, M. C., Sauder, U., Kammerer, R. A., Aebi, U., & Schoenenberger, C. A. (1999). Substitution of flight muscle-specific actin by human β-cytoplasmic actin in the indirect flight muscle of *Drosophila*. *Journal of Cell Science*, *112*(21), 3627–3639.

Brogiolo, W., Stocker, H., Ikeya, T., Rintelen, F., Fernandez, R., & Hafen, E. (2001). An evolutionarily conserved function of the *Drosophila* insulin receptor and insulin-like peptides in growth control. *Current Biology*, *11*(4), 213–221.

Brown, B. V. (2001). Flies, gnats, and mosquitoes. In S. A. Levin (ed.), *Encyclopedia of Biodiversity*. Academic Press, London, pp. 815–826.

Campbell, H. D., Fountain, S., Young, I. G., Claudianos, C., Hoheisel, J. D., Chen, K. S., & Lupski, J. R. (1997). Genomic structure, evolution, and expression of human FLII, a gelsolin and leucine-rich-repeat family member: Overlap with LLGL. *Genomics*, *42*(1), 46–54.

Carroll, S. B. (1995). Homeotic genes and the evolution of arthropods and chordates. *Nature*, *376*(6540), 479–485.

Carey, J. R., Papadopoulos, N., Kouloussis, N., Katsoyannos, B., Müller, H. G., Wang, J. L., & Tseng, Y. K. (2006). Age-specific and lifetime behavior patterns in *Drosophila melanogaster* and the Mediterranean fruit fly, *Ceratitis capitata*. *Experimental Gerontology*, *41*(1), 93–97.

Castle, W. E. (1906). Inbreeding, cross-breeding and sterility in *Drosophila*. *Science*, *23*(578), 153–153.

Chandler, P. J. (2014). *An Update of the 1998 Checklist of Diptera of the British Isles*. Dipterists Forum, Oxford, UK, p. 340. https://dipterists.org.uk/sites/default/files/pdf/BRITISH%20ISLES%20CHECKLIST%20 2023_03.pdf (accessed 23 December 2018).

Chambers, R. J., Sunderland, K. D., Stacey, D. L., & Wyatt, I. J. (1986). Control of cereal aphids in winter wheat by natural enemies: Aphid-specific predators, parasitoids and pathogenic fungi. *Annals of Applied Biology*, *108*(2), 219–231.

Chan, W. P., & Dickinson, M. H. (1996). In vivo length oscillations of indirect flight muscles in the fruit fly *Drosophila virilis*. *Journal of Experimental Biology*, *199*(12), 2767–2774.

Clement, S. L., Hellier, B. C., Elberson, L. R., Staska, R. T., & Evans, M. A. (2007). Flies (Diptera: Muscidae: Calliphoridae) are efficient pollinators of *Allium ampeloprasum* L. (Alliaceae) in field cages. *Journal of Economic Entomology*, *100*(1), 131–135.

Cole, L. R. & Harris, K. M. (2002). *Lestodiplosis* spp. (Dipt., Cecidomyiidae) predaceous on larvae of Lepidoptera and other insects on oaks (*Quercus robur* L.) in southern England. *Entomologists Monthly Magazine*, *138*, 1–10.

Conley, K. E., & Lindstedt, S. L. (2002). Energy-saving mechanisms in muscle: The minimization strategy. *Journal of Experimental Biology*, *205*(15), 2175–2181.

Coppel, H. C., House, H. L. & Maw, M. G. (1959). Studies on dipterous parasites of the spruce budworm, *Choristoneura fumiferana* (Clem.) (Lepidoptera: Tortricidae): VII. *Agria affinis* (Fall.) (Diptera: Sarcophagidae). *Canadian Journal of Zoology*, *37*, 817–830.

Courtney, G. W., & Merritt, R. W. (2008). Aquatic diptera: Part one: Larvae of aquatic diptera. In R. W. Merritt, K. W. Cummins and M. B. Berg (eds.), *An Introduction to the Aquatic Insects of North America,* 4th edition. Kendall/Hunt Publishing, Dubuque, Iowa, pp. 687–722.

Courtney, G. W., & Merritt, R. W. (2009). Diptera (non-biting flies). In G. E. Likens (ed.), *Encyclopedia of Inland Waters,* Volume 2. Elsevier Limited, Oxford, UK, pp. 288–298.

d'Almeida, J. M., & Lopes, H. D. S. (1983). Sinantropia de dípteros caliptrados (Calliphoridae) no Estado do Rio de Janeiro. *Arquivos da Universidade Federal Rural do Rio de Janeiro*, *6*(1), 31–38.

De Buck, N. (1990). Bloemboek en bestuivingsecologie van Zweevfliegen (Diptera, Syrphidae) in het bijzonder voor België. *Institut royal des Sciences naturelles de Belgique*, *60*, 1–167.

de Sousa, J. R. P., Esposito, M. C., da Silva Carvalho Filho, F., & Juen, L. (2014). The potential uses of sarco-saprophagous flesh flies and blowflies for the evaluation of the regeneration and conservation of forest clearings: A case study in the Amazon forest. *Journal of Insect Science*, *14*(215), 1–5.

Dennis, D. S., Barnes, J. K. & Knutson, L. (2013). Review and analysis of information on the biology and morphology of immature stages of robber flies (Diptera: Asilidae). *Zootaxa*, *3671*, 1–64.

Disney, R. H. L. (1983). Scuttle flies. Diptera, Phoridae (except Megaselia). *Handbooks for the Identification of British Insects*, *10*(6), 1–81.

Disney, R. H. L. (1989). Scuttle flies. *Diptera Phoridae genus Megaselia. Handbooks for the Identification of British Insects*, *10*(8), 1–155.

Dufek, M. I., Oscherov, E. B., Damborsky, M. P., & Mulieri, P. R. (2016). Assessment of the abundance and diversity of Calliphoridae and Sarcophagidae (Diptera) in sites with different degrees of human impact in the Iberá Wetlands (Argentina). *Journal of Medical Entomology*, *53*(4), 827–835.

Elberling, H., & Olesen, J. M. (1999). The structure of a high latitude plant-flower visitor system: The dominance of flies. *Ecography*, *22*(3), 314–323.

Endress, P. K. (2001). The flowers in extant basal angiosperms and inferences on ancestral flowers. *International Journal of Plant Sciences*, *162*(5), 1111–1140.

Englund, R. A., Wright, M. G., & Polhemus, D. A. (2007). Aquatic insect taxa as indicators of aquatic species richness, habitat disturbance, and invasive species impacts in Hawaiian streams. In N. L. Evenhuis and J. M. Fitzsimons (eds.), *Biology of Hawaiian Streams and Estuaries. Bishop Museum Bulletin in Cultural and Environmental Studies*, *3*, 207–232.

Esser, J. R. (1991). Biology of *Chrysomya megacephala* (Diptera: Calliphoridae) and reduction of losses caused to the salted-dried fish industry in south-east Asia. *Bulletin of Entomological Research*, *81*(1), 33–42.

Fast, E., & Wheeler, T. A. (2004). Faunal inventory of Brachycera (Diptera) in an old growth forest at Mont Saint-Hilarie, Quebec. *Fabreries*, *29*, 1–15.

Ferrar, P. (1987). A guide to the breeding habits and immature stages of Diptera Cyclorrhapha. *Entomonograph*, *8*, 1–907.

Free, J. B. (1970). *Insect Pollination of Crops*. Academic Press, London, New York, 555 pp.

Fritzsche, R. (1955). Phaoniatri maculata Bouchals Parasit des Groen Kohltriebrlers Ceuthorhynchus napi Gyll. und des Gefleckten Kohltriebrlers Ceuthorhynchus quadridens Panz. *Nachrichtenblattfr den DeutschenPflanzenschutzdienst*, *9*, 35–36.

Gagné, R. J. (2010). Update for a catalog of the Cecidomyiidae (Diptera) of the world. https://www.ars.usda.gov/ARSUserFiles/80420580/Gagne_Jaschhof_2021_World_Cat_5th_Ed.pdf (accessed 4 May 2021).

Galante, E., Marcos–Garcia, M. A. (2004). Decomposer insects. In *Encyclopedia of Entomology*. Springer, Netherlands, pp. 665–674.

Garibaldi, L. A., Carvalheiro, L. G., Vaissière, B. E., Gemmill-Herren, B., Hipólito, J., Freitas, B. M., & Zhang, H. (2016). Mutually beneficial pollinator diversity and crop yield outcomes in small and large farms. *Science*, *351*(6271), 388–391.

Good, J. A., & Speight, M. C. D. (1996). Saproxylic invertebrates and their conservation throughout Europe. In *Convention on the Conservation of European Wildlife and Natural Habitats*, Council of Europe, Strasbourg, 58 pp.

Hansen, M. (1983). Yuca (Yuca, Cassava). In D. Manzen (ed.), *Costa Rican Natural*. The University of Chicago Press, Chicago, IL, pp. 114–117.

Haines, C. P., &Rees, D. P. (1989). A field guide to the types of insects and mites infesting cured fish. *FAO Fisheries Technical Paper*, *303*, 1–33

Harris, K. M. (1966). Gall midge genera of economic importance (Diptera: Cecidomyiidae). Part 1: Introduction and subfamily Cecidomyiinae; supertribe Cecidomyiidi. *Transactions of the Royal Entomological Society of London*, *118*, 313–358.

Harris, K. M. (1973). Aphidophagous Cecidomyiidae (Diptera): Taxonomy, biology and assessments of field populations. *Bulletin of Entomological Research*, *63*, 305–325.

Harris, K. M. (1982). The apple midge: A brief history. *Antenna*, *6*, 286–289.

Harris, K. M. & Bennett, F. D. (2003). Records of gall midges (Diptera.: Cecidomyiidae) from the Isle of Man. *Entomologists Record and Journal of Variation*, *115*, 109–115.

Haslett, J. R. (1988). Qualitätsbeurteilung alpiner Habitate: Schwebfliegen (Diptera: Syrphidae) als Bioindikatoren für Auswirkungen des intensiven Skibetriebes auf alpinen Wiesen in Österreich. *Zoologischer Anzeiger*, *220*(3–4), 179–184.

Hennig, W. (1973). Diptera (Zweiflugler). *Handbuch der Zoologie*, *4*, 1–337.

Heath, A. C. G. (1982). Beneficial aspects of blowflies (Diptera: Calliphoridae). *New Zealand Entomologist*, *7*(3), 343–348.

Horiuchi, J., & Saitoe, M. (2005). Can flies shed light on our own age-related memory impairment? *Ageing Research Reviews*, *4*(1), 83–101.

Hövemeyer, K. (2000). Ecology of diptera. In L. Papp and B. Darvas (eds.), *Contributions to a Manual of Palaearctic Diptera,* Volume 1: General and Applied Dipterology. Science Herald, Budapest, Hungary, pp. 437–489.

Holloway, B.A. (1976). Pollen-feeding in hover-flies (Diptera: Syrphidae). *New Zealand Journal of Zoology*, *3*, 339–350.

Holston, K. C. (2005). Evidence for community structure and habitat partitioning in coastal dune stiletto flies at the Guadalupe-Nipomo dunes system, California. *Journal of Insect Science*, *5*(1), 42.

James, M. T. (1935). The genus Hermetia in the United States (Diptera: Stratiomyidae). *Bulletin of the Brooklyn Entomological Society*, *30*(4), 165–170.

Jenyns, L. (1832). Account of an extraordinary swarm of flies. *Annals and Magazine of Natural History*, *5*(series 1), 302.

Jones, M. G. (1969). The effect of weather on fruit fly and its predators. *Journal of Applied Ecology*, *6*, 425–441.

Karouna-Renier, N. K., & Zehr, J. P. (1999). Ecological implications of molecular biomarkers: Assaying sub-lethal stress in the midge *Chironomus tentans* using heat shock protein 70 HSP-70) expression. *Molecular Ecology of Aquatic Communities*, *401*, 255–264.

Kearns, C. A. (2002). Flies and flowers: An enduring partnership. *Wings*, *25*(2), 3–8.

Kearns, C. A. (1992). Anthophilous fly distribution across an elevation gradient. *American Midland Naturalist*, *127*, 172–182.

Kevan, P. (2002). Flowers, pollination, and the associated diversity of flies. *Biodiversity*, *3*(4), 16–18.

Kevan, P. G. (1972). Insect pollination of high arctic flowers. *The Journal of Ecology*, *60*, 831–847.

Klemm, D. J., Blocksom, K. A., Fulk, F. A., Herlihy, A. T., Hughes, R. M., Kaufmann, P. R., ... & Davis, W. S. (2003). Development and evaluation of a macroinvertebrate biotic integrity index (MBII) for regionally assessing Mid-Atlantic Highlands streams. *Environmental Management*, *31*, 0656–0669.

Kotrba, M. (2010). Massenauftreten der Gemeinen Rasenhalmfliege Thaumatomyianotata (Diptera, Chloropidae) an Gebuden. *Denisia*, *30*, 451–456.

Krivosheina, N. P. (2013). On the ecology of Phaonia larvae (Diptera, Muscidae). *Entomological Review*, *93*, 324–333.

Kuhlmann, U. (1995). Biology and predation rate of the sarcophagid fly, *Agria mamillata* a predator of European small ermine moths. *International Journal of Pest Management*, *41*(2), 67–73.

Kutty, S. N., Pont, A. C., Meier, R., & Pape, T. (2014). Complete tribal sampling reveals basal split in Muscidae (Diptera), confirms saprophagy as ancestral feeding mode, and reveals an evolutionary correlation between instar numbers and carnivory. *Molecular Phylogenetics and Evolution*, *78*, 349–364.

Labandeira, C. C. (1998). How old is the flower and the fly? *Science*, *280*(5360), 57–59.

Laurence, B. R. (1951). The prey of some tree trunk frequenting Empididae and Dolichopodidae (Dipt.). *Entomologist's Monthly Magazine*, *87*, 166–169.

Laurence, B. R. (1953). Some Diptera bred from cow dung. *Entomologist's Monthly Magazine*, *89*, 281–283.

Laurence, B. R. (1954). The larval inhabitants of cow pats. *Journal of Animal Ecology*, *23*(2), 234–260.

Laurence, B. R. (1955). Flies associated with cow dung. *Entomologist's Record and Journal of Variation*, *67*, 123–126.

Larson, B. M. H., Kevan, P. G., & Inouye, D. W. (2001). Flies and flowers: Taxonomic diversity of anthophiles and pollinators. *The Canadian Entomologist*, *133*(4), 439–465.

Leevers, S. J. (2001). Growth control: Invertebrate insulin surprises! *Current Biology*, *11*(6), R209–R212.

Lefebvre, V., Fontaine, C., Villemant, C., & Daugeron, C. (2014). Are empidine dance flies major flower visitors in alpine environments? A case study in the Alps, France. *Biology Letters*, *10*(11), 20140742.

Lenat, D. R. (1993). A biotic index for the southeastern United States: Derivation and list of tolerance values, with criteria for assigning water-quality ratings. *Journal of the North American Benthological Society*, *12*(3), 279–290.

Lyon, J. P., & Göldin, D. T. P. (1974). Les Syrphes predateurs de pucerons. In *Les Organismes Auxiliaires en Verger de Pommiers*. OILB-SROP, pp. 163–170.

MacFarlane, R. P. (1979). Notes on insects of the Chatham Islands. *New Zealand Entomologist*, *7*(1), 64–70.

Majer, J. D. (1987). Invertebrates as indicators for management. In D. A. Saunders, G. W. Arnold, A. A. Burbidge, and A. J. M. Hopkins (eds.), *The Role of Remnants of Native Vegetation*. Springer, New York, pp. 353–354.

Maret, T. R., Cain, D. J., MacCoy, D. E., & Short, T. M. (2003). Response of benthic invertebrate assemblages to metal exposure and bioaccumulation associated with hard-rock mining in northwestern streams, USA. *Journal of the North American Benthological Society*, *22*(4), 598–620.

Marshall, S. A. (2012). *Flies: The Natural History and Diversity of Diptera*. Firefly Books, New York, 616 pp.

Maughan, D., Moore, J., Vigoreaux, J., Barnes, B., & Mulieri, L. A. (1998). Work production and work absorption in muscle strips from vertebrate cardiac and insect flight muscle fibers. In H. Sugi and G. Pollack (eds.), *Mechanisms of Work Production and Work Absorption in Muscle*. Springer, New York, pp. 471–480.

McAlpine, J. F., Peterson, B. V., Shewell, G. E., Teskey, H. J., Vockeroth, J. R., & Wood, D. M. (1981). *Manual of Nearctic Diptera*, Volume 1: Research Branch, Agriculture Canada Monograph 27. 674 pp.

McAlpine, J. F., Peterson, B. V., Shewell, G. E., Teskey, H. J., Vockeroth, J. R., & Wood, D. M. (1987). *Manual of Nearctic Diptera*, Volume 2: Research Branch, Agriculture Canada Monograph 28. pp. 675–1332.

McLean, I. F. G. (2000). Beneficial Diptera and their role in decomposition. *Contributions to a Manual of Palaearctic Diptera (with Special Reference to Flies of Economic Importance)*, *1*, 491–517.

Michailova, P., Petrova, N., Sella, G., Ramella, L., & Bovero, S. (1998). Structural–functional rearrangements in chromosome G in *Chironomus riparius* (Diptera, Chironomidae) collected from a heavy metal-polluted area near Turin, Italy. *Environmental Pollution*, *103*(1), 127–134.

Milne, D. L. (1960). The gall midges (Diptera: Cecidomyidae) of clover flower-heads. *Transactions of the Royal Entomological Society of London*, *112*, 73–108.

Mitra, B., Parui, P., Banerjee, D., Mukherjeee, M., & Bhattacharya, K. (2005). A report on flies (Diptera : Insecta) as flower visitors and pollinators of Kolkata and it's adjoining areas. *Records of the Zoological Survey of India*, 105(3–4), 1–20.

Mitra, B., & Banerjee, D. (2007). Fly pollinators: Assessing their value in biodiversity conservation and food security in India. *Records of the Zoological Survey of India*, *107*, 33–48.

Mitra, B., (2010). Diversity of flower-visiting flies (Insecta: Diptera) in India and their role in pollination. *Records of the Zoological Survey of India*, pp.95–107.

Morris, H. M. (1922). On the larva and pupa of a parasitic phorid fly: *Hypocera incrassata* Mg. *Parasitology*, *14*(1), 70–74.

Milotic, T., Baltzinger, C., Eichberg, C., Eycott, A. E., Heurich, M., Ádám, R., … & Somay, L. (2018). Dung beetle assemblages, dung removal and secondary seed dispersal: Data from a large-scale, multi-site experiment in the Western Palaearctic. *Frontiers of Biogeography*, *10*(1–2). https://doi.org/10.21425/F5FBG37289

Mitchell, R. G., & Maksymov, J. K. (1977). Observations of predation on spruce gall aphids within the gall. *Entomophaga*, *22*(2), 179–186.

Morozova, T. V., Anholt, R. R., & Mackay, T. F. (2006). Transcriptional response to alcohol exposure in *Drosophila melanogaster*. *Genome Biology*, *7*, 1–10.

Moulton II, S. R., Carter, J. L., Grotheer, S. A., Cuffney, T. F., & Short, T. M. (2000). *Methods of Analysis by the US Geological Survey National Water Quality Laboratory-Processing, Taxonomy, and Quality Control of Benthic Macroinvertebrate Samples* (No. 2000-212). US Geological Survey.

Neff, J. L., Simpson, B. B., Evenhuis, N. L., & Dieringer, G. (2003). Character analysis of adaptations for tarsal pollen collection in the Bombyliidae (Insecta: Diptera): The benefits of putting your foot in your mouth. *Zootaxa*, *157*(1), 1–14.

Newton, G. L., Booram, C. V., Barker, R. W., & Hale, O. M. (1977). Dried *Hermetia illucens* larvae meal as a supplement for swine. *Journal of Animal Science*, *44*(3), 395–400.

Niccoli, A. & Fagnani, F. (1994). Indaginisull-andamentodelleinfestazioni di *Myzus varians* (Davidson) in peschetidella Toscana. *Redia*, *77*, 175–187.

Nichols, E., Spector, S., Louzada, J., Larsen, T., Amezquita, S., Favila, M. E., & Network, T. S. R. (2008). Ecological functions and ecosystem services provided by Scarabaeinae dung beetles. *Biological Conservation*, *141*(6), 1461–1474.

Nijveldt, W. (1969). *Gall Midges of Economic Importance*. Volume VIII. *Miscellaneous*. Crosby Lockwood & Son, London, UK, 221 pp.

Odat, N., Hasan, H. S., Obeidat, M., & Aladaileh, S. (2015). Relationships between species diversity and evenness of necrophagous Diptera and environmental conditions in three habitats of Jordan. *Journal of Entomology and Zoology Studies*, *3*, 89–94.

O'Hara, J. E., Floate, K. D., & Cooper, B. E. (1999). The Sarcophagidae (Diptera) of cattle feedlots in southern Alberta. *Journal of the Kansas Entomological Society*, 167–176.

Økland, B. (1994). Mycetophilidae (Diptera), an insect group vulnerable to forest practices? A comparison of clearcut, managed and seminatural spruce forests in southern Norway. *Biodiversity and Conservation*, *3*, 68–85.

Økland, B. (1996). Unlogged forests: Important sites for preserving the diversity of mycetophilids (Diptera, Sciaroidea). *Biological Conservation*, *76*, 297–310.

Økland, B. (2000). Management effects on the decomposer fauna of Diptera in spruce forests. *Studia Dipterologica*, *7*, 213–223.

Økland, B., Götmark, F., & Nordén, B. (2008). Oak woodland restoration: Testing the effects on biodiversity of mycetophilids in southern Sweden. *Biodiversity and Conservation*, *17*, 2599.

Økland, B., Götmark, F., Nordén, B., Franc, N., Kurina, O., & Polevoi, A. (2004). Regional diversity of mycetophilids (Diptera: Sciaroidea) in Scandinavian oak-dominated forests. *Biological Conservation*, *121*, 9–20.

Pape, T. (2009). Economic importance of Diptera. In B. V. Brown, A. Borkent, J. M. Cumming, D. M. Wood and M. Zumbado (eds.), *Manual of Central American Diptera*. Volume 1. NRC Research Press, Ottawa, Canada, pp. 65–77.

Papp, L. (1976). Ecological and zoogeographical data on flies developing in excrement droppings (Diptera). *Acta zoologica Hungarica*, *22*, 119–138.

Papp, L. (1985). Flies (Diptera) developing in sheep droppings in Hungary. *Acta zoologica Hungarica*, *31*, 367–379.

Papp, L., & Darvas, B. (eds.). (2000). *Contributions to a Manual of Palaearctic Diptera*. Volume 1. *General and Applied Dipterology*. Science Herald, Budapest, Hungary, 36 pp.

Parra, J. R. P. (2002). *Controle biológico no Brasil: Parasitóides e predadores*. Editora Manole Ltda, Sao Paulo, 609 pp.

Pellmyr, O. (1989). The cost of mutualism: Interactions between Trollius europaeus and its pollinating parasites. *Oecologia*, *78*, 53–59.

Prescher, S., & Buchs, W. (1998). Der Einfuabgestufter Extensivierungsmanahmenim Raps- und Erbsenanbau auf ntzlicheFliegen (Diptera, Brachycera). *Gesunde Pflanzen*, *50*, 213–218.
Priti, & Sihag, R. C. (1997). Diversity, visitation frequency, foraging behaviour and pollinating efficiency of insect pollinators visiting cauliflower (*B. oleracea L. var. botrytis* cv. *Hajipur local*) blossoms. *Indian Bee Journal*, 59(4), 230–237.
Priti, & Sihag, R. C. (1998). Diversity, visitation frequency, foraging behaviour and pollinating efficiency of different insect pollinators visiting carrot, *Daucus carotaL.var. Hc-l* blossoms. *Indian Bee Journal,* 59(4), 1–8.
Priti (1998). Abundance and pollination efficiency of insect visitors of onion bloom. *Indian Bee Journal*, 60(2), 75–78.
Resh, V. H., Meyers, M. M., & Hannaford, M. (1996). Use of biotic indices, habitat assessments, and benthic macroinvertebrates in evaluating environmental quality. In *Methods in Stream Ecology.* Academic Press, Orlando, FL, pp. 647–667.
Reiter, L. T., Potocki, L., Chien, S., Gribskov, M., & Bier, E. (2001). A systematic analysis of human disease-associated gene sequences in *Drosophila melanogaster*. *Genome Research*, *11*(6), 1114–1125.
Rojo, S., Pérez-Bañón, C., & Marcos-García, M. A. (1999). First observations on the biology of *Scaeva mecogramma* (Bigot, 1860) (Diptera, Syrphidae) and notes on some other syrphids preying on psyllids (Hemiptera, Aphalaridae and Triozidae). *Volucella*, *4*(1/2), 105–111.
Rosenberg, D. M., & Resh, V. H. (eds.). (1993). *Freshwater Biomonitoring and Benthic Macroinvertebrates*. Chapman and Hall, New York, 488 pp.
Rosenberg, D. M., Resh, V.H., & King, R. S. (2008). Use of aquatic insects in biomonitoring. In R. W. Merritt, K. W. Cummins and M. B. Berg (eds.), *An Introduction to the Aquatic Insects of North America.* 4th edition. Kendall/ Hunt Publishing, Dubuque, Iowa, pp. 123–137.
Rossi, J., Gamba, U., Pinna, M., Spagnolo, S., Visentin, C. & Alma, A. (2006). Hoverflies in organic apple orchards in north-western Italy. *Bulletin of Insectology*, *59*, 111–114.
Rotheray, G. E., Hancock, G., Hewitt, S., Horsfield, D., MacGowan, I., Robertson, D., & Watt, K. (2001). The biodiversity and conservation of saproxylic Diptera in Scotland. *Journal of Insect Conservation*, *5*, 77–85.
Saeed, S., Naqqash, M.N., Jaleel, W., Saeed, Q., & Ghouri, F. (2016). The effect of blow flies (Diptera: Calliphoridae) on the size and weight of mangos (*Mangifera indica* L.). *Peer Journal*, *4*, e2076.
Saether, O. A. (1979). Chironomid communities as water quality indicators. *Ecography*, *2*(2), 65–74.
Sakai, S., Kato, M., & Nagamasu, H. (2000). Artocarpus (Moraceae)–gall midge pollination mutualism mediated by a male-flower parasitic fungus. *American Journal of Botany*, *87*(3), 440–445.
Schneider, F. (1948). BeitragzurKenntnis der Generationsverhltnisse und Diapause rauberischer Schwebfliegen (Syrphidae, Dipt.). *Mitteilungen der Schweizenischen Entomologischen Gesellschaft*, *21*, 249–285.
Schowalter, T. D. (2016). Insect Ecology: *An Ecosystem Approach.* Academic Press, London, p. 774.
Schowalter, T. D., Noriega, J. A., & Tscharntke, T. (2018). Insect effects on ecosystem services: Introduction. *Basic and Applied Ecology*, *26*, 1–7.
Schwenke, W. (1974). Die Forstschädlinge Europas: Band II Käfer. Parey, Hamburg, Berlin, 468p.
Sheppard, D. C., Newton, G. L., Thompson, S. A., & Savage, S. (1994). A value added manure management system using the black soldier fly. *Bioresource Technology*, *50*(3), 275–279.
Sheppard, C. (1983). House fly and lesser fly control utilizing the black soldier fly in manure management systems for caged laying hens. *Environmental Entomology*, *12*(5), 1439–1442.
Skevington, J. H., & Dang, P. T. (2002). Exploring the diversity of flies (Diptera). *Biodiversity*, *3*(4), 3–27.
Skidmore, P. (1991). Insects of the British cowdung community. *Field Studies Council*, *Occasional Publication*, *21*, 1–160.
Sommaggio, D. (1999). Syrphidae: Can they be used as environmental bioindicators? *Agriculture*, *Ecosystems & Environment*, *74*(1–3), 343–356.
Soetavalta, O. (1947). The flight tone (wing stroke frequency) of insects. *Acta Entomologica Fennica*, *4*(1).
Sotavalta, O. (1953). Recordings of high wing-stroke and thoracic vibration frequency in some midges. *The Biological Bulletin*, *104*(3), 439–444.
Speight, M. C. D. (1986, August). Attitudes to insects and insect conservation. In *Proceedings of the 3rd European Congress of Entomology*, Volume 3. Amsterdam, pp. 369–385.
Speight, M. C. D. (2011). Species accounts of European Syrphidae (Diptera). In Glasgow (ed.), *The Database of European Syrphidae*, Volume 65. The Syrph Net Publications, Dublin, Ireland, 285 pp.
Ssymank, A., Kearns, C. A., Pape, T., & Thompson, F. C. (2008). Pollinating flies (Diptera): A major contribution to plant diversity and agricultural production. *Biodiversity*, *9*(1–2), 86–89.

Syme, D. A., & Josephson, R. K. (2002). How to build fast muscles: Synchronous and asynchronous designs. *Integrative and Comparative Biology*, *42*(4), 762–770.

Teskey, H. J. (1976). Diptera larvae associated with trees in North America. *Memoirs of the Entomological Society of Canada*, *100*, 1–53.

Thomson, J. R., Hart, D. D., Charles, D. F., Nightengale, T. L., & Winter, D. M. (2005). Effects of removal of a small dam on downstream macroinvertebrate and algal assemblages in a Pennsylvania stream. *Journal of the North American Benthological Society*, *24*(1), 192–207.

Togni, P. H., Venzon, M., Souza, L. M., Santos, J. P., & Sujii, E. R. (2019). Biodiversity provides whitefly biological control based on farm management. *Journal of Pest Science*, *92*, 393–403.

Toth, P., Tthov, M. & Tancik. J. (2004). First records of *Pemphigus fuscicornis* (Homoptera, Pemphigidae) from Slovakia. *Biologia*, *Bratislava*, *59*, 271–272.

Vigoreaux, J. O. (2001). Genetics of the *Drosophila* flight muscle myofibril: A window into the biology of complex systems. *Bioessays*, *23*(11), 1047–1063.

Waage, J. (1989). Population ecology of pest-pesticide-natural enemy interactions. In P. C. Jepson (ed.), *Pesticides and Non-Target Invertebrates*.

Wall, R., Howard, J. J., & Bindu, J. (2001). The seasonal abundance of blowflies infesting drying fish in south-west India. *Journal of Applied Ecology*, 38, 339–348.

Wiederholm, T. (1984). Incidence of deformed chironomid larvae (Diptera: Chironomidae) in Swedish lakes. *Hydrobiologia*, *109*(3), 243–249.

Wojciechowicz-Zytko, E., & Wnuk, A. (2012). The occurrence of Syrphidae in *Aphis fabae* Scop. (Hemiptera) colonies on broad bean intercropped with *Phacelia* (Part II). *Journal of Plant Protection Research*, *52*(2), 196–201.

Woodcock, T. (2012). *Pollination in the Agricultural Landscape: Best Management Practices for Crop Pollination*. Volume 113. NSERC-CANPOLIN, University of Guelph, Guelph, ON, Canada.

Wood, G. C. (1981). Asilidae. In J. F. McAlpine, G. E. Peterson and B. V. Shewell (eds.), *Manual of Nearctic Diptera*. Volume 1. Monograph No. 27. Research Branch Agriculture Canada, Ottawa Canada, pp. 549–573.

Yoder, C. O., & Rankin, E. T. (1998). The role of biological indicators in a state water quality management process. *Environmental Monitoring and Assessment*, *51*, 61–88.

Yang, L. H., & Gratton, C. (2014). Insects as drivers of ecosystem processes. *Current Opinion in Insect Science*, *2*, 26–32.

Young, A. M. (1986). Habitat differences in cocoa tree flowering, fruit-set, and pollinator availability in Costa Rica. *Journal of Tropical Ecology*, *2*(2), 163–186.

Young, A. M. (1994). *The Chocolate Tree: A Natural History of Cacao*. Washington, Smithsonian Institution Press, 200 pp.

5 Hoverflies in Agriculture

H. S. Venu, U. Amala, and T. M. Shivalingaswamy

LEARNING OBJECTIVES

1. Agriculturally important species of syrphids.
2. Life cycle and common rearing techniques of some common species of hoverflies.

5.1 INTRODUCTION

Syrphid flies, belonging to the family Syrphidae, are an economically important group of insects that contribute to both biological control of aphids and crop pollination. They are commonly encountered predators in any crop ecosystem with aphid infestations. Adults are frequently referred to as flower flies or hoverflies, as they constantly hover around flowers to collect nectar and pollen for their survival and mating. They exhibit distinct hovering behaviour around flowers and often mimic bees and wasps due to their morphological similarity. The agricultural significance of three different species of syrphids, namely, the drone fly *Eristalis tenax*, the yellow-shouldered hoverfly *Ischiodon scutellaris*, and the marmalade fly *Episyrphus balteatus*, is provided.

5.2 DRONE FLY, *ERISTALIS TENAX* (LINNAEUS, 1758)

Eristalis tenax (Linnaeus), commonly referred to as the drone fly or rat-tailed maggot, is migratory in habit, cosmopolitan in distribution (Skevington et al., 2019), and resembles as a mimic of the European honey bee *Apis mellifera* Linnaeus (Golding et al., 2001).

5.2.1 Taxonomic Classification

Kingdom: Animalia
Phylum: Arthropoda
Class: Insecta
Subclass: Pterygota
Order: Diptera
Family: Syrphidae
Genus: *Eristalis*
Species: *tenax*

5.2.2 Distribution

E. tenax is a cosmopolitan species widely distributed in the highest latitudes to the north (Metcalf, 1913), extreme southern latitudes, and in arid areas of Europe, Asia, and Africa.

5.2.3 Habitat

The immature stages of *E. tenax*, commonly referred to as the "rat-tailed maggot", are found in the aquatic habitats of heavily polluted manure, drainage ditches around dairy farms, and in the waste

DOI: 10.1201/9781003482581-7

lagoons of dairy, swine, and poultry farms. The adult fly feeds on pollen and nectar in different crop ecosystems and can be found throughout the year.

5.2.4 Life Cycle of *Eristalis tenax*

Egg: The egg appears white in colour, elongate in shape, and is covered with a sticky substance deposited in a sideward orientation perpendicular to the surface of the polluted substrate (Milne and Milne, 1980). The incubation period of the eggs is 2–3 days (Basley et al., 2018).

Larvae: The larvae of *E. tenax*, commonly referred to as "rat-tailed maggots", are aquatic in habit, requiring solid food to complete their development; hence, they prefer to live in water with high levels of organic matter (Day, 2008). The larva has a cylindrical shape with patches of horizontal folds that divide the body into segments. Two rows of flexible hairs occur in each segment. The larvae possess an elongated siphon on the posterior end that resembles a tail, which aids in respiration. The larva exhibits neoteny or paedogenesis, wherein each larva reproduces by copying itself, resulting in 7 to 30 daughter larvae (Ibrahim and Gad, 1978). The larval period ranges between 13 and 24 days depending upon the diet (Kamdem and Otomo, 2023).

Pupae: The mature larva moves towards the drier substratum for pupation. Pupation mostly occurs below the soil surface for a period of 8–10 days (Gilbert, 1986; Milne and Milne, 1980). The pupae appear grey-brown in colour with a pair of horn-like anterior spiracles and a caudal projection (Metcalf, 1913).

Adult: Adult flies feed on pollen and nectar upon emergence to obtain the necessary nutrients to complete reproduction and to gain energy for activity (Gilbert, 1986). They are reported to exhibit a forage preference for yellow-coloured flowers (Ilse, 1949). Male flies are reported to show territorial behaviour as they inhabit the same territory where they mate, feed, and groom, defending the area against other insects (Wellington and Fitzpatrick, 1981).

5.2.5 Sexual Dimorphism in *E. tenax*

Sexual dimorphism is well established in *E. tenax*, where male flies have lighter colour patterns than females (Heal, 1982). Male flies possess larger eyes that almost touch each other, whereas female flies have smaller eyes that are well spaced apart (Metcalf, 1913).

5.2.6 Overwintering in Adults

Adult flies are reported to be active during the months from late March to early December (Gilbert, 1986). During the late autumn months, adult females mate and seek a secure place for hibernation. The eggs remain in an underdeveloped condition within the female flies until spring; after the overwintering phase, the ovaries of the female flies become activated, and the oviposition cycle begins (Kendall and Stradling, 1972).

5.2.7 Laboratory Rearing and Long-Term Maintenance of *Eristalis tenax*

Nicholas et al. (2018) reported on the laboratory rearing and long-term culture maintenance techniques for the drone fly, *E. tenax*.

5.2.7.1 Rearing Steps

1. **Collection of mature larvae**: Second or third instar larvae can be collected from cattle farms.
2. The collected larvae can be released into containers with organically polluted water and semi-solid dung for feeding and survival.

3. Wood shavings can be added up to the height of the rim of the container to enable the mature larvae to crawl into the shavings and pupate.
4. The mature larvae and pupae in the container can be covered with a double-layered mosquito net to prevent the escape of emerging adult flies.
5. They should be kept at room temperature (21.5°C ± 2.5°C) with a light:dark cycle of 12-hour light and 12-hour darkness. Exposure of the larvae to 24 hours of light affects their rate of survival.
6. The duration of pupation may vary between 1 and 20 days, depending upon the maturity of the larvae at the time of collection.
7. Adult flies can be provided with bee pollen and honey feeding in cotton balls inside the enclosure cages. The feeding can be replaced every 2–3 days.

5.2.8 Housing and Long-Term Maintenance of *E. tenax*

1. Adult flies of *E. tenax* can be maintained in 30 cm × 45 cm plastic bags for smaller populations or in insect rearing cages (25 cm × 25 cm × 25 cm) for larger groups.
2. *Ad libitum* feeding of 10–20 grains of bee pollen and 2–3 mL of honey in cotton balls is required for the maintenance of adult flies.
3. The health and longevity of adult flies can be maintained by keeping them in a refrigerator at 8°C–10°C in complete darkness, removing them after 3–4 days, and allowing them to feed and groom at room temperature for 6 hours. The active flies are then again placed in the refrigerator at 8°C–10°C in complete darkness, and returned to normal temperature after 3–4 days. This is done to ensure the health and longevity of hoverflies during captivity.

5.2.9 Economic Importance of *E. tenax*

The larvae of *E. tenax* occasionally cause nuisance in livestock areas, where they are more abundant in manure lagoons and holding pits (Kaufman et al., 2000). Larvae migrate from feeding sites for pupation during the summer in massive numbers (Day, 2008). This massive migration causes nuisance and contamination in the livestock feed. Drone flies are reported to cause accidental myiasis when the larvae inadvertently inhabit a living host through the ingestion of contaminated food (Lakshminarayana et al., 1975; Aguilera et al., 1999). In humans, myiasis predominantly invades via intestinal or gastric, nasal, auricular, and anal routes, with intestinal or gastric being the most common (Rogers and Walker 1916; Herms, 1969).

Eristalis tenax is reported to be an effective pollinator for Pak choi (*Brassica rapa* spp. *chinensis*), kiwi fruit (*Actinidia deliciosa*), onion (*Allium cepa*) (Howlett and Gee, 2019), greenhouse sweetpepper (Arnaud et al., 1997), greenhouse tomato (Fernandez et al., 2021), and mango (Kusuma and Windriyanti, 2022).

5.2.10 Storage and Transportation of *Eristalis* sp.

Mass culture of syrphid flies is a challenging task as it demands year-round availability of host aphids. The storage and shipment of hoverflies present another major challenge that hinders the widespread utilisation of syrphid flies in pollination and biological control of aphids. Commercially available species of syrphid flies, such as drone flies, are well adapted to temperate and cool conditions. Drone flies exhibit strong foraging behaviour with rapid flying capacity and resistance to high temperatures (>36°C); thus, they facilitate cross-pollination that helps in the seed production of vegetables, oilseed crops, and ornamental crops. Drone flies are mass cultured and commercialized under the name of polyfly, with products like goldfly (*E. aeneus*) and queenfly (*E. tenax*) available in western countries for pollination services in crops grown under protected cultivation.

5.2.11 Procedure for Handling and Usage of *E. tenax*

1. Newly formed, 1-day-old pupae are stored in a refrigerator (>8°C), for a maximum of 1 week.
2. After 1 week, the pupae are shipped to the prescribed location, followed by the emergence of adult flies in 2–4 days. Acclimatization of pupae is required in cases of extreme temperatures.
3. The adult release recommendation is based on the number of individuals/m^2 in the crop ecosystem.
4. The first release of adult flies is done during the flowering period, followed by subsequent releases every 2 weeks after the initial release made during the flowering period.

5.3 Yellow-Shouldered Hoverfly, *Ischiodon scutellaris* (Fabricius, 1805)

The yellow-shouldered hoverfly, *Ischiodon scutellaris*, belongs to the family Syrphidae, and adult flies are reported to pollinate several crops, like *Coriandrum sativum*, *Cirsium arvense*, *Launaea procumbens*, *Prosopis juliflora*, *Allium cepa*, *Ranunculus muricatus* and *Daucus carota* (Sajjad and Saeed, 2010). The larvae of *I. scutellaris* are efficient predators of several species of aphids and are known as effective biological control agents for aphids.

5.3.1 Taxonomic Classification

Kingdom: Animalia
Phylum: Arthropoda
Class: Insecta
Subclass: Pterygota
Order: Diptera
Family: Syrphidae
Genus: *Ischiodon*
Species: *scutellaris*

5.3.2 Distribution

The species *I. scutellaris* is found in the Caucasus, Greece, Iran, Japan, Kazakhstan, and the Arabian Peninsula, extending south to the Indomalayan, Australasian, and Oriental regions (Mengual, 2018).

5.3.3 Hosts

The larvae of *I. scutellaris* are reported to feed on several species of aphids, namely, *Aphis craccivora* (Joshi et al., 1999), *Hyperomyzus carduellinus* (Amala et al., 2023b), *Brevicoryne brassicae* (Sharma and Bhalla, 1988), *Aphis gossypii*, *Myzus persicae* (Sharanabasappa et al., 2007), *Hyadaphis coriandri* (Amala et al., 2023a), and *Raphalosipum maidis* (Ghorpade, 1981).

5.3.4 Life Cycle of *I. scutellaris*

I. scutellaris is a holometabolous insect with four life stages: egg, larva, pupa, and adult.

Egg: The egg appears oblong-oval in shape, chalky white in colour with longitudinal ornamentations on the surface and blunt ends. It measures about 0.76–0.81 mm in length and 0.27–0.31 mm in width (Kumar et al., 1987). The adult female fly oviposits near prey aphid colonies to ensure prey availability for the larvae upon hatching. The incubation period of the eggs ranges between 3 and 4 days (Alfiler and Calilung, 1978).

Larvae: The larvae are voracious predators of aphids, with three instars and an increasing rate of predation trend towards the higher instars. The duration of the larval stage lasts for 5–7 days. The larvae appear greenish-brown in colour, with a median white line on the dorsal surface that runs along the entire body length, and brown spots flanking the median white line on the lateral sides. Mature larvae measure 9.6–10.8 mm in length and 2.2–2.3 mm in width (Kumar et al., 1987).

Pupae: Pupae of *I. scutellaris* are immobile and dark greenish in colour during the initial stages of pupation, attaining a brown colour nearing hatching. Mature pupae, approaching hatching, appear transparent, with abdominal bands resembling miniature adult flies enclosed in a puparium. The pupae measure 5.8–6.8 mm in length and 2.0–2.5 mm in width, with a total duration of 4–12 days.

Adults: Adult flies are slender, black in colour with yellow bands on the abdomen and distinct antennae. They actively hover around flowers foraging for pollen and nectar in the flower heads. The longevity of the adult flies varies by sex, with males living for 7–8 days and females for 11–22 days (Alfiler et al., 1978). Pollen feeding by female flies is a prerequisite for the maturation of the ovaries and fecundity (Iler et al., 2013). Adult flies are reported to exhibit Batesian mimicry.

5.3.5 Mass Culturing of *Ischiodon scutellaris*

5.3.5.1 Materials Needed

Eggs or Larvae: The eggs or larvae of *I. scutellaris* can be collected from plants infested with aphids.

Containers: Use small, well-ventilated containers for rearing. Plastic or glass containers with mesh lids work well. The containers should have enough space for larvae to move around the pupate.

Food: The larvae of syrphids feed on aphids. A steady supply of aphid culture is a prerequisite for rearing the aphids. Different species of aphids, such as the cowpea aphid (*Aphis craccivora*), fennel aphid, and maize aphid, can be cultured on their respective host plants to ensure a constant supply of aphids.

5.3.5.2 Oviposition Source for *I. scutellaris*

Host plants infested with aphids serve as an oviposition site for syrphid flies. Pollen pellets, honey, and yeast increase the fecundity of the flies. Cowpea seedlings infested with the aphid *Aphis craccivora* are the most suitable for successful oviposition and culture maintenance of adult flies of *Ischiodon scutellaris.*

5.3.6 Rearing of *Ischiodon scutellaris*

Collect or obtain eggs/larvae: Collect syrphid fly eggs or larvae from natural aphid-infested plants or from commercial suppliers. Mated adult female flies can be collected using sweep nets and caged with aphid-infested host plants for further oviposition.

Collect and introduce larvae: The larvae, after hatching from eggs, can be gently collected using a fine brush and introduced into rearing containers fitted with mesh, along with aphid-infested shoots for feeding.

Provide food: Successful establishment of syrphid culture depends upon a constant supply of fresh aphids. Unconsumed aphids, if any, can be removed, and containers should be cleaned at regular intervals to prevent mould and bacterial growth.

Pupation and emergence of adult flies: Mature larvae metamorphose into puparium inside the rearing container. From the pupae, adult flies emerge.

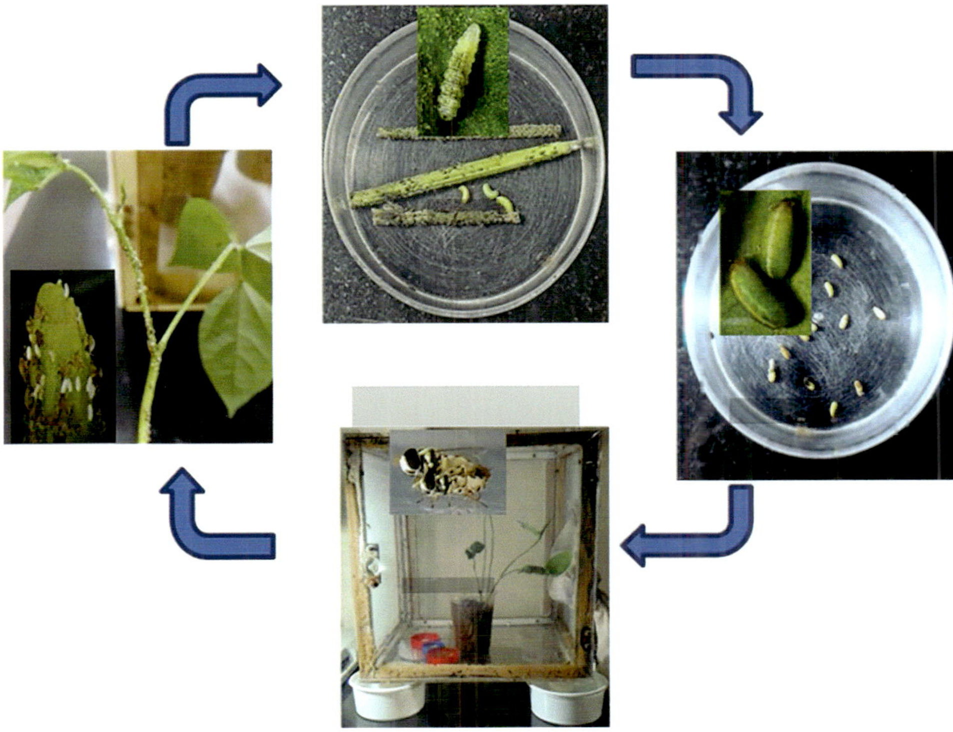

FIGURE 5.1 Rearing of life stages of *I. scutellaris*.

Release or use of adult syrphid flies: Adult flies can be released in the crop ecosystem for pollination, and larvae can be released on aphid-infested plants for predation and suppression of the aphid population. A flow chart for the laboratory rearing of *I. scutellaris* is depicted in Figure 5.1.

5.4 MARMALADE HOVERFLY, *EPISYRPHUS BALTEATUS* (DE GEER, 1776)

Episyrphus balteatus, commonly referred to as the Marmalade fly, is small in size, ranging from 9 to 12 mm, and is commonly observed hovering around flowers in gardens, parks, and sunny woodlands throughout the year. The larvae of *E. balteatus* are nocturnal predators of aphids and are widely used for the biological control of aphids on commercial crops.

5.4.1 Host

E. balteatus is a common hoverfly whose larvae feed on different species of aphids. Various species of aphid hosts, including *Aphis grossulariae* on willow-herb, *Cavariella* sp. on hogweed, *Macrosiphum rosae* on rose, *Brevicoryne brassicae* on cabbage (Mayadunnage et al., 2009), *A. fabae* on thistle, *Rhopalosiphum padi* on bird cherry (Sadeghi et al., 2014), *Hyadaphis coriandri* (Amala et al., 2023a), the green peach aphid, *Myzus persicae*, and the wheat aphid, *Schizaphis graminum* (Mushtaq et al., 2014), have been reported as larval feeding hosts of *E. balteatus*.

5.4.2 Taxonomic Classification

Kingdom: Animalia
Phylum: Arthropoda
Class: Insecta

Subclass: Pterygota
Order: Diptera
Family: Syrphidae
Genus: *Episyrphus*
Species: *balteatus*

5.4.3 Distribution

Episyrphus balteatus is found in the Palearctic region, which includes Europe, North Asia, and North Africa. This species is also widely distributed in the Oriental and Australasian regions but is not found in the Nearctic region.

5.4.4 Biology of Marmalade Hoverfly

E. balteatus is a holometabolous insect with four life stages: egg, larvae, pupae, and adult.

Egg: The egg appears pale white in colour, oval in shape, measuring 3.5 mm in length, and turns greyish in colour before hatching (Jalilian, 2015). The incubation period of the egg ranges between 2 and 3 days (Kumari, 2020).

Larvae: Larvae are the active feeding stage of *E. balteatus* that voraciously feed on aphids. Larvae pass through three instars and appear transparent with clearly visible black viscera throughout their bodies. The larval period lasts for 7–8 days during summer and 13–14 days during winter (Kumari, 2020; Singh et al., 2020). The mature third instar larva is transparent and pupates within a protective puparium.

Pupae: Pupae appear whitish to grey in colour, broad and rounded anteriorly, and narrow at the posterior end. The pupal period lasts for 8–9 days during the summer and 13–18 days during the winter.

Adults: Adult flies are active fliers, hovering around the flowers in search of nectar and pollen. The dorsal surface of the abdomen exhibits orange to yellow and black banded patterns with two or more identification characters: the presence of secondary black bands on the third and fourth dorsal plates, and the presence of faint greyish longitudinal stripes on the thorax (Jalilian, 2015). Sexual dimorphism is clear in *E. balteatus*, with males having holoptic compound eyes and females having dichoptic compound eyes. Adult female flies prefer to oviposit in heavily infested aphid colonies (Scholz and Poehling, 2003). Adults of *E. balteatus* pollinate fennel (presented in Figure 5.2).

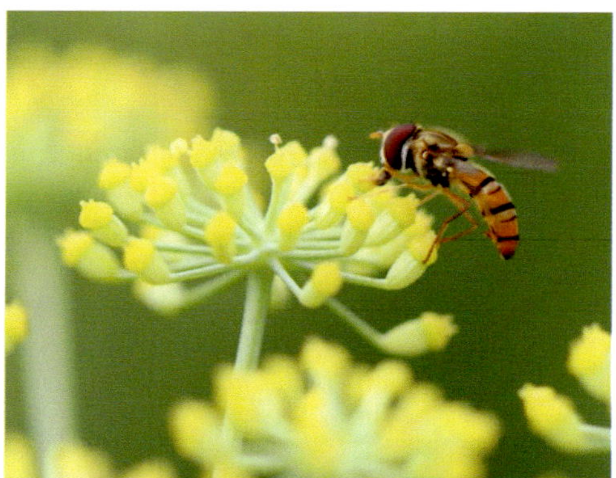

FIGURE 5.2 Adult of *E. balteatus* in fennel.

5.4.5 Rearing of *E. balteatus*

The rearing methodology and culture establishment of *E. balteatus* is reported by Moens (2011).

5.4.5.1 Steps Involved in the Culture of *E. balteatus*

1. Collect mature larvae or pupae of *E. balteatus* from the fields.
2. Release the emerged adults into insect rearing cages with fine nylon mesh around the sides and an opening at the front. Maintain the rearing cages at room temperature (23°C–25°C) and 70%–80% RH, with a 16-hour light and 8-hour dark photoperiod.
3. Provide bee-collected pollen and honey water (20%) soaked in cotton wool for adult feeding and replace the feed every 3 weeks to avoid fungal contamination.
4. Place 10–15 cm high broad bean plants (*Vicia faba*) infested with pea aphids (*Acyrthosiphon pisum*) inside the cages as oviposition sites for the syrphids.
5. Release 8- to 10-day-old adults into the cages and observe for mating and oviposition by the adult flies.
6. After oviposition, the plants containing syrphid eggs can be transferred to rearing containers and observed for hatching.
7. After hatching, *ad libitum* feeding of aphids can be provided to the newly hatched larvae. The larvae complete their development in 6–7 days, voraciously feeding on aphids, and the mature larvae turn into pupae, continuing the lifecycle.

Artificial diet for *E. balteatus*: Hideki et al. (2007) developed an artificial larval diet with powder from bee drone pupae as the main ingredient, autolysed brewer's yeast as an additive, and 5% sucrose as a phagostimulant. They reported a significant reduction in the survival rate (50%), a longer developmental period (12 days), and a smaller body length (9.5 mm) of *E. balteatus* compared to those replicates that were fed on aphids (81.80% survival; 12 mm length and 7.5 days developmental time).

5.5 CONCLUSION

Hoverflies are economically important insects. Most of them employ a "one stone, two birds" strategy, providing biotic benefits by pollinating crops as well as preying on phytophagous aphids in the fields. Laboratory rearing of economically important species, like *I. scutellaris*, *E. tenax*, and *E. balteatus* can be successfully achieved. Preparation of artificial diets, year-round storage, supply, and successful field utilization of hoverflies should be pursued.

5.6 POINTS TO REMEMBER

1. Syrphid flies have immense potential for utilization, as they provide the dual advantage of larvae as predators of aphids and adults as pollinators.
2. Maintenance of host aphids is a prerequisite for the successful establishment of syrphid cultures.

REFERENCES

Aguilera, A., Cid, A., Regueiro, B.J., Prieto, J. M., & Noya, M. (1999). Intestinal myiasis caused by *Eristalis tenax*. *Journal of Clinical Microbiology*, 37: 3082.

Alfiler, A. R. R., & Calilung, V. J. (1978). The life history and voracity of the Syrphid predator, *Ischiodon scutellaris* (F.) (Diptera: Syrphidae). *Philippine Entomologist*, 4(1/2): 105–117.

Amala, U., Chandramanu, K. G. R., Joshi, S., & Shivalingaswamy, T. M. (2023a). Studies to identify an alternative aphid host for culturing the predatory syrphid, *Ischiodon scutellaris* (Fabricius) (Diptera: Syrphidae). *Egyptian Journal Biological Pest Control*, 33: 39. https://doi.org/10.1186/s41938-023-00687-y

Amala, U., Chandramanu, K. G. R., Sunil, J., & Shivalingaswamy, T. M. (2023b). Fennel, *Foeniculum vulgare* as banker crop for syrphids to promote aphidophagy and myophily. *Current Science*, 124: 1469–1472.

Arnaud, J., Domingos, D. O., & Jean, G. (1997). Pollination by *Eristalis tenax* (Diptera: Syrphidae) and seed set of greenhouse Sweet Pepper, *Journal of Economic Entomology*, 90 (6): 1646–1649.

Basley, K., Davenport, B., Vogiatzis, K., & Goulson, D. (2018). Effects of chronic exposure to thiamethoxam on larvae of the hoverfly *Eristalis tenax* (Diptera, Syrphidae). *Peer Journal*, 6: e4258.

Day, E. R. (2008). Livestock area fly control. *Virginia Tech Extension*. https://ext.vt.edu/pubs/pmg/fc/LivestockAreaFlyControl.pdf.

Fernandez, F. J., Garay, J., Mori, T. F., Csiszar, V., Varga, Z., Lopez, I., Gamez, M., &Cabello, T. (2021). Theoretical foundation of the control of pollination by hoverflies in a greenhouse. *Agronomy*, 11: 167. https://doi.org/10.3390/agronomy11010167

Ghoepade, K. D. (1981). Insect prey of syrphidae (Diptera) from India and neighbouring countries: A review and bibliography. *Tropical Pest Management*, 27: 62–82.

Gilbert, F. S. (1986). *Hoverflies*. Cambridge University Press, Cambridge, England.

Golding, Y. C., Ennos, A. R., & Edmunds, M. (2001). Similarity in flight behaviour between the honeybee *Apis mellifera* (Hymenoptera: Apidae) and its presumed mimic, the dronefly *Eristalis tenax* (Diptera: Syrphidae). *The Journal of Experimental Biology*, 204: 139–145.

Heal, J. R. (1982). Colour patterns of Syrphidae: IV. Mimicry and variation in natural populations of *Eristalis tenax*. *Heredity*, 49(1): 95–109.

Herms, W. M. (1969). *Herms's Medical Entomology*, 6th ed. James, M. T., & Harwood, R. F. (eds.), The Macmillan Company, London, England.

Hideki, I., Keiko, N., & Mitsuo, M. (2007). An artificial diet for aphidophagous syrphids, *Episyrphus balteatus* (de Geer) and *Eupeodes bucculatus* (Rondani) (Diptera: Syrphidae) using drone honeybee brood powder, *Applied Entomology and Zoology*, 42(2): 167–172. https://doi.org/10.1303/aez.2007.167

Howlett, B., & Megan, G. (2019). The Potential Management of the Drone Fly (*Eristalis tenax*) As a Crop Pollinator in New Zealand. *New Zealand Plant Protection*, 72: 221–230.

Ibrahim, I. A., & Gad, A. M. (1978). The occurrence of paedogenesis in *Eristalis* larvae (Diptera, Syrphidae). *Journal of Medical Entomology*, 12: 268.

Iler, A. M., Inouye, D. W., Hoye, T. T., Miller-Rushing, A. J., Burkle, L. A., & Johnston, E. B. (2013). Maintenance of temporal synchrony between syrphid flies and floral resources despite differential phonological responses to climate. *Global Change Biology*, 19(8): 2348–2359.

Jalilian, F. (2015). Biology and larval feeding rate of *Episyrphus balteatus* (Dip.: Syrphidae) on *Aphis pomi* (Hom.: Aphididae) at laboratory conditions. *Biological Forum*, 7(1): 1395–1399.

Joshi, S., Ballal, C. R., Rao, N. S. (1999). Evaluation of biotic potential of syrphid predators *Ischiodon scutellaris* (Fabricius) and *Paragus serratus* (Fabricius) (Diptera: Syrphidae). *Journal of Aphid* 13: 9–16.

Kamdem, M. M. & Otomo, P. V. (2023). Developmental performance of *Eristalis tenax* larvae (Diptera: Syrphidae): Influence of growth media and yeast addition during captive rearing. *Journal of Experimental Zoology Part A: Ecological and Integrative Physiology*, 339: 503–513. https://doi.org/10.1002/jez.2696

Kaufman, P. E., Rutz, D. A., & Waldron, J. K. (2000). Common pest flies found in the urban/rural environment and their biological control agents. *IPM Fact Sheet* 1021PMFS1. Cornell Cooperative Extension.

Kendall, D. A., & Stradling, D. J. (1972). Some observations on the overwintering of the dronefly, *Eristalis tenax* (L.) (Syrphidae). *Entomologist*, 105: 229–230.

Kumar, A., Kapoor, V. C., & Laska, P. (1987). Immature stages of some aphidophagous syrphid flies of India (Insecta, Diptera, Syrphidae). *Zoologica Scripta*, 16(1): 83–88.

Kumari, M. (2020). Biology and feeding potential *Episyrphus balteatus* De Geer (Diptera: Syrphidae) on green apple aphid *Aphis pomi* De Geer (order Hemiptera: Aphididae) in Hills of Shimla (HP), India. *Environment Conservation Journal*, 21(1&2): 147–150.

Kusuma, R. M., & Windriyanti, W. (2022). Effective behavior of insects pollinators of flowers in Gadung Mango Clone 21 Variety. *Jurnal Ilmu Pertanian Indonesia*, 27(4): 596–605.

Mayadunnage, S., Wijayagunasekera, H. N. P., Hemachandra, K. S., & Nugaliyadda, I. (2009). Occurrence of aphidophagous syrphids in aphid colonies on cabbage (*Brassica oleracea*) and their parasitoids. *Tropical Agricultural Research*, 21(1): 99–109.

Mengual, X. (2018). A new species of *Ischiodon Sack* (Diptera, Syrphidae) from Madagascar. *African Invertebrates*, 59(1): 55–73.

Metcalf, C. L. (1913). The Syrphidae of Ohio. *Ohio State University Bulletin* 17: 1–123.

Milne, L., & Milne, M. (1980). *The Audubon Society Field Guide to North American Insects and Spiders*. Alfred A. Knopf, Inc., New York, NY.

Moens, J., De Clercq, P., &Tirry, L. (2011). Side effects of pesticides on the larvae of the hoverfly *Episyrphus balteatus* in the laboratory. *Phytoparasitica*, 39: 1–9.https://doi.org/10.1007/s12600-010-0127-3

Mushtaq, S., Akhtar, S., Rana, R. N., Maalik, S., & Ehsan, N. (2014). Developmental duration and predatory efficiency of *Episyrphus balteatus* on four aphid species in Pakistan. *International Journal of Agriculture and Biology*, 16(3): 614–618.

Nicholas, S., Thyselius, M., Holden, M., & Nordström, K. (2018). Rearing and long-term maintenance of *Eristalis tenax* hoverflies for research studies. *Journal of Visualized Experiments*: 135: 57711. https://doi.org/10.3791/57711

Rogers, J. S., & Walker, F. W. (1916). Syrphidae of maine. *Maine Experimental State Bulletin*, 253.

Sadeghi, H., Rotheray, G., Laska, P., & Gilbert, F. (2014). Host preferences of aphidophagous hoverflies from field distribution of their larvae. *Egyptian Journal of Biology*, 16: 1–16.

Sajjad, A., & Saeed, S. (2010). Floral host plant range of syrphid flies (Syrphidae: Diptera) under natural conditions in southern Punjab, Pakistan. *Pakistan Journal of Botany*, 42(2): 1187–1200.

Scholz, D., & Poehling, H. M. (2003). Oviposition site selection of *Episyrphus balteatus*. *Entomologia Experimentalis et Applicata*, 94: 149–158. 10.1046/j.1570-7458.2000.00615.x.

Sharanabasappa, D., Kulkarni, K, A., Mallapur, C. P., Gundannavar, K. P., & Kambrekar, D. K. (2007). Feeding potential of *Ischiodon scutellaris* (Fabricius) (Diptera: Syrphidae) on green peach aphid, *Myzus persicae* (Sultzer) (Homoptera: Aphididae). *Journal of Biological Control*, 21: 177–178.

Sharma, K. C., & Bhalla, O. P. (1988). Biology of six syrphid predators of cabbage aphid (*Brevicoryne brassicae*) on Caulifower (*Brassica oleracea* var. *botrytis*). *Indian Journal of Agricultural Sciences*, 58: 652–654.

Singh, P., Thakur, M., Sharma, K. C., Sharma, H. K., & Nayak, R. K. (2020). Larval feeding capacity and pollination efficiency of the aphidophagous syrphids, *Eupeodes frequens* (Matsmura) and *Episyrphus balteatus* (De Geer) (Diptera: Syrphidae) on the cabbage aphid (*Brevicoryne brassicae* L.) (Homoptera: Aphididae) on mustard crop. *Egyptian Journal of Biological Pest Control*, 30: 105. https://doi.org/10.1186/s41938-020-00300-6

Skevington, J. H., Locke, M. M., Young, A. D., Moran, K., Crins, W. J., & Marshall, S. A. (2019). *Field Guide to the Flower Flies of Northeastern North America*. Princeton University Press: Princeton, p. 512.

Wellington, W. G., & Fitzpatrick, S. M. (1981). Territoriality in the dronefly. *Eristalis tenax* (L.) (Syrphidae). *Canadian Entomologist* 113: 695–704.

6 Parasitic Flies

Meena Agnihotri, Rajnni Dogra, Radha Joshi, and Hassan Beg

LEARNING OBJECTIVES

1. To assess the potential of dipteran fly families as biological control agents against various pests, including their role in natural pest suppression and the benefits they offer in integrated pest management (IPM) systems.
2. To identify and list the host species targeted by these flies, providing insights into their specificity and the breadth of their impact on pest populations.
3. To explore the ecological roles of these fly families beyond pest control, including their contributions to nutrient cycling, decomposition, and maintaining ecosystem balance.
4. To highlight the importance of conserving these fly families due to their ecological and economic significance, and to promote biodiversity through sustainable pest management practices.
5. To identify gaps in current research on these families and propose areas for future study to enhance our understanding of their biology, ecology, and practical applications in pest management.

6.1 INTRODUCTION

In the order Diptera, there are approximately 16,000 described species of parasitoids, constituting around 20% of the species known to exhibit this particular lifestyle. The taxonomic distribution and evolutionary origins of the parasitoid lifestyle have been comprehensively examined by Eggleton and Belshaw (1992), who identified that parasitoids belong to 21 families of Diptera. The largest of these is the Tachinidae (some 9,200 species), followed by the Bombyliidae (some 4,500 species), along with the Pipunculidae and the Conopidae, which include parasitoidal genera such as *Stylogaster*. According to their hypothesis, this parasitic lifestyle has independently evolved more than 100 times within the order Diptera. The majority of dipteran parasitoids are believed to have descended from saprophagous predecessors, with both ancestors and hosts typically occupying habitats in close proximity to or within the soil surface (Feener Jr. and Brown, 1997). Dipteran parasitoids, including families such as Bombyliidae, Conopidae, Pipunculidae, and Tachinidae, play crucial roles in ecological and agricultural systems worldwide. These diverse families exhibit unique adaptations and strategies as parasitic insects, contributing significantly to the regulation of insect populations. Bombyliidae, commonly known as bee flies, are characterized by their robust bodies and hairy appearance, with larvae often parasitizing various stages of other insects, including beetles and solitary bees (Evenhuis, 1994). Conopidae, or thick-headed flies, are known for their parasitic larvae that develop within bees, wasps, and other Hymenoptera, impacting host populations through their specialized parasitism (Neff and Simpson, 1995). Pipunculidae, or big-headed flies, lay their eggs on or near Hemipteran hosts, such as leafhoppers and planthoppers, with larvae consuming the host from within, affecting pest populations in agricultural settings (Skevington and Marshall, 1998). Tachinidae, a large family of parasitoid flies, are highly diverse in their host range and life cycle strategies, often parasitizing caterpillars and other Lepidoptera, contributing significantly to natural pest control (Stireman et al., 2006). The life cycles of these dipteran parasitoids typically

DOI: 10.1201/9781003482581-8

involve complex interactions with their hosts. Bombyliidae larvae develop as internal parasites within hosts, such as the larvae of other insects or even within the pupae of bees, feeding on their host's tissues until they complete development (Evenhuis, 1994). Conopidae larvae are endoparasitic, with females depositing eggs on the body of the host insect, where the larvae then burrow into the host's body cavity, ultimately causing the host's death (Neff and Simpson, 1995). Pipunculidae follow a similar pattern, with females depositing eggs near or on their hemipteran hosts, leading to larvae that consume the host internally, impacting pest populations in both natural and agricultural environments (Skevington and Marshall, 1998). Tachinidae larvae also exhibit endoparasitic development, often targeting a wide range of insect hosts, where they consume the host's internal tissues before emerging to pupate (Stireman et al., 2006). Host specificity varies among these families, with Bombyliidae and Conopidae often displaying broader ranges, parasitizing various insects within their respective habitats. Pipunculidae are specialized in targeting specific Hemipteran hosts, primarily leafhoppers and planthoppers, which are significant agricultural pests due to their role in transmitting plant diseases (Skevington and Marshall, 1998). Tachinidae, with their extensive diversity, parasitize a wide array of insect hosts, including caterpillars, beetles, and true bugs, making them versatile agents in biological control programmes (Stireman et al., 2006). The biocontrol efficacy of these dipteran parasitoids is notable in both natural and managed ecosystems. Bombyliidae and Conopidae contribute to natural pest control by reducing populations of insect hosts, thereby influencing ecological balances within their habitats (Evenhuis, 1994; Neff and Simpson, 1995). Pipunculidae are recognized for their potential in IPM, particularly in agriculture, where they help mitigate populations of hemipteran pests, like leafhoppers and planthoppers, thus reducing crop damage and the spread of plant diseases (Skevington and Marshall, 1998). Tachinidae are extensively studied and utilized in biological control due to their effectiveness in targeting pest species across various agricultural and ecological contexts, contributing to sustainable pest management practices (Stireman et al., 2006). In summary, dipteran parasitoids belonging to families such as Bombyliidae, Conopidae, Pipunculidae, and Tachinidae represent diverse and ecologically significant groups of insects with unique life cycle adaptations and host interactions. Their roles in regulating insect populations, both as natural enemies and in integrated pest management strategies, underscore their importance in ecological studies and agricultural practices. Understanding their biology, life cycles, host interactions, and biocontrol efficacy is essential for harnessing their potential in sustainable pest management and conservation efforts globally.

6.2 FAMILY BOMBYLIIDAE

6.2.1 Introduction

The Bombyliidae, commonly known as bee flies, represent a highly diverse family encompassing species that exhibit parasitoid or predatory behaviour during their larval stage, while transitioning to a nectar-feeding diet as adults. Adults (excluding the few genera with non-functional mouthparts, like *Oestranthrax*) primarily consume nectar, while females rely on pollen intake from anthophilous plants as an essential component for egg development. Due to their pollen and nectar feeding habits, bombyliids frequently serve as significant pollinators for numerous flowering plants, particularly those found in arid regions of the Earth (Evenhuis and Greathead, 1999).

A significant number of species within this family act as endoparasites, targeting bees, solitary wasps, as well as the larvae and pupae of Lepidoptera and Coleoptera, and serving as hyperparasites of Diptera and Hymenoptera that develop within caterpillars. Furthermore, a select few species are recognized for parasitizing antlions. Notably, the Bombyliidae stand out as the sole Diptera family known to be specifically parasitic on antlions (Evenhuis and Greathead, 1999).

6.2.2 Systematic Position

Kingdom – Animalia
Phylum – Arthropoda
Class – Insecta
Order – Diptera

6.2.3 Diversity

The family Bombyliidae comprises a total of 6,163 species-group names, with 5,826 being valid nomenclaturally and 4,781 considered taxonomically valid (Evenhuis and Greathead, 1999).

6.2.4 Distribution

This family exhibits a global distribution, with the exception of Antarctica, boasting over 4,780 documented species (Evenhuis and Greathead, 1999). Species of Bombyliidae exhibit the highest abundance in regions characterized by a Mediterranean climate, potentially indicating a decrease in species richness as one moves towards tropical areas (Hull, 1973; Eggleton and Gaston, 1990). The Palaearctic Region boasts the highest diversity among all zoogeographical realms, with 1,478 species. The Afrotropical Region closely follows with 1,433 species. In contrast, the Neotropical and Oriental regions, despite having lower species counts, possess vast suitable habitats and host populations for bombyliids, suggesting a much greater species richness than currently documented. Bombyliid species are predominantly found in arid regions and represent a significant portion of fly diversity in desert areas. While some genera, such as *Euchariomyia*, *Ligyra s.* lat., *Palintonus*, and *Systropus*, exhibit a preference for tropical regions, they still hold potential as valuable indicators of biodiversity in arid regions (Evenhuis and Greathead, 1999).

The larvae of Bombyliidae demonstrate parasitoid or predatory tendencies towards the early developmental stages of various insects or egg masses of spiders. Certain species play a crucial role as natural predators of significant agricultural pests such as locusts, grasshoppers, armyworms, slug and nettle caterpillars, and tsetse flies. Some species parasitize the nests of solitary wasps and bees, occasionally causing harm by attacking bee larvae bred for crop pollination. Immatures are generally not well understood in their entirety, although a majority of those that have been studied are primarily parasitic on the immature stages of insects undergoing complete metamorphosis. Some species have been observed preying on the egg masses of orthopterans, while one particular species (*Petrorossiafeti*) has been found associated with spider egg masses.

6.2.5 Life Cycle

The adult bee flies commonly visit flowers to obtain nectar and pollen. Female bee flies typically have a modified terminalia that includes a specialized pouch located just behind the genital chamber. This pouch, known as the "sand chamber", is encircled by elongated setae and enlarged spines (Schremmer, 1964). The intricate oviposition behaviour demonstrated by most bee flies was initially highlighted by Painter (1932). The sand chamber, along with its associated vestiture, serves the purpose of collecting and retaining small particles of the substrate, which are subsequently affixed to the eggs prior to laying (Biliotti et al., 1965). In subfamilies where a sand chamber is present, the process of egg deposition usually takes place while the female is in a hovering position.

Female Bombyliidae may deposit eggs directly into the nests of potential hosts or scatter them more haphazardly on the substrate. Consequently, the initial instar (planidium) larva bears at least some responsibility for locating suitable hosts. The planidium primarily seeks hosts within the interface between leaf litter and soil, referred to as the substrate-zone habitat. Certain genera, such as Bechellus Greathead (Bombyliinae) and Antonia hew (Antoniiiae), have foregone the sand chamber, with their ovipositors adopting a tubular form. Although details regarding oviposition in these groups are scarce, behavioural adaptations have likely accompanied the significant morphological changes (Yeates and Greathead, 1997).

6.3 FAMILY CONOPIDAE

6.3.1 Introduction

The Conopidae, also known as thick-headed flies, belong to the infraorder Schizophora within the suborder Brachycera. This group of flies is intriguing but has not received much research attention, despite being found in almost every part of the world (Mitra et al., 2015). Conopids, comprising approximately 800 documented species, exhibit a global distribution with the exception of polar regions and numerous Pacific islands. The predominant conopid species display a coloration of black accented with yellow or orange markings and bands, often resembling their typical hosts, such as wasps or bees. The larvae of conopids, whose biological characteristics have been elucidated, function as internal parasites of various other insects (Schneider, 2010). Noteworthy instances of Hymenoptera mimicry are prevalent within two subfamilies, namely Conopinae and Dalmanniinae, with such mimicry potentially extending to certain conopids that mirror their plausible hosts (Gibson et al., 2014).

6.3.2 Systematic Position

Kingdom: Animalia
Phylum: Arthropoda
Class: Insecta
Order: Diptera
Family: Conopidae
Diversity and distribution: See Table 6.1.

6.3.3 Host

Documentation pertaining to host occurrences among Neotropical Conopidae is limited, encompassing a mere 5% of the total global species. Host verification is established for all conopids, excluding Stylogastrinae, which are associated with aculeate Hymenoptera. Stylogastrinae, on the

TABLE 6.1
Number of Subfamilies, Genera, and Species of Conopidae Reported from India

Subfamily	No. of Genera	No. of Species
Conopinae	7	35
Myopinae	3	10
Sicinae	1	3
Stylogastrinae	1	1
Zodioninae	1	3
Total	13	52

Source: Mitra et al. (2015).

other hand, exhibit confirmed associations with crickets and cockroaches belonging to Orthoptera and Blattodea (Gibson et al., 2014). It has been established that the hosts of these larvae include aculeate Hymenoptera, crickets, and cockroaches (Gibson and Skevington, 2013).

6.3.4 Life Cycle

The comprehensive life cycle documentation for the majority of species remains elusive; however, in cases where such information is available, the larvae exhibit an obligate endoparasitic relationship with other insect species (Gibson and Skevington, 2013). Eggs are deposited within the abdominal region of the host, giving rise to the larva responsible for consuming haemolymph and host tissues. Subsequent to the demise of the host, the larva undergoes pupation, leading to the emergence of the adult conopid from the remains of the deceased host. The presence of adults is predominantly noted in floral settings, with a proposed inclination towards nectar consumption (Gibson et al., 2014).

6.3.5 Biocontrol Efficacy (Table 6.2)

TABLE 6.2
Parasitoids of Subfamily Conopinae, Its Host, and Distribution in India

Parasitoids	Host	Distribution	References
Subfamily:*Conopinae*			
Archiconops erythrocephalus		Tamil Nadu, Maharashtra, Sikkim, Meghalaya, West Bengal, Gujarat	Zoological survey of India, Kolkata, India (2015)
Conops (Asiconops) nubeculosus	Bees and wasps	Sikkim, West Bengal	Zoological survey of India, Kolkata, India (2015), Schneider (2010), Mitra et al. (2015)
Conops (Asiconops) pactyas		Meghalaya	Zoological survey of India, Kolkata, India (2015); Mitra et al. (2015)
Conops (Conops) annulosus		Assam, Meghalaya, Uttar Pradesh, Himachal Pradesh	Zoological survey of India, Kolkata, India (2015), Mitra et al. (2015)
Conops (Conops) bigoti		Kerala	Zoological survey of India, Kolkata, India (2015), Mitra et al. (2015)
Conops (Conops) claripennis		Maharashtra	Zoological survey of India, Kolkata, India (2015), Mitra et al. (2015)
Conops (Conops) curtirostris		Sikkim	Zoological survey of India, Kolkata, India (2015), Mitra et al. (2015)
Conops (Conops) frontosus		Sikkim	Zoological survey of India, Kolkata, India (2015), Mitra et al. (2015)
Conops (Conops) indicus		Sikkim	Zoological survey of India, Kolkata, India (2015), Mitra et al. (2015)
Conops (Conops) maculiventris		Sikkim	Zoological survey of India, Kolkata, India (2015), Mitra et al. (2015)
Conops (Conops) nigriventris		Assam, Meghalaya	Zoological survey of India, Kolkata, India (2015), Mitra et al. (2015)
Conops (Conops) nigrofasciatus		Bihar	Zoological survey of India, Kolkata, India (2015), Mitra et al. (2015)
Conops (Conops) punctifrons		Sikkim	Zoological survey of India, Kolkata, India (2015), Mitra et al. (2015)

(Continued)

TABLE 6.2 (*Continued*)
Parasitoids of Subfamily Conopinae, Its Host, and Distribution in India

Parasitoids	Host	Distribution	References
Conops (Conops) rufofasciatus		Himachal Pradesh	Zoological survey of India, Kolkata, India (2015), Mitra et al. (2015)
Neobrachyceraea nigrita		India (not restricted to any area)	Zoological survey of India, Kolkata, India (2015), Mitra et al. (2015)
Physocephala annulifera	Bees and wasps	Assam	Zoological survey of India, Kolkata, India (2015), Mitra et al. (2015)
Physocephala argentifera		Bihar, Uttar Pradesh, Meghalaya	Zoological survey of India, Kolkata, India (2015), Mitra et al. (2015)
Physocephala assamensis		Assam	Zoological survey of India, Kolkata, India (2015), Mitra et al. (2015)
Physocephala aterrima		Sikkim	Zoological survey of India, Kolkata, India (2015), Mitra et al. (2015)
Physocephala aurantiaca		Bihar	Zoological survey of India, Kolkata, India (2015), Mitra et al. (2015)
Physocephala aureopygia		Sikkim	Zoological survey of India, Kolkata, India (2015), Mitra et al. (2015)
Physocephala calopa		Tamil Nadu, Uttar Pradesh, West Bengal, Arunachal Pradesh	Zoological survey of India, Kolkata, India (2015), Mitra et al. (2015)
Physocephala diffusa		Bihar, Karnataka	Zoological survey of India, Kolkata, India (2015), Mitra et al. (2015)
Physocephala limbipennis		India (not restricted to any area)	Zoological survey of India, Kolkata, India (2015), Mitra et al. (2015)
Physocephala munda		Gujarat (Deesa), Orissa.	Zoological survey of India, Kolkata, India, 2004, Mitra et al. (2015)
Physocephala nigrofasciata		India (not restricted to any area)	Zoological survey of India, Kolkata, India (2015), Mitra et al. (2015)
Physocephala paralleliventris		Kerala	Zoological survey of India, Kolkata, India (2015), Mitra et al. (2015)
Physocephala rufescens		Jammu and Kashmir	Zoological survey of India, Kolkata, India (2015); Mitra et al. (2015)
Physocephala rufipes	Hymenoptera-Bumble bees	Assam, Meghalaya	Zoological survey of India, Kolkata, India (2015), Otterstatter, et al. (2002), Mitra et al. (2015)
Physocephala scutellate	Bees and wasps	Uttarakhand, Mizoram, Meghalaya, Arunachal Pradesh, Himachal Pradesh	Zoological survey of India, Kolkata, India (2015), Mitra et al. (2015)
Physocephala tenella		Karnataka, Uttar Pradesh, Arunachal Pradesh, Himachal Pradesh	Zoological survey of India, Kolkata, India (2015), Mitra et al. (2015)
Physocephala Testacea		Tamil Nadu, West Bengal	Zoological survey of India, Kolkata, India (2015), Mitra et al. (2015)
Physoconops jutogensis		Himachal Pradesh	Zoological survey of India, Kolkata, India (2015), Mitra et al. (2015)
Physoconops sepulchralis		Assam, Meghalaya	Zoological survey of India, Kolkata, India (2015), Mitra et al. (2015)
Pleurocerinella dioctriaeformis		Himachal Pradesh	Zoological survey of India, Kolkata, India (2015), Mitra et al. (2015)

(*Continued*)

TABLE 6.2 (*Continued*)
Parasitoids of Subfamily Conopinae, Its Host, and Distribution in India

Parasitoids	Host	Distribution	References
Melanosomabella		Punjab	Zoological survey of India, Kolkata, India (2015), Mitra et al. (2015)
Myopa cincta	Solitary bees	India (not restricted to any area)	Zoological survey of India, Kolkata, India (2015), Mitra et al. (2015)
Myopa confusa		Jammu and Kashmir	Zoological survey of India, Kolkata, India (2015), Mitra et al. (2015)
Myopa curta		Uttar Pradesh	Zoological survey of India, Kolkata, India (2015), Mitra et al. (2015)
Myopa dorsalis		Bihar	Zoological survey of India, Kolkata, India (2015), Mitra et al. (2015)
Myopa nigriventris		Jammu and Kashmir, Uttar Pradesh, Uttarakhand	Zoological survey of India, Kolkata, India (2015), Mitra et al. (2015)
Myopa picta		India (not restricted to any area)	Zoological survey of India, Kolkata, India (2015), Mitra et al. (2015)
Myopatestacea		Jammu and Kashmir	Zoological survey of India, Kolkata, India (2015), Mitra et al. (2015)
Sicus abdominalis	Bumblee bees	India (not restricted to any area)	Zoological survey of India, Kolkata, India (2015), Mitra et al. (2015)
Sicus ferrugineus		Jammu and Kashmir, Sikkim	Zoological survey of India, Kolkata, India (2015), Mitra et al. (2015)
Sicus indicus		India: Himalayas	Zoological survey of India, Kolkata, India (2015), Mitra et al. (2015)
Thecophora atra	Bees	Uttar Pradesh, Himachal Pradesh	Zoological survey of India, Kolkata, India (2015), Mitra et al. (2015)
Thecophora flavipes		Maharashtra	Zoological survey of India, Kolkata, India (2015), Mitra et al. (2015)
Zodion cinereum		Uttar Pradesh, Himachal Pradesh	Zoological survey of India, Kolkata, India (2015), Mitra et al. (2015)
Zodion griseum		Jammu and Kashmir, Uttar Pradesh, Uttarakhand, Himachal Pradesh	Zoological survey of India, Kolkata, India (2015), Mitra et al. (2015)
Zodion montanum		West Bengal	Zoological survey of India, Kolkata, India (2015), Mitra et al. (2015)
Stylogaster orientalis		Assam, Kerala	Zoological survey of India, Kolkata, India (2015), Mitra et al. (2015)

6.4 FAMILY PIPUNCULIDAE

6.4.1 Introduction

Pipunculidae, or big-headed flies, are a family of over 1,400 parasitoid fly species within the order Diptera, exhibiting a wide array of morphological and behavioural adaptations that support their parasitic lifestyle (Rafael, 1998). These flies are globally distributed, thriving in diverse habitats from tropical rainforests to temperate regions, making them important for studying parasitic relationships in various ecological contexts (Skevington and Marshall, 1998). Their parasitism of pest insects such as leafhoppers and planthoppers highlights their potential for IPM, contributing to sustainable agriculture by reducing the need for chemical pesticides (Skevington, 2005).

6.4.2 Systemic Position

Pipunculidae belong to the order Diptera and are classified within the superfamily Syrphoidea. This family is closely related to Syrphidae (hoverflies) but can be distinguished by their distinct morphological features, such as their large, hemispherical heads, which house well-developed compound eyes (Skevington and Marshall, 1998).

6.4.3 Diversity and Distribution

The family Pipunculidae consists of over 1,400 described species, showcasing a diverse range of parasitoid flies. These species possess a variety of morphological and behavioural adaptations that support their parasitic way of life (Rafael, 1998). Pipunculidae are distributed globally, inhabiting a wide array of environments from tropical rainforests to temperate regions. This extensive distribution makes them valuable for studying parasitic relationships across different ecological settings (Skevington and Marshall, 1998). Due to their specialization in parasitizing pest insects that harm crops and spread plant diseases, Pipunculidae are highly promising for IPM programmes. Their use in IPM can help achieve more sustainable agricultural practices by reducing reliance on chemical pesticides (Skevington, 2005).

6.4.4 Biology

The Pipunculidae family undergoes a life cycle that includes a parasitic larval stage. Female Pipunculidae lay their eggs on or near host insects, which are typically leafhoppers or planthoppers. The larvae then grow inside the host, ultimately leading to the host's death as they reach maturity. This parasitic interaction is vital for managing host populations in both natural and agricultural environments (Rafael and De Meyer, 1992).

6.4.5 Host

Pipunculidae primarily target hemipteran insects, particularly leafhoppers (Cicadellidae) and planthoppers (Delphacidae). These host insects are significant agricultural pests, feeding on crops and transmitting plant pathogens. The specificity of Pipunculidae to these hosts underscores their potential in targeted biological control (Table 6.3).

6.4.6 Economic Importance

The parasitic nature of Pipunculidae makes them valuable agents in biological control programmes. By naturally reducing populations of pest insects, they help to minimize crop damage and decrease the need for chemical pesticides. Their effectiveness in various agricultural settings highlights their importance in sustainable pest management strategies (Skevington and Marshall, 1998).

6.5 FAMILY TACHINIDAE

6.5.1 Introduction

The Tachinidae constitute the second most extensive family in Diptera, following Tipulidae, encompassing nearly 10,000 documented species worldwide, many of which remain unidentified due to their remarkable diversity.

6.5.2 Systematic Position

Kingdom – Animalia
Phylum – Arthropoda
Class – Insecta
Order – Diptera

6.5.3 Diversity

The Tachinidae, a family composed entirely of parasitoids, is a sizable group encompassing close to 10,000 described species globally, showcasing significant morphological variations. All members of this family function as endoparasitoids of various arthropods, primarily targeting insects. While the majority focus on caterpillars (Lepidoptera), beetles (Coleoptera), true bugs (Heteroptera), and sawflies (Hymenoptera), some also parasitize hosts, like grasshoppers, cockroaches, earwigs, centipedes, and scorpions. Tachinids can exhibit either broad or specialized preferences in terms of the range of host species they target, demonstrating numerous adaptations concerning host localization, reproductive capacity, oviposition behaviour, and larval characteristics (O'Hara, 2010; Figure 6.1).

6.5.4 Distribution

Tachinids are found in Nearctic regions concerning two countries, namely the United States (*Cyzenis albicans*, *C. concinnata*, *Carcelialaxifrons*, and *Alsomyianidicola*) and Canada (*Lyphadubia*, *C. concinnata*, *Drino bobemica*, *Bigonicbaetasetipennis*, and *Siphonageniculata*). They are also

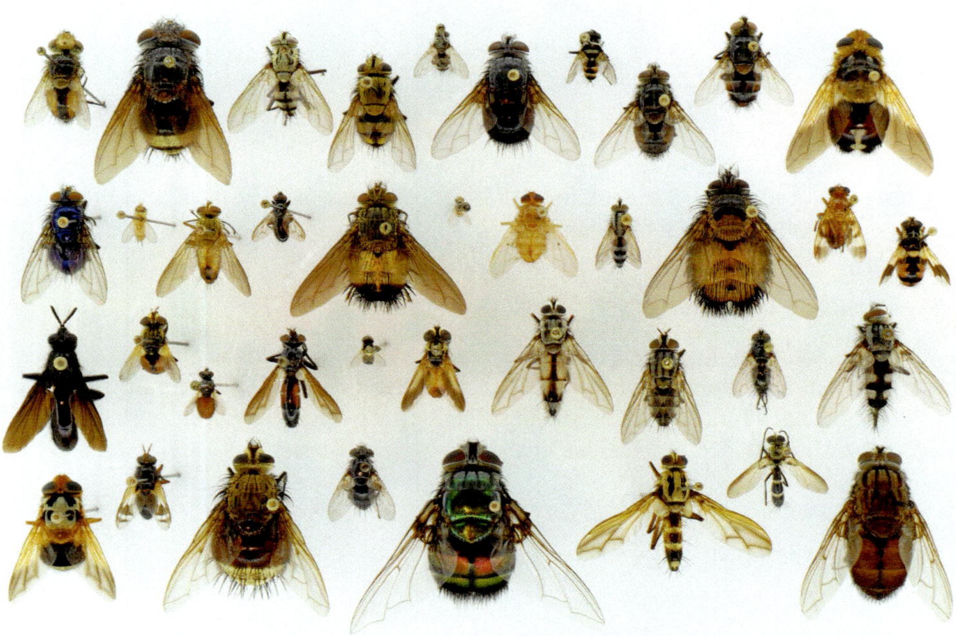

FIGURE 6.1 An assortment of world Tachinidae illustrating the great variation in size, shape, and coloration within the family. *Source*: O'Hara (2010).

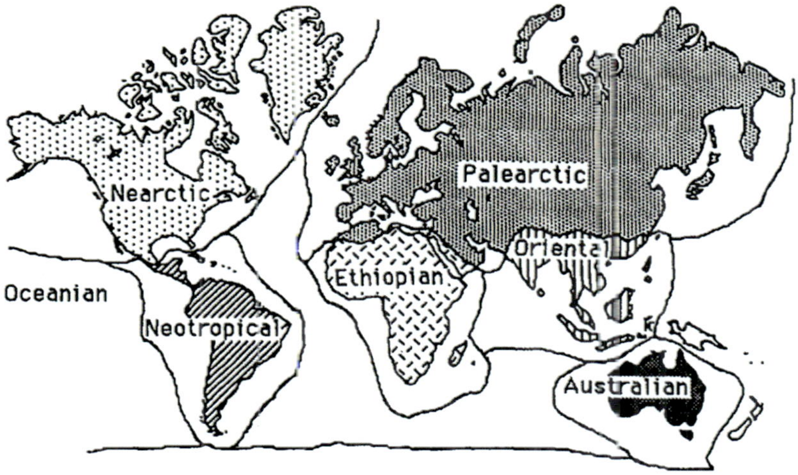

FIGURE 6.2 Main zoogeographic regions of the world (Ethiopian=Afrotropical; Oriental=Indomalayan). Source: Grenier (1988).

found in neotropical regions of the world, establishing in the West Indies, Brazil (*Lyphadiatraeae*), and Colombia, Mexico, Java, Sri Lanka, and the Indian subcontinent (*Exoristarossica, E. segregata*). The parasitoids were also imported to Australia – *Trichopodapennipes* against *N. viridula* and *Stomatomyialittoralis* for the coleopteran pest *Listroderes obliquus*. Oceanian regions include genera such as *Trichopodapennipes*, *Ceromasia (Lixophaga) sphenophori*, *Bonnetiaconta*, *Morphodexia nigra*, and *Dasyurornyia* sp., as well as some others in Palearctic regions (Grenier, 1988; Figure 6.2, Table 6.3).

6.5.5 Host

The parasitoids belonging to this family are more generalists than specialists. Tachinids exhibit endoparasitic behaviour towards approximately 15 orders of arthropods. Predominantly, these species parasitize the larval instars of Lepidoptera, Coleoptera, and Symphyta (Hymenoptera), in addition to adult beetles and Hemiptera (Arafa and Shestakov, 2020; Table 6.4).

For many insects, finding suitable hosts to lay their eggs is a crucial task for completing their life cycle. Numerous order of insects have developed systems that allow females to locate hosts by using olfactory and visual cues from those hosts. The visual and chemical signals that *Apocephalus paraponerae* (Diptera: Phoridae), a dipteran parasitoid, uses to locate and accept *Paraponera clavate* (Hymenoptera: Formicidae: Ponerinae), its host ant, have been described by Morehead and Feener (2000). *A. paraponerae* uses the visual cue of ant body size when locating hosts at short range, and these flies lay more eggs in ants that retain their surface chemicals than in ants with these chemicals removed.

Tachinids have a more diversified host range than any of their other dipteran counterparts. A strong inclination towards polyphagy within this particular family demonstrates a notable association with the capacity of larvae to evade the host's encapsulation response through the construction of a respiratory funnel or migration to anatomical sites that are not conducive to an encapsulation reaction (Belshaw, 1993).

Three basic forms of information that may be used to locate hosts partially overlap: signals that come from possible hosts' food plants or microhabitats, signals that are tangentially related to host activity in the microhabitat, and signals that come directly from the actual hosts. The accuracy and detection of the data in these areas vary over time. The most accurate signals for a host's location

TABLE 6.3
Parasitoids of Pipunculidae, Its Host and Distribution

Parasitoid Species	Host	Distribution	References
Pipunculus campestris	Leafhoppers (Cicadellidae)	Europe, North America	Skevington and Marshall (1998) and Rafael and De Meyer (1992)
Chalarus spurius	Planthoppers (Delphacidae)	Europe, North America	Skevington and Marshall (1998) and Skevington (2005)
Tomosvaryella littoralis	Leafhoppers (Cicadellidae)	Europe, Asia, North America	Rafael and De Meyer (1992)
Dorylomorpha albitarsis	Leafhoppers (Cicadellidae)	Europe, North America	Skevington and Marshall (1998)
Cephalops varipes	Leafhoppers (Cicadellidae)	Europe	Rafael and De Meyer (1992)
Nephrocerus flavicornis	Leafhoppers (Cicadellidae)	North America	Skevington and Marshall (1998)
Claraeola melanostola	Planthoppers (Delphacidae)	Europe, Asia	Skevington and Marshall (1998)
Eudorylas jenkinsoni	Leafhoppers (Cicadellidae)	Europe	Rafael and De Meyer (1992)
Pipunculu sfonsecai	Planthoppers (Delphacidae)	Europe	Skevington and Marshall (1998)
Eudorylas alternatus	Leafhoppers (Cicadellidae)	India	Maity et al. (2020)
Eudorylas subnitens	Planthoppers (Delphacidae)	India	Maity et al. (2020)
Tomosvaryella frontella	Leafhoppers (Cicadellidae)	India	Maity et al. (2020)
Pipunculus tenuirostris	Leafhoppers (Cicadellidae)	India	Maity et al. (2020)
Pipunculus aeratus	Leafhoppers (Cicadellidae)	India	Maity et al. (2020)
Cephalops semifumosus	Leafhoppers (Cicadellidae)	India	Maity et al. (2020)
Clistoabdominalis minor	Leafhoppers (Cicadellidae)	India	Maity et al. (2020)
Dorylomorpha rufipes	Leafhoppers (Cicadellidae)	India	Maity et al. (2020)
Tomosvaryella nigricosta	Planthoppers (Delphacidae)	India	Maity et al. (2020)
Jassidophaga villosa	Leafhoppers (Cicadellidae)	India	Maity et al. (2020)

TABLE 6.4
Number of Tachinid Species and Genera in each Biogeographic Region and the World

Biogeographic Region	Genera	Described Species
Neotropical	822	2,864
Nearctic	304	1,345
Palearctic	405	>1,600
Afrotropical	213	1,006
Oriental	264	725
Australasian	230	808
World	1,523	About 10,000

Source: O'Hara (2008).

and identification are those that are obtained directly from the source. Nevertheless, these signals are frequently too faint to be detected over great distances since hosts are always under selection pressure to reduce their prominence to natural foes (Hagen, 1964). On the other hand, cues coming from a potential host's food plant or microhabitat are often simpler to identify from a distance, but they do not provide much accurate information on the precise location and identity of the hosts. Consequently, signal detectability and dependability are frequently inversely correlated – a reliability–detectability problem (Feener and Brown, 1997).

Female parasitoids are able to recognize the signals from their hosts' "sexual communication system" and are attracted to these signals. Similar to *Ormia ochracea*, there is a tympanal hearing organ on the prothorax, which exhibits sexual dimorphism. The females' ears are more sensitive to male cricket songs than males, which helps the female to lay eggs near or on these males. Additionally, the parasitoid *Trichopoda pennipes* is attracted to males of *Nezara viridula* as they release aggregation pheromones (Harris and Todd, 1980). The subfamily Tachininae employs the strategy of host contact ambush, wherein recently hatched larvae utilize the chorion of the egg as a receptacle to perch. Positioned vertically, the larva pivots in response to mobile entities and affixes itself to a suitable host nearby. In the Goniini tachinid tribe, interaction with the host is passive during the egg stage. Eggs of microtype laid by the females persist inert in the surroundings until inadvertently consumed by a feeding host. Subsequently, the eggs are induced to emerge through a combination of salivary secretion, physical breakage, and elevated pH levels within the host's gastrointestinal tract (Hagen, 1964). Some tachinids are also parasites of beneficial insects, such as the mulberry silkworm, namely *Exorista bombycis*, which is harmful to cultivation and is considered a pest in silkworm rearing (Kumar et al., 1993; Narayanaswamy and Govindan, 2000) (Table 6.5).

6.5.6 Life Cycle

Some tachinids also have the ability to complete their life cycle by parasitizing the host without killing them. The larvae of *Platyprepia virginalis*, an arctiid moth, exhibited a remarkable ability to withstand the emergence of the tachinid *Thelaira bryanti*. Furthermore, these larvae demonstrated the capability to undergo metamorphosis into viable adult individuals capable of reproducing successfully (English et al., 1990).

6.5.7 Biocontrol Efficacy

More recently, the potential employment of tachinids for biological control remains to be assessed in diverse systems, including bromeliad weevils, palm weevils, the prickly pear cactus moth, and sugarcane borers (Arafa and Shestakov, 2020).

The frequencies of parasitism by tachinids were approximated to be 10% or higher within the extensive breeding initiatives of lepidopteran larvae (Stireman et al., 2017). When *C. concinnata* (77%) and *Carcelia laxifrons* (23%) were used against *Euproctis chrysorrhoea*, *T. pennipes* was used against *N. viridula* in Hawaii; *L. diatraeae* was used against *C. infuscatellus* in Taiwan, and *B. remota* was used against *L. iridescens* in the Fiji Islands, these gave a 70% success rate (Arafa and Shestakov, 2020).

6.6 CONCLUSION

The fly families Bombyliidae, Conopidae, Pipunculidae, and Tachinidae play significant ecological roles and hold considerable potential for biocontrol applications. Their systematic positions within Diptera reflect their evolutionary diversity and adaptability across various environments. These families exhibit a wide range of hosts and life cycle strategies, from parasitizing other insects to aiding in decomposition processes. The biocontrol efficacy of these flies, particularly in pest management and forensic science, underscores their importance. Continued research and conservation efforts are essential to harness their full potential and maintain ecological balance. Understanding the unique characteristics and interactions of these fly families can lead to more effective and sustainable pest management strategies, contributing to agricultural productivity and environmental health.

TABLE 6.5
Parasitoids, Host and Distribution of Tachinid Flies

Parasitoids	Host	Distribution	References
	Subfamily: *Dexiinae*		
Campylocheta (= Elpe) angustifrons		Oriental – India (Central)	O'Hara et al. (2019)
Billaea atkinsoni	Coleoptera (Cerambycidae, Lucanidae) or Lepidoptera (Pyralidae) hosts	India (North)	O'Hara et al. (2019)
Dexia caldwelli		India – Himanchal Pradesh, Punjab, India (Northwest, West)	Zhang, et al. (2010); O'Hara et al. (2019)
Dexia divergens		Karnataka (Ammatti, S. Coorg), Tamil Nadu (Naduvatam, Nilgiri Hills, Anamalai Hills)	Zhang, et al. (2010)
Dexia extendens		Assam, Shillong, India (Northeast)	Zhang, et al. (2010);
Dexia fulvifera		India (Central, North, Northeast, Northwest)	O'Hara et al. (2019)
Dexiaprakritiae		India	O'Hara et al. (2019)
Dexia quadristriata		India (Northeast)	O'Hara et al. (2019)
Dexiomimops rufipes		Karnataka, Kerala, and Tamil Nadu, Andhra Pradesh, and Orissa India (North and Northeast)	O'Hara et al. (2019)
Dinera orientalis	Coleoptera (Scarabidae)	India	Arnaud Jr. (1978) and O'Hara et al. (2019)
Estheria intermedia		India (North)	O'Hara et al. (2019)
Estheria magna		India (North and Northeast)	O'Hara et al. (2019)
Euthera fascipennis	Pentatomidae, Hemiptera (Heteroptera)	India (West)	Arnaud Jr. (1978) and
Euthera peringueyii		India (North)	O'Hara et al. (2019)
Halidaia luteicornis			
Hystricovoria bakeri		India (Central, Northwest, West)	O'Hara et al. (2019)

(Continued)

TABLE 6.5 (*Continued*)
Parasitoids, Host and Distribution of Tachinid Flies

Parasitoids	Host	Distribution	References
Periscepsia carbonaria	Lepidoptera, Noctuidae, Hymenoptera, Coleoptera	India (North, Northwest, West)	Arnaud Jr. (1978) and O'Hara et al. (2019)
Prosena facialis	Lepidoptera – Pieridae	India (Central)	Arnaud Jr. (1978) and
Prosena siberite	Coleoptera – Scarabaeidae	India (Central, North, Northeast)	O'Hara et al. (2019)
Rutilia (Chrysorutilia) rubriceps		India (Central)	O'Hara et al. (2019)
Thelairama cropus	Lepidoptera – ArctiidaeTineidae	India (North, Northeast, Northwest)	Arnaud Jr. (1978) and O'Hara et al. (2019)
Toroc camunda		India (Central, Northeast)	O'Hara et al. (2019)
Voria ruralis	Lepidoptera – Noctuidae, Tabanidae	India (Central, North, Northeast, Northwest, West)	Arnaud Jr. (1978) and O'Hara et al. (2019)
	Subfamily: Exoristinae		
Alsomyia anomala		India (Central, West)	O'Hara et al. (2019)
Alsomyia rufipes		India (Central, West)	O'Hara et al. (2019)
Aneogmena fischeri		India (North, West)	O'Hara et al. (2019)
Aneogmena lucifera		India (North)	O'Hara et al. (2019)
Aplomya flavisquama	Coleoptera – Curculionidae, Scarabaeidae	India	Arnaud Jr. (1978) and
Aplomya metallica	Hymenoptera – Cimbicidae, Pamphilidae Lepidoptera – Arctiidae, Agridae, Cimbicidae, Geometridae, Gracillariidae, Lasiocampidae, Lycaenidae, Lymantriidae, Noctuidae, Notodontidae, Olethreutidae, Pamphiliidae, Pyralidae, Tenebrionidae, Tortricidae	India (Central, North)	O'Hara et al. (2019)
Argyrophylax fransseni	Coleoptera – Chrysomelidae	India (Central)	Arnaud Jr. (1978) and
Argyrophylax nigrotibialis	Lepidoptera – Arctiidae, Notodontidae, Olethreutidae, Pyralidae, Saturnidae, Sphingidae	India	O'Hara et al. (2019)
Argyrophylax phoedus		India	
Austrophorocera grandis		India (Central)	

(*Continued*)

TABLE 6.5 (*Continued*)
Parasitoids, Host and Distribution of Tachinid Flies

Parasitoids	Host	Distribution	References
Bactromyia adiscalis		India (Central)	O'Hara et al. (2019)
Bactromyia aurora		India (Central)	
Bactromyia longifacies		India (Central)	
Bactromyiella ficta		India (Central)	
Bessa remota	Coleoptera – Scarabaeidae Lepidoptera – Acrididae, Argidae, Diprionidae, Tenthredinida, Geometridae, Gryllidae, Lymantriidae, Nymphalidae, Pyralidae, Tettigoniidae, Tortricidae Hymenoptera – Argidae, Diprionidae, Tenthredinidae	India (Central)	Arnaud Jr. (1978) and O'Hara et al. (2019)
Blepharella lateralis		India (Central, North, Northeast, Northwest)	O'Hara et al. (2019)
Blepharipa albocinta	Dermaptera – Forficulidae	India (Central)	Arnaud Jr. (1978) and O'Hara et al. (2019)
Blepharipa fusiformis	Lepidoptera – Lymantriidae, Lasiocampida, Noctuidae, Notodontidae, Pyralidae, Zygaenidae	India (North)	
Blepharipa jacobsoni		India	
Blepharipa orbitalis		India (Northeast)	
Blepharipa wainwrighti		India (Northeast)	
Blepharipa zebina		India (Central, North, Northeast, West)	
Blepharipa zebinamanipurensis			
Cadurcia vanderwulpi		India (North)	O'Hara et al. (2019)

(*Continued*)

TABLE 6.5 (*Continued*)

Parasitoids, Host and Distribution of Tachinid Flies

Parasitoids	Host	Distribution	References
Carcelia (Carcelia) caudata	Coleoptera – Carabidae, Scarabaeidae, Tenebrionidae Lepidoptera – Acrididae, Arctiidae, Gryllidae, Lasiocampidae, Limacodidae, Lymantriidae, Megalopygidae, Noctuidae, Notodontidae, Nymphalidae, Olethreutidae, Pyralidae, Saturniidae, Sphingidae, Tenthredinidae, Tortricidae	India (Central, North)	Arnaud Jr. (1978) and O'Hara et al. (2019)
Carcelia (Carcelia) corvinoides		India (Central, North, West)	
Carcelia (Carcelia) malayana		India (North)	
Carcelia (Carcelia) pilosella			
Carcelia (Carcelia) rasoides		India (Northeast)	
Carcelia (Euryclea) ceylanica		India (Central)	
Carcelia (Euryclea) delicatula		India (Northwest	
Chetogenaraoi		India (Central)	O'Hara et al. (2019)

(*Continued*)

TABLE 6.5 (*Continued*)
Parasitoids, Host and Distribution of Tachinid Flies

Parasitoids	Host	Distribution	References
Chaetexorista javana	Coleoptera – Curculionidae (*Conotrachelus naso*) Lepidoptera – Limacodidae (*Cnidocampa flauescens*), Tortricidae (*Choristoneura fumiferana*)	India (Central)	Arnaud Jr. (1978) and O'Hara et al. (2019)
Chaetexorista lushaiensis	Coleoptera, Lepidoptera		Arnaud Jr. (1978) and
Compsilura concinnata	Curculionidae (*Pissodes*); Cimbicidae (*Cimbex*); Diprionidae (*Diprion*); Pamphiliidae (*Neurotoma*); Tenthredinidae (*Croesus*, *Nematus*, *Pristiphora*, *Trichio campus*); Unidentified Hymenoptera (Sawfly (-flies), Tenthredinoidea; Arctiidae (*Diacrisia*, *Estigmene*, *Euchaetias*, *Halisidota*, *Hyphantria*, Unidentified Arctiidae); Bombycidae (*Bombyx*); Citheroniidae (*Anisota*); Ctenuchidae (*Ctenucha*); Danaidae (*Danaus*); Geometridae (*Biston*, *Cingilia*, *Ennomos*, *Eugonobapta*, *Hydria*, *Itame*, *Lambdina*, *Melanolophia*, *Nematocampa*, *Phigalia*, Unidentified Geometridae); Hesperiidae (*Epargyreus*, *Erynnis*, *Thymelicus*, Unidentified Hesperiidae); Lasiocampidae (*Epicnaptera*, Malacosoma, American tent caterpillar(-s)); Limacodidae (*Cnidocampa*); Lymantriidae (*Dasychira*, *Euproctis*, *Hemerocampa*, *Nygmia*, *Orgyia*, *Porthetria*, *Stilpnotia*, Tussock moth(-s), Unidentified Lymantriidae; Megalopygidae (*Megalopyge*); Noctuidae (*Acronicta*, *Alypia*, *Amphipyra*, *Calpe*, *Catocala*, *Ceramica*, *Euthisanotia*, *Lithophane*, *Phosphila*, *Plathypena*, *Plusiodonta*, *Polia*, *Pseudaletia*, *Rhodophora*, *Scoliopteryx*, *Simyra*, *Trichoplusia*, *Xylena*, Unidentified Catocalinae, Unidentified Noctuidae; Notodontidae (*Cerura*, *Datana*, *Fentonia*, *Heterocampa*, *Ichthyura*, *Nadata*, *Pheosia*, *Schizura*, *Symmerista*, Unidentified Notodontidae; Nymphalidae (*Agraulis*, *Chlosyne*, *Euphydryas*, *Limenitis*, *Nymphalis*, *Polygonia*, *Vanessa*, Unidentified Nymphalidae); Oecophoridae(*Dasy stoma*); Olethreutidae (*Eucosmaridingsana*), Papilionidae (*Battus*, *Papilio*, Unidentified Papilionidae; Pieridae (*Pieris*); Pterophoridae (*Oidaematophorus*) Pyralidae (*Euergestis*, *Ostrinia*); Saturniidae (*Anther aea*, *Automeris*, *Callosamia*, *Hemileuca*, *Platysamia*, Unidentified Saturniidae; Sp., Mngidae (*Ampeloeca*, *Amphion*, *Atreides*, *Ceratomia*, *Deidamia*, *Hemaris*, *Hyles*, *Manduca*, *Paonias*, *Pholus*, *Smerinthus*, *Sphecodina*, *Sphinx*, Tortricidae (*Archips*, *Choristoneura*); Lasiocampidae (*Malacosoma*)		Arnaud Jr. (1978);

(*Continued*)

TABLE 6.5 (*Continued*)

Parasitoids, Host and Distribution of Tachinid Flies

Parasitoids	Host	Distribution	References
Diglossocera bifida		India (Central)	O'Hara et al.,(2019)
Dolichocolon vicinum		India (Central, North)	O'Hara et al. (2019)
Drino (Drino) argenticeps	Diptera – Zygaenidae,	India	Arnaud Jr. (1978) and
Drino (Drino) facialis	Hymenoptera – Diprionidae, Tenthredinidae, Tipulidae	India (North, Northeast)	O'Hara et al. (2019)
Drino (Palexorista) biseriate	Lepidoptera – Citheroniidae, Geometridae, Hesperiidae, Lasiocampidae, Lymantriidae, Olethreutidae, Noctuidae, Notodontidae, Psychidae, Pyralidae, Saturniidae, Sphingidae, Sphinx, Tineidae		
Drino (Palexorista) dilaticornis			
Drino (Palexorista) laxa			
Drino (Palexorista) lucagus		India (Central)	
Drino (Palexorista) munda			
Drino (Palexorista) paraachrysops			
Drino (Palexorista) reclinata			
Drino (Palexorista) solennis		India (Central, North)	
Drino (Zygobothria) atropivora		India (Central, North, Northeast)	
Drino (Zygobothria) ciliata		India (Central, North, Northeast)	
Elodia atra	Lepidoptera – Arctiidae, Olethreutidae, Pterophoridae	India (Central)	Arnaud Jr. (1978) and O'Hara et al. (2019)
Eophyllophila elegans		India (Central)	O'Hara et al. (2019)
Eophyllophila filipes			
Eophyllophila includens		India (Central)	O'Hara et al. (2019)

(*Continued*)

TABLE 6.5 (*Continued*)

Parasitoids, Host and Distribution of Tachinid Flies

Parasitoids	Host	Distribution	References
Eurysthaea cinctella		India (Central)	O'Hara et al. (2019)
Eurysthaea leveriana		India (North)	O'Hara et al. (2019)
Exorista (Exorista) castanea	Coleoptera – Diprionidae, Gelechiidae, Scarabaeidae Hymenoptera – Tenthredinidae Lepidoptera – Arctiidae, Bombycidae, Danaidae, Geometridae, Glyphipterygidae, Hesperiidae, Lasiocampidae, Limacodidae, Lycaenidae, Lyman triidae, Megalopygidae, Noctuidae, Notodontidae, Nymphalidae, Olethreutidae, Pieridae, Pterophoridae, Pyralidae, Saturniidae, Sphingidae, Tortricidae, Yponomeutidae		Arnaud Jr. (1978) and O'Hara et al. (2019)
Exorista (Exorista) japonica		India (Central, North)	
Exorista (Exorista) larvarum		India (Northwest)	
Exorista (Exorista) psamathe			
Exorista (Exorista) rossica		India (Northwest)	
Exorista (Exorista) subnigra			
Exorista (Exorista) velutina		India (Central)	
Exorista (Podotachina) sorbillans		India	
Exorista (Ptilotachina) xanthapsis		India	
Frontina adusta	Hymenoptera – Apidae, Tenthredinidae Lepidoptera – Arctiidae, Bombycidae, Citheroniidae, Danaidae, Diprionidae, Geometridae, Gryllidae, Lasiocampidae, Lycaenidae, Lyman triidae, Megalopygidae, Noctuidae, Notodontidae, Nymphalidae, Papilionidae, Pieridae, Pyralidae, Saturniidae, Sphingidae, Yponomeutidae	India (North, Northwest)	Arnaud Jr. (1978) and O'Hara et al. (2019)
Hapalioloemus machaeralis		India (Central)	O'Hara et al. (2019)

(*Continued*)

TABLE 6.5 (*Continued*)
Parasitoids, Host and Distribution of Tachinid Flies

Parasitoids	Host	Distribution	References
Gonia chinensis	Coleoptera – Curculionidae, Meloidae, Scarabaeidae Hemiptera – Pentatomidae	India (Central, North, Northeast, Northwest, West)	Arnaud Jr. (1978) and O'Hara et al. (2019)
Gonia kalimpongensis	Lepidoptera – Arctiidae, Lymantriidae, Geometridae, Noctuidae, Phasmatidae, Pyralidae	India (North)	
Gonia klapperichi		India (North)	
Goniophthalmus halli		India (Central, West)	O'Hara et al. (2019)
Hygiella nigripes		India (North)	O'Hara et al. (2019)
Isochaetina dimorpha		India (Central)	O'Hara et al. (2019)
Isosturmia japonica		India	O'Hara et al. (2019)
Isosturmia picta		India (North, Northwest)	O'Hara et al. (2019)
Koralliomyia portentosa		India (Central)	O'Hara et al. (2019)
Nealsomyia rufella		India (North)	O'Hara et al. (2019)
Nealsomyia rufipes		India (Central, West)	O'Hara et al. (2019)
Pales murina	Coleoptera – Citheroniidae, Tenebrionidae Hymenoptera – Diprionidae Lepidoptera – Geometridae, Megathymidae, Notodontidae, Tortricidae	India	Arnaud Jr. (1978) and O'Hara et al. (2019)
Paradrino pilifacies		India (Northeast)	O'Hara et al. (2019)
Paratryphera longicornis		India (North)	O'Hara et al. (2019)
Phorina nigra			
Phorocerosoma vicarium		India	O'Hara et al. (2019)
Phryx epatruelis	Hymenoptera – Tenthredinidae Lepidoptera – Arctiidae, Danaidae, Forficulidae, Geometridae, Hesperiidae, Lymantriidae, Noctuidae, Notodontidae, Pieridae, Pyralidae, Saturniidae, Tortricidae	India (North)	Arnaud Jr. (1978) and O'Hara et al. (2019)
Polygasropteryx bicoloripes			

(*Continued*)

TABLE 6.5 (*Continued*)
Parasitoids, Host and Distribution of Tachinid Flies

Parasitoids	Host	Distribution	References
Prosopodopsis appendiculata		India (Central, North)	O'Hara et al. (2019)
Prosopodopsis orbitalis		India (North, West)	O'Hara et al. (2019)
Pseudogonia rufifrons		India (Central, Northeast, Northwest, West)	O'Hara et al. (2019)
Pseudoperichaeta indica	Coleoptera – Meloidae	India (Central, West)	Arnaud Jr. (1978) and O'Hara et al. (2019)
Pseudoperichaeta monochaeta	Lepidoptera – Meloidae, Noctuidae, Notodontidae, Olethreutidae, Pyralidae, Tortricidae	India	
Pseudoperichaeta roseanella		India (Central)	
Rhinomyodese mporomyioides		India (North)	O'Hara et al. (2019)
Senometopia excise	Lepidoptera – Noctuidae	India (Northwest)	Arnaud Jr. (1978) and O'Hara et al. (2019)
Senometopia illota		India (Central, North, West)	
Senometopia indica		India	
Senometopia prima		India (Central)	
Simomagra hami		India (North)	O'Hara et al. (2019)
Sisyropa formosa	Coleoptera – Chrysomelidae, Scarabaeidae	India (Central, North)	Arnaud Jr. (1978) and O'Hara et al. (2019)
Sisyropa heterusiae	Lepidoptera – Arctiidae, Lycaenidae, Lymantriidae, Megalopygidae, Noctuidae, Notodontidae, Nymphalidae, Saturniidae	India (Central, North)	
Sisyropa picta		India (Central)	
Sisyropa prominens		India (North)	
Sisyropa stylata		India (North)	
Sisyropa thermophila		India (North)	
Smidtia (=Timavia) atriventris		India	O'Hara et al. (2019)
Spallanzania hebes	Lepidoptera – Acrididae, Carabidae, Noctuidae	India (Northwest)	Arnaud Jr. (1978) and O'Hara et al. (2019)

(*Continued*)

TABLE 6.5 (*Continued*)
Parasitoids, Host and Distribution of Tachinid Flies

Parasitoids	Host	Distribution	References
Sturmia convergens	Diptera – Tipulidae Lepidoptera – Argidae, Citheroniidae, Diprionidae, Hesperiidae, Lymantriidae, Noctuidae, Notodontidae, Nymphalidae, Olethreutidae, Pyralidae, Saturniidae, Sphingidae, Tenthredinidae, Tipulidae, Tortricidae, Zygaenidae		Arnaud Jr. (1978) and
Sturmiopsis inferens		India (Central, North, Northeast, Northwest, West)	O'Hara et al. (2019)
Suensonomyia setinerva		India (Central)	O'Hara et al. (2019)
Takanomyia scutellata			
Thecocarcelia oculata			
Thecocarcelia parnarae		India	O'Hara et al. (2019)
Thecocarcelia sumatrana		India	O'Hara et al. (2019)
Thelairodrino gracilis		India (Central, North, Northwest, West)	O'Hara et al. (2019)
Trigonospila integra		India (Central)	O'Hara et al. (2019)
Trigonospila ludio		India	O'Hara et al. (2019)
Trigonospila transvittata		India (West)	O'Hara et al. (2019)
Trixomorpha indica		India (North, Northeast)	O'Hara et al. (2019)
Urodexia penicillum		India (Central, West)	O'Hara et al. (2019)
Winthemia mallochi	Coleoptera – Curculionidae Hymenoptera – Diprionidae Lepidoptera – Arctiidae, Bombycidae, Citheroniidae, Geometridae, Lasiocampidae, Lymantriidae, Noctuidae, Notodontidae, Satruniidae, Sphingidae	India	Arnaud Jr. (1978) and O'Hara et al. (2019)
Zenillia terrosa	Hymenoptera – Diprionidae Lepidoptera – Arctiidae, Bombycidae, Citheroniidae, Danaidae, Geomentridae, Lasiocampidae, Lymantriidae, Olethreutidae, Pieridae, Pyralidae, Megalopygidae, Noctuidae, Notodontidae, Nymphalidae, Saturniidae, Sphingidae, Tortricidae	India (Central, Northwest)	Arnaud Jr. (1978) and O'Hara et al. (2019)

(*Continued*)

TABLE 6.5 (*Continued*)
Parasitoids, Host and Distribution of Tachinid Flies

Parasitoids	Host	Distribution	References
	Subfamily: Phasiinae		
Bellina melanura		India	O'Hara et al. (2019)
Ecatocyptera evibrissata			
Eocyptera orientalis			
Ectophasia atripennis		India (Northeast)	O'Hara et al. (2019)
Cylindromyia orientalis	Hemiptera – Pentatomidae	India (Northeast)	Arnaud Jr. (1978) and
Cylindromyia wiedemanni	Hymenoptera – Diprionidae Lepidoptera – Peiridae, Noctuidae, Saturniidae Orthoptera – Acrididae		
Gymnosoma hamiense	Hemiptera – Pentatomidae	India	O'Hara et al. (2019)
Gymnosoma indicum	Lepidoptera – Peiridae, Pyralidae	India (Northwest)	O'Hara et al. (2019)
Hermyabeelzebul		India (Central, North, Northeast, Northwest)	O'Hara et al. (2019)
Hermyamicans		India (Northeast)	O'Hara et al. (2019)
Lophosiabicincta		India (North)	O'Hara et al. (2019)
Lophosia excise		India (Northwest)	O'Hara et al. (2019)
Lophosiafelderi		India	O'Hara et al. (2019)
Lophosiaimbuta		India	O'Hara et al. (2019)
Lophosia obscura		India	O'Hara et al. (2019)
Ocyptera fuscipennis	Lepidoptera – Pieridae, Saturniidae Orthoptera – Acrididae		Arnaud Jr. (1978) and
Pentatomophaga latifascia		India	O'Hara et al. (2019)
Perigymnosoma globulum		India	O'Hara et al. (2019)
Phasia indica	Hemiptera – Pentatomidae Lepidoptera – Lymantriidae, Tortricidae	India (North)	Arnaud Jr. (1978) and

(*Continued*)

TABLE 6.5 (*Continued*)
Parasitoids, Host and Distribution of Tachinid Flies

Parasitoids	Host	Distribution	References
	Subfamily: Tachininae		
Acemya indica	Coleoptera – Chrysomelidae Hemiptera – Pyrrhocoridae Orthoptera – Acrididae		Arnaud Jr. (1978) and
Actia mimetica	Lepidoptera – Arctiidae, Dioptidae, Drepanidae, Geometridae, Gelechiidae, Noctuidae, Notodontidae, Olethreutidae, Pieridae, Tortricidae	India (Central)	Arnaud Jr. (1978) and O'Hara et al. (2019)
Anthomyiopsis nigra		India (North, Northwest)	O'Hara et al. (2019)
Atylostoma javanum		India (Northwest)	O'Hara et al. (2019)
Ceromya mallochina			
Ceromya patellicornis		India (North)	O'Hara et al. (2019)
Clausicella triangulifera	Coleoptera – Curculionidae Hymenoptera – Apidae Lepidoptera – Geometridae, Lacosomidae, Noctuidae, Olethreutidae, Pyralidae, Tineidae	India (Northwest)	Arnaud Jr. (1978) and O'Hara et al. (2019)
Demoticoides pallidus		India (Central)	O'Hara et al. (2019)
Dexiosoma aristatum		India (Central, North)	O'Hara et al. (2019)
Dolichodexia albipilla			
Doleschalla elongata		India (Central)	O'Hara et al. (2019)
Eoucemyia errans		India	O'Hara et al. (2019)
Eurithia indica			
Gymnocheta porphyrophora	Lepidoptera – Arctiidae, Noctuidae	India (North)	Arnaud Jr. (1978) and O'Hara et al. (2019)
Janthinomyia felderi		India (North, Northwest)	O'Hara et al. (2019)
Leksia bezziana			
Linnaemya (Linnaemya) atriventris	Lepidoptera – Arctiidae, Lygaeidae, Noctuidae	India	Arnaud Jr. (1978) and O'Hara et al. (2019)

(*Continued*)

TABLE 6.5 (*Continued*)
Parasitoids, Host and Distribution of Tachinid Flies

Parasitoids	Host	Distribution	References
Linnaemya (Linnaemya) comta		India (Northwest)	
Linnaemya (Linnaemya) soror		India	
Linnaemya (Linnaemya) vulpinoides		India (North, West)	
Linnaemya (Ophina) omega		India (Northwest)	
Linnaemya (Ophina) picta		India (North)	
Macquartia tessellum	Coleoptera – Coleophoridae Lepidoptera – Arctiidae, Tortricidae	India (Northwest)	Arnaud Jr. (1978) and O'Hara et al. (2019)
Microphthalma europaea	Coleoptera – Scarabaeidae Dictyoptera – Blattidae Lepidoptera – Arctiidae	India	Arnaud Jr. (1978) and O'Hara et al. (2019)
Mikia apicalis			
Mikia tepens		India (North)	O'Hara et al. (2019)
Myostoma magnum			
Nemoraea echinata	Lepidoptera – Arctiidae, Noctuidae	India (Northeast)	Arnaud Jr. (1978) and O'Hara et al. (2019)
Nemoraea fenestrata		India (North, Northeast)	
Nemoraea grandis			
Nemoraea ornata		India (North, Northwest, West)	
Nemoraea raoi			
Nemoraea titan		India (North, Northeast)	
Peleteria iavana	Lepidoptera – Arctiidae, Gelechiidae, Lymantriidae, Noctuidae, Nymphalidae, Sphingidae	India (Central, North, Northeast, Northwest), Indonesia (Borneo, Jawa, Sulawesi, Sumatera), Malaysia (East Malaysia, Peninsular Malaysia)	Arnaud Jr. (1978) and O'Hara et al. (2019)
Peleteria varia			

(*Continued*)

TABLE 6.5 (*Continued*)
Parasitoids, Host and Distribution of Tachinid Flies

Parasitoids	Host	Distribution	References
Peribaea hyalinata		India	Arnaud Jr. (1978) and O'Hara et al. (2019)
Peribaea orbata		India (Central, North, Northeast, West)	
Peribaea suspecta		India (Central, North, West)	
Phasioormia bicornis		India (Northeast)	O'Hara et al. (2019)
Phytomyptera minuta	Lepidoptera – Endomychidae, Olethreutidae, Tortricidae	India (Central)	Arnaud Jr. (1978) and O'Hara et al. (2019)
Siphona (Aphantorhaphopsis) perispoliata	Diptera – Tipulidae Lepidoptera – Aegeriidae, Dioptidae, Noctuidae	India (Central, Northwest)	Arnaud Jr. (1978) and O'Hara et al. (2019)
Sumpigaster flavipennis		India	O'Hara et al. (2019)
Sumpigaster plumicornis		India (Central, West)	O'Hara et al. (2019)
Sumpigaster subcompressa		India (Northeast, Northwest)	O'Hara et al. (2019)
Tachina (Nowickia) polita	Coleoptera – Chrysomelidae, Cleridae	India	Arnaud Jr. (1978) and O'Hara et al. (2019)
Tachina (Tachina) fulva	Hemiptera – Cicadidae		
Tachina (Tachina) rufoanlis	Hymenoptera – Apidae Lepidoptera – Aegeriidae, Arctiidae, Bombycidae, Citheroniidae, Danaidae, Geometridae, Lasiocampidae, Lycaenidae, Lymantriidae, Megathymidae, Noctuidae, Notodontidae, Nymphalidae, Pieridae, Psychidae, Pyralidae, Saturniidae, Sphingidae, Tenthredinidae Orthoptera – Acrididae Phasmatodea – Phasmatidae	India	
Tachina (Tachina) sacontala		India (North, Northwest)	
Tachina (Tachina) sobria		India (North, Northeast, Northwest)	
Tachina (Tachina) subcinerea		India	
Tachina (Tachina) ursinoidea		India (North, Northeast, Northwest)	
Tachina (Tachina) tricolor		India	
Thelairoleskia longicornis		India	O'Hara et al. (2019)
Therobia abdominalis		India (North)	O'Hara et al. (2019)

6.7 POINTS TO REMEMBER

1. Dipteran parasitoids have a vast diversity containing about 16,000 described parasitoid species, constituting around 20% of species with this lifestyle, primarily in families like Tachinidae, Bombyliidae, Pipunculidae, and Conopidae.
2. Dipteran parasitoids play crucial roles in regulating insect populations, contributing significantly to the health of natural and agricultural ecosystems, and have ecological as well as agricultural importance. Adult Bombyliidae are important pollinators for many flowering plants, particularly in arid regions, enhancing their ecological significance beyond parasitism.
3. Host specificity and parasitism of these families are exhibited in the unique adaptations in their parasitic behaviours, targeting a variety of hosts from different insect orders, impacting pest populations in natural and agricultural settings.
4. The life cycles of these parasitoids involve complex interactions with their hosts, typically developing as internal parasites and exhibiting various strategies to find and parasitize hosts and adaptations accordingly.
5. The geographical distribution of these parasitoids is also important. Bombyliidae are found globally, especially in arid and Mediterranean climates; Conopidae and Pipunculidae are also globally distributed but with specific host preferences; Tachinidae are found across various regions, being one of the most diverse parasitoid families.
6. They have good biological control potential. Families such as Pipunculidae and Tachinidae have significant potential in IPM programmes, reducing the need for chemical pesticides and contributing to sustainable agriculture.
7. They have a diverse host range: Tachinidae exhibit a broad host range, parasitizing many insect orders, whereas Bombyliidae, Conopidae, and Pipunculidae have more specialized host preferences, targeting significant agricultural pests.
8. Research and conservation needs: Continued research on the biology, life cycles, and host interactions of these families is essential for harnessing their potential in sustainable pest management and conservation efforts, ensuring ecological balance and agricultural productivity.

REFERENCES

Arafa, E., and Shestakov, L. (2020). Overview of tachinid parasitoids classification (Tachinidae, diptera). *Research on Crops*, 21(2), 415–423.

Arnaud Jr, P. H. (1978). *A Host-Parasite Catalog of North American Tachinidae (Diptera)*. Science and Education Administration, United States Department of Agriculture, Washington, D.C., p. 868.

Belshaw, R. (1993). Tachinid flies (Diptera: Tachinidae). In O'Hara, J. (ed.), *Handbooks for the Identification of British Insects*, vol. 10(4a). Royal Entomological Society, London, pp. 1–169.

Biliotti, E., Demolin, G., and Du Merle, P. (1965, January). Parasitisme de la Processionnaire du pin par Villa quinquefasciata Wied, apud Meig.(Dipt. Bombyliidae). Importance du comportement de ponte du parasite. *Annales des Epiphyties*, 16, 279–288.

Eggleton, P., and Gaston, K. J. (1990). "Parasitoid" species and assemblages: Convenient definitions or misleading compromises? *Oikos*, *59*, 417–421.

English-Loeb, G. M., Karban, R., and Brody, A. K. (1990). Arctiid larvae survive attack by a tachinid parasitoid and produce viable offspring. *Ecological Entomology*, 15(3), 361–362.

Evenhuis, N. L. (1994). Catalogue of the Bombyliidae (Diptera) of the Neotropical Region. *Contributions on Entomology, International*, 1(4), 1–382.

Evenhuis, N. L., and Greathead, D. J. (1999). World catalog of bee flies (Diptera: Bombyliidae). Revised September (2015). http://hbs.bishopmuseum.org/bombcat/

Feener Jr, D. H., and Brown, B. V. (1997). Diptera as parasitoids. *Annual Review of Entomology*, 42(1), 73–97.

Gibson, J. F., and Skevington, J. H. (2013). Phylogeny and taxonomic revision of all genera of Conopidae (Diptera) based on morphological data. *Zoological Journal of the Linnean Society*, 167, 43–81.

Gibson, J. F., and Skevington, J. H. (2014). Conopidae (Diptera). *Biodiversidad de Artrópodos Argentinos*, 4, 159–165.

Grenier, S. (1988). Applied biological control with tachinid flies (Diptera, Tachinidae): A review. *Anzeiger für Schädlingskunde, Pflanzenschutz, Um*weltschutz, 61, 49–56.

Hagen, K. S. (1964). *Developmental Stages of Parasites*. Paul Biological Control of Insect Pests and Weeds, DeBach.

Harris, V. E., and Todd, J. W. (1980). Male-mediated aggregation of male, female and 5th-instar southern green stink bugs 1 and concomitant attraction of a tachinid parasite, *Trichopodapennipes*. *Entomologia Experimentalis et Applicata*, 27(2), 117–126.

Hull, F. M. (1973). *Bee Flies of the World: The Genera of the Family Bombyliidae*. Smithsonian Institution Press, Washington, DC.

Kumar, P., Manjunath, D., Prasad, K. S., Kishore, R., Kumar, V., and Datta, R. K. (1993). Integrated management of the uzi fly, Exoristabombycis (Louis) (Diptera: Tachinidae), a parasitoid of the silkworm, Bombyx mori L. *International Journal of Pest Management*, 39(4), 445–448.

Maity, A., Mukhopadhyay, E., Naskar, A., Hazra, S., Sengupta, J., Parui, P., and Banerjee, D. (2020). A checklist of Indian big-headed flies (Insecta: Diptera: Pipunculidae). *Zootaxa*, 4732(1), 1–52.

Mitra, B., Roy, S., Halder, S. Bhaumik, S., Biwas, O., and Mallick, K. (2015). Current status of the thick-headed flies (Conopidae: Diptera) in India. *The Journal of Zoology Studies*, 2(4): 29–37.

Morehead, S. A., and Feener, D. H. (2000). Visual and chemical cues used in host location and acceptance by a dipteran parasitoid. *Journal of Insect Behavior*, 13, 613–625.

Narayanaswamy, T. K., and Govindan, R. (2000). Mulberry Silkworm Ujifly, Exoristabombycis (Louis) (Diptera: Tachinidae). *Integrated Pest Management Reviews*, 5, 231–240.

Neff, S. E., and Simpson, B. B. (1995). Phylogenetic analysis of Conopidae (Diptera) based on molecular and morphological characters. *Systematic Entomology*, 20(4), 359–383.

O'Hara, J. E. (2008). Tachinid flies (Diptera: Tachinidae). *Encyclopedia of Entomology*, 4, 3675–3586.

O'Hara, J. E. (2010). Review of tachinid fly diversity in the gila national forest, New Mexico. *Natural History of the Gila*, 32. *The New Mexico Botanist*, Special Issue No. 3, October 2012.

O'Hara, J. E., Henderson, S. J., and Wood, D. M. (2019). *Preliminary Checklist of the Tachinidae (Diptera) of the World*. Canadian National Collection of Insects, Agriculture and Agri-Food Canada, 960 Carling Avenue, Ottawa, Ontario, Canada, p. 681.

Otterstatter, M. C., Whidden, T. L., and Owen, R. E. (2002). Contrasting frequencies of parasitism and host mortality among phorid and conopid parasitoids of bumble-bees. *Ecological Entomology*, 27, 229–237.

Painter, R. H. (1932). The Bombyliidae of China and nearby regions. *Lingnan Science Journal*, 11, 341–74.

Pape, T. (1996). Catalogue of the Sarcophagidae of the world (Insecta: Diptera). *Mem Entomol Inter*, 8, 1–558.

Pape, T., and Arnaud, P. H. (2001). *The world Tachinidae (Diptera) Inventory*. Myia.

Rafael, J. A. (1998). The pipunculidae (diptera) of the neotropical region: An overview. *Journal of Natural History*, 32(6), 843–880.

Rafael, J. A., and De Meyer, M. (1992). Pipunculidae (Diptera) as parasitoids of leafhoppers (Homoptera: Cicadellidae) in Argentina. *Revista Brasileira de Entomologia*, 36(3), 573–576.

Rotheray, G. E., and Gilbert, F. (2011). *The Natural History of Hoverflies*. CABI Publishing.

Schmid-Hempel, P. (1998). *Parasites in Social Insects*. Princeton University Press, Princeton.

Schneider, M. A. (2010). A taxonomic revision of Australian Conopidae (Insecta: Diptera). *Zootaxa*, 2581, 1–246.

Schremmer, F. (1964). GezielterAbwurfgetarnterEierbeiWoUschweberr (Dipt. Bombyliidae). *Verh DtschZoolGes*, 27, 291–303.

Skevington, J. H. (2005). Pipunculidae (Diptera) and biological control: Life history, host specificity, and efficacy. *Biological Control*, 32(2), 177–186.

Skevington, J. H., and Marshall, S. A. (1998). Pipunculidae of North America: Keys to genera and species. *Memoirs of the Entomological Society of Canada*, 165, 1–143.

Smith, K. G. V. (1989). An introduction to the immature stages of British flies: Diptera larvae, with notes on eggs, puparia and pupae. *Handbooks for the Identification of British Insects*, 10(14), 1–280.

Stireman III, J. O., Dyer, L. A., and Greeney III, H. F. (2017). Specialised generalists? Food web structure of a tropical tachinid-caterpillar community. *Insect Conservation and Diversity*, 10(5), 367–384.

Stireman, J. O. et al. (2006). Tachinidae: Evolution, behavior, and ecology. *Annual Review of Entomology*, 51, 525–555.

Wiegmann, B. M., Trautwein, M. D., Winkler, I. S., Barr, N. B., Kim, J.-W., Lambkin, C., … and Yeates, D. K. (2011). Episodic radiations in the fly tree of life. *Proceedings of the National Academy of Sciences*, 108(14), 5690–5695.

Yeates, D. K., and Greathead, D. (1997). The evolutionary pattern of host use in the Bombyliidae (Diptera): A diverse family of parasitoid flies. *Biological Journal of the Linnean Society*, 60, 149–185.

Zoological Survey of India (2004). Fauna of Gujarat. *State Fauna Series*, 8(Part-2), 1–427.

7 Tachinid Flies

Ramya Ramesan Syamala, Karamankodu Jacob David, Shivakumara Kadanakuppe Thammayya, and Ranjith Mohanrao

LEARNING OBJECTIVES

1. Understand the ecological significance of the family Tachinidae within the context of herbivore population regulation in diverse ecosystems.
2. Explain the diversity of oviposition strategies exhibited by tachinids and their adaptations for enhancing oviposition success.
3. Analyse the factors influencing host selection by tachinids, including ecological cues and sensory signals.
4. Evaluate the dynamic interactions between tachinids and their hosts, including tritrophic relationships and coevolutionary processes.
5. Discuss the challenges and opportunities associated with utilizing tachinids in biological control programmes, including the need for improved rearing techniques.
6. Identify future research directions aimed at enhancing our understanding of tachinid parasitoid biology and improving their utilization in biological control strategies.

7.1 INTRODUCTION

The family Tachinidae is highly diverse and comprises around 10,000 species worldwide, making it one of the most speciose families of Diptera (Irwin et al., 2003). These flies share a common characteristic in that all tachinids whose life histories are known are parasitoids of insects and other arthropods. In terms of their ecological importance as insect parasitoids and diversity, they are second only to parasitic Hymenoptera (such as Chalcidoidea and Ichneumonoidea). Tachinids predominantly parasitize the larval stage of Lepidoptera and other major groups of insect herbivores (such as Symphyta, Chrysomelidae, Heteroptera, and Scarabaeidae), and they contribute significantly to regulating herbivore populations and structuring both natural and managed ecological communities. Around 100 species have been utilized in the biological control programmes targeting crop and forest pests, and a significant number of these initiatives have achieved varying degrees of success (Greathead, 1986; Grenier, 1988; Stireman et al., 2006). Nevertheless, the introduction of tachinids has also been associated with destructive consequences for nontarget organisms (Boettner et al., 2000).

Tachinids can be found in various terrestrial environments worldwide, such as deserts, forests, grasslands, mountains, and tundra. In certain habitats, they represent a significant proportion of the fly population. Moreover, they are recognized as a relatively recent and actively radiating group of insects, currently undergoing an evolutionary expansion (Crosskey, 1976). Despite their widespread presence, diversity, and ecological significance, our understanding of the evolutionary history, ecology, and behaviour of tachinids remains limited. Even fundamental biological knowledge regarding their hosts, mating systems, and habitat preferences is available for fewer than half of the species, particularly in the most extensively studied regions, such as Europe (Mellini, 1990). The majority of knowledge about tachinids has been derived from extensive research focused on their potential utilization in pest control within managed agricultural and forest environments (Grenier, 1988). However, due to their ecological significance as parasitoids of herbivorous insects in natural ecosystems, tachinids are gaining increasing interest among researchers in basic ecology

DOI: 10.1201/9781003482581-9

(Gentry and Dyer, 2002; Stireman and Singer, 2003). Recent attention has also been directed towards the exploration of novel host location mechanisms exhibited by certain species, which have significant implications for the coevolution of host–parasitoid interactions (e.g. phonotaxis in response to the sexual calls of Orthoptera by the tribe Ormiini) (Gray and Cade, 1999). Furthermore, in recent times, systematic analyses of morphology and molecular phylogenetic studies have emerged, offering initial insights into the evolutionary relationships, historical biogeography, and the evolutionary development of host associations among tachinids. These studies serve as a foundational step towards a better understanding of these aspects of tachinid behaviour and biology.

7.2 SYSTEMATIC POSITION

Traditional Diptera classifications divided the order into two suborders, primarily based on distinctions in antenna type and body morphology: "Nematocera" (thread-horned flies) and "Brachycera" (short-horned flies). In modern classifications, there is a shift towards adopting a phylogenetic system that identifies five major groups, referred to as infraorders or suborders: Bibionomorpha, Brachycera, Culicomorpha, Psychodomorpha, and Tipulomorpha. Brachycera is further divided into clades, "Orthorrhapha" and "Cyclorrhapha" (Yeates, 2002). There are two divisions in Cyclorrhapha, which are "Aschiza" and "Schizophora". Schizophora is subdivided into the firmly established, monophyletic "Calyptratae" (McAlpine, 1989, Yeates and Wiegmann, 1999), with the remaining taxa believed to constitute the potentially paraphyletic "Acalyptratae" (Hennig, 1971, Yeates and Wiegmann, 1999; Wiegmann et al., 2011). Oestroidea is one of the superfamilies that belong to Calyptratae, and it includes all the families characterized by a vertically aligned row of bristles on the meron. Tachinidae, along with other families like Calliphoridae, Mesemberenellidae, Mystacinobiidae, Oestridae, Rhinidae, Rhinophoridae, and Sarcophagidae, belong to this superfamily.

7.3 CHARACTERISTIC FEATURES

Tachinids, which belong to the superfamily Oestroidea along with other groups such as flesh flies (Sarcophagidae), bottle flies (Calliphoridae), and bot flies (Oestridae), are muscoid calyptrate Diptera. These flies display a remarkable range of morphologies. Their sizes vary greatly, spanning from tiny specimens of around 2 mm (e.g. *Siphona* spp.) to impressively large individuals exceeding 20 mm (e.g. *Trixodes obesus* Coquillett). Many tachinid species exhibit vibrant colours, incorporating yellow, black, orange, and/or red markings, possibly serving as a form of mimicry resembling aculeate Hymenoptera. Some tachinid species showcase striking metallic hues, including vivid greens, blues, and other shades (e.g. the visually captivating Australian Rutiliini), while others, particularly those in the diverse subfamily Exoristinae, are relatively small, with grey or blackish colours that may appear inconspicuous at first glance. However, upon closer examination, these seemingly nondescript forms reveal a remarkable diversity of morphologies and patterns. These variations represent notable radiations within the tachinid family, as observed in the tribes Blondeliini, Eryciini, and Voriini (Stireman et al., 2006).

Their subscutellum (including the postscutellum and infrascutellum) is notably well-developed, appearing convex on both the upper and lower halves when observed from the side, although *Bezzimyia* presents an exception to this pattern. Additionally, these flies possess meral bristles.

Larvae are endoparasitic, living inside the bodies of other insects and occasionally in centipedes. There are even some unpublished reports of them parasitizing spiders and scorpions. In the first instar larval stage, they have an elongated, hook-like or axe-shaped labrum that is fused with the cephalopharyngeal skeleton and extends from it as a continuation. Their mandibles (lateral plates) are either reduced in size or not recognizable, and they lack hooked apices. During the second and third instar stages, these larvae develop well-developed paired mandibles, similar to those of most calyptrate flies. Additionally, the posterior end of the developing larva is typically encased in a respiratory funnel formed from the host's hypodermis (McAlpine et al., 1987).

7.4 OVERVIEW OF THE BIOLOGY OF TACHINID FLIES

All tachinid species exclusively function as parasitoids, specifically as internal (endo) parasitoids of other arthropods. As is customary for parasitoids, tachinids generally kill their hosts, although there are occasional exceptions (English-Loeb et al., 1990). While many tachinids emerge from their hosts' pupal stage, there is no record of any species attacking the pupae or eggs of their hosts. The majority of tachinid species target larval hosts, but a notable portion, approximately 5%–10% of species, parasitizes adults. Larval development takes 1–3 weeks, except for species that enter diapause within the host, which can extend over several months. Depending on the tachinid species, larvae develop either individually or gregariously, and they either pupate within the deceased host or abandon the host to pupate in the soil litter.

In contrast to parasitic Hymenoptera, tachinids do not possess a primitive piercing ovipositor. Consequently, except for a few groups where piercing structures have evolved from modified sternites (such as most Phasiinae and many Blondeliini), tachinids must lay their eggs externally on or near the host, and the newly hatched larvae must find a way to enter the host. This absence of an ovipositor also prevents the injection of paralysing toxins, mutualistic polyDNA viruses, and other supplementary substances that immobilize the host and/or its immune system. As a result, tachinids are categorized as koinobiont parasitoids (Askew and Shaw, 1986). This means that they allow their host to continue feeding and growing while the tachinid larvae develop inside, instead of arresting the host's development, as idiobionts do.

Tachinids exhibit a broad range of host targets, comparable to that of the more diverse parasitic wasps (Eggleton and Belshaw, 1993). The most commonly targeted hosts include phytophagous insects, primarily Lepidoptera, Coleoptera (Scarabaeidae and Chrysomelidae), Hymenoptera (Symphyta), Heteroptera, and Orthoptera. However, tachinids also attack hosts in at least six additional insect orders, such as Blattodea, Dermaptera, Diptera, Embioptera, Mantodea, and Phasmida. Certain tachinid genera even parasitize non-insect arthropods, specifically centipedes (e.g. *Loewia* and *Eloceria*) and scorpions (Williams et al., 1990). While there is a single instance of tachinid parasitism on a spider (Vincent, 1985), this family's remarkable breadth of host utilization is accompanied by wide host ranges within certain tachinid species. While parasitic Hymenoptera with comparable life histories (koinobiont endoparasitoids) typically exhibit high specialization towards specific hosts, many tachinid species, in contrast, are polyphagous and have been observed to parasitize a wide range of hosts spanning multiple families (Eggleton and Gaston, 1992). At the most extreme end, the tachinid species *Compsilura concinnata* Meigen targets nearly 200 host species, spanning multiple families and even orders (Lepidoptera, Hymenoptera, and Coleoptera) (Arnaud, 1978). The significant diversity in host range observed among Tachinidae species presents an excellent opportunity for exploring the evolutionary processes, ecological impacts, and behavioural underpinnings associated with host specificity.

Adult tachinids exhibit a wide distribution across various habitats, including leaves, tree trunks, flowers, rocks, and the ground. They are generally diurnal or crepuscular and display high activity levels, although exceptions also exist. Limited knowledge exists regarding tachinid mating behaviour, apart from sexual aggregations in many species at specific sites, such as hilltops and tree trunks (Wood, 1987; Alcock and Smith, 1995). Some groups, such as Phasiinae and Tachinini are frequently seen on flowers and may potentially serve as pollinators for diverse plant taxa, although this aspect remains largely unexplored. An intriguing example involves a highly specific tachinid species that pollinates *Trichoceros* orchids through pseudocopulation, where the female tachinid, while mimicking flowers, attracts male tachinids for attempted copulation, inadvertently aiding in pollination by acquiring pollinia (Dodson, 1962). The significance of adult resources, such as nectar, salts, leaf exudates, or protein sources like pollen, remains poorly understood, as does the understanding of adult dispersal patterns.

7.5 EVOLUTIONARY HISTORY AND PHYLOGENETIC RELATIONSHIPS OF TACHINIDAE

Our understanding of the early history of Tachinidae remains limited because of the scarcity of fossils, uncertainties surrounding the sister group, the region of initial evolution, and the basal relationships within the family. Despite the potential for significant discoveries in this vast taxon, it has been relatively understudied compared to smaller families that are more conducive to global-scale phylogenetic investigations (Stireman et al., 2006).

Tachinidae is the largest family within the Oestroidea superfamily, which includes other families such as Calliphoridae, Mesemberenellidae, Mystacinobiidae, Oestridae, Rhinidae, Rhinophoridae, and Sarcophagidae. The relationships among these families have been investigated by various researchers, but a firmly supported phylogenetic tree has yet to be established (McAlpine, 1989; Pape, 1992; Rognes, 1997). The Rhinophoridae (McAlpine, 1989; Wood, 1987) and Sarcophagidae (Pape, 1992; Rognes, 1997) have been proposed as potential sister groups to the Tachinidae. In earlier catalogues, the rhinophorids were classified as a subfamily of Tachinidae (Sabrosky and Arnaud, 1965; Guimaraes, 1971), but they have since been universally recognized as a distinct family following Crosskey's comprehensive review of the group (Crosskey, 1977). Recently, phylogenetic relationships within the Tachinidae were reconstructed using four nuclear loci (7,800 bp) by Stireman et al. (2018). The analysis strongly supported the placement of the Polleniinae (earthworm-parasitizing flies, formerly classified in Calliphoridae s.l.) as the sister group to Tachinidae.

The fossil record of the entire Oestroid lineage is notably scarce and generally does not provide significant information regarding the origins of the Oestroidea or Tachinidae. The earliest potential fossil within this lineage consists of puparia found in Alberta, Canada, dating back to the Upper Cretaceous period. Initially classified as Calliphoridae (McAlpine, 1970), this specimen is currently classified beyond the Schizophora (Grimaldi and Cumming, 1999) without further placement. All other identified Oestroidea fossils are from the Eocene epoch or later, and the oldest tachinid fossil is described from an Eocene compression fossil discovered in the United States (Evenhuis, 1994).

The monophyly of the Tachinidae family is well-established based on two synapomorphies: a well-developed subscutellum in adult flies and the fusion of the labrum with the cephalopharyngeal skeleton in first instar larvae (Rognes, 1986; Wood, 1987; Pape, 1992; Tschorsnig and Richter, 1998). While all tachinid flies exhibit obligate endoparasitism of arthropods, this trait may not be a reliable indicator of their monophyletic relationship.

Initially, efforts to categorize the Tachinidae into genera, tribes, and subfamilies primarily relied on the outward characteristics of adult specimens. This approach was predominantly employed by the highly productive C.H.T. Townsend, who introduced 1,555 new species names and 1,491 new generic names for Tachinidae throughout his career from the 1880s to the 1940s (Arnaud, 1958). Unfortunately, the external features of tachinids exhibit significant homoplasy, and many early researchers, including Townsend, placed excessive importance on these traits when constructing their higher-level classifications (Richter, 1987).

Townsend's classification of the Tachinidae was further affected by his tendency to create monotypic genera, where each genus consisted of only one species. Consequently, the organization of the Neotropical Tachinidae continues to be heavily influenced by Townsend's classification (Guimaraes, 1971). The Neotropical region is characterized by an excessive number of insignificant and minuscule genera, making it extremely challenging to compare its fauna with the more cohesive classifications found in other regions (Crosskey, 1976; Crosskey, 1980; Cantrell and Crosskey, 1989; Herting and Dely-Draskovits, 1993; O'Hara and Wood, 2004).

Currently, most researchers acknowledge the existence of four subfamilies within the Tachinidae: Exoristinae, Dexiinae, Phasiinae, and Tachininae (Herting, 1984; Wood, 1987; Herting and Dely-Draskovits, 1993; Tschorsnig and Richter, 1998; O'Hara and Wood, 2004). This recognition is partly due to advancements in our understanding of tachinid relationships and also because of a shared preference for a provisional classification until a more refined one is proposed.

The challenges posed by the characteristics that misled Townsend and other early researchers still persist for modern systematists. However, the composition of the four Tachinidae subfamilies is not entirely arbitrary. The Dexiinae is widely accepted as monophyletic due to distinctive traits in the male genitalia (Tschorsnig, 1985; Wood, 1987; Richter, 1992). The Phasiinae consists of a morphologically diverse group of species historically united by their parasitism of Heteroptera (Crosskey, 1973). However, the monophyly of the Phasiinae has been primarily supported by a specific characteristic of the male genitalia (Richter, 1992; Tschorsnig, 1985). While certain features unite the majority of Exoristinae and Tachininae, neither group can be unequivocally demonstrated to be monophyletic based on morphological criteria alone. Nevertheless, Tschorsnig (1985) suggested that the Exoristinae are likely monophyletic, and Stireman (2002c) provided some molecular evidence supporting the potential monophyly of this subfamily.

The resolution of relationships between tachinid subfamilies is complicated by several factors, including the possible para- or polyphyly of the Exoristinae and Tachininae subfamilies. Another complicating factor is the interpretation of oviparity/ovolarviparity and egg morphology within the different subfamilies. The presumed primitive condition in the Tachinidae is oviparity, which involves the laying of unincubated eggs without appreciable embryonic development. Oviparity is found in all Exoristini and Winthemiini (both within Exoristinae), a few Blondeliini and Eryciini (also within Exoristinae), and all Phasiinae (excluding Eutherini and Strongygastrini) (O'Hara and Wood, 2004; Wood, 1987), along with possibly other unexamined groups.

On the other hand, the ovolarviparous condition, which involves the laying of incubated eggs containing well-developed larvae, is present in the remaining Exoristinae subfamily and all members of Dexiinae and Tachininae. The interpretation of the relationships among subfamilies is influenced by whether ovolarviparity is believed to have evolved once or multiple times. Wood (1985) argued that ovolarviparity is associated with complex modifications of the female reproductive system and likely evolved only once. However, other authors have proposed that ovolarviparity developed at least twice, primarily based on egg morphology. This disagreement in interpretation has led to different phylogenetic hypotheses:

- Herting (1966, 1983) postulated the following intersubfamily relationships: Phasiinae + Exoristinae and Tachininae + Dexiinae.
- Richter (1992) modified Herting's interpretation to: Phasiinae – (Exoristinae + (Tachininae + Dexiinae)).
- Shima (1989) proposed: Phasiinae + Dexiinae and Exoristinae + Tachininae.

According to Herting's scheme (1966, 1983), the Tachinidae diverged early into two lineages. One lineage, comprising Phasiinae + Exoristinae, is characterized by eggs with a thickened and convex upper surface and a membranous lower surface (referred to as a "planoconvex" egg in tachinid literature). The other lineage, comprising Tachininae + Dexiinae, is characterized by eggs that are essentially membranous throughout.

The understanding of tachinid tribes is still evolving, and ongoing research is leading to refinements and reorganization of these tribes based on improved knowledge of their phylogenetic relationships. However, systematic studies have primarily focused on genera and species, resulting in limited revisions of regional or global faunas at the tribal level in recent decades. Over the past 30 years, significant revisions have been made to various tachinid tribes. These revisions have involved the Rutiliini (Crosskey, 1973), Uramyini (Guimaraes, 1980), Blondeliini (Wood, 1985), Siphonini (Andersen, 1983; O'Hara, 1989; Andersen, 1996), Dexiini (Barraclough, 1992), Winthemiini (Shima, 1996), and Polideini (O'Hara, 2002) tribes. It is worth noting that the two large tribes, Goniini (within Exoristinae) and Siphonini (within Tachininae), are currently recognized as monophyletic (having a common ancestor), primarily based on internal structures. Goniini is characterized by the production of microtype eggs, while Siphonini is distinguished by having two spermathecae in females instead of the typical three found in most tachinids. The monophyly of many other tribes still requires investigation, and the classification of World Tachinidae at all taxonomic levels is particularly in need of modernization.

Advancements in the suprageneric classification of Tachinidae will greatly benefit from integrating information from various sources. These include studies of eggs (Gaponov, 2003), first instars (Townsend, 1934–42; Thompson, 1968; O'Hara, 1988; Richter and Farinets, 1984, 1987, 1990), puparia (Ziegler, 1998), female (Herting, 1957) and male terminalia (Tschorsnig, 1985; Verbeke, 1962), molecular sequences (Stireman, 2002c), and host associations (Guimaraes, 1977; Arnaud, 1978; Shima, 1999). Additionally, it is important to interpret the external morphology of adult tachinids with caution.

Recently, molecular phylogenetic studies conducted by Stireman et al. (2018) using four nuclear loci, such as 28S, CAD, MAC, and MCS, successfully identified each of the four tachinid subfamilies and most recognized tribes, though exceptions were noted in the Dexiinae and Tachininae. Notably, the tachinine tribes Macquartiini and Myiophasiini formed a clade sister to all other Tachinidae, and a clade of Palpostomatini was reconstructed as sister to Dexiinae+Phasiinae. While many nodes received strong support, poorly resolved relationships were observed in lineages that underwent rapid episodes of diversification, such as basal Dexiinae and Tachininae, as well as Blondeliini. The reconstruction of host use evolution yielded equivocal results, but overall, it lent support to the hypothesis that the ancestral host of tachinids was a beetle. Subsequent host shifts to caterpillars may have coincided with accelerated diversification. Evolutionary reconstructions of reproductive strategy showed that the most probable scenario is that ancestral tachinids possessed unincubated, thick-shelled eggs, with incubated eggs evolving repeatedly, potentially expanding available host niches.

7.6 SPECIES DIVERSITY AND GEOGRAPHIC DISTRIBUTION

Tachinidae, a family of flies (Diptera), boasts a global presence and is considered one of the largest families within its order. The distribution of Tachinidae across various regions is detailed in Table 7.1, which summarizes tachinid species and genera in various biogeographic regions, along with the number and percentage of genera that are endemic to each region.

However, the actual number of species may be significantly higher than reported figures due to incomplete documentation. While the faunas of the Palearctic and Nearctic regions (Europe, North America, etc.) are relatively well-known, making up about 90% of documented faunas, the Neotropical region (Central and South America) stands out with a substantial number of described species, which is likely just a fraction of its true diversity, as numerous unidentified specimens continue to be found in collections. Moreover, the faunas of the Afrotropical (Africa), Oriental (Asia), and Australasian (Australia and neighbouring islands) regions are also underestimated and require further study to uncover their hidden richness. For instance, Australia, despite having nearly 500 described species (Cantrell and Crosskey, 1989) is believed to harbour a tachinid fauna of around 3,500–4,000 species (O'Hara et al., 2004). Considering the limited understanding of Tachinidae

TABLE 7.1
Distribution of Tachinid Genera and Species by Biogeographic Region (O'Hara and Henderson, 2020)

Number	World	Neotropical	Nearctic	Palaearctic	Afrotropical	Oriental	Australasian
Species	8,592	3,088	1,305	2,112	1,130	1,222	891
Genera	1,477	784	305	416	234	262	231
Endemic genera	1,053	595	52	141	104	37	124
Generic endemicity	–	76%	17%	34%	44%	14%	54%

worldwide, it is plausible that only half of the total species have been formally described, leaving ample room for future discoveries.

The geographic distribution of Tachinidae aligns with its sparse fossil record, which lacks evidence of an existence before the Tertiary period. If there was an earlier origin, it might be evident through sister group relationships among Southern Hemisphere tachinids, implying vicariance of ancient faunas during the late Cretaceous or early Cenozoic era. Such relationships would likely manifest at the generic level. However, no genera are exclusive to South America, Africa, and Australia, or to South America and Australia (Table 7.1). There is one genus, *Anacamptomyia*, known only from the Afrotropical and Australasian regions, but this apparent disjunction remains understudied, and the tachinid fauna of the intervening Oriental region is inadequately explored. Although Cortes (1983) suggested a relationship between the South American tribe Trichoprosopini and the New Zealand tribe Occisorini, this connection lacks thorough investigation from a phylogenetic standpoint. The region of origin of Tachinidae cannot be inferred from the available evidence. From a zoogeographic perspective, Tachinidae have radiated extensively worldwide. The faunas of neighbouring regions exhibit considerable overlap in generic composition (Table 7.1), and all regions harbour diverse major lineages. Nonetheless, each region also supports a significant endemic tachinid fauna.

7.7 DIVERSITY IN OVIPOSITION STRATEGIES AND EGG MORPHOLOGY

The wide array of oviposition strategies and associated egg morphologies in tachinids is one of their most remarkable characteristics. These strategies have been extensively discussed in the literature, and egg morphologies have undergone classification under various schemes (Townsend, 1911; Clausen, 1940; Wood, 1987; Belshaw, 1994; Tschorsnig and Richter, 1998). Notably, a significant division exists between species employing direct oviposition (laying eggs on the host) and those adopting indirect oviposition (laying eggs away from the host).

The direct oviposition category can be further subdivided based on whether eggs are laid externally or injected into the host, and whether the eggs undergo incubation (ovolarvipary) within a uterus, containing fully developed larvae upon deposition, or not (ovipary). Taxa belonging to Phasiinae, Exoristiini, Winthemiini, some Blondeliini, and *Aplomya* (Eryciini) lay eggs externally, but they are not incubated. Affixing an underdeveloped egg onto the host's skin is the most basic method of attacking an exposed host. This egg is relatively large, with an oval shape that is plano-convex, initially appearing translucent upon oviposition but later becoming white and conspicuous as it dries. Its flat ventral side is coated with a sticky substance, ensuring secure attachment to any part of the host's body. The embryo developing within this egg relies on numerous minute pores referred to as aeropyles, which are clustered at both ends of the egg. Upon reaching maturity and preparing to hatch, the larva follows one of two paths: it either dislodges the cap or operculum from the egg's anterior end and burrows into the host in front of it, or directly tunnels into the host through the egg's base. The species employing this egg deposition strategy lack a uterus, or ovisac, for retaining eggs in various stages of embryonic development. Consequently, these eggs exhibit minimal or no embryonic development and are described as unembryonated. Eggs left on the host's skin to undergo embryonic development remain vulnerable for an extended period. During this interval, they may be consumed by the host or misplaced when the host undergoes molting.

Numerous adaptations have emerged in specific taxa, like Phasiinae and Exoristiinae (e.g. Phorocera), to enhance the efficiency of larvae hatching and their subsequent entry into the host, thus enabling them to avoid the challenges outlined above. A departure from the basic placement of the planoconvex egg on the host's skin involves modifications to the female's abdominal sternites, facilitating the partial or complete insertion of unincubated eggs into the host's body. The genus *Phorocera* has devised mechanisms to partially or entirely embed their unembryonated eggs into the host's skin (Herting, 1983, Wood, 1972). While a few phasiines, like *Gymnosoma* and

Trichopoda, adhere planoconvex eggs to the surfaces of their hemipteran hosts, the abdominal sternites of most female Phasiinae have also developed intricate piercing structures to introduce their unembryonated eggs into their hosts.

Some genera employ distinct strategies to enable them to parasitize hosts that exhibit excessive aggressiveness, possess natural defences such as spines, hairs, or webbing, or are concealed and out of reach for adult flies. Perhaps the most significant advancement in their reproductive strategy, shared by the overwhelming majority of Tachinidae, involves the practice of storing eggs within an ovisac until the completion of embryonic development. The ovisac essentially serves as an expanded and elongated version of the common oviduct, equipped with an enhanced tracheal supply to ensure a sufficient oxygen supply for the maturing larvae. Consequently, a single female has the capacity to carry hundreds or even thousands of eggs, with those farthest from the ovaries poised to hatch upon deposition. In contrast to members of the Sarcophagidae family, which are entirely viviparous (meaning that eggs hatch within the female and active larvae are laid on the substrate), all Tachinidae species seem to follow an ovolarviparous approach, with eggs hatching after they have been laid. Occasionally, if a female perishes before her offspring, the larvae may subsequently hatch and emerge from her abdomen. In many species, however, eggs can hatch within moments of deposition, creating the illusion of larviparity. The advantage of swift hatching after oviposition is self-evident; the larva can immediately commence its penetration into the host.

Taxa belonging to Eryciini (Exoristinae), most Blondeliini, Voriini, and Strongygastrini exhibit an ovipositional strategy in which eggs are laid externally and undergo incubation. There are other taxa, such as Blondeliini (e.g. *Blondelia* and *Eucelatoria*) and Dexiinae (Palpostomatini), which inject incubated eggs into the host.

Meanwhile, taxa displaying indirect oviposition can be classified into two major groups: ovolarviparous species, where larvae hatch soon after egg-laying and either await passing hosts (e.g. many Tachininae) or actively search for suitable hosts (e.g. Dexiini), and species possessing "microtype" eggs. The details of all the above strategies are described in detail below.

An extensive category of species, which encompasses the majority of the Tachininae, employs a strategy of dispersing their eggs in locations that are likely to be frequented by their hosts. Typically, these locations are on food plants that have already suffered some form of damage. The larvae that hatch from these eggs adopt a patient approach, lying in wait until they can attach themselves to a suitable host that passes by and then burrow into it. To combat the risk of drying out, these larvae are equipped with tiny sclerites that interlock, creating a protective covering resembling a suit of armour. It is not surprising that this particular group of Tachininae boasts the broadest range of hosts, many of which are concealed during daylight hours. These hosts encompass a variety of organisms, including Orthoptera, Dermaptera, Embioptera, and Lepidoptera, as well as Chilopoda and Arachnida.

Within the Dexiini tribe, a similar strategy is employed whereby their eggs are widely dispersed. However, the hatched larvae take a different approach by burrowing into the substrate on which they were originally laid. This substrate can be soil, decaying wood, or even the excrement (frass) of the host if the host happens to be a burrower or miner. Once they have entered the substrate, the larvae actively search for their prospective host. A few genera within the Goniinae also utilize this method. For instance, newly hatched larvae belonging to *Lixophaga* and *Lydella* have been known to successfully parasitize wood and stem borers by depositing their eggs near openings created by the host. Subsequently, the first larval stage burrows through the host's frass to make direct contact.

The majority of potential hosts avoid direct attacks from ovipositing tachinids by adopting a strategy of remaining inaccessible during daylight hours when females are active. These potential hosts either take refuge in litter or soil, or they protect themselves with webbing. By doing so, they manage to evade direct contact with adult flies, which are primarily active during the day. Instead, they seek food at night, a time when the flies are less active and less likely to locate and parasitize them (McAlpine et al., 1987). Within Goniini and Blondeliini (e.g. *Anisia* and *Phasmophaga*), a clever solution has emerged to tackle the challenge of inaccessible hosts. This solution involves the production of tiny eggs designed for consumption by the host, referred to as "microtype eggs". Remarkably, these minute eggs manage to evade the host's mandibles, hatching within the foregut upon stimulation by digestive enzymes. Subsequently, they bore through the gut wall and enter the host's circulatory system, known as the haemocoel. In this scenario, all the fly needs to do is locate recently damaged foliage a suitable food plant and deposit its eggs there. This somewhat serendipitous approach, however, requires the deposition of a substantial number of eggs (McAlpine et al., 1987).

These diverse oviposition strategies have evolved in conjunction with host-searching and attack tactics, changes in fecundity, and the types of hosts targeted. As expected, indirect egg-laying species tend to exhibit high fecundities, sometimes numbering in the thousands of eggs, due to the higher likelihood of successful parasitization, while direct egg-layers typically have more moderate fecundities (Stireman et al., 2006).

It is intriguing that tachinids display a nearly equal distribution of taxonomic diversity across oviposition strategies. For instance, approximately 40% of Palearctic species adopt indirect modes of oviposition (Belshaw, 1994). Notably, the Tachinini (indirect "waiters"), Dexiini (indirect "searchers"), and Goniini (microtype) tribes rank among the most species-rich groups within Tachinidae. Moreover, these oviposition strategies might have been acquired or lost multiple times throughout the course of tachinid evolution.

Considering that nearly half of all tachinid species engage in indirect oviposition (Eggleton and Gaston, 1992), these strategies appear to be crucial innovations in the evolution of tachinids. Since tachinids typically target the active life stages of their hosts and lack paralytic poisons to subdue them, the hosts' behavioural and morphological defences can pose significant obstacles to oviposition. Host defences, such as biting, thrashing, stinging hairs or spines, and gregarious behaviour, may have initially driven the development of indirect oviposition strategies and facilitated the diversification of tachinid species employing these strategies. Moreover, the diurnal habits of most tachinid species and the absence of specialized ovipositors (unlike those in Hymenoptera) likely limited their access to concealed and/or nocturnal hosts during the early stages of their evolution. The emergence of host-searching first instars capable of burrowing through soil or into the galleries of concealed insects, as well as larvae that ambush nocturnally feeding caterpillars on their host plants, and microtype eggs that can be ingested by nocturnal or well-defended hosts, expanded the range of vulnerable hosts for tachinids to exploit. These innovations potentially opened up extensive adaptive opportunities for tachinids to colonize. However, it is important to note that most microtype Goniini and many Tachininae attack hosts that are seemingly accessible to direct oviposition (i.e. diurnal exophytic Lepidoptera). Thus, although indirect oviposition may have frequently been used to target inaccessible hosts, it could also be viewed as a strategy to reduce search time, handling time, and the potential for injuries associated with oviposition (Stireman and Singer, 2003).

7.8 EVOLUTIONARY PATTERNS OF HOST ASSOCIATIONS

Tachinids exploit a diverse range of hosts from various insect orders and families, as well as a few other arthropods. While some general associations of tachinid taxa with specific host orders and families have been identified, the host associations within the Tachinidae family are evolutionarily flexible, often showing significant variation even among closely related species. Most regions have documented detailed host associations of tachinid taxa (Herting, 1960; Crosskey, 1973; Crosskey, 1976; Guimaraes, 1977; Arnaud, 1978; Belshaw, 1993; Shima, 1999). Notable examples of strict associations include Phasiinae primarily parasitizing heteropterous hosts and Rutiliini being restricted to scarab hosts. Other broad associations involve Dexiini using Scarabaeidae as hosts, while most Tachininae and Exoristinae (including Voriini of Dexiinae) parasitizing Lepidoptera, and Ormiini target Orthoptera as hosts.

Most tachinids primarily target external caterpillars or other larvae of holometabolous insects that share ecological and morphological similarities with caterpillars, such as larval sawflies and chrysomelid beetles (Eggleton and Belshaw, 1992). The prevalence of these insects as hosts for tachinids can be attributed to their habit of feeding on the exterior of plants, relatively weak physical defenses, taxonomic diversity, suitable size, and notably, their specialized relationships with plants. Generally, the most diverse clades of parasitoids, including Tachinidae, Chalcidoidea, and Ichneumonoidea, tend to attack predominantly phytophagous insects, and the interactions between plants, phytophagous insects, and parasitoids may significantly influence the diversification of both herbivores and parasitoids. Plants indirectly affect parasitoids by facilitating their host location and serving as defensive mechanisms for herbivores (e.g. through sequestered secondary compounds). Consequently, this should lead to increased specialization and foster diversification among parasitoids. To comprehensively comprehend the patterns of tachinid host selection at both microevolutionary and macroevolutionary scales, it is crucial to explicitly consider the tritrophic framework involving host plants, herbivores, and tachinids.

7.8.1 Glimpse of the Host Range of Tachinids

At least eight different orders of insects, in addition to centipedes, act as hosts for tachinids. It is likely that the larvae of Lepidoptera are the major hosts for the Tachinidae family, with most species being associated with this group, especially within the vast subfamilies of Tachininae and Goniinae. When it comes to true bugs, specifically Pentatomidae, Coreidae, Nabidae, and Lygaeidae, they are primarily subject to parasitism by the Phasiinae subfamily. Interestingly, some exotic phasiines possess highly intricate egg-laying mechanisms. However, because all phasiines deposit unembryonated eggs or inject them, it is generally believed that this subfamily represents one of the more primitive groups within the Tachinidae family.

Various genera of tachinids utilize both adult and larval Coleoptera as their hosts. The first instars of Dexiini actively search for larvae belonging to Scarabaeidae, Cerambycidae, and Elateridae, which are typically found buried in soil or decaying wood. Adult scarabs, on the other hand, face attacks from members of the Palpostomatini tribe and also from the Blondeliine genus *Cryptomeigenia*. Carabidae adults can be parasitized by species of *Zaira* and *Freraea*. The first instars of *Cryptomeigenia* and *Zaira* possess serrated teeth along the anterior edge of their labrum, which presumably aids in cutting through the resilient cuticle of their hosts. Additionally, *Zaira eleodivora* (Walton) has been documented as emerging from tenebrionids, a beetle group renowned for their sturdy exoskeleton. The Chrysomelidae, both in their adult and larval stages, face significant parasitic pressure from various members of the Blondeliini tribe. Weevil larvae concealed within roots, stems, fruits, or nuts are actively sought out by the burrowing first instars of *Gnadochaeta*. Adult weevils, while feeding, can also be parasitized through their oral cavity by female *Rondania*.

Orthopteroid orders also serve as hosts for a diverse range of genera. One well-documented case involves the Acemyiini, which lay embryonated eggs directly onto grasshoppers. Among these, the tachinine genera *Ormia* and *Glaurocara* are known to be crepuscular or nocturnal, practising ovolarviposition on or near long-horned grasshoppers and crickets belonging to the Gryllidae, Gryllotalpidae, and Tettigoniidae families (Crosskey, 1965, Cade, 1975). Interestingly, female *Ormia* exhibit an attraction to the songs of singing males and can be drawn to an appropriate host's call notes (Cade, 1975). Meanwhile, species of the Blondeliine genus *Anisia* deposit incredibly small, fully embryonated eggs, each enclosed within a gelatinous capsule, on potential food sources of crickets and cave crickets.

While larvae of Diptera have generally avoided parasitism by tachinids, there are exceptions involving the larvae of Tipulidae and Tabanidae, both of which are known to dwell in soil and are frequent hosts for certain genera. Tipulid larvae encounter attacks from species of *Admontia* and *Siphona*, which seem to specifically target the exposed spiracular plates of their hosts, depositing their embryonated eggs directly on them. They are also targeted by members of *Allophorocera*, which lay microtype eggs, presumably when tipulid larvae are actively feeding. Additionally,

Phasiops flavus Coquillett and three species of *Billaea* have been successfully reared from *Tabanus* and *Hybomitra* larvae (Hayes, 1958; Teskey, 1969).

Among the Hymenoptera, various genera of tachinids have been discovered emerging from the leaf-feeding larvae of sawflies. Tachinids parasitize only a few other Hymenoptera species, including adult ants that fall victim to *Strongygaster globula* (Meigen). Additionally, colonial wasps suffer from infestations by members of the *Ophirion* genus and a *Lixophaga* species. In the case of *Ophirion*, it is presumed that they lay fully developed eggs near the entrances of the nests, allowing their newly hatched larvae to find their way to the brood chambers independently. In the Afrotropical, Oriental, and Australian regions, social wasps also experience parasitism by tachinid genera belonging to the Anacamptomyiini tribe (Crosskey 1973, 1976, 1980). Notably, all of these species that parasitize wasps exhibit a pale colouration, a characteristic commonly seen in various crepuscular and nocturnal tachinids. It is possible that they avoid their hosts' defenses by laying eggs during or after dusk.

Hyperparasitism involving one tachinid species attacking another tachinid species does not seem to have been documented previously. Nevertheless, instances of hyperparasitism have been documented in Japan, where tachinids, specifically *Nemorilla floralis* (Fallen) and *Bessa selecta* (Meigen), were observed hyperparasitizing an ichneumonid, *Cephaloglypta laricis* Momoi (Kamijo, 1973).

7.8.2 How Tachinids Manage to Have a Wide Host Range?

The variability in host use among most Tachinidae species may be attributed to their lack of specific adaptations to counter host physiological defenses. Larval tachinids are renowned for creating respiratory funnels using host defensive cells. Unlike many hymenopteran parasitoids that evade or destroy host hematocytes (Strand and Pech, 1995), tachinids often utilize them to form "breathing tubes". These structures allow many tachinids to have direct access to atmospheric air through their posterior spiracles, either via the host's external integument or major tracheal branches (Clausen, 1940). By capitalizing on the immune response and forming respiratory funnels, tachinids might gain flexibility in "exploring" new hosts, leading to dynamic evolution and diversification of host associations. This idea is supported by the observation that tachinids without respiratory funnels, free in the hemocoel, exhibit narrower host ranges compared to the family average.

Moreover, tachinids may possess relative tolerance to toxins actively or inadvertently consumed by their hosts, enabling broader evolutionary adaptability in host selection (Gauld et al., 1992; Mallampalli et al., 1996). This tolerance could be linked to preadaptations stemming from the ancestral saprophagous habits of the Oestroidea (Eggleton and Gaston, 1992). The larvae of Oestroidea, having dealt with highly toxic environments produced by bacteria and fungi, might have accumulated adaptations to endure these toxins. Additionally, the apparent tolerance of tachinids to host physiological defenses could also be related to the positioning of young larvae within the host. Instead of floating freely in the hemocoel, many early larval stages of tachinids embed themselves in specific tissues (Belshaw, 1994). For instance, *C. concinnata*, a highly polyphagous species, undergoes most of its larval development in the gut, between the peritrophic membrane and gut wall (Ichiki and Shima, 2003).

The notion that tachinids can overcome host physiological defenses through the formation of respiratory funnels, adaptations to toxic environments, or "hiding" in specific tissues has also been used to explain why many tachinid species have wide host ranges (Belshaw, 1994). Some tachinids, such as *C. concinnata, Exorista mella* (Walker), and *Lespesia aletiae* (Riley), exhibit unusually polyphagous behaviour by attacking numerous host species from different families. Notably, when analysing host records of Palearctic species, Eggleton and Gaston (1992) and Belshaw (1994) found a strong correlation between the number of tachinid rearings and the number of hosts, suggesting widespread polyphagy within Tachinidae. Consequently, this has led to a general perception that most, if not all, tachinids are polyphagous.

Tachinids possess several distinctive characteristics that enable them to have a wide range of host species. One such trait is their external oviposition strategy, which allows them to lay eggs on or near the host without exposing them to the host's immune defenses. Additionally, tachinid larvae develop rapidly, which may promote polyphagy, where they feed on multiple host species. While it was initially thought that species with indirect oviposition would have broader host ranges (Belshaw, 1994), specific tachinid–host communities have not supported this idea. Indirect ovipositing tachinids still demonstrate selectivity by depositing offspring on specific substrates, using fresh feeding damage by hosts as a cue for oviposition, and visually or otherwise locating hosts to lay eggs nearby. Interestingly, polyphagous tachinids are found across different lineages, often coexisting with genera that primarily consist of specialized species. This indicates that host range is not strictly conserved and is not closely linked to specific oviposition strategies or other major traits within the Tachinidae family. Consequently, tachinids offer a valuable opportunity to investigate the controversial hypothesis that host specialization drives diversification in parasitic insects.

7.8.3 Discovering Hosts and Determining Host Compatibility

In contrast to many hymenopteran parasitoids (Vinson and Iwantsch, 1980), tachinids do not appear to be significantly constrained by the physiological compatibility or defences of their potential hosts. Tachinids generally find most hosts physiologically acceptable, even though the so-called generalist tachinids utilize only a small fraction of the available hosts. One recurring observation regarding tachinid–host connections is that the hosts tachinids select seem to be more closely linked to ecological factors, such as habitat preferences, rather than to their evolutionary relationships (Belshaw, 1994; Crosskey, 1980; Eggleton and Gaston, 1992; Feener and Brown, 1997). Tachinids rely on relatively specific cues to locate suitable host habitats, such as host plant volatiles (Roland et al., 1995). Once in the appropriate habitat, they utilize relatively general cues to find and choose their hosts. Consequently, the processes of locating and selecting hosts, which govern immediate host choices, may ultimately shape broader ecological and evolutionary patterns of host utilization. This suggests that the cues guiding host selection determine which hosts are targeted, rather than the conventional perspective that the host itself dictates the cues used to locate it.

7.8.4 Selecting and Locating Hosts

The processes through which most tachinids locate and choose their hosts are not thoroughly understood. There is notably limited information available for species where the adult tachinids do not directly come into contact with the host. The available data from the small portion of species that have been studied suggests that tachinids can utilize a wide range of sensory cues, including olfactory, visual, auditory, and tactile chemosensory signals, in their host location efforts. For example, *C. concinnata* employs visual cues and the motion signals of its host, *Lymantria dispar* (Linnaeus), to locate it, whereas *Lixophaga diatraeae* (Townsend) utilizes a chemosensory approach, relying on the frass produced by its host, *Diatraea saccharalis* (Fabricius), for location (Roth et al., 1978; Weseloh, 1980). Other tachinid species, such as *Eucelatoria bryani* Sabrosky, *Drino bohemica* Mesnil *Exorista japonica* (Townsend), *E. mella*, *Cyzenis albicans* (Fallén), *Leschenaultia exul* (Townsend), and *Patelloa pachypyga* (Aldrich & Webber), employ an olfactory mode to detect cues from plant volatiles, helping them locate their respective hosts (Monteith, 1955; Hassell, 1968; Herrebout and vanden Veer, 1969; Roland et al., 1989, 1995; Martin et al., 1990; Mondor and Roland, 1997; Kainoh et al., 1999; Stireman, 2002a). There are also instances of tachinid species, like *Hemyda aurata* Robineau-Desvoidy, *Gymnoclytia occidentalis* Townsend, *Euclytia flava* (Townsend), and *Trichopoda pennipes* (Fabricius), relying on their olfactory senses to detect male pheromones emitted by their respective hosts for locating them (Harris and Todd, 1980; Aldrich and Zhang, 2002; Krupke and Brunner, 2003). Some tachinid species, like *Homotrixa alleni* Barraclough, *Ormia ochracea* (Bigot), and *Therobia leonidei* (Mesnil), make use of the auditory mode to locate the host through their sexual calls (Cade, 1975; Walker, 1993; Allen, 1995; Allen et al., 1999; Lehmann and Heller, 1998).

A closer look at these host location mechanisms reveals that many tachinids heavily rely on chemical signals originating from host plants, which are inhabited by their phytophagous insect hosts, or signals generated during interactions between the hosts and these plants (Monteith, 1955; Mondor and Roland, 1997; Roland et al., 1989). These cues appear to serve the purpose of attracting tachinids to the specific habitats or microenvironments where their hosts reside. Once in proximity to the hosts, more reliable close-range cues are employed to detect the presence of the host or signs of its presence. These close-range cues encompass scents directly associated with the host, substances produced by the host, like secretions or excretions (particularly frass), and visual identification of the hosts.

Several studies have demonstrated that female tachinids display oviposition behaviour in response to tactile chemosensory cues linked to the host's outer covering (cuticle), recently damaged leaves, and/or the presence of host frass (Burks and Nettles, 1978; Roth et al., 1978; Mondor and Roland, 1998). In these instances, females utilize chemosensory receptors located on their front tarsi, which might function similarly to the chemosensory receptors found on the long antennae of many hymenopteran parasitoids. This possibly explains behaviours like the "drumming" of tarsi on the host, which has been reported in *Exorista* species (Stireman, 2002b; Tanaka et al., 1999).

The utilization of visual cues appears to be a fundamental aspect of host identification and choice in numerous tachinids (Monteith, 1956; Stireman, 2002a; Stireman, 2002b; Weseloh, 1980; Yamawaki et al., 2002). In general, higher Diptera possess highly developed visual systems, particularly when it comes to detecting motion (Buschbeck and Strausfeld, 1997). This characteristic may have predisposed Tachinidae to depend on visual cues for locating and selecting hosts. Observable cues, such as volatile compounds linked to plants or plant damage, might act as attractants for female tachinids, drawing them to specific habitats. Once in these habitats, it is conceivable that many tachinids heavily rely on visually identifying host movement, which could lead to broad host preferences within a given habitat and potentially prompt swift evolutionary shifts in host selection.

One remarkable method employed by tachinids, which has garnered considerable attention in recent years, involves their phonotactic attraction to the mating calls of crickets and other Orthoptera. This behaviour is predominantly observed in tachinids belonging to the Ormiini tribe within the Tachininae subfamily (Cade, 1975; Walker, 1993; Muller and Robert, 2002). A well-documented example is the species *O. ochracea*, which conducts nocturnal host searches. This species possesses an "ear" located between its fore coxae, enabling it to detect and locate male crickets emitting mating calls, after which it proceeds to deposit eggs (Cade, 1975; Robert et al., 1996). Similar tactics are employed by other tachinid species when targeting nocturnal hosts that produce songs, such as katydids (Tettigoniidae) (Allen, 1995) and mole crickets (Gryllotalpidae) (Frank et al., 1996). This host-finding strategy is particularly intriguing because it creates a dilemma for male crickets: they simultaneously attract potential mates and potentially lethal parasitoids. Such conflicting pressures stemming from sexual selection and natural selection may lead to robust co-evolutionary interactions between ormiine tachinids and their host organisms (Zuk and Kolluru, 1998).

A similar utilization of sexual signals by tachinids has been reported in several members of the subfamily Phasiinae, which parasitize Heteroptera (Harris and Todd, 1980; Aldrich and Zhang, 2002). Tachinids, like *T. pennipes,* employ the volatile sexual pheromones emitted by their heteropteran hosts as cues for host detection through chemotaxis (Harris and Todd, 1980). In at least one instance, *E. flava*, it seems that the tachinid species consists of concealed "pheromone races" with varying sensitivity to specific pheromone components associated with different host species; sometimes even more sensitive than the hosts themselves (Aldrich and Zhang, 2002). Similar to the situation observed in Ormiini hosts, the conflicting selection pressures related to attracting mates and avoiding parasitoids may give rise to co-evolutionary "arms races". In these dynamics, hosts are continually selected to produce sexual signals that are unappealing to tachinids but attractive to potential mates (referred to as "new codes"), while tachinids are consistently selected to become more sensitive to these signals (referred to as "code-breakers"). Repetitive cycles of these interactions can potentially facilitate the process of speciation and the evolutionary diversification of both host and parasitoid. The reliance on host pheromones for host location likely extends widely within the Phasiinae, and this mechanism may have played a pivotal role in their evolutionary proliferation on heteropteran hosts.

7.9 INTERACTIONS BETWEEN TACHINIDS AND THEIR HOSTS IN ECOLOGICAL CONTEXT

The roles of tachinids as adversaries of native herbivores and their broader impacts on the structure and dynamics of natural ecosystems have remained largely unexplored. However, findings from various extensive caterpillar-rearing initiatives that concentrated on exophytic macrolepidoptera have revealed that tachinid-induced mortality is frequently on par with or even exceeds that caused by hymenopteran parasitoids. To illustrate, tachinids were accountable for over half of the caterpillar mortality attributed to insect parasitoids in rearing experiments conducted across diverse ecosystems, including the deserts of the southwestern United States (Stireman and Singer, 2003), forests in the northeastern United States (Sheehan, 1994), tropical dry forests in Costa Rica (Janzen, 1981), and tropical wet forests in Costa Rica (Gentry and Dyer, 2002).

Several associations between host characteristics and tachinid parasitism or diversity have been observed, with some of these patterns appearing consistent across various ecosystems. For instance, analyses from extensive caterpillar-rearing programmes conducted by Sheehan (1994) and Stireman and Singer (2003) have indicated that abundant, social, and host plant generalist caterpillars tend to be targeted by a higher number of tachinid species compared to their rarer, specialized, or solitary counterparts. Both studies proposed that this trend is linked to the process of locating suitable hosts. Additionally, Stireman and Singer (2003) noted that hairy caterpillars tend to host larger tachinid populations than smooth caterpillars. This observation, coupled with positive correlations between tachinid parasitism and traits, like gregariousness and shelter-building among caterpillars, has been used as evidence supporting the notion that the concept of "enemy-free space" (Jeffries and Lawton, 1984) may play a significant role in shaping tachinid host preferences (Gentry and Dyer, 2002; Stireman and Singer, 2003). In other words, hosts that possess strong defenses against predators might be particularly attractive to tachinid parasitoids, as these hosts reduce the risk of an immature parasitoid being consumed by a predator.

In-depth ecological investigations into the spatial distribution of parasitism have also uncovered that tachinids exhibit significant responses to the spatial layout of habitats or host plants (Cappuccino et al., 1998; Doak, 2000). A notable illustration of this phenomenon is found in the research conducted by Roland and Taylor (1997). These researchers demonstrated that the level of parasitism by three tachinid species and a pupal parasitoid from the sarcophagid family, targeting the forest tent caterpillar (*Malacosoma disstria* Hubner), varies markedly in response to forest structure. Larger-bodied parasitoids were found to be more sensitive to forest structure, and they were less likely to parasitize hosts in smaller fragments of forest. Based on these findings, the authors inferred that forest fragmentation could disrupt the regulation of host populations by this tachinid community.

Moreover, a study focusing on the insect community associated with a bracket fungus in old-growth forests also highlights a strong correlation between parasitism and habitat structure (Komonen et al., 2000). The primary parasitoid within this ecological chain, *Phytomyptera cingulata* (Robineau-Desvoidy), exhibited a decline in frequency as the age of forest fragments decreased and was entirely absent from the oldest fragments (ranging from 12–32 years). Given that tachinids occupy higher trophic levels and may be relatively sensitive to the structure and composition of their habitat, they (along with other parasitoids) could serve as valuable indicators of ecosystem health.

7.10 TRITROPHIC RELATIONSHIPS – EXPLORING THE COMPLEX WEB OF THREE LEVELS

The frequent observation that the rate of tachinid parasitism varies significantly across different habitats carries significant implications for the evolutionary trajectories of both tachinid flies and their primary plant-feeding hosts. Although a substantial portion of tachinid–plant interactions may be driven by cues provided by plants for host location, several investigations suggest that tritrophic interactions may also occur between larval tachinid flies, their hosts, and the plants serving as host food sources. A noteworthy instance involves the interplay between the arctiid caterpillar, *Arctia virginalis* (Boisduval), and the tachinid *Thelaira americana* Brooks. In this scenario, the host often manages to survive parasitism despite the emergence of mature *T. americana* larvae (English-Loeb et al., 1993). Nevertheless, the host's survival hinges significantly on the specific food plant it consumes. Parasitized larvae exhibit a preference for the plant *Conium maculatum* Linnaeus, which enhances their odds of surviving the parasitism process (Karban and English-Loeb, 1997).

The work conducted by Singer and collaborators (Singer and Stireman, 2003; Singer et al., 2004a, b) on the interactions between tachinid parasitoids and polyphagous arctiids provides compelling evidence of similar tritrophic relationships. In their studies, caterpillars demonstrated increased survival rates with reduced parasitism when their diets consisted of noxious plants, which were generally suboptimal for growth and survival when parasitoids were absent. These findings imply that some insects maintain their polyphagous feeding habits because certain food plants promote efficient growth ("good" plants), while others confer protection against parasitoids like tachinids ("nasty" plants) (Singer et al., 2004b). Furthermore, these results suggest that some tachinid species can be affected by host plant toxins ingested by their hosts.

Despite a recent surge in both basic and applied ecological studies, our understanding of the ecology of most tachinid species remains rudimentary at best. Currently, certain avenues of research are hindered by practical challenges, including the difficulty of breeding most tachinid species in laboratory settings. On the flip side, this lack of knowledge, the potential of tachinid–host interactions as model systems in the field, and the crucial role tachinids play as natural enemies of numerous agricultural and forest pests all indicate that ecological research involving tachinids presents vast opportunities and substantial rewards.

7.11 UTILIZATION OF TACHINID FLIES AS BIOCONTROL AGENTS

Compared to hymenopteran parasitoids, significantly less research has been conducted on dipterans, including the development of rearing technology; so far, only a handful of species have undergone mass production. Additionally, their relatively larger size, when compared to wasp parasitoids, is disadvantageous for mass production as it necessitates more resources and space to achieve production levels comparable to those achieved with hymenopterans. The potential for harnessing fly parasitoids in biological control hinges on the development of technology for their commercial-scale production.

Numerous attempts, whether successful or not, have been made to employ Tachinidae in classical and augmentative biological control programmes, particularly in the Nearctic and Neotropical regions, and to a lesser extent in the Australian and Oceanian regions. It's worth noting that examples of such programmes in the Palearctic region are almost non-existent. Failures in many instances were often attributed to insufficient knowledge about the biology, behaviour, and ecology of the species used, as well as improper rearing techniques and shipping procedures. The achievement of successful establishment did not depend on the quantity of flies released; instead, it was contingent on the climatic and ecological conditions prevalent in the introduced countries. Typically, optimal successes were observed in island environments.

Grenier (1988) documented various instances of classical and augmentative biological control programmes executed against forest lepidopterous defoliators and sawflies in North America using tachinid flies. One notable success involved the importation of *C. albicans* from Europe, which was subsequently released in Canada to control the winter moth *Operophtera brumata* (Linnaeus). The fly became established and contributed to the control of the target insect pest over several years (Hulme and Green, 1984; Horgan et al., 1999).

Two species, *Blepharipa pratensis* (Meigen) and *C. concinnata*, successfully established themselves in various states across the United States and were subsequently employed for augmentative releases targeting the gypsy moth (Blumenthal et al., 1979). Likewise, *Exorista larvarum* (Linnaeus) and *Parasetigena silvestris* (Robineau-Desvoidy), recognized as adversaries of *L. dispar* in Europe, were utilized in inoculative releases in the northern regions of the United States, where they became successfully established (Sabrosky and Reardon, 1976; Kenis and Lopez Vaamonde, 1998). Another tachinid of European origin, *Aphantorhaphopsis samarensis* (Villeneuve), was considered a promising candidate for the biological control of the gypsy moth due to its restricted host range, potentially minimizing the risk to nontarget lepidopterous species (Fuester et al., 2001). Despite repeated introductions in the northern United States and Canada, confirmation of its establishment has not been obtained (McManus and Csóka, 2007).

Similarly, *Lydella jalisco* Woodley, a parasitoid hailing from Mexico, underwent repeated introductions from its native habitat into Texas as part of classical control measures targeting the Mexican rice borer, *Eoreuma loftini* (Dyar) – a significant pest in Texas sugarcane cultivation. However, these introductions yielded limited success (Lauziére et al., 2001). In contrast, *L. diatraeae*, with its origins traced back to Cuba, stands out as a species effectively employed in both classical and augmentative biological control. Its prowess is particularly notable in combatting lepidopterous sugarcane borers of the *Diatraea* and *Chilo* genera, with a specific emphasis on *D. saccharalis*.

Archytas marmoratus (Townsend), a natural larval–pupal parasitoid of noctuids, was effectively mass-produced and utilized in augmentative field release trials against the corn earworm, *Helicoverpa zea* (Boddie), and the fall armyworm, *Spodoptera frugiperda* (J.E. Smith), in whorl-stage corn (Gross, 1990; Proshold et al., 1998). *Trichopoda pennipes,* indigenous to the southern United States and South America, serves as a parasitoid for the green vegetable bug, *Nezara viridula* (Linnaeus), and has been introduced to various countries worldwide for controlling the target insect, achieving variable success (Grenier, 1988; O'Hara, 2008).

In Florida, an extensive classical biological control initiative targeted the Mexican bromeliad weevil, *Metamasius callizona* Chevrolat, using the tachinid, *Lixadmontia franki* Wood and Cave. *Lixadmontia franki*, initially discovered in Honduras on a closely related species of bromeliad-eating weevil, underwent importation, extensive mass-rearing, and was subsequently released between 2007 and 2009. Despite these efforts, post-release monitoring detected only two F2 flies at one site, indicating minimal success (Cooper et al., 2011). Several factors were proposed to explain this limited success, including disparities in climate and elevation between the parasitoid's native and introduced regions, insufficient understanding of parasitoid biology, and challenges in rearing, which restricted the number of flies available for release.

7.12 ELEMENTS OF DIPTERAN PARASITOID BIOLOGY WITH PARTICULAR RELEVANCE TO PRODUCTION

A profound understanding of parasitoid biology, particularly regarding host range, oviposition strategies, and host–parasitoid interactions, serves as a pivotal tool to enhance the likelihood of successful rearing. Knowledge about the adopted oviposition strategy and the mechanisms influencing host selection is crucial for the parasitization process and the continuous *in vivo* culture of parasitoids, especially in the case of dipterans. Achieving the objective of continuous *in vitro* culture without the host also necessitates precise information about the parasitoid's oviposition strategy and factors triggering oviposition to induce direct oviposition on the artificial substrate.

Many tachinid larvae employ a strategy to evade the host immune response and exploit the host by constructing respiratory funnels, which are hardened folds around the hind part of their body. These funnels may be either primary, created by first instars upon entering the host integument, or secondary, formed by late-first or early-second instars in the host integument or tracheae. Tachinids that construct primary funnels, like *E. larvarum*, begin breathing atmospheric air from the onset of their development, facilitating rapid growth. In contrast, those forming secondary funnels, such as *E. bryani* and *Pseudogonia rufifrons* (Wiedemann), respire through their integument, resulting in slower growth until funnel formation.

Host–parasitoid relationships significantly impact the success of in vitro culture, as tachinids with developmental synchrony to the host have been shown to be challenging to rear on artificial media. Regardless of hormonal interactions, respiratory adaptations of parasitoid larvae substantially influence in vitro rearing methods. Species forming primary funnels require continuous contact with air from the first instar, making liquid media unsuitable for their culture. In vitro development may pose more challenges for parasitoids inducing the formation of secondary funnels, as opposed to primary funnels (Dindo, 2011).

7.13 TECHNIQUES FOR PRODUCING TACHINID PARASITOIDS

The classical method for the production of entomophagous insects is the natural tritrophic system, which includes the plant (or other natural food), host insect, and parasitoid. By simplifying the system, we can make parasitoid production easier.

The first step involves replacing the plant or other natural food with artificial diets to grow the insect hosts. There are many examples, especially with lepidopterous larvae used as hosts for parasitoid rearing (King and Leppla, 1984; Cohen, 2004). For instance, in Brazil, *Lydella minense* (Townsend) and *Billaea claripalpis* (van der Wulp) were reared on their natural host *Diatraea* spp., which was reared on an artificial diet to avoid the use of sugarcane (Rossi and Fowler, 2003). Systems based on rearing the natural host appear suitable for a number of tachinid species, including *C. concinnata*, *B. pratensis*, and other parasitoids of *L. dispar* (Odell and Godwin, 1979; Bourchier, 1991); *T. pennipes*, a parasitoid of *N. viridula* (Giangiuliani and Farinelli, 1995); and *L. franki*, a parasitoid of the weevil *Metamasius quadrilineatus* Champion (Suazo et al., 2006). The natural hosts of all these tachinids can be cultured without difficulties on either plants or artificial diets.

The fundamental qualitative requirements for dipteran parasitoids are generally similar to those of free-living insects, with some distinctions, particularly concerning aromatic amino acids and surfactants. Nitrogen sources can be supplied in the form of proteins, peptides, or free amino acids. Dipteran parasitoids, being carnivorous insects, undergo rapid growth during their larval stages (Grenier, 1980), especially when they have access to atmospheric oxygen through respiratory funnels. Consequently, a protein-rich medium with a well-balanced composition is essential to prevent the wastage of time and energy in metabolic conversion. While the standard 10 essential amino acids are necessary, additional amino acids prove highly beneficial for normal growth. In Tachinidae, aromatic amino acids are particularly required, especially towards the end of larval development for cuticle tanning (Bonnot et al., 1976). Commonly used sources of crude proteins or hydrolysates include casein, lactalbumin, ovalbumin, serum albumin, soybean extract, and yeast.

Lipids are primarily recognized as an energy source, and their inclusion in diets enhances the survival and fecundity of dipteran parasitoids. Certain polyunsaturated fatty acids are essential for both development and reproduction. Phospholipids are crucial as integral components of cell membranes and also function as molecular signals. All insects require dietary sterols (House, 1961). While lipids can be provided in the form of free fatty acids or triglycerides, their integration into aqueous-based formulations necessitates the use of surfactants. Carbohydrates are generally viewed as an energy source, and thus, a specific qualitative supply is not deemed necessary. Trehalose, the most prevalent nonreducing disaccharide in insects, plays a vital role in general metabolism (Thompson, 2003). Additionally, other nutrients, such as vitamins, organic acids, nucleic acids, and minerals, are essential in addition to the three basic nutrient types (proteins, lipids, and carbohydrates).

Tachinids have generally proven more challenging to rear artificially due to their intricate interactions with the host and more specific nutritional requirements. Limited success was achieved with species demonstrating developmental synchrony with the host. For instance, *Phryxe caudata* (Rondani) was only reared *in vitro* from the first to the third larval instar (Grenier et al., 1975). The medium composition was derived from the body composition of the fly larvae and potentially lacked protein. *Pseudogonia rufifrons* was reared from first-instar larva to adult, albeit with very low yields, on a subnatural medium based on *Galleria mellonella* (Linnaeus) pupal homogenate (Bratti and Monti, 1989). Additionally, it was reared on a medium containing bovine serum as the main ingredient, combined with trehalose, chicken egg yolk, and *G. mellonella* pupal haemolymph (Mellini et al., 1994).

Complete *in vitro* development on an insect-free artificial medium has been achieved solely for tachinids that lack developmental synchrony with their hosts. For instance, *L. diatraeae* marked the initial success in *in vitro* rearing of tachinids from the first instar to the adult stage, although only a few flies were obtained. This rearing process utilized an artificial medium gelled with agarose and comprised organic acids, inorganic salts, amino acids, B vitamins, fat-soluble vitamins, gelatin, protein hydrolysates, glycogen, adenosine triphosphate, lecithin, corn oil, and cholesterol (Grenier et al., 1978). Subsequently, *E. bryani* achieved *in vitro* rearing from the first-instar larva to the adult stage on a medium with a similar composition, supplemented with additional ingredients such as soy flour and chicken egg yolk (Nettles et al., 1980; Bratti and Nettles, 1992).

The most successful outcomes in rearing a tachinid parasitoid on artificial media have been observed with *E. larvarum*. Apart from exhibiting nonsynchronized development with the host, this parasitoid constructs primary integumental respiratory funnels, resulting in a simpler life cycle compared to species that form secondary funnels. These features, combined with polyphagy and gregarious behaviour, render this parasitoid especially well-suited for *in vitro* rearing (Dindo, 2007).

Factors, such as food, available space, and other abiotic conditions can influence adult survival, mating, fecundity, and the success of parasitoid rearing. While the nutritional needs of adult parasitoids are not fully understood, it is known that many of them feed on nectar or honeydew. These carbohydrate-rich food sources cater to their energy requirements (Thompson and Hagen, 1999). According to Wäckers (2003), nectar might also contribute to egg maturation and other physiological processes, despite its low content in amino acids, proteins, and lipids. In their natural habitat, some tachinids can feed on pollen (Campadelli, 1977). In captivity, adult tachinids are frequently provided with absorbent cotton soaked in honey– or sugar–water solutions and/or sugar cubes (Fusco et al., 1978; Kfir et al., 1989; Mason et al., 1991; Mellini and Coulibaly, 1991; Coulibaly and Fanti, 1992; Dindo et al., 1999, 2010; Sourakov and Mitchell, 2002).

Dipteran parasitoid adults typically exhibit proficient flying abilities. Parameters such as cage volume (available space) and adult density (number of individuals per cage) are critical considerations for survival and mating success, representing a pivotal phase in the completion of the life cycle. Successful mating was observed in *L. franki* adults when housed in spacious screen cages measuring $1.5 \times 1.5 \times 1.2\,m^3$, with a population consisting of 10 males and 10 females (Suazo et al., 2006). Additional crucial parameters influencing mating include sex ratio, age, and light intensity. For specific Tachinidae, adults are typically maintained within a restricted range of temperature and relative humidity (Coulibaly and Fanti, 1992; Dindo et al., 1999; Suazo et al., 2006). Mating often necessitates high light intensity. The commonly adopted photoperiod for adult rearing is 16:8 or 14:10 (L: D), although natural light conditions approximating 12:12 L:D were found suitable for *L. franki* (Suazo et al., 2006).

7.14 CONCLUSIONS AND FUTURE PROSPECTS

The production of dipteran parasitoids is intricately linked to their practical application in biological control. Future research endeavours should prioritize exploring the potential for more effective utilization of tachinid parasitoids in biocontrol strategies. Successful instances of biological control should serve as catalysts for expanding the use of proven effective species. For example, the successful applied biological control of lepidopterous sugarcane borers with *L. diatraeae* in the Americas could be replicated in other sugarcane-producing regions, such as China and other parts of Asia.

Furthermore, the notable achievements on a large scale with tachinids, particularly against sugarcane borers, should inspire renewed interest and investment in research and application programmes for *A. marmoratus*, *E. bryani*, and *Drino laxa* (Curran). These species showed promise for applied biological control and mass production, even *in vitro*, during the 1980s and 1990s but were later neglected. This neglect might be attributed to perceived programme expenses, especially in terms of rearing costs, as the larger size of tachinids compared to hymenopteran parasitoids demands more resources for mass production in terms of food and space. Additionally, some biological characteristics, such as the strong flying ability of adult flies leading to potential dispersal from release points, may have been considered unfavourable for inundative biological control.

Enhancing the utilization of dipteran parasitoids in applied biological control necessitates advancements in their rearing techniques to facilitate mass production. Future research in this domain could specifically address species identified as promising biological control agents, which, despite their potential, remain underutilized due to challenges in their rearing processes. Additionally, there is room for improving the rearing techniques of species already undergoing mass production, like *L. diatraeae*, by exploring the development of more efficient *in vitro* rearing procedures. In greenhouse environments, where the value of the crop is high, certain tachinids (like *E. larvarum*) might be valuable for the control of lepidopteran pests.

The positive outcomes achieved with tachinids against sugarcane borers could inspire the revival of programmes involving tachinids with similar biology and behaviour, acting as antagonists to lepidopterous pests of maize. Research aimed at refining rearing techniques and optimizing field release strategies could enhance the convenience and effectiveness of using tachinids. Additionally, future research should explore the identification of new dipteran parasitoid species suitable for biocontrol.

7.15 POINTS TO REMEMBER

1. **Global diversity**: Approximately 10,000 species worldwide.
2. **Parasitoid nature**: Tachinids parasitize insects and arthropods, contributing to ecosystem balance.
3. **Ecological importance**: Second only to parasitic Hymenoptera in insect parasitism and diversity.
4. **Utilization in biological control**: Over 100 species are used in pest control programmes with varying success rates.
5. **Habitat and distribution**: Found in diverse terrestrial environments worldwide.
6. Classified under the superfamily Oestroidea, along with other families like Calliphoridae and Sarcophagidae.
7. **Taxonomic divisions**: Divided into subfamilies such as Exoristinae, Dexiinae, Phasiinae and Tachininae.
8. **Phylogenetic studies**: Ongoing research uses molecular methods for a better understanding of evolutionary relationships.
9. **Morphological diversity**: Various sizes, colours, and body patterns are observed among tachinid species.
10. **Parasitic life cycle**: Larvae are endoparasitic, living inside the bodies of various insects and occasionally centipedes.
11. **Host range**: A broad range of hosts includes Lepidoptera, Coleoptera, Hymenoptera, and even non-insect arthropods.
12. **Reproductive strategy**: Categorized as koinobiont parasitoids, allowing hosts to continue developing while larvae develop inside.

13. Tachinids exhibit diverse oviposition strategies, which can be categorized into direct and indirect methods. Subcategories include external and internal oviposition, with or without egg incubation.
14. Tachinids utilize various sensory cues, such as olfactory, visual, auditory, and tactile chemosensory signals, to locate hosts.
15. Tritrophic interactions between larval tachinid flies, their hosts, and host plants contribute to the evolutionary trajectories of tachinids and their primary plant-feeding hosts.
16. Compared to hymenopteran parasitoids, research on dipteran parasitoids, including tachinids, has been relatively limited.
17. Several species of tachinids have been employed in classical and augmentative biological control programmes with varying degrees of success, often influenced by factors like species biology, behaviour, and rearing techniques.
18. Rearing techniques for tachinid parasitoids face challenges due to their complex interactions with hosts and specific nutritional requirements.
19. Future research should focus on enhancing the utilization of tachinid parasitoids in biocontrol strategies, building on successful instances of biological control.
20. Research efforts should prioritize refining rearing techniques and optimizing field release strategies to enhance the efficiency and effectiveness of using tachinids in pest management.

REFERENCES

Alcock, J. & Smith, A. (1995). Landmark defence and scramble competition mating systems in two Australian tachinid flies (Diptera). *Journal of the Kansas Entomological Society*, 68: 85–94.

Aldrich, J.R. & Zhang, A. (2002). Kairomone strains of *Euclytia flava* (Townsend), a parasitoid of stink bugs. *Journal of Chemical Ecology*, 28: 1565–1582.

Allen, G.R. (1995). The biology of the phonotactic parasitoid, *Homotrixia* sp. (Diptera: Tachinidae), and its impact on the survival of male *Sciarasaga quadrata* (Orthoptera: Tettigoniidae) in the field. *Ecological Entomology*, 20: 103–110.

Allen, G.R., Kamien, D., Berry, O., Byrne, P. & Hunt, J. (1999). Larviposition, host cues, and planidial behavior in the sound locating parasitoid fly *Homotrixa alleni* (Diptera: Tachinidae). *Journal of Insect Behavior*, 12: 67–79.

Andersen, S. (1983). Phylogeny and classification of Old World genera of Siphonini (Diptera: Tachinidae). *Scandinavian Entomology*, 14: 1–15.

Andersen, S. (1996). The Siphonini (Diptera: Tachinidae) of Europe. *Fauna Entomologica Scandinavica*, 33: 148.

Arnaud, P.H. Jr. (1958). The entomological publications of Charles Henry Tyler Townsend [1863–1944] with lists of his new generic and specific names. *Microentomology*, 23: 1–63.

Arnaud, P.H. Jr. (1978). A host-parasite catalog of North American Tachinidae (Diptera). *USDA Miscellaneous Publications*, 1319: 860.

Askew, R.R. & Shaw, M.R. (1986). Parasitoid communities: Their size, structure, and development. In: *Insect Parasitoids, 13th Symposium of the Royal Entomological Society of London* (eds. J.K. Waage & D. Greathead). Academic Press, London, pp. 225–264.

Barraclough, D.A. (1992). The systematics of the Australasian Dexiini (Diptera: Tachinidae: Dexiinae) with revisions of endemic genera. *International Journal of Invertebrate Taxonomy*, 6: 1127–1371.

Belshaw, R. (1993). Tachinid flies. Diptera: Tachinidae. Handbook for the identification of British Insects. *Royal Entomological Society of London, Part*, 4a(i): 170.

Belshaw, R. (1994). Life history characteristics of Tachinidae (Diptera) and their effect on polyphagy. In: *Parasitoid Community Ecology* (eds. B.A. Hawkins & W. Sheehan). Oxford University Press, New York, pp. 145–162.

Blumenthal, E.M., Fusco, R.A. & Reardon, R.C. (1979). Augmentative release of two established parasite species to suppress populations of the gypsy moth. *Journal of Economic Entomology*, 72: 281–288.

Boettner, G.H., Elkinton, J.S. & Boettner, C.J. (2000). Effects of a biological control introduction on three nontarget native species of saturniid moths. *Conservation Biology*, 14: 1798–1806.

Bonnot, G., Delobel, B. & Grenier, S. (1976). Composition corporelle en acides aminés du parasitoïde *Phryxe caudata* Rond. (Diptera) au cours de sa croissance larvaire. *Journal of Insect Physiology*, 22: 505–514.
Bourchier, R.S. (1991). Growth and development of *Compsilura concinnata* (Meigan) (Diptera: Tachinidae) parasitizing gypsy moth larvae feeding on tannin diets. *The Canadian Entomologist*, 123: 1047–1055.
Bratti, A. & Monti, M. (1989). Allevamento "in vitro" delle larve di *Pseudogonia rufifrons* Wied. (Dipt. Tachinidae) su omogeneizzato di crisalidi di *Galleria mellonella* L. (Lep. Galleriidae). *Bollettino dell'Istituto di Entomologia Guido Grandi della Università degli Studi di Bologna*, 43: 115–126.
Bratti, A. & Nettles Jr., W.C. (1992). In vitro rearing of *Eucelatoria bryani*: Improvement and evaluation of factors affecting efficiency. *Entomologia Experimentalis et Applicata*, 63: 213–219.
Burks, M.L. & Nettles, W.C. Jr. (1978). *Eucelatoria* sp. effects of cuticular extracts from *Heliothis virescens* and other factors on oviposition. *Environmental Entomology*, 7: 897–900.
Buschbeck, E.K. & Strausfeld, J. (1997). The relevance of neural architecture to visual performance: Phylogenetic conservation and variation in Dipteran visual systems. *Journal of Comparative Neurology*, 383: 282–304.
Cade, W. (1975). Acoustically orienting parasitoids: Fly phonotaxis to cricket song. *Science*, 190: 1312–1313.
Campadelli, G. (1977). Tecniche di allevamento per Ditteri Tachinidi con particolare riguardo agli adulti. *Bollettino dell'Istituto di Entomologia della Università degli Studi di Bologna*, 33: 215–240.
Cantrell, B.K. & Crosskey, R.W. (1989). Family Tachinidae. In: *Catalog of the Diptera of the Australasian and Oceanian Regions* (ed. N.L. Evenhuis). Bishop Museum Special Publications, Hawaii, p. 1155.
Cappuccino, N., Lavertu, D., Bergeron, Y. & Regniere, J. (1998). Spruce budworm impact, abundance and parasitism rate in a patchy landscape. *Oecologia*, 114: 236–242.
Clausen, C.P. (1940). *Entomophagous Insects*. Hafner, New York, p. 688.
Cohen, A.C. (2004). *Insect Diets: Science and Technology*. CRC Press, Boca Raton, FL.
Cooper, T.M., Frank, J.H., Cave, R.D., Burton, M.S., Dawson, J.S. & Smith, B W. (2011). Release and monitoring of a potential biocontrol agent, *Lixadmontia franki*, to control an invasive bromeliad-eating weevil, *Metamasius callizona*, in Florida. *Biological Control*, 59: 319–325.
Cortes, R. (1983). First record of transantarctic relationships in the Tachinidae (Diptera, Muscoidea, Calyptratae). *Revista Brasileira de Zoologia*, 1: 419–420.
Coulibaly, F. & Fanti, P. (1992). *Eucelatoria bryani Sabr.* (Diptera Tachinidae) rearing on the factitious host *Galleria mellonella* L. (Lepidoptera: Galleriidae): Effect of host age at exposure to the parasitoid females. *Bollettino dell'Istituto di Entomologia Guido Grandi della Università degli Studi di Bologna*, 46: 229–238.
Crosskey, R.W. (1965). The immature stages and affinities of the tachinid fly *Glaurocara flava*, a parasite of the African bush-cricket *Homorocoryphus nitidulus vicinus*. *Proceedings of the Zoological Society of London*, 144: 203–217.
Crosskey, R.W. (1973). A conspectus of the Tachinidae (Diptera) of Australia, including keys to the supra-specific taxa and taxonomic and host catalogues. *Bulletin of the British Museum (Natural History) Entomology Supplement*, 21: p. 221.
Crosskey, R.W. (1976). A taxonomic conspectus of the Tachinidae (Diptera) of the Oriental Region. *Bulletin of the British Museum (Natural History) Entomology Supplement*, 26: 357.
Crosskey, R.W. (1977). A review of Rhinophoridae (Diptera) and a revision of the Afrotropical species. *Bulletin of the British Museum (Natural History) Entomology*, 36: 66.
Crosskey, R.W. (1980). Family Tachinidae. In: *Catalogue of the Diptera of the Afrotropical Region*. (ed. R.W. Crosskey). British Museum of Natural History, London, pp. 822–882.
Dindo, M.L. (2007). Rearing the parasitoid *Exorista larvarum* (L.) (Diptera, Tachinidae) on artificial media. In: *Proceedings of the 11th Meeting of the Working Group Arthropod Mass Rearing and Quality Control-28/10/2007–1/11/2007* (eds. J.C. van Lenteren, P. De Clercq & M. Johnson). Canada Bulletin IOBC Global, Montreal, pp. 43–46.
Dindo, M.L. (2011). Tachinid parasitoids: Are they to be considered as koinobionts? *Biocontrol*, 56: 249–255.
Dindo, M.L., Farneti, R., Scapolatempo, M. & Gardenghi, G. (1999). In vitro rearing of the parasitoid *Exorista larvarum* (L.) (Diptera: Tachinidae) on meat homogenate-based diets. *Biological Control*, 16: 258–266.
Dindo, M.L., Stangolini, L. & Marchetti, E. (2010). A simplified artificial medium for the in vitro rearing of *Exorista larvarum* (Diptera: Tachinidae). *Biocontrol Science and Technology*, 20: 407–410.
Doak, P. (2000). The effects of plant dispersion and prey density on parasitism rates in a naturally patchy habitat. *Oecologia*, 122: 556–567.
Dodson, C.H. (1962). The importance of pollination in the evolution of the orchids of tropical America. *American Orchid Society Bulletin*, 31: 525–734.

Eggleton, P. & Belshaw, R. (1992). Insect parasitoids: An evolutionary overview. *Philosophical Transactions of the Royal Society of London Series B, Biological Sciences*, 337: 1–20.

Eggleton, P. & Belshaw, R. (1993). Comparisons of dipteran, hymenopteran and coleopteran parasitoids: Provisional phylogenetic explanations. *Biological Journal of the Linnean Society*, 48: 213–226.

Eggleton, P. & Gaston, K.J. (1992). Tachinid host ranges: A reappraisal (Diptera: Tachinidae). *Entomologist's Gazette*, 43: 139–143.

English-Loeb, G.M., Brody, A.K. & Karban, R. (1993). Host-plant-mediated interactions between a generalist folivore and its tachinid parasitoid. *Journal of Animal Ecology*, 62: 465–471.

English-Loeb, G.M., Karban, R. & Brody, A.K. (1990). Arctiid larvae survive attack by a tachinid parasitoid and produce viable offspring. *Ecological Entomology*, 15: 361–362.

Evenhuis, N.L. (1994). *Catalogue of the Fossil Flies of the World (Insecta: Diptera)*. Leiden, Backhuys, p. 600.

Feener, D.H. Jr, & Brown, B.V. (1997). Diptera as parasitoids. *Annual Review of Entomology*, 42: 73–97.

Frank, J.H., Walker, T.J. & Parkman, J.P. (1996). The introduction, establishment, and spread of *Ormia depleta* in Florida. *Biological Control*, 6: 368–377.

Fuester, R.W., Kenis, M., Swan, K.S., Kingsley, P.C., Lopez Vaamonde, C. & Hérard, F. (2001). Host range of *Aphantorhaphopsis samarensis* (Diptera: Tachinidae), a larval parasite of the gypsy moth (Lepidoptera: Lymantriidae). *Environmental Entomology*, 30: 605–611.

Fusco, R.A., Rhoads, L.D. & Blumenthal, M. (1978). *Compsilura concinnata*: Effect of temperature on laboratory propagation. *Environmental Entomology*, 7: 15–18.

Gaponov, S.P. (2003). *Morphology of Eggs of Tachinidae (Diptera)*. Voronezh State University, Voronezh, Russia, p. 87.

Gauld, I.D., Gaston, K.J. & Janzen, D.H. (1992). Plant allelochemicals, tritrophic interactions and the anomalous diversity of tropical parasitoids: The 'nasty' host hypothesis. *Oikos,* 65: 353–357.

Gentry, G. & Dyer, L.A. (2002). On the conditional nature of Neotropical caterpillar defenses against their natural enemies. *Ecology*, 83: 3108–3119.

Giangiuliani, G. & Farinelli, D. (1995). Technique for the laboratory rearing for *Trichopoda pennipes* F. (Diptera: Tachinidae), an adult parasitoid of the southern green stink bug, *Nezara viridula* (L.) (Hemiptera: Pentatomidae). *African Journal of Horticultural Science*, 5: 55–56.

Gray, D.A. & Cade, W.H. (1999). Sex, death and genetic variation: Natural and sexual selection on cricket song. *Proceedings of the Royal Society B: Biological Sciences*, 266: 707–709.

Greathead, D. (1986). Parasitoids in classical biological control. In: *Insect Parasitoids, 13th Symposium of the Royal Entomological Society of London* (eds. J.K. Waage & D. Greathead). Academic Press, London, pp. 289–318.

Grenier, S. (1980). Développement endoparasitaire et croissance pondérale larvaire du parasitoïde *Lixophaga diatraeae* (Dip.: Tachinidae) dans un hôte de substitution *Galleria mellonella* L. (Lep.: Pyralidae). *Entomophaga*, 25: 17–26.

Grenier, S. (1988). Applied biological control with tachinid flies (Diptera- Tachinidae): A review. *Anzeiger für Schädlingskunde, Pflanzenschutz, Umweltschutz*, 51: 49–56.

Grenier, S., Bonnot, G. & Delobel, B. (1975). Définition et mise au point de milieux artificiels pour l'élevage in vitro de *Phryxe caudata* Rond. (Diptera, Tachinidae). II—croissance et mues larvaires du parasitoïde en milieux définis. *Annales de Zoologie Ecologie Animale*, 7: 13–25.

Grenier, S., Bonnot, G., Delobel, B. & Laviolette, P. (1978). Développement en milieu artificiel du parasitoïde *Lixophaga diatraeae*. (Towns.) (Diptera, Tachinidae). Obtention de l'imago à partir de l'oeuf. *Comptes rendus de l'Académie des Sciences Paris Série D*, 387: 535–538.

Grimaldi, D. & Cumming, J. (1999). Brachyceran Diptera in cretaceous ambers and mesozoic diversification of the Eremoneura. *Bulletin of the American Museum of Natural History*, 239: 124.

Gross, H.R. (1990). Field release and evaluation of *Archytasmarmoratus* (Diptera: Tachinidae) against larvae of *Heliothis zea* (Lepidoptera: Noctuidae) in whorl-stage corn. *Environmental Entomology*, 19: 1122–1129.

Guimaraes, J.H. (1971). *Family Tachinidae (Larvaevoridae). In: A Catalogue of the Diptera of the Americas South of the United States*. Volume 104. Museum of Zoology of the University of São Paulo, São Paulo, p. 333.

Guimaraes, J.H. (1977). Host-parasite and parasite-host catalogue of South American Tachinidae (Diptera). *Arquivos de Zoologia*, 28: 1–131.

Guimaraes, J.H. (1980). Revision of the South American Uramyini (Diptera, Tachinidae). *Papéis avulsos do Departamento de Zoologia*, 33: 191–219.

Harris, V.E. & Todd, J.W. (1980). Male mediated aggregation of male, female, and 5th instar southern green stink bugs and concomittant attraction of a tachinid parasite, *Trichopoda pennipes*. *Entomologia Experimentalis et Applicata*, 27: 117–126.

Hassell, M.P. (1968). The behavioral response of a tachinid fly (*Cyzenis albicans* (Fall.)) to its host, the winter moth (*Operophtera brumata* (*L.*)). *Journal of Animal Ecology*, 37: 627–639.
Hayes, K.L. (1958). Descriptions of the larva and adult female of *Phorostoma tabanivora* (Hall) and notes on the biology of the species. *Annals of the Entomological Society of America*, 51: 552–553.
Hennig, W. (1971). Neue Untersuchungen über die Familien der Diptera Schizophora (Diptera: Cyclorrhapha). *Stuttgarter Beiträge zur Naturkunde aus dem Staatlichen Museum für Naturkunde in Stuttgart*, 226: 1–76.
Herrebout, W.M. & van den Veer, J. (1969). Habitat selection in *Eucarcelia rutilla* Vill III. Preliminary results of olfactometer experiments with females of known age. *Zeitschrift für Angewandte Entomologie*, 64: 55–61.
Herting, B. & Dely-Draskovits, A. (1993). Family tachinidae. In*: Catalogue of Palaearctic Diptera*: Volume 13: *Anthomyiidae-Tachinidae* (eds. A. Soos & L. Papp). Elsiver, Amsterdam, pp. 118–458.
Herting, B. (1957). Das weibliche Postabdomen der calyptraten Fliegen (Diptera) und sein Merkmalswert f¨ur die Systematik der Gruppe. *Zeitschrift für Morphologie und Ökologie Tiere* 45: 429–461.
Herting, B. (1960). Biologie der westpalarktischen westpalarktischen Raupenfliegen *Dipt., Tachinidae. Monographien zur angew Entomologie*, 16: 188.
Herting, B. (1966). Beitr¨age zur Kenntnis der europ¨aischen Raupenfliegen (Dipt. Tachinidae). *IX. Stuttgarter Beiträge zur Naturkunde*, 146: 12.
Herting, B. (1983). Phasiinae. In: Die Fliegen der palaearktischen Region (ed. E. Lindner). Schweiz. Verl, Stuttgart, pp. 1–88.
Herting, B. (1984). Catalogue of Palearctic Tachinidae (Diptera). *Stuttgarter Beiträge zur Naturkunde*. 369: 1–228.
Horgan, F.G., Myers, J.H. & Van Meel, R. (1999). *Cyzenis albicans* (Diptera: Tachinidae) does not prevent the outbreak of winter moth (Lepidoptera: Geometridae) in birch stands and blueberry plots on the lower mainland of British Columbia. *Environmental Entomology*, 28: 96–107.
House, H.L. (1961). Insect nutrition. *Annual Review of Entomology*, 6: 13–26
Hulme, M.A. & Green, G.W. (1984). Biological control of forest insect pests in Canada 1969–1980: Retrospect and prospect. In: *Biological Control Programmes Against Insects and Weeds in Canada 1969–1980* (eds. J.S. Kelleher & M.A. Hulme). Commonwealth Agriculture Bureaux, Slough, UK, pp. 215–227.
Ichiki, R. & Shima, H. (2003). Immature life of *Compsilura concinnata* (Meigen) (Diptera: Tachinidae). *Annals of the Entomological Society of America*, 96: 161–167.
Irwin, M.E., Schlinger, E.I. & Thompson, F.C. (2003). Diptera, true flies. In: *The Natural History of Madagascar* (eds. S.M. Goodman & J.P. Benstead) Chicago Press, Chicago, IL, p. 1728.
Janzen, D.H. (1981). The peak in North American ichneumonid species richness lies between 38o and 42o N. *Ecology*, 62: 532–537.
Jeffries, M.J. & Lawton, J.H. (1984). Enemy free space and the structure of ecological communities. *Biological Journal of the Linnean Society*, 23: 269–286.
Kainoh, Y., Tanaka, C. & Nakamura, S. (1999). Odor from herbivore-damaged plant attracts the parasitoid fly *Exorista japonica* Townsend (Diptera: Tachinidae). *Applied Entomology and Zoology*, 34: 463–467.
Kamijo, K. (1973). The parasite complex of *Choristoneura diversana* Hubner injurious to Todo-Fir, *Abies sachalinensis* Masters. *Japanese Journal of Applied Entomology and Zoology*, 17: 71–83.
Karban, R. & English-Loeb, G. (1997). Tachinid parasitoids affect host plant choice by caterpillars to increase caterpillar survival. *Ecology*, 78: 603–611.
Kenis, M. & Lopez Vaamonde, C. (1998). Classical biological control of the gypsy moth, *Lymantria dispar* (L.) in North America: Prospects and new strategies. Proceedings: Population dynamics, impact and integrated management of forest defoliating insects, *U.S. Department of Agriculture, Forest Service General Technical Reports*, p. 213–221.
Kfir, R., Graham, D.Y. & Van Vuuren, R.V. (1989). An improved method for mass rearing *Paratheresia claripalpis* for biological control of lepidopteran stalk borers. *Entomologia Experimentalis et Applicata*, 51: 37–40.
King, E.G. & Leppla, N.C. (1984). *Advances and Challenges in Insect Rearing*. Government Printing Office, Washington, DC, USA.
Komonen, A., Penttila, R., Lindgren, M. & Hanski, I. (2000). Forest fragmentation truncates a food chain based on an old-growth forest bracket fungus. *Oikos*, 90: 119–126.
Krupke, C.H. & Brunner, J.F. (2003). Parasitoids of the consperse stink bug (Hemiptera: Pentatomidae) in North Central Washington and attractiveness of a host-produced pheromone component. *Journal of Entomological Science*, 38: 84–92.

Lauzière, I., Legaspi, J., Legaspi, B. & Saldana, R. (2001). Field release of *Lydella jalisco* Woodley (Diptera: Tachinidae) in sugar-cane and other gramineous crops for biological control of *Eoreuma loftini* (Dyar) (Lepidoptera: Pyralidae) in Texas. *Subtropical Plant Science*, 49: 53–64.

Lehmann, G.U.C. & Heller, K.G. (1998). Bushcricket song structure and predation by the acoustically orienting parasitoid fly *Therobia leonidei* (Diptera: Tachinidae: Ormiini). *Behavioral Ecology and Sociobiology*, 43: 239–245.

Mallampalli, N., Barbosa, P. & Weinges, K. (1996). Effects of condensed tannins and catalpol on growth and development of *Compsilura concinnata* (Diptera: Tachinidae) reared in gypsy moth (Lepidoptera: Lymantriidae). *Journal of Entomological Science*, 31: 289–300.

Martin, W.R. Jr., Nordlund, A. & Nettles, W.C. Jr. (1990). Response of parasitoid *Eucelatoria bryani* to selected plant material in an olfactometer. *Journal of Chemical Ecology*, 16: 499–508.

Mason, C.F., Jones, R.L. & Thompson, M.M. (1991). Rearing *Lydella thompsoni* (Diptera: Tachinidae), a parasite of the European corn borer (Lepidoptera: Pyralidae). *Annals of the Entomological Society of America*, 84: 179–181.

McAlpine, J.F., Peterson, B.V., Shewell, G.E., Teskey, H.J., Vockeroth, J.R. & Wood, D.M. (1987). *Manual of Nearctic Diptera*. Volume 2. Monograph No. 28, Biosystematics Research Centre, Ottawa, Ontario, p. 668.

McAlpine, J.F. (1970). First record of calypterate flies in the Mesozoic era (Diptera: Calliphoridae). *The Canadian Entomologist*, 102: 342–346.

McAlpine, J.F. (1989). Phylogeny and classification of the Muscomorpha. In: *Manual of Nearctic Diptera.* Volume 3. Agriculture Canada, Monograph No. 32. (ed. J.F. McAlpine). Ottawa Research Branch, Ottawa, pp. 1397–1518.

McManus, M. & Csóka, G. (2007). History and impact of gypsy moth in North America and comparison to recent outbreaks in Europe. *Acta Silvatica et Lignaria Hungarica*, 3: 47–64.

Mellini, E. & Coulibaly, A.K. (1991). Un decennio di sperimentazione sul sistema ospite-parassita *Galleria mellonella* L.-*Pseudogonia rufifrons* Wied.: sintesi dei risultati. *Bollettino dell'Istituto di Entomologia Guido Grandi della Università degli Studi di Bologna*, 45: 191–249.

Mellini, E. (1990). Sinossi di biologia dei Ditteri Larvavoridi. *Bollettino dell'Istituto di Entomologia 'Guido Grandi', University of Bologna*, 45: 1–38.

Mellini, E., Campadelli, G. & Dindo, M.L. (1994). Possibile impiego di plasma bovino nell'allestimento di diete artificiali per le larve del parassitoide *Pseudogonia rufifrons* Wied. In: *M.A.F. Convegno Lotta Biologica, Acireale 1991* (ed. G. Viggiani). Sper. Pat. Veg., Roma, Italy, pp. 145–150.

Mondor, E.B. & Roland, J. (1997). Host locating behaviour of *Leschenaultia exul* and *Patelloa pachypyga*: Two tachinid parasitoids of the forest tent caterpillar, *Malacosoma disstria*. *Entomologia Experimentalis et Applicata*, 85: 161–168.

Mondor, E.B. & Roland, J. (1998). Host searching and oviposition by *Leschenaultia exul*, a tachinid parasitoid of the forest tent caterpillar, *Malacosoma disstria*. *Journal of Insect Behavior*, 11: 583–592.

Monteith, L.G. (1955). Host preferences of *Drino bohemica* Mesn. (Diptera: Tachinidae) with particular reference to olfactory responses. *The Canadian Entomologist*, 87: 509–530.

Monteith, L.G. (1956). Influence of host movement on selection of hosts by *Drino bohemica* Mesn. (Diptera: Tachinidae) as determined in an olfactometer. *The Canadian Entomologist*, 88: 583–586.

Muller, P. & Robert, D. (2002). Death comes suddenly to the unprepared: Singing crickets, call fragmentation, and parasitoid flies. *Behavioral Ecology*, 13: 598–606.

Nettles, W.C., Wilson, C.M. & Ziser, S.W. (1980). A diet and methods for the in vitro rearing of the tachinid *Eucelatoria* spp. *Annals of the Entomological Society of America*, 73: 180–184.

O'Hara, J.E. & Henderson, S.J. (2020).World genera of the Tachinidae (Diptera) and their Regional Occurrence. Version 11.0. https://www.uoguelph.ca/nadsfly/Tach/WorldTachs/Genera/Worldgenera.html

O'Hara, J.E. & Wood, D.M. (2004). Catalogue of the Tachinidae (Diptera) of America north of Mexico. *Memoirs on Entomology, International*, 18: 410.

O'Hara, J.E. (1988). Survey of first instars of the Siphonini (Diptera: Tachinidae). *Scandinavian Entomology*, 18: 367–382.

O'Hara, J.E. (1989). Systematics of the genus group taxa of the Siphonini (Diptera: Tachinidae). *Quaestiones Entomologicae*, 25: 1–229.

O'Hara, J.E. (2002). Revision of the Polideini (Tachinidae) of America north of Mexico. *Studia Dipterologica*, Suppl 10: 170.

O'Hara, J.E. (2008). Tachinid flies (Diptera: Tachinidae). In: *Encyclopedia of Entomology*. Second Edition (ed. J.L. Capinera). Springer, Dordrecht, pp. 3675–3686.

O'Hara, J.E., Skevington, J.H. & Hansen, D.E. (2004). A reappraisal of tachinid diversity in Carnarvon N.P., Australia, and estimation of the size of the Australian Tachinidae fauna. *Tachinid Times*, 17 8–10.
Odell, T.M. & Godwin, P.A. (1979). Laboratory techniques for rearing *Blepharipa pratensis*, a tachinid parasite of gypsy moth. *Annals of the Entomological Society of America*, 72: 632–635.
Pape, T. (1992). Phylogeny of the Tachinidae family-group. *Tijdschrift Voor Entomologie*, 135: 43–86.
Proshold, F.I., Gross, H.R. & Carpenter, J.E. (1998). Inundative release of *Archytas marmoratus* (Diptera: Tachinidae) against the corn earworm and fall armyworm (Lepidoptera: Noctuidae) in whorl-stage corn. *Journal of Entomological Science*, 33: 241–255.
Richter, V.A. (1987). Morphological parallelisms in the Tachinidae (Diptera). *Entomological Review*, 66(4): 66–86.
Richter, V.A. (1992). A new tribe, new and little known species of the tachinid flies (Diptera, Tachinidae) of the fauna of the USSR. *Entomological Review*, 70(8): 133–150.
Richter, V.A. & Farinets, S.I. (1984). The first instar larvae of tachinids of the subfam. Dexiinae (Diptera, Tachinidae). *Entomological Review*, 62(4): 142–165.
Richter, V.A. & Farinets, S.I. (1987). The first instar larvae of tachinids of the tribes Angiorhinini and Palpostomini (Diptera, Tachinidae) of the fauna of the USSR. *Entomological Review*, 66(2): 28–34.
Richter, V.A. & Farinets, S.I. (1990). Descriptions of first instar larvae of tachinids of the subfamilies Tachininae and Voriinae (Diptera, Tachinidae). *Entomological Review*, 69(5): 14–28.
Robert, D., Edgecomb, R.S., Read, M.P. & Hoy, R.R. (1996). Tympanal hearing in tachinid flies (Diptera, Tachinidae, Ormiini): The comparative morphology of an innovation. *Cell and Tissue Research*, 284: 435–448.
Rognes, K. (1986). The systematic position of the genus *Helicobosca* Bezzi with a discussion of the monophyly of the calyptrate families Calliphoridae, Rhinophoridae, Sarcophagidae and Tachinidae (Diptera). *Scandinavian Entomology*, 17: 75–92.
Rognes, K. (1997). The Calliphoridae (blowflies) (Diptera: Oestroidea) are not a monophyletic group. *Cladistics*, 13: 27–66.
Roland, J. & Taylor, P.D. (1997). Insect parasitoid species respond to forest structure at different spatial scales. *Nature*, 386: 710–713.
Roland, J., Denford, K.E. & Jimenez, L. (1995). Borneol as an attractant for *Cyzenis albicans*, a tachinid parasitoid of the winter moth, *Operopthera brumata L. (Lepidoptera: Geometridae). The Canadian Entomologist*, 127: 413–421
Roland, J., Evans, W.G. & Myers, J.H. (1989). Manipulation of oviposition patterns of the parasitoid *Cyzenis albicans* (Tachinidae) in the field using plant extracts. *Journal of Insect Behaviour*, 2: 487–503.
Rossi, M.N. & Fowler, H.G. (2003). Temporal patterns of parasitism in *Diatraea saccharalis* Fabr. (Lepidoptera: Crambidae) populations at different spatial scales in sugar-cane fields in Brazil. *Journal of Applied Entomology*, 127: 501–508.
Roth, J.P., King, E.G. & Thompson, A.C. (1978). Host location behavior by the tachinid, *Lixophaga diatraeae*. *Environmental Entomology*, 7: 794–798.
Sabrosky, C.W. & Arnaud, P.H. Jr. (1965). Family Tachinidae (Larvaevoridae). In: *A Catalog of the Diptera of America North of Mexico* (eds. A. Stone., C.W. Sabrosky, W.W. Wirth, R.H. Foote & J.R. Coulson). p. 1696, doi:10.1206/0003-0090(2004)283<0001:COTDDO>2.0.CO;2
Sabrosky, C.W. & Reardon, R.C. (1976). Tachinid parasites of the gypsy moth, *Lymantria dispar*, with keys to adults and puparia. *Miscellaneous Publications of the Entomological Society of America*, 10: 1–126.
Sheehan, W. (1994). Parasitoid community structure: Effects of host abundance, phylogeny, and ecology. In: *Parasitoid Community Ecology* (eds. B.A. Hawkins & W. Sheehan). Oxford University Press, New York, pp. 90–107.
Shima, H. (1989). Parasitic way of life in tachinid flies. *Insectarium*, 26: 4–9; 46–51; 88–94; 120–126.
Shima, H. (1996). Asystematic study of the tribe Winthemiini from Japan (Diptera, Tachinidae). *Beiträge zur Entomologie*, 46: 169–235.
Shima, H. (1999). Host-parasite catalog of Japanese Tachinidae (Diptera). *Makunagi Acta Dipterology Supplement*, 1: 108.
Singer, M.S. & Stireman, J.O. III. (2003). Does anti-parasitoid defense influence hostplant selection by a generalist caterpillar? *Oikos*, 100: 554–562.
Singer, M.S., Carriere, Y., Theuring, C. & Hartmann, T. (2004a). Disentangling food quality from resistance against parasitoids: Diet choice by a generalist caterpillar. *The American Naturalist*, 164: 423–429.
Singer, M.S., Rodrigues, D., Stireman, J.O. III. & Carriere, Y. (2004b). Roles of food quality and enemy-free space in host use by a generalist insect herbivore. *Ecology*, 85: 2747–2753.

Sourakov, A. & Mitchell, E.R. (2002). Laboratory biology of *Chetogena scutellaris* (Diptera: Tachinidae), a parasitoid of Noctuidae, reared on fall armyworm and cabbage looper. *Florida Entomologist*, 85, 341–343.

Stireman, J.O. III. (2002a). Host location and acceptance in a polyphagous tachinid parasitoid. *Entomologia Experimentalis et Applicata*, 103: 23–34.

Stireman, J.O. III. (2002b). Learning in the generalist tachinid parasitoid *Exorista mella* (Diptera: Tachinidae). *Journal of Insect Behavior*, 15: 715–732.

Stireman, J.O. III. (2002c). Phylogenetic relationships of tachinid flies in subfamily Exoristinae (Tachinidae: Diptera) based on 28S rDNA and elongation factor-1α. *Systematic Entomology*, 27: 409–435.

Stireman, J.O. III., Cerretti, P., O'Hara, J.E., Blaschke, J.D. & Moulton, J.K. (2018). Molecular phylogeny and evolution of world Tachinidae (Diptera). *Molecular Phylogenetics and Evolution*, https://doi.org/10.1016/j.ympev.2018.12.002.

Stireman, J.O. III & Singer, M.S. (2003). Determinants of parasitoid-host associations: Insights from a natural tachinid-lepidopteran community. *Ecology*, 84: 296–310.

Stireman, J.O., O'Hara, J.E. & Wood, D.M. (2006). Tachinidae: Evolution, behavior, and ecology. *Annual Review of Entomology*, 51: 525–555.

Strand, M.R. & Pech, L.L. (1995). Immunological basis for compatibility in parasitoid host relationships. *Annual Review of Entomology*, 40: 31–56.

Suazo, A., Arismendi, N., Frank, J.H. & Cave, R.D. (2006). Method for continuously rearing *Lixadmontia franki* (Diptera: Tachinidae), a potential biological control agent of *Metamasius callizona* (Coleoptera: Dryophthoridae). *Florida Entomologist*, 89: 340–353.

Tanaka, C., Kainoh, Y. & Honda, H. (1999). Physical factors in host selection of the parasitoid fly *Exorista japonica* Townsend (Diptera: Tachinidae). *Applied Entomology and Zoology*, 34: 91–97.

Teskey, H.J. (1969). Larvae and pupae of some eastern North American Tabanidae (Diptera). *Memoirs of the Entomological Society of Canada*, 63: 1–141.

Thompson, S.N. & Hagen, K.S. (1999). Nutrition of Entomophagous Insects and Other Arthropods. In: *Handbook of Biological Control* (eds. T.S. Bellows & T.W. Fisher). Academic Press, San Diego, pp. 594–652.

Thompson, W.R. (1968). The tachinids of Trinidad. *VIII. Phorocerines. Memoirs of the Entomological Society of Canada*, 56: 207.

Thompson, S.N. (2003). Trehalose - the insect 'blood' sugar. *Advances in Insect Physiology*, 31: 205–285.

Townsend, C.H.T. (1911). Review of work by Pantel and Portchinski on reproductive and early state characters of muscoid flies. *Proceedings of the Entomological Society of Washington*, 13: 151–170.

Townsend, C.H.T. (1934–42). *Manual of Myiology in Twelve Parts*. Townsend & Filhos, Sao Paulo.

Tschorsnig, H.P. (1985). Taxonomie forstlich wichtiger Parasiten: Untersuchungen zur Struktur des m¨annlichen Postabdomens der Raupenfliegen (Diptera, Tachinidae). *Stuttgarter Beiträge zur Naturkunde Ser. A*, 383: 1–137.

Tschorsnig, H.P. & Richter, V.A. (1998). Family Tachinidae. In: *Contributions to a Manual of Palaearctic Diptera (with Special Reference to Flies of Economic Importance): Higher Brachycera*. Volume 3. (eds. L. Papp & B. Darvas). South African National Biodiversity Institute, Pretoriap, pp. 691–827.

Verbeke, J. (1962). Contribution `a l'´etude des Tachinidae africains (Diptera). *Scientific Results from Exploration Hydrobiological, lakes Kivu, Edward and Albert*, 3(4): 77–187.

Vincent, L.S. (1985). The first record of a tachinid fly as an internal parasitoid of a spider (Diptera: Tachinidae; Araneae: Antrodiaetidae). *The Pan-Pacific Entomologist*, 61: 224–225.

Vinson, S.B. & Iwantsch, G.F. (1980). Host regulation by insect parasitoids. *The Quarterly Review of Biology*, 55: 143–165.

Wäckers, F.L. (2003). The parasitoids' needs for sweets: Sugar in mass rearing and biological control. In: *Quality Control and Production of Biological Control Agents- Theory and Testing Procedures* (ed. J.C. van Lenteren). CABI Publishing, Oxon, UK, pp. 59–72.

Walker, T.J. (1993). Phonotaxis in female *Ormia ochracea* (Diptera: Tachinidae), a parasitoid of field crickets. *Journal of Insect Behavior*, 6: 389–410.

Weseloh, R.M. (1980). Host recognition behavior of the tachinid parasitoid, *Compsilura concinnata. Annals of the Entomological Society of America*, 73: 593–601.

Wiegmann, B.M., Trautwein, M.D., Winkler, I.S., Barr, N.B., Kim, J.W., Lambkin, C., Bertone, M.A., Cassel, B.K., Bayless, K.M., Heimberg, A.M., Wheeler, B.M., Peterson, K.J., Pape, T., Sinclair, B.J., Skevington, J.H., Blagoderov, V., Caravas, J., Kutty, S.N., Schmidt-Ott, U., Kampmeier, G.E., Thompson, F.C.,

Grimaldi, D.A., Beckenbach, A.T., Courtney, G.W., Friedrich, M., Meier, R. & Yeates, D.K. (2011). Episodic radiations in the fly tree of life. *Proceedings of the National Academy of Sciences*, 108: 5690–5695.

Williams, S.C., Arnaud, P.H. & Lowe, G. (1990). Parasitism of *Anuroctonus phaiodactylus* (Wood) and *Vaejovis spinigerus* (Wood) (Scorpiones: Vaejovidae) by *Spilochaetosoma californicum* Smith (Diptera: Tachinidae), and a review of parasitism in scorpions. *Myia*, 5: 11–27.

Wood, D.M. (1972). A revision of the New World Exoristini (Diptera: Tachinidae) I. *Phorocera subgenus Pseudotachinomyia. Canadian Entomologist*, 104: 471–503.

Wood, D.M. (1985). A taxonomic conspectus of the Blondeliini of North and Central America and the West Indies (Diptera: Tachinidae). *Memoirs of the Entomological Society of Canada*, 132: p. 130.

Wood, D.M. (1987). Tachinidae. In *Manual of Nearctic Diptera*. Volume 2. (eds. J.F. McAlpine, B.V. Peterson, G.E. Shewell, H.J. Teskey, J.R. Vockeroth & D.M. Wood). Canada Communication Group – Publishing, Ottawa, Canada, 28, pp. 1193–1269.

Yamawaki, Y., Kainoh, Y. & Honda, H. (2002). Visual control of host pursuit in the parasitoid fly *Exorista japonica*. *Journal of Experimental Biology*, 205: 485–492.

Yeates, D.K. & Wiegmann, B.M. (1999). Congruence and controversy: Toward a higher-level classification of Diptera. *Annual Review of Entomology*, 44: 397–428.

Yeates, D.K. (2002). Relationships of the lower Brachycera (Diptera): A quantitative synthesis of morphological characters. *Zoologica Scripta*, 31: 105–121.

Ziegler, J. (1998). Die Morphologie der Puparien und der larvalen Cephalopharyngealskelette der Raupenfliegen (Diptera, Tachinidae) und ihre phylogenetische Bewertung. *Stud. Dipterology Supplement*, 3: p. 244.

Zuk, M. & Kolluru, G.R. (1998). Exploitation of sexual signals by predators and parasitoids. *The Quarterly Review of Biology*, 73: 415–438.

8 Scuttle Flies (Phoridae)

Kailash Chandra

LEARNING OBJECTIVES

1. Understanding the biology and taxonomy of scuttle flies belonging to the family Phoridae within the order Diptera.
2. Analysing the geographical distribution of these species within India and comparing it with their distribution globally.
3. Evaluating the roles of Phoridae species in various ecosystem services.
4. Deciphering the role of scuttle flies as biocontrol agents.
5. Exploring the medical and forensic implications of scuttle flies.

8.1 INTRODUCTION

Members of the family Phoridae are commonly referred to as scuttle flies because of their ability to run quickly in short bursts. They are also known as coffin flies because their larvae enter coffins to feed on bodies. These humpbacked flies share similarities with fruit flies and are considered one of the most biologically diverse families of insects (Disney, 1994). Phorids are widely distributed across the globe. The smallest known species of fly belong to this family; for instance, the world's smallest fly, *Euryplatea nanaknihali*, measuring 0.4 mm in size, was documented in Thailand (Brown, 2012).

8.2 CHARACTERISTIC FEATURES

The representatives of the Phoridae family have the characteristic of rapidly running across surfaces. They possess a distinctive humped back appearance, with a small, low head and eyes (Amoudi et al., 1989). Their head is usually rounded and sometimes narrowed in front, covered with a group of bristles. The ocellar callus in some species is swollen and highly raised above the vertex of the head. Their eyes are generally black or brown and dichoptic in both males and females, with closer-set eyes in males and wider-set eyes in females (Brown, 2012). The third segment of the antenna is large and rounded or elongated, bearing a long apical or dorsal arista directed sideways. The arista is either glabrous or feathered. There is notable sexual dimorphism in the size and shape of the third segment, which is longer in males. The proboscis is usually short and elongated, sometimes with enlarged labella. Maxillary palpi vary in shape. Two pairs of supra-antennal bristles are sometimes completely reduced, and three bristles are spaced along the margin of the eyes: anterolateral, mid-lateral, and posterolateral. Immediately before the ocellar callus, there are two preocellar bristles. The ocellar callus bears a pair of bristles, and in some genera, two additional intermediate bristles occur between the antennae and the preocellar bristles. The mesonotum is convex and covered with hairs and rows of bristles. The anterior spiracles are located on the pleura of the thorax, which is a characteristic feature of the group. The metapleuron may be entire or divided by a suture into two halves, sometimes along with a few long bristles, glabrous or pubescent. Their legs have stout femora, with hind femora often laterally compressed. Their wings are clear with a slight tinge and rarely have markings. The wing venation is reduced, with strong radial veins ending in the costa about halfway along the wing. The medial veins are not very prominent, usually

DOI: 10.1201/9781003482581-10

diagonal, often parallel, and without cross-veins (Brown, 2012). The abdomen consists of six visible segments. In males, segments VII to X form the genitalia (hypopygium), while in females, these segments comprise the terminalia. Some genera have females with segments VII to X highly sclerotized and extended into a tube ("ovipositor") (Amoudi et al., 1989). The larvae are small, typically less than 10 mm in length, with 12 visible segments. Their shape ranges from fusiform (spindle-shaped) to short, broad, and flattened, often featuring noticeable projections. They are typically whitish, yellowish-white, or grey. The first larval instar is metapneustic, while later instars are amphipneustic (Amoudi et al., 1989). The puparium (pupal case) is oval and pointed at the ends, with the second abdominal segment bearing a dorsal pair of long, slender pupal respiratory horns (Pallavi et al., 2023).

8.2.1 Life Cycle

The flies represent the typical holometabolous development, comprising four distinct stages, namely, eggs, larvae, pupa, and adult. The phorid fly passes through three distinct larval instars, with the last instar usually lasting longer, as it then changes to pupa and subsequently into a fly. The development of flies depends on various environmental conditions, feeding, and the host. First and second instars last 1–2 days, whereas the third instar lasts 3–4 days, followed by another 1–2 days before pupation. The male fly matures 2 days before the females, gaining the advantage of early feeding and maturation of sperm before the female emerges. The female reproduces through oviposition and lays relatively large eggs due to extended periods (Disney, 1994).

8.2.2 Species Diversity

The Phoridae is one of the largest families of the insect order Diptera, belonging to the superfamily Phoroidea and infraorder Aschiza of the suborder Brachycera. Altogether, 156,968 living species of Diptera have so far been recorded worldwide. Hitherto, 4,798 species belonging to 271 genera of the family Phoridae are known globally, mostly belonging to the genus *Megaselia* (Catalogue of life, 2024). Presently, 67 species belonging to four subfamilies, namely Metopininae, Aenigmatiinae, Termitoxeniinae, and Phorinae, comprising 18 genera, have been recorded from India, representing about 1.6% of global species (Table 8.1) (Mitra et al., 2016). Fewer than 50% of the total species are endemic to India. Among the states, Maharashtra has the highest number of species with 15, followed by West Bengal with 13 species. Karnataka has seven species, Assam has three species, Meghalaya four species, Bihar three species, and Kerala two species. Other states and Union territories, including the Andaman & Nicobar Islands, Chandigarh, Himachal Pradesh, Punjab, Tamil Nadu, and Uttarakhand, are each represented by only one species (Mitra et al., 2016).

8.3 HISTORICAL ACCOUNT

Wasmann (1902), Brues (1905, 1907), Brunetti (1912, 1924), Schmitz (1912, 1913a,b, 1914, 1915, 1924, 1926a,b, 1938), and Senior-White (1922, 1924) initiated the work on Phoridae in India, leading to the description of several new species. Later, Disney (1981, 1988, 1990, 1992, 1994, 1995, 2001) made substantial contributions towards the discovery of many species of Phoridae from India. Besides, Colyer (1961), Papp (1982), Sandhu and Bhattal (1987), and Mostovski (2002) have also described some new species from India. Approximately 20 species that were described as new from neighbouring countries, previously known to be part of British India and outside India, have also been reported from India through various publications (Loew, 1866; Meigen, 1804, 1830; Brues, 1909, 1936; Annandale, 1912; Wasmann, 1913; Schmitz, 1927; Beyer, 1950, 1967; Disney, 2002).

Disney (1994) in his exclusive book on "Scuttle Flies" has collated the natural history of the family Phoridae. The user-friendly illustrated identification keys were also provided in the book for

229 genera globally. The book also reviews the biology of Phoridae, including eggs, oviposition, larval habitats (such as saprophagous, kleptoparasites, fungus breeders, plant feeders, predators, parasitoids, parasites, and enemies), pupae and their enemies, development, and adult habits (including feeding, special associations, courtship, mating, phoretic mites, and enemies), as well as ecological aspects and a complete bibliography. The taxonomic account of the family Phoridae (Diptera) has been followed as per Pape et al. (2010).

In addition, Mercedes and Hardy (1977) published a catalogue on phorid flies of the oriental region. Brues (1906, 1915) and Brown (1992, 1993, 2012) made a valuable contribution to the group. The phorid flies of the states of Uttarakhand and Maharashtra were reported by Mitra and Bhattacharya (2010) and Dutta et al. (2012), respectively. Chakraborti et al. (2013) published an account of scuttle flies from India.

8.4 HABIT AND HABITAT

Phorid flies are cosmopolitan and distributed in tropical and subtropical regions. Their populations predominantly thrive in moist, unsanitary vicinities, such as trash containers, dumpsters, vegetable remains, homes, sewer pipes, rotting meat, and public washrooms. Adults primarily feed on sugary substances, while larvae feed on decaying animal and plant materials (Sukontason, 2003). They possess a wide range of feeding adaptations and are by nature carnivores, fungus feeders, herbivores, parasitoids, scavengers, and true parasites. They are typically parasitic, infesting the nests of wasps, bees, ants, termites, molluscs, and diplopods (Wakid, 2008). The phorids play an important role in the ecosystem, acting as scavengers, biocontrol agents, and forensic indicators of human and wildlife crimes.

8.5 IMPORTANCE AS PEST

Phorid flies are common pests in homes, restaurants, orchards, gardens, hotels, bars, and even restrooms, as they can thrive in any organic material available in drains, pipes, garbage, or food sources such as fruits, vegetables, and animal waste. Some of these flies are becoming serious pests. Recently, phorid flies have been globally considered as a minor pest, particularly in mushrooms, and their populations have been increasing, with yield losses ranging between 10% and 40% reported (Navarro et al., 2021).

8.6 IMPORTANCE AS BIOCONTROL AGENT: PARASITE AND PARASITOID

When an organism attacks any developmental stage of its host, characterized by its larvae, which grow on or inside the host and always kill it as part of its life cycle (Godfray and Shimada, 1999; Machkour-M'Rabet et al., 2015) it is called a parasitoid. Numerous studies have been conducted on various organisms as parasites and parasitoids for biological control. *Megaselia scalaris*, a polyphagous saprophage, is a widely distributed species in the family Phoridae. This easily cultured fly species is an emerging model organism in the fields of genetics and developmental biology. This species has been transported around the world by humans (Disney, 1994). Bragança et al. (2002) studied the characteristics of two phorid fly species' parasitism in relation to their host, the leaf-cutting ant, *Atta laevigata* (Hymenoptera: Formicidae), which is one of the forestry and agricultural pests in Brazil. There are emerging threats to honey bee populations from the parasitic phorid fly, *Apocephalus borealis* (Core et al., 2012). Remadevi et al. (1980) reported the phorid fly *Megaselia* sp. (Diptera: Phoridae) as a newly recorded parasite of *Nephantis serinopa* Meyrick (Lepidoptera: Xylorictidae) from India. Lloyd (2000) studied the biology of *Pseudaction* (Diptera: Phoridae) ant parasitoids and found that this phorid fly has the potential to control *Solenopsis* fire ants (Hymenoptera: Formicidae).

The American cockroach, *Periplaneta americana* (Linnaeus, 1758), is one of the most common household pest species widely distributed across the world. They survive in diverse environments

TABLE 8.1
List of Species of the Family Phoridae and Their Distribution

S.N.	Family/Subfamily/Tribe/Genus/Subgenus/ Species	Distribution in States and Union Territories of India	Distribution Outside India
	Family – Phoridae Curtis, 1833		
	Subfamily – Aenigmatiinae		
	I. Genus *Assmutherium* Schmitz, 1924		
1.	*Assmutherium rostratum* Schmitz, 1924: 300	Karnataka	
	Subfamily – Metopininae		
	Tribe – Metopinini		
	II. Genus *Apocephalus* Coquillett, 1901		
	Subgenus *Apocephalus* Coquillett, 1901		
2.	*Apocephalus (Apocephalus) caudatarius* Schmitz, 1915	Maharashtra	
	III. Genus *Bolsiusia* Schmitz, 1913		
3.	*Bolsiusia termitophila* Schmitz, 1913: 268	Maharashtra	
	IV. Genus *Chonocephalus* Wandolleck, 1898		
4.	*Chonocephalus collini* Disney, 2002	India	Thailand
5.	*Chonocephalus fletcheri* Schmitz, 1912: 727	Bihar, West Bengal	Thailand
6.	*Chonocephalus* similis Brues, 1905: 554	Maharashtra	Thailand
	V. Genus *Megaselia* Rondani, 1856		
7.	*Megaselia apposita* Brues, 1936: 449	India	Japan, Philippines
8.	*Megaselia chlumetiae* Disney, 1992:	Maharashtra	
9.	*Megaselia curtineura* (Brues, 1909):	West Bengal	Africa, Australia, Israel, Malaysia, New Zealand, Philippines, Taiwan, Takao, USA
	Synonyms *(Aphiochaeta) Aphiochaeta insulata* Brues, 1911: 542 *Aphiochaeta subfurcata* Brunetti, 1912: 508 *Aphiochaeta variata* Malloch, 1912: 515		
10.	*Megaselia malaisei* Beyer, 1958:	India	Myanmar
11.	*Megaselia pallicornis* (Brunetti, 1912)	West Bengal	
12.	*Megaselia palpella* (Beyer, 1967)	India	Micronesia
13.	*Megaselia pleurota* Disney, 1994	Chandigarh	Indonesia
14.	*Megaselia ruficornis* (Meigen, 1830)	India	Canary, Madeira, Estonia, Europe, USA, Russia
15.	*Megaselia rufipes* (Meigen, 1804): 313 *(Trineura)*	India	Arab, Atlantic Islands, Canary Islands, Europe, USA
16.	*Megaselia rutilipes* Beyer, 1958: 67	India	Myanmar
17.	*Megaselia sandhui* Disney, 1981: 509	Punjab	
18.	*Megaselia scalaris* (Loew, 1866): 53 *(Phora)*	Assam, West Bengal	Java, Philippines, Saudi Arabia, Sri Lanka, Subtropics and Tropic Regions of the world.

(Continued)

TABLE 8.1 (*Continued*)
List of Species of the Family Phoridae and Their Distribution

S.N.	Family/Subfamily/Tribe/Genus/Subgenus/ Species	Distribution in States and Union Territories of India	Distribution Outside India
	Synonyms		
	Aphiochaeta banksi Brues, 1909: 5		
	Aphiochaeta circumsetosa de Meijere, 1911: 348		
	Megaselia ferruginea Brunetti, 1912: 84		
19.	*Megaselia tamilnaduensis* Disney, 1995: 516	Tamil Nadu	South Africa
20.	*Megaselia tetricifrons* Beyer, 1967	India	Bonin Island, Japan, Micronesia
21.	*Megaselia apicalis* (Brues, 1905): 401 (*Aphiochaeta*)	Maharashtra	
22.	*Megaselia approximata* (Brunetti, 1912): 507 (*Aphiochaeta*)	West Bengal	
23.	*Megaselia flavifacies* (Brunetti, 1912): 509 (*Aphiochaeta*)	West Bengal	
24.	*Megaselia flavifacioides* (Senior-White, 1922): 153 (*Aphiochaeta*)	Meghalaya	
25.	*Megaselia inaequalis* (Brunetti, 1912): 511 (*Aphiochaeta*)	India	Nepal
26.	*Megaselia latifasciata* (Brunetti, 1912): 508 (*Aphiochaeta*)	Bihar, West Bengal	Pakistan
27.	*Megaselia pseudoscalaris* (Senior-White, 1922): 399 (*Aphioc haeta*)	Bihar	Sri Lanka
28.	*Megaselia tibialis* (Brues, 1905): 545 (*Aphiochaet a*)	Maharashtra	
29.	*Megaselia trilineata* (Brunetti, 1912): 510 (*Aphiochaeta*)	West Bengal	
	VI. Genus *Metopina* Macquart, 1835		
30.	*Metopina ciceri* Disney, 1988: 611	Peninsular Region	Nearctic Region
	VII. Genus *Phalacrotophora* Enderlein, 1912		
	Subgenus *Omapanta* Schmitz,1932		
31.	*Phalacrotophora (Omapanta) indiana* Colyer, 1961: 93	India	
32.	*Phalacrotophora* (*Omapanta*) *marginata* (Brunetti, 1912): 512 (*Hypocera*)	Kerala	
	VIII. Genus *Puliciphora* Dahl, 1897		
33.	*Puliciphora anceps* Schmitz, 1915: 324	Karnataka	
34.	*Puliciphora borinquenensis* Wheeler, 1906	India	South Africa
35.	*Puliciphora matheranensis* Brues, 1907: 409	Maharashtra	
36.	*Puliciphora termitum* Schmitz, 1926: 15	Uttarakhand	
37.	*Puliciphora velocipes* (Schmitz, 1913): 13 (*Termitophora*)	Maharashtra	
	IX. Genus *Rhynchomicropteron* Annandale, 1912		
38.	*Rhynchomicropteron brevipes* Papp, 1982	Meghalaya	
39.	*Rhynchomicropteran caecutiens* Schmitz, 1914: 519	Maharashtra	

(*Continued*)

TABLE 8.1 (*Continued*)
List of Species of the Family Phoridae and Their Distribution

S.N.	Family/Subfamily/Tribe/Genus/Subgenus/ Species	Distribution in States and Union Territories of India	Distribution Outside India
40.	*Rhynchomicropteron dudichi* Papp, 1982	West Bengal	
41.	*Rhynchomicropteron nudicosta* (Brues, 1907):	Maharashtra	
42.	*Rhynchomicropteron nudiventer* Papp, 1982	Meghalaya	Hungary, Thailand
43.	*Rhynchomicropteron puliciforme* Annandale, 1912: 86	India	Sri Lanka
	X. Genus *Woodiphora* Schmitz. 1925		
	Subgenus *Triemisticha* Schmitz, 1925		
44.	*Woodiphora* (*Trimisticha*) *limbata* (Brues, 1905): 546 (*Aphiochaeta*)	Maharashtra	Seychelles
	Subfamily – Phorinae		
	XI.Genus *Conicera* Meigen, 1830		
45.	*Conicera kempi* Brunetti, 1924: 106	Meghalaya	
	XII. Genus *Diplonevra Lioy*, 1864		
46.	*Diplonevra assmuthi* (Schmitz, 1915): 322 (*Dohrniphora*)	Karnataka, Maharashtra	Widely distributed
47.	*Diplonerva basalis* (Brunetti, 1912): 500 (*Phora*)	Assam	Widely distributed
48.	*Diplonevra rufithorax* (Brunetti, 1912): 502 (*Phora*)	India	Widely distributed
	Subgenus *Tristoechia* Schmitz, 1927		
49.	*Diplonevra (Tristoechia) bifasciata* (Walker, 1860)	Assam	Eat Asia, Japan and Taiwan
	XIII. Genus *Dohrniphora* Dahl, 1898		
50.	*Dohrniphora aequidistans* Brunetti, 1912: 501 (*Phora*)	West Bengal	
51.	*Dohrniphora cornuta* (Bigot, 1857): 348 (*Phora*)	West Bengal	Cuba, Philippines, Taiwan, USA
	Synonyms		
	Phora cleghorni Bigot, 1890: 191		
	Phora mordax Brues, 1911: 531		
52.	*Dohrniphora geetae* (Disney, 2001): 216 (*Megaselia*)	Karnataka	
53.	*Dohrniphora indiae* (Disney, 2001: 215	West Bengal	
54.	*Dohrniphora orientalis* (Schiner, 1868): 224 (*Phora*)	Andaman and Nicobar	
55.	*Dohrniphora transformata* Schmitz, 1915: 312	Karnataka	Sumatra
56.	*Dohrniphora vorax* Schmitz, 1915: 318	Karnataka, Maharashtra	Sulawesi, Sumatra
	XIV. Genus *Hypocera* Lioy,1864		
57.	*Hypocera marginata* Brunetti,1912	Kerala	
	XV. Genus *Phora* Latreille, 1796		
58.	*Phora bullata* Schmitz, 1927: 158	India	England
59.	*Phora himachalensis* Mostovski, 2002: 237	Himachal Pradesh	
	Subfamily – Termitoxeniinae		
	XVI. Genus *Ceylonoxenia* Schmitz, 1936		

(*Continued*)

TABLE 8.1 *(Continued)*

List of Species of the Family Phoridae and Their Distribution

S.N.	Family/Subfamily/Tribe/Genus/Subgenus/ Species	Distribution in States and Union Territories of India	Distribution Outside India
60.	*Ceylonoxenia. bugnioni* (Wasmann, 1913): 20 (*Termitoxenia*)	India	Sri Lanka
61.	*Ceylonoxenia butteli* (Wasmann, 1913): 20 (*Termitoxenia*)	India	Sri Lanka
62.	*Ceylonoxenia flavescens* Schmitz, 1938: 59	India	Java
63.	*Ceylonoxenia heimi* (Wasmann, 1902): 602 (*Termitoxenia*)	Maharashtra	
64.	*Ceylonoxenia wasmanni* Schmitz, 1938: 56	India	
	XVII. Genus *Clitelloxenia* Kemner, 1932		
65.	*Clitelloxenia assmuthi* (Wasmann, 1902): 151 (*Termitoxenia*)	Maharashtra	Java, Malaysia, Sri Lanka
66.	*Clitelloxenia marshalli* Schmitz, 1938: 35	Karnataka	
	XVIII. Genus *Termitosphaera* Wasmann, 1913		
67.	*Teretomitosphaera fletcheri* (Wasmann, 1913): 17 (*Termitoxenia*)	West Bengal	Myanmar

*Checklist source–Mitra et al. (2016).

and carry various pathogens, causing critical threats to public health and the ecosystem. There are observations of decapitated American cockroaches as a result of infestation with scuttle fly (*Megaselia scalaris*) parasitoids (Arafat et al., 2024). The behavioural alterations in the form of zombification-like behaviour observed in cockroaches reared in the laboratory before being decapitated imply that the insect targets cockroach heads (Arafat et al., 2024). This endoparasitoid acts as a novel biocontrol agent against adult American cockroaches (Arafat et al., 2024).

The larvae of scuttle flies have also been reported as parasitoids of hawk moths (Lepidoptera: Sphingidae) and their frugivory on avocado (Souza et al., 2020); on mango shoot borer, *Chlumetia transversa* (Lepidoptera:Noctuidae), and reared from *Spodoptera exigua* (Hübner, 1808) (Lepidoptera: Noctuidae) feeding on cauliflower (Disney et al., 2024). There is a record of a parasitoid of the fall armyworm, *Spodoptera frugiperda* (J. E. Smith) (Lepidoptera: Noctuidae) from India (Deshmukh et al., 2021) attracting parasitic flies (Diptera: Phoridae) to injured workers of the giant ant, *Dinoponera gigantea* (Hymenoptera: Formicidae) (Costa and Moutinho, 1996). In South India, it has been reported that the edible oyster mushroom cultivated there is attacked by the larvae of the phorid fly, *Megaseliata milnaduensis*. These larvae feed on the mycelium, reducing the yield of sporophores from 400–500 g to 200–350 g (Mohan and Disney, 1995).

A comprehensive review covered the morphological and behavioural characteristics of 190 scuttle fly species that are termitophilous or associated with termites worldwide. This review provided a complete list of these phorids along with their termite hosts (Dupont and Pape, 2009). The review also explored how various factors, including egg size, batch size, developmental cycles, wing reduction, winglessness, egg-laying behaviours, and other morphological adaptations, are related to the lifestyle associated with termites. It is suggested that endoparasitism could be a beneficial strategy for numerous phorids associated with termites (Dupont and Pape, 2009).

8.7 IMPORTANCE TO FORENSIC ENTOMOLOGY

Coffin flies, or scuttle flies, are most commonly found in buried human bodies after years of burial, and they become active on exposed bodies after butyric fermentation and when the corpse starts to dry. They are capable of completing several life cycles beneath the ground. However, in the case of enclosed indoor areas, much smaller flies (scuttle flies) can enter the corpse and deposit their eggs. The colonisation time of the flies can be analysed to calculate the post-mortem interval (PMI), aiding in estimating the time of death. These studies were conducted in various indoor settings, where determining the age of PMI was found to be more accurate (Chakroborty et al., 2016; Reibe and Madea, 2010). Greenberg and Wells (1998), Kar et al. (2023), Disney (2005, 2006), Disney and Manlove (2005), Manlove and Disney (2008), Boehme et al. (2010), Disney et al. (2014), and Zuha et al. (2016) have contributed on phorid flies relevant to forensic investigations.

8.8 IMPORTANCE TO MEDICAL SCIENCE

The phorid fly, *Megaselia scalaris*, is also of medical importance as it causes myiasis and various problems in human beings. The female fly lays its eggs in fruits, vegetables, decaying matter, debris, wet food articles, and faeces. Sporadic cases of facultative human myiasis caused by *Megaselia scalaris* have been reported in many parts of the world (Carpenter and Chastain, 1992), which may result in cutaneous, pneumonic, nasal, gastrointestinal, urogenital, and ophthalmic myiasis (Carpenter and Chastain, 1992). The maggots of *Megaselia scalaris* were also reported from the urine sample of a 5-year-old Saudi girl (Wakid et al., 2008). Protozoan flagellates were obtained from the gut of the larvae and were found to be a causative agent of urinary human myiasis in Saudi Arabia (Wakid et al., 2008). In India, Disney and Kurahashi (1978), Singh and Rana (1988) and Singh et al. (1988) reported cases of urogenital myiasis and intestinal myiasis, respectively, with the causative agent being the phorid fly, *Megaselia scalaris*.

8.9 CONCLUSIONS

To conclude, the importance of phorid flies, both studied in their natural habitats and extensively reared for biological control, has been emphasized. The application of the scuttle fly as a biological control agent for managing American cockroach populations and their respective complications is discussed elsewhere. Their role as parasites and parasitoids can be utilized in controlling various insect pest species. Estimating the PMI using the developmental times of scuttle flies can provide a reliable alternative to determining blowfly larval age. Scuttle flies are found in enclosed environments with varying temperatures, where blowflies are typically inactive. The scuttle fly (*Megaselia scalaris*) can be easily cultured in laboratories, and due to its diverse habitat, it is emerging as a model organism for studies in genetics, developmental biology, and biocontrol.

8.10 POINTS TO REMEMBER

1. Phorid flies are commonly known as scuttle flies due to their ability to run quickly in short bursts and are widely distributed across the globe.
2. One of the most biologically diverse families of insects, scuttle flies share similarities with fruit flies.
3. The distinctive humped back appearance is a characteristic feature of scuttle flies.
4. Males and females can be distinguished based on the differences in size and shape of the third antennal segment.
5. In India, there are 67 species in 18 genera and four subfamilies: Metopininae, Aenigmatiinae, Termitoxeniinae, and Phorinae.

6. In South India, the larvae of the phorid fly *Megaseliata milnaduensis* attack edible oyster mushrooms, reducing yield.
7. Various life stages of scuttle flies serve as biological agents, controlling the populations of pests.
8. Scuttle flies, common in buried human bodies where they can complete their life cycles underground, are useful in calculating the PMI in forensic investigations.
9. Phorid fly, *Megaselia scalaris*, is of medical importance as it causes myiasis and various other health issues in humans.
10. The scuttle flies are easily cultured in laboratories and are emerging as a model organism for genetics, developmental biology, and biocontrol studies due to their diverse habits and habitats.

ACKNOWLEDGEMENTS

The author is grateful to the Director of the Zoological Survey of India for the facilities. The author also thanks Dr Sumana Halder, Research Associate, and Mr P. Parui, Retd. Scientist of the Zoological Survey of India, for their inputs.

REFERENCES

Amoudi, M.D., Diab, F.M., & Abu-Fannah, S.S. (1989). The occurrence of *Megaselia scalaris* (Loew) (Diptera: Phoridae) in Saudi Arabia with some aspects on the life history and distribution in Ryiadh province. *Journal of King Saud University* Science 1–2: 43–51.

Annandale, N. (1912). Description of a micropterous fly of the family Phoridae associated with ants Spolia Zeylanica, *Colombo* 8: 85–89.

Arafat, E.A., Lamia, M. Samad, El, Mohamed A., & Hassan, M.A. (2024). Scuttle fly *Megaselia scalaris* (Loew) (Diptera: Phoridae) endoparasitoid as a novel biocontrol agent against adult American cockroaches (*Periplaneta americana*). *Scientific Reports* 14: 9762.

Beyer, E.M. (1967). *Diptera Phoridae Insects of Micronesia* 13: 329–360.

Bigot, J.M.F. (1890). New species of Indian Diptera. *Indian Museum Notes* 1: 191–195.

Boehme, P, Amendt, J, Disney R.H.L., & Zehner R. (2010). Molecular identification of carrion-breeding scuttle flies (Diptera: Phoridae) using COI barcodes. *International Journal of Legal Medicine* 124: 577–581.

Bragança M.A.L., Tonhasca, J.A. & Moreira D.D.O. (2002). Parasitism characteristics of two phorid fly species in relation to their host, the leaf-cutting ant, *Atta laevigata* (Smith) (Hymenoptera:.Formicidae). *Neotropical Entomology* 31: 241–244.

Brown, B.V. (1992). Generic revision of Phoridae of the Nearctic Region and phylogenetic classification of Phoridae, Sciadoceridae, and Ironomyiidae (Diptera: Phoroidea). *Memoirs of the Entomological Society of Canada* 164: 1–144.

Brown, B.V. (1993). Taxonomy and preliminary phylogeny of the parasitic genus *Apocephalus*, subgenus *Mesophora* (Diptera: Phoridae). *Systematic Entomology* 18: 191–230.

Brown, B.V. (2012). Small size no protection for acrobat ants: World's smallest fly is a parasitic phorid (Diptera: Phoridae). *Annals of the Entomological Society of America* 105(4): 550–554.

Brues, C.T. (1906). Diptera, Fam Phoridae. *Genera Insectorum* 44: 1–21.

Brues, C.T. (1907). A remarkable new phorid from Cape Colony. *Entomological News* 18: 430.

Brues, C.T. (1909). Some further remarks on the affinities of the Phoridae, with descriptions of two North American species. *Bulletin of the Wisconsin Natural History Society* 7: 103–108.

Brues, C.T. (1915). A synonymic catalogue of the dipterous family Phoridae. *Bulletin of theWisconsin Natural History Society* 12: 85–152.

Brues, C.T. (1936). Philippine Phoridae from Mount Apo region in Mindanao. *Proceedings of the American Academy of Arts and Sciences* 70: 365–466.

Brunetti, E. (1912). Description of a hitherto undescribed species of Phoridae that causes Myasis in man. *Records Indian Museum* 7: 83–86.

Brunetti, E. (1924). Diptera of the Siju Cave, Garo Hills, *Assam*. 1. Tipulidae, Tabanidae, Anthomyidae, Acalyptratae, Muscidae and Phoridae. *Records of the Indian Museum, Calcutta* 26: 99–106.

Carpenter, T.L. & Chastain, D.O. (1992). Facultative Myiasis by *Megaselia* sp. (Diptera: Phoridae) in Texas: A case Report. *Journal of Medical Entomology* 29(3): 561–563.
Chakraborty, A, Naskar, A, Hazra, S, Maity, A, & Banerjee, D. (2013). Indian Scuttle Flies (Insecta: Diptera: Phoridae). www.zsi.gov.in/check_list.html (accessed on December 2, 2015).
Chakraborty, A, Naskar, A, Parui, P., & Banerjee D. (2016). Developmental Variation of Indian Thermophilic Variety of Scuttle Fly *Megaselia (Megaselia) scalaris* (Loew, 1866) (Diptera: Phoridae) on Different Substrates. *Scientifica (Cairo)* 2: 1–9.
Colyer, C.N. (1954). The 'coffin fly', *Conicera tibialis* Schmitz (Dipt., Phoridae). *Journal of the Society for British Entomology* 4: 203–206.
Colyer, C.N. (1961). A new species of *Phalacrotophora* (Diptera, Phoridae) from India. *Brotena* 30: 93–97.
Core, A., Runckel, C., Ivers, J., Quock, C., & Siapno, T. (2012). A New Threat to Honey Bees, the Parasitic Phorid Fly, *Apocephalus borealis*. *PLoS One* 7(1): e29639. doi:10.1371/journal.pone.0029639.
Costa, A. & Moutinho, P. (1996). Attracting parasitic flies (Diptera: Phoridae) to injured workers of the giant ant, *Dinoponera gigantea* (Hymenoptera: Formicidae). *Entomological News* 107(2): 93–98.
Deshmukh, S.S., Kiran, S., Naskar, A., Pradeep, P., Kalleshwaraswamy, C.M., & Sharat, K.N. (2021). First record of a parasitoid, *Megaselia (M.) scalaris* (Diptera: Phoridae) of fall armyworm, *Spodoptera frugiperda* (J.E. Smith) (Lepidoptera: Noctuidae) from India. *Egyptian Journal of Biological Pest Control* 31: 94.
Disney, R., & Henry, L. (2002). Revisionary notes on *Chonocephalus* Wandolleck (Diptera: Phoridae) with keys to species of the Holarctic Region. *Zootaxa* 60: 1–36.
Disney, R.H.L. (1981). Megaselia *sandhui* sp. nov. (Diptera: Phoridae), a pest of cultivated mushrooms in India. *Bulletin of Entomological Research* 71: 509–512.
Disney, R.H.L. (1988). A remarkable new species of scuttle fly (Diptera: Phoridae) whose larvae infest chick-pea root nodules in India. *Journal of Natural History* 22(3): 611–616
Disney, R.H.L. (1990). A key to *Diplonevra* males of the Australasian and Oriental Regions, including two new species (Diptera, Phoridae). *Entomologica Fennica* 5: 33–39.
Disney, R.H.L. (1994). *Scuttle Flies: The Phoridae*. Chapman-Hall, London, pp. 1–467.
Disney, R.H.L. (2001). Two new species of Phoridae (Diptera) from India. *Entomologist's Monthly Magazine* 137: 215–218.
Disney, R.H.L. (2005). Duration of development of two species of carrion breeding scuttle flies and forensic implications. *Medical and Veterinary Entomology* 19: 229–235.
Disney, R.H.L. (2006). Scuttle flies (Diptera: Phoridae). Part I: All genera except *Megaselia*. *Fauna of Arabia* 22: 473–521.
Disney, R.H.L. (2008). Six new species of *Megaselia* Rondani (Diptera: Phoridae) from mainland Australia. *Zootaxa* 1899: 57–68.
Disney, R.H.L, & Kurahashi, H. (1978). A case of urogenital myiasis caused by a species of *Megaselia* (Diptera: Phoridae). *Journal of Medical Entomology* 14: 717.
Disney, R.H.L., & Manlove, J.D. (2005). First occurrences of the phorid, *Megaselia abdita*, in forensic cases in Britain. *Medical and Veterinary Entomology* 19: 489–491.
Disney R.H.L., & Michailovskaya, M.V. (2001). New species and new records of *Puliciphora* Dahl (Phoridae: Diptera) from Russia, India and the Seychelles. *Fragmenta Faunistica (Warsaw)* 44(2): 329–340.
Disney, R.H.L., Khochare, N.N., & Godase, S.K. Jr. (1992). A new parasitoid (Diptera: Phoridae) of the mango shoot borer, *Chlumetia transversa* (Lepidoptera: Noctuidae), in India. *Bulletin of Entomological Research* 82(2): 191–195.
Disney, R.H.L., Garcia-Rojo, A., Lindström, A., & Manlove, J.D., (2014). Further occurrences of *Dohrniphora cornuta* (Bigot) (Diptera, Phoridae) in forensic cases indicate likely importance of this species in future cases. *Forensic Science International* 241: 20–22.
Disney, R.H.L., Karimzadeh, J., Besharatnejad, M.H., Gilasian, E., & Sheikhigarjan, A. (2024). Scuttle flies (Diptera: Phoridae) reared from *Spodoptera exigua* (Hübner, 1808) (Lepidoptera: Noctuidae) in Iran. *Zootaxa* 5448(2): 292–300.
Dupont, S., & Pape, T. (2009). A review of termitophilous and other termite-associated scuttle flies worldwide (Diptera: Phoridae). *Terrestrial Arthropod Reviews* 2(1): 3–40.
Dutta Saha, P., Sharma, R.M., & Mitra, B. (2012). Insecta: Diptera in Fauna of Maharashtra. Zoological Surviey of India, *State Fauna Series* 20(2): 531–538.
Godfray, H.C.J., & Shimada, M. (1999). Parasitoids as model organism for ecologists. *Researches on Population Ecolgy* 41: 3–10.

Greenberg, B., & Wells, J.D. (1998). Forensic use of *Megaselia abdita* and *Megaselia scalaris* (Phoridae: Diptera): Case studies, development rates, and egg structure. *Journal of Medical Entomology* 35: 205–209.

Kar, O., Naskar, A., Pramanik, D., Mukherjee, K., Sarkar, S., Mukherjee, A., Ghosh, D., & Banerjee, D. (2023). A checklist of forensic flies from India. *Records of the Zoological Survey of India* 122(4): 387–392.

Loew, H. (1866). Diptera *America se septentrionalis indigena.*Centuria Septima. *Berliner Entomologische. Zeiteschrift* 10: 1–54.

Lloyd, W.M. (2000). Biology of *Pseudaction* (Diptera: Phoridae) ant parasitoids and their potential to control *Solenopsis* fire ants (Hymenoptera: Formicidae). *Recent Research Developments in Entomology* 3: 1–13.

Machkour-M'Rabet, S., Dor, A., & Henaut, Y. (2015). *Megaselia scalaris* (Diptera: Phoridae): An opportunistic endoparasitoid of the endangered Mexican redrump tarantula, Barchypelma vagans (Araneae:Theraphosidae). *The Journal of Arachnology* 43: 115–119.

Manlove, J.D., & Disney, R.H.L. (2008). The use of *Megaselia abdita* (Diptera: Phoridae) in winter forensic entomology. *Forensic Science International* 175: 449–451.

Meigen, J.W. (1804). *Klassifikazion und Beschreibung der europaischenz zweifliegelingen Insekten*. (Diptera Linn.) *Erster Band Abt.* I.xxviii: 1–152. Abt.II. vi+pp.153–314.

Meigen, J.W. (1830). *Systematische Beschreibung bekannten europaeischenz zweifliegelingen Insekten* Hamm, 6(IV): 1–401.

Mercedes, D.D., & Hardy, D.E., (1977). Phoridae. In: *A catalog of the Diptera of the oriental region, Suborder Brachycera through Division Aschiza, Suborder Cyclorrahapha*. The University Press of Hawaii, Honolulu, pp. 261–295.

Mohan, S. & Disney, R.H.L. (1995). A new species of scuttle fly (Diptera: Phoridae) that is a pest Oyster mushrooms (Agaricales:Pleurotaceae) in India. *Bulletin of Entomological Research* 85(4): 515–518.

Mitra, B, & Bhattacharya, K. (2010). Diptera: Insecta. Director, Zoological Survey of India, *Fauna of Uttrakhand State Fauna Series*, 18(2): 361–411.

Mitra, B., Roy, S., Halder, S., Roy, S., & Mukhopadhyay, S. (2016). Diversity and distribution pattern of scuttle flies (Diptera: Phoridae) in India. *International Journal of Entomological Research* 1(3): 33–38.

Mostovski, M.B. (2002). Two new species of *Phora* (Dipt., Phoridae) from Tajikistan and India. *Entomologist's Monthly Magazine* 138(1660–1663): 237–240.

Navarro, M.J., Escudero-Colomar, L.A., Carrasco, J., & Gea, F.J. (2021). Mushroom phorid flies: A review. *Agronomy* 11(1958): 1–16.

Pallavi, J., Snehal, H., Kolipakala, R.S., Salazar, D., Hanbar, M., Chiramel, L.B., Jha, K.A., Venkatesh, S.B.L., Shetty, T.D., Madhusudan, N., Mohan, A., John, A., D'Souza, N.D., Sheet, P., & Nagarajan, D. (2023). A complete morphological characterization of all life stages of the phorid fly. *Megaselia Scalaris, Scientific Reports* 13: 22933.

Papp, L. (1982). Three new species of *Rhynochomicropteron* from India (Diptera: Phoridae). *Acta Zoologica Academiae Scientiarum Hungaricae* 2: 125–131.

Pape, T., Blagoderov, V., & Mostovski, M.B. (2011). Order DIPTERA Linnaeus, 1758. In: Z.Q. Zhang (Ed.) Animal Biodiversity: An outline of higher-level classification and survey of taxonomic richness. *Zootaxa* 3148: 222–229.

Reibe, S., & Madea, B. (2010). Use of *Megaselia scalaris* (Diptera: Phoridae) for post-mortem interval estimation indoors. *Parasitology Research* 106(3): 637–640.

Remadevi, O.K., Mohamed, U.V.K., & Abdurahiman, U.C. (1980). Notes on *Megaselia* sp. (Diptera: Phoridae) a newly recorded parasite of *Nephantis serinopa* Meyrick (Lepidoptera: Xylorictidae). *Current Science (*Bangalore*)* 49(12): 491–492.

Sandhu, G.S., & Bhattal, D.S. (1987). Biology of Phorid Fly, *Megaselia sandhui* Disney (Diptera: Phoridae) on Temperate Mushroom. *Developments in Crop Science* 10: 395–404.

Schmitz, H. (1913a). Eine neuetermitophile Phoriden-Gattung und -Art, *Bolsiusia termitophila* n.g. n. sp. *aus Ostindien Zoologlscher Anzelger* 42: 268–273.

Schmitz, H. (1913b). Beschreibung von *Termitophora velocipes* (Wasmanninlitt.), einertermitophilen Phoride de ausVorderindien. *Entomologiske Meddelelser* 10: 9–16.

Schmitz, H. (1915). Neue Britragezurzur Kenntnis der myrmecophilen und termitophilen Phoriden. (No. 16-22) Neue Phoridenaus Vorderindien, gesammelt von J Assmuth S J, Bombay. *Weiner. Entomologische Zeitung* 34: 311–330.

Schmitz, H. (1924). Dreineue Platyphorinen (Phoridae, Diptera) und eineneue Wirtstermite. *Zoologischer Anzeiger* 59: 289–304.

Schmitz, H.H. (1926a). Sauter's Formosa-Ausbeute: Phoriden (Dipt.). *Entomologische Mitteilungen* 15(1): 46–57.

Schmitz, H. (1926b). A new termitophilous phorid from India. *Entomologist's Monthly Magazine* 62: 15–16.

Schmitz, H. (1927). Eine neue myrmecophile *Metopina*, nebstanderenneuen Artendieser Gattung. *Zoologischer Anzeiger* 74: 241–248.

Schmitz, H. (1938). Phoridae: In E. Lindner (ed.), *Die Fliegen der palaearktischen Region* 4(33). (Lieferung 123): 1–64.

Senior-White, R.A. (1922). Notes on Indian Diptera. *Menl. Department of Agriculture India* (ent. ser.). 7: 1–169.

Senior-White, R.A. (1924). The Muscidae Testaceae of the Oriental Region (with descriptions of those found within Indian limits). *Spolia Zeylanica* 12: 294–314.

Singh, N.B., Singh, T.K., Singh, Y.I., & Razaque, M.A. (1988). Intestinal myiasis caused by *Megaselia scalaris* (Diptera: Phoridae): A case report. *Journal of Medical Entomology* 20 163.

Singh, T.S., & Rana, D. (1988). Urogenital myiasis caused by *Megaselia scalaris* (Diptera: Phoridae): A case report. *Journal of Medical Entomology* 26: 228–229.

Souza, T.S., Fernandes, V.J., Aguiar-Menezes, E.L., Resende, A.L.S., Pereira, T.P.L., Gazal, V.S., & Menezes, E.B. (2020). Larvae of Megaselia Rondani, 1856 (Diptera:Phoridae) as parasitoid of Sphingidae (Lepidoptera) and its frugivory on avocado. *Entomological Communications* 2: 1–3.

Sukontason, K., Sukontason, K.L., Piangjai, S., Boonchu, N., Chaiwong, T., & Vogtsberger, R.C. (2003). Mouthparts of *Megaselia scalaris* (Loew) (Diptera: Phoridae). *Micron* 34(8): 345–50.

Tonhasca, A. Jr. (1996). Interactions between a parasitic fly, *Neodohrniphora declinata* (Diptera: Phoridae), and its host, the leaf-cutting ant, *Atta sexdensrubropilosa* (Hymenoptera: Formicidae). *Ecotropica* 2: 157–164.

Wakid, M.H. (2008). A laboratory-based study for first documented case of urinary myiasis caused by larvae of *Megaselia scalaris* (Diptera: Phoridae) in Saudi Arabia. *Korean Journal of Parasitology* 46(1): 33–36.

Wasmann, E. (1902). Termiten, Termitophilen und Myrmekophilen, gesammelt auf Ceylon, mitandernostindischen Material bearbeitet. *Zoologische JahrbucherAbteilungfor Systematik* 17: 99–164.

Wasmann, E. (1913). Revision der Termitoxenunae von Ostindien und Ceylon. *Annales de la Societe Entomologique de Belgique* 57: 16–22.

Zuha, R.M., Ankasha, S.J., Henry, R.L., Disney, R.H.L., & Omar, B. (2016). Indoor decomposition study in Malaysia with special reference to the scuttle flies (Diptera: Phoridae). *Egyptian Journal of Forensic Science* 6(3): 216–222.

Section II

Flies of Medical, Veterinary, and Forensic Importance

9 Flies of Public Health Importance

L. Rajesh Chowdary, Giri Naga Harish, Ashok Kumar Karedla, and Keerthi Manikyanahalli Chandrashekara

LEARNING OBJECTIVES

1. Recognize the various families, genera, and species of flies that impact human and animal health.
2. Identify the ecological niches and geographical ranges of sand flies, tsetse flies, house flies, stable flies, bot flies, horse flies, and screwworm flies.
3. Describe the life cycle stages of each fly species, from egg to adult.
4. Evaluate the role of these flies as vectors of diseases such as leishmaniasis, trypanosomiasis, and myiasis.
5. Understand the epidemiology of diseases spread by these vectors.
6. Learn about various control measures, including environmental management, chemical interventions, and biological control methods.
7. Stay updated on recent advancements in entomological research related to medically important flies.
8. Explore innovative control strategies and their potential applications.

9.1 SAND FLIES

Sand flies are insects belonging to the order Diptera (two-winged flies), specifically the suborder Nematocera, family Psychodidae, and subfamily Phlebotominae. Globally, around 1,000 species and subspecies of sand flies have been identified, with 98 species known to act as vectors for human leishmaniasis (Cecílio et al., 2022). Sand flies display diverse ecological and behavioural patterns. Some prefer to rest indoors, while others are typically found outdoors. Certain species inhabit active rodent burrows in plains, while others thrive in mountainous regions. Nocturnal by nature, sand flies are highly susceptible to dehydration, seeking refuge in caves, rock crevices, animal burrows, tree holes, and human dwellings (Gherbi et al., 2020). They are characterized by weak flight capability, moving short distances close to the ground. Although their typical flight range extends to approximately 300 m, certain desert species can travel up to 2,300 m. Due to their limited flight range, adults generally remain close to their larval development sites. In the New World, sand flies are commonly found near tree holes and caves, whereas in the Old World, they are associated with contaminated soils found in animal shelters, rodent burrows, termite mounds, and the earthen floors of human habitations (Wijerathna and Gunathilaka, 2020).

Distribution: *Phlebotomus* species primarily inhabit warm, humid, and tropical climates, often in savannah and semi-desert regions, although some are present in temperate zones. They can colonize rural, peri-urban, and urban areas. Sand flies require a humid microclimate for egg development, and their larvae thrive in cool, moist habitats with decaying organic matter (Tichá et al., 2021). Adult sand flies typically inhabit rock crevices, caves, and rodent burrows, and in peridomestic settings, they seek shelter in cool, dark, and humid

DOI: 10.1201/9781003482581-12

corners of animal shelters or human dwellings. Both rodent burrows and peridomestic environments provide access to blood meals and protection from adverse weather conditions. Phlebotomine sand flies are distributed across tropical, subtropical, and temperate zones. *Phlebotomus* species are found in Africa, where they serve as significant vectors in certain regions, as well as in Europe (particularly the Mediterranean), the Middle East, and Asia (especially the Indian subcontinent) (Trájer et al., 2018). Sand flies are restricted to areas where temperatures remain above 15.6°C for at least three months each year. In regions where temperatures drop below 10°C, sand flies enter a dormant state to survive winter, thereby reducing the breeding population (Muñoz et al., 2021). Adequate environmental moisture is crucial for egg survival; however, excessive rainfall can diminish sand fly numbers by reducing suitable resting sites for adults, limiting flight activity, and killing immature stages (Akhoundi et al., 2016).

Biology: Sand flies undergo a four-stage life cycle: egg, larva, pupa, and adult. Eggs typically hatch within 4–20 days, though cooler temperatures can delay this process. Larval development includes four instars and lasts for 20–30 days, depending on species, temperature, and nutrient availability. Extreme environmental conditions (e.g. heat, cold, or drought) can induce larvae to enter diapause, prolonging development for several months. Larvae primarily scavenge on organic matter, such as fungi, decaying leaves, animal faeces, and decomposing arthropods. The pupal stage lasts for 6–13 days before adult sand flies emerge. Adult sand flies mate soon after emergence. Males locate females at resting sites or on vertebrate hosts using pheromones. Female sand flies typically lay 30–70 eggs per gonotrophic cycle, depositing them in cracks and holes in the ground, in buildings, within animal burrows, and among tree roots. Eggs require a humid microhabitat for survival but are not laid in water. Generally, one blood meal is sufficient for producing a single batch of eggs (Wale and Shearer, 1997; Cecílio et al., 2022).

Both male and female sand flies feed on sugary secretions from fruits, flowers, and plant juices, using carbohydrates as their primary energy source. Females also require blood to produce eggs. Sand flies use their mouthparts to probe exposed skin, creating a pool of blood for feeding. Sand fly saliva contains pharmacologically active components that facilitate the feeding process. Female sand flies must feed on blood to complete egg development; however, some species are autogenous and can lay eggs without a blood meal. Feeding behaviour is influenced by temperature, humidity, and air movement, as sand flies are weak fliers, and even light winds can hinder flight and reduce biting activity. Most species feed at dusk and during the night when temperatures drop and humidity rises. While most sand flies feed outdoors, daytime biting may occur indoors in darkened rooms or shaded vegetation, particularly when disturbed by human activity. Anthropophilic sand flies often bite humans outside their tents, homes, and accommodations (Akhoundi et al., 2016).

9.1.1 Disease Transmission

Sand flies, particularly those of the Phlebotominae subfamily, are significant vectors of various pathogens responsible for numerous diseases affecting humans and animals. The most notable diseases transmitted by sand flies are various forms of leishmaniasis, caused by protozoan parasites of the genus *Leishmania*. Visceral leishmaniasis, often termed kala-azar, is a severe form of the disease caused by *Leishmania donovani* and *Leishmania infantum*, which are transmitted by species *Phlebotomus alexandri* (Studentsky et al., 2023). This disease can be fatal if untreated and primarily affects internal organs, like the liver and spleen. Cutaneous leishmaniasis, another form of the disease, results in severe skin lesions and is caused by species such as *Leishmania major* and *Leishmania tropica*. These parasites are transmitted by sand flies, like *Phlebotomus papatasi* and *Lutzomyia longipalpis* (Cecílio et al., 2022). The transmission dynamics involve sand flies acquiring the parasite through blood meals from infected hosts and subsequently transmitting it to new hosts. In addition to leishmaniasis, sand flies are vectors for other pathogens, including various viruses within the *Phlebovirus* genus, which can cause diseases like sand fly fever. Furthermore, the bacterium *Bartonella bacilliformis*, responsible for Carrion's disease, is also transmitted by sand flies (Benallal et al., 2022).

The geographical distribution of these diseases is extensive, with significant occurrences in tropical, subtropical, and some temperate regions. For instance, in the Maghreb region of North Africa, leishmaniasis is prevalent and poses a considerable public health challenge (Benallal et al., 2022). Similarly, in parts of the Middle East, Asia, and Latin America, sand fly-borne diseases continue to affect thousands annually, highlighting the need for ongoing surveillance and vector control measures. In conclusion, the role of sand flies as vectors for a variety of significant pathogens underscores the importance of understanding their biology and ecology to implement effective control strategies against the diseases they transmit. Regular updates and verification of sand fly data are essential for guiding public health interventions and mitigating the impact of these vector-borne diseases.

9.1.2 Management

Effective management of sand flies, particularly those responsible for the transmission of leishmaniasis, requires a multi-faceted approach. One of the primary strategies is environmental management, which involves modifying habitats to reduce sand fly breeding sites. This can include measures such as plastering the bases of walls with cement and fly ash to eliminate resting sites for sand flies, like *Phlebotomus argentipes*, a vector for visceral leishmaniasis (Dinesh et al., 2017; Figure 9.1). Insecticide-based interventions are also crucial. Indoor residual spraying (IRS) with insecticides, like α-cypermethrin, has shown significant effectiveness in reducing sand fly populations and the incidence of cutaneous leishmaniasis. Additionally, insecticide-treated bed nets have been evaluated for their potential in providing individual protection against sand fly bites, though their effectiveness for large-scale vector control needs further validation (Faraj et al., 2016). Monitoring and surveillance of sand fly populations are essential for effective management. The use of synthetic attractants, such as 1-octen-3-ol in combination with light traps, has been recommended for the effective monitoring of sand fly populations, aiding in the early detection and control of outbreaks

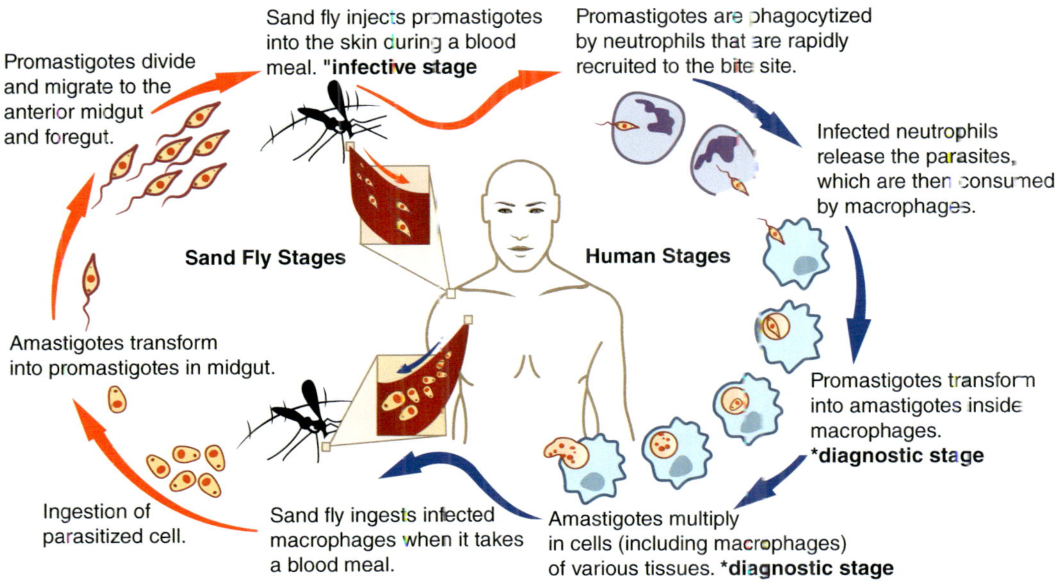

FIGURE 9.1 Leishmaniasis life cycle.

(Mikery et al., 2022).Biological control methods and the use of biological agents to target sand fly larvae and adults are also under exploration. These methods can be complementary to chemical control strategies and can help reduce the reliance on insecticides, thereby mitigating the risk of resistance development (Sharma and Singh, 2008).In conclusion, the management of sand flies involves an integrated approach that combines environmental management, chemical and biological control, monitoring and surveillance, and the consideration of climatic factors. These strategies are essential for controlling sand fly populations and reducing the transmission of leishmaniasis.

9.2 TSETSE FLIES

Tsetse flies (Diptera: Glossinidae) encompass all species within the genus *Glossina*, classified in their own family, Glossinidae. They are distinguishable from other large flies by two prominent features. Tsetse flies fold their wings completely when at rest, overlapping them over their abdomens in a scissor-like configuration. They also possess a long proboscis extending forwards, attached by a distinct bulb beneath their heads (Hordofa and Haile, 2017). Tsetse flies are slender-bodied, ranging from yellow to dark brown, and measure between 6 and 13.5 mm in length. Their thorax exhibits a dull greenish hue with subtle spots or stripes, while the abdomen appears light to dark brown with six visible segments from a dorsal view (Akhoundi et al., 2016).

Tsetse flies spend most of their resting time in shaded areas within forested regions, favouring the lower woody parts of vegetation where many hide in tree trunk holes and among roots. They actively seek food for brief periods during the day, often resting near food sources (Taylor et al., 2007). Common risk areas for tsetse fly bites include forest trails near water sources and vegetation near bathing and water collection sites along riverbanks (Janinin, 1999).

Distribution: Their distribution is specific, influenced by climate, vegetation, and soil conditions critical for larval deposition and pupal survival. Tsetse flies are endemic to the African continent, residing between latitudes 5°N and 20°S. They avoid areas of extreme drought in the north, cold temperatures in the south, and high-altitude regions. Their presence is restricted to regions where the average annual temperature exceeds 20°C, with 25°C being optimal for their survival (Radostits et al., 2007).

Covering an estimated 10 million square kilometres, tsetse flies inhabit regions from the semi-arid Sahel margins through tropical rainforests to subtropical savannahs, like those in KwaZulu-Natal, South Africa. Three main groups are recognized: the forest (*fusca*) group in west, central, and east African forests; the savannah (*morsitans*) group in west, east, and southern African savannahs; and the riverine (*palpalis*) group, with its five species found mainly in west and central African forests and riparian areas. Their habitat preferences include dense forests, bushlands, and savanna grasslands, providing shelter from sunlight and wind (Hordofa and Haile, 2017).

Biology: The life cycle of tsetse flies is unusual as they do not lay eggs externally. Instead, inseminated females develop eggs and young larvae within their uterus, depositing mature (third stage) larvae into moist soil or sand in shaded areas, often under fallen bushes, logs, large stones, and buttress roots (Janinin, 1999). Larvae quickly burrow underground, beginning pupation within 60 to 90 minutes, and emerge as adults 20–45 days later, depending on temperature (pupal development fails below 17°C or above 32°C). Each female produces one offspring at a time, with up to 12 offspring during her typical 2–3 month adult lifespan. Consequently, the intrinsic population growth rate of tsetse flies remains low, with estimates suggesting a maximum increase of 10–15 times per year (Kuzoe and Schofield, 2004). Even minor increases in daily mortality rates can lead to population declines, and sustained reductions of 2%–4% can result in population extinction.

Both male and female tsetse flies are obligate blood-feeders, relying solely on vertebrate blood for survival. Adults feed every 2–3 days, creating a pool of blood at the bite site into which they inject saliva through their long proboscis. This saliva contains potent anticoagulants that keep the blood fluid, facilitating continuous feeding (Okhoya, 2004). Tsetse flies predominantly feed during daylight hours, rarely flying for more than 30 minutes daily, with dispersal distances of up to approximately 1 km per day. They spend most of their time resting on vegetation, with engorged flies tilting their heads upwards to excrete excess water away from their bodies. When hungry, flies often rest horizontally, dorsal side down (Mullen and Durden, 2009). Host attraction and recognition are mediated by visual and olfactory cues, with host odours shown to attract tsetse flies from distances of up to 100 m.

Disease Transmission: Key species, such as *G. morsitans*, *G. palpalis*, *G. longipalpalis*, *G. pallidipes*, and *G. austeni*, serve as significant vectors of African trypanosomiasis. Exclusively blood feeders, tsetse flies acquire and transmit trypanosome species responsible for diseases, like nagana among animals and humans, which can be potentially fatal if untreated. Infection rates among tsetse flies are typically low (1–20%), yet infected flies remain carriers for life, posing substantial challenges to livestock rearing due to disease transmission (Krafsur, 2009; Figure 9.2). African trypanosomiasis profoundly impacts tropical countries' economic development, impacts the economic development of tropical countries, and indirectly by reducing productivity in terms of milk, meat, manure, and traction (FAO, 2000).

Management: Various tsetse fly management techniques have been deployed to reduce populations, replacing earlier, less effective methods with ecologically sound strategies. Bush clearance to eliminate shaded resting and larval deposition sites and extensive wildlife shooting to remove wild blood sources has been attempted (Hocking et al., 1963). However, these methods were ecologically disruptive and challenging to sustain. Current approaches

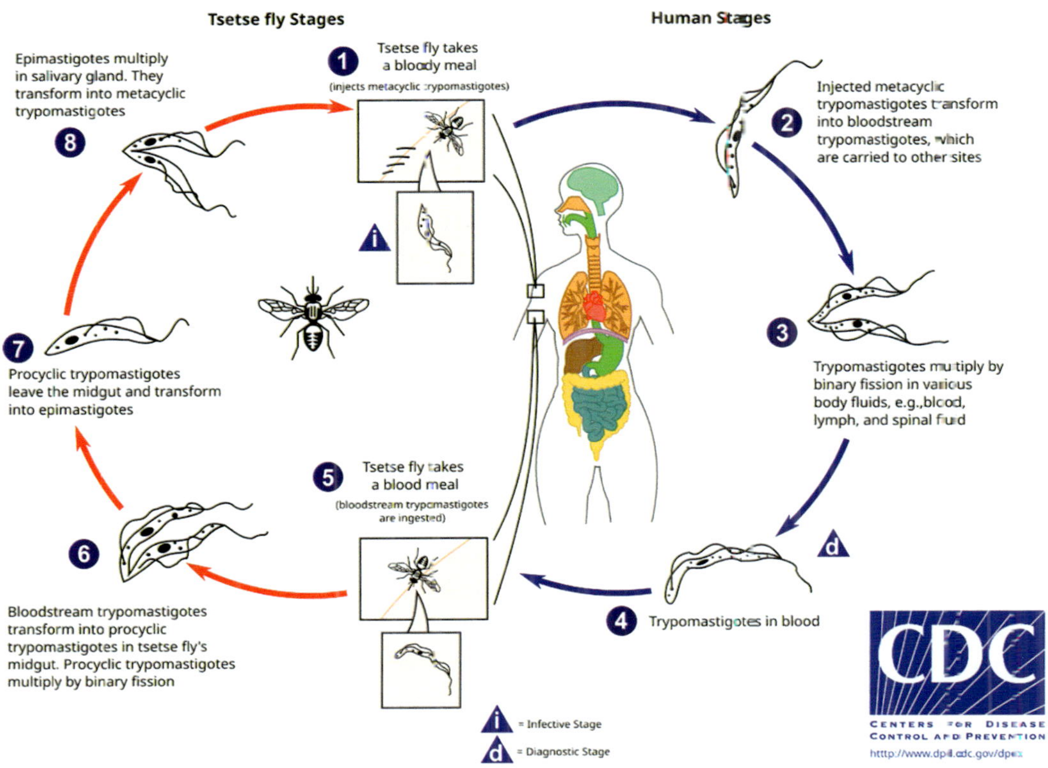

FIGURE 9.2 Life cycle of the *Trypanosoma brucei*.

include the direct application of insecticides to cattle via dip, spray, or pour-on formulations. For example, a deltamethrin spray solution at 5 mL/L of water can be applied using a knapsack sprayer over the animal's entire body. Tsetse traps and targets, using biodegradable insecticides, attract and eliminate flies that land on them, contributing to population reduction efforts (Kuzoe and Schofield, 2004).

9.3 HOUSE FLY

The house fly, *Musca domestica* L. (Diptera: Muscidae), is the most prevalent and widespread fly species globally. This synanthropic insect has thrived by colonizing organic substrates provided by humans. Economically significant, it can transmit disease-causing organisms, like *Salmonella* and *Escherichia coli*, and is a nuisance around farms and homes. Believed to have originated from the savannahs of Central Asia, it has spread worldwide, thriving in both rural and urban areas of tropical and temperate climates (Hussein et al., 2014; Ommi et al., 2015). Its habitat is cosmopolitan, found everywhere humans live as well as in the wild (Figure 9.3).

Biology: The house fly is the most common fly species (Kettle, 1995). Diurnal by nature, its activities include seeking food and water, feeding, mating, resting, and laying eggs. House flies are multivoltine, producing 10–12 generations annually in temperate regions, with population peaks in summer. They do not migrate seasonally or enter diapause in winter, instead surviving and breeding in refuges (Malik et al., 2007).

Each female lays 75–150 eggs per cluster, totalling 350–900 eggs in her lifetime. Eggs are laid 4–12 days after emerging from the pupal case in moist materials, like fresh manure (less than a day old), manure mixed with hay or straw, and waste grains. These moist materials provide ideal breeding sites for house flies and other pests. Maggots emerge in

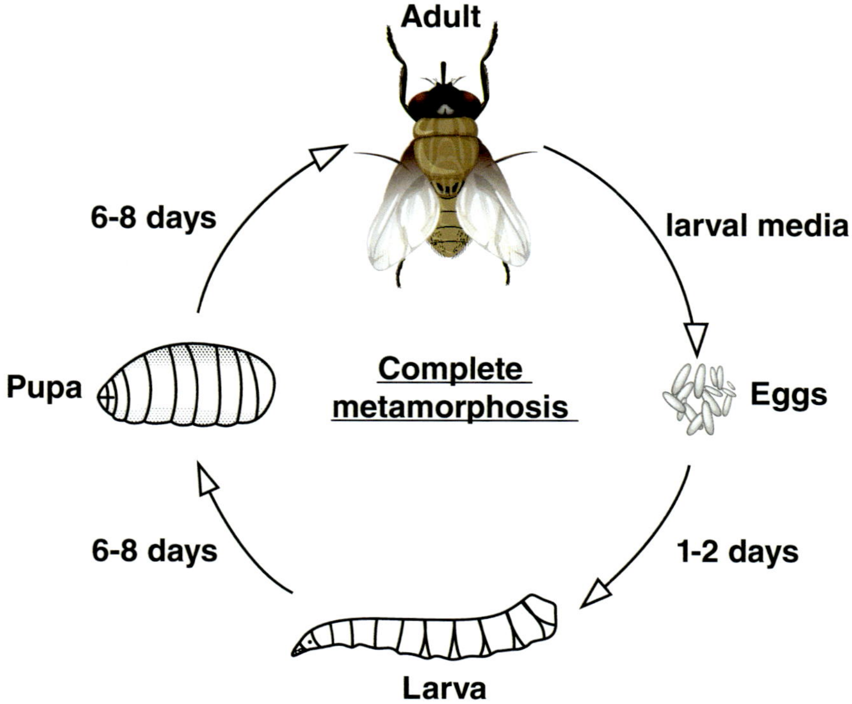

FIGURE 9.3 Life cycle of house fly.

8–20 hours and start feeding. Under favourable conditions, larvae develop through three stages in 3–7 days. Before pupating, larvae migrate to drier areas at the edge of their breeding habitat. Depending on temperature and humidity, adults emerge from the pupal case in three days to four weeks, resulting in six to eight generations per year (Naycuch and Burrus, 2017).

Adult house flies have sponging mouthparts, requiring liquid food or the regurgitation of crop contents onto solid foods to soften them before ingestion. "Bubbling", where flies exude a droplet of regurgitate, helps eliminate excess water (Stoffolano, 2019). During feeding, flies regurgitate, depositing any bacteria present in the crop onto food sources (Graczyk et al., 2001). They also frequently defecate on food, spreading microbes from the rectum (Sasaki et al., 2000; Graczyk et al., 2001).

Disease Transmission: A global pest of public health importance, house flies have plagued humans throughout history (West, 1951). Their ability to develop in various organic larval substrates enables them to thrive in any human-inhabited area (Lietze et al., 2011). Concerns about food-borne illnesses have increased documentation of flies spreading pathogens, like *Escherichia coli*, *Shigella* spp., and *Salmonella* spp. (Macovei et al., 2008; Holt et al., 2007). Pathogen-carrying flies can contaminate food items, like milk, steak, and potato salad (Ahmad et al., 2007; Macovei et al., 2008). They are commonly found around waste and landfills, dispersing to areas of human activity. *M. domestica* can transmit bacterial infections, like shigellosis, salmonellosis, cholera, and Campylobacter infection. Additionally, they carry eggs and cysts of intestinal worms, including *Ascaris* spp., hookworms, and tapeworms, and contribute to the spread of trachoma, epidemic conjunctivitis, and skin infections (Huang et al., 2009).

Management: Cultural management, such as maintaining animal manure, can control house flies in poultry farms. Jacobs (2013) noted that good sanitation, exclusion, and cultural controls effectively reduce fly populations. Tomberlin (2006) highlighted that proper drainage and garbage management, along with household hygiene, are effective control methods. Large sticky traps have been successfully used on farms to capture adult flies (Kaufman et al., 2005). Hertz et al. (2011) used chemically treated cords (natural and synthetic) with insecticides, like fipronil or indoxacarb. Dichlorvos EC and diflubenzuron granules are effective larvicides (Tilak et al., 2010). Pospischil et al. (2005) recommended using baits with oral chemical controls. Black and white colours attract flies, while white is least effective when used with baits (Ahmed et al., 2005). Ojianwuna et al. (2011) found basil oil to be a cost-effective control measure. Biological control agents, such as wasp species (*Spalangia nigroaenea*, *Muscidifurax raptor*, *Muscidifurax zaraptor*, and *Spalangia cameroni*), are also used; the wasps lay eggs in house fly pupae, and their larvae feed inside the fly until it dies (Tomberlin, 2006).

Beauveria bassiana is an effective biopesticide. Chemicals, like Cry1B, 1,8-cineole, pulegone, limonene, menthol, and certain oils, are also effective biopesticides (Geden, 2012). Although UV lights can kill house flies to some extent, they do not significantly reduce populations, as they do not address key growth sources. Electronic baits (fly catchers) are considered highly effective for fly control (Smallegange, 2004).

9.4 STABLE FLIES

Stable flies, commonly referred to as biting filth flies, barn flies, biting house flies, dog flies, power mower flies, or beach flies, belong to the family Muscidae and the genus *Stomoxys*. Some of these names describe their habitats; for instance, beach flies are associated with outbreaks on leisure beaches, dog flies parasitize dogs, and lawn or power mower flies refer to larvae that develop in the dampness beneath matted grass, such as under lawn mowers. The term "biting house flies" is misleading, although it became popular due to its superficial resemblance to the house fly (Rochon et al., 2021).

About 18 species are described within the genus *Stomoxys*, all of which widely distributed in tropical regions, except for *Stomoxys calcitrans*, which has a worldwide distribution due to human and European livestock introductions (Zumpt, 1973). Adult stable flies are 5–7 mm long, with a forward-projecting proboscis and a greyish abdomen adorned with seven circular black spots.

Distribution: They are native to Africa, Europe, and Asia; however, during colonial times and livestock introductions, they spread widely to tropical and temperate regions globally. Stable flies breed continuously in tropical and subtropical climates, whereas in temperate regions, they hibernate in immature stages in unfrozen larval substrates. Both male and female flies inflict painful bites on warm-blooded animals, including humans, primarily around the ankles.

Biology: Mating in adult stable flies occurs after acquiring blood from warm-blooded animals. One blood meal is sufficient before mating for males aged 1–2 days, whereas females aged 3–4 days require 2–3 blood meals. However, during the post-mating period, females require 3–4 blood meals to develop a batch of eggs. Consequently, they deposit an average of 100 eggs during each ovarian cycle and can oviposit up to 600–800 eggs in their lifetime (Jones et al., 1999). Females prefer to oviposit around rotting straw, manure, or other decomposing materials. Hatching occurs within 12–24 hours after oviposition. Newly hatched larvae prefer to develop in cattle manure, soil and compost mixtures, and various crop by-products, such as peanut hulls and sugarcane bagasse, as well as substrates with fibrous materials, like straw bedding, wet hay, algal mats, and wet grass clippings.

The developmental period from egg to pupation takes about 12–13 days, with adults emerging from pupae in 7 days, completing their life cycle in an average of 3 weeks (Lysyk, 1998). Adults survive for approximately 14 days and persist throughout the year in some locations, although their population declines if the maximum temperature exceeds 30°C or the minimum temperature drops below freezing. Managing stable flies is challenging due to their preference for larval habitats with accumulated decomposing vegetation. Moreover, many cultural practices in agricultural and urban environments support these habitats. Additionally, adults are highly mobile with slight disturbance (Rochon et al., 2021).

Disease Transmission: Literature suggests that while stable flies prefer livestock and they can become significant pests to humans when livestock populations are low (Hogsette and Ose, 2017). During periods of higher adult populations, they feed from various parts of animals, disrupting their feeding, reproductive, and resting behaviours. Affected individuals exhibit defensive behaviours to avoid being bitten. These flies reduce livestock production directly by causing blood loss and lowering milk yield, and indirectly by transmitting various disease-causing pathogens, especially where these diseases are invasive and have global transmission potential. The decrease in cattle productivity due to stable fly infestation alone was estimated at $2.66 billion annually in the U.S., $6.8 million in Mexico, and $340 million in Brazil.

Compared to other flies such as mosquitoes, tsetse flies, and horseflies, stable flies have poor disease transmission efficiency to livestock, primarily mechanical. After acquiring blood from a pathogen-infected animal, they must initiate blood-feeding from uninfected animals within a short period. While stable flies do not transmit diseases to humans, higher populations can disrupt human recreational activities. Due to their adaptability to climate and agronomic changes, they sustain themselves, leading to population increases that threaten livestock in various regions, including outbreaks in North America (Rochon et al., 2021). Nonetheless, they are significant from public and animal health perspectives due to their nuisance feeding behaviour.

Management: Integrated pest management approaches are preferable for stable fly management. Cultural practices include frequent removal of manure, typically every two weeks, which has been documented to reduce populations by 30%–50% (Thomas et al., 1996). This, along with well-maintained drainage, prevention of water system leaks, and proper waste management around livestock production areas, underscores that sanitation reduces immature stable fly development, forming the basis for comprehensive management. Similarly, timely removal and appropriate disposal of stall litter and other fly habitats help mitigate population growth Commercially available traps, such as Starbar Bite Free and the Knight Stick, can also reduce population levels. However, careful consideration of trap placement, the number per unit area, and management is essential. Various biological control agents, including predators like macrochelid mites and staphylinid and histerid beetles, have shown significant effects on immature stable fly populations (Azevedo et al., 2018). Currently, only the poultry house pill beetle, *Carcinops pumilio*, is commercially available for the biocontrol of stable fly larvae. Many chemical agents used to control adult and immature stages of other livestock pests can effectively reduce stable fly populations. Treatments with ultralow volume (ULV) insecticides on cattle feeding pastures and surrounding breeding sites have been shown to provide short-term relief for up to 24 hours. Insecticide-treated blue-black fabric targets, which attract and kill stable flies, have remained effective in the field for four months, using 0.1% lambda-cyhalothrin or 0.1% zeta-cypermethrin.

9.5 BOT FLIES

Bot flies, also known as warble flies, gad flies, and heel flies, belong to the family Oestridae and the superfamily Oestroidea. Globally, approximately 130 species of these flies are classified under 26 genera. In India, however, 13 species representing 10 genera and 3 subfamilies – Gasterophilinae, Hypodermatinae, and Oestrinae – have been documented. The limited evolutionary diversification of bot flies is attributed to their obligate animal parasitism, which restricts their niche and thus limits opportunities for diversification. Since the domestication of hoofed animals, they have become a significant problem for livestock.

Bot flies are parasitic, with larvae developing on the skin, flesh, nasal passages, ophthalmic regions, and alimentary tracts of goats, sheep, cattle, and horses, causing obligatory myiasis. While many bot fly species are not host-specific, some demonstrate host specificity. Current information indicates that 5% of human myiasis cases are caused by the human bot fly, *Dermatobia hominis*, which is the only known bot fly species primarily parasitic on humans. However, other species can incidentally become parasitic when humans are in close proximity to livestock (Banerjee and Bhattacharya, 2012).

9.5.1 Distribution

Bot flies (family Oestridae) exhibit a distinct geographical distribution that is closely linked to the availability of suitable hosts and specific environmental conditions conducive to their life cycles. The distribution of various genera within the family Oestridae, such as *Cuterebra*, *Dermatobia* and *Gasterophilus*, demonstrates significant regional variation. Cuterebra species are predominantly found in North America. These bot flies parasitize rodents and lagomorphs, and their presence is noted across diverse habitats within this region. For instance, species, like *Cuterebra americana*, *C. buccata*, *C. emasculator*, and *C. fontinella* have broad distributions throughout North America, while *C. cuniculi* is more restricted, being primarily found in southern Georgia and Florida (Slansky, 2006).

Dermatobia hominis, known as the human bot fly, is widespread in Central and South America. This species is particularly prevalent in regions with dense forests and humid climates, such as the Amazon Basin. The life cycle of *D. hominis* is intricately tied to the tropical environment, which provides the necessary conditions for its development and propagation. *Gasterophilus* species, which primarily parasitize equines, have a more cosmopolitan distribution. These bot flies are found in both temperate and tropical regions worldwide, including parts of Europe, Asia, Africa, and the Americas. The global distribution of *Gasterophilus* reflects their adaptability to a variety of climatic conditions, although they are most commonly found in regions where their equine hosts are prevalent (Marchiori, 2021). The geographical distribution of bot flies is not static; it is influenced by both natural factors and human activities. Environmental changes, such as deforestation and urbanization, can impact the distribution and prevalence of bot flies by altering the habitats of their host species and introducing new ecological dynamics. As a result, some bot fly species have adapted to new areas and hosts, demonstrating the intricate relationships between parasites, hosts, and the environment (Marchiori, 2021). In summary, the distribution of bot flies is a complex interplay of ecological and environmental factors, with each genus showing distinct geographical patterns reflect their specific host associations and environmental requirements.

Biology: Ovipositing females deposit small, faint yellowish-coloured eggs directly on the host; in the case of *D. hominis*, these eggs are attached to the ventral surface of the body. Animal parasites often utilize intermediate hosts, such as houseflies and mosquitoes, while *D. hominis* uses ticks. Species colonizing the digestive tract and other internal parts reach these areas after the host licks surfaces containing eggs. Fertilized females relying on intermediate hosts or phoretic insects for transportation attach to the wings of these insects, depositing about 15–30 eggs on the insect's abdomen, where they incubate. This process repeats similarly throughout the female's adult lifespan of 8–9 days, during which she deposits 100–400 eggs. Upon reaching a suitable substrate on the host, thermal cues stimulate hatched larvae to burrow into the skin or other infested parts (Drees and Jackman, 1999). The larvae that grow in burrowed skin cause myiasis or tissue damage, although they do not kill the animals and are considered true parasites. The parasitic larva on mammalian hosts does not significantly impact their skeletal anatomy. Fully grown larvae drop from infested skin and pupate in the soil; species developing in the intestine reside there for about 10–12 months before passing out through faeces.

Human bot fly appears bumblebee-like, with large and dense hairs on each body segment. This species is geographically restricted to Central and South America. The eggs of *D. hominis* attach to the ventral surface of blood-sucking insects, such as mosquitoes or ticks, and through phoresis, they are transported to the host's skin surface where they hatch in response to the host's temperature cues. The larval stage has three morphologically distinctive instars: the first instar is worm-like, the second instar is bottle-neck shaped, and the third instar is cylindrical. After complete development, the larvae crawl out and pupate in the soil. Adults emerge within 2–3 weeks, with the entire life cycle averaging about 5–12 weeks.

Disease Transmission: Those involved in equine farming face challenges with certain species that prefer to infest the front legs, knees, nose, and throat, depending on species behaviour. In cattle, lesions caused by botflies pave the way for the entry of the bacterium, *Mannheimia granulomatis*, which causes *Lechiguana*, a disease characterized by rapidly growing hard lumps beneath the infested animal. This disease can lead to pneumonia and haemorrhagic septicaemia in cattle and other livestock. Adult flies emerge in two to three months, continuing the infestation cycle as described previously. Various dewormers, such as ivermectin, trichlorfon, and dichlorvos, are effective in mitigating infestation. However, when infestation is coupled with other disease-causing microbial pathogens, antibiotic treatment is essential; otherwise, the stressed animal may die within 3–11 months (Riet-Correa et al., 2000). Some macaws and wild parrots have been reported to be infested by botfly species of the genus *Philornis*. Botfly larvae can be mechanically removed from the skin using a reverse syringe design snake bite extractor (Olah et al., 2013).

The larval stage of this species inhabits the subcutaneous layer and is known to cause myiasis, resulting in pustules on the skin that secrete fluids. Raised lesions on the skin become hard and often cause extreme pain to affected mammals. However, the infestation is not reported to transmit any disease-causing pathogens, and individuals migrating from Central and South America are occasionally diagnosed with myiasis associated with *D. hominis*. Common hosts, apart from humans, include dogs, monkeys, cattle, buffalo, and other warm-blooded animals (Larrick et al., 2008).

Management: In conventional methods, petroleum jelly is applied around the wound, causing larvae to suffocate due to asphyxiation. The larvae can then be removed with pincers or, after local anaesthesia is administered, with a scalpel by cutting the infested wound. Sometimes, pressure is applied around the wound to encourage the larvae to emerge. Many individuals have reported that lidocaine injections beneath the wound create pressure, allowing the larvae to emerge. After removing the larvae from the host, antibiotics must be administered to prevent infection (Larrick et al., 2008). Besides various physical and mechanical methods, oral administration of ivermectin has been documented as highly effective. This non-invasive treatment also induces larvae to exit the wound.

9.6 HORSEFLIES

Horseflies, also known as deer flies, belong to the family Tabanidae, within the superfamily Tabanoidea. Approximately 4,455 species have been described under Tabanidae across 1,500 genera, with 1,300 species placed in the genus *Tabanus*. Among these genera, species under *Tabanus* and *Hybomitra* (horseflies), *Haematopota* (clegs), and *Chrysops* (deer flies) are the only ones known to cause harm to various animals.

Adults are medium to large-sized, ranging from 5 to 25 mm, and are robust flies with a wingspan of up to 60 mm. They are swift fliers, typically active in the morning under sunlight, avoiding shady and dark areas. Flying horseflies are attracted to polarized reflections on water, and thus, large numbers may congregate around water pools, causing a nuisance. Many species of tabanids exhibit agile flying mechanisms, with notable species, like *Hybomitra* observed performing aerial manoeuvers comparable to those of fighter jets. Research has documented horseflies as the fastest flying insects, with speeds of up to 145 km per hour (90 mph) recorded in male *Hybomitra hinei* during nuptial flight.

The genus *Tabanus*, commonly known as horseflies, is large (up to 25 mm) with a dark brown body and eyes exhibiting a metallic sheen. Many species are characterized by their protruding compound eyes, which can be dichoptic (widely separated) or holoptic (almost touching), and brightly coloured eyes. The body and antennae are covered in short hairs, with no bristles present. Unlike many other species, the classification of *Tabanus* species does not rely on genital variations but rather on differences observed in antennae, frons, and maxillae (head appendages), wing venation, last abdominal segment, and body patterning, often associated with variations in hair distribution (Bradley et al., 2022).

Adults of this species primarily feed on plant exudates, such as nectar, while some are specialized pollinators. Female horseflies possess well-developed mouthparts and are anautogenous, requiring blood meals from vertebrates, including humans. In contrast, males have weak mouthparts and feed solely on plant-based sources. This dietary distinction is crucial as females require protein for egg production, with the digestion of a blood meal taking an average of 6 days before they seek another.

Distribution: Tabanids are widely distributed, predominantly found in warm regions, but they can be observed worldwide except in certain locations, such as the Polar Regions (Hawaii, Greenland, Iceland). Their presence has been noted at altitudes of up to 3 300 m (10,800 feet) above sea level (Hansens and Rabin, 1981).

Biology: Mating in many tabanid species occurs in swarms at locations like hilltops or aquatic ecosystems, with variations in timing, habitats, and times of day among species. Females obtain a blood meal post-mating from warm-blooded animals to support egg development, typically depositing around 1,000 eggs in clusters in suitable aquatic or semi-aquatic habitats, including vegetation floating on water. Initially white, these eggs darken to brown before hatching within six days, aided by hatching spikes on developing larvae.

Larvae detach from the substrate and fall into water or moist areas, where their semi-aquatic habitats make them predators of aquatic fauna. Most species have legless grubs with small, white heads, cylindrical bodies tapering at both ends, and 11–13 segments, featuring respiratory siphons at the posterior end. Larvae are adorned with warty outgrowths (tubercles) known as pseudopods and possess a bulbous Graber's organ at the posterior end for respiration. Pupal stages exhibit clusters of tubercles resembling spines. Several Tabanidae species are predatory, feeding on various arthropods, worms, and occasionally displaying cannibalistic behaviour in captivity. Their larval development includes moulting between six and 13 times over a period of a year or more, with temperate species undergoing diapause in winter while tropical species may be multivoltine. After completing larval development, they pupate outside water in damp places, constructing mud cases where they metamorphose over about two weeks. Adults emerge by splitting open the pupal case along the thorax, typically with males emerging first, followed by females. Mating occurs in flight before descending to the ground, continuing the life cycle of many tabanids. Adults can live for up to one month, with species succession commonly observed. Depending on the species, their entire life cycle may range from two months to two years.

Disease Transmission: The bite of tabanids is notably painful and immediately noticeable to large mammal hosts, unlike the bites of related blood-sucking insects, such as mosquitoes, which can initially go undetected due to the delayed onset of pain caused by injected saliva. Despite this, many large animals are often unable to dislodge horseflies during the 4-minute blood-feeding period. Evolutionary biologists argue that tabanids, while feeding, have not evolved mechanisms to evade detection or minimize pain as effectively as other blood-sucking insects.

The significant blood loss caused by numerous tabanids feeding on hosts can amount to up to 300 mL per day, weakening animals and potentially leading to fatalities. Moreover, their feeding behaviour, which relies on multiple hosts, such as cattle, horses, camels, and deer, facilitates disease transmission. Tabanids act as vectors for 35 pathogenic agents, including bacteria, viruses, protozoa, and blood-borne worm diseases. In endemic areas, diseases transmitted by horsefly vectors include the anaemia virus, anthrax in sheep and cattle, tularemia in rabbits and humans, as well as certain trypanosomes and the filarial worm *Loa* in humans (Foil, 1989; Service, 1980).

This underscores the critical role of tabanids in livestock production, although there are instances where they also transmit diseases to humans. Diseases transmitted by tabanids are reported to reduce milk output in livestock and directly cause damage through blood loss and reduced body weight, especially in the absence of adequate shelter to mitigate such effects.

Management: Managing tabanid flies presents challenges due to their complex biology and feeding habits. Unlike other blood-sucking insects, tabanids often feed on the undersides of animals or around their lower legs, areas that are difficult to reach with chemical treatments. Traps, such as the Malaise trap, utilizing baits like carbon dioxide or octanol, are employed to capture them, with variations, such as the Manitoba trap being adaptations. Chemicals like pyrethroids, applied to cattle, act as repellents and insecticides, supplemented by insecticide-impregnated ear tags or collars for effective management (Bradley et al., 2022).

9.7 SCREWWORM FLIES

Screwworm flies belong to the family Calliphoridae, genus *Cochliomyia*, and are well known as blowflies. This genus is referred to as New World screwworm flies in the literature, distinguishing them from Old World screwworm flies known as *Chrysomya bezziana*. Four species described under this genus are *C. macellaria*, *C. hominivorax*, *C. aldrichi*, and *C. minima*. The first two species live in tropical areas, with *C. hominivorax* identified as the primary screwworm because it feeds on the living tissues of animals and causes myiasis. Especially in the Neotropics, it is a parasite of livestock, wildlife, pets, and, sporadically, humans and other warm-blooded animals (Knipling, 1992; Wyss, 2000; Vargas-Teran et al., 2005; Mastrangelo and Welch, 2012). This species has been documented as a severe problem in Mexico, Central and South America, and the southern parts of the USA (Bushland et al., 1955; Knipling, 1992; USDA, 2012). Infections by *C. hominivorax* and *C. bezziana* in the umbilicus of neonate calves are common. Practices in animal husbandry, such as dehorning, shearing, castrating, and branding, promote injuries that lead to increased invasion by screwworm flies and other parasites (Bushland et al., 1955; Knipling, 1992; Wyss, 2000).

Distribution: The screwworm flies, *Cochliomyia hominivorax*, are native to South and Central America and are also present in the southern USA. The adult flies oviposit near wounds on various animal body parts. The larvae typically hatch within a day, penetrate the outer layer of the skin, enter deeper layers, and feed on healthy tissues. External disturbances to the larvae cause them to burrow deeper. A larva typically completes development in a few days and then pupates outside in the ground by burrowing out of the infected tissues. Severe myiasis associated with *Cochliomyia* can be fatal to animals and can be diagnosed by the larval morphological characteristics. Taxonomic characteristics, such as the size and dimensions of the spiracles and mouthparts, are useful for identifying the causal organism associated with myiasis. The screwworm larvae are clearly segmented with ring-shaped thicker parts, hence the name "screwworm".

Biology: The infection process starts when mated female flies are attracted to the fresh wounds of warm-blooded animals and oviposit about 100–200 eggs near the wound. Immediately after oviposition, gravid females start feeding on the wound site to acquire protein for producing the next egg mass, resulting in an average female laying around 1,000 eggs in her lifetime. The diet restricted to fresh wounds avoids interspecific competition from other animal parasites, and the constant body heat of warm-blooded animals promotes growth and development in a shorter period. Less acidic host tissue favours better digestion compared with carrion-feeding maggots. Besides, predation by ants and other predators is more prevalent in carcasses than in living flesh. The average incubation period lasts about 10–20 hours, after which freshly hatched larvae start feeding on the fresh open wound for only 4–12 days to complete their development. Fully grown larvae fall to the ground for pupation, spend about one week in that stage, and then adults emerge, mate, and continue acquiring protein from animals, thereby continuing the infection cycle. Adult screwworm flies resemble houseflies but are twice the size, with blue-green bodies, orange eyes, and three dark stripes on their backs. The average life cycle lasts about 2–3 weeks (Bushland et al., 1955; Knipling, 1992; Wyss, 2000).

Disease Transmission: As a result of the infection process, the damage to animals is profound, with deep, pocket-like lesions appearing on the skin. The secondary screwworm species, *C. macellaria*, causes facultative myiasis, although they are close relatives of primary screwworms. Their invasion of host tissues follows that of primary myiasis-causing flies, and the two species often do not coexist. *C. macellaria* is known as the secondary screwworm because it feeds on necrotic tissue and produces myiasis (Bushland et al., 1955; Knipling, 1992; Wyss, 2000).

Management: Timely and appropriate management options are essential for screwworms, as infections are often fatal to animals. Invasions into vital organs can result in septicaemia due to the maggots' feeding on living tissue or secondary infections. Screwworm infections in tropical areas are continuous, while in temperate regions, they are often restricted to mild winters, as adult survival depends on warm spells (Bushland et al., 1955; Knipling, 1992; Wyss, 2000). Treatment starts with cleaning the affected parts by shaving and then washing with antiseptic shampoo. The wounds are flushed to remove the screw-worm larvae as early as possible. Chemicals belonging to the avermectin and nitenpyram classes are highly effective against fly larvae (Bushland et al., 1955; Knipling, 1992; Wyss, 2000).

The sterile insect technique (SIT) was tested and implemented using *C. hominivorax*. This technique was conceptualized and developed by Dr. Emory Cushing, Dr. Edward F. Knipling, and Dr. Raymond C. Bushland. They performed basic analyses and created techniques that could be exploited for successful pest management. The successful demonstration of SIT in *C. hominivorax* is attributed to the unselective sexual behaviour of males and solitary mating behaviour of females (Knipling, 1992). The eradication of *C. hominivorax* with the SIT programme began in 1957 in Florida and later spread to various parts of the USA and other countries (USDA, 2012). As a result of SIT, the geographical spread of this species has been restricted in many tropical and temperate regions of the New World and has been eliminated from the Nearctic (Tables 9.1–9.7).

TABLE 9.1
List of Various Diseases Transmitted through Sand Flies

Common Name	Family	Order	Scientific Name	Disease	Causal Organism
Sand fly	Psychodidae	Diptera	*Phlebotomus nogouchi*	Carrion disease	*Bartonella bacilliformis*
			Phlebotomus intermedius	American Leishmaniasis	*Leishmania brasiliensis*
			Phlebotomus argentipes	Leishmaniasis/ Kalaazar/ Dumdum fever/ Black fever	*Leishmania donovaani*
			Phlebotomus serganti	Oriental sore	*Leishmania tropica*
				Sand fly fever	Virus

TABLE 9.2
List of Various Diseases transmitted through Tsetse Fly

Common Name	Family	Order	Scientific Name	Disease	Causal Organism
Tsetse fly	Glossidae	Diptera	*Glossina palpalis*	Gambian sleeping sickness or African sleeping sickness	*Trypanosoma gambiensis*
			Glossina morsitans	Rhodesian sleeping sickness or Rhodesian trypanosomiasis	*Trypanosoma rhodesiense*

TABLE 9.3
List of Various Diseases Transmitted through House Flies

Common Name	Family	Order	Scientific Name	Disease	Causal Organism
House flies	Muscidae	Diptera	*Musa* sp.	Dysentery	*Shigella dysentariae*
			Musa sp.	Typhoid fever	*Eberthella typhosa*
			Musa sp.	Chlorea	*Vibrio comma*
			Musa sp.	Poliomyelitis	Virus
			Musa sp.	Tuberculosis	*Myobacterium tuberculosis*
			Musa sp.	Typhoid fever	*Salmonella typhi*
			Musa sp.	Amoebiasis	*Entamoeba histolytica*

TABLE 9.4
Diseases Transmitted through Stable Fly

Common Name	Family	Order	Scientific Name	Disease	Causal Organism
Stable flies	Muscidae	Diptera	*Stomoxys calcitrans*	Onchocerca	*Habronema microstoma*

TABLE 9.5
Diseases Transmitted through Bot Fly

Common Name	Family	Order	Scientific Name	Disease	Causal Organism
Bot flies	Oestridae	Diptera	*Dermatobia hominis*	*Lechiguana*	*Mannheimia granulomatis*

TABLE 9.6
List of Various Diseases Transmitted through Horse Flies

Common Name	Family	Order	Scientific Name	Disease	Causal Organism
Horse flies	Tabanidae	Diptera	*Tabanus* spp.	Tularemia	*Pasteurella tularensis*
			Tabanus spp.	Anthrax	*Bacillus anthracis*
			Tabanus spp.	Loiasis	*Parasitic Roundworm*

TABLE 9.7
Diseases Transmitted through Screw Worms

Common Name	Family	Order	Scientific Name	Disease	Causal Organism
Screw worms	Calliphoridae	Diptera	*Chrysomya bezziana*	Myiasis	*C. macellaria*

Amongst the successful and exceptional achievements in insect pest management programmes was the elimination of New World screwworms, *C. hominivorax*, from continental North America to the Panama–Colombia border. Research efforts by USDA-ARS (US Department of Agriculture-Agricultural Research Service) scientists demonstrated the effectiveness of the sterile insect technique (SIT), resulting in the eradication of screwworms from the USA. Thereafter, SIT was deployed in Mexico, Central America, and Libya with the support of USDA-ARS and collaborators (Mastrangelo and Welch, 2012). The efficient control of screwworms has benefitted the livestock industry by at least $1.3 billion (Vargas-Teran et al., 2005), with substantial benefits to humans, pets, and wildlife.

9.8 CONCLUSION

The study of various fly species reveals their unique roles in ecosystems and their significant impact on human and animal health. Sand flies, part of the Psychodidae family, are key vectors for diseases like leishmaniasis and thrive in habitats ranging from caves to human dwellings. Their limited flight range and specific environmental preferences highlight localized management challenges. Tsetse flies adapt to diverse African landscapes and are known for their unique wing-folding behaviour and specialized proboscis. They are vectors for trypanosomiasis, affecting wildlife and livestock in forests, savannahs, and riparian zones. The house fly, *Musca domestica*, is a globally distributed species that directly impacts human health through disease transmission. Its adaptability to human environments and rapid reproduction present challenges for population control and health risk mitigation. Stable flies (*Stomoxys* spp.) and bot flies (Oestridae) add further complexities to livestock management; stable flies cause pain and irritation through biting, while bot flies cause parasitic damage. Understanding their regional distributions and life cycle dynamics is essential for effective management.

Horse flies (Tabanidae) and screwworm flies (*Cochliomyia* spp.) also pose significant challenges. Horse flies are known for their painful bites, while screwworm flies prevent severe health risks through myiasis. Their habitat preferences and life cycle intricacies require integrated pest management approaches to reduce economic losses and health impacts. In conclusion, the diversity, distribution, ecological roles, and health impacts of these fly species emphasize the need for integrated pest management strategies that combine ecological, biological, and chemical methods. Addressing these challenges necessitates collaborative efforts across various disciplines, including entomology and public health, to mitigate the adverse effects of these insects on human and animal populations worldwide.

9.9 POINTS TO REMEMBER

1. Medically important flies include species from families such as Psychodidae (sand flies), Glossinidae (tsetse flies), Muscidae (house flies and stable flies), Oestridae (bot flies), Tabanidae (horse flies), and Calliphoridae (screwworm flies).
2. Sand flies inhabit tropical, subtropical, and temperate regions, favouring humid environments.
3. Tsetse flies are found in sub-Saharan Africa, particularly in forested areas and savannahs.
4. House flies are ubiquitous, thriving in human environments globally.
5. Stable flies, bot flies, and horse flies are widespread in both tropical and temperate regions.
6. Screwworm flies are native to the Americas and are prominent pests in tropical regions.
7. Sand flies are vectors of leishmaniasis.
8. Tsetse flies transmit trypanosomiasis.
9. House flies and stable flies spread pathogens causing diseases like salmonellosis and shigellosis through mechanical transmission.
10. Bot flies cause myiasis, infesting the skin and tissues of their hosts.

11. Horse flies and screwworm flies also cause significant health issues through painful bites and myiasis, respectively.
12. These flies have a profound impact on public health, agriculture, and livestock production. Effective control measures are essential to mitigate economic losses and health risks associated with their presence.
13. IPM strategies include a combination of environmental management, chemical controls, biological agents, and monitoring.
14. Approaches involve habitat modification, insecticide application, traps, and biological control measures.
15. Regular monitoring of fly populations is crucial for early detection and effective outbreak control.
16. Surveillance methods include the use of light traps, synthetic attractants, and population sampling techniques.
17. Ongoing research and innovation are enhancing pest management strategies and biocontrol agents.

REFERENCES

Ahmad, A., Nagaraja, T. G., & Zurek, L. (2007). Transmission of *Escherichia coli* O157: H7 to cattle by house flies. *Preventive Veterinary Medicine*, *80*(1), 74–81.

Akhoundi, M., Kuhls, K., Cannet, A., Votýpka, J., Marty, P., Delaunay, P., & Sereno, D. (2016). A historical overview of the classification, evolution, and dispersion of *Leishmania* parasites and sandflies. *PLoS Neglected Tropical Diseases*, *10*(3), e0004349.

Azevedo, L. H., Ferreira, M. P., de Campos Castilho, R., Cançado, P. H. D., & de Moraes, G. J. (2018). Potential of *Macrocheles* species (Acari: Mesostigmata: Macrochelidae) as control agents of harmful flies (Diptera) and biology of *Macrochele sembersoni* Azevedo, Castilho and Berto on *Stomoxys calcitrans* (L.) and Musca domestica L.(Diptera: Muscidae). *Biological Control*, *123*, 1–8.

Banerjee, D., & Bhattacharya, K. K. (2012). *Checklist of Botflies (Insecta: Diptera: Oestridae) from India*. Zoological Survey of India, Kolkata, pp. 1–3.

Benallal, K. E., Garni, R., Harrat, Z., Volf, P., & Dvorak, V. (2022) Phlebotomine sand flies (Diptera: Psychodidae) of the Maghreb region: A systematic review of distribution, morphology, and role in the transmission of the pathogens. *PLOS Neglected Tropical Diseases*, *16*(1), e0009952. https://doi.org/10.1371/journal.pntd.0009952

Cecílio, P., Cordeiro-da-Silva, A., & Oliveira, F. (2022). Sand flies: Basic information on the vectors of leishmaniasis and their interactions with *Leishmania* parasites. *Communications Biology*, *5*, 305. https://doi.org/10.1038/s42003-022-03240-z

Dinesh, D. S., Kumari, S., Hassan, F., Kumar, V., Singh, V. P., & Das, P. (2017). Efficacy and evaluation of environmental management system to control sandfly vector of Kala-azar. *Journal of Environmental Management*, *201*, 366–368.

Drees, B., & Jackman, J. (1999). *Horse Bot Fly: Field Guide to Texas Insects*. Houston, TX.

FAO (2000). *Training Manual for Tsetse Control Personnel*. Food and Agriculture Organization of the United Nations, Rome, Italy, p. 1.

Faraj, C., Yukich, J., Adlaoui, E. B. et al. (2016). Effectiveness and cost of insecticide-treated bed nets and indoor residual spraying for the control of cutaneous leishmaniasis: A cluster-randomized control trial in Morocco. *The American Society of Tropical Medicine and Hygiene*, *94*(3), 679–685. doi:10.4269/ajtmh.14-0510

Geden, C. J. (2012). Status of biopesticides for the control of houseflies. *Journal of Biopesticides*, *4*(2), 33–37.

Gherbi, R., Bounechada, M., Latrofa, M. S., Annoscia, G., Tarallo, V. D., Dantas-Torres, F. et al. (2020). Phlebotomine sand flies and *Leishmania* species in a focus of cutaneous leishmaniasis in Algeria. *PLOS Neglected Tropical Diseases*, *14*(2), e0008024, https://doi.org/10.1371/journal.pntd.0008024

Graczyk, T. K., Knight, R., Gilman, R. H., & Cranfield, M. R. (2001). The role of non-biting flies in the epidemiology of human infectious diseases. *Microbes and Infection*, *3*(3), 231–235.

Hertz, J. C., Pereira, R. M., & Koehler, P. G. (2011). House fly (diptera: muscidae) resting preference on various cords and potential of fipronil-or indoxacarb-impregnation on cords for fly control. *Journal of Entomological Science*, *46*(4), 325–334.
Hocking, K. S., Lamerton, J. F., & Lewis, E. A. (1963). Tsetse-fly control and eradication. *Bulletin of the World Health Organization*, *28*(5–6), 811.
Hogsette, J. A., & Ose, G. A. (2017). Improved capture of stable flies (Diptera: Muscidae) by placement of knight stick sticky fly traps protected by electric fence inside animal exhibit yards at the Smithsonian's National Zoological Park. *Zoo Biology*, *36*(6), 382–386.
Holt, P. S., Geden, C. J., Moore, R. W., & Gast, R. K. (2007). Isolation of *Salmonella enterica serovar* Enteritidis from houseflies (*Musca domestica*) found in rooms containing *Salmonella serovar* Enteritidis-challenged hens. *Applied and Environmental Microbiology*, *73*(19), 6030–6035.
Hordofa, K. S., & Haile, G. (2017). A review on epidemiological distribution, impacts and integrated control approach of tsetse fly. *Journal of Parasitology and Vector Biology*, *9*(9), 122–131.
Huang, J. G., Zhou, L. J., Xu, H. H., & Li, W. O. (2009). Insecticidal and cytotoxic activities of extracts of *Cacalia tangutica* and its two active ingredients against *Musca domestica* and *Aedes albopictus*. *Journal of Economic Entomology*, *102*(4), 1444–1447.
Hussein, S. A., & John, L. C. (2014). Housefly, *Musca domestica* Linnaeus (Insecta: Diptera: Muscidae). *Institute of Food and Agricultural Sciences*, *47*, 1–7.
Jacobs, S. B. (2013). *Entomological Notes*.The Pennsylvania State University, Pennsylvania.
Jannin, J. (1999). Tsetse biology and ecology: Their role in the epidemiology and control of trypanosomiasis. *Bulletin of the World Health Organization*, *77*(5), 450.
Jones, C. J., Isard, S. A., & Cortinas, M. R. (1999). Dispersal of synanthropic Diptera: Lessons from the past and technology for the future. *Annals of the Entomological Society of America*, *92*(6), 829–839.
Kaufman, P. E., Rutz, D. A., & Frisch, S. (2005). Large sticky traps for capturing house flies and stable flies in dairy calf greenhouse facilities. *Journal of Dairy Science*, *88*(1), 176–181.
Kettle, D. S. (1995). Muscidae and fanniidae. In: *Medical and Veterinary Entomology*. CABI Publishing, New York, pp. 248–267.
Killick-Kendrick, R., & Rioux, J. A. (2002). Mark-release-recapture of sand flies fed on leishmanial dogs: The natural life-cycle of Leishmania infantum in *Phlebotomus ariasi*. *Parassitologia*, *44*(1–2), 67–71.
Knipling, E. F. (1992). *Principles of Insect Parasitism Analyzed from New Perspectives: Practical Implications for Regulating Insect Populations by Biological Means* (No. 693). Department of Agriculture Research Service.
Krafsur, E. S. (2009). Tsetse flies: Genetics, evolution, and role as vectors. *Infection, Genetics and Evolution*, *9*(1), 124–141.
Macovei, L., Miles, B., & Zurek, L. (2008). Potential of houseflies to contaminate ready-to-eat food with antibiotic-resistant enterococci. *Journal of Food Protection*, *71*(2), 435–439.
Malik, A., Singh, N., & Satya, S. (2007). House fly (*Musca domestica*): A review of control strategies for a challenging pest. *Journal of Environmental Science and Health Part B*, *42*(4), 453–469.
Marchiori, C. H. (2021). Study of the biology of the Tachinidae family. *Open Access Research Journal of Multidisciplinary Studies*, *2*(1), 52–58. doi:10.53022/oarjms.2021.2.1.0052.
Mikery, O., Rojas, J. C., Rebollar-Téllez, E. A., Valle-Mora, J., & Castillo, A. (2022). Assessment of synthetic chemicals for the anthropophilic sandfly *Lutzomyia cruciata* attraction to light-baited traps. *International Journal of Pest Management*, *70*, 1–11.
Mullen, G. R., & Durden, L. A. (2009). Medical and veterinary entomology. In: *Tsetse Flies (Glossinidae)* (Ed. W. L. Krinsky, 2nd edition). Academic Press, London, pp. 288–299.
Muñoz, C., Risueño, J., Pérez-Cutillas, P., Bernal, L. J., Ortiz, J. M., Ruiz de Ybáñez, R., Sánchez-López, P. F., Martínez-Carrasco, C., Del Río, L., De la Rúa, P., García-Martínez, J. D., Gonzálvez, M., Murcia, L., Collantes, F., Goyena, E., Spitzova, T., Elshanat, S., & Berriatua, E. (2021). Density assessment and reporting for *Phlebotomus perniciosus* and other sand fly species in periurban residential estates in Spain. *Parasitology Research*, *120*, 3091–3103.
Nayduch, D., & Burrus, R. G. (2017). Flourishing in filth: House fly–microbe interactions across life history. *Annals of the Entomological Society of America*, *110*(1), 6–18.
Ojianwuna, C. C., Edafemakor, A. G., & Iloh, A. C. (2011). Toxicity of *Ocimum suave* (wild basil) leaf oil on adult housefly (*Musca domestica*). *International Research Journal of Agricultural Science and Soil Science*, *10*(1), 417–420.
Olah, G., Vigo, G., Ortiz, L., Rozsa, L., &Brightsmith, D. J. (2013). *Philornis* sp. bot fly larvae in free living scarlet macaw nestlings and a new technique for their extraction. *Veterinary Parasitology*, *196*(1–2), 245–249.

Ommi, D., Mohammadreza Hashemian, S., Tajbakhsh, E., & Khamesipour, F. (2015). Molecular detection and antimicrobial resistance of *Aeromonas* from houseflies (*Musca domestica*) in Iran. *Revista MVZ Córdoba*, *20*, 4929–4936.

Radostits, O. M., Gay, C. C., Hinchcliff, K. W., & Constable, P. D. (2007). *Veterinary Medicine- A Textbook of the Diseases of Cattle, Horse, Sheep, Pigs and Goats*. 10th Edition. Saunders Elsevier, Edinburgh, pp. 1531–1540.

Riet-Correa, F., Ladeira, S. L., Andrade, G. B., & Carterb, G. R. (2000). *Lechiguana* (focal proliferative fibro-granulomatous panniculitis) in cattle. *Veterinary Research Communications*, *24*, 557–572.

Sasaki, T., Kobayashi, M., & Agui, N. (2000). Epidemiological potential of excretion and regurgitation by *Musca domestica* (Diptera: Muscidae) in the dissemination of *Escherichia coli* O157: H7 to food. *Journal of Medical Entomology*, *37*(6), 945–949.

Sharma, U., & Singh, S. (2000) Insect vectors of *Leishmania*: Distribution, physiology and their control. *Journal of Vector Borne Diseases*, *45*(4), 255–272. Retraction in: J Vector Borne Dis. 2012 Mar; *49*(1), 54.

Shimabukuro, P. H. F., de Andrade, A. J., & Galati, E. A. B. (2017). Checklist of American sand flies (Diptera, Psychodidae, Phlebotominae): Genera, species, and their distribution. *ZooKeys*, *660*, 67.

Slansky, F. (2006). Cuterebra bot flies (Diptera: Oestridae) and their indigenous hosts and potential hosts in Florida. *Florida Entomologist*, *89*(2), 152–160.

Smallegange, R. C. (2004). Fatal attraction. Control of the housefly (*Musca domestica*). *Entomologische Berichten*, *63*, 87–92.

Stoffolano, J. G. (2019). Fly foregut and transmission of microbes. *Advances in Insect Physiology*, *57*, 27–95.

Studentsky, L., Orshan, L., Akad, F., Avi, I. B., Diaz, D., Elbaz, S., Zagron, G., Valinsky, L., Davidovich-Cohen, M., & Baneth, G. (2023). *Leishmania donovani* transmission cycle associated with human infection, *Phlebotomus alexandri* sand flies, and hare blood meals, Israel. *Emerging Infectious Diseases*, *29*(5), 945.

Taylor, M. A., Coop, R. L., & Wall, R. (2015). *Veterinary Parasitology*. John Wiley & Sons, New York.

Thomas, G. D., Berry, I. L., Berkebile, D. R., & Skoda, S. R. (1989). Comparison of three sampling methods for estimating adult stable fly (Diptera: Muscidae) populations. *Environmental Entomology*, *18*(3), 513–520.

Ticha, L., Kykalova, B., Sadlova, J., Gramiccia, M., Gradoni, L., & Volf, P. (2021). Development of various *Leishmania (Sauroleishmania) tarentolae* strains in three *Phlebotomus* species. *Microorganisms*, *9*(11), 2256.

Tilak, R., Verma, A. K., & Wankhade, U. B. (2010). Effectiveness of Diflubenzuron in the control of houseflies. *Journal of Vector Borne Diseases*, *47*(2), 97.

Tomberlin, J. K. (2006). *Controlling Houseflies*. Agrilife Extension, Texas A&M Universaity System, Texas.

Trájer, A. J., Hammer, T., & Padisák, J. (2018). Reflection of the Neogene–Quaternary phylogeography in the recent distribution limiting climatic factors of eight Mediterranean *Phlebotomus* species (Diptera: Psychodidae). *Journal of Natural History*, *52*(27–28), 1763–1784.

Vargas-Teran, M., Hofmann, H. C., & Twiddle, N. E. (2005). Impact of screwworm eradication programmes using the sterile insect technique, pp. 629–650. In: *Sterile Insect Technique: Principles and Practices in Area-Wide Integrated Pest Management* (Eds. V. A. Dyck, J. Hendrichs, & A. S. Robinson). Springer, Dordrecht, The Netherlands.

Wall, R., & Shearer, D. (1997). *Veterinary Entomology: Arthropod Ectoparasites of Veterinary Importance*. Springer, New York.

Wijerathna, T., & Gunathilaka, N. (2020). Diurnal adult resting sites and breeding habitats of phlebotomine sand flies in cutaneous leishmaniasis endemic areas of Kurunegala District, Sri Lanka. *Parasites & Vectors*, *13*, 1–10.

Wyss, J. H. (2000). Screwworm eradication in the Americas. *Annals of the New York Academy of Sciences*, *916*(1), 186–193.

Zumpt, F. (1973). *The Stomoxyine Biting Flies of the World. Diptera: Muscidae. Taxonomy, Biology, Economic Importance and Control Measures*. Gustav Fischer Verlag, Stuttgart.

10 Flesh Flies (Sarcophagidae)

Shuvra Kanti Sinha and Nandan Jana

LEARNING OBJECTIVES

1. Comprehend the taxonomy, bionomics and faunal diversity of Sarcophagidae.
2. Illustrate the diagnostic morphology of adult flies within the three subfamilies.
3. Explore the life cycle of *Liosarcophaga choudhuryi* Sinha & Nandi, 2002 and the life history strategies of gravid females across the three subfamilies.
4. Gain insight into the ecological roles and their feeding habits.
5. Assess the forensic and medico-veterinary implications of adults and larvae, focusing on their role in myiasis and infestations in host animals.
6. Deliberate on taxonomic research of Sarcophagidae within the context of India, particularly regarding species diversity.

10.1 INTRODUCTION

Flies of the family Sarcophagidae, commonly known as flesh flies, constitute a diverse group of calyptrate flies within the order Diptera. They are widespread, found all over the world except in the Arctic and Antarctic regions (Ramos et al., 2022). They are generally greyish in appearance, medium to large in size (3.5–20 mm). The dorsal part of the thorax is covered with three dark longitudinal stripes. The abdomen usually has a black and white checkered pattern, and the hypopleura is hairy, which can easily distinguish them from other calyptrate flies.

Adult flesh flies are usually observed in and around the dead bodies of different animals, garbage, animal dung, fresh and rotten fish, meat, and in vegetable markets. Some flies are found around flowering plants. A few are synanthropic in nature, found in and around human habitations (Ren et al., 2018).

Feeding habits of sarcophagid flies are diverse; most of them lean towards **necrophagous** (feed on carcasses or corpses of various vertebrate and invertebrate animals) (Ren et al., 2018). Some are specialized **saprophagous** (i.e. they feed on decaying organic matter like rotten fruits and vegetables). Some are **coprophagous** (i.e. they feed on freshly deposited dung of different animals). Some play roles as **pollinators** (i.e. they feed on nectar from flowers and help in pollination) (Buenaventura et al., 2020).

Adult flies usually deposit first instar larvae on different breeding media, i.e. carrion, decaying organic matter, and dung. Larvae consume decomposing matter and play a crucial role in ecological processes as **scavengers**. Beyond ecological significance, flesh flies play a vital role in forensic criminal investigations, helping to determine **post-mortem time interval** (PMI) (Ren et al., 2018).

In addition, there are some species with medical and veterinary importance. They can cause **myiasis**, an infestation of vertebrate tissues by maggots (Diptera larvae). Adult flies are mostly attracted to wounds, blood, injured areas, and open orifices such as the nose, mouth, ears, anus, and vagina (Ramos et al., 2022). Myiasis induced by Sarcophagidae includes ophthalmomyiasis, urogenital myiasis, oral myiasis, nasal myiasis, and cutaneous myiasis (Ren et al., 2018). Members of this family also serve as potential vectors for several bacterial, viral, protozoan, and helminth diseases, including amoebic dysentery, typhoid, cholera, and tuberculosis in humans and animals (Greenberg, 1971).

DOI: 10.1201/9781003482581-13

10.2 TAXONOMY OF FLESH FLIES (SARCOPHAGIDAE)

Senior-White et al. (1940) classified flesh flies as the subfamily Sarcophaginae within the family Calliphoridae. Later, Lehrer (1970) elevated the status of the subfamily Sarcophaginae to that of a separate family, alongside two other families, that is Calliphoridae and Rhiniidae. Faunal diversity of Sarcophagidae is extensive, with more than 3,000 described species over 173 genera worldwide (Pape et al., 2011). The family ranks as the second most diverse calyptrate group in the superfamily Oestroidea, following Tachinidae, which encompasses 9,626 valid species (Pape et al., 2011). Flies of this family are widely distributed, but most species are found in tropical regions (Pape, 1996; Mello-Patiu, 2016). Identification of adult flies in this group is based on various morphological features including;

1. Chaetotaxy (arrangement of bristles primarily on the head, thorax, abdomen, and legs)
2. Wing venation
3. Markings on the thorax and abdomen
4. Male genitalia

The global fauna of Sarcophagidae is divided into three subfamilies: Miltogramminae, Paramacronychiinae, and Sarcophaginae (Pape, 1996).

10.2.1 Subfamily–Miltogramminae (Figure 10.1)

The subfamily Miltogramminae within the family Sarcophagidae is notably diversified with around 600 species documented worldwide (Verves, 1989; Nandi, 2002), including 29 recorded in India (Barták et al., 2019). Flies of this subfamily show a worldwide distribution, with particularly high species diversity found in African and Asian countries (Pape, 1996). Adults are typically small to medium in size, with length ranges between 5 and 10 mm. The body is characterised by a greyish to pale blackish colouration with transverse dark marginal bands on the abdomen. The dorsal surface of the thorax usually bears three dark longitudinal stripes, and the head capsule is relatively large.

10.2.2 Subfamily–Paramacronychiinae (Figure 10.2)

Paramacronychiinae is the least diversified subfamily within the family Sarcophagidae, comprising 97 species worldwide (Buenaventura et al., 2020) and three from India (Barták et al., 2019). Despite its limited diversity, members of this group exhibit a widespread distribution, except for regions of Australasia (Pape, 1996; Nandi, 2002). Flies in this subfamily are characterised by small to large

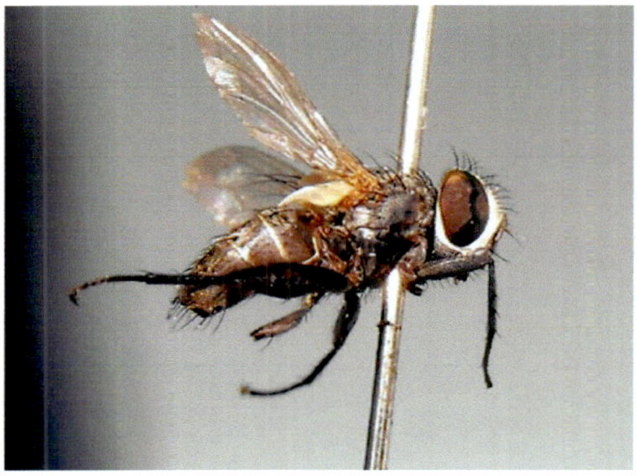

FIGURE 10.1 *Senotainia albifrons* (Rondani, 1859) (Miltogramminae fly) (Source Sinha, 2012a).

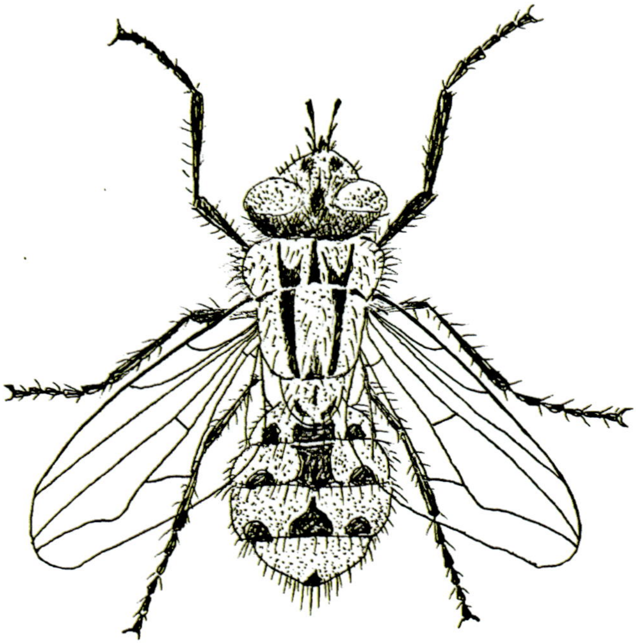

FIGURE 10.2 Paramacronychiinae fly.

bodies (3.5–20 mm). The thorax and abdomen are coated with dense blackish to greyish pollen. The abdomen is usually checkered with dark median and lateral bands.

10.2.3 Subfamily–Sarcophaginae (Figure 10.3)

Sarcophaginae stands out as the most diverse subfamily of the family Sarcophagidae, nearly 2,300 species worldwide (Buenaventura et al., 2020). In India, the faunal diversity of Sarcophaginae

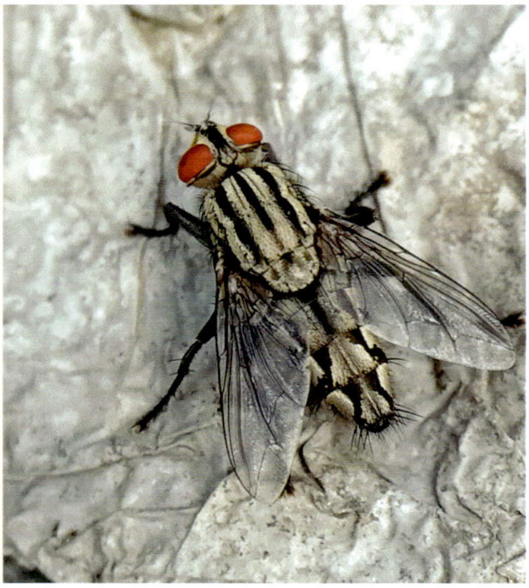

FIGURE 10.3 Male *Sarcophaga* sp. (Sarcophaginae fly).

includes 107 species under 36 genera (Barták et al., 2019; Sinha et al., 2023). Flies of this subfamily usually exhibit a uniform greyish colouration with three dark longitudinal stripes on the thorax. The body typically appears robust with a checkered greyish abdomen. The notopleura disc is characterised by four distinct bristles (two primary and two secondary), distinguishing them from flies of the other two subfamilies.

10.3 BIONOMICS OF FLESH FLY (SARCOPHAGIDAE)

Flesh flies are mostly **larviparous**, i.e. they directly deposit first instar larvae on breeding substrate instead of laying eggs (Ren et al., 2018). A gravid female may deposit larvae on different media, including dung, garbage, and the living and dead bodies of spiders, snails, turtles, snakes, reptiles, birds, bats, rabbits, mammals, and even human beings (Nandi, 1980; Sinha & Nandi, 2010; Chakraborty et al., 2014). Moreover, immature stages of some flies (e.g. *Sarcophaga sarraceniae* Riley, 1874; *Fletcherimyia* spp.) have been reported at the bottom of the pitcher tube of pitcher plants (Dahlem & Naczi, 2006; Zhang et al., 2014). Some larvae are parasitoids (larvae develop on or within a host, feeding on its tissues or body fluids and ultimately killing the host), and a few are kleptoparasitoids (i.e. some female Miltogrammines deposit larvae on the paralysed prey, captured by wasp mothers for their progeny). Three subfamilies of Sarcophagidae flies display varied feeding habits, life history strategies, ecological roles, and other behaviours.

10.3.1 Miltogramminae

Flies in this group are primarily kleptoparasitic in nature, with wasps and bees (Hymenoptera) often being targeted. Females may deposit their larvae on paralysed prey carried by wasps before they are taken into the nest or brood chamber. Alternatively, flies may directly larviposit by searching entrances of wasp nests (Pape, 1996). Some are flower visitors to a variety of flowering plants and act as good pollinators. A few are capable of inducing wound and intestinal myiasis in human beings (Nandi, 1998). Larvae of some species also serve as bio-controlling agents on various agricultural pests, playing an active role in pest management.

10.3.2 Paramacronychiinae

Adults of this subfamily breed on decaying fish, amphibians, and snails. Adult and larval feeding behaviour ranges from coprophagous and saprophagous to necrophagous. Some species (e.g. *Wohlfahrtia* sp.) are known to cause myiasis in humans and other mammals, being attracted to wounds and open orifices. Moreover, certain species within this group are active predators and parasites on snails, as well as various insect groups including Lepidoptera, Orthoptera, Coleoptera, and Hymenoptera (Pape, 1996; Nandi, 1998).

10.3.3 Sarcophaginae

Adult flies of this subfamily inhabit diverse habitats, such as carcasses, decaying fish and meat, garbage, animal dung, and human settlements (Nandi, 1998). Larvae of some species of the genera *Bercaea* and *Parasarcophaga* grow on faeces. Larval feeding habits are predominantly necrophagous and often lead to myiasis in humans and vertebrate animals. Some are coprophagous, carnivorous, parasitic, and predaceous on other animals. Species of the genus *Sarcophaga* within this group hold immense forensic importance, with notable species including *Parasarcophaga albiceps* (Meigen); *Liosarcophaga dux* (Thomson); *Sarcophaga ruficornis* (Fabricius); and *Sarcophaga peregrina*

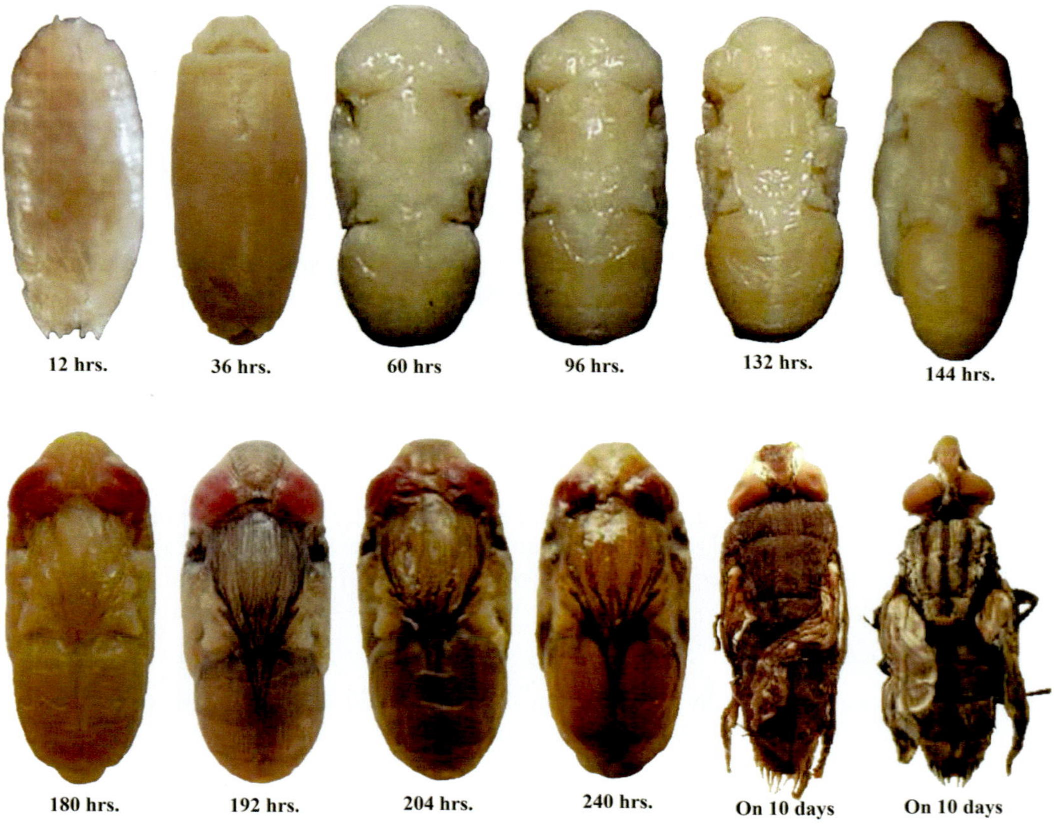

FIGURE 10.4 Intra-puparial development of *Liosarcophaga dux* (Thomson, 1869) (Source Sinha & Mahato, 2016).

(Robineau-Desvoidy) (Chakraborty et al., 2014). The sequential intra-puparial development (time duration taken by the pupa up to adult emergence) of some forensically important Sarcophaginae flies has provided valuable insights in the field of criminal investigations (Figure 10.4) (Sinha & Mahato, 2016; Li et al., 2023; Shang et al., 2023).

10.4 LIFE CYCLE OF *LIOSARCOPHAGA CHOUDHURYI* SINHA & NANDI, 2002 (FIGURE 10.5) (*SOURCE*: SINHA & NANDI, 2010)

Liosarcophaga choudhuryi Sinha & Nandi, 2002 is known for its parasitoid nature, which breeds in intertidal snail, *Littoraria* (*Palustorina*) *melanostoma* Gray, 1839 (Gastropoda: Littorinidae). This species follows an ovoviviparous life cycle, consisting of three larval instars, pupa, and adult. The larva undergoes three moults (first, second, and third instar) within the snail host before pupation. Under ambient conditions (temperature 24°C ± 4°C; relative humidity 66% ± 4%), the entire life cycle (from larviposition to adult emergence) spans nearly 11–12 days. Throughout their lifespans, they may infest up to 30 snails. The male and female flies exhibit average lifespans of 27 and 36 days, respectively.

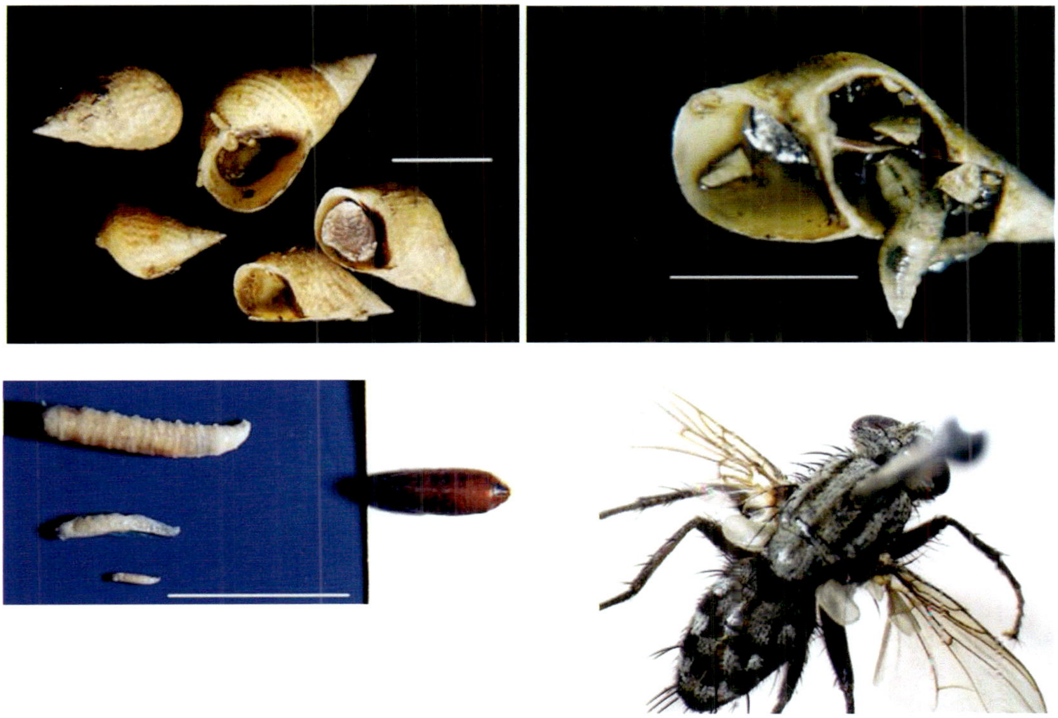

FIGURE 10.5 Life cycle of *Liosarcophaga choudhuryi* Sinha & Nandi, 2002 on intertidal snail *Littoraria* (*Palustorina*) *melanostoma* Gray, 1839 (Source Sinha & Nandi, 2010).

1. **Mating**: Females engage in mating with males approximately 3–5 days after emergence, with an average mating duration of 18 minutes. Females often mate multiple times throughout their life cycle.
2. **Larviposition**: After mating, gravid females usually lay their first instar larvae on snails around 14 days after emergence, in several batches. Females deposit 1–3 larvae on each snail, with larviposition reported up to 30 days post-emergence. In a single mating cycle, females can produce over 70 first instar larvae.
3. **First instar larvae**: The first instar larvae are creamy white, consist of 12 segments, and measure about 1.5 and 2.0 mm in length. They possess weakly-developed posterior spiracles, unevenly sclerotised incomplete cephaloskeleton and a small curved mouth hook. Anterior spiracles are indistinct.
4. **Second instar larvae**: The second instar larvae usually appear approximately 6–7 hours after larviposition, measuring about 5–7 mm in length, with well-developed anterior and posterior spiracles. Pair posterior spiracles consist of two slit-like openings in a deep cavity. Cephaloskeleton is more sclerotised and mouth hook ventrally curved.
5. **Third instar larvae**: The third instar larvae emerge around 14–15 hours after larviposition. The length is about 12–14 mm, and segments 2–11 features with complete anterior bands. Mouth hook is strong and well-developed, pointed downward. Cephaloskeleton is highly sclerotised. Anterior and posterior spiracles are prominent.
6. **Puparium**: Third instar larvae are transformed into pupae within the puparia around 76–77 hours after larviposition, with the pupal stage remaining an average of 192 hours. The puparia are capsule-like structures, brownish in colour, and measure about 7.0–7.5 mm in length.

7. **Emerged adult**: Adults can emerge from the puparia approximately 11–12 days later. Within 1–2 hours of emergence, they can fly and become ready to mate 3–5 days afterwards.

10.5 FLESH FLY LARVAL INFESTATION OF DIFFERENT ANIMALS

Members of the family Sarcophagidae are the most opportunistic flies, completing their life cycle on a diverse range of substrates. Their larval feeding habits are mostly necrophagous, since gravid females strategically deposit first instar larvae on various living and dead organisms to ensure their nourishment and successive larval development. Subsequently, the larval stages consume necrotic or fresh tissues, often leading to myiasis or even death. Some interesting instances of Sarcophagidae larval infestation are as follows:

10.5.1 Larval Infestation of Snails (Figure 10.6)

The parasitoid sarcophagid fly *Liosarcophaga choudhuryi* Sinha & Nandi, 2002, commonly found in the Sundarbans Biosphere Reserve, India, is known to infest and breed on the intertidal snail *Littoraria* (*Palustorina*) *melanostoma* Gray, 1839 (Gastropoda: Littorinidae). Following mating, gravid females generally lay 1–3 first instar larvae on the operculum when the snail emerges from its shell to feed. The larvae then penetrate the host's body, begin to feed on fresh tissues, and ultimately cause the host's death (Sinha & Nandi, 2010). Besides *L. choudhuryi*, several flies of the family Sarcophagidae, such as *L. dux* and *Sarcorohdendorfia megafilosia* Pape, Mckillup & Mckillup, 2000 have been documented as predators of various freshwater and seawater snails, including *Indoplanorbis exustus* (Dashayes, 1834) and *Littoraria filosa* (G. B. Sowerby I, 1832) (Sinha & Nandi, 2010).

10.5.2 Larval Infestation of Spiders

Sarcophagidae larvae are generally parasitic in nature, utilizing invertebrate and vertebrate animals as hosts for their development. Larval infestation of Sarcophagidae on spiders represents a conspicuous ecological interaction. Flesh flies (e.g. *Metopia* sp.) have been observed as parasites on spiders. The association of Sarcophagidae larvae on spiders is seen as kleptoparasitism. Gravid females may occasionally deposit their first instar larvae onto paralysed spiders captured by wasps (Schwendinger & Pape, 2000). The larvae then penetrate the spider's body and consume its fluids and tissues for nourishment.

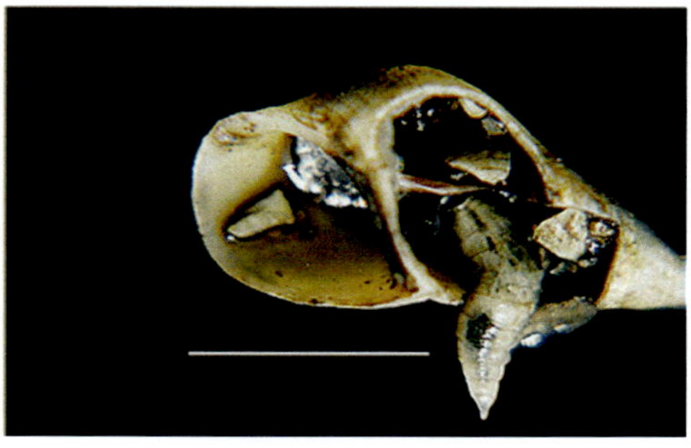

FIGURE 10.6 *Littoraria* (*Palustorina*) *melanostoma* Gray, 1839 infested by larvae of *Liosarcophaga choudhuryi* Sinha & Nandi, 2002 (Source: Sinha & Nandi, 2010).

10.5.3 Larval Infestation of Wasp Nests

Infestation by Sarcophagidae larvae on wasps, or kleptoparasitism, represents a fascinating example of parasitic interaction. The process usually begins when female sarcophagid flies, primarily Miltogramminae, deposit their first instar larvae within the nests of Hymenopteran wasps (Vespidae and Sphecidae) and bees. In subsequent larval depositions, the predatory maggots steal and consume the provisioned food sources collected by wasps to nourish their own offspring, ultimately leading to the death of the host either directly or indirectly (Maqbool et al., 2022).

10.5.4 Larval Infestation of Frogs

Amphibians are still subject to infestation by fly larvae belonging to members of four Diptera families, including Muscidae, Calliphoridae, Chloropidae, and Sarcophagidae. Case reports from various regions of the world have documented instances of myiasis in amphibians caused by sarcophagid larvae, particularly members of the genus *Lepidodexia* (*Notochaeta*) (Hagmen et al., 2005; Vázquez-Corzas et al., 2018; Mulieri et al., 2018).

10.5.5 Larval Infestation of Turtle Nests

Sarcophagidae is a family of flies known for their attraction to various decaying matters, including remains found in turtle nests containing dead eggs or hatchlings. Turtles usually deposit a number of eggs in buried nests without providing any parental care. Nests containing dead eggs or decaying matter are often infested by larvae of various dipteran flies, particularly the maggots of flesh flies. One of the most common Sarcophagidae species that infest freshwater turtle nests is *Tripanurga importuna* Walker (Geller, 2022).

10.5.6 Larval Infestation of Birds (Figure 10.7)

In general, birds are susceptible to various kinds of ectoparasites, such as lice, fleas, mites, etc., but infestation by Sarcophagidae larvae is extremely uncommon. Birds that visit garbage or feed on decaying organic matter infested with larvae may be at risk of infestation. For instance, a case report of larval infestation by Sarcophagidae on a common Pariah Kite (*Milvus migrans* Boddaert, 1783), documented by Sinha et al. (2017), suggested that infestation occurred during the bird's visit to corpses infested with Sarcophagidae maggots.

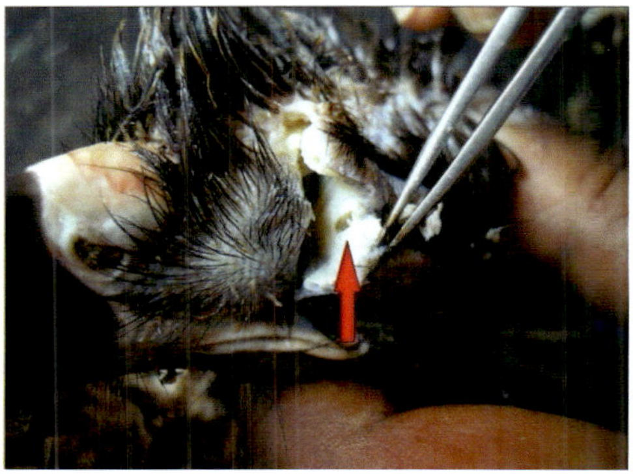

FIGURE 10.7 Larval infestation by Sarcophagidae on the common Pariah Kite (*Milvus migrans* Boddaert, 1783) (*Source*: Sinha et al., 2017).

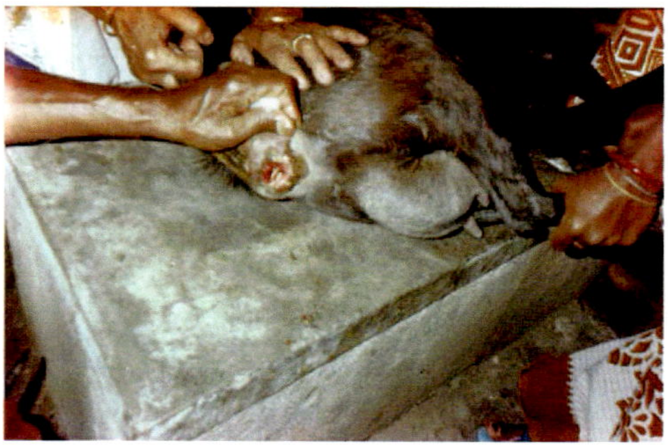

FIGURE 10.8 Vaginal myiasis in a goat caused by larval infestation of *Sarcophaga reciproca* Walker, 1856 (*Source*: Sinha, 2012b).

10.5.7 Larval Infestation of Mammals (Figure 10.8)

Feeding habits of Sarcophagidae larvae are mostly necrophagous; development often depends on carrion or dead bodies of vertebrate and invertebrate animals. Gravid females of Sarcophagidae primarily deposit their first instar larvae on dead animals or carcasses. However, in certain situations, such as open wounds, sores, blood, and orifices like the nose, ears, mouth, anus, and vagina, a foul smell attracts gravid females for larviposition. Sarcophagids can infest a wide range of mammals, including cattle, sheep, goats, pigs, dogs, cats, and wild animals. After larviposition, maggots usually invade host tissues and cause severe myiasis (Sinha, 2012b; Bonacci et al., 2013; Salant et al., 2020; Singh, 2020).

10.5.8 Larval Infestation of Humans

Infestation of humans by dipterous larvae, known as myiasis, primarily involves members of the families Calliphoridae, Muscidae, Oestridae, and Sarcophagidae (Robbins & Khachemoune, 2010). Following Calliphoridae, infestation by Sarcophagidae larvae on humans is particularly common in tropical and subtropical countries with poor hygiene. Female Sarcophagidae may deposit first instar larvae on human bodies in certain situations, such as untreated wounds, moist open orifices, or on immobile persons such as the elderly or infants living in unsanitary conditions. Larvae feed on necrotic and fresh tissues in infested regions, leading to severe pathological conditions that sometimes cause death (Philip et al., 2007; Giangaspero et al., 2017; Najjari et al., 2020; Zhou et al., 2021).

10.6 STATUS OF FLESH FLY RESEARCH IN INDIA

The pioneer research work on Indian Sarcophagidae was initiated by Senior-White (1924). Subsequently, a number of taxonomists who have contributed significantly to the knowledge of Indian flesh flies (Sarcophagidae) include Dr. B. Dasgupta (1927–2009), Dr. B.C. Nandi (1947–present), Dr. A.N.T. Joseph (1936–present), P. Parui (1938–2024), and Dr. S.K. Sinha (1975–present).

The comprehensive research on Sarcophagidae in India was conducted by Dr. B.C. Nandi in his monograph "The Fauna of India and the Adjacent Countries Diptera, Sarcophagidae (Vol. X, 2002)". He mentioned a total of 163 species, of which 119 species under 39 genera were documented from India across three subfamilies: Sarcophaginae, Miltogramminae, and Paramacronychiinae. Thereafter, Barták et al. (2019) revised the Indian flesh flies and reported 138 known species, including the first record of *Sarcolomonia shinonagai* (Kano & Sooksri, 1977) from the country. Among them, the genus *Liosarcophaga* was identified as the most speciose genus, comprising 21 species (Table 10.1). Recently, Sinha et al. (2023) reported an additional species, *Parasarcophaga (Sinonipponia) baruai* Segiyama, 1988 from West Bengal, which increased the total number of known species in India to 139.

The number of known species in India represents around 4% of globally described species, and among them, 55% are indigenous (Chakraborty et al., 2017). However, flesh flies in India remain poorly understood. More field-based taxonomic surveys are needed to explore this group further, and many species are awaiting discovery.

TABLE 10.1
List of Sarcophagidae Species Recorded in India

Subfamily	Species
Miltogramminae	*Senotainia (Arrenopus) albifrons* (Rondani, 1859)
	Senotainia (Arrenopus) anamalaica (Verves, 1988)
	Senotainia (Arrenopus) navigatrix (Meijere, 1910)
	Eremasiomyia macularis (Wiedemann, 1824)
	Protomiltogramma nandii Verves, 1979
	Protomiltogramma obscurior (Villeneuve, 1916)
	Protomiltogramma rufiventris (Baranov, 1938)
	Pterella krombeini Verves, 1979
	Cylindrothecum angustifrons (Townsend, 1933)
	Cylindrothecum ibericum (Villeneuve, 1912)
	Miltogramma testaceifrons (Roser, 1840)
	Miltogrammidium taeniatum (Meigen, 1824)
	Craticulina diffusa Villeneuve, 1934
	Craticulina tabaniformis (Fabricius, 1805)
	Hoplocephalomima nathani Verves, 1988
	Krombeinomyia indica Verves, 1988
	Krombeinomyia mirabilis Verves, 1979
	Phylloteles hyalipennis (Baranov, 1934)
	Amobia auriceps (Baranov, 1935)
	Amobia signata (Meigen, 1824)
	Metopia argentata Macquart, 1850
	Metopia campestris (Fallén, 1810)
	Metopia nudibasis (Malloch, 1930)
	Metopia sauteri (Townsend, 1933)
	Metopia tshernovae Rohdendorf, 1955
	Phrosinella (s. str.) *fedtshenkoi* (Rohdendorf, 1925)
	Sphenometopa (Asiaraba) jacobsoni Rohdendorf, 1967
	Sphenometopa (Euaraba) fastuosa (Meigen 1824)
	Taxigramma heteroneura (Meigen, 1830)
Paramacronychiinae	*Brachicoma devia* (Fallén, 1820)
	Wohlfahrtia nuba (Wiedemann, 1830)
	Wohlfahrtia trina (Wiedemann, 1830)
Sarcophaginae	*Blaesoxipha bhutanensis* Nandi, 1992
	Blaesoxipha karnataka Pape, 1994
	Blaesoxipha nathani Lopes, 1990
	Blaesoxipha pygmaea (Zetterstedt, 1844)

(*Continued*)

TABLE 10.1 (*Continued*)
List of Sarcophagidae Species Recorded in India

Subfamily	Species
	Blaesoxipha redempta (Pandellé, 1896)
	Blaesoxipha rishikeshi Nandi, 1990
	Blaesoxipha rufipes (Macquart, 1839)
	Blaesoxipha valangae (Aldrich, 1932)
	Ravinia pernix (Harris, 1780)
	Alisarcophaga sawainensis (Nandi, 1989)
	Asioboettcheria papei (Nandi, 1994)
	Helicophagella (Parabellieria) melanura (Meigen, 1826)
	Dravidia cavangarei (Nandi, 1988)
	Karnatakia aldrichi (Nandi, 1992)
	Kozlovea lopesi Nandi, 1976
	Kozlovea peshelicis (Senior-White, 1930)
	Nagpuria vervesi (Nandi, 1993)
	Discachaeta smithi (Nandi, 1990)
	Leucomyia alba (Schiner, 1868)
	Asceloctella (s. str.) *calicifera* (Böttcher, 1912)
	Girnaria girnarensis (Nandi, 1992)
	Pseudobellieriomima wyatti (Nandi, 1994)
	Pseudothyrsocnema dasguptai (Nandi, 1979)
	Pseudothyrsocnema indica (Shinonaga & Lopes, 1975)
	Pseudothyrsocnema longistylata (Shinonaga & Lopes, 1975)
	Pseudothyrsocnema lushainensis (Nandi, 1992)
	Pseudothyrsocnema nicobarensis (Nandi, 1989)
	Thyrsocnema kentejana Rohdendorf, 1937
	Harpagophalla kempi (Senior-White, 1924)
	Iranihindia futilis (Senior-White, 1924)
	Iranihindia indica Nandi, 1979
	Iranihindia jamesi Nandi, 1979
	Iranihindia martellata (Senior-White, 1924)
	Iranihindia martellatoides (Baranov, 1931)
	Iranihindia mengraia Lehrer, 2008
	Iranihindia nepalensis Kano & Shinonaga, 1969
	Nandimyia panchganiensis (Nandi, 1993)
	Sarconandia madrasiola Lehrer, 2005
	Ampilicercomyia amplicercus (Shinonaga & Tumrasvin, 1979)
	Ampilicercomyia ballardi (Senior-White, 1924)
	Bercaea africa (Wiedemann, 1824)
	Curvosarcophaga curvata (Nandi, 1989)
	Fengia kaimaraensis Nandi, 1992
	Fengia ostindicae (Senior-White, 1924)
	Hosarcophaga auricauda (Ho, 1938)
	Liopygia (s. str.) *ruficornis* (Fabricius, 1794)
	Liopygia (Thomsonea) argyrostoma (Robineau-Desvoidy, 1830)
	Liosarcophaga (Curranea) yunnanensis (Fan, 1965)
	Liosarcophaga (Jantiella) coei (Rohdendorf, 1966)

(*Continued*)

TABLE 10.1 (*Continued*)
List of Sarcophagidae Species Recorded in India

Subfamily	Species
	Liosarcophaga (*Jantiella*) *djakonovi* (Rohdendorf, 1937)
	Liosarcophaga (*Jantiella*) *javana* (Macquart, 1851)
	Liosarcophaga (s. str.) *choudhuryi* (Sinha & Nandi, 2002)
	Liosarcophaga (s. str.) *dux* (Thomson, 1869)
	Liosarcophaga (s. str.) *geetai* (Fahd & Zambare, 2016)
	Liosarcophaga (s. str.) *harpax* (Pandellé, 1896)
	Liosarcophaga (s. str.) *idmais* (Séguy, 1934)
	Liosarcophaga (s. str.) *jaipurensis* (Nandi, 1990)
	Liosarcophaga (s. str.) *josephi* (Nandi, 2002)
	Liosarcophaga (s. str.) *kohla* (Johnson & Hardy, 1923)
	Liosarcophaga (s. str.) *parkeri* (Rohdendorf, 1937)
	Liosarcophaga (s. str.) *portschinskyi* (Rohdendorf, 1937)
	Liosarcophaga (s. str.) *sarupi* (Nandi, 1979)
	Liosarcophaga (s. str.) *scopariiformis* (Senior-White, 1927)
	Liosarcophaga (s. str.) *tuberosa* (Pandellé, 1896)
	Liosarcophaga (*Pandelleisca*) *assamensis* (Nandi, 1982)
	Liosarcophaga (*Pandelleisca*) *bainbriggei* (Senior-White, 1925)
	Liosarcophaga (*Pandelleisca*) *hui* (Ho, 1936)
	Liosarcophaga (*Pandelleisca*) *kurahashii* (Nandi, 1992)
	Parasarcophaga (*Baranovisca*) *banksi* (Senior-White, 1924)
	Parasarcophaga (*Baranovisca*) *cantrelli* *Verves*, 1991
	Parasarcophaga (s. str.) *albiceps* (Meigen, 1826)
	Parasarcophaga (s. str.) *hirtipes* (Wiedemann, 1830)
	Parasarcophaga (s. str.) *macroauriculata* (Ho, 1932)
	Parasarcophaga (s. str.) *misera* (Walker, 1849)
	Parasarcophaga (s. str.) *taenionota* (Wiedemann, 1819)
	Parasarcophaga (*Sinonipponia*) *bengalensis* (Nandi, 1977)
	Parasarcophaga (*Sinonipponia*) *smarti* (Nandi, 1990)
	Parasarcophaga (*Sinonipponia*) *baruai* Sugiyama, 1988
	Robineauella (*Digitiventra*) *walayari* (Senior-White, 1924)
	Sarcorohdendorfia *desaii* (Nandi, 1978)
	Sarcorohdendorfia *flavinervis* (Senior-White, 1924)
	Sarcorohdendorfia *ghaiae* Nandi, 1979
	Sarcorohdendorfia *inextricata* (Walker, 1860)
	Sarcorohdendorfia *mysorensis* Nandi, 1983
	Sarcorohdendorfia *pusana* (Senior-White, 1924)
	Sarcosolomonia (*Parkerimyia*) *andamanensis* Nandi, 1989
	Sarcosolomonia (*Parkerimyia*) *chambaensis* Nandi, 1989
	Sarcosolomonia (*Parkerimyia*) *crinita* (Parker, 1917)
	Sarcosolomonia (*Parkerimyia*) *indica* Nandi, 1976
	Sarcosolomonia (*Parkerimyia*) *kaushanensis* Nandi, 1990
	Sarcosolomonia (*Parkerimyia*) *nathani* Lopes & Kano, 1969
	Sarcosolomonia (*Parkerimyia*) *rohdendorfi* Nandi, 1976
	Sarcosolomonia (s. str.) *shinonagai* Kano & Sooksri, 1977

(*Continued*)

TABLE 10.1 (*Continued*)
List of Sarcophagidae Species Recorded in India

Subfamily	Species
	Boettcherisca bengalensis Nandi, 1992
	Boettcherisca karnyi (Hardy, 1927)
	Boettcherisca nathani Lopes, 1961
	Boettcherisca nepalensis Kano & Sugiyama, 1983
	Boettcherisca peregrina (Robineau-Desvoidy, 1830)
	Lioproctia (Burmanomyia) beesoni (Senior-White, 1924)
	Lioproctia (Coonoria) lothianensis Sinha & Nandi, 2002
	Lioproctia (Coonoria) pattoni (Senior-White, 1924)
	Phallosphaera gravelyi (Senior-White, 1924)
	Rosellea khasiensis (Senior-White, 1924)
	Saputaramyia saputaraensis (Nandi, 1992)
	Seniorwhitea annandalei (Senior-White, 1924)
	Seniorwhitea mantiae Nandi, 2002
	Seniorwhitea princeps (Wiedemann, 1830)

Source: Barták et al. (2019) & Sinha et al. (2023).

10.7 CONCLUSION

Family Sarcophagidae is taxonomically divided into three subfamilies: Miltogramminae, Paramacronychiinae, and Sarcophaginae, with a notable diversity of over 3,000 species worldwide. The diverse feeding behaviours of both adults and larvae underscore their significance as scavengers, pollinators, and potential carriers of several diseases, with some species implicated in tissue myiasis among vertebrate animals. Some also contribute to forensic investigations. The faunal diversity of Sarcophagidae in India, with 139 species, represents around 4% of the global described species.

10.8 POINTS TO REMEMBER

1. Flesh flies belonging to the family Sarcophagidae are medico-veterinary important calyptrate Diptera, classified into three subfamilies: Miltogramminae, Paramacronychiinae, and Sarcophaginae.
2. The faunal diversity of Sarcophagidae comprises over 3,000 species worldwide, with 139 species found in India.
3. They have significant forensic importance, aiding in the estimation of PMI in criminal investigations. Females deposit first-instar larvae on dead bodies, becoming crucial indicators for forensic entomologists to ascertain the time of death.
4. Both adults and larvae contribute to a diverse range of ecological roles as scavengers, primarily associated with carrion, decaying organic matter, dung, and even flowering plants as pollinators.
5. Flesh flies possess medical and veterinary significance, capable of causing myiasis in vertebrate animals, including humans. Some also serve as potential vectors for several diseases.

REFERENCES

Barták, M., Khrokalo, L. & Verves, Y. (2019). New records, synonyms and combinations for oriental Sarcophagidae (Diptera), with updated checklists for Cambodia, India, Taiwan, Thailand and Vietnam. *Journal of Asia-Pacific Entomology*, 22: 44–55.

Bonacci, T., Greco, S., Whitmore, D. & Curcio, U. (2013). First data on myiasis caused by *Wohlfahrtia magnifica* (Schiner, 1862) (Insecta: Diptera: Sarcophagidae) in Calabria, southern Italy. *Life: The Excitement of Biology*, 1(4): 197–201.

Buenaventura, E., Szpila, K., Cassel, B., Wiegmann, B.M. & Pape, T. (2020). Anchored hybrid enrichment challenges the traditional classification of flesh flies (Diptera: Sarcophagidae). *Systematic Entomology*, 45: 281–301.

Chakraborty, A., Ansar, W., Ghosh, S. & Banerjee, D. (2014). The first of the life cycle of *Sarcophaga* (L.) *dux* on dead reptilian carcass: Their application as forensic indicators. *Scholars Academic Journal of Biosciences*, 2(2): 731–739.

Chakraborty, A., Hora, G., Parui, P., Saha, G.K. & Banerjee, D. (2017). A biosystematic species inventory of Indian Sarcophagidae (Insecta: Diptera: Sarcophagidae). *Journal of Entomology and Zoology Studies*, 5(1): 465–473.

Dahlem, G.A. & Naczi, R.F.C. (2006). Flesh flies (Diptera: Sarcophagidae) associated with North America Pitcher plants (Sarraceniaceae), with descriptions of three new species. *Systematics*, 99(2): 218–240.

Geller, G.A. (2022). Notes on Flesh fly (Diptera: Sarcophagidae) presence at Ouachita Map turtle (*Graptemys ouachitensis* Cagle, 1953) nests along the lower Wisconsin River, USA. *Herpetology Notes*, 15: 27–32.

Giangaspero, A., Marangi, M., Balotta, A., Venturelli, C., Szpila, K. & Palma, A.D. (2017). Wound myiasis caused by *Sarcophaga* (*Liopygia*) *argyrostoma* (Robineau-Desvoidy) (Diptera: Sarcophagidae): Additional evidences of the morphological identification dilemma and molecular investigation. *Hindawi the Scientific World Journal*, 1–9. doi:10.1155/2017/9064531

Greenberg, B. (1971). *Flies and Diseases*. Vol. 1. Princton University Press: New Jersey.

Hagman, M., Pape, T. & Schulte, R. (2005). Flesh fly myiasis (Diptera, Sarcophagidae) in Peruvian poison frogs genus *Epipedobates* (Anura, Dendrobatidae). *Phyllomedusa*, 4(1): 69–73.

Lehrer, A.Z. (1970). Consideration phylogenetiques et taxobomiques sur la famile Calliphoridae (Diptera: Calliphoridae). *Annotations Zoologicae et Botanicae Bratistlava*, 61: 1–51.

Li, L., Zhang, Y., Chen, Y., Guo, Y., Wang, Y., Hu, G., Kang, C., Wang, [illegible]. & Wang, Y. (2023). Intrapuparial development and age estimation of *Sarcophaga peregrina* (Diptera: Sarcophagidae) for postmortem interval estimation. *Journal of Asia-Pacific Entomology*, 26(2).

Maqbool, A., Maqbool, I., Banu, A.N., Rather, S.U. & Wachkoo, A. (2022). First record of *Amobia quatei* (Diptera: Sarcophagidae: Miltogramminae) from Indian subcontinent as kleptoparasite of *Anterhychium flavomarginatum* (Hymenoptera: Vespidae: Eumeninae). *Revista de la Sociedad Entomologica Argentina*, 81(3): 62–69.

Mello-Patiu, C.A.D. (2016). Family Sarcophagidae. *Zootaxa*, 4122(1): 884–903.

Mulieri, P.R., Schaefer, E.F., Dure, M.L. & González, C.E. (2018). A new flesh fly species (Diptera: Sarcophagidae) parasitic on leptodactylid frogs. *Parasitology Research*, 117: 809–818.

Najjari, M., Dik, B. & Pekbey, G. (2020). Gastrointestinal Myiasis Due to *Sarcophaga argyrostoma* (Diptera: Sarcophagidae) in Mashhad, Iran: A case report. *Journal of Arthropod- Borne Disease*, 14(3): 317–324.

Nandi, B.C. (1980). Studies on the larvae of flesh flies from India (Diptera: Sarcophagidae). *Oriental Insects*, 14(3): 303–323.

Nandi, B.C. (1998). Biodiversity and Flesh Flies (Diptera: Sarcophagidae) in India. *Proceeding of the Zoological Society*, 51(1): 79–85.

Nandi, B.C. (2002). *Fauna of India and the Adjacent Countries- Diptera (Volume X) Sarcophagidae*. Zoological survey of India, Kolkata, pp. 1–608.

Pape, T. (1996). Catalogue of the Sarcophagidae of the world (Insecta: Diptera). *Memiors on Entomology, International*, 8, 557.

Pape, T., Blagoderov, V. & Mostovski, M.B. (2011). Order Diptera Linnaeus, 1758. In: Z.Q. Zhang (ed.), Animal biodiversity: An outline of higher-level classification and survey of taxonomic richness. *Zootaxa*, 3148(1): 222–229.

Philip, J., Matthews, R. & Scipio, J.E. (2007). Larvae in the mouth. *British Dental Journal*, 203: 174–175.

Ramos, R.L., Trindade-Santos, M.E., Pamponet, F.M., Lopes, D.S., de Mello-Patiu, C.A. & de Oliveira, F.F. (2022). New records of *Sarcophaga* Meigen (Diptera: Sarcophagidae: Sarcophaginae) for the Northeast region of Brasil. *Scientia Plena*, 18(9): 1–8.

Ren, L., Shang, Y., Chen, W., Meng, F., Cai, J., Zhu, G., Chen, L., Wang, Y., Deng, J. & Guo, Y. (2018). A brief review of forensically important flesh flies (Diptera: Sarcophagidae). *Forensic Sciences Research*, 3(1): 16–26.

Robbins, K. & Khachemoune, A. (2010). Cutaneous myiasis: A review of the common types of myiasis. *International Journal of Dermatology*, 49: 1092–1098.

Salant, H., Mumcuoglu, K.Y. & Baneth, G. (2020). Myiasis in a dog in Jerusalem. *Israel Journal of Veterinary Medicine*, 75(4): 221–224.

Schwendinger, P.J. & Pape, T. (2000). *Metopia sinensis* (Diptera, Sarcophagidae), an unusual predator of *Liphistius* (Araneae, Mesothelae) in Northern Thailand. *The Journal of Arachnology*, 28: 353–356.

Senior-White, R. (1924). A revision of the subfamily Sarcophaginae in the Oriental Region. *Records of the Indian Museum*, 26(3): 193–283.

Senior-White, R., Aubertin D. & Smart, J. (1940). *The Fauna of British India, Including the Remainder of the Oriental Region, Diptera. Family Calliphoridae*. Taylor & Francis, London, p. 300.

Shang, Y., Yang, F., Ngando, F.J., Zhang, X., Feng, Y., Ren, L. & Guo, Y. (2023). Development of Forensically important *Sarcophaga peregrina* (Diptera: Sarcophagidae) and Intra-Puparial age estimation ultilizing multiple methods at constant and fluctuating temperatures. *Animals*, 13(1607): 1–16.

Singh, A. (2020). Canine myiasis and its causal agents in India. *Journal of Biomedical Research and Environmental Sciences*, 1(5): 150–153.

Sinha, S.K. & Mahato, S. (2016). Intra-puparial development of the flesh fly *Sarcophaga dux* (Thomson) (Diptera, Sarcophagidae). *Current science*, 111(6): 1063–1070.

Sinha, S.K., Mahato, S., Hazari, P., Ojha, S., Jana, N., Pandya, N., Hajra, A., Ghosh, U. & Bhattacharyya, S. (2023). Flies in the high for floral hike? Altitudinal variation in species diversity and composition of Diptera (Insecta) in the eastern Himalaya, India. *Journal of Threatened Taxa*, 15(11): 24241–24254.

Sinha, S.K. & Nandi, B.C. (2010). Life history of *Liosarcophaga choudhuri* (Sinha & Nandi) (Diptera: Sarcophagidae), a parasitoid of the intertidal snail *Littoraria melanostoma* (Gray) (Gastropoda: Littorinidae). *Tijdschrift voor Entomologische*, 153: 85–90.

Sinha, S.K. (2012a). Report of some satellite flies (Diptera, Miltogramminae) in West Bengal, India, for the first time. *North Bengal University Journal of Animal Science*, 6: 1–7.

Sinha, S.K. (2012b). Myiasis in domestic animals: New records of calyptrate Diptera. *Journal of Parasitic Disease*, 36(2): 277–279.

Sinha, S.K., Sinha, A.P., De, P. & Bhakat, S. (2017). Larval infestation in a common Pariah Kite *Milvus migrans (Boddaert). Journal of Parasitic Diseases*, 41(1): 199–201.

Vázquez-Corzas, F.G., Sandoval-Comte, A., Hernández-López, P., Ibáñez-Bernal, S. & Pineda, E. (2018). First records of parasitoidism by Sarcophagidae flies (Diptera) on three amphibian species in Mexico. *Journal of Natural History*, 52(35–36): 2339–2350.

Verves, Y.G. (1989). The phylogenetic systematics of the Miltogramminae flies (Diptera: Sarcophagidae) of the world. *Japanese Journal of Medical Science and Biology*, 42: 111–126.

Zhang, M., Chen, J.L., Gao, X.Z., Pape, T. & Zhang, D. (2014). First description of the female of *Sarcophaga* (*Sarcorohdendorfia*) *gracilior* (Chen, 1975) (Diptera, Sarcophagidae). *Zookeys*, 396: 43–53.

Zhou, M., Cao, K., Huang, H., Luo, X., Wang, Y., Ma, W. & Lv, Z. (2021). Neonatal oral myiasis caused by the larvae of *Sarcophaga ruficornis* (Diptera: Sarcophagidae): A case report. *BMC Infectious Disease*, 21(1067): 1–4.

11 Mosquitoes of Public Health and Veterinary Importance

Rajander S. Sharma

LEARNING OBJECTIVES

1. To understand mosquito vectors of human and veterinary public health importance
2. Distribution of malaria vectors
3. Biology and ecology of *Aedes* vectors
4. Learn the mode of transmission

11.1 INTRODUCTION

Mosquitoes are members of the family Culicidae. Important genera include *Aedes*, *Anopheles*, *Culex*, *Culiseta*, and *Psorophora*. Although they are tiny, fragile dipterans, mosquitoes are perhaps some of the most voracious blood-feeding arthropods. Approximately 300 species have been described worldwide, with ~150 species found in the temperate regions of North America. Mosquitoes are found in such diverse areas as salt marshes of the coastal plains, snow pools at elevations above 14,000 ft (4,300 m), and gold mines at 3,600 ft (1,100 m) below sea level. The volume of water in which mosquitoes breed varies from that within an empty can or tree hole to large shallow pools of accumulated, standing water from either rain or snowmelt.

The mosquito, whose name comes from the Spanish word meaning "small fly", is a type of insect that belongs to the family Culicidae. There are thousands of species of mosquitoes, but a distinguishing characteristic is that the female possesses tube-like mouthparts, called a proboscis, which pierces the skin of the host to draw blood. Female mosquitoes require the nutrients (mainly vitamins) in blood to produce eggs.

Mosquitoes feed primarily on vertebrates, including humans and other mammals, as well as birds, reptiles, and others. Most species have a preference for either humans or certain animals as the source of their blood meal. They are attracted by body odours, carbon dioxide, and heat emitted by a person or animal. Most mosquitoes prefer biting at certain hours, such as dusk or dawn. Different species also vary in their preferred places to feed or rest; some prefer natural vegetative habitats, while others favour urban environments, particularly trash or receptacles in yards.

While obtaining a blood meal from a host, the female mosquito releases some of its own saliva into the skin. The saliva contains anticoagulants and anti-inflammatory substances that prevent the host's blood from clotting, so that the proboscis does not become trapped in the host. Upon detecting a foreign substance, the immune system of the host releases histamine and cytokines, substances that cause the itching and wheals associated with mosquito bites (Levin, 2014).

11.2 HISTORICAL ASPECTS OF MEDICAL – VETERINARY ENTOMOLOGY

Englishman Patrick Manson (1844–1922) (Figure 11.1a) was the first to demonstrate pathogen transmission by a blood-feeding arthropod. Working in China in 1877, he showed that the mosquito *Culex pipiens fatigans* is a vector of *Wuchereria bancrofti,* the causative agent of *Bancroftian filariasis.* After this landmark discovery, the role of various blood-feeding arthropods in transmitting pathogens was recognized in relatively rapid succession. In 1891, Americans Theobald

DOI: 10.1201/9781003482581-14

Smith (1859–1934) (Figure 11.1b) and Frederick L. Kilbourne (1858–1936) implicated the cattle tick, *Rhipicephalus (Boophilus) annulatus*, as a vector of *Babesia bigemina,* the causative agent of Texas cattle fever (bovine babesiosis). This paved the way for a highly successful *R. annulatus* eradication programme in the United States directed by the US Department of Agriculture (USDA). The eradication of this tick resulted in the projected elimination of indigenous cases of Texas cattle fever throughout the southern United States. In 1898, Englishman Sir Ronald Ross (1857–1932), working in India, demonstrated the role of mosquitoes as vectors of avian malarial parasites from diseased to healthy sparrows. Also in 1898, the cyclical development of malarial parasites in anopheline mosquitoes was described by Italian Giovanni Battista Grassi (1854–1925). In the same year, Frenchman Paul Louis Simond (1858–1947), working in Pakistan (then part of India), showed that fleas are vectors of the bacterium that causes plague.

In 1848, American physician Josiah Nott (1804–1873) of Mobile, Alabama, published circumstantial evidence that led him to believe that mosquitoes were involved in the transmission of the yellow fever virus to humans. In 1881, the Cuban-born Scottish physician Carlos Finlay (1833–1915) presented persuasive evidence for his theory that what we know today as the yellow fever mosquito, *Aedes aegypti*, was the vector of this virus. However, it was not until 1900 that American Walter Reed (1851–1902) led the US Yellow Fever Commission in Havana, Cuba, which proved *Aedes aegypti* to be the principal vector of the yellow fever virus.

11.2.1 Vector Mosquitoes

Vectors are living organisms that can transmit infectious pathogens between humans or from animals to humans. Information regarding the immature aquatic and adult stages of vectors is useful for identifying and differentiating vectors from non-insect vectors (NVBDCP, 2015). Understanding the morphology and biology of a vector is an important skill for planning vector control and surveillance. While feeding on a host (human or animal), vector mosquitoes ingest pathogens, which are replicated or transformed and later transmitted to a new host (Becker, 2010). Once a vector becomes infectious, it is capable of transmitting the pathogen for the rest of its life during each subsequent bite or blood meal. The ecology of vectors is therefore a prerequisite for eradicating or eliminating VBDs and will be essential for sustaining long-term success (Sharma, 1982, 1983).

Mosquitoes are arthropods classified under the class Insecta. They belong to the order Diptera and the family Culicidae. There are approximately 3,600 species of mosquitoes, which are divided into three subfamilies:

1. Toxorhynchitinae
2. Anophelinae
3. Culicinae

The most important vector species belong to the genera *Anopheles, Culex, Aedes* and *Mansonia.* The *Anopheles* species are vectors of malaria; *Aedes* species are important vectors of dengue, chikungunya, and Zika; *Culex* species transmit *Wuchereria bancrofti*, as well as arboviruses causing Japanese encephalitis (JE), and *Mansonia* species transmit *Brugia malayi.*

11.2.2 Classification of Mosquito

Phylum: Arthropoda
Superclass: Hexapoda
Class: Insecta
Order: Diptera
Family: Culicidae

11.2.2.1 Subfamilies

1. Anophelinae includes *Anopheles*.
2. Culicinae includes *Culex, Aedes,* and *Mansonia*.

11.2.2.2 Characters of Subfamilies

- **Subfamily Anophelinae**: The sterna and terga are wholly or largely devoid of scales.
- **Subfamily Culicinae**: The abdominal terga and sterna are densely covered by scales.

11.2.3 Morphological Characters of Mosquitos

Mosquitoes are distinguished from flies of a somewhat similar shape and size by: (i) the possession of a conspicuous forward-projecting proboscis; (ii) the presence of numerous appressed scales on the thorax, legs, abdomen and wing veins; (iii) a fringe of scales along the posterior margin of the wings; (iv) a characteristic wing venation, that is, the second, fourth and fifth longitudinal veins are branched; (v) they possess a pair of functional wings known as forewings and a pair of hindwings, which are represented by a pair of small, knob-like halteres. The mosquito body is mainly divided into the head, thorax and abdomen (Figure 11.1).

11.2.4 Head and Mouthparts

All sensory organs, like compound eyes, antennae, palpi, and mouthparts (proboscis), are located in the head. A pair of filamentous and segmented antennae is situated between the eyes. Mosquitoes can be identified as male or female by examining their antennae. Individuals with feathery, plumose antennae are males, while those with only short and rather inconspicuous antennal hairs or pilose antennae are females.

The appendages of the mouthparts, which are associated with the oral cavity, are commonly known as the proboscis. In female mosquitoes, piercing and sucking mouthparts are present, while male mosquitoes lack these mouthparts. The proboscis is long and projects conspicuously forwards in both sexes. The largest components of the mouthparts are the mandibles, hypopharynx, maxillae, labrum, and labium. The uppermost structure, that is, the labrum, is slender, pointed, and grooved along its ventral surface. The flexible gutter-shaped labium, which terminates in a pair of small flap-like structures, is called labella. In cross section, the labium is seen to almost encircle all the other components of the mouthparts and serves as a protective sheath (Figures 11.1 and 11.2).

11.2.5 Thorax

The thorax is divided into three parts known as the prothorax, mesothorax, and metathorax. They are covered dorsally and laterally with scales, which may be dull or shiny, white, brown, or black, depending on the species. Wings and halteres both arise from the thorax. The wings are long and relatively narrow. When resting, mosquitoes place their wings across each other over the abdomen, resembling a closed pair of scissors. The hind (metathoracic) wings are modified into a dumb-bell shape, called the halteres. Each pair of legs is associated with each thoracic segment. The legs are long, slender, and covered with scales, which are usually brown, black, or white and may be arranged in patterns, often in the form of rings. The thoracic legs are composed of the coxa, trochanter, femur, tibia, and tarsus.

11.2.6 Abdomen

The abdomen is composed of ten segments, but only the first seven or eight are visible. Mosquitoes in the subfamily Culicinae usually have their abdomen covered dorsally and ventrally with mostly brown, blackish, or whitish scales. In the Anophelinae, however, the abdomen is almost entirely

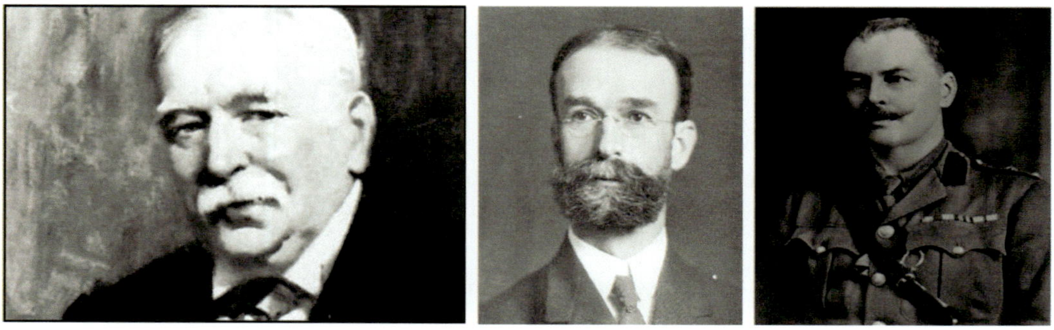

(a) (b) (c)

FIGURE 11.1 Historical figures in medical-veterinary entomology: (a) Patrick Manson (1844–1922), (b) Theobald Smith (1859–1934), and (c) Ronald Ross (1857–1932).

devoid of scales. Small openings called spiracles line both sides of the abdomen, allowing the mosquitoes to breathe. The last abdominal segment of a female mosquito terminates in a pair of small finger-like cerci, whereas in the male there is a pair of prominent claspers, which comprise part of the male external genitalia. The abdomen is thin and slender in unfed mosquitoes, but after females have taken a blood meal from a suitable host (only females bite), the abdomen resembles an oval red balloon and becomes greatly distended.

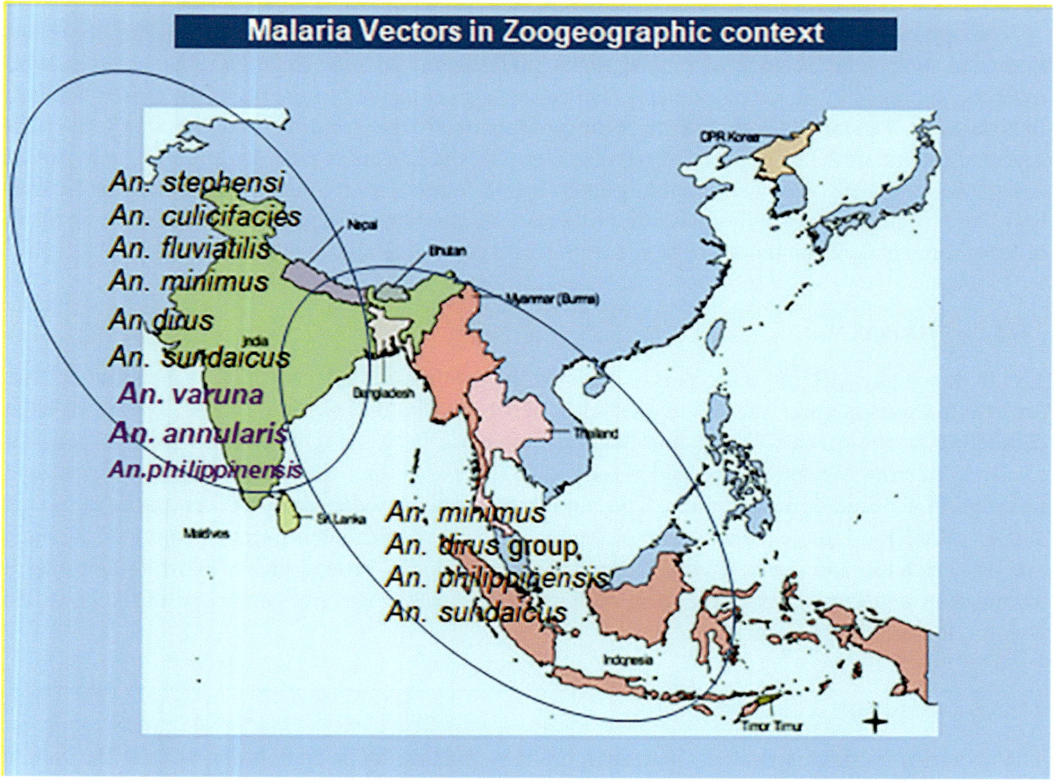

FIGURE 11.2 Geographical distributions of malaria vectors.

11.3 MOSQUITO LIFE CYCLE

The cycle of mosquitoes is completed in water and partly in the terrestrial environment. Knowing the different stages of a mosquito's life helps prevent mosquitoes around your home and also assists you in choosing the right pesticides for your needs, if you decide to use them. All mosquito species go through four distinct stages during their life cycle:

- **Egg**: hatches when exposed to water.
- **Larva**: (plural: larvae) "wriggler" lives in water; moults several times; most species surface to breathe air.
- **Pupa**: (plural: pupae) "tumbler" does not feed; this stage occurs just before emerging as an adult.
- **Adult**: flies a short time after emerging and after its body parts have hardened.

The first three stages occur in water, while the adult is an active flying insect. Only the female mosquito bites and feeds on the blood of humans or other animals. After obtaining a blood meal, the female mosquito lays the eggs directly on or near water, in soil, and at the base of some plants in places that may fill with water. The eggs can survive dry conditions for a few months. The eggs hatch in water, resulting in a mosquito larva or "wriggler". The length of time to hatch depends on water temperature, food, and the type of mosquito. The larva lives in the water, feeds, and develops into the third stage of the life cycle called a pupa or "tumbler". The pupa also lives in the water but no longer feeds. Finally, the mosquito emerges from the pupal case after 2 days to a week in the pupal stage. The life cycle typically takes about 2 weeks, but depending on conditions, it can range from 4 days to as long as a month. The adult mosquito emerges onto the water's surface and flies away, ready to begin its life cycle (Crans, 2004, Figure 18, EPA, CDC 2024).

11.4 MOSQUITOES OF PUBLIC HEALTH IMPORTANCE

Although the itching can be very irritating, the much more serious risk from mosquitoes is their ability to serve as vectors, or carriers, for a number of diseases, including malaria, dengue, chikungunya, Zika virus, yellow fever, and JE

Mosquitoes are responsible for the transmission of many medically important pathogens and parasites, such as viruses, bacteria, protozoans, and nematodes, which cause serious diseases like malaria, dengue, Zika, yellow fever, encephalitis, or filariasis. Transmission can be mechanical (e.g. myxoma virus causing myxomatosis in rabbits) or biological. The latter is more complex because it involves an obligatory period of replication and/or development of the pathogen or parasite in the vector insect. Due to their blood-sucking behaviour, mosquitoes are able to acquire the pathogens or parasites from one vertebrate host and pass them to another if the mosquito's ecology and physiology are appropriate for transmission (Sharma, 1983, 1984, 1985, 1992, & 1997). Highly efficient vectors must be closely associated with the hosts, and their longevity must be sufficient to enable the pathogens and parasites to proliferate and/or to develop to the infective stages in the vector. For successful transmission, multiple blood meals are usually necessary (Mike, 2012, Christopher, 1933).

11.5 MOSQUITO-BORNE DISEASES

Mosquito	Disease Caused	Type of Pathogen
Aedes	Dengue, chikungunya, Yellow fever, Zika	Virus
Culex	Lymphatic filariasis, Japanese encephalitis	Parasite virus
Anopheles	Malaria	Protozoan parasite

11.5.1 Mosquito-Borne Parasitic Diseases

11.5.1.1 Human

Causative agent: *P. falciparum, P. vivax, P. malariae*
Vector: *Anopheles* species

B: Zoonotic Malaria (Reservoir: Monkey)
Causative Agent: *P. cynomolgi* (*vivax*-like)
Vector: *Anopheles sundaicus*
Causative Agent: *P. knowlesi*(*Pf*-like)
Vector: *Anopheles* species

11.5.2 Lymphatic Filariasis

Causative agent: *Wuchereria bancrofti, Brugia malayi* – Nocturnal periodicity

- **Vector**: Culex *quinquefasciatus* and *Mansonia* species.
  Causative agent: *W. bancrofti,* Diurnal periodicity
- **Vector**: *Aedes niveus*
  Andaman and Nicobar Islands

11.5.3 Non-Filarial Elephantiasis

Causative agent: Silica crystals
Endemicity: Rajasthan
(Barefoot walking)

11.5.4 Mosquito-Borne Viral Diseases

Dengue Fever
Causative agent: Flavivirus (serotypes 1–4)
Vectors: *Aedes aegypti, Aedes albopictus*
Chickungunya
Causative agent: Alphavirus.
Vectors: *Aedes aegypti, Aedes albopictus.*
Zika
Causative agent: Flavivirus (JE)
Vectors: *Aedes aegypti, Aedes albopictus.*
Japanese Encephalitis
Causative agent: Flavivirus (JE)
Vectors: *Culex tritaeniorhyncus. Culex vishnui complex* (Reddya Naik et al., 2023)

11.6 BIONOMICS AND DISTRIBUTION OF MALARIA VECTORS

The term bionomics is defined as the inter-relationship of an organism to its biotic and abiotic environment. Climatic factors play an important role in species distribution, behaviour, survival, and vectorial status. The relative number of vector species in an area determines the transmission of pathogens to the human population. An understanding of vector bionomics is important in the epidemiology of VBDs and planning methods of vector control (Crans, 2004, Tyagi, 1994, 2002, 2006, 2007, 2008). The environments of immature species and adult vectors are interdependent since the adult vector must have access to water for egg laying. The aerial environment is necessary for mating and dispersal. The terrestrial environment provides habitats for feeding, resting, and completion of the life cycle of ovarian development from blood meal to egg laying.

The transmission dynamics are governed by environmental factors that affect the vector–human–pathogen interaction. IVM relies on several factors, but foremost is the selection of proven vector control methods based on knowledge of local vector biology and ecology, disease transmission, and morbidity. The details on different vectors are explained below:

The major ecosystems where malaria is endemic in the country include forests, rural plains, urban areas, coastal regions, and arid zones. There is a strong relationship between ecosystem and the prevalence of vector and parasite species in malaria transmission in an area. Vector species have a distinct distribution pattern in the country, which is governed by land use patterns and the types of breeding sites available. For example, topography and climatic conditions in forest ecosystems, in addition to influencing the prevalence of vector species, also affect the longevity of the vectors. In laboratory studies at 27°C–28°C and 70%–80% relative humidity *P. falciparum* takes longer to complete its sporogonic cycle than *P. vivax* in vectors (Figures 11.2 and 11.3)

11.6.1 Malaria Vectors in India

In India, out of 58 species of *Anopheles* mosquitoes, nine species are known vectors of malaria:

1. *Anopheles culicifacies*
2. *Anopheles fluviatilis*
3. *Anopheles minimus*
4. *Anopheles baimaii (dirus)*
5. *Anopheles stephensi*

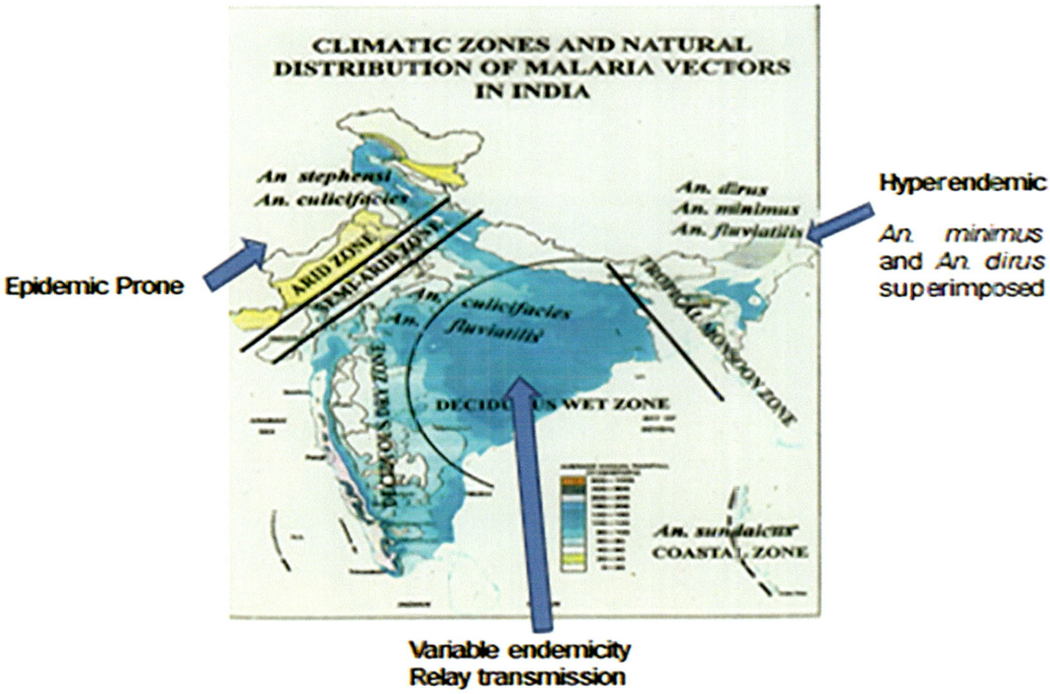

FIGURE 11.3 Distribution of malaria vector in different climatic zones.

6. *Anopheles epiroticus (sundaicus)*
7. *Anopheles annularis*
8. *Anopheles philippinensis*
9. *Anopheles varuna*

An. culicifacies, An. fluviatilis, An. minimus, An. dirus (baimaii), An. Stephensi, and *An. sundaicus (epiroticus)* have been considered primary vectors of malaria, whereas three species are secondary vectors: *An. annularis*, *An. philippinensis*, and *An. varuna*, which are of local importance in the transmission of the disease. (Sharma, 1995, 1999, 2014), whereas the remaining vectors play their role in rural areas.

11.6.1.1 *An. culicifacies*

Distribution: The species is widely distributed in India.

Breeding places: It breeds in rainwater pools and puddles, borrow pits, riverbed pools, irrigation channels, seepage, rice fields, wells, pond margins, and sluggish streams with sandy margins. Extensive breeding of An. culicifacies is generally encountered after the monsoon (Figure 11.4).

11.6.1.2 *An. fluviatilis*

Distribution: The species is widely distributed in the foothill areas including both peninsular and northeast India. It plays a major role especially in Odisha (Figure 11.5).

Breeding places: It typically breeds in slow-running streams, seepages, and irrigation channels; it is also recorded from rice fields and shallow wells. During heavy rains, breeding is often disrupted.

Resting habits: It rests indoors in human dwellings and cattle sheds.

Biting time: Generally, the vector species enters houses at dusk and completes feeding before midnight, with a peak from 09:00 to 11:00 hours.

Feeding preferences: This species is generally highly anthropophilic; however, a zoophilic nature has also been reported from northern India.

Flight range: It has a limited flight range.

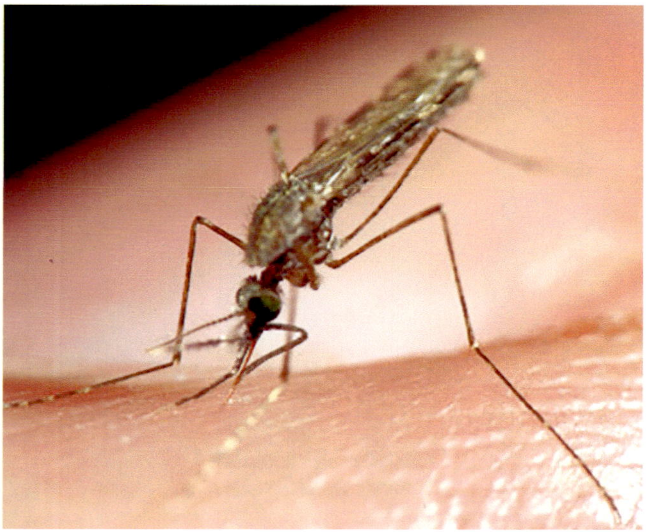

FIGURE 11.4 *Anopheles culicifacies.*

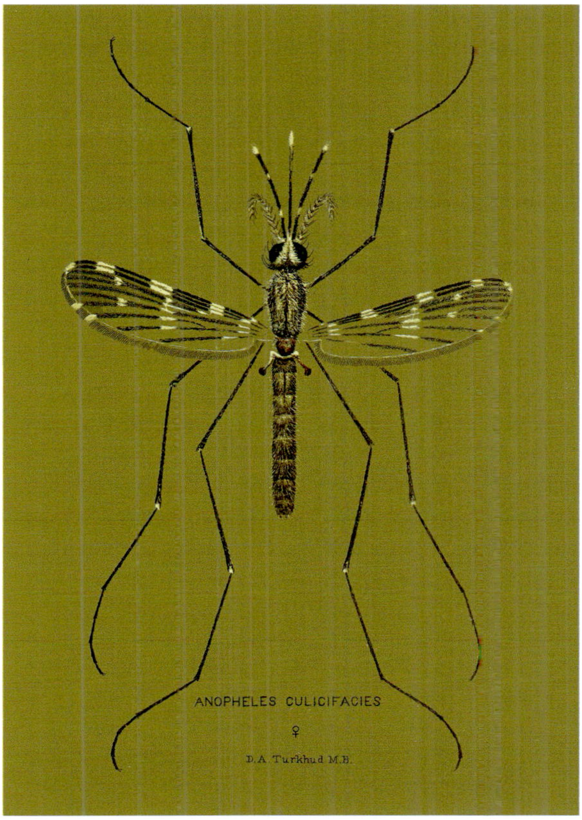

FIGURE 11.5 *Anopheles fluviatilis.*

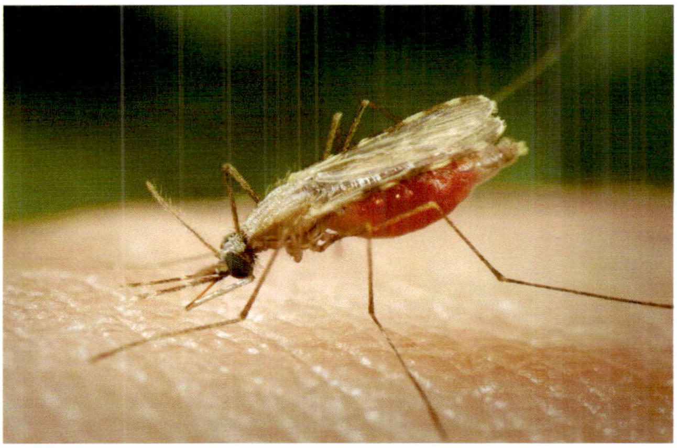

FIGURE 11.6 *Anopheles minimus.*

11.6.1.3 *An. minimus*

Distribution: The species has a restricted distribution to the northeastern states. This species was thought to have been eliminated because of insecticidal spraying in the 1950s and 1960s but reappeared in the late 1970s (Figure 11.6).

Breeding places: *An. minimus* breeds in shaded, slow-flowing streams with grassy margins, swamps, ditches, channels, and shallow earth wells; it is occasionally found breeding in borrow pits, rice fields, and seepage from flowing water.

Resting habits: It rests inside houses, preferring to rest on the lower portions of walls.

Biting time: Peak biting activity occurs from 18:00 to 19:00 hours outdoors and from 24:00 to 02:00 hours indoors. Biting times may vary from one locality to another and seasonally.

Feeding habits: A highly anthropophilic species, and therefore a very efficient vector of malaria.

Flight range: Normally 0.5 km but can disperse up to 2 km from the original location.

11.6.1.4 *An. baimii (dirus)*

Distribution: Its distribution is restricted to the forested areas of the northeastern states (Figure 11.7).

Breeding places: Breeds in pools, rainwater collections in deep forest, forest fringes, and stream margins with decaying organic matter and animal footprints during the monsoon.

Resting habits: Enters human dwellings to bite and rest but tends to leave houses soon after a blood meal.

Biting time: The peak biting activity is from 22:00 to 02:00 hours.

Feeding habits: High preference for human blood but also bites monkeys, other primates, and cattle.

Flight range: Flight range varies from 1 to 2.5 km in forests.

11.6.1.5 *An. stephensi*

Distribution: This species is distributed across India, except at higher altitudes; it is found sporadically in the northeast (Figure 11.8).

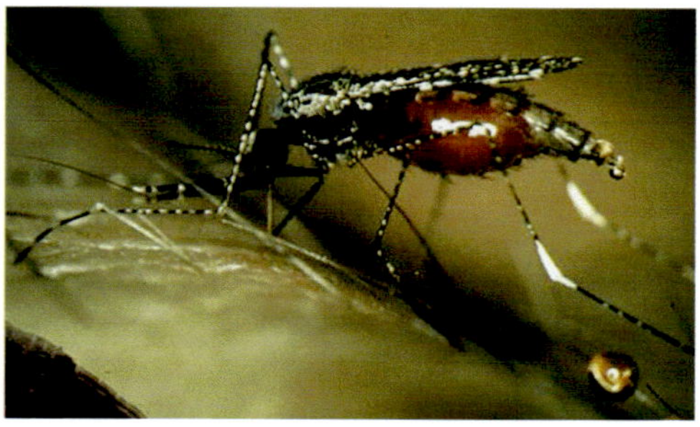

FIGURE 11.7 *Anopheles baimii* (dirus).

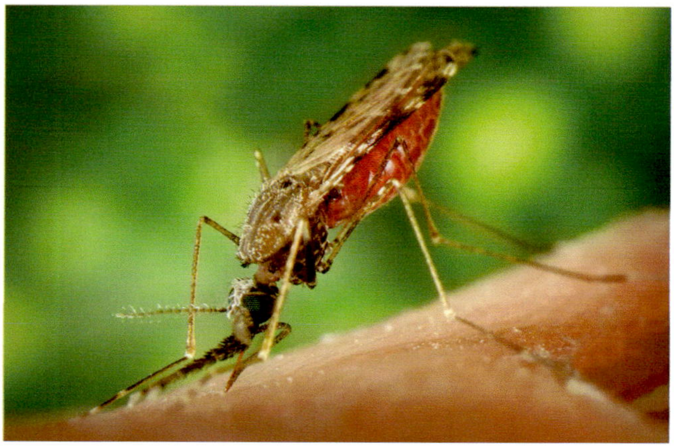

FIGURE 11.8 *Anopheles stephensi*.

Breeding places: Breeds in wells, overhead and ground-level water tanks, cisterns, rainwater collections in roof gutters, peri-domestic containers, and underground water storage tanks. In Rajasthan's desert, it breeds and rests in the water storage tanks called tankas in rural areas.

Resting habits: Rests in human dwellings and cattle sheds. Inside human dwellings, it may rest on hanging objects, behind curtains, etc. Outdoor resting has been observed in wells and underground cement tanks.

Biting time: Biting varies from area to area and seasonally, but peak biting activity is generally from 22:00 to 24:00 hours.

Feeding habits: An indiscriminate feeder that bites both humans and animals.

Flight range: Limited flight range in urban areas, but in rural areas, the flight range may be up to 3 km.

11.6.1.6 *An. epiroticus(sundaicus)*

Distribution: Reported from coastal Odisha, Andhra Pradesh, and West Bengal in 1950s. At present, it is restricted to the Andaman and Nicobar Islands (Figure 11.9).

Breeding places: Breeds in brackish water pools with algae, margins of mangroves, lagoons, and swamps. *An. epiroticus (sundaicus)* can tolerate salinity levels from 0.08% to 2.6% and pH from 7.7 to 8.5.

Resting habits: Rests indoors in human dwellings, cattle sheds, and mixed dwellings.

Biting time: Biting occurs throughout the night, but peak biting is from 20:00 to 02:00 hours.

Feeding habits: An opportunistic feeder that prefers to bite humans.

Flight range: About 1–3 km.

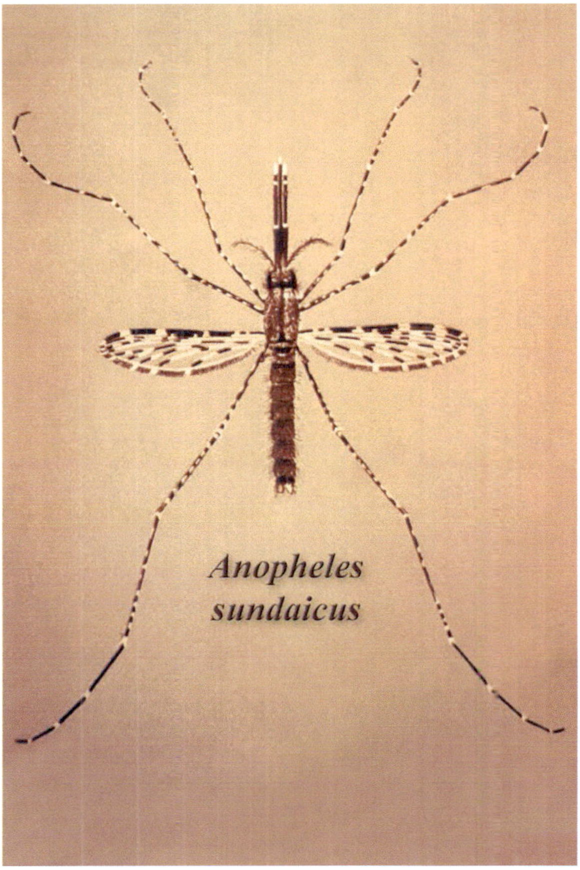

FIGURE 11.9 *Anopheles sundaicus.*

11.6.1.7 *An. annularis*

Distribution: This species is found all over the country.

Breeding places: Breeds in still waters with abundant vegetation in a variety of water bodies; also breeds in wells, moats (a deep, wide ditch surrounding a castle or fort filled with water), tanks, borrow pits, rice fields, and other water bodies such as lakes and stream margins with vegetation (Figure 11.10).

Resting habits: During daytime, it rests in houses, cattle sheds, and mixed dwellings, and also rests outdoors in small numbers.

Biting time: Peak biting activity takes place from 22:00 to 24:00 hours.

Feeding habits: Azoophilic mosquito; biting humans is infrequent.

Flight range: Normally up to 1 km.

11.6.1.8 *An. philippinensis*

Distribution: This species is distributed in West Bengal, northeastern states. It was reported from Andaman and Nicobar Islands.

Breeding places: Breeds in tanks, swamps, ditches, rice fields, pools, leaf axils, shaded lake margins, inundated drains, and water bodies generally with good growth of vegetation (Figure 11.11).

Resting habits: During day time, adults rest in cattle sheds and human dwellings.

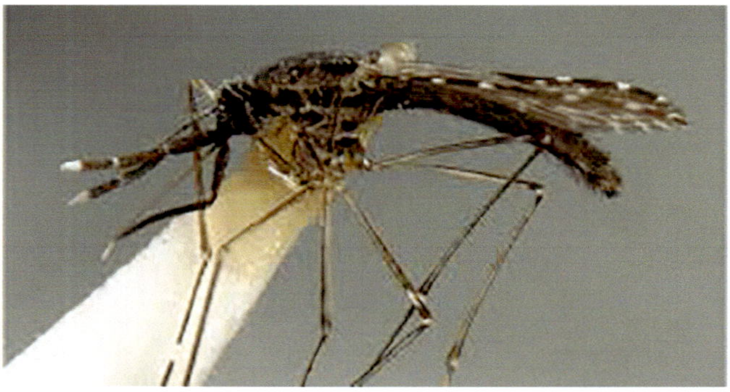

FIGURE 11.10 *Anopheles annularis.*

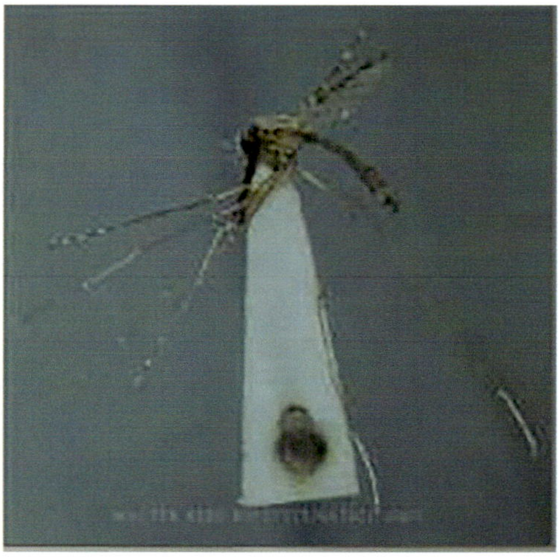

FIGURE 11.11 *Anopheles philippinensis.*

Biting time: Biting occurs outdoors and indoors throughout the night, with two peaks from 20:00 to 22:00 and 02:00 to 04:00 hours.

Feeding habits: Predominantly zoophagic but may also bite humans.

Flight range: Normally up to 0.8 km.

11.6.1.9 *An. varuna*

Distribution: Distributed widely across the country from the northeastern plains to peninsular India and the Lakshadweep Islands.

Breeding places: Breeds in rainwater pools, tanks, ponds, rice fields, drains, irrigation channels, wells, and slow-moving streams with ample shade provided by overhanging vegetation (Figure 11.12).

Resting habits: Rests indoors during the daytime in human dwellings, cattle sheds, and mixed dwellings. It also rests outdoors near stream banks.

Biting time: Biting occurs throughout the night, but peak biting activity is from 24:00 to 02:00 hours.

11.7 VECTORS OF DENGUE AND CHIKUNGUNYA

11.7.1 *Aedes aegypti*

Aedes aegypti is a common vector for dengue and chikungunya (Sharma, 2006, 2008).

Distribution: In India, the density of *Aedes* mosquitoes is higher during the monsoon and post-monsoon seasons. In dry or water-scarcity areas, the vector density is linked to water storage practices (Figure 11.13).

Breeding places: *Ae. aegypti* is the main vector in urban, semi-urban, and rural areas. *Ae. aegypti* mosquitoes prefer to breed in man-made containers, such as water storage containers, water tanks (cement tanks, overhead tanks, underground tanks), exterior extensions of buildings, coolers, discarded buckets, bottles, tyres, coconut shells, etc., in which water stagnates for more than a week (Sharma, 1982, 1983, 1984, 1994, 1998, 1999, 2001, 2003, 2014).

In unfavourable conditions, the eggs can remain viable for over a year in dry conditions, allowing the mosquito to re-emerge after winter or dry spells. The eggs (up to 100–120) are laid singly on damp surfaces just above the waterline.

Resting habits: *Ae. aegypti* prefers to rest in dark corners of houses, on dark clothing, umbrellas, under furniture and beds, on shelves, in coolers, behind hangings, shoes, alongside household articles, and curtains, but rarely on walls.

Biting time: A day-biting mosquito has to bite many times to complete its blood meal as, during the daytime, humans are mostly active. This is also known as an indiscriminate feeder.

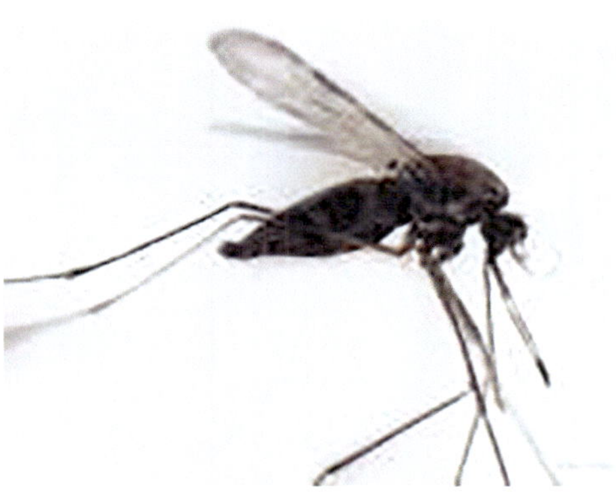

FIGURE 11.12 *Anopheles varuna.*

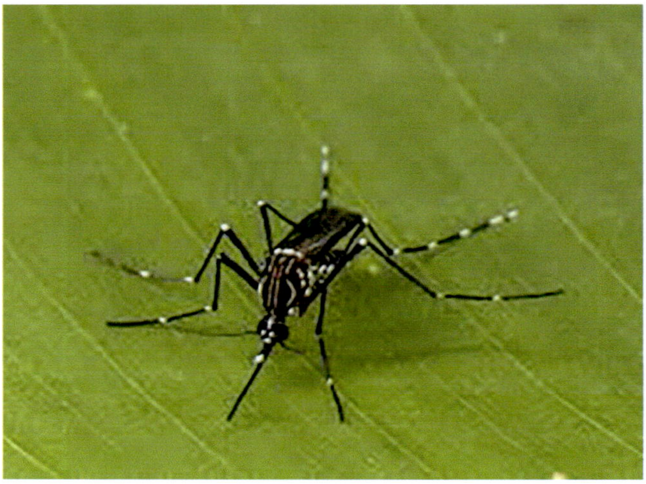

FIGURE 11.13 *Aedes aegypti*.

Feeding habits: The species is strongly anthropophilic, showing a high preference for human blood.

Flight range: The average flight range of *Aedes* is 100–300 m. The flight range for *Aedes* is generally 100 m, but it can fly up to 400 m (WHO, 2011).

11.7.2 *Aedes albopictus*

Distribution: It is the secondary vector in sylvatic areas. It is a feral species that spreads the disease in built-up areas, particularly in parks and gardens. It also co-breeds in peridomestic water collections. The species feeds on humans and other animals (Figure 11.14).

Breeding places: *Ae. albopictus* mosquitoes prefer to breed in natural habitats, such as tree holes, latex collection cups of rubber plantations, leaf axils of pineapple plants, and coconut shells, etc.

Resting habits: *Ae. albopictus* mosquitoes rest outdoors in bushes, shrubs, and long grasses in and around peri-domestic situations. They are sometimes found in domestic conditions as well.

Biting habits: *Ae. albopictus* feeds on different vertebrate hosts, including humans (NVBDCP, 2020, Tyagi, 2003, 2015). It is also a day-biter.

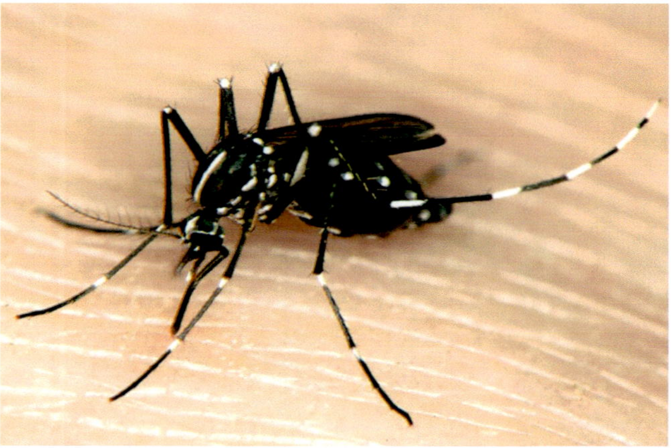

FIGURE 11.14 *Aedes albipictus*.

Flight range: The flight range for *Ae. albopictus* is up to 400 m It may also disperse to newer areas through passive transportation, especially eggs.

11.8 VECTORS OF JE

Culex vishnui subgroup mosquitoes, composed of *Cx. tritaeniorhynchus, Cx. Vishnui,* and *Cx. pseudovishnui,* have been implicated as major vectors of JE in India. *Cx. tritaeniorhynchus* is the primary vector. *Cx. pseudovishnui, Cx. whitmorei, Cx. gelidus, Cx. epidesmus, Anopheles subpictus, An. Peditaeniatus,* and *Mansonia uniformis* are suspected to play some role in the epidemiology of JE (Kanojia, 2003, 2005, Tyagi, 2023; Figure 11.15).

Distribution: These mosquitoes are usually found in rural rice-growing and pig-farming regions, but they can also be found in canals on the outskirts of cities in close proximity to human populations.

Breeding places: They prefer to breed in rice fields. A conducive ecosystem comprising irrigation canals, rice fields, ponds, ditches, and lakes favours JE vector breeding, particularly in rural areas. However, in semi-urban areas, the breeding of *Culex vishnui* group mosquitoes can be found in small ponds and ditches with water hyacinth and other aquatic plants.

Resting habits: The main vectors of JE rest outdoors.

Biting time: JE vectors bite during the night.

Feeding habits: JE vectors are mainly exophilic and exophagic in nature.

Flight range: The flight range varies from 1 to 3 km.

11.9 VECTORS OF LYMPHATIC FILARIASIS

Distribution: *Culex quinquefasciatus* breeds in association with human habitations. It is the most common house-frequenting mosquito.

Breeding places: Breeds in many types of habitats including fresh, clear, brackish, turbid, and polluted water with decayed organic matter from garbage and human waste accumulations in ground pools, ditches, drains, sewages, septic tanks, etc. Various kinds of artificial containers (bottles, cans, flower pots, vases, bowls, jars, cement tanks, etc.) both indoors and outdoors are also preferred breeding sites (Figure 11.16).

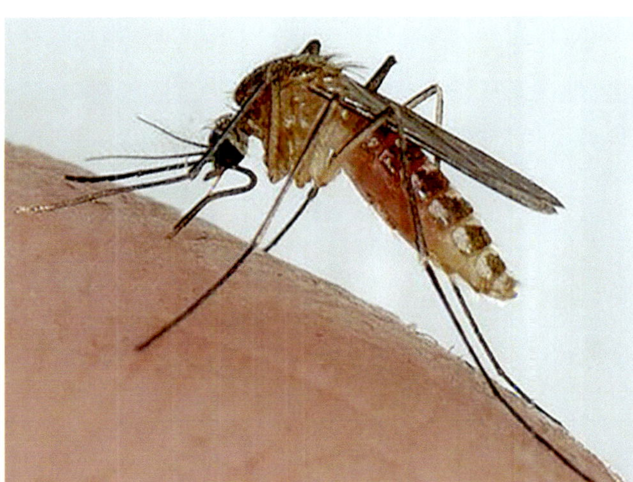

FIGURE 11.15 *Culex triataeniorhynchus.*

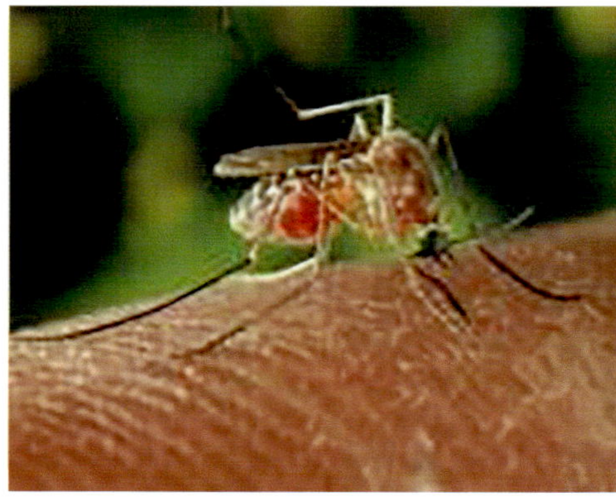

FIGURE 11.16 *Culex quiquefasciatus.*

Resting habits: Enters houses for feeding at night and for resting during the daytime, that is, endophilic and endophagous. Rests in dark corners of walls, hanging objects, cobwebs, inside shoes, cupboards, under cots, tables and chairs, bathrooms, etc.

Biting time: Blood feeding takes place within 24–48 hours after mating from sunset until dawn. The highest peak is in the late night or third-quarter night. It is endophagous as well as exophagous (Reubenet al., 1994).

Feeding habits: Highly anthropophilic; may also feed on birds and other domestic animals.

Flight range: The average flight range of *Cx. quinquefasciatus* is about 2–3 km. Males are weak fliers.

11.10 MANSONIA SPECIES

Important species: *Mn. annulifera, Mn. uniformis,* and *Mn. indiana*

Distribution: *Mn. annulifera* is the main vector, but *Mn. uniformis* also plays a role. Both species are found throughout the year, but with slightly higher densities during June–August. *Mn. uniformis* density is higher where Salvinia host plants are completely replaced by Pistia (Service, 1980a–c; Apiwathnasorn, 2006; Figure 11.17).

Breeding places: Breeding of *Mansonia* species is restricted to freshwater ponds, lakes, swamps, and channels with floating vegetation and high organic pollution with a pH range of 6.2–6.8. *Pistia*

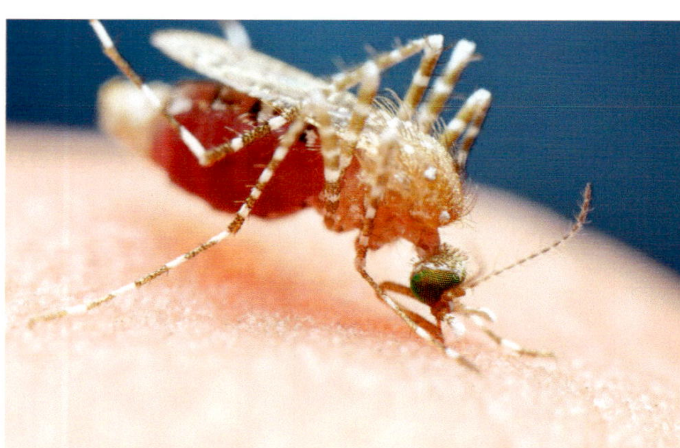

FIGURE 11.17 *Mansonia annulifera.*

stratiotes is the most preferred plant for breeding of *Mn. annulifera*, but the Salvinia plant is preferred by *Mn. uniformis*. *Mansonia* species lay eggs in clusters of 80–120 on the undersurfaces of floating water plants. The tips of the pupal breathing trumpets are modified for attachment to the plant (Sallum, 2007). Larvae and pupae obtain oxygen from the air spaces of the floating vegetation (Mattingly, 1972, Mike, 2008, 2012).

Resting habits: *Mn. annulifera,* endophilic and endophagous, rests in dark corners of houses.

Mn. indiana is mostly confined to cattle sheds and other outdoor situations.

Biting time: Active throughout the night, with peak biting activity in the first and second quarters of the night. Endophagous in nature.

Feeding habits: *Mn. annulifera* is highly anthropophilic; *Mn. uniformis* is more zoophilic.

Flight range: Not strong fliers, easy to catch due to hopping, like sandflies. Silent in flight with a limited flight range.

11.11 BIOLOGICAL TRANSMISSIONS

11.11.1 Cyclico-Developmental and Propagative

A disease-producing organism, like the malaria parasite, undergoes development by multiplication in the body of the *Anopheles* mosquito, and mosquitoes spread the disease from one person to another.

11.11.2 Cyclico-Developmental

A disease-causing organism, such as microfilaria, undergoes development in the body of the *Culex quinquefasciatus* mosquito but does not multiply in the vector (Mishra, 2014).

11.11.3 Propagative

A disease-causing organism may simply multiply in the vector, such as the dengue virus, which multiplies in *Ae. aegypti* mosquitoes, and *Pasteurella pestis*, which multiplies in rat fleas; these vectors spread these organisms to healthy humans.

- **Trans-ovarion transmission**: The disease organism is transmitted to eggs through the ovary of an infected female. *Orientalis tsutsugamushi*, the agent for scrub typhus, is transmitted by the trombiculid mite *Leptotrombidium deliense*.
- **Trans-stadial transmission**: The disease-causing organism is transmitted from one stage to another; for example, the tick typhus organism Rickettsia conorii is transmitted from infected larva to nymph to adult (Rehman et al., 1989).

11.12 MOSQUITO-BORNE VIRUSES OF ANIMALS

Large populations of mosquitoes can cause irritation and extensive blood loss to livestock; this can result in reduced productivity and sometimes even death. Mosquitoes have been implicated in carrying many different disease pathogens and viruses that infect vertebrates (ICMR-VCRC, 2010).

11.12.1 Eastern Equine Encephalomyelitis

Eastern equine encephalomyelitis (EEE) virus is an important cause of mortality in horses and other equids, caged pheasants, whooping cranes and emus. The virus occurs in endemic areas of the US, particularly in Texas, along the Gulf Coast and Atlantic seaboard to Massachusetts. If a horse contracts the virus, it will succumb to the infection within 2–5 days. Signs of infection begin with abnormal behaviour and a high fever; the horse will then drop to the ground and lapse into a coma before death. Few horses will survive an infection that presents with these acute symptoms. EEE has also been reported in dogs and pigs. Cases of EEE begin to occur in Texas in spring and summer. Immunizations are available to reduce the chances of horses contracting EEE.

11.12.2 Western Equine Encephalomyelitis

Western equine encephalomyelitis (WEE) virus occurs in horses almost every summer within the virus's range. Immunizations are available to reduce the chances of horses contracting WEE. The last outbreak in Texas occurred in Hale County in 1965.

11.12.3 Venezuelan Equine Encephalomyelitis

Venezuelan equine encephalomyelitis (VEE) complex typically does not occur in the US but is common in Mexico. VEE is transmitted by many species of mosquitoes to horses, burros, and mules. An interesting aspect of VEE is that mosquitoes can acquire the complex from horses and transmit it to another horse or equid; this differs from WEE and EEE, in which the mosquito gets the virus from a bird and transmits it to horses, the dead-end host. Dog heartworm is caused by the transmission of the filarial nematode, *Dirofilaria immitis*, by mosquitoes. The adult worm lives in the right ventricle of the canine heart and the pulmonary arteries. The worms can grow to 31 cm long and form aggregations that sometimes extend into the right atrium of the heart. The worms living in the heart lead to changes in the endothelium and the integrity of the walls. These changes result in decreased cardiac output to the lungs, weakness, lethargy, chronic coughing, and ultimately congestive heart failure. An untreated dog may die. A dog becomes infected when an infected mosquito takes a blood meal. The larva of the worm breaks out of the mosquito's mouthparts during feeding and drops onto the dog's skin. The larva then enters the skin through the hole made by the mosquito. In 70–90 days, the larva reaches the dog's heart, where it stays and develops into an adult. Preventative measures are the best way to control dog heartworm; drugs can be administered after infection, but these are costly and very painful for the animal.

11.12.4 Rift Valley Fever

Rift Valley fever was first recognised in the Rift Valley in East Africa, with a virus known as Wesselsbron virus isolated from a dead lamb and later also from human blood. The same virus was isolated from mosquitoes in sheep, lambs, and cattle. In 1951, a severe epizootic occurred among the Western Orange Free State, Southern Transvaal, and adjoining districts of northwestern Cape Province. Another epizootic occurred among sheep in southwestern Orange. The virus was isolated from two abundant mosquito species: *Aedes caballus*, *Aedes circumluteus*, and *Taeniorhynchus uniformis*.

Other diseases in which mosquitoes play a minor role are fowl pox and myxomatosis. In the case of fowl pox, mosquitoes act as mechanical transmitters. Myxomatosis of rabbits has been reported in England, Europe, and Australia. In Australia, the principal transmitting mosquitoes are various species of *Aedes*, *Anopheles annulipes*, and *Culex annulirostris. Anopheles annulipes* feeds on rabbits above ground at night and also attacks them in burrows during the day, whereas *Culex annulirostris* bites only at night.

11.12.5 St. Louis Encephalitis Virus

This virus was identified as the causative agent of disease during an outbreak of encephalitis-like illness in Paris, Illinois (USA) in 1932, and St. Louis, Missouri (USA) in 1933. It was isolated from a patient with encephalitis in the Yakima Valley of Washington (USA) in the early 1940s and found to be a frequent cause of human illness in the Central Valley of California during the 1930s and 1940s. This virus is distributed widely in North America and also occurs in parts of Mexico, Central America, the Caribbean, and South America as far south as Argentina (Figure 15.27). The encephalitic illness caused by the St. Louis encephalitis (SLE) virus shows a bimodal age distribution, with children and elderly people most frequently affected. Attack rates during epidemics range from 5 to 800 per 100,000 population, depending on location, year, strain virulence, and population immunity resulting from earlier epidemics. In the eastern United States, mortality rates have ranged from about 3% to 20% of laboratory-diagnosed cases, while in the western United States, mortality rates have been lower. In North America, three enzootic cycles of the SLE virus have been described. In the eastern United States, north of Florida but including Texas, the primary vectors are *Culex pipiens* and *Cx. quinquefasciatus* (Figure 15.29). The former mosquito occurs in a more northerly distribution, whereas the latter is more southerly, with a hybrid zone at about the latitude of Memphis, Tennessee (USA). Females of both species feed on birds. In addition, *Cx. quinquefasciatus* females frequently feed on mammals as the summer progresses. Whether these mosquitoes alone or other vectors play a role in transmission to humans depends on the abundance of these two species and other competent vectors. House sparrows are significant vertebrate amplifier hosts in peridomestic settings. In the western United States, a mosquito-bird-mosquito cycle similar to that of western equine encephalomyelitis virus, involving *Cx. tarsalis,* has been elucidated. In addition, in California, both *Cx. pipiens and Cx. quinquefasciatus*, and possibly *Cx. stigmatosoma*, function secondarily as either enzootic or epidemic vectors. In Florida, *Cx. nigripalpus* apparently serves as the enzootic, epizootic, and epidemic vector of the SLE virus. In Latin America and the Caribbean basin, the SLE virus has been isolated from many different species of *Culex, Sabethes, Mansonia, Wyeomyia,* and other genera, as well as from a wide variety of birds and mammals. In these areas, human SLE is generally rare. There is some evidence of virus persistence in overwintering, diapausing female mosquitoes. The history of SLE in North America has been characterized by epidemics, either local or widespread, interspersed with years when there was apparently no virus activity or epidemics, and either no or only a few isolated human cases (William, 1973). The first epidemic, in the early 1930s in St. Louis, Missouri, was accompanied by hot and dry weather, which favoured the development of populations of mosquitoes in the *Culex pipiens* complex, the larvae of which develop in water rich in sewage or other organic matter. The epidemic involved about 1,100 human cases and 200 deaths. Since that time, there have been approximately 50 outbreaks of SLE in the United States. Human cases have also occurred in Manitoba and Ontario, Canada. These epidemics have occurred in both rural and urban settings. A very large outbreak occurred in 1975, involving 30 states and the District of Columbia, with over 1,800 cases reported. More recently, epidemics have arisen in such diverse locations in the United States as Pine Bluff (Arkansas), Florida, Los Angeles (California), Houston (Texas), New Orleans (Louisiana), and Grand Junction (Colorado). A total of 4,437 human cases of SLE infection were reported to the CDC from 1964 to 1995, with an average of 139 cases per year. From 2007 to 2016, there were 95 diagnosed cases and five deaths (Monath, 1980). The historical distribution of human cases of SLE neuroinvasive disease (encephalitis and/or meningitis) in the United States is shown, along with the average annual incidence by county of residence per 100,000 population between 2007 and 2016.

11.12.6 Murray Valley Encephalitis Virus

This virus has been associated with encephalitis-type illness in humans in the eastern and western parts of Australia and in New Guinea (Marshall, 1988; Figure 15.27). Mortality rates vary greatly during outbreaks, ranging from 18% to 80%, with long-term neurological effects occurring in 30% to 50% of survivors. Epidemics of encephalitis in Australia in 1917, 1918, 1922, and 1925 were probably caused by the Murray Valley encephalitis (MVE) virus. It was isolated from the brain of a human in 1951 and from a pool of *Culex annulirostris* in 1960. Later periods of transmission were detected in Australia in 1956, 1971, 1974, 1978, 1981, and 1984. A resurgence of virus activity and human infections occurred in 2011, the first outbreak of significance since 1974. The enzootic cycle involves *Cx. annulirostris* as the vector and birds as vertebrate reservoir and amplifier hosts. Epidemics appear to be associated with excessive rainfall, which allows an increase in mosquito populations to high densities and the immigration of wading birds. Kunjin virus is closely related to MVE virus. It is also mosquito-borne but is rarely associated with human disease in Australia Zika (ZIK) virus. This virus was first isolated from a sentinel rhesus monkey in Zika Forest, Uganda, in 1947, and soon after in the mosquito *Aedes africanus* in that forest. Human cases were first documented in Africa in 1952. However, the first major outbreak in humans occurred much later, in Micronesia in 2007. It has now spread through nearly all of equatorial Africa.

11.13 CONCLUSION

The future of mosquito-borne diseases will depend on the improvements and implementation of chemotherapy and vaccination. Regular entomological surveillance in different ecotypes will help in devising vector control plans in time and space. Studies on new formulations of larvicides and insecticides should continue for vector control. Other control measures include parasitoids, nematodes, larvivorous fish, *Toxorhynchites* mosquitoes, insect viruses, growth hormones, sex attractants, natural products, sanitation, and water management. Vector control should be combined with personnel training and carried out on an international scale using biological and integrated control measures.

11.14 POINTS TO REMEMBER

1. Mosquitoes are vectors of malaria, dengue, chikungunya, Zika, and JE.
2. Mosquitoes also transmit diseases in animals, such as equine encephalomyelitis, Rift Valley fever, and St. Louis encephalitis (SLE) virus.
3. Dr Ronald Ross was awarded the Nobel Prize in Physiology & Medicine for his work on the transmission of the malarial parasite by mosquitoes in 1897.
4. The modes of transmission are cyclico-developmental and propagative. A disease-causing organism like the malaria parasite undergoes development, including multiplication, in the body of the *Anopheles* mosquito, which spreads the disease from one person to another. In cyclico-developmental transmission, a disease-causing organism, such as microfilaria, undergoes development in the body of the *Culex quinquefasciatus* mosquito but does not multiply in the vector. In propagative transmission, a disease-causing organism may simply multiply in the vector, such as the dengue virus, which multiplies in *Ae. aegypti* mosquitoes, and *Pasteurella pestis*, which multiplies in rat fleas. These vectors then spread these organisms to humans.

Acknowledgements

The author is thankful to Dr. Laxman Kanekhar and Dr. Gujju Gandhy for the illustrations used in this manuscript.

REFERENCES

Apiwathnasorn, C., Samung, Y., Prummongkol, S., Asavanich, A., Komalamisra, N., & Mccall, P. (2006). Bionomics studies of Mansonia mosquitoes inhabiting the peat swamp forest. *Southeast Asian Journal of Tropical Medicine and Public Health*, 37(2), 272–278.

Barnitharan, M., Gokulakrishnan, J., & Sridhar, N. (2018). *Introduction of Vector Mosquito*. Lambert Academic Publishing, Saarbrucken, Germany, p. 148.

Becker, N., Petric, D., Zgomba, M., Boase, C., Madon, M., Dahl, C., & Kaiser, A. (2010). *Mosquitoes and their Control*, 2nd edition. Springer, New York.

Carroll, K. C., Funke, G., Jorgensen, J. H., Louise Landry, M., Warnock, D. W. (2011). *Manual of Clinical Microbiology*. Wiley, New York. https://doi.org/10.1128/9781555816728.ch146.

Christopher, S. R. (1933). *The Fauna of British India: Family Culicidae Tribe Anophelinae*, Vol. IV. Taylor & Francis, London, p. 371.

Crans, W. J. (2004). A classification system for mosquito life cycles: Life cycle types for mosquitoes of the northeastern United States. *Journal of Vector Ecology*, 29(1), 1–10.

Environmental Protection Agency. (2024). *CDC Mosquito Life Cycle*. https://www.cdc.gov/mosquitoes/about/life-cycle-of-anopheles-mosquitoes.html

Ferguson, H. M., Dornhaus, A., Beeche, A., Borgemeister, C., Gottlieb, M., Mulla, M. S., Gimnig, J. E., Fish, D., & Killeen, G. F. (2010). Ecology: A prerequisite for malaria elimination and eradication. *PLoS Medicine*, 7(8), 1000303.

Godfray, H. C. J. (2013). Mosquito ecology and control of malaria. *Journal of Animal Ecology*, 82(1), 15–25.

ICMR-Vector Control Research Centre (2010). *Annual Report*. https://vcrc.res.in/Iannino

Kanojia, P. C., & Geevarghese, G. A. (2005). New mosquito records of an area known for Japanese encephalitis hyperendemicity, Gorakhpur District, Uttar Pradesh, India. *Journal of the American Mosquito Control Association,* 21(1), 1–4.

Kanojia, P. C., Shetty, P. S., & Geevarghese, G. A. (2003). Long-term study on vector abundance & seasonal prevalence in relation to the occurrence of Japanese encephalitis in Gorakhpur district, Uttar Pradesh. *Indian Journal of Medical Research*, 117, 104–110.

Kaul, S. M., Sharma, R. S., Sharma, S. N., Panigrai, N., Phukan, P. K., & ShivLal (1998). Preventing dengue/dengue haemorrhagic fever: The role of entomological surveillance. *Journal of Affective Disorders,* 30(3), 197–192.

Lamino, F., Sulli, N., Maitino, A., Pascucci, I., Pampiglione, G., & Salucci, S. (2017). Species, biology and flea-borne diseases. *Veterinariaitaliana*, 53(4), 277–288.

Levin, M. L. (2014). Medical entomology. *Emerging Infectious Disease,* 20(8), 14–28.

Manimegalai, K., & Sukanya, S. (2014). Biology of the filarial vector Culexquinquefasciatus (Diptera: Culicidae). *International Journal of Current Microbiology and Applied Sciences*, 3(4), 718–724.

Mattingly, P. F. (1972). Mosquito eggs XIX. Genus *Mansonia* (subgenus *Mansonioides* Theobald). *Mosquito Systematics*, 4(2), 50–59.

Mike, S. (2008). *Medical Entomology for Students*, 4th edition. USA Cambridge Univiversity Press, Cambridge p. 314.

Mishra, C. (2014). Culex mosquito: Vector of Filariasis. *Odisha Review*, 2–3, 95–98.

NVBDCP. (2015). *Operational Manual for Integrated Vector Management in India*. www.nvbdcp.gov.in, pp. 1–248. IVM-Manual-Draft-2015.pdf (mohfw.gov.in)

NVBDCP. (2020). *Guideline on Mosquito and Other Vector Control Response*. pp. 1–98. https://ncvbdc.mohfw.gov.in/Doc/Guidelines-Mosquito-and-other-vector-control-response-2020.pdf

OECD. (2018). *Consensus Document on the Biology of Mosquito Aedes aegypti: Unclassified ENV/JM/MONO*. OECD Publishing, Paris, p. 23.

Reddya Naik, B., Tyagi, B. K., & Xue, R.-D. (2023). Mosquito-borne diseases in India over the past 50 years and their global public health implications: A systematic review. *Journal of the American Mosquito Control Association,* 39(4), 258–277.

Reuben, R., Tewari, S. C., Hiriyan, J., & Akiyama, J. (1994). Illustrated keys to species of *Culex (Culex)* associated with Japanese encephalitis in SoutheastAsia (Diptera: Culicidae). *Mosquito Systematics*, 26(2), 75–96.

Sallum, M. A. M. (2007). *Mansonia (Mansonia) iguassuensis* sp. nov. (Diptera:Culicidae) from Brasil. *Zootaxa*, 1527, 45–52.

Sam, R., & Telford III (2011). *Arthropods of Medical Importance*. pp. 2505–2525. https://doi.org/10.1128/9781555817381.ch148.

Service, M. W. (1980a).Culicine mosquitoes (order diptera: Family culicidae, subfamily Culicinae). In: *A Guide to Medical Entomology*, 53–70. doi:10.1007/978-1-349-16334-2_6.

Service, M. W. (1980b). Anopheles mosquitoes (order) Diptera: Family culicidae, subfamily anophelinae). In: *A Guide to Medical Entomology*, 44–52. doi:10.1007/978-1-349-16334-2_5.

Service, M. W. (1980c). Fleas (order siphonaptera: Families pulicidae, leptopsyllidae and ceratophyllidae). In: *A Guide to medical Entomology*. pp. 127–135. doi:10.1007/978-1-349-16334-2_15.

Sharma, R. S. (1982). Analysis of mosquito collection in the Dengue fever infected localities of Gurgaon Urban, Haryana State. *Entomon*, 8, 197–188.

Sharma, R. S. (1984). Seasonal density and natural survival rate of filariasis vector *Culex quinquefasciatus* (Diptera:Culicidae) in Gurgaon. *Entomon,* 9(4), 257–260.

Sharma, R. S. (1995). Urban malaria and its vector *Anopheles stephensi* and *Anopheles culicifacies* (Diptera Culicidae) in Gurgaon India. *South East Journal of Medicine,* 26(1), 172–176.

Sharma, R. S. (1997). Seasonal prevalence of *Anopheles culicifacies, Anopheles stephensi, Culexquinquefaciatus* and *Aedes aegypti* (Diptera: Culicidae) in urban Gurgaon. In: *Proceeding of the Second symposium on Vector and Vector Borne Diseases*, Paris, France, pp. 277–231.

Sharma, R. S. (2006). Entomological studies during outbreak of Chikungunya in Marathwada region of Maharashtra (India). *Indian Journal for the Practisi*

ng Doctor 3(5), 34–36.

Sharma, R. S. (2008). Entomological studies during outbreak of Chikungunya in Lakshdweep island. *WHO Dengue Bulletin,* 32, 178–18.

Sharma R. S., & Dahiya, B. S. (1983). Prevalence of adult and larvae of bancroftian Filariasis vector *Culex fatigans* (Diptera:Culicidae) in Gurgaon U.P. *Journal of Zoology*, 3, 154–156.

Sharma, R. S., Kaul, S. M., & Sokhay, J. (2005). Seasonal fluctuations of dengue fever vector. *Aedes aegypti* (Diptera:Culicidae) in Delhi, India. *Southeast Asian Journal of Tropical Medicine and Public Health,* 36(1), 1–5.

Sharma, R. S., Kumari, R., Srivastava, P. K., Barua, K., & Chauhan, L. S. (2014). Emergence of dengue problem in India: A public health challenge. *Journal of Communicable Diseases*, 46, 1745.

Sharma, R. S., Panigrai, N., & Kaul, S. M. (2001). *Aedes aegypti* prevalence in hospitals and schools the priority sites for DHF transmission in Delhi, India. *WHO-Dengue Bulletin,* 25, 107–108.

Sharma, R. S., Panigraai, N., Kaul, S. M., Lal, S., Barua, K., & Bharadwaj, M. (1999). Status report on DH/DHF during 1998 in the National Capital Territory of Delhi, India, WHO. *Dengue Bullitien*, 23, 109–112.

Sharma, R. S., Rakesh, K., Kumar, K., & Kuldip Singh, G. (2003). Seasonal prevalence of *Aedes aegypti*, a vector of Dengue/Dengue hemorrhagic fever, in different zones of Delhi, India. *Journal of Environmental Sciences*, 7(2), 163–167.

Sharma, R. S., & Sharma, K. (1984). Density of potential vector of Dengue Hemorrhagic fever *Aedes aegypti* (Diptera: Culicidae). *Entomon,* 9(2), 93–95.

Sharma, R. S., & Shrivastava, P. K. (1995). Seasonal trends in population density of malaria vector *Anopheles culicifacies* and *Anopheles fluviatilis* (Diptera: Culicidae) Mos. *Born. Disease Bullitien,* 10(2), 39–42.

Sharma, R. S., Shrivastava, P. K., Kaul, S. M., & Lal, S. (1999). Urban malaria control in India including control of Malaria and Dengue in the NCT. *Delhi Farm Medicine,* 3(3), 42–45.

Sharma, R. S., Singh, I., & Dahiya, B. S. (1984). Breeding places and seasonal abundance of Bancroftian filarial vector *Culex fatigans* (Diptera:Culicidae in Gurgaon. *Entomon,* 9, 65–67.

Sharma, R. S. et al. (2014).Urban Malaria: A growing threat to public health in India. *Journal of Affective Disorders,* 46, 17–45.

Tyagi, B. K. (1994). Distribution of arthropod vector-borne communicable diseases and control. *Indian Review of Life Science,* 14, 223–243.

Tyagi, B. K. (2002). *Malaria in the Thar Desert: Facts, Figures and Future*. Agrobios, Jodhpur, India, p. 165.

Tyagi, B. K. (2003). *Medical Entomology: A Handbook of Medically Important Insects and Other Arthropods Handbook of Medical Entomology*. Scientific Publishers Jodhpur, India, p. 262.

Tyagi, B. K. (2007). Chikungunya in India. *Bulletin de la Societe de Pathologie Exotique,* 100, 321.

Tyagi, B. K. (2008). *Vector-Borne Diseases: Epidemiology and Control*. Scientific Publishers, Jodhpur, India.

Tyagi, B. K. (2023). *Mosquitoes of India*. Taylor and Francis, London, United Kingdom.

Tyagi, B. K., Munirathinam, A., & Venkatesh, A. (2015). A catalogue of Indian mosquitoes. *International Journal of Mosquito Research*, 2(2), 50–97.

William, N. B. (1973). Control of arthropods of medical and veterinary importance. *Advances in Parasitology*, 11, 115–192.

World Health Organization, Regional Office for South-East Asia. (2011). *Comprehensive Guideline for Prevention and Control of Dengue and Dengue Haemorrhagic Fever*. Revised and expanded edition. WHO Regional Office for South-East Asia. https://iris.who.int/handle/10665/204894

12 Blackflies, *Simulium* spp. (Diptera: Simuliidae)

Vijay Veer

LEARNING OBJECTIVES

1. To learn about the biodiversity, biology, and pestiferous role of blackflies in India.
2. To learn about various diseases transmitted by blackflies to humans and animals.
3. To learn about the transmission of the disease onchocerciasis (river blindness) in humans.

12.1 INTRODUCTION

The biting flies of the dipteran insects of the family Simuliidae are of medical, veterinary, and ecological importance. These flies are popularly known as *blackflies* worldwide over; however, not all of them are black or grey in colour, as many are also yellow or orange. These flies are also known as *buffalo gnats* because they have a *hump* on their thorax. These flies are found in and around hilly areas and foothills near flowing water, ranging from almost stationary to rapid waters, as their larvae have the *most remarkable biological feature of filtering out the food materials* from moving water while remaining stationary (sessile) on a substratum.

Blackflies are notorious pests of birds, livestock, wild animals, and humans due to their biting nuisance and disease transmission. They rank second as the most harmful group of insects after mosquitoes in terms of their impact on human health, as they transmit two important human diseases (onchocerciasis, or *river blindness*, and mansonellosis) in addition to causing biting annoyance. Human onchocerciasis is an eye and skin disease and represents a significant public health problem, caused by a filarial nematode, *Onchocerca volvulus*, which infects about 37 million people in the central belt of Africa, Yemen, and Central and South America (Figure 12.1).

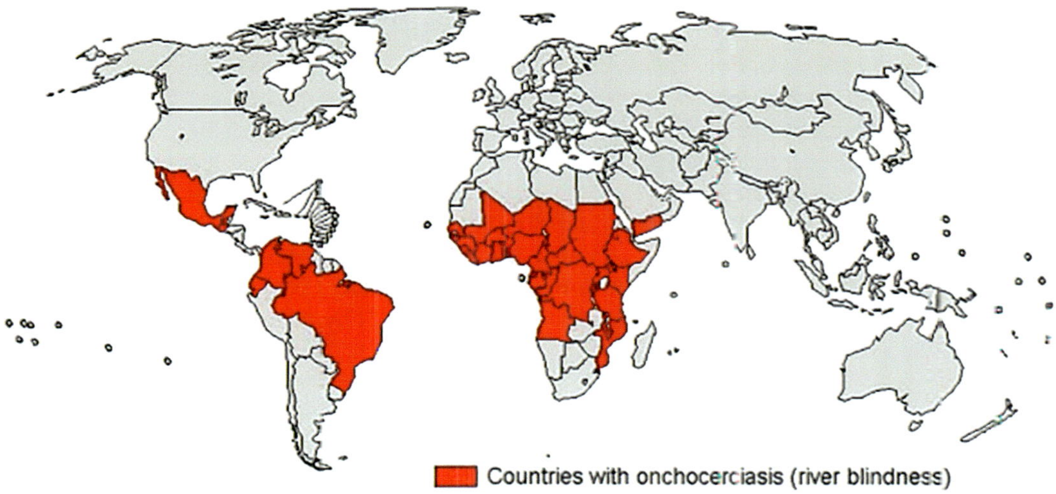

FIGURE 12.1 World map showing Onchocerciasis-affected countries. (After WHO.)

DOI: 10.1201/9781003482581-15

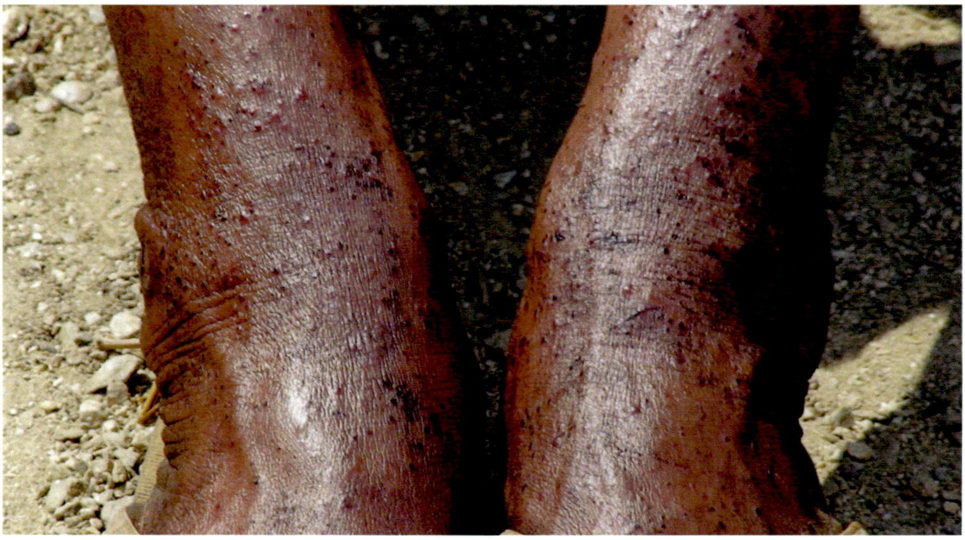

FIGURE 12.2 Black scars and skin hyperpigmentation due to secondary infection in human legs in Salari, Arunachal Pradesh, India. This condition is quite common among the locals (Adopted from Dhiman et al. (2014), *Journal of Environmental Biology*, 35 (2), 421–425.)

Of these, 4 million people suffer from skin disease, and 2 million are blind or severely visually impaired. Additionally, they are known to transmit several other parasites and pathogens to domestic animals and wildlife. In India, blackflies inflict painful bites and cause intense annoyance to humans during outdoor activities. These bites result in irritation, itching, localized tissue damage, dermatitis, inflammation, formation of blisters, followed by secondary infection that leaves black scars on the body (Figure 12.2), as well as allergic reactions (known as *blackfly fever)*. They are quite common in the North-east part of the country, where they are commonly referred to as *dim-dam flies*. However, onchocerciasis has not been reported in India, except for one unconfirmed case from Assam. Recently, Vijay Veer (2022) published a book on Indian blackflies. This chapter is largely based on that book.

12.2 TAXONOMIC POSITION AND BIODIVERSITY

Simuliidae represents a relatively small and morphologically homogeneous family within the order Diptera. Therefore, morphological species differentiation is very difficult, and there are a large number of isomorphic species (sibling species) and species complexes. Blackflies are most closely related to other dipteran families, such as Ceratopogonidae (biting midges), Chironomidae (non-biting midges), and Thaumaleidae (solitary midges), as members of these families share similarities in the form of larval mouthparts. These four families, including Simuliidae, collectively form a superfamily, Chironomoidea (previously, Simuliidae was placed with mosquitoes in the superfamily Culicoidea), within the infraorder Culicomorpha of the suborder Nematocera within the order Diptera. Blackflies can be easily distinguished from mosquitoes by the absence of scales on their wings and their elongated mouthparts.

12.2.1 Classification

Phylum – Arthropoda
Class – Insecta
Order – Diptera

Suborder – Nematocera
Family – Simuliidae
Subfamily – Simuliinae
Tribe – Simuliini
Genus – *Simulium* Latreille, 1802

The family Simuliidae is represented by 2,311 extant and 16 fossil species across 30 genera occurring worldwide (Adler & Crosskey, 2017). The species are further divided into two subfamilies: Parasimuliinae and Simuliinae. The subfamily Parasimuliinae contains only one tribe, Parasimuliini, while the subfamily Simuliinae comprises two tribes: Prosimuliini and Simuliini. The tribe Parasimuliini is known by one genus with only four species. The tribe Prosimuliini of the subfamily Simuliinae is known by six genera and 143 living species, while the tribe Simuliini consists of 23 genera containing 2,164 living species.

Family: **Simuliidae**

I. Subfamily: **Parasimuliinae**
   1. Tribe: Parasimuliini (1 genus, 4 spp.)
   2. Genus: *Parasimulium* (4 spp.)

II. Subfamily: **Simuliinae**
   1. Tribe: Prosimuliini (6 genera, 143 spp.)
   2. Genera: *Gymnopais* (12 spp.), *Helodon* (36 spp.), *Levitinia* (3 spp.), *Prosimulium* (79 spp.), *Twinnia* (10 spp.), *Urosimulium* (3 spp.)
   3. Tribe: Simuliini (23 genera, 2,164 spp.)
   4. Genera: *Araucnephia* (3 spp.), *Araucnephioides* (1 spp.), *Austrosimulium* (30 spp.), *Bunyipellum* (1 sp.), *Cnephia* (7 spp.), *Cnesia* (3 spp.), *Cnesiamima* (1 sp.), *Crozetia* (2 spp.), *Ectemnia* (4 spp.), *Ectmenoides* (6 spp.), *Gigantodax* (65 spp.), *Greniera* (13 spp.), *Lutzsimulium* (4 spp.), *Metacnephia* (57 spp.), *Nothogreniera* (2 spp.), *Paracnephia* (14 spp.), *Paraustrosimulium* (3 sp.), *Pedrowygomyia* (4 spp.), *Protaustrosimulium* (4 spp.), *Simulium* (1,886 spp.), *Stegopterna* (14 spp.), *Sulcicnephia* (24 spp.), and *Tlalocomiya* (16 spp.).

The biodiversity of blackflies in India is poorly known. In India, all species of blackflies belong to a single tribe, *Simuliini*, and a single genus, *Simulium*. So far, 76 nominal species and 17 unnamed species in seven genera are known. These seven genera are *Asiosimulium* Takaoka & Choochote, 2005, *Eusimulium* Roubaud, 1906, *Gomphostilbia* Enderlein, 1921, *Montisimulium* Rubtsov, 1974, *Nevermannia* Enderlein, 1921, *Simulium* Latreille, 1802, and *Wilhelmia* Enderlein, 1921. The genus *Asiosimulium* was recently reported from Arunachal Pradesh by the author in his monograph on Indian blackflies from Assam. Meanwhile, 140 species and 33 unnamed species in nine subgenera are known from the Indian subregion (India and neighbouring countries), and in the Oriental Region, there are 492 species of blackflies in ten subgenera.

12.3 BIOLOGY

Blackflies are very different in appearance from other biting dipteran insects, such as mosquitoes, midges, gnats, stableflies, hornflies, horseflies, and deerflies. Adult blackflies are usually small in size (5–15 mm long), stout-bodied, and *humpbacked*; black to grey in colour with short, porrect, horn-like antennae (mostly 11-segmented), with piercing and sucking mouthparts, and large compound eyes. Females have dichoptic eyes, which are markedly separated by the frons, whereas males have holoptic eyes that meet at the midline. The wings are hyaline, without any scales, and have a broad wingspan of 6–10 mm with strong costa, subcosta and radius veins. The first tergum of the abdomen is modified as a basal scale fringed with long hairs.

12.3.1 Habitat

Blackflies are distributed worldwide except in polar regions, high mountains, deserts, and islands where flowing water is not available. In India, the Himalayan region provides excellent hilly terrain with varied abiotic and biotic conditions for the propagation of blackflies, having plenty of freshwater rivers, streams, rivulets, water channels, etc., with different water flow speeds. The immature stages occupy every conceivable running-water habitat, from tiny headwater trickles to mighty rivers, and from hot springs to glacial melt waters.

12.3.2 Life Cycle

The simuliid flies are holometabolous insects, as they exhibit distinct metamorphosis in their life cycle, which passes through aquatic egg, larva, and pupa to become the adult fly (Figure 12.3). The length of the life cycle varies with species and environmental conditions. Common Indian species are multivoltine and may have 3–6 generations per year. Species living at high altitudes in temperate climates have one or two generations per year and are univoltine or bivoltine in nature. Tropical African species, *S. damnosum* (vector of *river blindness*) have continuous breeding and complete their life cycle in less than 2 weeks.

Female blackflies are ready to mate usually after an emergence period of 1–2 hours, but stenogamous females may mate immediately after emergence. Males emerge earlier than females. Mating occurs in the vicinity of the breeding site, mostly during the afternoon. Some species mate throughout the day, depending on their emergence patterns. In some species, mating takes place on the

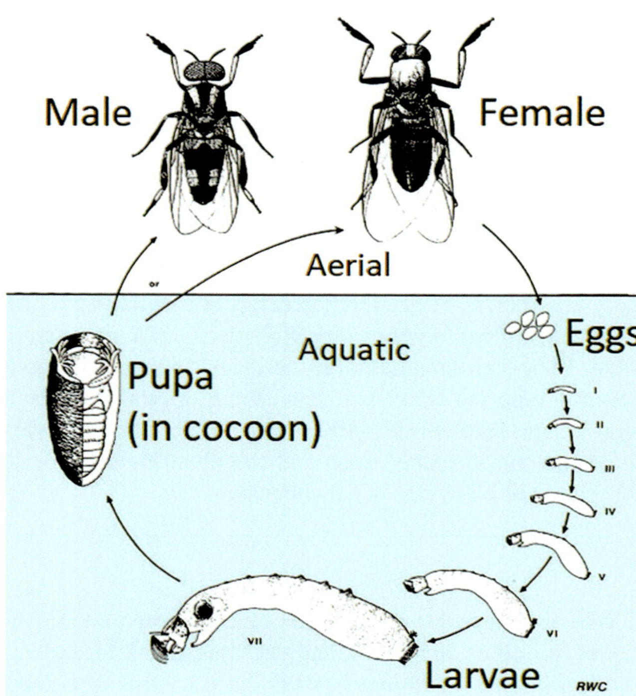

FIGURE 12.3 Life cycle of blackfly.

ground, while for the majority, mating occurs on the wing when a female enters a male swarm. Males form small swarms in association with some visual markers, which may be located on the top of 1–3 m tall trees, beside rivers, or 2–3 m above the ground. Copulating pairs settle on nearby vegetation. Mating usually lasts for 5–8 minutes at temperatures of 27°C–32°C, but mating duration may vary from a few seconds to hours across different species. Blackfly males can mate 2–3 times, but females mostly mate once; however, females of some species may mate a second time as well. Females also feed on nectar, similar to males, who do not feed on vertebrate blood. Most females require blood meal proteins for egg maturation before each gonotrophic cycle and are classified as anautogenous species. Some species lay their eggs without a blood meal and are non-blood feeding, with poorly developed mouthparts; they are known as autogenous species. There are other species that lay the first batch of their eggs without a blood meal but require a blood meal for the development of subsequent batches of eggs. Such flies are known as primiparous autogenous. *S. aureohirtum* is a widespread species in both Palaearctic and Oriental regions and has normal biting mouthparts, being mammalophilic and ornithophilic in India; however, females in Japan, the Philippines, and Taiwan are found emerging with mature eggs (Takaoka & Noda, 1979). This species exhibits primiparous autogeny.

12.3.3 Oviposition

Adult flies are found abundantly on sunny days near their breeding habitats of flowing streams and rivers. Egg laying varies with the species except that all females lay their eggs in running water. Blackflies adopt different strategies for oviposition among different species, ensuring that their eggs survive and progeny develop. Egg laying is performed by mainly four methods in India: either (i) by dropping eggs while flying above the water, (ii) by tapping the abdomen through the water while hovering, (iii) by tapping the abdomen into the water while crawling on the emergent wetted substratum, or (iv) by crawling under the water (up to 15 cm below the water surface) on the submerged substrates. Eggs may be laid in long strings of beads or untidy egg masses within a gelatinous matrix by a female, or in several layers of thousands of eggs by multiple females on a single substrate. The eggs are usually laid in masses on submerged or emergent live or dead vegetation or settle into sediments at the bottom of the flowing watercourses. The peak period of oviposition is normally in the evening before sunset, and oviposition may last for 1–2 days for a gonotrophic cycle. Generally, blackflies oviposit in water currents of 0.3–0.9 m/s. Some flies lay their eggs in almost still water. Different species select different watercourses for oviposition. Communal oviposition in blackflies is common, as several conspecific gravid females aggregate to deposit their eggs on a suitable site or substratum under the attraction of pheromone stimuli. Recently, three compounds (cis-9-tetradecen-1-ol, 1-pentadecene, and 1-tridecene) have been identified from eggs, which can induce an oviposition response in female flies (McGaha et al., 2015). Similar reproductive behaviour is seen in other medically important species of the order Diptera, and it has been observed that volatiles produced by eggs, larvae, habitat, microbes, infusion, and plants influence the oviposition behaviour of gravid females. Communal oviposition behaviour in the *Culex quinquefasciatus* mosquito and *Lutzomyia longipalpis* sand fly is largely stimulated by egg oviposition pheromones, erythro-6-acetoxy-5-hexadecanolide and dodecanoic acid, respectively. A cuticular hydrocarbon, heneicosane, produced by conspecific larvae in water, has been identified as attracting conspecific gravid females of the dengue mosquito, *Aedes aegypti*, and egg-derived dodecanoic and (Z)-9-hexadecenoic acids also show significant positive ovipositional responses from females of *A. aegypti*.

Simuliids also use visual cues to identify suitable oviposition sites, as observed in various studies (Golini & Davies, 1975). It was observed that females oviposited more on green, yellow, and white than on purple, blue, orange, and red strips.

12.3.4 Eggs

Eggs are minute (0.1–0.5 mm long), sub-triangular or roughly ovoid with a bulge on one side, with or without a micropyle. The surface of the egg is smooth, whitish to light orange or yellowish in colour when freshly laid but darkens during embryogenesis. The chorionic surface may exhibit a latticework of polygonal cellular imprints or be almost smooth. The microstructure pattern of the endochorion may be useful in taxonomic identification, as it is an important diagnostic feature in other dipterans. Eggs hatch within 1–2 days, which may be extended up to 1 week in North-east India. Eggs hatching in species with several generations per year can take from 4 to 30 days. Species with one generation per year often enter diapause at the egg stage; therefore, hatching can take as long as 7 months.

12.3.5 Larvae

Larvae are aquatic, worm-like and lead a sessile life, as they remain attached to the submerged substrates in the water current, which brings food to them. Sessile larvae filter food from the water current through their two extendable cephalic fans and feed on small organic particles, algae, and bacteria. Larvae play a major role as detritivores in lotic ecosystems. The larvae are light to deep in colour, poorly segmented, and distinguishable by a brownish-black head with a prominent pair of cup-like cephalic fans (labral fans) or feeding brushes. The larval body has two prolegs, one on the prothorax and another on the terminal abdominal segment (IX). The larva uses tiny hooks present on the posterior circlet of the abdominal proleg for attachment to a silk pad, which is spun by the anterior proleg from their massive silk glands, and the pad is glued to a substratum. This attachment allows the larva to remain in flowing water. When disturbed or if the silken pad deteriorates, it can move to another place by releasing its hooklets from the silken pad and drifting downstream using the silk thread. The mature larva is about 6–7 mm long, cylindrical, and swollen posteriorly. The mature larva is recognized by the presence of dark gill histoblasts or spots on each side of the thorax. These gill spots develop into respiratory gills. In fact, the mature larva is a pharate pupa, which is a feeding and moving stage that spins a silk cocoon for pupation. This is a unique feature of blackflies.

In India, the larval life of *Simulium* species undergoes 6–7 moults, rarely nine moults, and is completed in 12–15 days. The larval period varies with the temperature of the breeding water, as well as the quality and quantity of food. Normally, the larval stage occupies nearly 20–25 days; for example, *Simulium praelargum, Simulium gracilis,* and *S. grisescens* overwinter in the larval stage in upland streams in the Darjeeling area of West Bengal.

12.3.6 Larval Feeding

In the normal feeding position, larvae orient themselves by anchoring posteriorly to the stable substratum and stretching out in the direction of the current with their heads downstream. The body is twisted through 90°–180° to face the fans and mouthparts towards the surface of the water. Continuous water current is diverted by the proleg and directed towards the cup-like cephalic fans, which strain suspended particles from the passing water. Cibarium glands produce a sticky secretion that helps the fans capture fine particulate matter from the water and transfer it to the cibarium by the mandibular brushes for ingestion. The cephalic fans are held open and retracted at intervals in the current for cleaning with the mandibles. The larvae ingest bacteria, diatoms, algae, vegetable detritus, sand, and silt (most commonly 10–100 µm diameter particles) as food. Larvae feed indiscriminately and ingest particulate matter without any preference, but a high concentration (50 mg/L) of particles may cause feeding inhibition. Some species of simuliids are not filter feeders, and cephalic fans are absent in species of the genera *Gymnopais* and *Twinnia* occurring in subarctic streams; instead, they feed by scraping algal matter from the substrate with the help of the labrum and the chisel-like teeth of the hypostomium (Smith, 1973).

12.3.7 Phoretic Association

Larvae and pupae of several species of blackfly attach themselves to nymphs of mayflies (Ephemeroptera) and crabs and prawns (crustaceans) for transport and protection in the fresh waters of Africa and Asia. This association is known as phoretic association. This relationship is termed phoresis, also called phoresy, derived from the Greek word meaning "to carry". It is an inter-species biological interaction, and neither organism is physiologically dependent on the other. Phoresis is an adaptive association of blackfly larvae that allows them to survive and secure a pupation site in fast-flowing rivers, where violent water movements frequently displace stones or sand, leading to disorientation, which may crush or bury them. Eggs are not laid on the crabs or mayfly nymphs; it is the young larva that finds its own phoretic partner. This association, it seems, is a biological prerequisite for the survival of the simuliid species, without which the concerned species has no future (Crosskey, 1990).

In India, a phoretic association was found between mayfly nymphs and blackflies. However, no such association between crustaceans and blackflies has been reported so far from this region. Phoresis has been reported from the north-east Himalaya (Kurseong) and north-western Himalaya (Kangan (J&K), Uttarakhand, Himachal Pradesh). Stauder & Kiel (2004) have studied the phoretic association of two blackfly species, *S. ephemerophilum* and *S. rashidi,* with mayfly nymphs of the family Heptageniidae in fast-flowing streams in Kullu Valley, Himachal Pradesh. They found five species of mayflies carrying larvae and pupae of these phoretic blackflies. These mayfly species were *Epeorus bispinosus*, *Electrogena eatoni*, *Iron martensi*, *Iron psi,* and *Rhithrogena tianshanica*. They reported that blackfly larvae were preferably attached to the thorax and the pupae to the wings of their carriers. Singh & Bisht (1988) found larvae of *Simulium* sp. on mayfly nymphs at the Bhagirathi River at Gangotri (3,048 m altitude) in a 1–1.5 m deep stream with a 1–2 m/s water current on 28 May 1985. The water was turbid due to melting snow. Simulium larvae were mostly found attached at the base of the abdomen, just below the coxa of the hind leg of nymphs.

12.3.8 Blackflies as Ecological Indicator

Larvae live in running water and are aquatic filter feeders, as they are able to capture suspended particulate organic matter classified as "dissolved organic matter" (DOM). The blackfly larvae capture bacteria and diatoms with a pair of extendable cephalic fans. Because of this habit, blackflies can be considered good environmental indicators for assessing the ecological health of both watercourses and surrounding landscapes. This activity of blackflies has necessitated the study of the ecology of larvae. Many species of blackflies can be considered indicator species (IS) as ecological indicators for monitoring environmental changes, assessing environmental integrity and health, as well as pollution and climate change. In the lotic ecosystem, blackfly adults and larvae constitute an essential food resource in the food web of aquatic animals such as Trichoptera, dragonflies, birds, and fish. Blackfly larvae grow in massive numbers under favourable conditions in streams, attaining population densities of millions of individuals per metre, which allows them to collect considerable amounts of fine particulate organic matter in streams. The massive amount of faecal matter produced by them acts as crucial fodder for micro-invertebrates and microorganisms.

12.3.9 Pupa

The pupa is immobile, more or less ovoid in shape, and remains partially enclosed in a cocoon fixed to the substrate of the breeding habitat. The pupal shape is almost similar to that of the developing adult, with the appendages closely applied to the body. The head of the pupa lies below the thorax, with two large eyes on either side. The head and thorax are usually provided with simple or branched setae called trichomes. The thorax bears a pair of variously branched filamentous, inflated, or bulbous gills on its anterolateral corners, generally directed forwards or upwards, but rarely downwards. These pupal gills are cuticular projections and respiratory organs, varying in number. The filament surface may be annulated or reticulated. These gills are the most diverse structures in the family and are heavily used as *key characteristics for species diagnosis.* The pupal abdomen has nine visible segments and usually bears transverse rows of various hooks and spines on tergites and sternites. Most conspicuous are eight recurved hooks along the posterior margin of tergites III and IV. The pupa has a pair of strong recurved terminal hooks, known as grapnel hooks, for locking itself in the cocoon, which has diagnostic value.

Cocoons are variously shaped. The salivary glands secrete silk strands, which are woven differently in different species. Thus, pupal cocoons vary in shape, complexity, thickness of strands, density of weave, and colour. Cocoons with a definitive structure are either slipper-shaped if they lack a collar at the anterior margin or boot-shaped if the anterior margin has a collar. These are further subdivided into seven different types. The cocoon case may be woven closely or loosely, with or without windows or interspaces, and may feature anterodorsal projections and ridges. Ecdysis of the larva–pupa takes place within this cocoon.

12.3.10 Adults Emergence and Prevalence

After 2–6 days of pupation, adult flies emerge, mostly in large numbers. The adult flies are known to travel up to 16–20 km from their breeding sites in search of a host for a blood meal. The adult females are attracted to humans mainly through the chemical cue carbon dioxide, which we exhale. The blackflies are also attracted to dark-coloured clothing, perfume, and sweat. They pupate underwater and then emerge in a bubble of air as flying adults. They are often preyed upon by trout during emergence. The adults of both sexes feed on plant nectar, pollen from flowers, honeydew, or plant juice. Most females also suck blood from vertebrates, including humans, for the protein required for the development of ovaries and maturation of eggs.

Blackflies develop in running water; therefore, they have well-defined altitudinal and seasonal distributions, with different river zones occupied by various blackfly species or species groups. The distribution of blackfly larvae largely depends on water velocity and stable, smooth substrata, including riverbed stones, rocks, vegetation, and other submerged objects. In contrast, in low-lying areas, the abundance of species is largely determined by water quality. In addition, several environmental factors are directly affected by human pressures on the river ecosystem, such as the loss of riparian vegetation, hydro-morphological modifications of the riverbed, and chemical and physico-chemical impairments of water and the surrounding landscape of streams and rivers.

12.4 DISEASE VECTORS AND TRANSMISSION

Female blackflies are haematophagous and pestiferous to humans, poultry, livestock, and wildlife, transmitting at least 15 protozoans, 12 filarial nematodes, and one virus (Adler, 2005), causing physical, psychological, and monetary losses to humans. They cause nuisance and biting problems, trauma, and pathogen transmission to warm-blooded vertebrates, notably *Onchocerca* spp. to humans, swine, deer, dogs, cattle, and buffalo; *Mansonella* to humans; *Leucocytozoon* and *Trypanosoma* to birds; and *Dirofilaria* to bears, splendidofilaria in ducks, as well as viruseslike Rift Valley fever and vesicular stomatitis in horses and cattle; and chlamydial bacteria that cause blindness in sheep and abortion in cattle. Furthermore, blackfly bites also cause other problems for humans, such as pain, localized swelling, chronic dermatitis, inflammation, and allergic reactions accompanied by intense irritation that lasts for several days or even weeks. Man-biting flies are included in four genera of the Simuliidae family: *Simulium*, *Prosimulium*, *Austrosimulium*, and *Cnephia*. However, the genus *Simulium* is the most widespread and includes most disease vector species for several diseases, including human onchocerciasis or *river blindness*.

12.4.1 Pestiferous Flies

Female adults of blackflies are voracious outdoor biters during daylight and dusk. Adult females of the subgenus *Simulium* are typically mammalophilic (feeding on mammals), but some are anthropophilic (feeding on) humans, possessing toothless claws while their larvae lack ventral tubercles. Females of the two subgenera *Nevermannia* and *Gomphostilbia* are ornithophilic (taking blood from birds) and have toothed claws adapted for movement through feathers.

In India, at least 21 species of blackflies are known to bite humans; 13 species are pests of livestock, and two species are pests of poultry (Table 12.1). Blackflies come into contact with humans during travel, hunting, fishing, honey gathering, construction activities, firewood collection, forestry activities, cultivation, and insurgency operations in North-east India. Blackflies were also

TABLE 12.1

Blackflies species regarded as biting and nuisance pest of humans, livestock and poultry in India

Species	Disease	Area
	Humans (21 spp.)	
Simulium (Simulium) alajense	Biting nuisance	Kashmir, Ladakh , North Pakistan
Simulium (Simulium) asishi	Biting nuisance	Darjeeling (West Bengal)
Simulium (Nevermannia) aureohirtum	Biting nuisance	Northeast India
Simulium (Simulium) barnesi	Biting nuisance	Arunachal Pradesh
Simulium (Simulium) barraudi	Biting nuisnace	North and Western Himalaya of India.
Simulium(Simulium) christophersi	Biting nuisance	Arunachal Pradesh
Simulium (Simulium) grisescens	Biting nuisance, dermetitis	Wide spread in hilly regions of India, Pakistan, Bhutan
Simulium (Simulium) himalayense	Dermetitis, allergic reaction	southern foot of the Himalaya, from Pakistan through India and Nepal to Myanmar and southern China
Simulium (Simulium) indicum	Dermetitis, Simulosis (allergic reactions,)	Wide sprad and common species in Himalayan mountains from Afghanistan and Pakistan in the west through India and Nepal, Tibet, Bhutan, Bangladesh to Myanmar
Simulium (Simulium) kapuri	Biting nuisance	North east India
Simulium(Gomphostilbia)) metatarsale	Biting nuisance	Wide spread in north east India and dominant in Mizoram
Simulium (Wilhelmia) pseudequinum	Biting nuisance	Kashmir
Simulium (Simulium) nilgiriricum	Biting nuisance	Tamil Nadu, Sri lanka
Simulium (Simulium) nitidithorax	Biting nuisance	Arunachal Pradesh

(*Continued*)

TABLE 12.1 (*Continued*)
Blackflies species regarded as biting and nuisance pest of humans, livestock and poultry in India

Species	Disease	Area
Simulium (*Simulium*) *nodosum*	Biting nuisance	Assam, West Bengal, Myanmar, southern china, Thailand, Vietnam
Simulium (*Simulium*) *novolineatum*	Biting nuisance	North east India, Myanmar
Simulium (*Nevermannia*) *praelargum*	Biting nuisance	North east India
Simulium (*Simulium*) *rufibasis*	Biting nuisance	Pakistan, north east India, Nepal, Myanmar
Simulium (*Simulium*) *stevensoni*	Biting nuisance	Kashmir, Ladakh, North Pakistan
Simulium (*Simulium*) *striatum*	Biting nuisance	Himalayan Region
Simulium (*Gomphostilbia*) *tenuistylum*	Biting nuisance	Himalayan Region
Livestock (13 spp.)		
Simulium (Nevermannia) *aureohirtum*	Biting nuisance,	North east India
Simulium (Simulium) *barraudi*	Biting nuisance	Wide spread in north east India
Simulium (Simulium) *himalayense*	Biting nuisance, blood loss. Affect milk production	Wide spread and abundant in Arunachal Pradesh, north east India
Simulium (Simulium) *indicum*	Biting nuisance, blood loss. Affect milk production	Wide spread and abundant in north east India
Simulium (Simulium) *kapuri*	Biting nuisance	Wide spread in north east India
Simulium (Simulium) *metatarsale*	Biting nuisance	Wide spread in north east India
Simulium (*Wilhelmia*) *pseudequinum*	Biting nuisance	Kashmir
Simulium (Simulium) *nilgiricum*	Biting nuisance	Wide spread in north east India
Simulium (Simulium) *nodosum*	Vector of zoonotic onchocerciasis in Thailand	Wide spread in north east India
Simulium (Simulium) *novolineatum*	Biting nuisance	
Simulium (Simulium) *rufibasis*	Biting nuisance	Wide spread in north east India
Simulium (Simulium) striatum	Biting nuisance	Himalayan Region, Sri lanka
Simulium (Simulium) stevensoni	Biting nuisance	Ladakh (Jammu & Kashmir)
Poultry (2 spp.)		
Simulium (*Nevermannia*) *aureohirtum*	Biting nuisance	Wide spread in India, Pakistan, Nepal, Bhutan, Sri Lanka
Simulium (*Gomphostilbia*) *tenuistylum*	Biting nuisance	North east India

troublesome to forest workers in the Tehri division (Uttarakhand), Himachal Pradesh, and Kashmir in the past. There is a need for a current assessment of the blackfly biting problem in this area (Table 12.1).

The following six species of blackflies (*S.* (*Nevermania*) *aureohirtum*, *S.* (*Simulium*) *grisescens*, *S.* (*Simulium*) *himalayense*, *S.* (*Simulium*) *indicum*, *S.* (*Simulium*) *rufibasis*, and *S.* (*Simulium*) *striatum*) are considered serious pests in India. Details on their distribution, bioecology, and economic importance are provided below.

12.4.1.1 *Simulium (Nevermannia) aureohirtum* Brunetti, 1911

Distribution: *Simulium* (*Nevermannia*) *aureohirtum* is one of the most widespread and abundant species in the Oriental Region and extends into the Palearctic and Australasian Regions. **India**: Assam, Andhra Pradesh, Arunachal Pradesh, Haryana, Himachal Pradesh, Karnataka, Maharashtra, Manipur, Meghalaya, Mizoram, Tamil Nadu, and West Bengal. **Elsewhere**: Bhutan, China, Guam, Indonesia (Flores, Java, Kalimantan, Maluku, Sulawesi, Sumatra), Japan, Malaysia (Malaya, Sabah, Sarawak), Nepal, Myanmar, Pakistan, Philippines (Bohol, Luzon, Mindanao, Negros, Palawan, Panay), Sri Lanka, Taiwan, Thailand, and Vietnam.

Bioecology: The blackfly species, *S. aureohirtum,* is geographically widespread and utilizes diverse habitats. It is the only autogenous species in the Oriental Region, in which the female can develop its first batch of eggs without a blood meal. The pupae and larvae of this species appear to be highly adapted to relatively high water temperatures (as high as 33°C), slow-flowing, and even somewhat muddy or polluted waters, where most other simuliid species do not occur. Ecologically, this species occurs in small, shallow streams often associated with outlets from human-made ponds or irrigation channels but may also breed in water rapids. In lowland areas, the fly is common during the rainy season. These capabilities, together with environmental factors, may explain why this species is so widely distributed in the Oriental Region and extends into the Palearctic and Australasian regions.

The fly is found in tributaries, paddy fields, semi-permanent streams, and man-made irrigation channels. The fly overwinters in the larval stage and is univoltine, at least at high altitudes (1,380–1,450 Shillong, Meghalaya). Females oviposit in slow water currents (0.2–0.5 m/s) but never in waters with high velocities, by (i) tapping the abdomen through the water while hovering over a substratum, which is constantly splashed with water or overlain by slow-moving water, and (ii) crawling underwater and laying their eggs on the undersurface of the substratum. A female can lay up to 225 eggs. Larvae are herbivorous, feeding on algae, diatoms, sand grains, and vegetable debris, and are rarely cannibalistic. They are frequently found on decaying leaves or grasses in small streams or trickles of water in the study areas of Manipur, Meghalaya, Mizoram, and Arunachal Pradesh.

Economic importance: The species *aureohirtum* is commonly found biting birds (ornithophilic) and animals (zoophilic), and less frequently humans. The man-biting activity of this species has been reported in Arunachal Pradesh and Assam (North-east India) It is one of the most dominant and abundant blackfly species in India. Insights into its biting behaviour remain to be studied.

12.4.1.2 Simulium (Simulium) grisescens Brunetti, 1911

Distribution: **India**: Arunachal Pradesh, Assam, Himachal Pradesh, Karnataka, Kerala, Maharashtra, Manipur, Meghalaya, Nagaland, Punjab, Sikkim, Tamil Nadu, and West Bengal (Darjeeling, Kurseong). **Elsewhere**: Bhutan, Pakistan, and Taiwan.

Bioecology: *S.* (*S.*) *grisescens* is distributed throughout India. In the Darjeeling area, this species is moderately abundant and breeds in both lowland and upland rivers. In lowland rivers, it undergoes hibernation in the egg stage and completes three generations in a year; while in upland streams, it hibernates in the larval stage and completes only one generation in a year.

Economic importance: The fly *S.* (*S.*) *grisescens* bites humans and animals. Fly bites cause dermatitis in humans.

12.4.1.3 *Simulium (Simulium) himalayense* Puri, 1932

Distribution: **India**: Arunachal Pradesh, Bihar, Himachal Pradesh, Manipur, Sikkim, and West Bengal. **Elsewhere**: Myanmar, Nepal, Pakistan, and China (Tibet).

Bioecology: *S.* (*S.*) *himalayense* preferably breeds in seepage water in North-east India.

Economic importance: The black fly species *himalayense* is mammalophilic and preferably bites ungulates. It also frequently bites tourists, farmers, and field workers in the north-east, especially in Arunachal Pradesh. The *himalayense* is the most prominent species in Arunachal Pradesh. It preferably bites the teats of cows and sheep and the lower parts of the legs of humans.

12.4.1.4 *Simulium (Simulium) indicum* Becher, 1885, Figure 12.4

Distribution: **India**: Himachal Pradesh, Kashmir, Manipur, Meghalaya, Nagaland, Sikkim, Uttar Pradesh, Uttarakhand, and West Bengal. The present author also found Simulium indicum specimens (two pupae) from the Mussoorie (Uttarakhand) area during October. **Elsewhere**: Afghanistan, Bangladesh, Bhutan, China (Tibet), Nepal, Myanmar, and Pakistan-occupied Kashmir (Balistan, Kashmir).

Species complex: The species *S.* (*S.*) *indicum* (Figure 12.4) is reported as a variable species. Cytological and molecular studies may prove that it comprises more than one species and that the species *S. kashmiricum* may be resurrected from synonymy as a valid species in future studies. It is generally believed that a wide geographical distribution of a species signals the presence of more than one species. The same may be true in the case of species *indicum*.

Bioecology: The *indicum* fly is a mountain and shade-loving species and is widespread in India. *S. indicum* is evidently a mountain and woodland species, ranging up to 3,000 m altitude but extending down to 900 m. Moreover, this species is comparable in many ways with the African subgenus *Lewisellum*, which includes *S. neavei* Roubaud, a vector of onchocerciasis (river blindness) in central Africa. The possibility of *S. indicum* being a potential vector of human onchocerciasis cannot be ruled out. Thus, the need for further investigation into its disease transmission becomes of paramount importance.

The fly *indicum* occurs from February to June, with the peak appearance of these flies during the dry season from April to June. It disappears during the rainy months. Herbal and synthetic repellents were evaluated for personal protection against blackfly bites.

Economic importance: The species *S.* (*S.*) *indicum* is primarily anthrophilic but also feeds on other mammals (zoophilic). The bites cause inflammation and scarring on the skin of tourists, field workers, and farmers. The fly can bite throughout the day inside forests or shaded locations. Generally, flies avoid sunny areas for biting. Biting by fly indicum just before dawn (1,820–1,830 hours) in Chilas in Pakistan-occupied Kashmir has been reported.

It is one of the notorious biting species in North-east India, especially in Arunachal Pradesh, Assam, Manipur, and Nagaland. Fly *indicum* has been noted as the most dominant species in Manipur and Nagaland while studying the biting behaviour of blackflies in North-east India; this

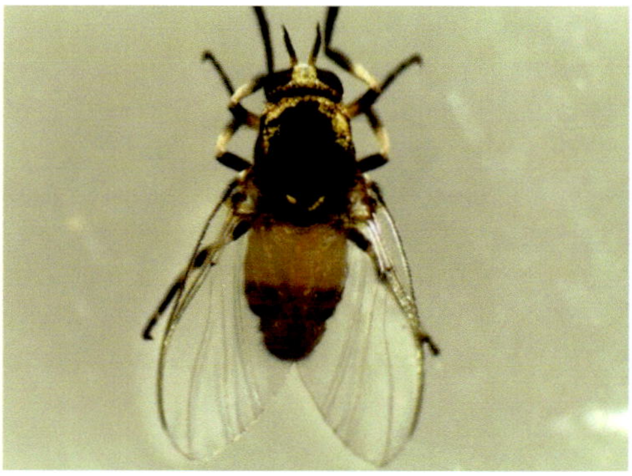

FIGURE 12.4 *Simulium indicum* female – a serious biting blackfly in India. It is more common in North-east India. (After Vijay Veer, 2022.)

study employed three baits: human volunteers, cows (*Bos taurus*), and sheep (*Ovis aries*). Cows and sheep are bitten more on those body parts where little or no pelage, wool, or fur is present, such as the eyes, teats, udder, and underbelly. However, teats were the most preferred by the flies.

There are various reports of biting on humans and animals by this pestiferous fly from Arunachal Pradesh, Assam, Himachal Pradesh, Kashmir, Manipur, Meghalaya, Nagaland, Uttar Pradesh (the hilly part now in Uttarakhand), and West Bengal (the Himalayan region).

The present author has also collected a large number of biting females of fly *indicum* from team members in October during midday hours (12:00–14:00 hours) at a roadside tea shop at Durga Mandir on the way to Tawang (NH-13) before Sessa village in Arunachal Pradesh. Several times, I was bitten on my hands by this fly during field visits to various parts of Arunachal Pradesh. Bites resulted in intense itching and scratching, muscle pain, and swelling in the bitten area of the hand the following day. A detailed study of the biology and disease transmission of fly *indicum* is urgently warranted in India due to its medical and veterinary importance.

12.4.1.5 *Simulium (Simulium) rufibasis* Brunetti, 1911

Distribution: **India**: Arunachal Pradesh, Himachal Pradesh, Manipur, Meghalaya, Sikkim, West Bengal (Darjeeling). **Elsewhere**: China, Japan, South Korea, Myanmar, Nepal, Pakistan, Taiwan, Thailand, Vietnam.

Bioecology: The fly *rufibasis* was found in moderate abundance while carrying out ecological studies on 16 species of blackflies in the Darjeeling area. Females laid eggs mostly in small upland streams, although a few ditches also harboured immature stages of this species. Females of *rufibasis* oviposited in shallow water on grass blades by the side of the watercourse; after selecting a spot, each female simultaneously settled down separately on the plant. Ultimately, they began to crawl to the parts of the plant just touching the water surface, where they laid eggs by dipping the tip of their abdomen into the water. They seldom oviposit on stones. Oviposition occurs in the late afternoon. Hibernation occurs in the egg stage. Larvae were absent from late October and appeared again in early March. The water temperature during hibernation was up to 6°C and was generally above 10°C when masses of eggs hatched. Three generations (trivoltine) occurred per year. Larvae and pupae were found to occur in rather slow watercourses having water currents of 0.3–0.5 m/s, and they attached themselves to decaying leaves, twigs, green grasses, or other leaves submerged in water.

In Korea, the larvae and pupae were mainly collected from moderate to fast-flowing streams with well-developed trailing grasses, leaves, and twigs, but large numbers were collected from the trailing grasses, leaves, and twigs in forest streams. Larvae were infrequently infected with unidentified microsporidian and *Coelomycidium simulii* fungus. Nine larval instars were identified for this species based on measurements of the head capsules of laboratory-reared individuals.

Economic importance: The species *rufibasis* is a multiple-host blood-feeding blackfly and is reported to bite and feed on the blood of humans, cows, and sheep in North-east India, as well as in Arunachal Pradesh and Assam. This species is known to feed on the blood of birds, horses, and humans in Japan. It is both mammalophilic and ornithophilic.

12.4.1.6 *Simulium (Simulium) striatum* Brunetti, 1912

Distribution: **India**: Andaman & Nicobar Islands, Arunachal Pradesh, Karnataka, Kerala, Maharashtra, Meghalaya, Tamil Nadu. **Elsewhere**: Bhutan, Sri Lanka.

Bioecology: The blackfly *striatum* is quite common and widespread in South India. The effect of hierarchical dynamics (spatio-temporal patterns) on the distribution of immatures in 24 streams of the Western Ghats in South India was studied by Anabalagan et al. (2018), and they found that species striatum is abundantly present (15.1%) and most frequently distributed (62.5%) among the 16 species of blackflies occurring in the study area.

Economic importance: It is a mammalophilic blackfly. It frequently bites humans in South India and Sri Lanka. This blackfly has also been reported for biting humans in Arunachal Pradesh.

12.4.2 Adults Biting Periodicity

Adult flies are exophilic and exophagic. The blood-feeding behaviour of blackflies is determined by type, and it is difficult to dislodge the fly once blood sucking has started until it is fully engorged. Fly orientation during blood feeding may be parallel or at an angle of 45°–60° to the host's skin and may also extrude diuretic fluid from the anus, as found in other blood-sucking insects like Anopheles mosquitoes. This is a mechanism for rapidly concentrating the blood meal. During field studies on simuliids in Arunachal Pradesh, India, the author experienced that the bites of S. indicum are painless, and the fly may remain adhered to the host's skin for up to 2–5 minutes. Oozing blood from the biting sites is usual after the fly leaves, and a haemorrhagic spot develops, with pain and itching lasting for about a month.

They feed abundantly during the day, especially on sunny days. Their biting activity starts after the sun rises above the horizon, but at mid-day, their activity is minimized. The flies are again active in the afternoon until twilight. Different species may have different biting periodicities, which may be unimodal or bimodal, and these may vary in the same species during different seasons and geographical locations. In India, the author has observed that *S. indicum* has a bimodal biting pattern in open areas but has a unimodal behaviour inside forested areas, with maximum biting occurring around 12:00–14:00 hours. *S. indicum* moves to shaded areas to avoid high temperatures outside in the open. It is also observed that during the winter months, blackflies in lowland areas of Arunachal Pradesh have one biting peak around 11:00–14:00 hours.

The posture preference of simuliids was studied by offering human subjects in standing, sitting, and lying positions in Arunachal Pradesh. It was found that blackflies are mostly attracted to the sitting position (56.8%), followed by standing (42.6%) and lying positions (0.6%).

Visual stimuli of simuliid flies play the most important role in locating hosts for their blood meals. Simuliids are known to be positively phototropic insects. It is also known that colour plays an important role in the selection of the host for biting. Simuliids are more attracted to dark colours than light colours, and it is suggested to avoid wearing dark blue clothing, particularly as this colour attracts the most. Popular notions indicate that some people are more attractive to blackflies than others, and these differences may be accounted for by individual production rates of breath CO_2.

The study revealed the greatest collection on black garments, followed by red; the lowest being on yellow. It has been concluded that the attractiveness of simuliids to colour decreases with increased reflectivity, that is, black < red < green < olive green < white < yellow.

12.4.3 Host Location and Blood Feeding

Females of some species of blackflies may actively search for hosts, whereas other species may wait until hosts come within range of detection and adopt a sit-and-wait strategy. They appear in small groups after a gap of 10–15 minutes. Host location and subsequent feeding involve a series of steps in which habitat features and host-specific attributes play a role in host selection. Flies use a combination of physical, visual, olfactory, and thermal cues to locate their hosts. Once a fly approaches a host, it uses the host's CO2 emissions, colour, and body movements as the most important factors that keep swarming females in close proximity until landing cues are received. The fly is ultimately attracted to specific parts of the host's body based on stimuli such as light, temperature, humidity, skin and hair/feather colour and texture, and odours from whole blood. The fly uses various host-derived volatile chemicals to locate its host and preferred body part for feeding. Gravid females detect oviposition pheromones by using odour receptors on their antennae, as well as contact chemoreceptors on their tarsi, mouthparts, and antennae. These chemicals are identified in the host's breath and body odour. These chemicals are a kind of kairomone, as the receiving individuals of different species (flies) benefit. The kairomones include CO2, acetophenone, decanal, hexanal, hexanoic acid, nonanoic acid, octanoic acid, 1-octen-3-ol, and 1-octonol, which are broadly attractive to *S. ochraceum s.l.* and *S. damnosum s.l.*, vectors of onchocerciasis. These studies are helpful for developing broad-based attractant baits for blackfly trapping. These traps replace the standard practice of human landing collection to monitor the effectiveness of vector populations in various control programmes. Such traps may also be used for the mass trapping and killing of flies to reduce the vector population and, in turn, aid in disease control.

Blood from fresh wounds attracts more females to wound areas and stimulates biting behaviour in others. This may be due to phagostimulants, such as adenosine phosphate (ATP), occurring in the blood. Blackflies attack all exposed human body parts, such as near the eyes, ears, nostrils, wrists, arms, and legs, with a preference for the legs and hands of humans in India. In contrast, flies prefer to feed on teats, udders, mouths, and areas near the eyes in cattle. Blackflies are mostly diurnal and outdoor biters; however, there are some crepuscular and nocturnal biting species as well. Many species feed indiscriminately on both avian and mammalian hosts, suggesting they may be opportunistic feeders. Smith (1973) stated that the feeding of blackflies on humans is an incidental form of feeding by species that are widely zoophilic, and no species is exclusively anthropophilic.

Female flies, upon landing on a host, crawl and probe for some time before biting, unlike mosquitoes, which bite rapidly after settling. After settling, the fly pulls out its labella and small teeth, along with spines at the apex of the labrum and hypopharynx. The bite is accomplished by first stretching the skin using the teeth on the apex of the labrum for easy laceration of the skin through a snipping action with the maxillae and mandibles, rupturing fine capillaries to allow the labrum, hypopharynx, and laciniae to enter the wound. The laciniae enable the fly to anchor the wound with the help of its backwardly directed teeth. During biting, the laceration of the host's skin by the fly's mouthparts results in the formation of a reservoir of oozing blood, which the fly imbibes. Their bites are shallow, and they are pool feeders (telmophagous), unlike mosquitoes, which feed directly on blood from capillaries (solenophagous). Feeding is facilitated by a powerful anticoagulant in the flies' saliva, which also partially numbs the site of the bite, reducing the host's awareness of being bitten and thus extending the flies' feeding time. The mandibles, maxillae, and hypopharynx penetrate the host's tissue to a depth of 120–150 µm. Blood is imbibed through a food channel enclosed interiorly by the labrum and posteriorly by the anterior one of the paired overlapping mandibles. At this point, the fly may transmit any pathogen that it carries and, in turn, may pick up pathogens from its host's peripheral blood. Ingested blood is stored in the midgut.

Blood-feeding dipterans have developed an extraordinary array of pharmacologically active salivary proteins to overcome hosts' haemostatic barriers, cause maximum and prolonged vasodilation of peripheral blood vessels, and suppress inflammatory and immunological reactions. Blackflies introduce secretions into the feeding lesion that act in a coordinated manner on three arms of the vertebrate haemostatic system, including platelet aggregation, coagulation, and vasoconstriction. Saliva contains various components that act as local anaesthetics, vasodilator enhancers, and anti-platelet aggregation agents (with high apyrase activity) as well as anti-blood coagulation factors. These help the fly to stop the host's immune system response while it is feeding. The saliva of blackflies contains anti-thrombotic, anti-coagulant, and immunomodulating effects (suppressing serum IL-6, IL-10, and tumour necrosis factor) and induces anaphylaxis and acute cardiotoxicity. The bite can also cause a systemic reaction (*blackfly fever*) that precipitates headaches, fever, nausea, vomiting, malaise, and generalized lymphadenopathy. This systemic vasculitis is known as Kawasaki disease (KD). Active substances released at the site of the bite include histamine, leukotrienes, prostaglandins, anti-platelet-activating factors, and eosinophilic chemotactic factors. A potent anticoagulant molecule in the saliva of blackflies has been identified as simukunin, which preferentially inhibits Factor Xa and also inhibits other enzymes, such as elastase and cathepsin G. This further suggests that the simukunin protein may modulate inflammation, which could potentially affect pathogen transmission.

12.5 PUBLIC HEALTH IMPORTANCE

The importance of blackflies to humans is largely due to their nuisance problem, biting habit, and disease transmission. About 1.5% of all species are vectors of human diseases. Of the nine simuliid-borne animal diseases, only two, mansonellosis and onchocerciasis, afflict humans. Onchocerciasis is a debilitating disease infecting an estimated 37 million people in Africa, Latin America, and Yemen, whereas mansonellosis is a mild disease in the Neotropics.

12.5.1 Swarming Nuisance

Simuliid adults create a nuisance by persistently flying around a person and often entering the eyes, ears, nose, and even mouth while walking, and crawling on the skin. Fly nuisance forces a person to leave the area. Some flies may also bite when they land on the body, depending on the species. Several non-biting species even form swarms or fly in clouds, which can make outdoor activities unpleasant and intolerable, especially in the wetter parts of North-east India from late April to July when blackfly populations swell. This becomes a nuisance to humans engaging in common outdoor activities such as gardening, boating, camping, and backpacking.

12.5.2 Biting and Allergic Reaction

Female blackflies are determined feeders, not easily interrupted while feeding, and will not leave until they consume their own weight in the host's blood or are satiated. Feeding in most species lasts for about 3–6 minutes and involves taking 5–10 mg of blood, depending on the species. A female fly may live for up to a month. Blackflies exhibit a wide variation in host selection. It has been observed that bites from anthropophilic species are usually painless to humans, compared to the bites of zoophilic species. This difference may be due to the presence of powerful anaesthetic molecules in the saliva of human-biting species or due to the biochemical differences in the saliva of these flies.

In blackfly-infested areas, dermatitis or simuliosis is a common problem in humans and animals. It is characterized by clinical features such as intense itching, which accompanies the repetitive eruption of papules and vesicles, resulting in excoriations, scarring, and permanent hyperpigmentation, leading to disfigurement of the skin. A histopathological study of dermatitis from Northeast India revealed the characteristic features of the *Simulium* bite reaction, such as vesicles filled with serous fluid, dermal oedema, and perivascular infiltrates rich in eosinophils and lymphocytes. The clinical manifestations and severity of *Simulium* dermatitis are serious concerns for hypersensitive persons, although variable clinical forms have been described (oedematous, erythematous, erysipeloid, inflammatory-indurative, phlegmonoid, and haemorrhagic). Insect bite hypersensitivity represents an immunoglobulin E (IgE)-mediated hypersensitivity to salivary antigens, and severe reactions are quite rare. The severity of *Simulium* dermatitis in hypersensitive persons is an important concern for daily practice, as the risk of anaphylaxis and acute cardiotoxicity exists, although this is unusual.

12.5.3 Human Onchocerciasis or River Blindness

Human onchocerciasis (Figure 12.5) was a severe public health problem, responsible for blindness and visual impairment, debilitating skin disease, and relentless itching in millions of people. The disease had serious socio-economic consequences, including depopulation of fertile river valleys and reduced productivity of affected persons. It is caused by the parasite *Onchocerca volvulus* (Leuckart) (Nematoda: Kinetoplastida: Onchocercidae). Symptoms of the disease include severe itching, small papules (dermatitis), various skin changes, visual impairment, and blindness. It is caused by the migrating progeny of microfilariae of the *O. volvulus* parasite in subcutaneous tissues and induces intense inflammatory responses upon their death. Microfilariae are released by

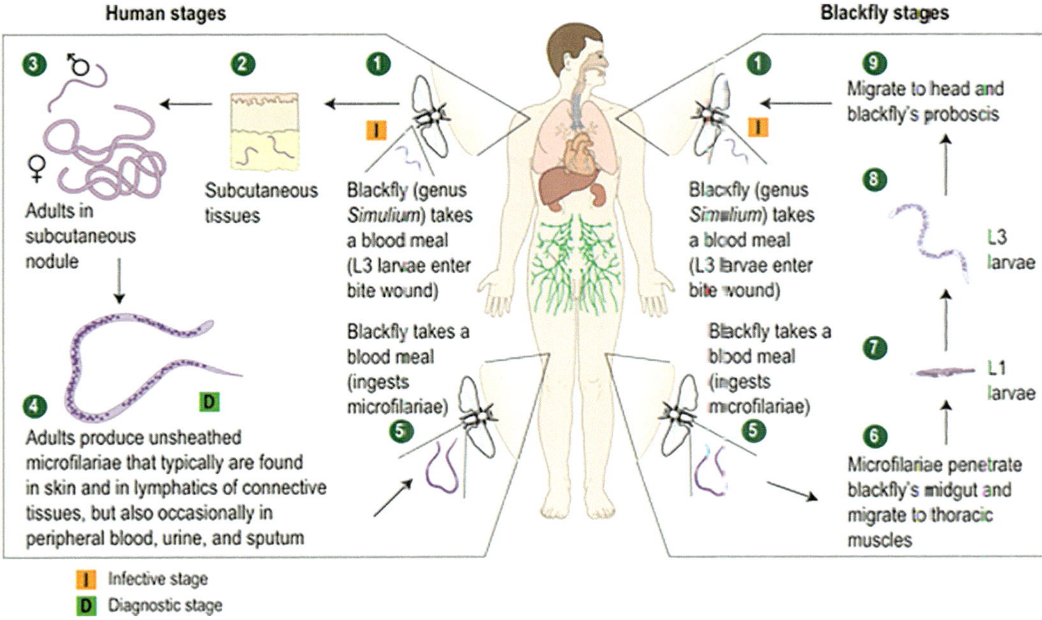

FIGURE 12.5 Life cycle of *Onchocerca volvulus*. (Adapted from the Centre for Disease Control and Prevention DPDx.)

adult females residing in subcutaneous nodules (also known as onchocercomata). Individuals with onchocerciasis can have several hundred nodules on their skin. The nodules vary in size, with some measuring up to 15 cm in diameter. They can cause discomfort but are usually not painful. Onchocerciasis is affecting 37 million people living in 38 countries. Of these, 4 million have skin manifestations, and 2 million are blind or severely visually impaired. This accounts for an estimated global loss of 1 million disability-adjusted life years. The affected countries include Angola, Benin, Burkina Faso, Burundi, Cameroon, Central African Republic, Chad, Republic of Congo, Côte d'Ivoire, Democratic Republic of the Congo, Equatorial Guinea, Ethiopia, Gabon, Ghana, Guinea, Guinea-Bissau, Kenya, Liberia, Malawi, Mali, Mozambique, Niger, Nigeria, Rwanda, Senegal, Sierra Leone, South Sudan, Sudan, Togo, Uganda, and the United Republic of Tanzania. Onchocerciasis is transmitted in six South American countries (Brazil, Colombia, Ecuador, Guatemala, Mexico, and the Bolivarian Republic of Venezuela) and also occurs in pockets in Yemen. Onchocerciasis was probably introduced during the slave trade, as it has a patchy distribution in South American countries. In Latin American countries, the disease has been eliminated in most affected countries, except for Brazil and Venezuela, where the Yanomami people still need treatment.

The parasite *O. volvulus* completes its entire life cycle in two hosts: humans and blackflies of the genus *Simulium*; the latter is its obligatory vector. Humans are its definitive hosts, as they represent the dead end for blood-circulating microfilariae of the parasite unless they are ingested along with a blood meal by the intermediate host or vector fly for further development into infective microfilariae (L3 stage), which can then be passed on by the intermediate host (blackfly) to another person during successive bites. Thus, a fly acts inadvertently as the transmitting agent or vector of the parasite.

When a blackfly bites an infected person and ingests the blood meal, microfilariae (220–360 μm long) penetrate the gut wall of the fly and make their way to the thoracic muscles, where they lose their motility and transform into first-stage larvae, which then moult into second-stage larvae and then into third-stage larvae. The third-stage larva is the infective stage and migrates to the fly's head and mouthparts for transmission to another individual (Figure 12.6). The entire development

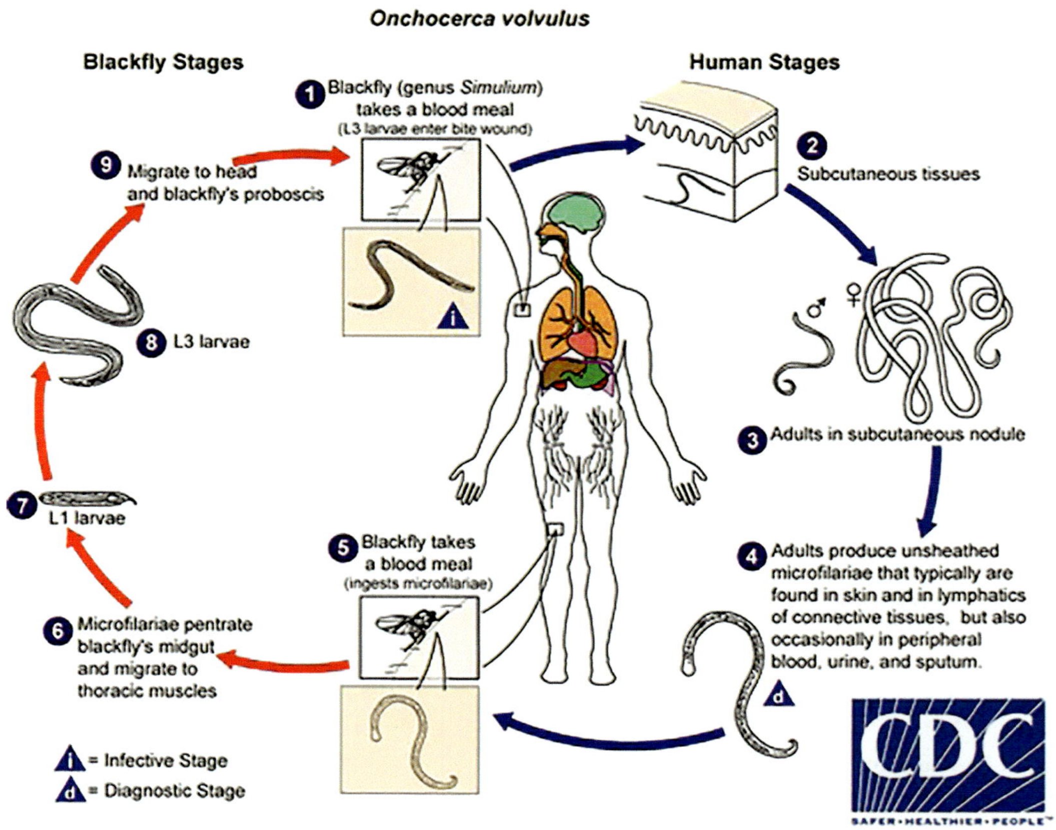

FIGURE 12.6 Migration route of ingested microfilariae (mf) to the thorax to develop into the infective stage (L3) before migrating to the mouthparts for infection. Inset showing cibarium without (a) and with (a) and with (b) cibarial armature.

of the parasite in the fly takes about 6–12 days, depending on the ambient temperature and vector species. For successful transmission, the blackfly requires successive blood meals, which it takes after 3–5 days from an earlier blood meal. Thus, the blackfly may be successful in pathogen transmission only after the third meal and when the fly is 8–10 days old. A female blackfly usually lives for up to 30 days.

The infective microfilariae (L_3), after invading the human skin, disperse from the site of the bite into the subcutaneous tissues of the human body and develop into fourth-stage and then mature worms within 12–18 months, becoming ready for reproduction. The adult worms are mostly encapsulated in fibrous cellular nodules of varying sizes, from 0.5 to 10 cm, which are produced in response to the body's defence mechanism to isolate the parasites and cause no inflammation or great discomfort to the host. These nodules can form in subcutaneous tissues or deep in connective tissues. The adult worm's body is white, and its surface has closely arranged annular ridges. The female worm is large, measuring 30–80 cm long, while the male worm is smaller, at 19–42 mm long, and entwined in the nodules. Mating and reproduction occur inside the nodules. The adult female worm produces large numbers (about a thousand) of tiny microfilariae daily, which migrate to the skin, eyes, and various other organs of the human host. Microfilariae present in the skin can be acquired by the blackfly while blood-feeding. Onchocerciasis can also be diagnosed by the presence of hundreds of microfilariae in skin snips. As a female worm can live for 12–14 years and continuously produce microfilariae, an infected person may have microfilariae for a long period for transmission. Microfilariae can live for 1–2 years.

12.5.3.1 Skin Disease

The manifestation of skin disease depends on the load of microfilariae in infected individuals. In cases of low transmission, the disease may be asymptomatic, but over several years, a heavy load of microfilariae can produce the most severe aspects of the disease, such as intense itching, skin rashes, swelling, inflammation, dermal lesions, nodules, patches of depigmentation ("leopard skin"), leathery skin (lizard skin), loss of skin elasticity, fibrosis coupled with lymphatic reactions, and ocular problems. Heavy infestation of microfilariae in the dermis, in addition to intolerable itching, also leads to bleeding, secondary bacterial infections, loss of sleep, fever, headache, and even suicidal thoughts. In Yemen, the itching symptoms of the disease are commonly known as *sowda*. The lymphatic nodes are also affected by the microfilariae, especially in the groin and thigh regions, leading to hanging groin.

12.5.3.2 Eye Blindness

The eye disease gives onchocerciasis its common name – river blindness. The eye problems are the most severe manifestation of the disease. Invasion of microfilariae into the eyes leads to ocular pathology, affecting all tissues of the eye. Ocular problems are associated with the presence of both live and dead microfilariae, causing an inflammatory response. This results in cataracts, retinal haemorrhages, corneal opacities, secondary glaucoma, sclerosing keratitis, and optic neuritis. Thus, various forms of visual impairment occur, such as night blindness and reduction in peripheral vision, with the most severe consequence being irreversible blindness with complete loss of light perception. Ophthalmic signs often appear several years after the infection, and blindness usually takes several years to occur. That is why it is rarer in young infected persons than in older persons aged 50 years and above, when half of the infected victims may be blind. Long-term inflammation of the cornea, or keratitis, leads to thickening of the corneal stroma, ultimately resulting in blindness. The prevalence of blindness is highest in the savannahs of West Africa, with some villages experiencing rates as high as 10%–15% blindness, where up to 100% of adults are infected. The socioeconomic effects of the disease are often far-reaching, destabilizing communities and causing the abandonment of entire villages. Recent studies on onchocerciasis revealed that the major inflammatory response in the cornea is caused by an intracellular endosymbiotic bacterium (*Wolbachia* sp.) harboured in *Onchocerca volvulus*, which suggests that antibiotic treatments might prevent ocular damage. *Wolbachia* bacteria are released after the death of the microfilariae, which triggers the immunogenic response. The inflammatory response to dying filarial microfilariae in the skin and eyes, and the release of their bacterial endosymbiotic *Wolbachia*, is the basis of onchocercal dermatitis and ocular keratitis (*river blindness*) immunopathology. These endobacteria play an important role in the development, viability, and fertility of the filarial Onchocerca volvulus and in the pathogenesis of filariasis.

In Africa, the savannah strain with moderate parasite burdens of *O. volvulus* is more likely to cause ocular disease, while the rainforest strain, despite high parasitic loads, is not responsible for causing blindness. The prevalence of ocular disease due to the savannah strains has been correlated with higher quantities of *Wolbachia* DNA, as determined by PCR probes.

12.5.3.3 Symptoms

An infected person may be asymptomatic, with approximately 10% of infected persons completely without symptoms. Symptoms may usually consist of one or more of the following three manifestations: skin rash, subcutaneous nodules under the skin, and eye lesions.

a. **Early symptoms**: The first signs that a person has been infected with the *O. volvulus* parasite include fever, neuralgic pain in the joints, and temporary hives on the trunk and face.
b. **Dermatological symptoms**: The two main symptoms of onchocerciasis that involve the skin are onchocercal dermatitis and onchocercomas.
   i **Onchoceral dermatitis** is the most common symptom of the disease. The condition can appear anywhere on the body and includes alterations in skin pigmentation, scratching, and itching. The pattern of itching can vary from intermittent to constant, depending on the individual. A rash consisting of patches of papules can appear on the body at any time and often leads to incessant scratching. In West Africa, this condition is known as craw-craw.
   ii **Onchocercomas** are subcutaneous, fibrous nodules where adult worms dwell and breed. These nodules are most easily felt when they form over a bony part of the body. Deep nodules around the groin region can be harder to detect, but identifying every nodule is important for the appropriate treatment of the disease. Having more nodules does not necessarily indicate a more severe microfilarial load. The location of the nodules on the body depends on the site of the fly bite, which varies by region. In the Americas, nodules are found mostly on the upper body, particularly in the head and neck region, in contrast to Africa, where nodules are mostly located on the lower body, especially in the groin region.

12.5.3.4 Diagnosis

The diagnosis of onchocerciasis can be difficult in light infections, which are more common in persons who have travelled to but are not residents of affected areas. There are multiple ways through which the diagnosis can be made. The most common method is a skin biopsy to identify larvae, which emerge from the skin when placed in physiological solutions (e.g. normal saline). Typically, six snips are taken from different areas of the body. Polymerase chain reaction (PCR, using the O-150 PCR technique) of the skin should be performed for diagnosis if the larvae are not visualized.

12.5.3.5 Socio-Cultural Impact

Onchocercal skin disease has a significant adverse socio-cultural impact on society. People with the disease often experience low self-esteem, social isolation, and a worry that they will never marry. Children are distracted in school due to constant itching. The socioeconomic importance of the disease was the main reason for the creation of the Onchocerciasis Control Programme in West Africa (OCP) in 1974. Blindness affected up to 50% of adults in some areas of the West African savannah, leading people to abandon fertile river valleys in fear of contracting the disease. Poverty and famine increased. In the 1970s, economic losses were estimated at US$30 million, and onchocerciasis became a major obstacle to socioeconomic development.

12.5.3.6 Onchocerciasis-Associated Epilepsy

Onchocerciasis-associated epilepsy was reported in previously healthy children between the ages of 5 and 18 years from all the regions where onchocerciasis (river blindness) is endemic and poorly controlled, such as Uganda, Tanzania, Cameroon, and the Democratic Republic of the Congo. A high prevalence and incidence of epilepsy have been reported in areas with significant onchocerciasis transmission. This syndrome is characterized by head-nodding, an atonic seizure, and is often followed by tonic–clonic seizures (also called grand mal seizures), declining cognitive and motor function, psychiatric problems, stunted growth, physical deformities, and early death. Until recently, the cause of the syndrome was unknown. Therefore, no strategy for prevention or cure was possible.

12.5.3.7 Vector Species of Human Onchocerciasis

There are at least 25 species of *Simulium* known as vectors of onchocerciasis. Previously, *S. damnosum* was considered the main vector of the disease in Africa. However, the *Simulium damnosum* sensu lato species complex is now known to consist of several cytoforms, making it the largest sibling complex of any vector. These cytoforms differ in their ecologies and vectorial roles, and at least 63 cytoforms are recognized. Some cytotypes are probably cytospecies or sibling species, while others are likely geographical races. *S. damnosum s.l.* is responsible for more than 95% of onchocerciasis cases globally. These cytoforms are sibling species that are morphologically similar but represent reproductively isolated populations. Many cytoforms are now designated as valid species, thanks to morpho-cyto-molecular studies. There are currently 33 important vectors of onchocerciasis recognized. The principal vectors in West Africa are *S. damnosum s.s.* and *S. sirbanum*, which are more widespread and common in savannah zones and are capable of long-distance migration; *S. sanctipauli*, *S. soubrense*, and *S. yahense* are mostly found in forests, while *S. squamosum* occurs in highland areas. Currently, the *damnosum* species complex contains 17 cytotypes and six morphospecies. In Central and East Africa, the principal vectors of the disease are members of *Simulium neavei* and *S. albivirgulatum*. The larvae and pupae of *Simulium neavei* live in a phoretic association with freshwater crabs. In Central and South America, at least nine species or complexes are vectors of the disease. The important vector species include *Simulium exiguum*, *S. limbatum*, *S. incrustatum*, *S. guianense*, *S. metallicum*, *S. ochraceum*, and *S. oyapockense*.

12.5.3.8 Human Onchocerciasis in the Oriental Region?

So far, there is no report of human onchocerciasis transmission from the Oriental region despite the prevalence of man-biting blackflies. The parasite *Onchocerca volvulus* and human onchocerciasis do not occur naturally in this region, perhaps because the environment and vectors are not suitable for the pathogen. It is reported that Japanese parasitologists contracted onchocerciasis while studying this disease in endemic areas during their mission. Perhaps human onchocerciasis has been introduced and established in South America through the slave trade. However, onchocerciasis has also been introduced in the USA several times but has been unable to establish there in the absence of appropriate vector species. There are several case reports of human infection with zoonotic onchocerciasis from Albania, Austria, Canada, Crimea, Hungary, Kuwait, Japan, Switzerland, Turkey, and the USA, which suggest that some species of zoonotic *Onchocerca* spp. can be potential causative agents of zoonotic onchocerciasis in humans as well.

In India, so far there is no report of worm isolation from blackflies, including two common man-biting species, *S. indicum* and *S. nodosum*. However, worms were isolated from *S. nodosum* in northern Thailand. *S. indicum* is regarded as a potential vector of onchocerciasis, and it has been opined that some infected people from Africa or tropical America may bring *Onchocerca volvulus* infection to India. The present author shares this opinion because, in addition to foreign travellers, a good number of Indians are currently visiting those countries where onchocerciasis is prevalent. Thus, the possibility of the invasion of this disease in the near future in India cannot be ruled out. Recently, an indigenous case of ocular onchocerciasis was reported from Assam, which marks the first record in India. However, this case is under debate and requires a thorough study in North-east India for the detection and confirmation of *Onchocerca volvulus* in humans as well as in *Simulium* species. In view of the above facts, it is urgently required to carry out studies on the prevalence of onchocerciasis and its vectors prior to its possible establishment in North-east India. Such a study will be helpful to combat onchocerciasis if it were to be established in India in the future.

12.5.4 Mansonellosis

Mansonellosis is caused by three filarial nematode species, *Mansonella perstans*, *M. streptocerca*, and *M. ozzardi*, in humans. Biting midges of the genus *Culicoides* can transmit all three species effectively, while blackflies transmit *Mansonella ozzardi* only in South America and Panama. It is transmitted by several species of blackflies in the rainforests of Northern South America and Panama. These include the *Simulium amazonicum* complex, *S. argentiscutum*, and *S. sanguineum*, reported in endemic sites of Colombia; *S. amazonicum*, *S. argentiscutum*, and *S. oyapockense* have been implicated as the main vectors in the Amazon Basin of Brazil; *S. sanchezi* in Venezuela; *S. sanguineum* in Panama; and *S. minusculum* in Guyana.

Human infection with *M. ozzardi* (Figure 12.7) is highly prevalent in some of the Caribbean islands, among riverine communities in the Amazon Basin, and on both sides of the border between Bolivia and Argentina. The prevalence of *M. ozzardi* in Brazil is very high; about 44–52% of Brazilian farmers are infected with it. It is also prevalent among the American Indian population. The disease is asymptomatic. *M. ozzardi* may cause symptoms that include skin rashes, headaches, fever, pruritus, lymphoedema (swelling of the arms or legs), and joint pain. Recently, ocular manifestations (especially keratitis) have been associated with mansonellosis, opening an important area of investigation.

The life cycle of *M. ozzardi* is similar to that of *O. volvulus* in blackflies. Adults of *M. ozzardi* occur in the subcutaneous tissue of humans, and the microfilariae are found in the peripheral

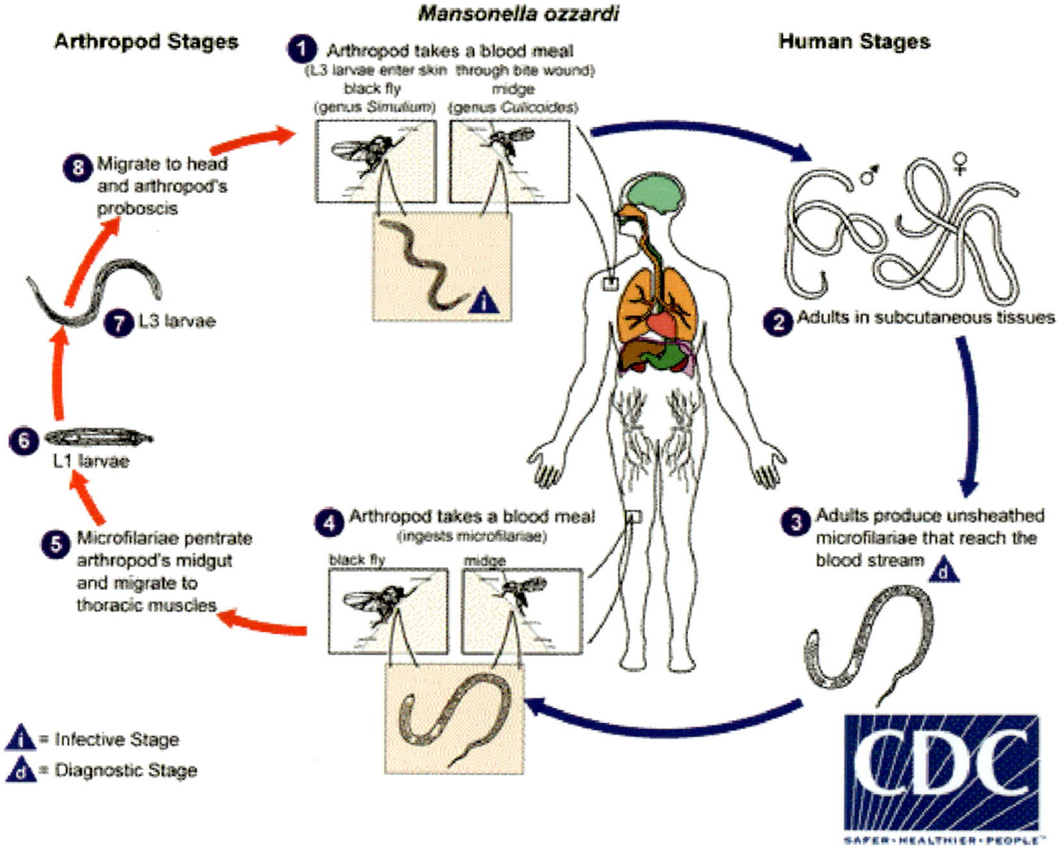

FIGURE 12.7 Life cycle of *Mansonella ozzardi* nematode parasite in man and blackfly. (Adopted from CDC).

blood, from where they are acquired by the blood-feeding females that transfer third-stage filarial larvae onto the skin of another person during subsequent blood meals. They develop into adults that commonly reside in subcutaneous tissues. Adults produce unsheathed and non-periodic microfilariae that enter the bloodstream. The microfilariae, after ingestion during a blood meal, migrate from the arthropod's midgut through the hemocoel to the thoracic muscles. There, the microfilariae develop into first-stage larvae and subsequently into third-stage infective larvae, which migrate to the arthropod's proboscis and can infect another human when the arthropod takes a blood meal.

12.6 VETERINARY IMPORTANCE/ZOONOTIC DISEASES

Blackflies are of veterinary importance, as they transmit pathogens and cause biting nuisance and swarming. Flies harm poultry, swine, cattle, horses, mules, sheep, goats, dogs, deer, and wild animals. They transmit several diseases to animals, such as leucocytozoonosis (avian malaria) in poultry, animal onchocerciasis, animal trypanosomiasis, and myxomatosis in rabbits. Persistent attacks by flies cause unruly host behaviour, weight loss, reduced egg and milk production, malnutrition in young animals, dermatitis and epidermal necrosis, impotence, delayed pregnancy, and stress-related diseases. Ornithophilic blackflies attacking birds make them agitated and exhausted in their attempts to escape. Flies feed on body parts where feathers are absent, including the eyelids, cere, corners of the beak, neck, underwings, and auricular openings. Sometimes, flies kill nestlings.

12.6.1 Leucocytozoonosis

Ornithophilic blackflies transmit leucocytozoonosis, a malaria-like disease caused by protozoan species of the genus *Leucocytozoon* (Apicomplexa: Plasmodiidae) in poultry, especially ducks, geese, and turkeys in North America. Blackflies are the vectors of 12 species of *Leucocytozoon* out of 100 known species. Turkeys are affected by *L. smithi*, with its primary vectors being *S. meridionale* and *S. slossonae*. Ducks and geese are parasitised by *L. simondi*, whose primary vectors are *Cnephia ornithophilia*, *S. anatinum*, and *S. rugglesi*. Infections with *Leucocytozoon* spp. are most often subclinical but can occasionally cause clinical and even fatal disease. Mortality varies greatly with the strain of parasite, species, degree of exposure, age, immune status, and other factors. Outbreaks of leucocytozoonosis have been reported in chickens (Asia, Africa), turkeys (North America), waterfowl (North America, Europe, Asia), and a number of free-living and captive avian species throughout the world. In the past, disease outbreaks occurred in the poultry industry in North America, causing the death of entire flocks and the shutdown of production facilities in South Carolina and Manitoba. Birds with chronic infections developed depressed immune systems and decreased reproductive capacity. Infections can lead to emaciation, dehydration, and convulsions that may result in death. Mortality in birds can range from 5% to 100%. However, to date, the transmission of leucocytozoonosis by blackflies has not been studied in India, though the disease is quite common in chickens in this region.

The parasite, *Leucocytozoon* species, undergoes a malaria-like life cycle involving two hosts: the blackfly and the bird. Female blackflies acquire gametocytes of the parasite along with the blood of an infected bird. The parasite then undergoes sexual and asexual development in the fly over 3–4 days. The infected fly transmits the parasites as sporozoites to another healthy bird for further asexual and gametocyte formation.

12.6.2 Zoonotic Onchocerciasis

Blackflies also transmit *Onchocerca* parasites among both bovines and non-bovine animals and cause zoonotic onchocerciasis in domesticated animals almost worldwide. At least eight species of *Onchocerca* are transmitted by blackflies. Infected animals show dermatitis and inflammation of the skin and connective tissues; though the impact of parasites is not very high, the infection rate is quite significant in animals. A high rate of parasite infection could pose a threat to meat-producing animals and cause economic losses to the meat and dairy industries. In Asia, zoonotic onchocerciasis associated with blackflies has been reported from Japan and Thailand. Seven species of blackflies are identified as natural and experimental vectors of six *Onchocerca* species in Japan. *Simulium bidentatum* is a natural vector of *O. dewittei japonica*, a parasite of wild boar, and has been reported to infect humans in Japan. Three species of blackfly, *S. nodosum*, *S. asakoae*, and *S. nigrogilvum*, which feed on water buffaloes and humans, are implicated as vectors of three unidentified filarial species in Thailand. The fly *S. nodosum* also occurs in India. In India, three species – *Onchocerca armillata*, *O. gutturosa*, and *O. gibsoni* – are common filarial parasites; however, no blackfly species has been reported as a vector so far. Therefore, a detailed blackfly survey for the isolation of parasites is required to establish the blackfly–parasite relationship in this region.

Elsewhere in the world, *Onchocerca lienalis* is the most widespread parasite in cattle and is vectored by *S. jeningsi* in the USA and the *S. ornatum* complex in the Palearctic region. The microfilariae of *O. lienalis* are concentrated in the umbilical region of the host, from where they are picked up by the blackfly during blood feeding, ingested, and developed to the third stage in the fly's muscles, which are then transmitted to another animal during subsequent blood feeding. Another species of parasite, *O. gutturosa*, common in the Palearctic region, has its microfilariae found in the skin of the neck and back of cattle and is transmitted by *S. erythrocephalum* in Ukraine. In Africa, *O. ochengi* is transmitted to cattle by the *S. damnosum* species complex, and *O. dukei* is transmitted by *S. bovis*. Both species of parasites produce nodules. In non-bovine hosts, *O. cervipedis* in North America and *O. tarsicola* in Europe infect the connective tissues of the legs of deer and moose. Therefore, sometimes this disease is referred to as leg worms. *O. ramachandrini* is a parasite of warthogs and is transmitted by members of the *S. damnosum* species complex in West Africa.

Another important and emerging parasite, *Onchocerca lupi*, was originally isolated from the eye of a wolf in 1967 in Russia. It has come into focus as several sporadic cases of ocular infection, specifically subconjunctival onchocerciasis in dogs, have been reported from the USA and Europe. Recently, more than six human infections with *Onchocerca lupi* have been reported from Europe, the USA, Iran, Turkey, and Tunisia, causing infections in subconjunctival, orbital, spinal, and subdermal regions. *O. lupi* causes ocular, dermatological, or neurological disease. It is transmitted by *S. tribulatum* in California. The vector fly in other locations is not known. Infection in humans with zoonotic parasites is accidental and transmitted through the bites of those flies, which feed on both animals and humans. The symptoms of zoonotic disease are mostly manifested as nodule formation, harbouring mature or immature worms. There is no further microfilariae production, but *O. lupi* can cause ocular infection in canines and humans. Studies on simuliid flies should be encouraged, considering their role as vectors of zoonotic *Onchocerca* spp. infecting humans and animals. Several of today's anthropogenic diseases, for example, TB and HIV, originally emerged from animals.

12.6.3 Vesicular Stomatitis (VSN)

The vesicular stomatitis virus is transmitted to livestock, cattle, horses, and pigs by blackflies. This virus is contagious and characterized by the formation of lesions in various epithelial tissues, especially in the mouth, which subsequently leads to a reduction in weight and milk production in affected animals. The New Jersey virus strain of vesicular stomatitis is the causative agent of epidemics of vesicular stomatitis, an economically important disease in the United States, as it affects cattle, horses, swine, and pigs, and is responsible for economic losses of millions of dollars. The virus has been isolated from biting flies and non-biting dipterans during outbreaks, suggesting that insects serve as both mechanical and biological vectors of VSN-NJ. Biological transmission of VSN NJ by blackflies to mice, domestic swine, and domestic cattle has been demonstrated.

12.6.4 Simuliotoxicosis

Blackflies cause simuliotoxicosis in animals, which is a diseased condition resulting from the toxic effects of bites from blackfly swarms. Many blackfly attacks have been massive and virulent, causing high morbidity and mortality in livestock and poultry. Deaths may be due to injected salivary constituents, which lead to acute toxemia, anaphylactic shock, or exsanguination (bleeding out). Cattle, especially calves, are highly susceptible to simuliotoxicosis. The blackfly, *S. (Simulium) colombaschense* (Scopoli), is considered the most destructive blackfly in history, as it was once responsible for killing as many as 22,000 livestock per year in the Danube River in Europe. In the northern hemisphere, vast areas are rendered nearly uninhabitable due to the biting rates. Recently, an avian simuliotoxicosis outbreak involving the fly *Simulium meridionale* occurred in Louisiana, USA, killing several captive psittacine (parrot family) birds, including macaws. Fly strikes caused necrosis, eosinophilic dermatitis, severe oedema, and vasculitis in the birds, with their deaths resulting from cardiopulmonary collapse and anaphylactoid reactions.

12.7 MANAGEMENT

The blood-feeding females are serious biting pests and obligate vectors of several vertebrate parasites and pathogens. This is amply emphasized in the preceding pages of this chapter. To manage blackfly-borne nuisance and disease, two main approaches are required: fly population control and treatment of disease with antiparasitic drugs. Blackfly control is difficult because the flies are day biters and their immature larvae live in running fresh waterways. The larvae, while remaining stationary on a substratum, filter food from flowing water and often form a large proportion of the benthic biomass in well-oxygenated sections of streams, rivers, waterfalls, and spillways. Therefore, immature stages of blackflies are preferably targeted in disease control programmes. Control practices largely depend on periodical treatment of streams and rivers with safe larvicides, along with environmental modification. The larvicide is applied to the breeding site, which is then carried downstream to kill the larvae.

The commonly used larvicides are either synthetic organophosphate insecticides or biological ones such as temephos (Abate®) and the bacterial larvicide (*Bacillus thuringiensis israelensis,* serotype H-14). However, any treatment effect is limited in duration because females of pest species are capable of flying long distances from other larval developmental sites and may soon re-infest the treated areas. Other measures include personal and area protection from the biting flies by using insect repellents and fine mesh netting material, which prevents contact between humans and blackflies, thus helping to interrupt the transmission of parasite microfilariae to hosts.

For the treatment of onchocerciasis, the drug ivermectin (Mectizen®) has been successfully used in mass treatment since 1987. It is quite safe and, unlike previous treatments with DEC, which had serious side effects including patient death,ivermectin gradually kills or paralyser the microfilariae of the parasite *O. volvulus* in infected persons. Treatment with ivermectin relieves intense skin itching and halts the progression of blindness. It does not kill the adult female worm but suppresses its capacity to produce microfilariae. Ivermectin increases the permeability of the cell membranes of muscle and nerve cells of microfilariae to chloride ions by binding to glutamate-gated chloride ion channels. This results in hyperpolarization of the cell, leading to paralysis and death of the microfilariae. Ivermectin also disrupts GABA-mediated central nervous system (CNS) neurosynaptic transmission.

Under onchocerciasis control programmes, the affected countries have successfully employed a combined strategy of vector control and mass treatment with the antiparasitic drug ivermectin (annually or semi-annually) to interrupt onchocerciasis transmission. There are, however, some more recent developments in blackfly control that are effective and eco-friendly. The following multipronged approach against blackflies will be very effective in the protection and containment of the disease. This includes

1. Personal protection from fly bites
2. Larvae control
3. Mass trapping of adult blackflies
4. Biological control
5. Onchocerciasis treatment.

12.7.1 WHO Onchocerciasis Programs

The World Health Organization (WHO) has implemented various programmes since 1974 to control onchocerciasis by using insecticides for vector control and mass chemotherapy with the anti-helminthic drug ivermectin for parasite control, achieving success in the interruption of disease transmission. The first such programme was the Onchocerciasis Control Programme (OCP, 1975–2002) in 11 savannah countries of West Africa. Initially under OCP operations, aerial spraying of insecticide (temephos as a larvicide) was conducted over the breeding sites of blackflies to kill their larvae; later, in 1987, control operations were changed, and vector control was combined with ivermectin treatment (in the form of Mectizan tablets donated by Merck & Co., Inc.) or, in some areas, ivermectin treatment alone. In 1995, WHO launched another programme, the African Programme for Onchocerciasis Control (APOC), in 19 non-OCP African countries with endemic onchocerciasis. The principal strategy was the development of sustainable community-directed treatment with ivermectin (CDTI) for at least 15 years. However, CDTI has not halted the transmission of the parasite in highly endemic foci in Africa. Later, it was decided that all possible intervention tools, which are appropriate and cost-effective, should be used to interrupt disease transmission and not just ivermectin, including vector control. APOC was closed in 2015 but was replaced by another programme, the Expanded Special Projects for Elimination of Neglected Tropical Diseases (ESPEN), in 2016 to promote an integrated approach to controlling onchocerciasis along with four other high-burden neglected tropical diseases, including lymphatic filariasis, trachoma, schistosomiasis, and soil-transmitted helminthiases.

12.8 CONCLUSION

The biodiversity of Indian blackflies has not been thoroughly studied. To address this gap, it is crucial to conduct extensive and intensive surveys, particularly in the Western Himalayan and Aravali hill regions. India's unique temperate, subtropical, and tropical settings across diverse ecoregions present an excellent opportunity for such biodiversity studies. Blackflies are highly isomorphic. To distinguish them, a morpho-cyto-molecular approach is required. DNA sequence studies of 16S rRNA and ITS-1 have significantly advanced our understanding of blackfly biodiversity. Data collected from three mitochondrial genes (COI, ND4, and 16S rRNA) and two segments of the nuclear 28S ribosomal RNA (the D1 to D2 and the D4 expansion regions) have provided valuable insights into the identification and classification of pest species and species complexes. Therefore, intensive multi-gene molecular systematic studies are essential for a comprehensive understanding of genus taxonomy, phylogenetic relationships, and evolutionary history.

Research on the role of Indian blackflies in disease transmission to humans, domestic animals, and wildlife is urgently needed, as there is currently no information on their involvement in such processes. With diagnostic tools for onchocerciasis now available, it is crucial to initiate these investigations promptly to understand and mitigate potential health risks.

Research on the composition and isolation of pharmacologically active compounds from the saliva of blood-feeding blackflies could facilitate the development of new vasodilators and other drugs. Like other blood-sucking arthropods, blackflies have evolved effective mechanisms to inhibit haemostatic responses, such as blood clotting, platelet aggregation, and vasoconstriction in their vertebrate hosts. The saliva of blackflies contains a vast array of these pharmacologically active compounds, primarily proteins and peptides (sialotranscriptomes), which are responsible for their antihaemostatic effects and enable them to feed on blood. Understanding these compounds is particularly valuable, as platelet aggregation and vasoconstriction are crucial haemostatic responses, especially in small wounds.

The development of trapping devices for blackfly collection is essential to replace the common but criticized practice of human landing collection for monitoring fly populations. To create an effective trap, it is necessary to study the vision and chemical cues that attract blackflies. Research on semiochemicals will be particularly valuable in identifying suitable compounds that can serve as chemical cues for trap development. There is a need to develop suitable guidelines for the control of blackflies in India.

12.9 POINTS TO REMEMBER

1. Blackflies belong to the order Diptera, family Simuliidae, and are known by 76 species in seven genera from India and by 2,311 species in 30 genera worldwide.
2. They are biting pests and transmit various diseases of medical and veterinary importance.
3. They are the second most harmful group of insects after mosquitoes in affecting human health, as they transmit two important human diseases (onchocerciasis, or river blindness, in Central Africa, South America, and Yemen, and mansonellosis in South America and Panama).
4. Out of 76 known species, six species are serious biting pests in India and are popularly known as dim-dam flies in the north-east parts of the country. These are *Simulium*. (*Nevermania*) *aureohirtum*, *S.* (*Simulium*) *grisescens*, *S.* (*Simulium*) *himalayense*, *S.* (*Simulium*) *indicum*, *S.* (*Simulium*) *rufibasis,* and *S.* (*Simulium*) *striatum*. *S.* (*Simulium*) *indicum* is a serious human-biting blackfly in India
5. Larvae are aquatic, sessile, and live in flowing water, where they filter out their food with the help of two labral fans, thus helping to clean the water and playing an important role as ecological indicators.

Acknowledgements

I am highly thankful to all those authors and publishers for adopting figures and photos from their publications.

REFERENCES

Adler, P.H. (2005). Black flies, the Simuliidae. In W. C. Marquardt (ed.). *Biology of Disease Vectors*, 2nd edn. Elsevier, California, pp. 127–140.

Adler, P.H., & Crosskey, R.W. (2017). World blackflies (Diptera: Simuliidae): A comprehensive revision of the taxonomic and geographical inventory, www.clemson.edu/cafls/departments/esps/biomia/pdfs/blackflyinventory1.pdf

Crosskey, R.W. (1990). The *Natural History of Blackflies*. John Wiley & Sons, Chichester, pp. I-ix +711.

Dhiman, D., Hazarika, S., Rabha, B., Das, N.G., Bhola, R.K., Vijay, V., & Singh, L. (2014). Black fly (*Simulium sp.*) composition, daytime biting activity and possible onchocerciasis infection in north-east, India. *J. Environ. Biol.*, **35** (2): 421–425.

Golini, V. I., & Davies, D. M. (1975). Relative response to colored substrates by ovipositing blackflies (Diptera: Simuliidae). I. Oviposition by *Simulium* (*Simulium*) *verecundum* Stone and Jamnback. *Canad. J. Zool.* **53** (5): 521–535.

McGaha Jr, T.W., Young, R.M., Burkett-Cadena, N.D, Iburg, J.P., Beau, J.M., Hassan, S., Katholi, C R., Cupp, E.D., Baker, B.J., Unnasch, T.R., & Noblet, R. (2015). Identification of communal oviposition pheromones from the black Fly *Simulium vittatum*. *PLoS One,* **10** (3): e0118904.

Singh, H. R., & Bisht, B.S. (1988) Phoretic association between Simulium and Mayfly nymph in the river Bhagirathi. *Environ. Ecol.* **6** (2): 451–454.

Smith, K. G. V. (1973). *Insects and Other Arthropods of Medical Importance*. The Trustees of the British Museum (Natural History), London, pp. 109–153.

Stauder, A., & Kiel, E. (2004). New observations on phoretic associations of Simuliidae (Diptera) with Heptageniidae (Ephemeroptera) in India. *Acta Zool. Univ. Comen.* **46**(1): 15–21.

Takaoka, H., & Noda, S. (1979). Autogeny of the Black Fly *Simulium* (*Eusimulium*) *aureohirtum* (Diptera: Simuliidae), *J. Med. Entomol.* **15** (2):183–184.

Vijay, V. (2022). *Biology, Diagnosis and Management of Indian Pestiferous Blackflies. DRDO Monographs/ Special publications Series.* Defence Scientific Information & Documentation Centre, Metcalfe House Delhi, pp. xvi+309.

13 Flies of Forensic Importance

Mani Chellappan, Ranjith Matta Thodikayil,
Jasti Sri Vishnu Murthy, and Naveena Unnikrishnan

LEARNING OBJECTIVES

1. To provide comprehensive knowledge on flies for precise species identification.
2. To enhance understanding of the global distribution patterns, habitats, and life cycle durations of these flies.
3. To grasp the economic significance of these flies in forensic science, veterinary public health, and waste management sectors.

13.1 INTRODUCTION

The insect world is a vast and diverse realm, with dipteran flies reigning supreme as a group of remarkable creatures renowned for their aerial prowess and widespread presence across diverse habitats worldwide (Yeates et al., 2007; Wiegmann et al., 2011). Diptera is the most diverse order and is commonly called true flies, with an estimated 240,000 species, including sand flies, house flies, gnats, midges, and mosquitoes (Yeates and Wiegmann, 2005). Boasting an astonishing diversity, with over 120,000–150,000 identified species, flies hold pivotal roles in ecosystems, serving as vital components of food webs and ecological processes (Brown, 2001; Thompson, 2006; Alikhan et al., 2018; Raguso, 2020). Dipteran flies fulfil a plethora of ecological functions, ranging from essential pollinators of flowering plants to efficient decomposers of organic matter (Retka, 2021). Their ability to traverse various landscapes and adapt to a myriad of environmental conditions underscores their resilience and adaptability. However, in certain instances, flies can also pose challenges as pests, affecting agricultural crops and human health. There are around 86,000 species of flies, excluding mosquitoes (Castner, 2009). Dipterans are crucial for nutrient recycling in terrestrial ecosystems as they accelerate the decomposition of microbes and facilitate the breakdown of animal tissues (Savage, 2002). These flies are necrophagous and are primarily vital scavengers of decaying flesh. In addition, they serve as a prominent category of insects commonly employed in legal investigations (Catts and Goff, 1992). The blow flies (Calliphoridae), flesh flies (Sarcophagidae), and house flies (Muscidae and Fannidae) are considered to be significant in forensic entomology (Savage, 2002). They are crucial because they consume human and animal corpses, making them indispensable for forensic investigations. These families are important in forensic investigations due to their decaying and synanthropic traits. These flies also have significant implications for public health and hygiene for both humans and animals. Mosquitoes, sand flies, black flies, and house flies are believed to be the cause of considerable human and animal distress, occasionally leading to lethal outcomes. Many of these flies are potential vectors of dreadful diseases (Carvalho and Mello-Patiu, 2008). By unraveling the intricacies of these fascinating insects, we aim to gain a deeper understanding of their roles in forensic and public health (Tables 13.1 and 13.2).

DOI: 10.1201/9781003482581-16

TABLE 13.1
Dipteran Flies of Forensic Importance and Public Health Importance

Higher Taxa	Family	Genus	Forensically Important Species
Suborder Brachycera			
Oestroidea	Calliphoridae	*Calliphora*	*Calliphora vomitoria* (Linneaus, 1758); *C. vicina* Robineau-Desvoidy, 1830; C. *graham* Aldrich, 1930; C. *erythrocephala* Macquart, 1834
		Lucilia	*Lucilia ampullacea* Villeneuve, 1922; *L. cuprina* (Wiedemann, 1830); *L. illustris* (Meigen, 1826); *L. papuensis* Macquart, 1844; *L. porphyrina* (Walker, 1856); *L. sericata* (Meigen, 1826)
		Chrysomya	*C. albiceps* (Wiedemann, 1819); *C. bezziana Villeneuve*, 1914; *C. defixa* (Walker, 1857) *C. indiana* (Algalil and Zambare, 2017); *C. megacephala* (Fabricius, 1794); *C. nigripes* Aubertin, 1932; *C. pinguis* (Walker, 1858) *C. phaonis* (Séguy, 1928); *C. putoria* (Wiedemann, 1830); *C. rufifacies* (Macquart, 1843) *C. saffranea* (Bigot, 1877); *C. thanomthini* Kurahashi and Tumrasvin, 1977; *C. villeneuvi* Patton, 1922
		Phormia	*P. regina* (Meigen, 1826)
	Sarcophagidae	*Sarcophaga*	*Sarcophaga haemorrhoidalis* (Fallen); *S. bullata* (Parker, 1916); *S. princeps* (Wiedemann, 1830); *S. misera* (Walker, 1849); *S. albiceps* (Meigen, 1826); *S. dux* (Thomson, 1869); *S. fuscicauda* (Böttcher, 1912); *S. hainanensis* (Ho, 1934); *S.hirtipes* (Wiedemann, 1830); *S. brevicornis* (Ho 1934); *S. ruficornis* (Fabricius, 1794); *S. dux* (Thomson, 1869); *S. orientaloides* (Senior-White, 1924)
Calyptratae	Muscidae	*Musca*	*Musca domestica* (Linnaeus, 1758); *M. sorbens* (Wiedemann, 1830); *M. confiscate* (Speiser, 1924); *M. autumnalis* (De Geer, 1776); *M. lucens* (Villeneuve, 1922); *M. ventrosa* (Wiedemann, 1830)
		Fannia	*Fannia canicularis; F. scalaris* (Fabricius)
		Hydrotaea	*H. armipes Fallén*, 1825; *H. capensis* Wiedemann, 1818; *H. chalcogaster* (Wiedemann, 1824)
Platypezoidea	Phoridae	*Megaselia*	*Megaselia rupifes* (Meign, 1804); *M. scalaris* (Loew, 1866)

13.2 ORDER DIPTERA (FLIES)

13.2.1 Family Calliphoridae (Blow Flies)

Calliphoridae is one of the largest families, encompassing more than 1,900 recognized species across the world (Benecke, 2021; Retka, 2021). Calliphorids are commonly known as blow flies. The term "blow fly" originates from the behaviour of these insects, which lay eggs on fresh meat, resulting in the meat becoming "fly blown". The family has three important genera: *Calliphora* (blue bottle flies), *Lucilia* (green bottle flies), and *Cochliomyia* (screwworm flies). Blowflies are the first insects to arrive on carrion within seconds to minutes of death (Mondor et al., 2012; Bharti and Singh, 2017; Wang et al., 2017). The attraction of blowflies to excrement and their tendency to inhabit food sources, along with their strong flying abilities, raise concerns regarding their potential as vectors

TABLE 13.2

Taxonomic Classification and Families of Diptera Relevant to Medical and Veterinary Entomologists

Higher Taxa	Family	Common Name
Suborder Brachycera		
Oestroidea	Oestridaea (Cuterebrinae, Gasterophilinae, and Hypodermatinae)	Botflies, warble flies
	Calliphoridae	Blow flies
	Sarcophagidaea	Flesh flies
Cyclorrhapha	Syrphidae	Flower flies, hover flies
Platypezoidea	Phoridae	Humpbacked flies
Schizophora	Chloropidae	Chloropid flies, eye gnats
Tephritoidea	Piophilidae	Skipper flies
Ephydroidea	Drosophilidae	Small fruit flies, vinegar flies
Calyptratae	Muscidaea	Houseflies, stable flies, and allies
	Glossinidaea	Tsetseflies
	Hippoboscidaea	Louse flies
	Nycteribiidaea	Spider-like bat flies
	Streblidaea	Bat flies
Suborder Nematocera		
Infraorder Tabanomorpha	Tabanidaea	Horseflies, deerflies
	Rhagionidae	Snipe flies
	Athericidae	Athericid flies
Infraorder Stratiomyomorpha	Stratiomyidae	Soldier flies
Infraorder Tipulomorpha	Tipulidae	Crane flies
Infraorder Bibionomorpha	Bibionidae	March flies
	Mycetophilidae	Fungus gnats
	Sciaridae	Dark-winged fungus gnats
Infraorder Psychodomorpha	Psychodidaea	Moth flies, sand flies
Infraorder Culicomorpha	Chaoboridae	Phantom midges
	Corethrellidae frog-biting midges	Frog-biting midges
	Culicidaea	Mosquitoes
	Simuliidaea	Blackflies
	Ceratopogonidaea	Biting midges
	Chironomidae	Chironomid midges

of pathogens for humans and animals (Hall, 1948; Prado et al., 2021). These significant insect species provide accurate, reliable information for estimating the post-mortem interval (PMI), along with muscid and sarcophagid flies. Additionally, blowflies are important in community ecology and nutrient recycling due to their role in the removal and decomposition of vertebrate carcasses. Adult blowflies are medium-sized insects characterised by their robust build and varying lengths, ranging from 6 to 14mm. They possess striking metallic-coloured bodies, which can range from vibrant green and blue to deep black, often accentuated by conspicuous bristles. Their antennae, adorned with distinctive bristle-like structures known as aristae, aid in identification, complemented by large reddish-brown eyes. Typically, they exhibit fascinating behaviours, such as congregating in groups on warm surfaces like fences and buildings to bask in the sun, and occasionally visiting flowers for nectar consumption (Bharti and Singh, 2022). The larvae of blowflies, commonly known as maggots, present a distinct appearance with their yellowish-white coloration and lack of a head capsule, thriving in environments rich in decaying organic matter. Blowfly larvae range in length from 8 to 23 mm. The larval abdominal terminal segment has six or more cone-shaped tubercles around its perimeter and a pair of posterior spiracles (Bunchu et al., 2012). Adult blowflies are the first to deposit eggs on carcasses, using their telescopic ovipositor. Several batches of eggs are typically inserted in the nose and mouth, as well as in other natural openings (if exposed). Open wounds are often used for egg insertion (Bharti and Singh, 2003). Different species of flies are found visiting carcasses at different times of the year, and their life stages are described in Table 13.3. For example, in India, flies from the genus *Calliphora* are considered winter flies, whereas *Chrysomya* can be found associated with carcasses all year (Bharti and Singh, 2003). Warm-weather species, on the other hand, belong to the genus *Lucilia*. In this exploration of blowflies, we will delve into their ecological forensic significance and potential implications for public health (Figure 13.1).

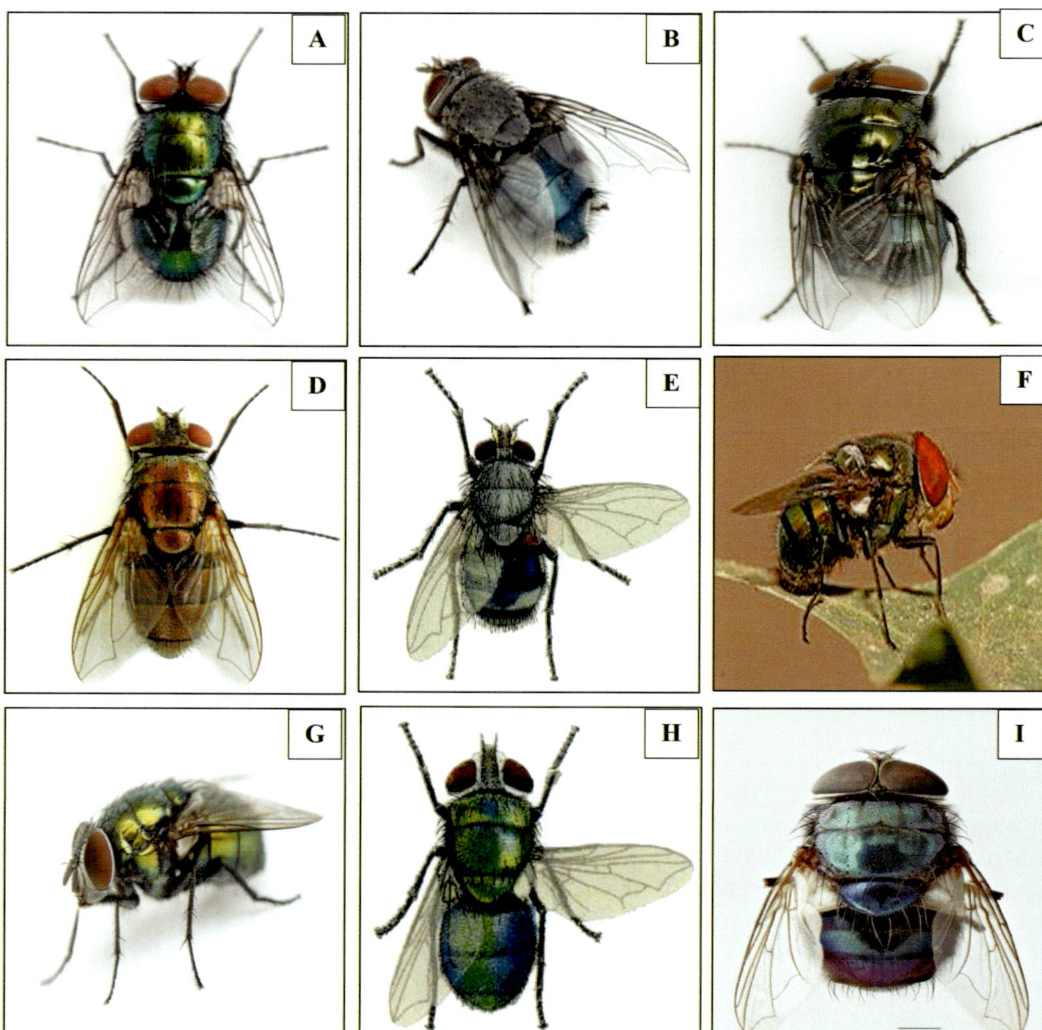

FIGURE 13.1 Important blow fly species. (a) Green bottle fly, *Lucilia sericata*; (b) blue bottle fly, *Calliphora vomitoria*; (c) black blow fly, *Phormia regina*; (d) red-tailed green bottle fly, *L. cuprina*; (e) *Calliphora vicina*; (f) common oriental latrine fly, *Chrysomya megacephala*; (g) *Chrysomya rufifacies*; (h) black blow fly, *L. caesar*); (i) *Cochliomyia hominivorax*.

TABLE 13.3
Life Stages Description of Different Species

Species	Egg	Larva	Pupa	Adult
Lucilia sericata	Eggs hatches within 18–21 hours	Larval development spans three instars and typically lasts 3–4 days.	Brown, oval-shaped. Form in soil or pupation site. Pupal development typically lasts 7–10 days.	Metallic green or blue. Adult female lays 150–200 eggs laid on decaying matter or wounds
Calliphora vomitoria	Egg hatching takes 12–24 hours	Approximately 5–7 days	Typically lasts 7–10 days	Adult stage lasts up to 7–10 days. Metallic blue or green. Feed on nectar and decaying matter.
Phormia regina	Hatches within hours	Larvae develop in 3–5 days	Typically lasts 7–10 days.	Adult lays eggs in batches of up to 300
Lucilia cuprina	Approximately 8–20 hours	Around 4–5 days	Usually lasts 5–6 days	Lasts upto 7 days
Calliphora vicina	Approximately 1–3 days	Around 3–10 days	Usually lasts 6–14 days	Adult stage lasts upto 7–10 days
Chrysomya megacephala	1–2	4–7	6–10	Adult stage lasts upto 7–10 days
Chrysomya rufifacies	1–2	4–7	6–10	Adult stage lasts upto 7–10 days.
Lucilia caesar	1–2	3–5	5–7	Adult stage lasts upto 7–10 days
Cochliomyia hominivorax	1–2	4–7	6–10	Adult stage lasts upto 7–10 days

13.2.1.1 Genus *Calliphora*

13.2.1.1.1 *Calliphora vomitoria*

Calliphora vomitoria, also known as the blue bottle fly, typically measures between 10 and 14 mm in length, featuring a metallic blue abdomen with a dull grey head and thorax. These flies are characterized by red eyes, sponging mouthparts, and a body covered in bristle-like hairs (Figure 13.1). The maggots of this species are white, ranging from 10 to 16 mm in length, devoid of legs and eyes, and equipped with hooks at their head region (Hall, 1948; Greenberg, 1971; Erzinclioglu, 1985). Commonly found in urban environments, *C. vomitoria* is a key contributor to forensic entomology studies due to its predictable colonization patterns on decomposing remains (Triplehorn et al., 2005; Smith and Whitman, 2007). *C. vomitoria* exhibits predictable colonization behaviour on cadavers and tends to prefer shaded environments. By analysing the development of *C. vomitoria* larvae found on a body and comparing it with known developmental rates under specific environmental conditions, forensic entomologists can estimate the PMI. This species is commonly encountered as the predominant blow fly species on buried or concealed corpses. Its larvae have been utilized to estimate the time of decapitation of a body, with fly infestation occurring after the head was severed from the body (James, 1947; Hall and Townsend, 1977; Smith, 1986; Anderson, 1997)

13.2.1.1.2 *Calliphora vicina*

Calliphora vicina, similar in appearance to *C. vomitoria*, is also known for its metallic blue coloration and is commonly found in urban and rural environments (Figure 13.1). It plays a significant role in forensic entomology as a colonizer of human remains (cabicompendium, 2022). *C. vicina* is recognized as one of the most significant blow flies from a forensic standpoint, as highlighted by Erzinclioglu (1983), Smith (1986), and Introna et al. (1991). It has been noted to occasionally enter residential homes during the cooler months (Anderson, 1995). In the region of Punjab, it typically emerges as a winter fly, active from December to March. This temporal pattern could serve as a crucial indicator if larvae are detected on a body during midsummer, suggesting an unusual occurrence for that season. Greenberg (1995) conducted a study where the minimum time since death of a nine-year-old girl, discovered deceased in the bathroom of an abandoned apartment, was estimated using pupae of this fly collected from the bathroom floor. Similarly, Nolte et al. (1992) identified death resulting from cocaine poisoning in a severely decomposed body where conventional tissue analysis was unfeasible. Toxicological examination of larvae from this fly found on the body provided crucial insights. Lord et al. (1992) encountered a case where conventional methods failed to accurately determine the PMI. Larvae and pupae of *C. vicina* were abundant around the body, presenting an opportunity to estimate the PMI accurately. The temperature at the site was 19°C, consistent with standard laboratory rearings, facilitating the correlation of environmental data with laboratory findings for precise PMI calculation (James, 1947; Hall, 1948; Payne, 1965; Greenberg, 1971; Hall and Townsend, 1977; Nuorteva, 1977; Erzinclioglu, 1985; Smith, 1986).

13.2.1.2 Genus *Lucilia*

13.2.1.2.1 ***Lucilia sericata*** (Meigen)

The *Lucilia sericata* (Meigen), commonly known as the sheep blow fly, is most common, with a worldwide distribution, especially in the Holarctic (Byrd and Castner, 2001). *L. sericata* prefers moist climate and coastal distribution (Australian Museum, 2009). It is approximately 8–10 mm long and is recognized for its vibrant green metallic coloration (Figure 13.1). It possesses red eyes and sponge-like mouthparts, and its body is covered in bristle-like hairs. Maggots, on the other hand, are white, smooth, and range from 1 to 18 mm in length. They lack legs and eyes but have hooks located at their head region. *L. sericata* is a frequent visitor to carrion, excrement, and garbage, and it plays an important role in forensic, medical, and veterinary science (Strikewise, 2007; Rueda et al., 2010). The development of *L. sericata*, from egg to adult, varies with temperature, taking approximately 21 hours to hatch at 21°C and 18 hours at 27°C for eggs, and progressing through three larval instars over four days at 20°C to three days at 27°C (Anderson, 2000). The development is influenced by factors such as food source and humidity (Tarone et al., 2006). After the larvae leave the host, pupal development lasts around 10 days at 21°C and seven days at 27°C, culminating in adult emergence. Females lay clusters of up to 200 eggs, allowing for multiple generations annually (Strikewise, 2007).

13.2.1.2.2 *Forensic and Public Health Importance*

L. sericata is most prevalent in various habitats and exhibits predictable colonization patterns on decomposing remains. It plays a crucial role in forensic science by estimating the minimum PMI using its immature flies, as they are among the first insects to arrive at a corpse, typically within minutes of death (Byrd and Castner, 2009; Rueda et al., 2010). Despite the typical daytime ovipositing behaviour of *L. sericata*, it has been observed to oviposit in cool nocturnal conditions, influenced by factors such as the local presence of flies near a corpse and the availability of artificial lighting. Estimating PMI using dipteran larvae, including *L. sericata*, traditionally involves determining the developmental stage of the collected larvae; however, Tarone and Foran (2010) have developed a more precise method using gene expression analysis, improving the accuracy and precision of PMI estimation. In nearly every province of China, case reports have successfully utilized *L. sericata* to infer the minimum PMI, with estimates differing from the true time of death by only 0.5 days in some instances (Wang et al., 2019). Additionally, *L. sericata* larvae are frequently associated with myiasis cases and act as ectoparasites in sheep across various temperate regions worldwide, rendering them economically significant insects. Furthermore, due to maggots' capability to consume necrotic tissue, eliminate bacteria, and facilitate wound healing, they are also employed in maggot therapy (Sherman et al., 2000).

13.2.1.2.3 Medical and Veterinary Importance

L. sericata is widely employed in human wound treatment for injuries that conventional therapies fail to heal (Rueda et al., 2010). This practice, known as maggot therapy, is increasingly utilized. Under medical supervision, *L. sericata* larvae are applied to the wound, which is then covered, allowing the larvae to consume necrotic tissue and bacteria present in infected wounds. Their activity promotes healthy tissue growth by not only consuming decomposing tissue but also secreting antimicrobial enzymes while in the wound (Horobin et al., 2002). Most patients undergoing maggot therapy experience minimal discomfort. Initially, concerns regarding wound contamination existed, but the proper use of sterile maggots has mitigated any risk of transmitting microorganisms (Sherman et al., 2000).

13.2.1.2.4 ***Lucilia illustris*** (Meigen, 1826)

This species is part of a group commonly referred to as the green bottle fly. *L. illustris* has a widespread distribution across the Holarctic region. In North America, it is particularly abundant, ranging from Mexico to southern Canada and throughout the American Midwest. Adult specimens typically measure between 6 and 8 mm in length, with a gleaming greenish-blue thorax and abdomen, complemented by black legs. Known as a "warm weather species", *L. illustris* thrives in open woodlands during the summer months. Adult flies are mainly drawn to fresh carrion, although they can occasionally be found on excrement. The larvae feed on both carrion and fecal materials, although they are most commonly found on carrion (Hall, 1948; Greenberg, 1971; Hall and Townsend, 1977; Smith, 1986). *L. illustris* is a medium-sized metallic green sarco-saprophagous fly frequently found in urban and suburban areas (Anderson, 1995). In a study by Lord et al. (1986), maggots of this species played a pivotal role in resolving a complex case involving conflicting estimates of the PMI provided by medical examiners. By collecting and rearing maggots from the body to the adult stage and considering the ambient temperature of the area, the developmental time of this species was calculated, leading to an accurate determination of the PMI.

13.2.1.3 Genus *Chrysomya*

13.2.1.3.1 ***Chrysomya megacephala*** (Fabricius, 1784)

Chrysomya megacephala is a tropical blow fly with a wide distribution across Asia and the Pacific regions. Adults typically measure around 1/2 inch (12.0 mm) in length (Figure 13.1). Their head is predominantly grey, featuring large red eyes. It is found in tropical and subtropical regions worldwide and is often associated with human habitations, particularly in areas with poor sanitation (Williams and Villet, 2006). With a global distribution, *C. megacephala* remains active throughout the year in the state of Punjab. Goff (1992) utilized this species to estimate the PMI of a corpse discovered wrapped in a blanket. Similarly, Goff et al. (1988) utilized data on the life history of this species to resolve three homicidal cases occurring in different habitats (mixed vegetation, scrub, and swamp). Despite variations in environmental factors, such as temperature and moisture, PMI estimates based on entomological evidence consistently aligned with circumstantial evidence, falling within a range of 4–5.5 days.

13.2.1.3.2 ***Chrysomya rufifacies*** (Macquart, 1842)

Chrysomya rufifacies adult flies are sturdy and display a metallic green hue, appearing distinctly blue under bright sunlight, particularly evident in the brilliant blue posterior margins of the abdominal tergites (Baumgartner et al., 1993) (Figure 13.1). The larvae, referred to as "hairy maggots", earned this name due to the presence of fleshy tubercles along each body segment imparting a slightly hairy appearance despite lacking true hairs (Baumgartner, 1986). *C. rufifacies* is among the first species to colonize remains, with oviposition continuing for the initial 4–5 days of decomposition. As a result, it serves as a valuable forensic indicator, as its maggots often exhibit the longest association with the cadaver. Goff et al. (1986) calculated the PMI of a body found in a drainage ditch by utilizing knowledge of its developmental time, corroborating findings from other investigative methods. Additionally, Goff and Odom (1987) successfully resolved another case involving a body discovered in an apartment closet, with *C. rufifacies* providing crucial evidence.

13.2.1.4 Genus *Phormia*

13.2.1.4.1 *Phormia regina*

The black blow fly exhibits a Holarctic distribution and is widespread throughout the United States, except for southern Florida. Adult flies typically measure between 7 and 9 mm in length. They have a dark green to olive-coloured thorax and abdomen, with black legs, though the entire body may appear black under certain lighting conditions. A distinctive feature of this species is the presence of bright orange hairs surrounding the anterior thoracic spiracle, aiding in its identification. Considered a cold weather fly, the black blow fly is most abundant in the spring and fall across most of the U.S., with populations persisting throughout the winter months. In the southern U.S., it predominates during the winter and is absent during hot summers (James, 1947; Hall, 1948; Kamal, 1958; Zumpt, 1965). The larvae primarily develop in carrion and are known producers of myiasis. Historically, this species has been utilized in maggot therapy for wound cleansing. *P. regina,* characterized by its deep black coloration (Figure 13.1c), is often associated with carrion and is an important tool in estimating PMIs in forensic investigations (Greenberg, 1971; Denno and Cothran, 1975; Hall and Townsend, 1977; Smith, 1986). These flies are employed in maggot therapy for wound debridement, yet they can also pose a pest threat, causing secondary myiasis in animals and potentially transmitting diseases through mechanical means as adult flies (James, 1947; Hall, 1948).

13.2.1.4.2 Case Studies in India

Several investigations across India have used blow fly species to estimate PMIs. Babu et al. (2022) found *C. megacephala* and *C. rufifacies* on highly decomposed corpses, estimating a PMI of 5.5 days for a male body in Modakpal village, Chhattisgarh. Similarly, in Bastar district, they estimated a PMI of 3.5 days for a headless male fetus using *C. rufifacies* (Babu et al., 2013). Palavesam et al. (2022) estimated minimum PMI in Tamil Nadu using *C. megacephala* and *C. rufifacies* with thermal summation constants. A 45-year-old male corpse in Ludhiana, Punjab, had numerous second-instar larvae of *C. megacephala*, with a PMI of 9.6 days estimated using the accumulated degree hours method (Sharma and Bala, 2016). In another study in Sangrur, a decapitated 38-year-old male was found with third-instar *C. megacephala*, assessing a PMI of 9 days (Bala and Sharma, 2015). During autopsies, Sharma et al. (2018) examined insects on five bodies (4 males and 1 female). They found *C. megacephala* maggots, pupae, adults, and egg batches, as well as *C. rufifacies* larvae and adults, *C. albiceps* maggots, and adults of *P. regina*.

13.2.2 Family Sarcophagidae (Flesh Flies)

Sarcophagids are commonly known as flesh flies, with a global distribution. They encompass over 100 genera and 2,600 species, of which about 800 species belong to the genus *Sarcophaga*. The dominant species vary significantly by geographic region and climate, which has led to recent studies on the succession of insect fauna, including flesh flies, on decaying carcasses. Adults typically feed on sweet substances, like honeydew or nectar. However, their maggots consume animal flesh; as a result, they are known as flesh flies (Pape, 1996; Povolny, 1997; Hu, 2000; Chen, 2013; Tomberlin and Benbow, 2015). In addition to animal flesh, maggots also feed on excrement and exposed meat. Flesh flies cause myiasis and serve as mechanical vectors for disease transmission. Many species of flesh flies are parasitic on other insects, particularly bees and wasps. However, with respect to forensic entomology, at least some species are beneficial to humans. Flesh flies are medium-sized, measuring between 2 and 14 mm in length (Singh and Bharti, 2022). In adults, especially on the thorax, grey and black longitudinal stripes are present, and on the abdomen, a tessellated pattern is present, lacking metallic coloration. In flesh flies, the antennae are plumose only at their base. Sarcophagid bodies typically have bristles, and their eyes are noticeably spaced apart in both males and females. In certain species, the eyes are vividly red, and the genitalia at the end of the abdomen are prominently visible. The maggots possess posterior spiracles situated within a pit or depression at the tip of the abdomen, bordered by fleshy tubercles. This character differentiates flesh fly larvae from blow fly larvae (Byrd and Castner, 2010; Singh and Bharti, 2022). Sarcophagid species share similarities in both adult and larval stages, making species-level identification notoriously challenging. To accurately identify the species, maggots must be reared to adulthood (Szpila et al., 2015). Flesh flies are drawn to carrion in various conditions, including sun, shade, dry, wet, indoors, and outdoors, and are present throughout all stages of decomposition. Females deposit living larvae directly onto decomposing remains, rather than laying eggs. When determining the PMI using flesh fly evidence, the duration required for egg development must also be excluded from consideration. *Sarcophaga* flies typically arrive on human remains alongside or slightly after blow flies, sometimes being the first to arrive, even in harsh weather conditions. They often enter indoor environments, leading to larvae being recovered from human remains in homes. These are the predominant flies recovered from human corpses situated in indoor habitats (Aldrich, 1916; Arnett and Jacques, 1981; Bland and Jacques, 1978; Borror and White, 1970; Borror et al., 1989; Castner et al., 1995; Greenberg, 1971; Hall and Doisy, 1993; Hogue, 1993; James, 1947; James and Harwood, 1969; Knipling, 1936; Payne, 1965; Peterson, 1979; Shewell, 1987; Smith, 1956, 1975, 1986). The important species are described below.

13.2.2.1 Sarcophaga

13.2.2.1.1 *Sarcophaga haemorrhoidalis* (Fallen) (Figure 13.2)

S. haemorrhoidalis, also known as the red-tailed flesh fly, has a cosmopolitan distribution. This species is found worldwide and is commonly associated with human and animal carcasses. They are characterized by well-developed lower calypteres, which are associated with their wings (Byrd 1998–2011; Madubunyi, 1986). The maggots typically infest carcasses in various stages of decomposition, often arriving at the scene along with blow flies (Aldrich, 1916; James, 1947; Zumpt, 1952; Greenberg, 1971; Smith, 1975, 1986).

Description: Adult *S. haemorrhoidalis*, resembling house flies but larger and more robust (8–14 mm), can be distinguished by three dark longitudinal stripes on the thorax. *S. haemorrhoidalis* has a black body covered with a whitish, powder-like substance that gives it a greyish tint, as well as a checkerboard pattern on the abdomen. The species name is derived from the red-coloured external genitalia at the tip of the abdomen. They possess large compound eyes, long antennae with plumose bases, and a row of frontal bristles on the head. Their mouthparts are adapted for lapping liquids. The dorsal mesothorax has longitudinal bristles, though those anterior to the scutum are rudimentary or absent (Byrd and Castner, 2001).

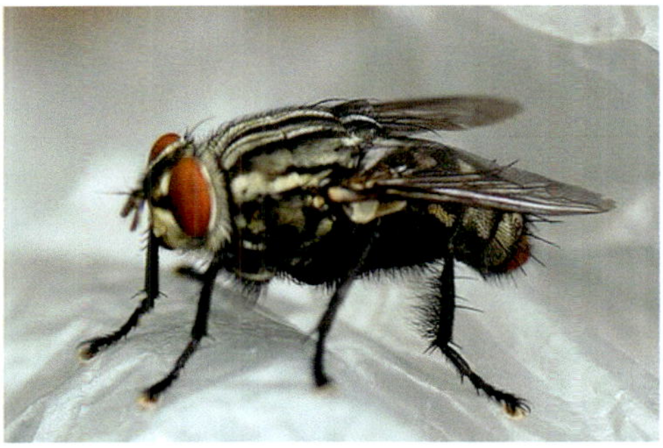

FIGURE 13.2 *Sarcophaga haemorrhoidalis.*

Larvae: They are white to slightly yellow, worm-like, and larger than other fly larvae, reaching 10–22 mm before pupation. They have strong mandibles for feeding, and the spiracles on the posterior end are located in a cavity fringed with triangular tubercles. The number of slits in each spiracle helps determine the larval instar (Byrd and Castner, 2001).

13.2.2.1.2 Forensic Importance

S. haemorrhoidalis is significant in forensic sciences because it is one of the first insects to arrive at a corpse. This species is known for its strong flying capabilities, allowing it to navigate and reach remains even in adverse weather conditions when other arthropod species cannot do so. It is commonly associated with corpses found indoors, particularly during the summer months in the south-eastern United States. Similar to blowflies, sarcophagid flies, including *S. haemorrhoidalis*, are used in forensic investigations to determine the PMI. The short development cycle of this species makes it especially useful for estimating PMI within the first three to four weeks following death. Additionally, *S. haemorrhoidalis* has been utilized for PMI estimations on severely burnt remains, demonstrating its versatility and value in forensic contexts. These characteristics make it a critical tool for forensic entomologists in death investigations (Aldrich, 1916; James, 1947; Zumpt, 1952; Greenberg, 1971; Smith, 1975; Introna et al., 1986, 1998; Byrd and Castner, 2001).

13.2.2.1.3 Medical and Economic Importance

S. haemorrhoidalis, known to cause gastrointestinal myiasis, infests living tissue, leading to medical and economic issues in livestock. Myiasis occurs due to its attraction to feces and indoor larviposition. Females deposit larvae on rectal mucosal tissues, particularly in immobile subjects. Myiasis can result from ingesting contaminated food and is common in overcrowded, unsanitary conditions but can also occur in hospitals and nursing homes. Symptoms include intestinal pain, itching, and inflammation. Other forms include nasal and aural infestations. This species also transmits diseases, like *E. coli*, *Shigella dysenteriae*, *Streptococcus*, *Salmonella*, tapeworms, and the poliovirus (Smith and Whitman 1992; Braverman et al. 1994; Byrd and Castner 2001; Mullen and Durden 2002; Turhan et al. 2007).

13.2.3 Family Muscidae (Muscid Flies)

Muscid flies belong to a large, globally distributed family with over 1,000 species worldwide. They are typically small to medium-sized, ranging from 3 to 10 mm in length, and are generally dull grey to dark in colour, though some species exhibit a metallic sheen (Greenberg and Kunich, 2002). They can be distinguished from bottle flies and blow flies (family Calliphoridae) by specific wing and head characteristics. Unlike sarcophagid and calliphorid flies, adult muscids are usually less bristly, and their antennae have a plumose arista throughout their length, a trait they share with calliphorids (Grzywacz and Pape, 2014). Muscid flies are ubiquitous and occupy a wide range of terrestrial habitats. Many species are synanthropic, meaning they are closely associated with human environments. This association has led to their unintentional transport and introduction to regions beyond their natural ranges. Their presence in domestic settings contributes significantly to their medical and forensic relevance. They infest dead bodies after the arrival of flesh flies and blow flies, often laying eggs in natural body openings, wounds, or soiled clothing. While their larvae primarily feed on carrion, some species prey on the eggs and larvae of other carrion-feeding insects, affecting the composition of the carrion's insect fauna (Grzywacz et al., 2017). Common genera of muscid flies found on carrion include *Hydrotaea* (bronze dump fly), *Musca* (house fly), *Atherigona* (shoot fly), and *Neomyia*. Common members of the Muscidae family include house flies, stable flies, horn flies, and latrine flies. The tsetse fly, a vector for African sleeping sickness, is also part of this family. The feeding habits of adult muscid flies are diverse; they may consume decaying plant and animal matter, dung, excrement, pollen, or blood. Stable and horn flies, which feed on blood, can be significant nuisances to both humans and livestock. Species that breed in and feed on garbage, sewage, and human waste can mechanically transmit diseases, such as typhoid, anthrax, dysentery, and yaws. House flies, for instance, regurgitate digestive fluids onto food, facilitating the spread of these diseases (James and Harwood, 1969; Borror and White, 1970; Bland and Jacques, 1978; Peterson, 1979; Arnett and Jacques, 1981; Borror et al., 1989; Castner et al., 1995; Hogue, 1993; Huckett and Vockeroth, 1987).

13.2.3.1 *Musca*

13.2.3.1.1 *Musca domestica*

The house fly, *Musca domestica*, is found worldwide, including throughout the U.S. and Canada, though it may not be the dominant fly species in every region. Adults are 6–7 mm long and grey with black longitudinal stripes on the thorax that extend onto the abdomen. This species is almost always found near human habitation and is a major nuisance due to its movement from garbage, carrion, and excrement to human food. House flies are vectors for over a hundred disease-causing pathogens. Both adults and larvae prefer excrement and decomposing vegetable matter. Adults are also attracted to sweet foods and meat, and larvae can develop well in these materials. They readily enter homes to colonize decomposing remains and are among the first flies attracted to excrement and carrion, usually arriving after blow flies. House flies are present year-round but are most abundant during summer. In temperate zones, their populations peak in spring and late summer, while in tropical and subtropical regions, they are most numerous during the hot summer months. It is rare to find house flies on a fresh corpse unless excrement is present or gut contents are exposed (Chapman, 1944; James, 1947; Greenberg, 1971; Smith, 1986).

13.2.3.2 *Fannia*

13.2.3.2.1 *Fannia canicularis*

The lesser house fly, also known as the little house fly, is found worldwide. This small, slender fly typically measures 6–7 mm in length. It has a black to dark brown thorax and an abdomen covered with a silvery-grey powder. Its legs are yellowish, and the thorax features three longitudinal brown stripes that do not extend onto the abdomen. Most abundant during the warm summer months, the lesser house fly is the most common *Fannia* species involved in myiasis. It is often found on excrement, decomposing vegetable matter (such as fruits), dairy products, and urine-saturated materials. It is frequently recovered from decomposing human remains, especially where excrement or gut contents are exposed. The larvae thrive on liquefying decomposing substances. Adapted to such habitats, the larvae are flattened with branched protuberances that help them float in semi-liquid environments. While similar in appearance to *F. scalaris* larvae, *F. canicularis* larvae have fewer branched protuberances and can grow longer than those of the latrine fly. When ready to pupate, the larvae migrate to drier areas. Adults often enter indoor environments, where they hover in mid-air or fly erratically, becoming nuisances as they gather in large numbers during certain times of the year. They are strongly attracted to carrion and excrement (James, 1947; Payne, 1965; Greenberg, 1971; Wasti, 1972; Nuorteva, 1974; Smith, 1986).

13.2.3.2.2 *Fannia scalaris* (Fabricius)

The latrine fly, also known as *Fannia scalaris*, is cosmopolitan in distribution, found worldwide. Similar in appearance to the lesser house fly, adult latrine flies measure 6–7 mm in length. They are black with a dusty silver-grey coating on the thorax and abdomen, giving them a superficial resemblance to small houseflies. The larvae are small, flattened, and typically do not exceed 6 mm in length (James, 1947; Greenberg, 1971; Nuorteva, 1974). Each body segment of the larvae has a pair of lateral feathered processes (tubercles) that may assist in flotation within their preferred habitat of semi-liquid fecal matter. Eggs are laid in human or animal dung and decaying vegetable materials. The larvae can develop in a variety of environments, including dung, carrion, bird nests, other insect nests, and human cadavers, especially where excrement or exposed gut contents are present. They

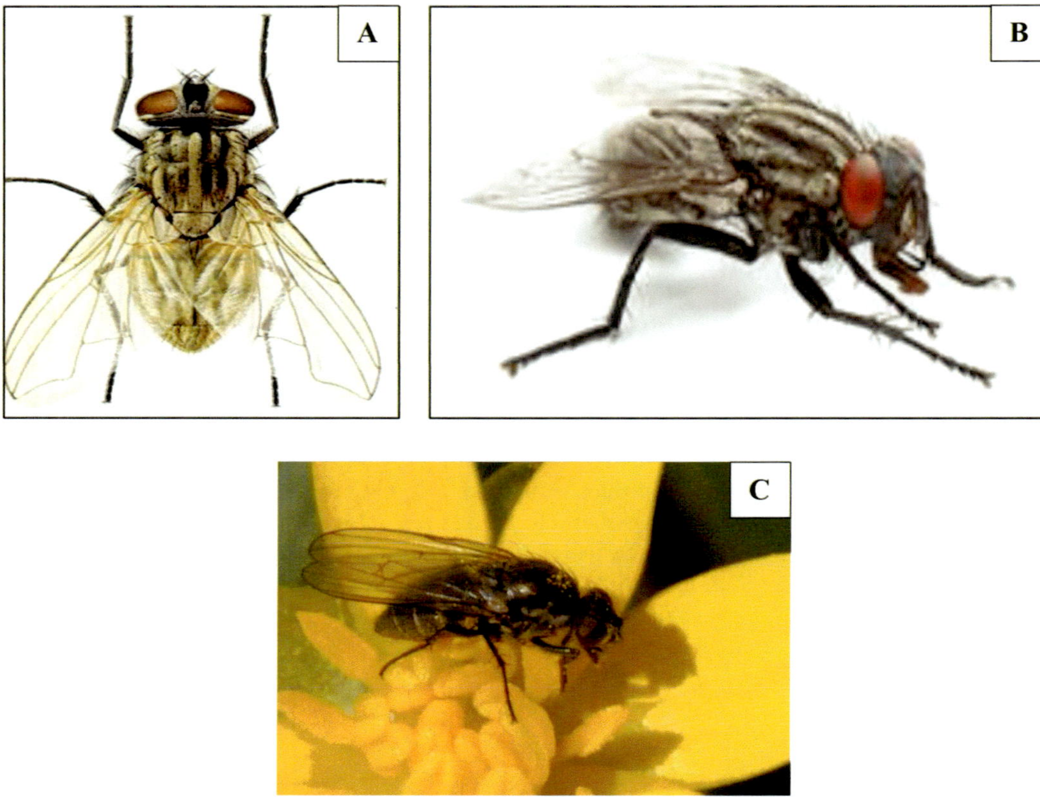

FIGURE 13.3 Important forensic house flies: (a) *Musca domestica*; (b) *Fannia canicularis*; and (c) *Fannia scalaris*.

are commonly found on urine-soaked clothing and other soiled materials. Unlike the lesser house fly, *F. scalaris* is less likely to enter indoor habitats. However, when found indoors, the presence of latrine flies usually indicates unsanitary conditions (James, 1947; Greenberg, 1971; Nuorteva, 1974; Smith, 1986) (Figure 13.3).

13.2.4 Family Psychodidae (Moth Flies, Sand Flies, and Owl Midges) (Figure 13.4)

Moth flies, part of the family Psychodidae, are found globally, with over 90 species identified in the United States and Canada. These tiny flies are typically 3–4 mm long as adults. Their bodies and wings are covered in scales, giving them a moth-like appearance. The wings taper to a point and have prominent longitudinal veins. Moth fly larvae thrive in moist environments and can grow up to 10 mm in length. Within the Psychodidae family, two subfamilies are of medical importance:

1. **Phlebotominae** (sand flies): These flies have non-aquatic larvae, and the adults do not hold their wings roof-like over their bodies. Found in the southern United States and tropical regions, female sand flies feed on blood and are vectors for diseases such as leishmaniasis.
2. **Psychodinae** (moth flies or owl midges): Their larvae are typically aquatic and develop in the slime found in sewers and drains. Adult moth flies hold their wings roof-like over their bodies and are commonly found in warm, damp environments, such as restrooms or showers. Although they do not feed on blood, they can be a nuisance due to their large numbers. These flies exhibit distinctive behaviour, running and flying rapidly in an erratic manner. Psychodid flies rarely make up a significant portion of the arthropods that colonize

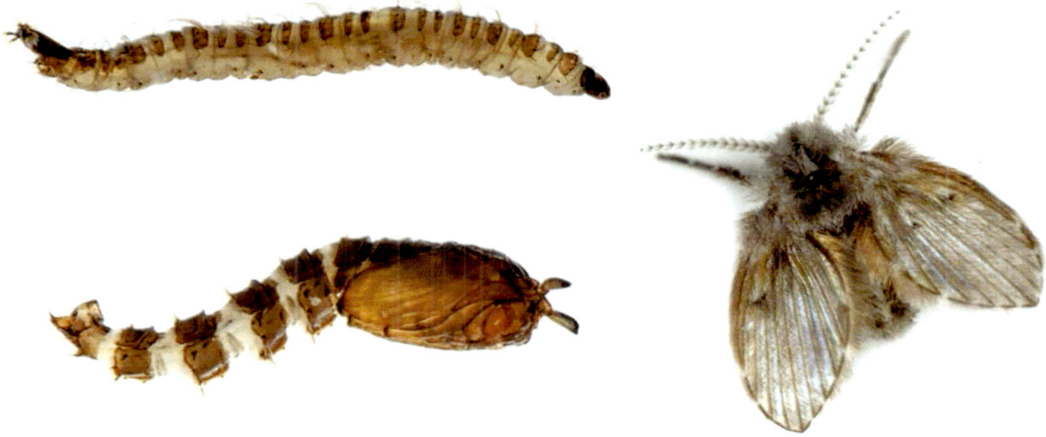

FIGURE 13.4 Psychodidae (moth flies, sand flies, and owl midges).

human remains. However, adult moth flies are sometimes attracted to carrion and are commonly found indoors and associated with humans (James and Harwood, 1969; Borror and White, 1970; Bland and Jacques, 1978; Peterson, 1979; Arnett and Jacques, 1981; Quate and Vockeroth, 1981; Borror et al., 1989; Hogue, 1993; Castner et al., 1995).

13.2.5 Family Sepsidae (Black Scavenger Flies) (Figure 13.5)

Black scavenger flies, also known as sepsids, are found worldwide and encompass a diverse group of at least 240 species. These small flies are typically shiny black, purple, or red and measure no more than 3.5 mm in length. They possess a distinct body shape characterized by a rounded head and a narrowing of the abdomen at the base. One of the key identifying features of sepsid flies is their behaviour of flicking their wings outwards as they walk, earning them the common name "waggle flies". This behaviour is unique to this group and aids in their recognition. These flies are often encountered in large numbers and are commonly found on dung. The larvae of sepsid flies develop in various decomposing organic materials, including carrion, excrement, and even decaying seaweed. Mature larvae are relatively small, typically ranging from 3 to 6 mm in length. (James and Harwood, 1969; Borror and White, 1970; Bland and Jacques, 1978; Peterson, 1979; Arnett and Jacques, 1981; Streyskal, 1987; Borror et al., 1989; Hogue, 1993; Castner et al., 1995)

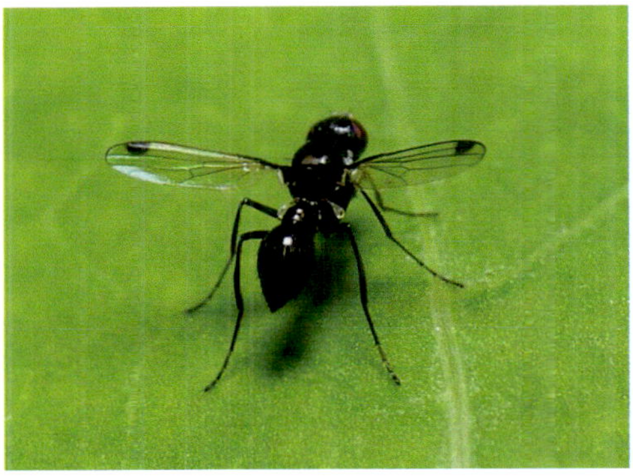

FIGURE 13.5 Sepsidae (black scavenger flies).

13.2.5.1 *Sepsis* spp.

Black scavenger flies of the genus *Sepsis* spp. are distributed worldwide, including throughout the U.S. and Canada. These shiny black flies exhibit the characteristics typical of the Sepsidae family, such as a rounded head and a narrowed abdomen base. Additionally, adult *Sepsis* species feature a dark spot near the wing tip along the front margin. These flies are attracted to various decaying matter, including carrion and excrement. Due to their small size and narrow "waist", they are sometimes mistaken for ants. Black scavenger flies are often abundant on carcasses, particularly during advanced stages of decay, as well as on excrement and other decaying materials (Greenberg, 1971; James, 1947; Smith, 1975, 1986).

13.2.6 Family Scathophagidae (Dung Flies) (Figure 13.6)

Dung flies are often classified as a separate family, although some references may place them under the families Muscidae or Anthomyiidae. The name "Scathophagidae" means "dung-eating", but they are also sometimes referred to as "Scatophagidae". There are over 250 species, predominantly found in the Holarctic region, with about 150 species in temperate North America, especially in southern Canada. Common dung flies are typically red or yellow and densely hairy. While many species are drawn to excrement or decaying plant material, with larvae commonly found in dung, other species vary significantly. Some are dark as adults, with larvae that act as leaf miners, pests of flower heads, parasites, predators, or even live in aquatic environments. Larvae of the genus *Scatophaga* primarily feed on dung but are also found on decaying seaweed (James and Harwood, 1969; Borror and White, 1970; Bland and Jacques, 1978; Peterson, 1979; Arnett and Jacques, 1981; Streyskal, 1987; Vockeroth, 1987; Borror et al., 1989; Hogue, 1993; Castner et al., 1995).

13.2.6.1 Scatophaga

13.2.6.1.1 ***Scatophaga stercoraria*** *Linnaeus*

The common dung fly, found across the U.S. and Canada, is a slender insect measuring 7–10 mm in length. Although its body is black, it is covered with dense yellow or yellow-brown hairs, giving it a bright yellow appearance. The thorax features several long black hairs, and the wings are typically held flat over the back when at rest. Adults are active from spring through late fall. The larvae thrive in various habitats and can be found on cadavers, especially when excrement or gut contents are exposed.

13.2.7 Family Piophilidae (Skipper Flies) (Figure 13.7)

Skipper flies, a small family of only 69 species, are found worldwide, with their greatest diversity in temperate regions. Adults are metallic blue or black and typically range from 2.5 to 4.5 mm in

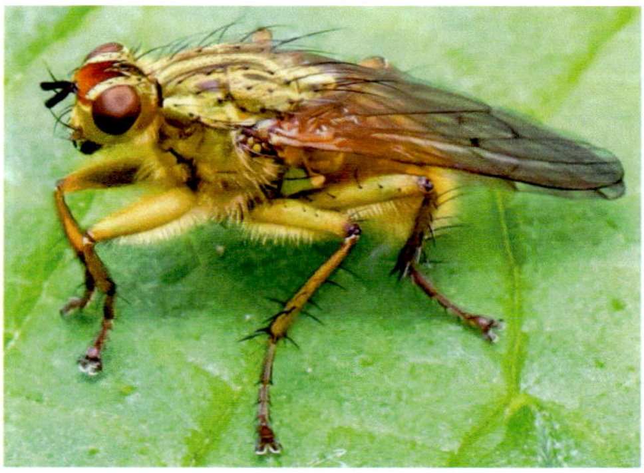

FIGURE 13.6 Scathophagidae (dung flies).

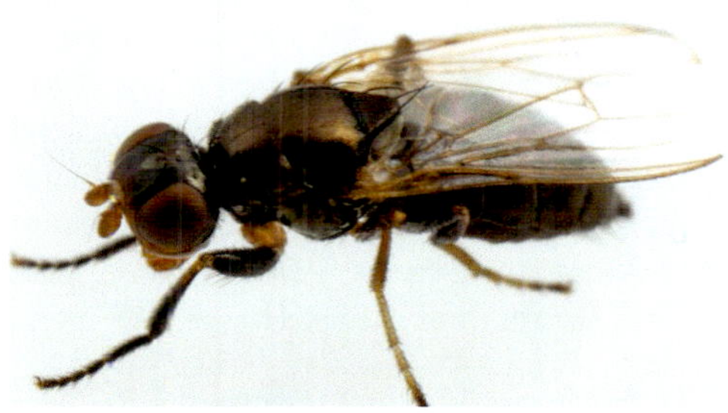

FIGURE 13.7 Piophilidae (skipper flies).

length. These flies inhabit a variety of environments, including carrion, human waste, bones, skin, and fur, and are commonly associated with dry, protein-rich food sources. The name "skipper" originates from the unique behaviour of the larvae of some species, such as the cheese skipper (*Piophila casei*). These larvae can propel themselves into the air by gripping small protrusions on their anal segment with their mouth hooks and then suddenly releasing. This action can fling the larvae 3–4 inches high and 6–8 inches laterally, serving as an effective escape mechanism and aiding in larval migration. Additionally, they move in a traditional creeping manner, like most fly larvae. Skipper fly larvae are primarily scavengers, feeding on the same types of decaying food materials as the adults. Some species specialize in rotting fungi, while a European species has larvae that are blood-sucking ectoparasites of young birds. The larvae are often larger than the adults, usually ranging from 5 to 10 mm in length (James and Harwood, 1969; Borror and White, 1970; Bland and Jacques, 1978; Peterson, 1979; Arnett and Jacques, 1981; Steyskal, 1987; McAlpine, 1987; Vockeroth, 1987; Borror et al., 1989; Hogue, 1993; Castner et al., 1995).

13.2.7.1 *Piophila*

13.2.7.1.1 *Piophila casei* (Linnaeus)

Cheese skippers, found globally, are small (2.5–4.5 mm) shiny black flies with yellow legs. Adults frequent carrion, excrement, and garbage, preferring darker, shaded areas, and resting with their wings flat over their backs. The larvae develop on almost any protein-rich food source, making them a significant pest in the food industry. Adults lay eggs on cheese, bacon, smoked fish, and cured meats, often leading to the ingestion of larvae by humans. Remarkably, the larvae can survive and pass through the human digestive system, causing enteric pseudomyiasis. Cheese skippers are typically found on human bodies after active decay, as the body begins to dry. Adults can appear on remains just 3–4 days after death, but the presence of an adult does not necessarily indicate egg-laying. Although they prefer dry substrates, they are also found on bodies in aquatic environments. Notably, their puparia have been recovered from human organs in a 2000-year-old Egyptian mummy (Cockburn et al., 1975; Simmons, 1927).

13.2.8 Family Stratiomyidae (Soldier Flies)

Soldier flies belong to the family Stratiomyidae and encompass over 250 described species, ranging in size from 5 to 20 mm. The coloration of adult soldier flies varies, with many common species resembling wasps in appearance. Their antennae consist of three segments, with the last segment often elongated or rounded, featuring a long hair protrusion. Adult soldier flies are frequently found around flowers and are commonly observed in wooded areas, on vegetation in moist environments, and near decomposing plant or animal matter. The family name "soldier flies" originates from the presence of spines on the adults of certain species, giving them a resemblance to armed soldiers. Mature soldier fly larvae exhibit significant variation in length, ranging from 4 to 40 mm, depending on the species. Some larvae are purely aquatic, while others inhabit terrestrial environments. Terrestrial larvae typically develop in decomposing plant or animal materials, with some species exhibiting predatory behaviour. Habitats for these larvae include rotting wood, compost piles, and excrement. Aquatic forms of soldier fly larvae can thrive in unexpected environments, such as hot springs or extremely saline waters. In some instances, soldier fly larvae may be ingested through the consumption of infested fruit, leading to cases of enteric pseudomyiasis (James and Harwood, 1969; Borror and White, 1970; Bland and Jacques, 1978; Peterson, 1979; Arnett and Jacques, 1981; Streyskal, 1987; Vockeroth, 1987; Borror et al., 1989; Hogue, 1993; Castner et al., 1995).

13.2.8.1 Black Soldier Fly (*Hermetia illucens*) (Figure 13.8)

The Black Soldier Fly, scientifically known as *Hermetia illucens*, originates from the Neotropical region but has spread to temperate and tropical areas worldwide, likely through contaminated food transportation. It is prevalent throughout the United States and Canada, particularly abundant in the southeastern U.S. and less common in the Northwest. These flies closely resemble wasps in both appearance and behaviour, earning them the nickname "wasp fly". Adult black soldier flies measure approximately 15–20 mm in length, with females displaying a blue-black coloration and males having a slightly brown abdomen. Their wings, held flat over the back when at rest, contribute to their wasp-like appearance. Characteristic behaviours, such as rapid movement of their antennae,

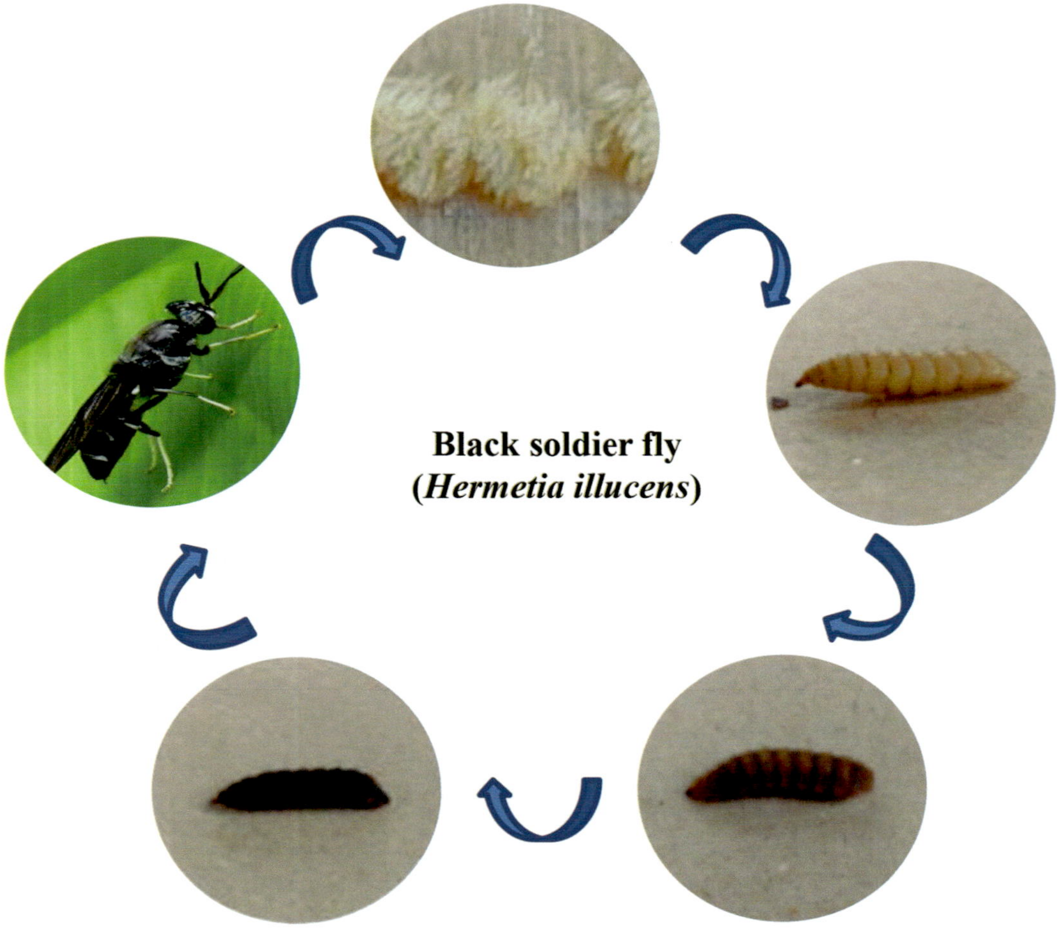

FIGURE 13.8 Life stages of the black soldier fly.

agitated running, and occasional mimicry of stinging behaviour, further enhance their resemblance to wasps. The larvae of the black soldier fly are broad, flattened, and distinctly segmented, featuring a narrow, prominent "head" and rows of stout hairs along each body segment. Grey to brown in colour, the larvae have a hard, thick surface with a unique cobblestone texture, termed "shagreened", under magnification. This texture results from an outer layer of calcium carbonate deposited on the skin, providing protection from desiccation during dry periods. Black soldier fly larvae develop on various decaying organic materials, making them versatile scavengers. They are considered beneficial in certain contexts, as they can suppress house fly populations by competing for the same food sources. Common habitats for larvae include rotting fruits and vegetables, compost and refuse, excrement, and carrion. When associated with human remains, black soldier fly larvae are typically found during the advanced to dry stages of decay, contributing to the decomposition process (Bohart and Gressitt, 1951; Dunn, 1916; Greenberg, 1971; James, 1947; Lord et al., 1994; Payne and King, 1970; Reed, 1958; Smith, 1975, 1986).

13.2.9 Family Sphaeroceridae (Small Dung Flies and Minute Scavenger Flies)

Small dung flies, belonging to the family Sphaeroceridae, are widely distributed worldwide, with over 240 species found in North America alone. They are commonly encountered throughout the U.S. and Canada. These flies are typically small, ranging from 1 to 5 mm in length, and are often dull black or brown in colour. Taxonomic characteristics of their hind legs and wing venation are used for identification at the family level. Both adult and larval stages of Sphaerocerid flies are associated with dung and excrement. They are frequently found in cow dung, often alongside larger dung flies (family Scathophagidae) and black scavenger flies (family Sepsidae). Besides animal waste, they may also inhabit carrion, refuse, seaweed, fungi, and other decaying organic matter. The presence of excrement or soiled clothing on human remains increases the likelihood of encountering small dung flies in association with the remains. However, there has been limited research on the developmental times of these flies (James and Harwood, 1969; Borror and White, 1970; Bland and Jacques, 1978; Peterson, 1979; Arnett and Jacques, 1981; Streyskal, 1987; Vockeroth, 1987; Borror et al., 1989; Hogue, 1993; Castner et al., 1995) (Figure 13.9).

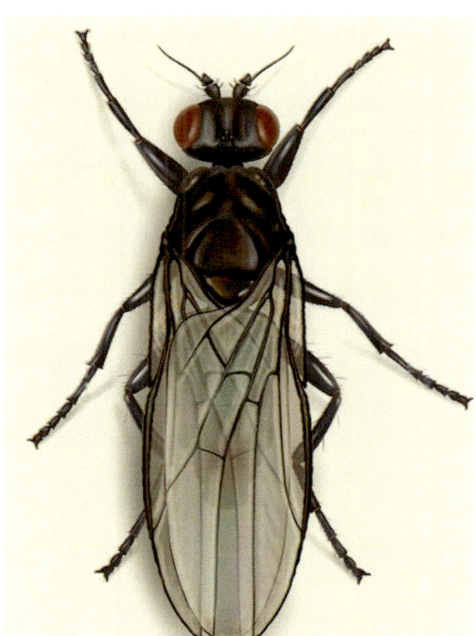

FIGURE 13.9 Sphaeroceridae (small dung flies and minute scavenger flies).

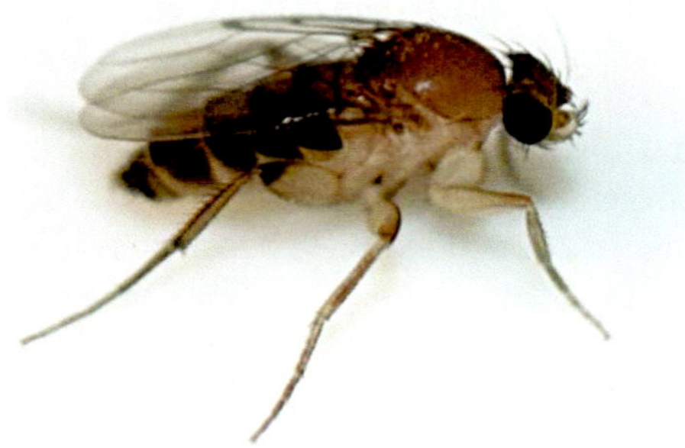

FIGURE 13.10 Phoridae (humpbacked flies or scuttle flies).

13.2.9.1 Small Dung Fly, *Poecilosomella angulata* (Thomson)

This species of small dung fly measures only 2–3 mm in length. It is infrequently found on human remains unless there is the presence of excrement or excrement-soiled clothing. Occasionally, they may also be attracted to exposed gut contents or soil saturated with gut contents. They are commonly found around large vertebrate carcasses, particularly bovines, where substantial amounts of gut contents are exposed during decomposition. *Poecilosomella angulata* has been implicated in cases of intestinal myiasis.

13.2.10 Family Phoridae (Humpbacked Flies or Scuttle Flies) (Figure 13.10)

Humpbacked flies, also known as scuttle flies, belong to the diverse Phoridae family, which includes over 2,500 species worldwide. Nearly half of these species are from the genus *Megaselia*. In the United States, around 226 species have been documented, with approximately 350 species identified in North America. These flies are notable for their distinctive humpbacked appearance, especially noticeable from the side. Key identifying features include the flattened femora of their hind legs and prominent veins at the base of their anterior wing margin. Their coloration varies, with individuals appearing black, brown, or yellow. Adult phorid flies are found in a wide range of environments, frequently inhabiting decaying plant matter and often being considered persistent pests in live insect colonies. Their rapid and erratic movement has earned them the nickname "scuttle flies". The larvae of these flies thrive in decomposing organic matter of all kinds, including human, animal, and vegetative sources. The puparia are easily identified by their flattened shape and often feature horns or "breathing trumpets" at the front end. While some species are predatory or parasitic, others have commensal relationships with ants and termites or develop in fungi. Humpbacked flies are essential decomposers in ecosystems, aiding in the breakdown of organic matter.

13.3 MYIASIS

Myiasis is a parasitic infestation caused by the larvae (maggots) of various fly species, including blow flies. These larvae feed on living or necrotic tissue, resulting in tissue damage and potential secondary infections. They typically deposit their eggs on open wounds, mucous membranes, or body cavities of animals. Upon hatching, the larvae feed on the host's tissue, causing distress and potential health complications (Saari et al., 2018).

Myiasis can manifest in different forms:

1. **Cutaneous Myiasis**: This occurs when larvae infest the skin, causing painful lesions and ulceration.
2. **Nasal Myiasis**: Larvae infest the nasal passages, sinuses, or nasopharynx, resulting in irritation, discharge, and respiratory symptoms.

3. **Ophthalmomyiasis**: This condition involves larvae infesting the eyes, causing discomfort, inflammation, and potential damage to ocular tissues.
4. **Aural Myiasis**: Larvae infest the ears, leading to pain, inflammation, and potential hearing impairment.

Blow fly myiasis can affect a wide range of hosts, including mammals (such as livestock, pets, and humans), birds, and even reptiles. Certain species of blow flies may exhibit preferences for specific hosts or environmental conditions. Symptoms of myiasis vary depending on the affected body part but may include pain, itching, swelling, discharge, and fever. If left untreated, myiasis can lead to secondary infections, tissue necrosis, and systemic illness. Preventive measures for blow fly myiasis include maintaining good hygiene, promptly treating wounds, and using insect repellents in areas with high fly activity. Treatment typically involves the removal of larvae, wound cleaning, and the administration of antibiotics or other medications to manage secondary infections. Blow fly myiasis can have significant economic implications in agriculture, veterinary medicine, and healthcare. Infestations in livestock can lead to reduced productivity, loss of meat or milk quality, and increased treatment costs. Understanding the lifecycle, types, symptoms, and preventive measures associated with blow fly myiasis is essential for the effective management and control of this parasitic infestation. Prompt identification and treatment are crucial to mitigate the impact of myiasis on both individual health and economic well-being (Saari et al., 2018).

13.3.1 Maggot Therapy

Maggot therapy, also referred to as larval therapy or biosurgery, utilizes the natural scavenging abilities of blow fly larvae to facilitate wound healing, primarily by debriding the wound. Administered within sterile dressings to chronic or infected wounds, the larvae consume necrotic tissue, exudate, and bacteria, fostering a clean environment conducive to healing. This therapy proves particularly effective for treating chronic wounds, such as diabetic foot ulcers, pressure ulcers, and venous leg ulcers, as well as in cases of osteomyelitis or infected wounds unresponsive to conventional treatments. Clinical studies have validated its efficacy in reducing wound size, encouraging the formation of granulation tissue, and expediting wound closure. While generally well-received, potential adverse effects may include pain, discomfort, or transient erythema at the wound site, underscoring the necessity of clinical oversight and patient monitoring throughout treatment. Maggot therapy presents a cost-effective and clinically supported approach to wound management, contributing to enhanced outcomes and improved quality of life for patients grappling with complex wounds (Saari et al., 2018).

13.4 VETERINARY IMPORTANCE

The well-being of wild and domestic animals is directly affected by Diptera in many ways. As vectors of pathogens, flies are responsible for spreading 186 Medical and Veterinary Entomology viruses, such as those that cause bluetongue disease in sheep and cattle and haemorrhagic disease in deer; rickettsial infections, such as anaplasmosis; protozoans, such as those causing avian malaria; and metazoan infections, such as canine heartworm. *Trypanosoma*-caused nagana, vectored by tsetse flies, has eliminated most animal agriculture throughout large areas of Africa. In many parts of the world, infestations of living tissue with fly larvae, called myiasis, can be a problem for livestock and other domestic or wild animals. At one time, myiasis caused by screwworms constituted a major impediment to cattle, hog, and sheep production in the southern United States, Mexico, and Central America and was a significant mortality factor among wildlife, especially deer. With the success of sterile-male releases and other anti-screwworm measures, this species is no longer a significant problem in North America. Other myiasis-causing flies in North America include cattle and reindeer grubs, sheep nose bots, deer and reindeer nose bots, rabbit and rodent bots, and stomach bots of horses and other equids. In most localities, species of blowflies that cause myiasis have a direct summertime impact on most types of livestock and pets. These flies can invade wounds, sores, or body orifices, such as unhealed navels of newborns and vaginal tissues of postpartum females. The condition is perhaps best recognized by the sheep industry as fly-strike or sheep strike and has had an extensive impact, particularly in Australia and New Zealand. Blood-feeding flies can affect the productivity and profitability of livestock operations by causing exsanguination and, in extreme cases, anaemia. Although the biting rates of diurnal species are obvious to livestock producers (e.g. horseflies), those of crepuscular or nocturnal species are largely unappreciated. Livestock on pasture or in production systems where large numbers of animals are artificially confined may be subject to intense biting rates from flies. Bunching, kicking, and other avoidance behaviours by animals under attack from biting flies can interfere with grazing time, feed consumption, and the efficiency of energy conversion. The enormous numbers of non-biting flies associated with livestock and livestock facilities can constitute an annoyance factor. The feeding spots and faecal spots made by flies can create sanitary and aesthetic problems. In the poultry industry, fly specks on chicken eggs are a major economic problem. Flies produced in one location may affect animals in another. For example, stable flies emanating from cattle feedlots may immigrate to nearby farmsteads where they feed on pets and companion animals. Flies, such as stable flies and eye gnats, breeding adjacent to dog kennels may annoy dogs and other animals even at considerable distances from the breeding sites (Alikhan et al., 2018).

13.5 CONCLUSION

Dipteran flies, also known as true flies, are incredibly diverse, with an estimated 240,000 species. These include sand flies, house flies, gnats, midges, and mosquitoes. Identified species range from 120,000 to 150,000, showcasing their pivotal roles in ecosystems. Dipteran flies are essential pollinators of flowering plants. They act as efficient decomposers, aiding in the breakdown of organic matter. They facilitate nutrient recycling in terrestrial ecosystems by accelerating microbial decomposition and breaking down animal tissues. Flies can traverse various landscapes and adapt to diverse environmental conditions, highlighting their resilience. Dipteran flies, particularly blow flies (Calliphoridae), flesh flies (Sarcophagidae), and house flies (Muscidae and Fannidae), are crucial in forensic entomology. They are vital for investigating human and animal corpses due to their necrophagous and synanthropic traits. Flies, like mosquitoes, sand flies, black flies, and house flies, can cause significant distress to humans and animals, sometimes leading to lethal outcomes. Many flies are potential vectors for serious diseases, impacting public health and hygiene.

13.6 POINTS TO REMEMBER

1. Dipteran flies, also known as true flies, are incredibly diverse, with an estimated 240,000 species. These include sand flies, house flies, gnats, midges, and mosquitoes. Identified species range from 120,000 to 150,000, showcasing their pivotal roles in ecosystems.
2. Dipteran flies are essential pollinators of flowering plants. They act as efficient decomposers, aiding in the breakdown of organic matter. They facilitate nutrient recycling in terrestrial ecosystems by accelerating microbial decomposition and breaking down animal tissues. Flies can traverse various landscapes and adapt to diverse environmental conditions, highlighting their resilience.
3. Dipteran flies, particularly blow flies (Calliphoridae), flesh flies (Sarcophagidae), and house flies (Muscidae and Fannidae), are crucial in forensic entomology. They are vital for investigating human and animal corpses due to their necrophagous and synanthropic traits.
4. Flies like mosquitoes, sand flies, black flies, and house flies can cause significant distress to humans and animals, sometimes leading to lethal outcomes. Many flies are potential vectors for serious diseases, impacting public health and hygiene.

REFERENCES

Aldrich, J. M. (1916). *Sarcophaga and Allies in North America,* Vol. 1. Thomas Say Foundation, La Fayette, 356 pp.

Alikhan, M., Al Ghamdi, K., Mahyoub, J. A., & Alanazi, N. (2018). Public health and veterinary important flies (order: Diptera) prevalent in Jeddah Saudi Arabia with their dominant characteristics and identification key. *Saudi Journal of Biological Sciences*, 25(8), 1648–1663.

Anderson, G. S. (1995). The use of insects in death investigations: An analysis of cases in British Columbia over a five year period. *Canadian Society of Forensic Science Journal*, 28(4), 277–292.

Anderson, G. S. (1997). The use of insects to determine time of decapitation: A case-study from British Columbia. *Journal of Forensic Sciences*, 42(5), 947–950.

Anderson, G. S. (2000). Minimum and maximum development rates of some forensically important Callophoridae (Diptera). *Journal of Forensic Science,* 45, 824–832.

Arnett, R. H., & Jacques, R. L. (1981). *Simon and Schuster's Guide to Insects: A Fireside Book Nature Guide Series*. Simon and Schuster, New York, 512 pp.

Australian Museum. (November 2009). *Decomposition: Fly Life Cycle and Development Times*. https://australianmuseum.net.au/Decomposition-fly-life-cycles/ (30 August 2011)

Babu, B. S., Kumar, R., El-Sharnouby, M., Salah, M., Sayed, S., Alhazmi, A., Hemeg, H. A., Asdaq, S. M. B., & Bala, M. (2022). Calliphorids as forensic indicator to facilitate PMI estimation: A case study from Chhattisgarh, India. *Journal of King Saud University-Science*, 34(1), 101709.

Babu, B. S., Sharma, H., Bharti, M., & Colony, B. (2013). Estimation of post mortem interval by rearing *Chrysomya rufifacies* (Macquart, 1842) (Diptera: Calliphoridae): A case study from central India. *Anil Aggrawal's Internet Journal of Forensic Medicine and Toxicology*, 14, 1–11.

Bala, M., & Sharma, A. (2015). A case study of decapitated 38 years old male corpse from Punjab (India): Image Article. *Journal of Forensic Research*, 6(2), 1.

Baumgartner, D. L. (1986). The hairy maggot blow fly *Chrysomya rufifacies* (Macquart) confirmed in Arizona. *Journal of Entomological Science*, 21, 130–132.

Baumgartner, D. L. (1993). Review of *Chrysomya rufifacies* (Diptera: Calliphoridae). *Journal of Medical Entomology*, 30(2), 338–352.

Baumgartner, D. L., & Greenberg, B. (1984). The genus *Chrysomya* (Diptera: Calliphoridae) in the new world. *Journal of Medical Entomology*, 21(1), 105–113.

Benecke, M. (2021). Blow flies (Diptera: Calliphoridae, polleniidae, rhinidae). *Handbook for the Identification of British Insects,* Vol. 10. Part 16 by Olga Sivell. Paperback, 2021, 206 pp. Published by the Royal Entomological Society. ISBN 9781910159064. *Entomologist's Monthly Magazine*, 157(4), 258–260.

Bharti, M., & Singh, B. (2017). DNA-based identification of forensically important blow flies (Diptera: Calliphoridae) from India. *Journal of Medical Entomology*, 54(5), 1151–1156.

Bharti, M., & Singh, D. (2003). Insect faunal succession on decaying rabbit carcasses in Punjab, India. *Journal of Forensic Sciences*, 48(5), JFS2001358.

Bharti, M., & Singh, D. (2022). Insects in forensic investigations. In: Omkar (ed.), *Insects as Service Providers*. Springer Nature, Singapore, pp. 165–182.

Bland, R. G., & Jaques, H. E. (1978). *How to Know the Insects*. W. C. Brown, Dubuque, IA, 409 pp.

Borror, D. J., & White, R. E. (1970). *A Field Guide to Insects: America North of Mexico* (Vol. 19). Houghton Mifflin Harcourt, 404 pp.

Borror, D. J., Triplehorn, C. A., & Johnson, N. F. (1989). *An Introduction to the Study of Insects*, 6th edn. Saunders College, Saunders, 875 pp.

Braverman, I., Dano, I., Saah, D., & Gapany, B. (1994). Aural myiasis caused by flesh fly larva, *Sarcophaga haemorrhoidalis*. *The Journal of Otolaryngology*, 23(3), 204–205.

Brian, V. (2001). Brown, flies, gnats, and mosquitoes. In S. A. Levin (ed.), Encyclopedia of Biodiversity. Elsevier, Amsterdam, pp. 815–826.

Bunchu, N., Thaipakdee, C., Vitta, A., Sanit, S., Sukontason, K., & Sukontason, K. L. (2012). Morphology and developmental rate of the blow fly, *Hemipyrellia ligurriens* (Diptera: Calliphoridae): Forensic entomology applications. *Journal of Parasitology Research*, 1–10. doi:10.1155/2012/371243.

Byrd, J. H. (1998–2011). *Forensic Entomology: Insects in Legal Investigations*. Natonal History Museum, 681 pp.

Byrd, J. H., & Butler, J. F. (1998). Effects of temperature on *Sarcophaga haemorrhoidalis* (Diptera: Sarcophagidae) development. *Journal of Medical Entomology*, 35(5), 694–698.

Byrd, J. H., & Castner, J. L. (2009). Insects of forensic importance. In. J. H. Byrd & J. L. Castner (eds.), *Forensic Entomology: The Utility of Arthropods in Legal Investigations*, 2nd edn. CRC Press, Boca Raton, FL, pp. 43–45.

CABICompendium. (2022). Cabicompendium, 10950, *Calliphora vicina*. doi:10.1079/cabicompendium.10950.
Carvalho, C. J. B. D., & Mello-Patiu, C. A. D. (2008). Key to the adults of the most common forensic species of Diptera in South America. *Revista Brasileira de Entomologia*, 52, 390–406.
Castner, J. L. (2009). General entomology and insect biology. In J. H. Byrd & J. L. Castner (eds.), *Forensic Entomology,* 2nd edn. CRC Press, Boca Raton, FL, pp. 17–38.
Castner, J. L., Byrd, J. H., & Butler, J. F. (1995). *Forensic Insect Field Identification Cards*. Forensic Sciences Foundation, Colorado Springs.
Catts, E. P., & Goff, M. L. (1992). Forensic entomology in criminal investigations. *Annual Review of Entomology*, 37(1), 253–272.
Chapman, R. K. (1944). An interesting occurrence of *Musca domestica* L. larvae in infant bedding. *The Canadian Entomologist*, 76(11), 230–232.
Chen, L. S. (2013). *Necrophagous flies in China*. Guizhou Science and Technology Press, Guiyang, China, pp. 267–270.
Cockburn, A., Barraco, R. A., Reyman, T. A., & Peck, W. H. (1975). Autopsy of an Egyptian mummy: A mummy can be a scientific treasure chest; to unlock its secrets, a multidisciplinary approach is needed. *Science*, 187(4182), 1155–1160.
Cragg, J. B. (1956). The olfactory behaviour of *Lucilia* species (Diptera) under natural conditions. *Annals of Applied Biology*, 44(3), 467–477.
Davis, W. T. (1928). Lucilia flies anticipating death. *Bulletin of the Brooklyn Entomological Society*, 23, 118.
Denno, R. F., & Cothran, W. R. (1975). Niche relationships of a guild of necrophagous flies. *Annals of the Entomological Society of America*, 68(4), 741–754.
Dunn, L. H. (1916). *Hermetia illucens* breeding in a human cadaver (Dipt.). *Entomol News*, 17(2), 59–61.
Erzinçlioğlu, Y. Z. (1985). Immature stages of British *Calliphora* and *Cynomya*, with a re-evaluation of the taxonomic characters of larval Calliphoridae (Diptera). *Journal of Natural History*, 19(1), 69–96.
Erzincllioĝlu, Y. Z. (1983). The application of entomology to forensic medicine. *Medicine, Science and the Law*, 23(1), 57–63.
Goff, M. L. (1992). Problems in estimation of postmortem interval resulting from wrapping of the corpse: A case study from Hawaii. *Journal of Agricultural Entomology*, 9(4), 237–243.
Goff, M. L., & Odom, C. B. (1987). Forensic entomology in the Hawaiian Islands: Three case studies. *The American Journal of Forensic Medicine and Pathology*, 8(1), 45–50.
Goff, M. L., Odom, C. B., & Early, M. (1986). Estimation of post-mortem interval by entomological techniques: A case study from Oahu, Hawaii. *Bulletin of the Society for Vector Ecology*, *11*, 82–93.
Goff, M. L., Omori, A. I., & Gunatilake, K. (1988). Estimation of postmortem interval by arthropod succession: Three case studies from the Hawaiian Islands. *The American Journal of Forensic Medicine and Pathology*, 9(3), 220–225.
Greenberg, B. (1971). *Flies and Disease* (2 Vol.). Princeton University Press, Princeton, NJ, 464 pp.
Greenberg, B. (1985). Forensic entomology: Case studies. *Bulletin of the ESA*, 31(4), 25–28.
Greenberg, B., & Kunich, J. C. (2002). *Entomology and the Law: Flies as Forensic Indicators*. Cambridge University Press, Cambridge, 315 pp.
Grzywacz, A., & Pape, T. (2014). Larval morphology of Atherigonaorientalis (Schiner)(Diptera: Muscidae): A species of sanitary and forensic importance. *Acta Tropica*, 137, 174–184.
Grzywacz, A., Hall, M. J., Pape, T., & Szpila, K. (2017). Muscidae (Diptera) of forensic importance—an identification key to third instar larvae of the western Palaearctic region and a catalogue of the muscid carrion community. *International Journal of Legal Medicine*, 131, 855–866.
Hall, D. G. (1948). *The Blowflies of North America*. The Thomas Say Foundation, Lafayette, 477 pp.
Hall, R. D., & Doisy, K. E. (1993). Length of time after death: Effect on attraction and oviposition or larviposition of mid summer blow flies (Diptera: Calliphoridae) and flesh flies (Diptera: Sarcophagidae) of medicolegal importance in Missouri. *Annals of the Entomological Society of America*, 86(5), 589–593.
Hall, R. D., & Townsend, L. H. (1977). *The Blow Flies of Virginia (Diptera: Calliphoridae)*. Virginia Polytechnic Institute and State University, Research Division, 56 pp.
Hogue, C. L. (1993). *Latin American Insects and Entomology*. University of California Press, California, 281 pp.
Horobin, A. J., Pritchad, D. L., & Shakesheff, L. M. (2002). How do larvae of *Lucilia sericata* initiate human wound healing. *European Cells & Materials*, 4(Suppl 2), 70–71.
Hu, C. (2000). *Forensic Entomology*. Chongqing Publishing House, Chongqing, 230 pp.
Introna, F., Suman, T. W., & Smialek, J. E. (1991). Sarcosaprophagous fly activity in Maryland. *Journal of Forensic Sciences*, 36(1), 238–243.
Introna, Jr, F., Campobasso, C. P., & Di Fazio, A. (1998). Three case studies in forensic entomology from southern Italy. *Journal of Forensic Sciences*, 43(1), 210–214.

James, M. T. (1947). *The Flies that Cause Myiasis in Man*. Miscellaneous Publication of the U.S. Department of Agriculture, Washington, D.C., pp. 631:1–175.

James, M. T. (1981). Manual *of Nearctic Diptera*, Vol. 1, Monograph No. 27. Canadian Government Publishing Centre, Hull, Quebec, 674 pp.

James, M. T., & Harwood, R. F. (1969). Ticks and tick-borne diseases. In: *Herm's Medical Entomology,* 6th edn. Collier-Macmillan Ltd., London, pp. 323–324.

Kamal, A. S. (1958). Comparative study of thirteen species of sarcosaprophagous Calliphoridae and Sarcophagidae (Diptera) I. Bionomics. *Annals of the Entomological Society of America*, 51(3), 261–271.

Knipling, E. F. (1936). A comparative study of the first-instar larvae of the genus *Sarcophaga* (Calliphoridae, Diptera), with notes on the biology. *The Journal of Parasitology*, 22(5), 417–454.

Lord, W. D., Adkins, T. R., & Catts, E. P. (1992). The use of *Synthesic myianudesita* [sic](Van Der Wulp) (Diptera: Muscidae) and *Calliphora vicina* (Robineau-Desvoidy)(Diptera: Calliphoridae) to estimate the time of death of a body buried under a house. *Journal of Agricultural Entomology*, 9(1), 227–235.

Lord, W. D., Goff, M. L., Adkins, T. R., & Haskell, N. H. (1994). The black soldier fly *Hermetia illucens* (Diptera: Stratiomyidae) as a potential measure of human postmortem interval: Observations and case histories. *Journal of Forensic Sciences*, 39(1), 215–222.

Madubunyi, L.C. (1986). Laboratory life history parameters of the red-tailed fleshfly, *Sarcophaga haemorrhoidalis* (Fallen) (Diptera: Sarcophagidae). *International Journal of Tropical Insect Science*, 7, 617–621.

McAlpine, J. F. (1987). *Manual of Nearctic Diptera*, Vol. 2, Monograph No. 28. Canadian Government Publishing Centre, Hull, Quebec, 584 pp.

McAlpine, J. F., Peterson, B. V., Shewell, G. E., Teskey, H. J., Vockeroth, J. R., & Wood, D. M. (1981). *Manual of Nearctic Diptera*, Vol. 1, Monograph No. 27. Research Branch Agriculture Canada, Ottawa, 1003 pp.

Mondor, E. B., Tremblay, M. N., Tomberlin, J. K., Benbow, E. M., Tarone, A. M., & Crippen, T. L. (2012). The ecology of carrion decomposition. *National Educatioon Knowledge*, 3, 21.

Mullen, G. R., & Durden, L. A. (Eds.). (2009). *Medical and Veterinary Entomology*. Academic Press, London, 794 pp.

Nolte, K. B., Pinder, R. D., & Lord, W. D. (1992). Insect larvae used to detect cocaine poisoning in a decomposed body. *Journal of Forensic Sciences*, 37(4), 1179–1185.

Nuorteva, P. (1974). Age determination of a blood stain in a decaying shirt by entomological means. *Forensic Science*, 3, 89–94.

Nuorteva, P. (1977). Sarcosaprophagous insects as forensic indicators, in Forensic Medicine: A study in trauma and environmental hazards. In: C. G. Tedeschi, W. G. Eckert, & L. G. Tedeschi (eds.), Physical Trauma, Vol. II. Saunders, Philadelphia, 1072 pp.

Palavesam, A., Selvakumar, R., Latha, B. R., Soundararajan, C., Jyothimol, G., & Harikrishnan, T. J. (2022). Occurrence of necrophagous flies of forensic importance in medico-legal cases in Tamil Nadu State, India. *Egyptian Journal of Forensic Sciences*, 12(50), 1–12.

Pape, T. (1996). *Catalogue of the Sarcophagidae of the world (Insecta: Diptera). Associated Publishers*, 8, 1–558.

Payne, J. A. (1965). A summer carrion study of the baby pig *Sus scrofa* Linnaeus. *Ecology*, 46(5), 592–602.

Peterson, A. (1979). *Larvae of insects (Part II)*. Lithographed by Edwards Brothers, Inc., Ann Arbor, MI, 416 pp.

Povolny, D. (1997). The flesh-flies of Central Europe (Insecta, Diptera, Sarcophagidae). *Spixiana Supplments*, 24, 1–260.

Pradoe Castro, C., & Ameixa, O. M. C. C. (2021). Blow flies (Diptera: Calliphoridae) promising candidates as animal feed ingredients. *Journal of Insects as Food and Feed*, 7(7), 1065–1076.

Raguso, R. A. (2020). Don't forget the flies: Dipteran diversity and its consequences for floral ecology and evolution. *Applied Entomology and Zoology*, 55(1), 1–7.

Retka, O. (2021). *Blow Flies:(*Diptera: Calliphoridae, Polleniidae, Rhiniidae). Royal Entomological Society, London, 208 pp.

Rueda, L. C., Ortega, L. G., Segura, N. A., Acero, V. M., & Bello, F. (2010). *Lucilia sericata* strain from Colombia: Experimental colonization, life tables and evaluation of two artifcial diets of the blowfy *Lucilia sericata* (Meigen) (Diptera: Calliphoridae), Bogotá, Colombia strain. *Biological Research*, 43(2), 197–203.

Saari, S., Näreaho, A., & Nikander, S. (2018). *Canine Parasites and Parasitic Diseases*. Academic Press, London, 271 pp.

Savage, J. (2002). Cleaning up the world: Dipteran decomposers. *Biodiversity*, 3(4), 12–15.

Sharma, A., & Bala, M. (2016). Case study and PMI estimation of male corpse from Ludhiana, Punjab, India: An implication of ADH method. *Indian Journal of Forensic Medicine & Toxicology*, 10(2), 28–33.

Sharma, A., Bala, M., & Singh, N. (2018). Five case studies associated with forensically important entomofauna recovered from human corpses from Punjab, India. *Journal of Forensic Sciences & Criminal Investigation*, 7, 1–6.

Sherman, R. A., Hall, M. J. R., & Thomas, S. (2000). Medicinal maggots: An ancient remedy for some contemporary afflictions. *Annual Review of Entomology*, 45(1), 55–81.

Simmons, P. (1927). *The Cheese Skipper as a Pest in Cured Meats* (No. 1453). US Department of Agriculture, Washington, DC, 64 pp.

Smith, E., & Whitman, R. (1992). *Flesh Flies*: *Field Guide to Structural Pests*, Vol. 4. National Pest Control Association. Fairfax, VA, 800 pp.

Smith, E. H., & Whitman, R. C. (2007). Flies (non-biting)-Blow Flies. In: *NPMA Field Guide of Structural Pests*, Vol. 6.1.1. National Pest Management Association International, Fairfax, VA, pp. 1–54.

Smith, K. G. (1956). On the diptera associated with the stinkhorn {phallus impudicus pers.) with notes on other insects and invertebrates found on this fungus. In *Proceedings of the Royal Entomological Society of London. Series A, General Entomology,* 31(4–6), 49–55.

Smith, K. G. (1975). The faunal succession of insects and other invertebrates on a dead fox. *Entomological Gazette*, 26, 277–287.

Smith, K. G. V. (1986). *A Manual of Forensic Entomology*. Cornell University Press, Ithaca, NY, 102 pp.

Strikewise. (2007). Blowfly strike.

Szpila, K., Richet, R., & Pape, T. (2015). Third instar larvae of flesh flies (Diptera: Sarcophagidae) of forensic importance: Critical review of characters and key for European species. *Parasitology Research*, 114, 2279–2289.

Tarone, A. M., & Foran, D. R. (2006). Components of developmental plasticity in a Michigan population of *Lucilia sericata* (Diptera: Calliphoridae). *Journal of Medical Entomology*, 43(5), 1023–1033.

Tarone, A. M., & Foran, D. R. (2011). Gene expression during blow fly development: Improving the precision of age estimates in forensic entomology. *Journal of Forensic Sciences*, 56, 112–122.

Thompson, F.C. (2006). *Nomenclator Status Statistics*. The Biosystematic Database of world Diptera. https://bonn.leibniz-lib.de/dateien/dokumente/279-295_studia_dipt-suppl-23_thompson_-_mengual_et_al._279-295.pdf

Tomberlin, J. K., & Benbow, M. E. (Eds.). (2015). *Forensic Entomology: International Dimensions and Frontiers*. CRC Press, Boca Raton, FL, 468 pp.

Turhan, V., Aydin, A. F., Eyigun, C. P., Araz, E., Tanyuksel, M., & Pahsa, A. (2007). An intestinal myiasis case of flesh fly (*Sarcophaga haemorrhoidalis*). *The Anatolian Journal of Clinical Investigation*, 1(8), 270–272.

Vockeroth, J. R. (1987). *Manual of Nearctic Diptera*, Vol. 2, Monograph No. 28, Canadian Government Publishing Centre, Hull, Quebec.

Wang, M., Chu, J., Wang, Y., Li, F., Liao, M., Shi, H., … & Wang, J. (2019). Forensic entomology application in China: Four case reports. *Journal of Forensic and Legal Medicine*, 63, 40–47.

Wasti, W. S. (1972). A study of the carrion of the common fowl, *Gallus domseticus*, in relation to arthropod succession, *Journal of the Georgia Entomological Society,* 7, 221–229.

Whitworth, T. (2019). Keys to the genera and species of blow flies (Diptera: Calliphoridae) of America, North of Mexico. *Proceedings of the Entomological Society of Washington*, *108*, 3.

Wiegmann, B. M., Trautwein, M. D., Winkler, I. S., Barr, N. B., Kim, J. W., Lambkin, C., ... & Yeates, D. K. (2011). Episodic radiations in the fly tree of life. *Proceedings of the National Academy of Sciences*, 108(14), 5690–5695.

Williams, K. A., &Villet, M. H. (2006). A new and earlier record of *Chrysomya megacephala* in South Africa, with notes on another exotic species, *Calliphora vicina* (Diptera: Calliphoridae). *African Invertebrates*, 47(1), 347–350.

Yeates, D. K., & Wiegmann, B. M. (2005). Phylogeny and evolution of Diptera: Recent insights and new perspectives. In: D. K. Yeates & B. M. Wiegmann (eds.), *The Evolutionary Biology of Flies*. Columbia, New York, pp. 14–44.

Yeates, D. K., Wiegmann, B. M., Courtney, G. W., Meier, R., Lambkin, C., & Pape, T. (2007). Phylogeny and systematics of Diptera: Two decades of progress and prospects. *Zootaxa*, 1668(1), 565–590.

Zumpt, F. (1965). *Myiasis in Man and Animals in the Old World. A Textbook for Physicians, Veterinarians and Zoologists*. Embrapa Informação Tecnológica, Brasília, 279 pp.

Zumpt, F., & Patterson, P. M. (1952). Flies visiting human faeces and carcasses in Johannesburg, Transvaal. *South African Journal of the Chinese Science Cape Town (incorporating Chinese Proceedings)*, 3(2), 92–106.

14 Flies in Forensic Investigations

Bhanvi Wadhawan and Devinder Singh

LEARNING OBJECTIVES

1. To understand the significance of flies in forensic science.
2. To acquaint oneself with important fly orders that assist in forensic investigations.
3. To recognize the diversity of fly species with forensic importance in India.
4. To gain a comprehensive understanding of the life cycles of blow flies and flesh flies.
5. To understand the relationship between fly development stages and techniques used for post-mortem interval (PMI) estimates

14.1 INTRODUCTION

Carrion represents a highly dynamic and patchy microhabitat with a rich nutrient content and intense biological activity, distinctly different from the surrounding environment. These habitats, characterized by rapidly changing physicochemical conditions, serve as key points for nutrient cycling and invertebrate congregation. Such aggregations facilitate the release of water, energy, and nutrients, which are crucial for the long-term functioning of ecosystems. These resource islands provide niches, influence the spatial and temporal distribution of invertebrate biodiversity, and act as corridors for their dispersal within and across ecosystems (Garcia-Moya and Mckell, 1970; Mummey and Stahl, 2003; Matuszewski et al., 2011). In the case of human cadavers, decomposition is often delayed or prevented by hygienic practices, such as burial or cremation. However, certain circumstances, such as criminal activities or sudden deaths, can expose human bodies to natural environmental effects, including invertebrate invasion.

A corpse, whether human or animal, undergoes a series of significant physical, biological, and chemical transformations driven by tissue autolysis and the activity of bacteria and fungi from both the intestine and the external environment (Coe and Curran, 1980; Introna and Campobasso, 2000; Amendt et al., 2004; Anderson, 2010). These transformations include livor mortis, algor mortis, rigor mortis, postmortem cooling, changes in body chemistry, autolysis, and putrefaction within the early PMI, that is, 0–72 hours post-death (Kashyap and Pillay, 1989; Gennard, 2012). In the later decomposition stage, starting approximately 30–72 hours post-death (depending on ambient temperature), the corpse progresses through fresh, bloated, active decay, advanced decay, dry decay, and remains stages (Bornemissza, 1957; Reed, 1958; Payne, 1965).

Each decomposition stage attracts different groups of sarcosaprophagous arthropods, each with a specific life strategy suited to a particular niche. These arthropods are more consistently associated with decomposing bodies than any other resource (Putman, 1983). Co-existence among these arthropods is facilitated by succession on a single corpse and resource partitioning. Some are strongly attracted to the corpse for food or oviposition, while others are drawn by the large aggregation of other arthropods they prey upon (Schoenly and Reid, 1987; Wells and Greenberg, 1994). Insects dominate the arthropod decomposer fauna in both species diversity and individual numbers. According to Smith (1986), four ecological guilds can be identified in a corpse community:

DOI: 10.1201/9781003482581-17

1. **Necrophagous species**: These feed directly on the carrion.
   a. **Sarcosaprophages**: Consume decomposing flesh and body fluids, for example, Calliphoridae, Sarcophagidae, Muscidae, and Dermestidae.
   b. **Coprophages**: Attracted to stomach/intestinal contents, for example, Scarabaeidae, Muscidae.
   c. **Dermatophages**: Feed on dried skin, hair, ligaments, and bones, for example, Dermestidae, Tineidae.
2. **Predators and parasites of necrophages**: This group includes Coleoptera: Silphidae, Staphylinidae, Histeridae, and Diptera (Calliphoridae and Stratiomyidae). It also contains schizophagous species that initially feed on carrion but may become predatory in later larval stages.
3. **Omnivorous species**: Wasps, ants, and some beetles that feed on both the corpse and its inhabitants.
4. **Adventive species**: These use the corpse as an extension of their habitat, for example, Collembola (springtails), and spiders (which may become incidental predators). Acari feeding on fungi and moulds growing on the corpse may also be included.

Flies and beetles constitute most of these assemblages. It is estimated that Diptera and Coleoptera make up 60% of the fauna associated with decomposing corpses (Moretti et al., 2008), with Diptera being richer in species and having a higher biomass in most ecosystems compared to other insect decomposers (McLean, 2000).

In forensic entomology, precise identification of insect and arthropod species is crucial. It allows for the application of accurate developmental data and distribution ranges in investigations. Errors in species determination can compromise the reliability of estimated PMIs. The aim of this chapter is to offer a concise summary of the taxonomic traits, behavioural patterns, and biological characteristics of the order Diptera significant in forensic contexts.

14.2 DIPTERA OF FORENSIC IMPORTANCE

The order Diptera encompasses flies and includes over 1,50,000 described species, making it one of the largest insect orders (Capinera, 2008; Sarwar, 2020). Flies inhabit nearly every environment and are distinguished by having a single pair of wings, with the second pair reduced to knob-like structures called halteres, which help to stabilize them in flight. Flies possess large compound eyes and various types of mouthparts, although most flies associated with corpses have sponging mouthparts. Fly larvae, commonly known as maggots, are typically cream-coloured, soft, legless, and lack a visible head. Aquatic larvae, such as those of midges and mosquitoes, are slender and have a discernible head. Flies play a crucial role as scavengers, removing decomposing plant and animal materials from the environment. Some species are predators or parasites of other insects, while others contribute to plant pollination.

Most flies commonly linked with the colonization of deceased organisms belong to the Infraorder Muscomorpha, which is part of the Suborder Brachycera within the Order Diptera (Calliphoridae, Sarcophagidae, Muscidae, Fanniidae, Piophilidae, Phoridae, Scathophagidae, Sepsidae, Ulididae). This group is characterized by having a sleek, compact appearance, a three-part antenna featuring a thick hair-like projection called an arista on the third segment, and a puparium (as shown in Figures 14.1 and 14.2) from which the adult fly emerges through a round opening. Very few species belong to the Infraorder Stratiomyomorpha (Stratiomyidae) of the Suborder Brachycera and the Infraorder Psychodomorpha of the Suborder Nematocera (Psychodidae). This chapter focuses on the dipteran species that are necrophagous and are usually encountered on corpses.

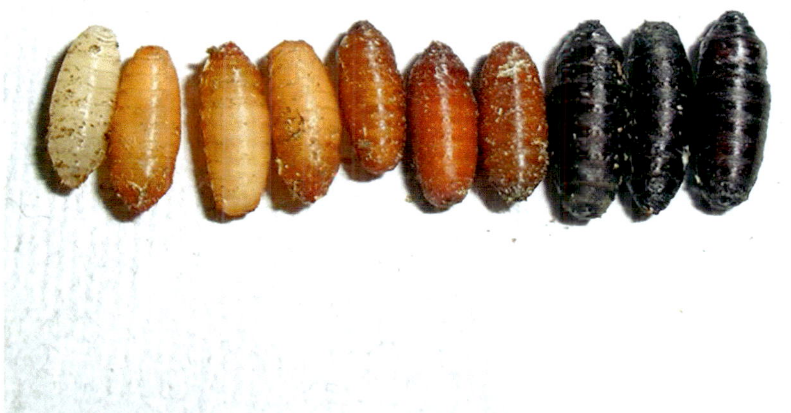

FIGURE 14.1 Stages in the maturation of pupa.

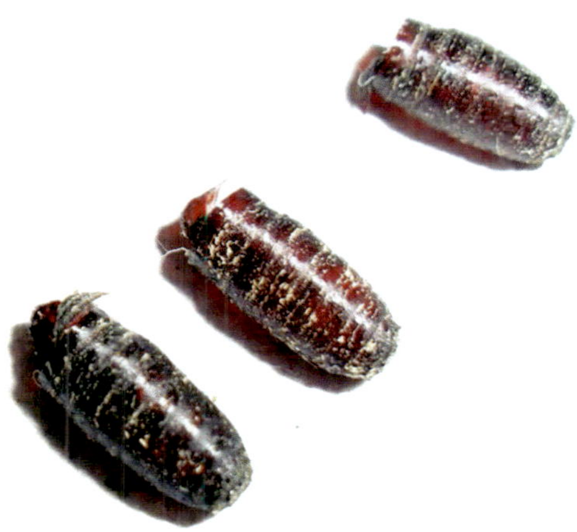

FIGURE 14.2 Fly puparia.

14.2.1 Calliphoridae

This extensive family of medium-sized flies includes over 1,500 species worldwide (Merrit et al., 2009). Attracted to carrion and excrement, some calliphorid species also exploit open wounds. This family includes well-known green bottle flies (*Lucilia*), blue bottle flies (*Calliphora*), and screwworm flies (*Cochliomyia*). Besides their forensic significance, they play a vital role in nutrient recycling and community ecology through the decomposition of vertebrate carcasses.

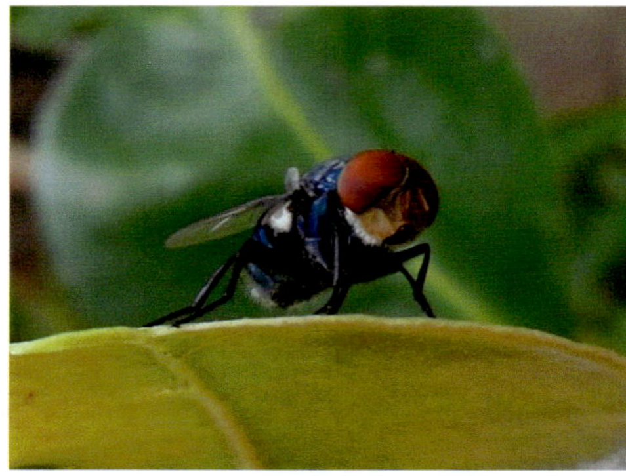

FIGURE 14.3 Adult Calliphorid.

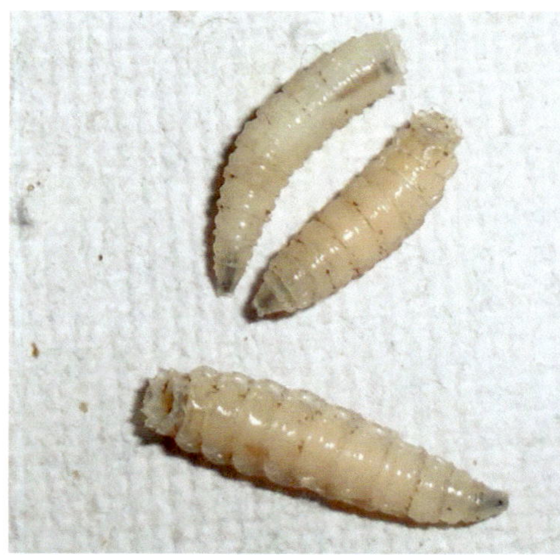

FIGURE 14.4 Calliphorid larvae.

The name of this family, Calliphoridae, originates from the characteristic shiny appearance of its adult flies, which often display various metallic blue and green hues (Calliphoridae=jewel-bearing) (Figure 14.3). The larvae of these flies (as depicted in Figure 14.4) are commonly known as maggots and typically exhibit a creamy white coloration with a tapered cylindrical shape. Mature larvae of blow flies range from 8 to 23 mm in length and are usually white or cream-coloured. The narrower end of the maggot, which houses the mouth-hooks used for feeding, serves as the feeding point, while the broader end contains the spiracular plate, functioning as the primary respiratory opening for the larva. There is also a small fan-shaped anterior spiracle near the tapered or head end of larger or later instar larvae. While most larvae in this family are smooth, some may feature tubercles (spiny projections), for example, *Chrysomya rufifacies*, which are highly useful for identification purposes.

Adult calliphorids typically range from 6 to 14 mm in length and are usually metallic in appearance, with colours varying from green to blue, bronze, or black. These adults have three-segmented antennae with a hair-like arista on the last segment, which is plumose or hairy along its entire length.

Blow flies are generally the first to colonize dead bodies, drawn by the odours produced during decomposition (Wall and Warnes, 1994). They can detect these odours from great distances

(Braack, 1981; Erzinclioglu, 1996). Compounds rich in ammonia and hydrogen sulphide serve as key stimulants for their oviposition, alongside moisture, certain pheromones, and tactile cues (Ashworth and Wall, 1994). In addition to olfactory stimuli, visual cues, colour, and the presence of other flies on the body also attract them (Wall and Fisher, 2001). Blow flies are attracted to decomposing bodies because they provide a protein source for both the flies and their offspring (Smith and Wall, 1997). The female's abdomen extends to form an ovipositor for egg laying, typically placing large numbers of eggs in the nose, mouth, and other natural body openings. Open wounds are also preferred for egg deposition, leading to maggot mass formations and uneven defleshing of bodies, which can indicate premortem or perimortem trauma (Liu and Greenberg, 1989).

Beyond their role in nutrient recycling and community ecology through the breakdown of vertebrate carcasses, blow flies are crucial forensic indicators during the initial stages of decomposition (Lord and Goff, 1997), as they complete all stages of their life cycle on the carcasses (Putman, 1983). Baseline knowledge of blow fly activity on dead bodies is extensively utilized in forensic entomology (Greenberg, 1991; Byrd and Castner, 2009).

Worldwide, members of the genus *Calliphora* spp. share the common life history trait of being associated with cooler temperatures and temperate latitudes. During the transition from winter to spring in temperate regions, this species is among the first to become active in the seasonal succession of fly species. In India, *Calliphora* species are active during the winter months, while species of *Chrysomya* are found associated with carcasses year-round (Bharti and Singh, 2003). *Lucilia* has a widespread distribution in temperate regions worldwide and is considered a warm-weather species. Interestingly, *L. sericata* is widely utilized for maggot debridement therapy, as its larvae secrete substances with notable antibacterial properties (Kerridge et al., 2005). *Lucilia sericata* is capable of inducing myiasis and is pertinent for estimating the time of colonization on decomposing remains.

Chrysomya rufifacies holds significance as a facultative predator of other larval flies. While *Chrysomya rufifacies* has been implicated in cases of wound myiasis, it is not considered a major myiasis-causing fly species in its introduced range (Baumgartner, 1993). Adults of this species display a metallic blue-green coloration without any stripes on the body. Larvae are morphologically distinctive, covered in pointed tubercles arranged in lines parallel to the long axis of the larval body. The ease of identifying larvae, combined with available developmental data (Byrd and Butler, 1997), and its frequent presence during the hottest periods of the year, makes it an important species for estimating the PMI.

Chrysomya megacephala is widespread across the Oriental regions, South Africa, and South America, and has become well-established in North America (Greenberg, 1988; Wells, 1991). Adults have short, stout bodies and noticeably larger heads. Their unusually large eyes are a prominent shade of red, making the flies easily identifiable in the field. The eyes cover most of the head, particularly in males, where they meet along the midline (holoptic condition) (Figure 14.5). In females, the eyes do not meet (dichoptic condition) (Figure 14.6). Additionally, in males, the facets of the compound eyes change their orderly pattern on the lower third of the ocular surface.

Both male and female *C. megacephala* are attracted to carrion, fruit, sweet foods, urine, and faecal material, earning them the common name Oriental latrine fly. This species shows a pronounced activity peak during the heat of the afternoon but is also among the first to become active in the early morning and one of the last to leave carrion at nightfall. Because of this activity pattern, *C. megacephala* is often the first to arrive at human and animal remains and typically the first to deposit eggs. Once they have settled on dead bodies, they are not easily disturbed and are therefore frequently collected, even in low numbers (Wells and Kurahashi, 1994).

14.2.2 Sarcophagidae

Flesh flies constitute a vast family comprising over 2,600 species (Merrit et al., 2009) distributed worldwide, with most species inhabiting tropical or warm temperate regions. Sarcophagidae

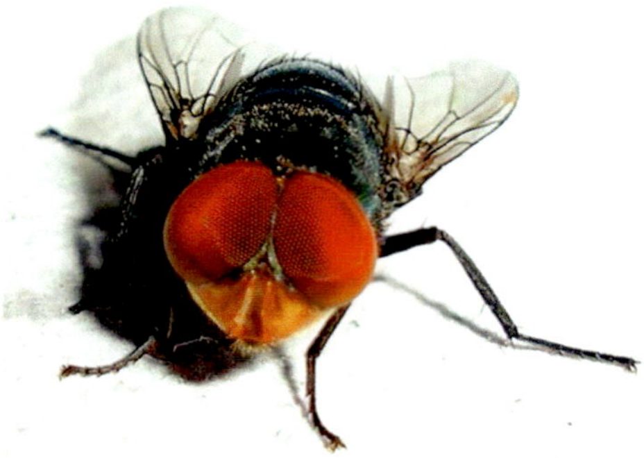

FIGURE 14.5 Male *Chrysomya megacephala.*

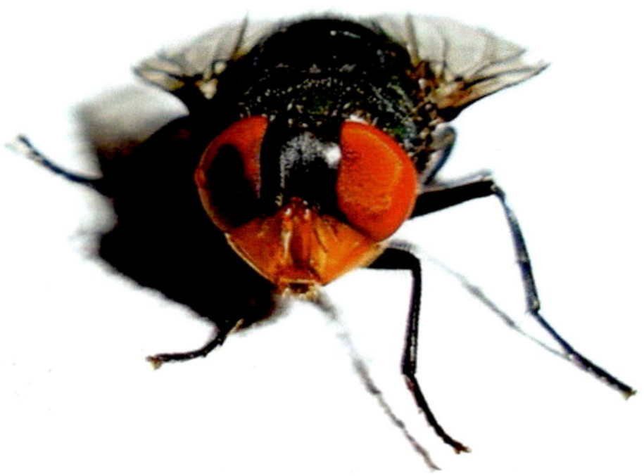

FIGURE 14.6 Female *Chrysomya megacephala.*

(depicted in Figure 14.7) are commonly larger than blow flies (Calliphoridae), with a less shiny appearance that may include tessellation (a pattern resembling a black and white checkerboard) on the abdomen, and black and white stripes on the thorax. A notable difference in life history between flesh flies and other flies associated with myiasis and decomposition is that female sarcophagids retain eggs within their bodies, allowing them to develop into the first instar before laying them in a wound or on decomposing flesh (ovoviviparity).

Adult flesh flies are commonly encountered on flowers, where they are attracted to nectar. They also feed on other sweet substances, such as sap and honeydew. The family's Latin name, "Sarcophagidae", translates to "flesh-eating", reflecting the larvae's typical diet of animal material, including carrion, excrement, or exposed meat. Flesh flies are known to cause myiasis and may be involved in transmitting diseases. Some species are parasitic on other insects, particularly bees and wasps.

Medium-sized, ranging from 2 to 14 mm in length, flesh flies typically lack metallic colouration. Additionally, the arista of their antennae is plumose only at the base, while in calliphorids, it is plumose throughout its length. Their bodies are often bristly, and the eyes are relatively widely

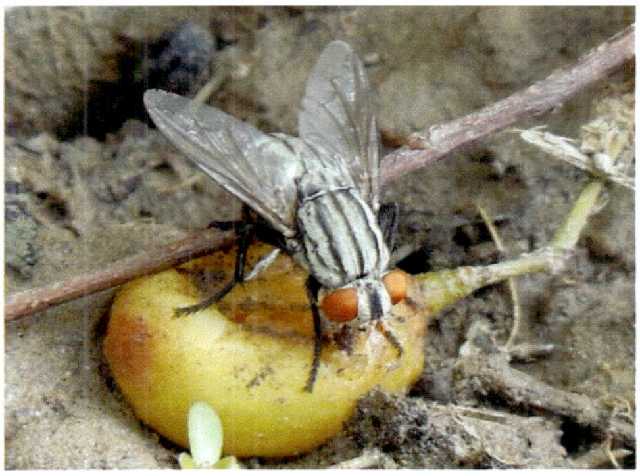

FIGURE 14.7 Sarcophagid fly.

separated in both sexes. In some species, the eyes and the highly visible genitalia at the tip of the abdomen are bright red.

The larvae of flesh flies have posterior spiracles located in a pit or depression at the tip of the abdomen, bordered by fleshy tubercles. This feature distinguishes them from blow fly larvae. However, identifying species within the family Sarcophagidae can be challenging, as they are similar to one another in both adult and larval stages. Therefore, maggots should be reared to the adult stage for accurate species identification.

Flesh flies of the genus *Sarcophaga* typically arrive on human remains concurrently or slightly after blow flies. They are known to fly under adverse conditions, which may allow them to be the first species to arrive at carrion (Nandi, 2002). These flies often enter indoor habitats, and thus, their larvae are frequently recovered from human remains found in homes. Females have a greater potential to disperse their offspring across multiple habitats compared to calliphorid females, who typically deposit all their eggs in a single large mass. Therefore, flesh flies may have a better opportunity to inhabit small wounds, and because they are already equipped to feed upon arrival at a wound site or carrion (females deposit larvae rather than eggs), these maggots can penetrate tissues more rapidly and complete development faster than their presumed competitors, the blow flies. Female flesh flies deposit living first instar larvae on decomposing remains, rather than laying eggs (Spzila and Pape, 2007). Therefore, fly egg masses found on human remains cannot be attributed to sarcophagids, and the time required for egg development must be considered when estimating the PMI based on flesh fly evidence. Flesh flies are part of the entomological fauna associated with both myiasis and decomposing remains, and literature detailing larval development is available if accurate identification can be reliably achieved (Byrd and Castner 2009).

14.2.3 Muscid Flies (Family Muscidae)

Muscid flies belong to a vast family found worldwide, comprising 5,150 species (Merrit et al., 2009). These species are ubiquitous and closely associated with human habitats (synanthropic behaviour), inadvertently spreading to areas beyond their native ranges. This close association with human environments contributes significantly to their medical and forensic relevance. Common members of the family Muscidae include the house fly, stable fly, horn fly, and latrine fly. Muscid flies exhibit diverse biology and habits, with adults feeding on decaying plant and animal matter, dung, pollen, and even blood. Stable flies and horn flies, for instance, can become troublesome pests for both humans and livestock when they feed on blood. Certain species within the family Muscidae breed and feed on garbage, sewage, and human waste, potentially serving as mechanical vectors for disease transmission.

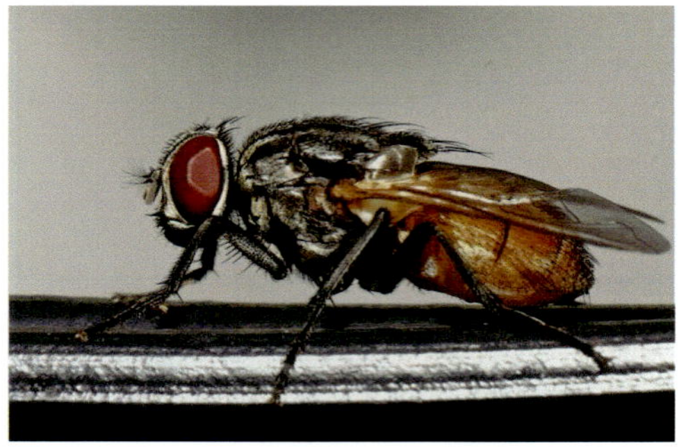

FIGURE 14.8 Muscid fly.

Typically small to medium-sized, ranging from 3 to 10 mm in length, muscid flies often exhibit dull grey to dark colouring, although some species may have a metallic sheen (Figure 14.8). They can be distinguished from blow flies and bottle flies (family Calliphoridae) by specific taxonomic features of the wings and head. Adult muscid flies generally lack the bristliness observed in sarcophagid and calliphorid flies. The arista of their antennae is plumose throughout its length, a characteristic shared with the family Calliphoridae. Most muscid larvae have the typical cylindrical shape of maggots, tapering from the tail end towards the head. Mature larvae range from 5 to 12 mm in length and are typically white, yellow, or cream-coloured.

The muscid family encompasses several of the most prevalent pest flies, such as the house fly (*Musca domestica*), horn fly (*Haematobia irritans*), stable fly (*Stomoxys calcitrans*), face fly (*Musca autumnalis*), and numerous others. These flies are commonly associated with filth and the decomposition of faecal matter. Myiasis caused by these flies is rare and often linked to infected wounds or accidental introduction. Unlike the Calliphoridae and Sarcophagidae, which are regarded as early colonizers of decomposing remains, the Muscidae are typically viewed as late-stage decomposition colonizers, usually found during the highly moist advanced decay stages (Byrd and Castner, 2009).

The genus *Musca* spp. comprises the most prevalent muscids, notably *M. domestica*, recognized as a synanthropic fly, meaning it thrives in close association with humans. Myiasis caused by *Musca* spp. appears to predominantly occur through accidental introduction and is less frequent compared to blow flies or flesh flies. These species are typically not associated with the early stages of decomposition unless faeces or gut contents are exposed. Instead, they are often observed in the later succession of insects associated with advanced decay. *Musca* spp. are generally brown to black flies, slightly smaller on average than Calliphoridae. Their larvae are usually very light in colour, nearly translucent white in some instances, and tend to be smaller and more slender than blow fly larvae (Byrd and Castner, 2009). As they mature, muscid larvae may exhibit predatory behaviour, influencing the composition of insect fauna on remains by preying on the eggs and larvae of other carrion-feeding flies.

Muscid flies commonly encountered on carrion belong to genera such as *Hydrotaea* (bronze dump fly), *Musca* (house fly), *Atherigona* (shoot fly), *Muscina*, and others. Muscid flies hold significant forensic importance due to their widespread distribution, presence in human environments, and tendency to associate with carrion (Grzywacz et al., 2017).

14.2.4 Lesser Houseflies (Family Fanniidae)

Flies belonging to the genus *Fannia* spp., also referred to as lesser house flies, share similarities with *Musca* spp. in that they are not typically associated with early decomposition stages but can colonize during advanced decomposition stages, commonly found in filth and faeces. *Fannia* flies are not considered significant myiasis-causing flies, and instances where they are documented to cause infestation are suspected to be accidental (Byrd and Castner, 2009). Adult *Fannia* closely resemble house flies but appear smaller. Morphologically, *Fannia* larvae are distinctive due to their dorso-ventrally flattened shape and lateral projections or tubercles running in a single line along both sides of the larva. Although the Fanniidae are less frequently utilized, many of their species are commonly found in decomposing carcasses and corpses (Matuszewski et al., 2010a,b, 2011; Aballay et al., 2012).

14.2.5 Skipper Flies (Family Piophilidae)

Skipper flies belong to a relatively small family comprising only 80 species (Merrit et al., 2009), yet they are distributed worldwide, with the highest diversity found in temperate regions. Adults of skipper flies typically exhibit metallic blue or black coloration and measure between 2.5 and 4.5 mm in length. These flies inhabit various environments, including carrion, human waste, bones, skin, and fur. They are commonly associated with protein-rich dry food sources. The name "skipper" originates from a peculiar behaviour observed in the larvae of certain species, such as the cheese skipper (*Piophila casei*). These larvae use their mouth hooks to show jumping behaviour, which serves as an effective escape mechanism and is also utilized during larval migration. However, skipper fly larvae also exhibit the more conventional creeping movement observed in most fly larvae. Primarily scavengers, skipper fly larvae feed on decaying food materials similar to those on which the adults are found. Skipper fly larvae can significantly exceed the adults in size, ranging from 5 to 10 mm in length. Regarding their attraction to carrion, piophilids are typically associated with carcasses in advanced stages of decay, and their presence on human corpses has been documented as early as the initial stages of decomposition. Despite their frequent mention in forensic entomology reviews and their recognition as important forensic indicators, the biological understanding of this group remains limited. Consequently, the forensic potential of the family Piophilidae is likely underutilized (Martin-Vega, 2011).

14.2.6 Humpbacked Flies or Scuttle Flies (Family Phoridae)

Humpbacked flies, also known as scuttle flies, are a diverse family comprising more than 4,000 species worldwide (Merrit et al., 2009). Nearly half of these species belong to the genus *Megaselia*. These flies are small, typically ranging from about 1.5–6 mm in length. They are easily identifiable by their humpbacked appearance, particularly noticeable when viewed from the side. Other taxonomic characteristics aiding in their identification include the flattened femora of the hind legs and the prominent veins at the base of the anterior wing margin. Phorid flies can exhibit black, brown, or yellow colouration.

Adult phorid flies are found in various environments, commonly associated with decaying plant matter and frequently regarded as unwanted yet widespread pests in areas where live insect colonies are present. Their distinctive behaviour of running swiftly and erratically has earned them the nickname "scuttle flies". Larvae of phorid flies typically develop in decomposing organic matter of diverse origins, including human, animal, or vegetative matter. While some species are predatory or parasitic, others may inhabit ant or termite nests, or develop in fungi. In forensic entomology, the earliest sarcosaprophagous insect to colonize an indoor corpse can serve as a primary indicator for estimating the PMI. In enclosed spaces and obscured environments, this often refers to the small scuttle flies (Diptera: Phoridae), which can penetrate narrow openings to access a concealed corpse. Scuttle flies are recognized as insects of forensic importance, and their presence on a human corpse can be a crucial indicator for determining the minimum PMI (Greenberg and Wells, 1998; Campobasso et al., 2004; Reibe and Madea, 2010; Zuha et al., 2016).

14.2.7 Dung Flies (Family Scathophagidae)

Dung flies, considered a distinct family, are named Scathophagidae, which translates to "dung-eating". With over 360 species (Smith, 1989) worldwide, dung flies exhibit considerable diversity. Common dung fly species are usually red or yellow and densely covered in hairs. While some species are attracted to excrement or decaying plant material, their larvae are predominantly found in excrement. Other species exhibit various ecological roles, such as leaf miners, flower head pests, parasites, predators, and even aquatic forms. The larvae of the genus *Scathophaga* primarily feed on dung but are also commonly found on decaying seaweed. These flies can also be present at crime scenes where excrement or gut contents are exposed (Matuszewski et al., 2008; Abd El-Gawad et al., 2019).

14.2.8 Black Scavenger Flies (Family Sepsidae)

Black scavenger flies, also known as sepsids, are distributed worldwide and encompass at least 375 species (Merrit et al., 2009). These small flies typically exhibit shiny black, purple, or red coloration and are usually no longer than 3.5 mm in length. They possess a distinct shape characterized by a rounded head and a narrowing of the abdomen at the base. Despite their miniature size, they are easily recognizable due to their unique behaviour of flicking their wings outwards as they move, earning them the nickname "waggle flies". Often found in large numbers, they are particularly common on dung. The larvae of sepsid flies develop in various decomposing organic matter, including carrion, excrement, and even decaying seaweed. Mature larvae are small, ranging from 3 to 6 mm in length. Sepsids are rarely encountered on corpses (Gill, 2005; Recinos-Aguilar,2020) and are of minor importance.

14.2.9 Soldier Flies (Family Stratiomyidae)

Soldier flies comprise a diverse group of over 2,700 species (Woodley, 2001), ranging in size from 5 to 20 mm. The coloration of adults varies, with many common species resembling wasps. Soldier flies have antennae consisting of three segments, with the last segment elongated or rounded, often bearing a long hair. Adults are commonly found near flowers, in wooded areas, and on vegetation in wet environments, as well as on decomposing plant or animal tissues. The family name originates from the spines present on the adults of certain species, giving them a resemblance to "armed" soldiers.

Mature larvae of soldier flies exhibit significant variation in length, ranging from 4 to 40 mm, depending on the species. Some species are exclusively aquatic, while others inhabit terrestrial environments. Terrestrial larvae typically develop in decomposing plant or animal materials, although some may exhibit predatory behaviour. Common habitats for soldier fly larvae include rotting wood, compost piles, and excrement. Aquatic soldier fly larvae are capable of thriving in harsh conditions, like hot springs or highly saline waters. Occasionally, soldier fly larvae may be ingested through the consumption of infested fruit, leading to cases of enteric pseudomyiasis. This species also breeds in cadavers and can serve as a bioindicator in forensic entomology, such as for determining the PMI in criminal cases (Lord et al., 1994; Pujol-Luz et al., 2008; Michalski et al., 2021).

14.2.10 Moth Flies (Family Psychodidae)

Moth flies, belonging to the family Psychodidae, are distributed worldwide with 2,900 species (Merrit et al., 2009). These flies are very small as adults, usually measuring no more than 3–4 mm in length. They have bodies and wings covered with scales, giving them a moth-like appearance, with wings ending in a pointed tip and prominent straight longitudinal veins. Within the family

Psychodidae, the subfamily Psychodinae includes moth flies, whose larvae are typically aquatic and develop in slime found in sewers and drains. Adult flies hold their wings roof-like over their bodies and do not feed on blood but can be considered pests due to their abundance. Commonly found in warm, damp environments, they are often seen indoors, especially in restrooms or showers, running and flying quickly in a distinctive, erratic manner. While psychodid flies usually constitute a minor portion of the arthropod fauna colonizing human remains, adult moth flies are occasionally attracted to carrion and are frequently encountered indoors, particularly in association with human activities. The family Psychodidae has been identified as forensically significant (Schoenly et al., 2007) and is frequently observed in decomposition surveys (Eberhardt and Elliot, 2008; Horenstein et al., 2012; Azmiera et al., 2021). However, detailed information on species interactions with human cadavers is limited. Some studies on decomposition provide insights into the ecological preferences of moth flies, suggesting that specific microhabitat conditions are critical for their biology. For instance, *Psychoda pseudoalternata* was found only during the post-decay stage of decomposition in Hawaii, USA (Tullis and Goff, 1987). Other *Psychoda* species were observed exclusively in winter (Tantawi et al., 1996), during the dry season (Ahmad and Ahmad, 2009), or on unwrapped carcasses rather than wrapped ones (Ahmad et al., 2011). Further research is needed to elucidate the ecological nuances of Psychodidae in relation to their use of carrion.

14.2.11 Picture-Winged Flies (Family Ulidiidae)

The family Ulidiidae (picture-winged flies), comprising 700 species worldwide (Merrit et al., 2009), a large group of small to medium-sized flies often characterized by wings with black, brown, or yellowish markings. These flies typically have a white band on their forelegs, and their bodies are often shiny and metallic green. They are commonly found in moist environments and are particularly abundant in tropical regions. Their larvae feed on plant materials, while others live in decaying matter. These flies are known to visit carrion, particularly during the fresh, bloated, and early decay stages (from Day 1 to Day 4). As a result, their presence on dead animal carcasses indicates the early stages of decomposition, which can be useful in forensic investigations. Rumiza et al. (2010), Al-Mesbah et al. (2012), and Sawaby et al. (2018) reported *Physiphora* from animal carcasses, while Tuccia et al. (2021) reported *Physyphora alceae* from human remains.

Table 14.1 presents a compilation of forensically significant flies in India, derived from an extensive review of the literature available in the country (White et al., 1940; Emden, 1965; Nandi, 2002; Bharti, 2008a,b; Sinha, 2009; Mitra et al., 2010; Bharti, 2011; Bhagat, 2016; Abd Algalil, 2017; Chakraborty et al., 2017a,b; Roy et al., 2018; Barták et al., 2019; Bharti, 2019; Kaur et al., 2020; Achint and Singh, 2021; Dar and Mir, 2022; Kar et al., 2022a,b; Palavesam et al., 2022).

14.3 FORENSIC ENTOMOLOGY

Forensic entomology, which includes various subdisciplines, uses insect evidence to assist in civil and criminal legal investigations. This broad field encompasses three main areas: urban, stored product, and medico-legal entomology (Hall and Huntington, 2001).

1. **Urban entomology** focuses on arthropod infestations in human-made structures, such as termite damage to buildings and fly breeding in indoor livestock facilities (Catts and Goff, 1992).
2. **Stored product entomology** investigates contaminated food products, including insect infestations in stored grains and kitchen products.
3. **Medicolegal entomology** also known as forensic entomology (Lord and Stevenson, 1986), involves drawing significant conclusions from the examination of arthropods collected from or near cadavers.

TABLE 14.1
List of Forensically Important Flies of India

Family	Superfamily	Subfamily	Tribe	Genus	Subgenus	Species	Distribution
Calliphoridae	Ameniinae	Calliphorinae	Calliphorini	*Calliphora* Robineau-Desvoidy, 1830		*C. vomitoria* (Linneaus, 1758)	West Bengal, Himachal Pradesh, Meghalaya, Sikkim, Punjab
					Calliphora Robineau-Desvoidy, 1826	*C. (C.) erythrocephala* Macquart, 1834	Himachal Pradesh
						C. (C.) grahami Aldrich, 1930	West Bengal
						C. (C.) vicina Robineau-Desvoidy, 1830	West Bengal, Himachal Pradesh, Sikkim, Uttar Pradesh, Punjab
		Luciliinae	Luciliini	*Hemipyrellia* Townsend, 1917		*H. ligurriens* (Wiedemann, 1830)	West Bengal, Bihar, Sikkim, Tamil Nadu
						H. pulchra (Wiedemann, 1830)	West Bengal, Bihar, Orissa, Punjab, Tamil Nadu, Uttar Pradesh, Pondicherry
				Lucilia Robineau-Desvoidy, 1830		*L. ampullacea* Villeneuve, 1922	West Bengal, Kerala
						L. cuprina (Wiedemann, 1830)	West Bengal
						L. illustris (Meigen, 1826)	West Bengal, Sikkim, Punjab
						L. papuensis Macquart, 1844	West Bengal, Kerala, Arunachal Pradesh, Kashmir
						L. porphyrina (Walker, 1856)	West Bengal, Kashmir, Arunachal Pradesh, Himachal Pradesh, Sikkim

(*Continued*)

TABLE 14.1 (*Continued*)
List of Forensically Important Flies of India

Family	Superfamily	Subfamily	Tribe	Genus	Subgenus	Species	Distribution
						L. sericata (Meigen, 1826)	West Bengal
		Chrysomyinae	Chrysomyini	*Chrysomya* Robineau-Desvoidy, 1830		*C. albiceps* (Wiedemann, 1819)	West Bengal, Arunachal Pradesh
						C. bezziana Villeneuve, 1914	All over India
						C. defixa (Walker, 1857)	West Bengal
						C. indica Sinha, 2004	West Bengal
						C. indiana (Abd Galil and Zambare, 2016)	Maharashtra
						C. megacephala (Fabricius, 1794)	All over India
						C. nigripes Aubertin, 1932	West Bengal, Assam, Tamil Nadu, Meghalaya, Arunachal Pradesh, Himachal Pradesh
						C. pinguis (Walker, 1858)	All over India
						C. phaonis (Séguy, 1928)	West Bengal, Sikkim, Nicobar Islands
						C. putoria (Wiedemann, 1830)	Himachal Pradesh
						C. rufifacies (Macquart, 1843)	All over India
						C. saffranea (Bigot, 1877)	Maharashtra
						C. thanomthini Kurahashi and Tumrasvin, 1977	Himachal Pradesh
						C. villeneuvi Patton, 1922	All over India

(*Continued*)

TABLE 14.1 (*Continued*)
List of Forensically Important Flies of India

Family	Superfamily	Subfamily	Tribe	Genus	Subgenus	Species	Distribution
			Phormiini	*Phormia* Robineau-Desvoidy, 1830		*P. regina* (Meigen, 1826)	All over India
Sarcophagidae	Miltogrammatinae	*sarcophaginae*	Amobiini	*Sarcophaga* Meigen, 1826	*Boettcherisca* Rohdendorf, 1937	*S. (B.) peregrina* (Robineau-Desvoidy, 1830)	Assam, Bihar, Kerala, Uttar Pradesh, Madhya Pradesh, Himachal Pradesh, Tamil Nadu, West Bengal, Tripura, Mizoram, Manipur, Nagaland
					Harpagophalla Rohdendorf, 1937	*S. (H.) kempi* (Senior-White, 1924)	All over India
					Iranihindia Rohdendorf, 1961	*S. (I.) martellata* (Senior-White, 1924)	West Bengal, Bihar, Karnataka
					Lioproctia Enderlein, 1928	*S. (L.) annandalei* (Senior-White, 1924)	West Bengal, Bihar, Gujarat, Uttar Pradesh
						S. (L.) pattoni (Senior-White, 1924)	Tamil Nadu, Mizoram
					Liopygia Enderlein, 1928	*S. (L.) ruficornis* (Fabricius, 1794)	All over India
					Liosarcophaga Enderlein, 1928	*S. (L.) aegyptica* Salem, 1936	Punjab
						S. (L.) dux Thomson, 1869	All over India
					Parasarcophaga Johnston and Tiegs, 1921	*S. (P.) albiceps* (Meigen, 1826)	All over India
						S. (P.) hirtipes (Wiedemann, 1830)	All over India

(*Continued*)

TABLE 14.1 (*Continued*)
List of Forensically Important Flies of India

Family	Superfamily	Subfamily	Tribe	Genus	Subgenus	Species	Distribution
						S. (P.) macroauriculata (Ho, 1932)	Manipur, West Bengal, Nagaland, Sikkim, Uttar Pradesh, Meghalaya
						S. (P.) misera (Walker, 1849)	All over India
						S. (P.) taenionota (Wiedemann, 1819)	All over India
					Seniorwhitea Rohdendorf, 1937	*S. (S.) princeps* Wiedemann, 1830	All over India
					Sinonipponia Rohdendorf, 1965	*S. (S.) bengalensis* (Nandi, 1977)	West Bengal, Maharashtra
						S. (S.) hainanensis Ho, 1936	All over India
					Uroxanthisca Rohdendorf, 1963	*S. (U.) calicifera* Böttcher, 1912	Bihar, Haryana, Himachal Pradesh, Karnataka, Maharashtra, Nagaland, Tamil Nadu, West Bengal, Uttar Pradesh, Andaman And Nicobar Islands
Muscidae		Muscinae	Muscini	*Musca* Linnaeus, 1758	*Byomya* Robineau-Desvoidy, 1830	*M. (B.) conducens* Walker, 1859	Andhra Pradesh, Assam, Madhya Pradesh, Orissa, Punjab, Uttar Pradesh, West Bengal
						M. (B.) confiscata Speiser, 1924	Andhra Pradesh, Madhya Pradesh, Uttar Pradesh, West Bengal
						M. (B.) pattoni Austen, 1910	Andhra Pradesh, Assam, Bihar, Tamil Nadu, Uttar Pradesh, West Bengal
						M. (B.) sorbens Wiedemann, 1830	Andhra Pradesh, Assam, Bihar, Tamil Nadu, Goa, Uttar Pradesh, West Bengal

(*Continued*)

TABLE 14.1 (*Continued*)
List of Forensically Important Flies of India

Family	Superfamily	Subfamily	Tribe	Genus	Subgenus	Species	Distribution
						M. (B.) ventrosa Wiedemann, 1830	Punjab
					Musca Linnaeus, 1758	*M. (M.) domestica* Linnaeus, 1758	All over India
				Muscina Robineau-Desvoidy, 1830		*M. stabulans* (Fallén, 1817)	Himachal Pradesh, Kashmir
				Hydrotaea Robineau-Desvoidy, 1830		*H. armipes* Fallén, 1825	Kashmir
						H. capensis Wiedemann, 1818	Punjab, Karnataka, Madhya Pradesh
						H. chalcogaster (Wiedemann, 1824)	All over India
				Ophyra Robineau-Desvoidy, 1830		*O. capensis* (Wiedemann, 1818)	Assam, Himachal Pradesh, Kerala, Tamil Nadu, Maharashtra, Goa, Uttar Pradesh, West Bengal
				Synthesiomyia Brauer and Bergenstamm, 1893		*S. nudiseta* (van der Wulp, 1883)	West Bengal
			Atherigonini	*Atherigona* Rondani, 1865		*A. savia* Pont and Magpayo, 1995	Punjab
					Acritochaeta Grimshaw, 1901	*A. (A.) orientalis* Schiner, 1868	All over India
Fanniidae				*Fannia* Robineau – Desvoidy, 1830		*F. canicularis* (Linnaeus, 1761)	Kashmir, Himachal Pradesh, Bihar, Tamil Nadu
Piophilidae				*Piophila* Fallen, 1810		*P. flavifacies* Brunetti, 1909	West Bengal

(*Continued*)

TABLE 14.1 (*Continued*)
List of Forensically Important Flies of India

Family	Superfamily	Subfamily	Tribe	Genus	Subgenus	Species	Distribution
						P. casei (Linnaeus, 1758)	Punjab, Himachal Pradesh
				Stearibia Lioy, 1864		*S. nigriceps* Meigen, 1826	All over India
Phoridae	Phoroidea	Metopininae	Metopinini	*Megaselia* Rondani, 1856	*Megaselia* Rondani, 1856	*M. (M.) rupifes* (Meigen, 1804)	All over India
						M. (M.) scalaris (Loew, 1866)	Assam, West Bengal
				Conicera Meigen, 1830		*C. kempi* Brunetti, 1924	Assam, Meghalaya
Scathophagidae				*Scathophaga* Meigen, 1803		*S. mellipes* Coquileet, 1898	Kashmir, Sikkim, West Bengal
						S. stercocaria (Linnaeus, 1758)	Himachal Pradesh, Sikkim, Kahmir, Uttar Pradesh
Sepsidae				*Themira* Robineau-Desvoidy, 1830		*T. bifida* Zuska, 1974	Punjab, Himachal Pradesh
Stratiomyidae		Hermetiinae		*Hermetia* Linnaeus, 1758		*H. illucens* (Linnaeus, 1758)	All over India
						H. laeta Meijere, 1904	West Bengal
Psychodidae		Psychodinae	Psychodini	*Psychoda* Latreille, 1796		*P. alternata* Say, 1824	West Bengal
						P. nigripennis Brunetti, 1908	Himachal Pradesh, West Bengal
Ulidiidae		Ulidiinae	Ulidiini	*Physiphora* Fallen, 1810		*P. clausa* (Macquart, 1844)	All over India
						P. flavipes Karsch, 1888	Punjab

Forensic entomology provides crucial evidence in forensic investigations:

- It can help determine the *time of death and the time elapsed since death* for humans and animals, including livestock or protected species (Anderson, 1999).
- It can reveal if a *body was moved* after death. The presence of live fly larvae or insect remnants at a location without a body indicates that the corpse was relocated (Campobasso and Introna, 2001; Wells and Škaro, 2014).
- Human DNA extracted from the gut material of fly larvae and its molecular analysis can help *identify a victim* when the body is missing (Benecke and Wells, 2001; Wells et al., 2001; Benecke et al., 2004).
- *Entomotoxicology*, another medicolegal application, involves analysing the gut contents of flies from human remains for toxins.
- Infestation of living humans by fly larvae (*myiasis*) may indicate neglect, abuse, or sexual molestation (Anderson and Huitson, 2004).
- Insects typically invade corpses through natural orifices. An unusually large number of insects in areas of the body suggests *antemortem trauma* and should be closely examined (Campobasso et al., 2001).

These pieces of evidence can support and verify various stages of the judicial process, providing vital clues about the time, place, and cause of death. They can also help establish or refute the alibis of witnesses and suspects during judicial trials.

14.4 FLY DEVELOPMENT

In the early stages of decomposition, the fly development method is typically used to assess PMI. This involves estimating the age of immature insects (larvae, pupae) feeding on the body, usually blowflies (Figure 14.9), which are the primary colonizers, and flesh flies, which appear later. The age of the oldest fly eggs, larvae, or pupae present is determined and used to calculate the PMI (Catts and Goff, 1992; Goff, 1993). Development data, varying by species and environmental factors, can suggest a PMI ranging from under a day to more than a month (Smith, 1986; Wells and LaMotte, 2001).

For accurate PMI estimation using fly development, several prerequisites must be met:

1. Correct identification of fly species.
2. Availability of baseline development data for the species at various temperatures and geographic locations.

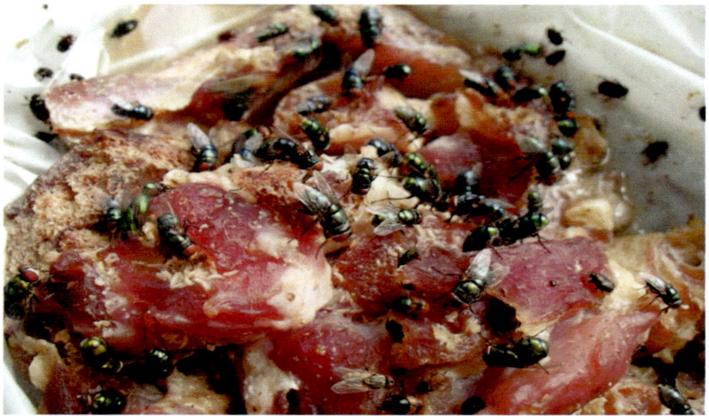

FIGURE 14.9 Fly assemblage on carrion.

3. Access to meteorological data for the area where the body was found.
4. Determination of the age of the oldest immature insects present in or around the remains.

Comparisons are made with other death investigations or through experiments replicating case conditions (Goff, 1992; Introna et al., 1989). Typically, previously published datasets are consulted. When scene conditions closely match those used in baseline laboratory studies, the likelihood of error in estimating the PMI is minimized (Wells and LaMotte, 2001). Knowledge of the fly life cycle and the duration of each stage is essential for estimating the PMI.

14.4.1 Life Cycle of a Blow Fly

The generalized life cycle of a blow fly, shown in Figure 14.10, is similar across calliphorid species and includes two moults (ecdysis), three feeding stages called instars, a pupal stage, and an adult stage. Adult female blow flies typically lay their eggs in wounds or natural openings, like the mouth and nose. The first instar larvae, which hatch from these eggs, are very small and lack the strength to

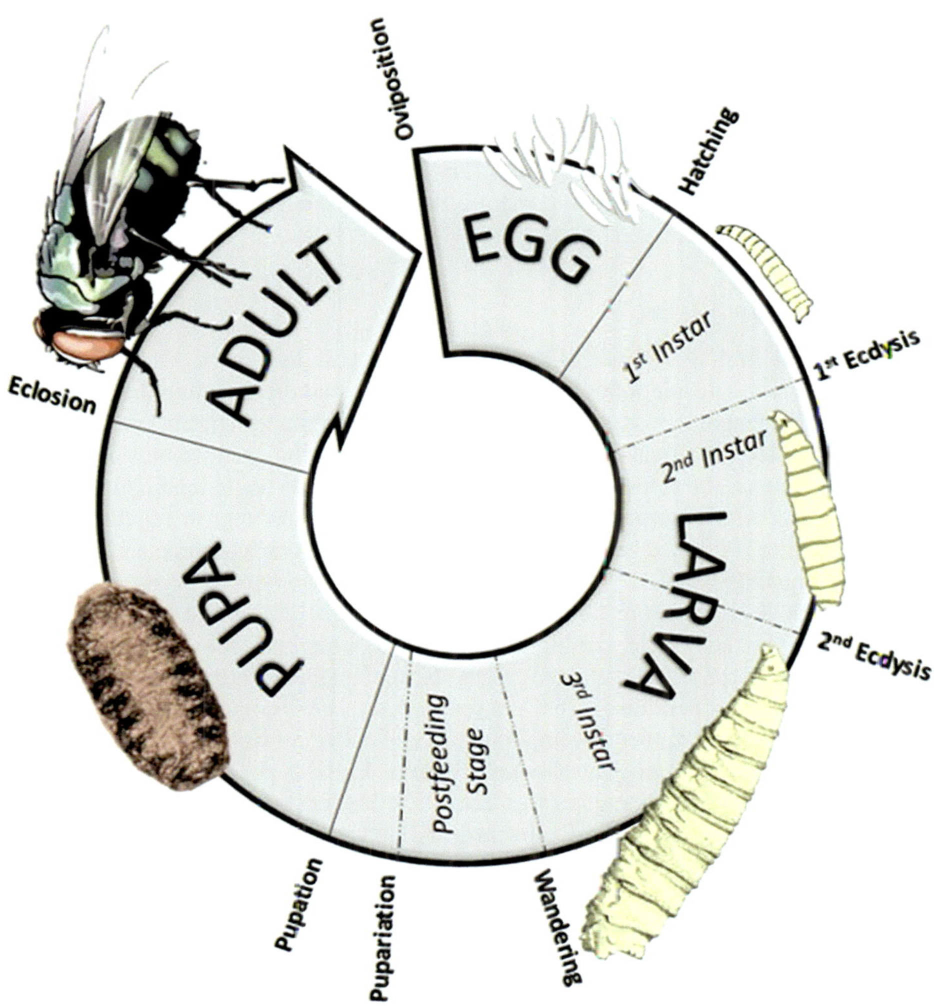

FIGURE 14.10 A Generalised Blowfly life cycle.

pierce tough external tissues, like unbroken skin. Their flexible cuticle allows for significant expansion within each stage to accommodate rapid growth due to intensive feeding. As the larvae grow, they need to shed their outer skin, a process known as moulting (ecdysis). After the first moult, they become second instar larvae, which feed more than the first instars. By this stage, the pH of the decomposing tissue usually becomes more alkaline, aiding in the breakdown of connective tissues and making it easier for the larvae to feed. During the second instar, the crop (a food storage organ) becomes visible and enlarges as the larvae consume more food than they digest.

The second instar larvae moult again to become third instar larvae. The third instar has two distinct phases: the feeding stage, where the larvae feed aggressively and grow to their maximum size, and the post-feeding stage, where they stop feeding and search for a safe place to pupate. During the post-feeding stage, the larvae use the stored food in their crops, which gradually shrink. An opaque layer of fat develops under the cuticle, changing the larvae's colour to an opaque, creamy whitish-yellow. After several days, the larvae start pupariation, transforming their soft, whitish-yellow cuticle into a hard, brownish-black protective shell.

Pupariation involves significant morphological and physiological changes, including slowed movement, muscle contraction, cuticle shrinkage, and hardening (tanning) of the cuticle. The prepupal stage, which marks the start of pupariation, is brief. During this stage, the third instar larva's skin, now called the puparium, hardens and darkens, leading to pupation. During pupation, the insect detaches from the puparium's inner surface in a process called larval–pupal apolysis. Approximately 40% of a fly's development time is spent in pupariation and pupation (Catts, 1992). When metamorphosis is complete, adult flies emerge from the puparia with soft cuticles, small abdomens, and unexpanded wings. Within a few hours, their cuticles harden, and their wings and abdomens expand, making them teneral adults. These adults are not yet reproductively mature and typically require protein consumption to mature their reproductive organs (Rasso and Fraenkel, 1954).

14.4.2 Life Cycle of a Flesh Fly

The life cycle of the flesh fly (Figure 14.11) consists of several distinct stages: larviposition, larval development, pupation, and adulthood. Flesh flies are ovoviviparous, meaning that the eggs develop and hatch within the female's body. Instead of laying eggs, the female deposits live first instar larvae directly onto a suitable host, such as decaying meat, carrion, or the open wounds of living animals. This process is known as larviposition. Once deposited, the larvae begin feeding immediately. The larval stage consists of three instars. Second instar larvae continue to grow rapidly and moult into the third instar. Third instar is the final larval stage, where the larvae consume a significant amount of food, growing quickly before they prepare to pupate. This stage typically lasts about 5 days under optimal conditions. After reaching the third instar, the larvae leave the host to find a suitable pupation site, usually in the soil. Here, they form a puparium, a hard protective shell. The pupal stage involves significant morphological changes as the larva transforms into an adult fly. This process takes about 1 week at a temperature of 25°C. In some species, environmental cues can trigger a state called diapause, where development is temporarily halted under unfavourable conditions. Adult flies emerge from the puparium after approximately 10 days. Initially, the adults have soft bodies and unexpanded wings, but within a few hours, their cuticle hardens, wings expand, and they become fully functional adults. These adults are capable of flying, mating, and beginning the cycle anew by seeking out suitable locations for larviposition.

14.5 PMI ESTIMATION

Under normal circumstances, determining the PMI of a body is the responsibility of a forensic pathologist. They use various parameters, such as lividity, rigor mortis, postmortem cooling, changes in the chemical constituents of the body, tissue autolysis, and decomposition due to bacterial activity.

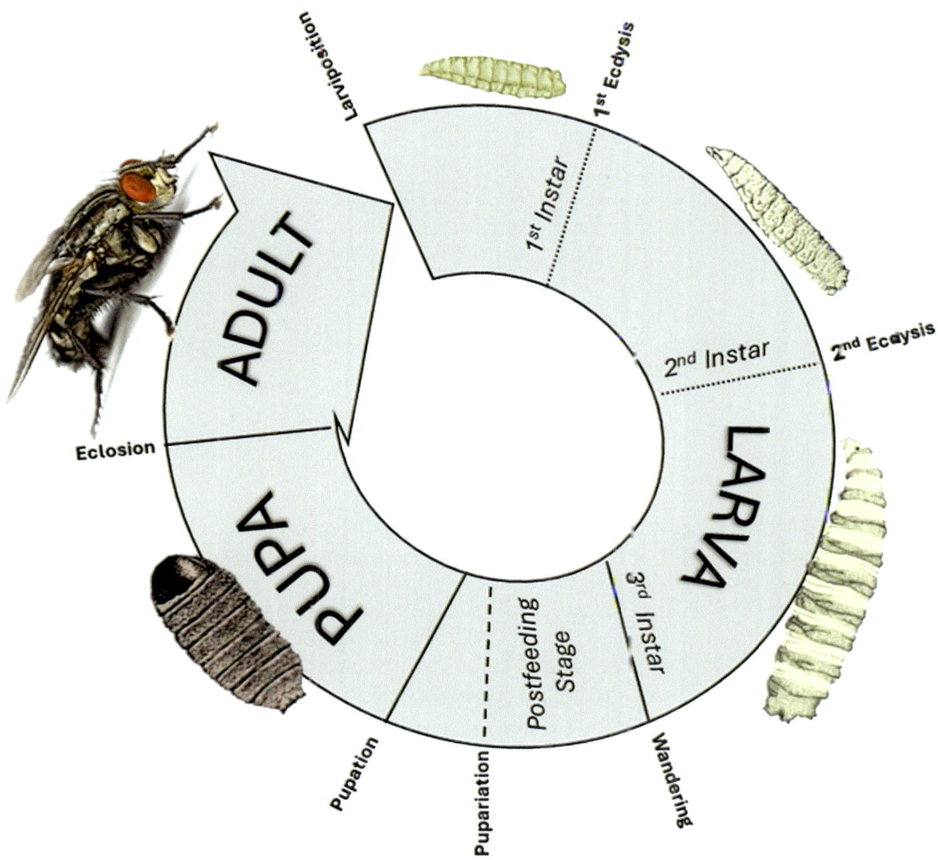

FIGURE 14.11 A Generalised Fleshfly life cycle.

However, these methods become unreliable beyond 72 hours after death. Forensic entomologists, on the other hand, use insects, especially flies and their immature stages, as biological indicators to determine the PMI, which is particularly effective for times greater than 72 hours postmortem (Kashyap and Pillay, 1989; Tempelman-Kluit, 1993). Numerous forensic cases have utilized flies to calculate the PMI, often corroborating time intervals established by pathologists (Smith, 1986; Catts and Haskell, 1990).

14.5.1 Eggs

Blowfly eggs sampled from remains shortly after death can be reared in the laboratory, and the time to incubation and first instar hatching can determine a short PMI (Bourel et al., 2003). Gene expression in blowfly eggs (bcd, sll, cs) can also predict age (Tarone et al., 2007).

14.5.2 Larvae

Estimating the age of insects can be done by examining their physical development or the stages they have reached (such as first, second, third instar, post-feeding stage, and pupa). Factors like length, weight, or width are used to determine the age of fly larvae (Byrd and Butler, 1996, 1997, 1998; Anderson, 2001; Byrd and Allen, 2001; Grassberger and Reiter, 2001, 2002a,b;

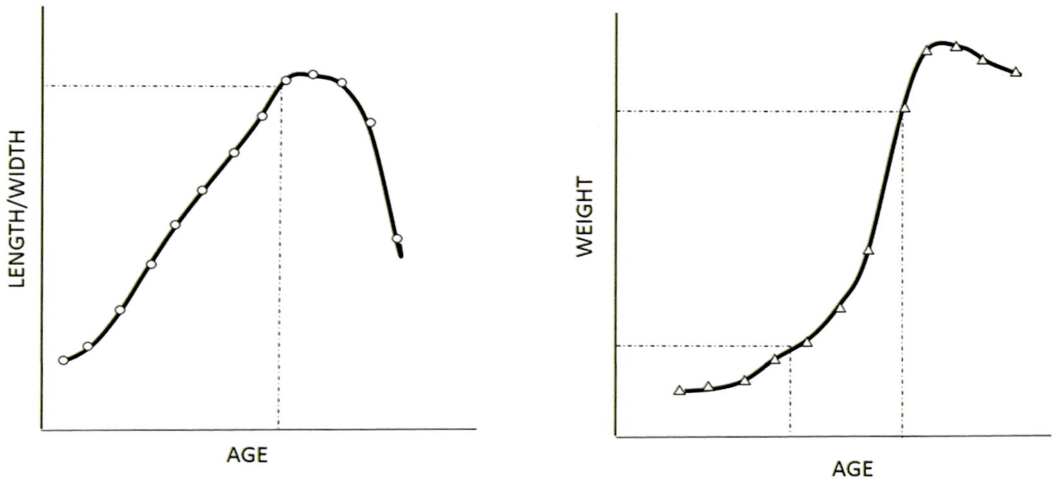

FIGURE 14.12 Theoretical growth patterns for fly larvae (at a specific temperature) depicting the usual trends in length/width and weight changes from egg hatching to pupariation. Dotted lines represent projected age estimations based on size.

Day and Wallman, 2006). For instance, during an investigation, a larva of an unknown age from a specific fly species might be collected from a body. Growth curves for that species from the same geographic area, derived from literature datasets, show length, weight, or width as a function of age (Figure 14.12). These growth curves, which account for similar environmental conditions (season, temperature, humidity, photoperiod), serve as a reference. Typically, these curves are sigmoidal, indicating slow growth in the first two larval instars, rapid growth during the third instar, and slowed growth after feeding ceases. The collected larvae are preserved and measured similarly to those in the reference literature. These measurements are then compared to the growth curve to estimate age. Additionally, significant morphological changes at stages like pupariation, metamorphosis, and adult eclosion can also aid in age estimation (Greenberg, 1991). Another method involves expressing development in terms of accumulated degree-hours or degree-days, known as thermal summation (Higley and Haskell, 2001; Richards and Villet, 2009), which is used to create simulated computer models of insect growth.

The simplest method for aging insects is the "isomorphen diagram," which plots the time from egg hatching to adult emergence against a constant temperature, showing developmental landmarks. The "isomegalen diagram" plots larval size (length, weight) against temperature, offering finer time resolution compared to developmental milestones (Grassberger and Reiter, 2001). Thermal summation models use linear regression analysis to relate temperature to development. The development rate (1/D) is plotted against temperature, assuming linearity between the upper and lower developmental thresholds. Development is measured in "degree days" or "degree hours". Each life stage (egg, larva, pupa) requires a specific amount of accumulated degree hours/days to progress to the next stage. In practice, insects sampled from remains are reared in the laboratory, and the time needed to develop until adult emergence is recorded in ADD/ADH units. This laboratory development time is subtracted from the total time for the species' development to determine the insect's age at sampling (Nabity et al., 2006). However, linear models can be too simplistic and may not account for nonlinearity at extreme temperatures. Curvilinear models are more accurate as they incorporate nonlinearity at temperature extremes when the development rate is plotted against temperature. However, these models are complex and impractical for field use, with no universal curvilinear model proving superior to linear models. Thus, the linear thermal summation model remains preferred for estimating insect age and PMI.

After blowfly maggots complete feeding and reach maximum length, they begin to wander (post-feeding stage) to find a pupation site, with the anterior part of their intestine remaining empty during this time. Radiological examination of intestinal contents can help estimate PMI (Reiter and Hajek, 1984). If larval length is unreliable due to shrinkage in the postfeeding stage or improper handling, the width at the junction of the fifth and sixth abdominal segments can be used to estimate age (Day and Wallman, 2006). The weight of blowfly larvae and pupae can be used for age estimation. Statistical models showing the distribution of larval and pupal weights versus age allow for comparison and inverse prediction to estimate PMI (Wells and LaMotte, 1995). Analysis of volatile compounds released by blowfly larvae and pupae, using gas chromatography–mass spectrometry, can supplement PMI estimation (Frederickx et al., 2012a,b).

14.5.3 Pupae

Hydrocarbons in the fly puparium cuticle change composition over time and can be analysed using gas chromatography–mass spectrometry to estimate age and PMI from puparial shells (Ye et al., 2007; Drijfhout, 2010). Gene expression analysis can establish reliable ageing methods for the intra-puparial stage to accurately estimate the minimum PMI. Differential gene expression during pupal development can indicate age (Wang et al., 2018). Histological techniques can study the internal morphology of fly pupae. Differences in thoracic muscles and brain development with age can indicate PMI (Davies and Harvey, 2013). Micro-computed tomography describes internal and external morphological changes in blowfly pupae during metamorphosis. This method can estimate pupal age and PMI with high precision (Richards et al., 2012). Hyperspectral imaging allows non-destructive analysis of insect specimens, aiding in age prediction. This technique has shown promise in determining pupal age with high accuracy (Voss et al., 2017). Quantitative analysis of ecdysteroid levels in insect pupae can provide precise age information. Ecdysteroid levels during pupal development indicate developmental maturity (Gaudry et al., 2006).

14.5.4 Adults

The initial emergence of adult flies at a crime scene can have significant forensic implications, making it important to determine their age. Newly emerged flies are identifiable by their shrunken wings, small abdomen, dull grey colour, and a ptilinum that inflates and deflates rhythmically. Within a few hours, these young adults undergo sclerotization and may appear similar to mature flies. Although methods like pteridine fluorescence and lipofuscin accumulation are effective for aging adult flies, they are not suitable for larvae or pupae (Ettershank et al., 1983; Wall et al., 1990; Cammack et al., 2017).

14.6 CONCLUSIONS

This chapter delves into the realm of forensic entomology, focusing on the significance of various Diptera families, such as Calliphoridae, Sarcophagidae, and Muscidae, in forensic investigations. By meticulously tabulating the species of forensic importance in India and elucidating the life cycles of blowflies and flesh flies, this study provides a comprehensive understanding of their role in estimating PMI. The detailed examination of the developmental stages of flies and their correlation with PMI estimation underscores the importance of accurate species identification and understanding of insect biology in forensic entomology. Although forensic entomology holds promise, it encounters various obstacles in India, such as a lack of awareness among law enforcement and forensic professionals, the absence of standardized procedures and techniques, and inadequate infrastructure and resources for conducting entomological examinations.

While this chapter is a primer for understanding the forensic significance of flies, there are numerous avenues for future research and exploration. Conducting extensive surveys to catalogue the diversity of Diptera across various regions of India would deepen our comprehension of species distribution and abundance, thus refining techniques for estimating PMIs. Investigating the impact of diverse environmental factors, such as temperature, humidity, habitat types, and seasonal fluctuations on insect colonization patterns and developmental rates would enhance the precision of PMI estimates tailored to Indian conditions. Exploring the integration of cutting-edge technologies, such as DNA analysis, gene expression studies, cuticular hydrocarbon analysis, hyperspectral imaging, and machine learning algorithms into forensic entomology methodologies could enhance the accuracy and reliability of PMI estimates. Advocating for the integration of forensic entomology evidence into the legal framework and raising awareness among law enforcement agencies, the judiciary, and forensic experts about its utility and significance in criminal investigations are crucial steps forward. In conclusion, by collaborating across disciplines, leveraging technological advancements, and establishing a strong legal framework, the field of forensic entomology in India has the potential to evolve and make significant contributions to the administration of justice and forensic science practice.

14.7 POINTS TO REMEMBER

1. Forensic entomology utilizes knowledge of insect biology to aid in legal investigations.
2. Forensically important fly families include Calliphoridae, Sarcophagidae, Muscidae, Fanniidae, Piophilidae, Phoridae, Scathophagidae, Sepsidae, Stratiomyidae, Ulidiidae, and Psychodidae.
3. Cadavers represent a small temporal and spatial niche, and compared to other ecosystems, they undergo a distinct faunal succession. Families, like Calliphoridae (blow flies) and Sarcophagidae (flesh flies) are often the first to arrive at a corpse. After the initial colonizers, other species, like Muscidae (house flies) and Fanniidae (lesser house flies), arrive. Families such as Piophilidae (skipper flies) and Phoridae (humpbacked flies) often arrive during later stages of decomposition, particularly when the body is in a more advanced state.
4. Estimating the PMI, the time elapsed since death, is a vital aspect of forensic investigations. Forensic entomologists use insects, especially flies and their immature stages, as biological indicators to determine the PMI, which is particularly effective for times greater than 72 hours postmortem.
5. To accurately estimate the PMI using fly development, several conditions must be satisfied: precise identification of the fly species, availability of baseline development data for the species across different temperatures and geographical areas, access to meteorological data from the location where the body was discovered, and determination of the age of the oldest immature insects found on or near the remains.
6. Apart from PMI, insect evidence can help indicate if a body was relocated post-mortem. Extracting and analysing human DNA from the gut contents of fly larvae can aid in identifying a missing victim. Entomotoxicology, a field within forensic science, examines the gut contents of flies from human remains to detect toxins. Infestation of living individuals by fly larvae (myiasis) may be indicative of neglect, abuse, or sexual assault. An abnormal number of insects in parts of the body other than natural orifices can suggest antemortem injury.

REFERENCES

Aballay, F. H., Domínguez, M. C., & Campón, F. F. (2012). Adult Fanniidae associated to pig carcasses during the winter season in a semiarid environment: Initial examination of their potential as complementary PMI indicators. *Forensic Science International*, *219*(1–3): 284–e1.

Abd Algalil, F. M. (2017). Molecular identification of forensically important flesh flies (Diptera: Sarcophagidae) using COI Gene. *Journal of Entomology and Zoology Studies*, *5*(2): 263–267.

Abd El-Gawad, A., Badawy, R. M., Abd El-Bar, M. M., & Kenawy, M. A. (2019). Successive waves of dipteran flies attracted to warfarin-intoxicated rabbit carcasses in Cairo, Egypt. *The Journal of Basic and Applied Zoology*, *80*: 1–10.

Achint, R., & Singh, D. (2021). Application of COI gene for identification of some economically and forensically important muscid flies of India (Diptera: Muscidae). *International Journal of Tropical Insect Science*, *41*(4): 3023–3029.

Ahmad, A., & Ahmad, A. H. (2009). A preliminary study on the decomposition and dipteran associated with exposed carcasses in an oil palm plantation in Bandar Baharu, Kedah, Malaysia. *Tropical Biomedicine*, *26*(1): 1–10.

Ahmad, N. W., Lim, L. H., Dhang, C. C., Chin, H. C., Abdullah, A. G., Mustaffa, W. N. W., Kian, C. W., Jeffery, J., Hashim, R., & Azirun, S. M. (2011). Comparative insect fauna succession on indoor and outdoor monkey carrions in a semi-forested area in Malaysia. *Asian Pacific Journal of Tropical Biomedicine*, *1*(2): S232–S238.

Al-Mesbah, H., Moffatt, C., El-Azazy, O. M., & Majeed, Q. A. (2012). The decomposition of rabbit carcasses and associated necrophagous Diptera in Kuwait. *Forensic Science International*, *217*(1–3): 27–31.

Amendt, J., Krettek, R., & Zehner, R. (2004). Forensic entomology. *Naturwissenschaften*, *91*: 51–65.

Anderson, G. S. (1999). Wildlife forensic entomology: Determining time of death in two illegally killed black bear cubs. *Journal of Forensic Sciences*, *44*(4): 856–859.

Anderson, G. S. (2001). Forensic entomology in British Columbia: A brief history. *Journal of the Entomological Society of British Columbia*, *98*: 127–136.

Anderson, G. S. (2010). Decomposition and invertebrate colonization of cadavers in coastal marine environments. In: J. Amendt, M. Lee Goff, C. P. Campobasso & M. Grassberger (eds.), *Current Concepts in Forensic Entomology*. Springer, New Yorl, pp. 223–272.

Anderson, G. S., & Huitson, N. R. (2004). Myiasis in pet animals in British Columbia: The potential of forensic entomology for determining duration of possible neglect. *The Canadian Veterinary Journal*, *45*(12): 993–998.

Ashworth, J. R., & Wall, R. (1994). Responses of the sheep blowflies *Lucilia sericata* and *L. cuprina* to odour and the development of semiochemical baits. *Medical and Veterinary Entomology*, *8*(4): 303–309.

Azmiera, N., Low, V. L., & Heo, C. C. (2021). Colonization of rabbit carcasses by drain fly larvae, *Psychoda* sp. (Diptera: Psychodidae): The first report. *Acta Parasitologica*, *66*: 706–709.

Barták, M., Khrokalo, L., & Verves, Y. (2019). New records, synonyms and combinations for oriental Sarcophagidae (Diptera), with updated checklists for Cambodia, India, Taiwan, Thailand and Vietnam. *Journal of Asia-Pacific Entomology*, *22*(1): 44–55.

Baumgartner, D. L. (1993). Review of *Chrysomya rufifacies* (Diptera: Calliphoridae). *Journal of Medical Entomology*, *30*(2): 338–352.

Benecke, M., Josephi, E., & Zweihoff, R. (2004). Neglect of the elderly: forensic entomology cases and considerations. *Forensic Science International*, *146*: S195–S199.

Benecke, M. & Wells, J. D. (2001). DNA techniques for forensic entomology. In: J. H. Byrd & J. K. Tomberlin (eds.), *Forensic Entomology: Utility of Arthropods in Legal Investigations*. CRC Press, Boca Raton, FL, pp. 341–352.

Bhagat, R. C. (2016). Biodiversity of dipterous flies (Insecta) of myiasis causing importance in animals and human of Jammu, Kashmir and Ladakh Himalayas (India). *Journal of Global Biosciences*, *5*(7): 4341–4349.

Bharti, M. (2008a). Current status of family Muscidae (Diptera) from India. *Journal of Entomological Research*, *32*(2): 171–176.

Bharti, M. (2008b). Diptera: Calliphoridae, Rhiniidae from India. *Journal of Entomological Research*, *32*(1): 79–82.

Bharti, M. (2011). An updated checklist of blowflies (Diptera: Calliphoridae) from India. *Halteres*, *3*: 34–37.

Bharti, M. (2019). New records of *Chrysomya putoria* and *C. thanomthini* (Diptera: Calliphoridae) from India, with a revised key to the known Indian species. *Journal of Threatened Taxa*, *11*(1): 13188–13190.

Bharti, M., & Singh, D. (2003). Insect faunal succession on decaying rabbit carcasses in Punjab, India. *Journal of Forensic Sciences*, *48*(5): 1133–1143.

Bornemissza, G. F. (1957). An analysis of Arthropod succession in Carrion and the effect of its decomposition on the soil fauna. *Australian Journal of Zoology*, *5*(1): 1–12.

Bourel, B., Callet, B., Hédouin, V., & Gosset, D. (2003). Flies eggs: A new method for the estimation of short-term post-mortem interval? *Forensic Science International*, *135*(1): 27–34.

Braack, L. E. O. (1981). Visitation patterns of principal species of the insect-complex at carcasses in the Kruger National Park. *Koedoe*, *24*(1): 33–49.

Byrd, J. H., & Allen, J. C. (2001). The development of the black blow fly, *Phormia regina* (Meigen). *Forensic Science International*, *120*(1–2): 79–88.

Byrd, J. H., & Butler, J. F. (1996). Effects of temperature on *Cochliomyia macellaria* (Diptera: Calliphoridae) development. *Journal of Medical Entomology*, *33*(6): 901–905.

Byrd, J. H., & Butler, J. F. (1997). Effects of temperature on *Chrysomya rufifacies* (Diptera: Calliphoridae) development. *Journal of Medical Entomology*, *34*(3): 353–358.

Byrd, J. H., & Butler, J. F. (1998). Effects of temperature on *Sarcophaga haemorrhoidalis* (Diptera: Sarcophagidae) development. *Journal of Medical Entomology*, *35*(5): 694–698.

Byrd, J. H., & Castner, J. L. (2009). *Forensic Entomology: The Utility of Arthropods in Legal Investigations*. CRC press, Boca Raton, FL, 705 pp.

Cammack, J. A., Reiskind, M. H., Guisewite, L. M., Denning, S. S., & Watson, D. W. (2017). Quantifying pteridines in the heads of blow flies (Diptera: Calliphoridae): Application for forensic entomology. *Forensic Science International*, *280:* 44–48.

Campobasso, C. P., & Introna, F. (2001). The forensic entomologist in the context of the forensic pathologist's role. *Forensic Science International*, *120* (1–2): 132–139.

Campobasso, C. P., Di Vella, G., & Introna, F. (2001). Factors affecting decomposition and Diptera colonization. *Forensic Science International*, *120*(1–2): 18–27.

Campobasso, C. P., Henry, R., Disney, L., & Introna, F. (2004). A case of *Megaselia scalaris* (Loew)(Dipt., Phoridae) breeding in a human corpse. *Anil Aggrawal's Internet Journal of Forensic Medicine and Toxicology*, *5*(1): 3–5.

Capinera, J. L. (Ed.). (2008). *Encyclopedia of Entomology*. Springer Science & Business Media, New York.

Catts, E. P. (1992). Problem in estimating the postmortem interval in death investigations. *Journal of Agricultural Entomology*, *9*(4): 245–255.

Catts, E. P., & Goff, M. L. (1992). Forensic entomology in criminal investigations. *Annual Review of Entomology*, *37*(1): 253–272.

Catts, E. P., & Haskell, N. H. (Eds.). (1990). *Entomology & Death: A Procedural Guide*. Joyce's Print Shop Inc., Clemson, p. 182.

Chakraborty, A., Hora, G., Parui, P., Saha, G. K., & Banerjee, D. (2017a). A biosystematic species inventory of Indian sarcophagidae (Insecta: Diptera: Sarcophagidae). *Journal of Entomology and Zoology Studies*, *5*(1): 465–473.

Chakraborty, A., Saha, G. K., & Banerjee, D. (2017b). Biosystematic Approach: To inventorization of ubiquitious myiasis causing flies of veterinary importance in India. *Research in: Agricultural & Veterinary Sciences*, *1*: 116–134.

Coe, J. I., & Curran, W. J. (1980). Definition and time of death. In: W. J. Curran & A. L. McGarry (eds.), *Modern Legal Psychiatry and Forensic Science*. FA Davis Co, Philadelphia, p. 1310.

Dar, T. A., & Mir, A. H. (2022). Checklist of blowflies (Diptera: Calliphoridae) of Indian subcontinent. *Journal of Entomological Research*, *46*(4): 907–916.

Davies, K., & Harvey, M. L. (2013). Internal morphological analysis for age estimation of blow fly pupae (Diptera: Calliphoridae) in postmortem interval estimation. *Journal of Forensic Sciences*, *58*(1): 79–84.

Day, D. M., & Wallman, J. F. (2006). Width as an alternative measurement to length for post-mortem interval estimations using *Calliphora augur* (Diptera: Calliphoridae) larvae. *Forensic Science International*, *159*(2–3): 158–167.

Drijfhout, F. P. (2010). Cuticular hydrocarbons: A new tool in forensic entomology? In: J. Amendt, M. Lee Goff, C. P. Campobasso & M. Grassberger (eds.), *Current Concepts in Forensic Entomology*. Springer, New York, pp. 179–203.

Eberhardt, T. L., & Elliot, D. A. (2008). A preliminary investigation of insect colonisation and succession on remains in New Zealand. *Forensic Science International*, *176*(2–3): 217–223.

Erzinçlioğlu, Z. (1996). *Blowflies*. Richmond Publishing Co. Ltd., Oxford, UK, ii+71 pp.

Ettershank, G., Macdonnell, I., & Croft, R. (1983). The accumulation of age pigment by the fleshfly, *Sarcophaga bullata* Parker (Diptera: Sarcophagidae). *Australian Journal of Zoology*, *31*(2): 131–138.

Frederickx, C., Dekeirsschieter, J., Brostaux, Y., Wathelet, J. P., Verheggen, F. J., & Haubruge, E. (2012a). Volatile organic compounds released by blowfly larvae and pupae: New perspectives in forensic entomology. *Forensic Science International*, *219*(1–3): 215–220.

Frederickx, C., Dekeirsschieter, J., Verheggen, F. J., & Haubruge, E. (2012b). Responses of Lucilia sericata-Meigen (Diptera: Calliphoridae) to cadaveric volatile organic compounds. *Journal of Forensic Sciences*, *57*(2): 386–390.

Garcia-Moya, E., & McKell, C. M. (1970). Contribution of shrubs to the nitrogen economy of a desert-wash plant community. *Ecology*, *51*(1): 81–88.

Gaudry, E., Blais, C., Maria, A., & Dauphin-Villemant, C. (2006). Study of steroidogenesis in pupae of the forensically important blow fly *Protophormia terraenovae* (Robineau-Desvoidy) (Diptera: Calliphoridae). *Forensic Science International*, *160*(1): 27–34.

Gennard, D. (2012). *Forensic Entomology: An Introduction*. John Wiley & Sons, New York, 272 pp.

Gill, G. J. (2005). *Decomposition and Arthropod Succession on above Ground Pig Carrion in Rural Manitoba* (Master's thesis), 215 pp.

Goff, M. L. (1992). Problems in estimation of postmortem interval resulting from wrapping of the corpse: A case study from Hawaii. *Journal of Agricultural Entomology*, *9*(4): 237–243.

Goff, M. L. (1993). Estimation of postmortem interval using arthropod development and successional patterns. *Forensic Science Review*, *5*: 81–94.

Grassberger, M., & Reiter, C. (2001). Effect of temperature on *Lucilia sericata* (Diptera: Calliphoridae) development with special reference to the isomegalen-and isomorphen-diagram. *Forensic Science International*, *120*(1–2): 32–36.

Grassberger, M., & Reiter, C. (2002a). Effect of temperature on development of the forensically important holarctic blow fly *Protophormia terraenovae* (Robineau-Desvoidy)(Diptera: Calliphoridae). *Forensic Science International*, *128*(3): 177–182.

Grassberger, M., & Reiter, C. (2002b). Effect of temperature on development of *Liopygia (= Sarcophaga) argyrostoma* (Robineau-Desvoidy)(Diptera: Sarcophagidae) and its forensic implications. *Journal of Forensic Sciences*, *47*(5): 1332–1336.

Greenberg, B. (1991). Flies as forensic indicators. *Journal of Medical Entomology*, *28*(5): 565–577.

Greenberg, B., & Wells, J. D. (1998). Forensic use of *Megaseliaabdita* and *M.* scalaris (Phoridae: Diptera): Case studies, development rates, and egg structure. *Journal of Medical Entomology*, *35*(3): 205–209.

Grzywacz, A., Hall, M. J., Pape, T., & Szpila, K. (2017). Muscidae (Diptera) of forensic importance—an identification key to third instar larvae of the western Palaearctic region and a catalogue of the muscid carrion community. *International Journal of Legal Medicine*, *131*: 855–866.

Hall, R. D., & Huntington, T. E. (2001). Introduction: Perceptions and status of forensic entomology. In: H Byrd & J. K. Tomberlin (eds.), *Forensic Entomology: The Utility of Arthropods in Legal Investigations* CRC Press, Boca Raton, pp. 1–15.

Higley, L. G., & Haskell, N. H. (2001). Insect development and forensic entomology. In: H. Byrd & J. K Tomberlin (eds.), *Forensic Entomology: The Utility of Arthropods in Legal Investigations*. CRC Press, Boca Raton, FL, pp. 287–302.

Horenstein, M. B., Rosso, B., & García, M. D. (2012). Seasonal structure and dynamics of sarcosaprophagous fauna on pig carrion in a rural area of Cordoba (Argentina) Their importance in forensic science. *Forensic Science International*, *217*(1–3): 146–156.

Introna Jr, F., Altamura, B. M., Dell'Erba, A., & Dattoli, V. (1989). Time since death definition by experimental reproduction of *Lucilia sericata* cycles in growth cabinet. *Journal of Forensic Sciences*, *34*(2): 478–480.

Introna, F., & Campobasso, C. P. (2000). Forensic dipterology. In: L. Papp & B. Darvas (eds.). *Manual of Palaeartic Diptera*, Vol. 1, Science Herald, pp. 793–846.

Kar, O., Naskar, A., Pramanik, D., Mukherjee, K., Sarkar, S., Mukherjee, A., Ghosh, D. & Banerjee, D. (2022a). A checklist of forensic flies from India. *Records of the Zoological Survey of India*, 387–392.

Kar, O., Naskar, A., Pramanik, D., Mukherjee, K., Sarkar, S., Mukherjee, A., Ghosh, D. & Banerjee, D. (2022b). An inventory of necrophagous flies from India. *Uttar Pradesh Journal of Zoology*, *43*(23): 79–108.

Kashyap, V. K., & Pillay, V. V. (1989). Efficacy of entomological method in estimation of postmortem interval: A comparative analysis. *Forensic Science International*, *40*(3): 245–250.

Kaur, P., Bala, M., & Al Galil, F. M. A. (2020). First report of *Boettcheris canathani* Lopes, 1961 and *Boettcherisca bengalensis* Nandi, 1992 (Sarcophagidae: Diptera) from northwest India. *International Journal of Tropical Insect Science*, *40*: 441–447.

Kerridge, A., Lappin-Scott, H., & Stevens, J. R. (2005). Antibacterial properties of larval secretions of the blowfly, *Lucilia sericata*. *Medical and Veterinary Entomology*, *19*(3): 333–337.

Liu, D., & Greenberg, B. (1989). Immature stages of some flies of forensic importance. *Annals of the Entomological Society of America*, *82*(1): 80–93.

Lord, W. D., Goff, M. L., Adkins, T. R., & Haskell, N. H. (1994). The black soldier fly *Hermetia illucens* (Diptera: Stratiomyidae) as a potential measure of human postmortem interval: Observations and case histories. *Journal of Forensic Sciences*, *39*(1): 215–222.

Lord, W. D. & Stevenson, J. R. (1986). *Directory of Forensic Entomologists*. Defense Pest Management Information Center, Walter Reed Army Medical Center Washington, Washington, DC, pp. 1–42.

Lord, W. D., Virginia, Q., & Goff, M. L. (1997). Forensic entomology: Insects in the investigation of violent crime. In: D. W. Kaplan & C. Denver (eds.), *Managing Death Investigations*. S Karger AG, Basel, pp. 155–163.

Martín-Vega, D. (2011). Skipping clues: Forensic importance of the family Piophilidae (Diptera). *Forensic Science International*, *212*(1–3): 1–5.

Matuszewski, S., Bajerlein, D., Konwerski, S., & Szpila, K. (2008). An initial study of insect succession and carrion decomposition in various forest habitats of Central Europe. *Forensic Science International*, *180*(2–3): 61–69.

Matuszewski, S., Bajerlein, D., Konwerski, S., & Szpila, K. (2010a). Insect succession and carrion decomposition in selected forests of Central Europe. Part 1: Pattern and rate of decomposition. *Forensic Science International*, *194*(1–3): 85–93.

Matuszewski, S., Bajerlein, D., Konwerski, S., & Szpila, K. (2010b). Insect succession and carrion decomposition in selected forests of Central Europe. Part 2: Composition and residency patterns of carrion fauna. *Forensic Science International*, *195*(1–3): 42–51.

Matuszewski, S., Bajerlein, D., Konwerski, S., & Szpila, K. (2011). Insect succession and carrion decomposition in selected forests of Central Europe. Part 3: Succession of carrion fauna. *Forensic Science International*, *207*(1–3): 150–163.

McLean, I. F. G. (2000). Beneficial Diptera and their role in decomposition. *Contributions to a Manual of Palaearctic Diptera (with special reference to flies of economic importance)*, *1*: 491–517.

Merritt, R. W., Courtney, G. W., & Keiper, J. B. (2009). Diptera:(flies, mosquitoes, midges, gnats). In: V. H. Resh & R. T. Cardé (eds.), *Encyclopedia of Insects*. Academic Press, USA, pp. 284–297.

Michalski, M., Gadawski, P., Klemm, J., & Szpila, K. (2021). New species of soldier fly—*Sargusbipunctatus* (Scopoli, 1763)(Diptera: Stratiomyidae), recorded from a human corpse in Europe: A case report. *Insects*, *12*(4): 302.

Mitra, B. Banerjee, D., & Parui, P. (2010). Diversity and distribution of true flies (Insecta: Diptera) in the Andaman and Nicobar Islands. In: T. M. Ramakrishna, C. Raghunathan, & C. Sivaperuman C (eds.), *Recent Trends in Biodiversity of Andaman & Nicobar Islands*. Zoological Survey of India, Kolkata, pp. 467–493.

Moretti, T. D. C., Ribeiro, O. B., Thyssen, P. J., & Solis, D. R. (2008). Insects on decomposing carcasses of small rodents in a secondary forest in Southeastern Brazil. *European Journal of Entomology*, *105*(4): 691–696.

Mummey, D. L., & Stahl, P. D. (2003). Spatial and temporal variability of bacterial 16S rDNA-based T-RFLP patterns derived from soil of two Wyoming grassland ecosystems. *FEMS Microbiology Ecology*, *46*(1): 113–120.

Nabity, P. D., Higley, L. G., & Heng-Moss, T. M. (2006). Effects of temperature on development of *Phormia regina* (Diptera: Calliphoridae) and use of developmental data in determining time intervals in forensic entomology. *Journal of Medical Entomology*, *43*(6): 1276–1286.

Nandi, B. C. (2002). *The Fauna of India and the Adjacent Countries: Diptera*: Vol. X Sarcophagidae. Zoological Survey of India, Delhi, India.

Palavesam, A., Selvakumar, R., Latha, B. R., Soundararajan, C., Jyothimol, G., & Harikrishnan, T. J. (2022). Occurrence of necrophagous flies of forensic importance in medico-legal cases in Tamil Nadu State, India. *Egyptian Journal of Forensic Sciences*, *12*(1): 1–12.

Payne, J. A. (1965). A summer carrion study of the baby pig *Sus scrofa* Linnaeus. *Ecology*, *46*(5): 592–602.

Pujol-Luz, J. R., Francez, P. A. D. C., Ururahy-Rodrigues, A., & Constantino, R. (2008). The Black Soldier-fly, Hermetiaillucens (Diptera, Stratiomyidae), used to estimate the postmortem interval in a case in Amapá State, Brazil. *Journal of Forensic Sciences*, *53*(2): 476–478.

Putman, R. J. (1983). *Carrion and dung: The decomposition of animal wastes*. The Institute of Biology's Studies in Biology No. 156, Edward Arnold, London, 61 pp.

Rasso, S. C., & Fraenkel, G. (1954). The food requirements of the adult female blow-fly, *Phormia regina* (Meigen), in relation to ovarian development. *Annals of the Entomological Society of America*, *47*(4): 636–645.

Recinos-Aguilar, Y. M., García-García, M. D., Malo, E. A., Cruz-López, L., Cruz-Esteban, S., & Rojas, J. C. (2020). The succession of flies of forensic importance is influenced by volatiles organic compounds emitted during the first hours of decomposition of chicken remains. *Journal of Medical Entomology*, *57*(5): 1411–1420.

Reed Jr, H. B. (1958). A study of dog carcass communities in Tennessee, with special reference to the insects. *American Midland Naturalist*, *59*:213–245.

Reibe, S., & Madea, B. (2010). Use of *Megaseliascalaris* (Diptera: Phoridae) for post-mortem interval estimation indoors. *Parasitology Research*, *106*: 637–640.

Reiter, C., & Hajek, P. (1984). Age-dependent changes in the intestinal contents of blowfly maggots: A study method in the framework of forensic determination of the time of death. *Zeitschrift fur Rechtsmedizin. Journal of Legal Medicine*, *92*(1): 39–45.

Richards, C. S., Simonsen, T. J., Abel, R. L., Hall, M. J., Schwyn, D. A., & Wicklein, M. (2012). Virtual forensic entomology: Improving estimates of minimum post-mortem interval with 3D micro-computed tomography. *Forensic Science International*, *220*(1–3): 251–264.

Richards, C. S., & Villet, M. H. (2009). Data quality in thermal summation development models for forensically important blowflies. *Medical and Veterinary Entomology*, *23*(3): 269–276.

Roy, S., Chakraborty, S. K., Parui, P., & Mitra, B. (2018, June). Taxonomy of soldier flies (diptera: Stratiomyidae) of sunderban biosphere reserve, India. *Proceedings of the Zoological Society*, *71*, 121–126.

Rumiza, A. R., Khairul, O., Zuha, R. M., & Heo, C. C. (2010). An observation on the decomposition process of gasolineingested monkey carcasses in a secondary forest in Malaysia. *Tropical Biomedicine*, 27(3): 373–383.

Sarwar, M. (2020). Typical flies: Natural history, lifestyle and diversity of Diptera. In: M. Sarwar (ed.), *Life Cycle and Development of Diptera*, IntechOpen, London, UK, pp. 1–50. https://doi.org/10.5772/intechopen.91391.

Sawaby, R. F., Hamouly, H. E., & Abo-El Ela, R. H. (2018). Diagnosis and keys of the main dipterous families and species collected from rabbit and guinea pig carcasses in Cairo, Egypt. *The Journal of Basic and Applied Zoology*, *79*: 1–14.

Schoenly, K., & Reid, W. (1987). Dynamics of heterotrophic succession in carrion arthropod assemblages: Discrete seres or a continuum of change? *Oecologia*, *73*: 192–202.

Sinha, S. K. (2009). Sarcophagidae, calliphoridae and muscidae (diptera) of the sundarbans biosphere reserve, West Bengal, India. *Occasional Paper-Records of the Zoological Survey of India*, *308*: 1–46.

Smith, K. E., & Wall, R. (1997). Asymmetric competition between larvae of the blowflies Calliphora vicina and Lucilia sericata in carrion. *Ecological Entomology*, *22*(4): 468–474.

Smith, K. G. V. (1986). *A Manual of Forensic Entomology*. Cornell University Press, Ithaca, p. 205.

Smith, K. G. V. (1989). An introduction to the immature stages of British flies. *Handbooks for the Identification of British Insects*, 10: 1–280.

Szpila, K., & Pape, T. (2007). Rediscovery, redescription and reclassification of *Beludzhiaphylloteliptera* (Diptera: Sarcophagidae: Miltogramminae). *European Journal of Entomology*, *104*(1): 119.

Tantawi, T. I., El-Kady, E. M., Greenberg, B., & El-Ghaffar, H. A. (1996). Arthropod succession on exposed rabbit carrion in Alexandria, Egypt. *Journal of Medical Entomology*, *33*(4): 566–580.

Tarone, A. M., Jennings, K. C., & Foran, D. R. (2007). Aging blow fly eggs using gene expression: A feasibility study. *Journal of Forensic Sciences*, *52*(6): 1350–1354.

Tuccia, F., Giordani, G., Cattaneo, C., Mazzarelli, D., & Vanin, S. (2021). First record of Physyphoraalceae (Preyssler, 1791)(Diptera, Ulidiidae) from a forensic case in Northern Italy: Description of immature stages, DNA barcoding and phylogenetic analysis. *The European Zoological Journal*, *88*(1): 1071–1083.

Tullis, K., & Goff, M. L. (1987). Arthropod succession in exposed carrion in a tropical rainforest on O'ahu Island, Hawai'i. *Journal of Medical Entomology*, *24*(3):332–339.

Van Emden, F. 1965. *Fauna of India: Diptera Vol. III Muscidae Part-I*. Baptist Mission Press, Calcutta.

Voss, S. C., Magni, P., Dadour, I., & Nansen, C. (2017). Reflectance-based determination of age and species of blowfly puparia. *International Journal of Legal Medicine*, *131*: 263–274.

Wall, R., & Fisher, P. (2001). Visual and olfactory cue interaction in resource-location by the blowfly, *Lucilia sericata. Physiological Entomology*, *26*(3):212–218.

Wall, R., & Warnes, M. L. (1994). Responses of the sheep blowfly *Lucilia sericata* to carrion odour and carbon dioxide. *Entomologiaexperimentalis et Applicata*, *73*(3): 239–246.

Wall, R., Langley, P. A., Stevens, J., & Clarke, G. M. (1990). Age-determination in the old-world screw-worm fly *Chrysomya bezziana* by pteridine fluorescence. *Journal of Insect Physiology*, *36*(3): 213–218.

Wang, Y., Gu, Z. Y., Xia, S. X., Wang, J. F., Zhang, Y. N., & Tao, L. Y. (2018). Estimating the age of *Lucilia illustris* during the intrapuparial period using two approaches: Morphological changes and differential gene expression. *Forensic Science International*, *287*:1–11.

Wells, J. D. (1991). *Chrysomya megacephala* (Diptera: Calliphoridae) has reached the continental United States: Review of its biology, pest status, and spread around the world. *Journal of Medical Entomology*, *28*(3): 471–473.

Wells, J. D., & Greenberg, B. (1994). Resource use by an introduced and native carrion flies. *Oecologia*, *99*: 181–187.

Wells, J. D., & Kurahashi, H. (1994). *Chrysomya megacephala* (Fabricius) (Diptera: Calliphoridae) development: Rate, variation and the implications for forensic entomology. *Medical Entomology and Zoology*, *45*(4): 303–309.

Wells, J. D., & LaMotte, L. R. (1995). Estimating maggot age from weight using inverse prediction. *Journal of Forensic Sciences*, *40*(4): 585–590.

Wells, J. D., & LaMotte, L. R. (2019). Estimating the postmortem interval. In: J. H. Byrd & J. K. Tomberlin (eds.), *Forensic Entomology*. CRC Press, Boca Raton, FL, pp. 213–224.

Wells, J. D., & Škaro, V. (2023). Application of DNA-based methods in forensic entomology. In: D. Primorac & M. Schanfield (eds.), *Forensic DNA Applications*. CRC Press, Boca Raton, FL, pp. 285–304.

Wells, J. D., Introna Jr, F., Di Vella, G., Campobasso, C. P., Hayes, J., & Sperling, F. A. (2001). Human and insect mitochondrial DNA analysis from maggots. *Journal of Forensic Sciences*, *46*(3): 685–687.

White, R. S., Aubertin, D., & Smart, J. (1940). *Fauna of British India, Diptera*, Vol. VI. Family Calliphoridae. Taylor and Francis, London.

Woodley, N. E., & Thompson, F. C. (2001). *A world catalog of the Stratiomyidae (Insecta: Diptera)* (Vol. *11*). *North American Dipterists' Society*, 11(8):1–475.

Ye, G., Li, K., Zhu, J., Zhu, G., & Hu, C. (2007). Cuticular hydrocarbon composition in pupal exuviae for taxonomic differentiation of six necrophagous flies. *Journal of Medical Entomology*, *44*(3): 450–456.

Zuha, R. M., Ankasha, S. J., Disney, R. H. L., & Omar, B. (2016). Indoor decomposition study in Malaysia with special reference to the scuttle flies (Diptera: Phoridae). *Egyptian Journal of Forensic Sciences*, *6*(3): 216–222.

Subject Index

Note: Bold page numbers refer to tables; *italic* page numbers refer to figures.

For Product Safety Concerns and Information please contact our EU representative GPSR@taylorandfrancis.com Taylor & Francis Verlag GmbH, Kaufingerstraße 24, 80331 München, Germany

Batch number: 10733639

Printed by Printforce, the Netherlands